Occupational Therapy
in the
Promotion of
Health and Wellness

Occupational Therapy
in the
Promotion of Health and Wellness

Marjorie E. Scaffa, PhD, OTR/L, FAOTA
Professor
Department of Occupational Therapy
University of South Alabama
Mobile, AL

S. Maggie Reitz, PhD, OTR/L, FAOTA
Professor and Chair
Department of Occupational Therapy and Occupational Science
Towson University
Towson, MD

Michael A. Pizzi, PhD, OTR/L, FAOTA
Founder
Touching Humanity, Inc.
www.touchinghumanityinc.org
Wellness Consultant
New York City, NY

 F.A. Davis Company • Philadelphia

F. A. Davis Company
1915 Arch Street
Philadelphia, PA 19103
www.fadavis.com

Copyright © 2010 by F. A. Davis Company

Printed in the United States of America

Last digit indicates print number: 10 9 8 7 6 5 4 3 2 1

Publisher: Margaret Biblis
Senior Acquisitions Editor: Christa Fratantoro
Manager of Content Development: George W. Lang
Developmental Editor: Peg Waltner
Art and Design Manager: Carolyn O'Brien
Cover image: Courtesy of Brand X Pictures

Library of Congress Cataloging-in-Publication Data

Scaffa, Marjorie E.
  Occupational therapy in the promotion of health and wellness / Marjorie E. Scaffa, S. Maggie Reitz, Michael A. Pizzi.
    p. ; cm.
  Includes bibliographical references and index.
  ISBN-13: 978-0-8036-1193-1
  ISBN-10: 0-8036-1193-5
1. Health promotion. 2. Occupational therapy. I. Reitz, S. Maggie. II. Pizzi, Michael, III. Title.
  [DNLM: 1. Occupational Therapy. 2. Health Behavior. 3. Health Promotion. WB 555 S278o 2010]
  RA427.8.S23 2010
  613—dc22

                                                                                2009012275

In our own daily occupations, we have many people who teach us about life, health, wellbeing, and what it is to be a productive member of society. This book is dedicated to those who have taught us, and continue to teach us, to believe in the limitless power of occupational engagement to promote health and wellbeing and prevent and reduce disability. It is our fervent hope that this book will inspire and instruct us all to live full, productive, and healthy lives.

Marjorie dedicates this book to the memory of her mother, Doris R. Scaffa, and grandmother, Marjorie M. Scaffa, who lived lives of love, laughter, and commitment, and inspired her to do the same.

Maggie dedicates this book to her parents, Mr. William Ross & Mrs. Patricia Thomson; sister, Heather L. Gratton; daughter, Jessica L. Reitz; and last but not least, her life partner Fred, for their efforts to facilitate her development as an individual committed to social and occupational justice.

Michael dedicates this book to the memory of his parents, who, despite chronic illness and disenfranchisement, taught him the lesson of being fully human and fully alive and to face life's obstacles with great compassion, understanding, and dignity. Michael also dedicates this book to his partner and legal spouse, Kenneth Brickman, who provides a nurturing, loving, and supportive environment in which he can create.

Preface

The three of us have known each other for over 20 years, first as practitioners and then as educators. In 2002, over dinner during the American Occupational Therapy Association conference, Michael suggested that the foundation for wellness and health promotion in occupational therapy was finally solidifying but that there were no significant occupational therapy textbooks specifically committed to the subject. Thus, a project that held great importance to the three of us was born!

We, the editors and chapter authors, share a strong commitment, passion, and urgency to further the profession and strengthen the groundwork that was laid decades ago but was never properly acknowledged or fully developed. Wilma West, Geraldine Finn, and Ruth Brunyate Wiemer are three of the prominent pioneers on whose shoulders we stand.

> *In order for a profession to maintain its relevancy it must be responsive to the trends of the times. The trend today in health services is toward the prevention of disability. Occupational therapists are being asked to move beyond the role of the therapist to that of health agent. This expansion in role identity will require a reinterpretation of current knowledge, the addition of new knowledge and skills, and the revision of the educational process.*[1(p59)]

Finn made that prophetic statement in 1972. What happened? An attachment to medicalizing what we do transformed our profession for decades. Health care has undergone major shifts and continues to dramatically change. It is time to reclaim our rightful place in prevention of disability and the promotion of health and healthy lifestyles. As a profession, we risk losing an opportunity to be world leaders as the health agents about which Finn spoke so eloquently. The shift to health agent takes little effort—it does, however, take tremendous dedication, passion, and commitment to the values of occupational therapy and to the power of occupation in daily life. Wellness and health promotion, combined with occupation, can expand the scope and impact of occupational therapy in the future.

We are grateful for this opportunity to share our vision for the future of occupational therapy. We welcome our colleagues, students, and friends to share their own visions of wellbeing, health promotion, and prevention; to build bridges between those visions and current practice; and to create new and insightful strategies that support productivity and wellbeing for individuals, families, communities, and society. Together we can become leading health agents of the 21st century!

Marjorie E. Scaffa, PhD, OTR/L, FAOTA
S. Maggie Reitz, PhD, OTR/L, FAOTA
Michael A. Pizzi, PhD, OTR/L, FAOTA

[1]Finn, G. (1972). The occupational therapist in prevention programs. *American Journal of Occupational Therapy, 26*(2), 59–66.

Contributors

Melba J. Arnold, MS, OTR/L
Assistant Professor
Department of Occupational Science and
Occupational Therapy
Saint Louis University
St. Louis, MO

Angela Blair-Newton, OTR
Occupational Therapist
Tyler, TX

Bette R. Bonder, PhD, OTR/L, FAOTA
Dean and Professor
College of Science
Cleveland State University
Cleveland, OH

Kimberly Mansfield Caldeira, MS
Faculty Research Associate
Center for Substance Abuse Research
University of Maryland
College Park, MD

Regina Michael Campbell, MS, OTR, FAOTA
Associate Professor
School of Occupational Therapy
Texas Woman's University
Dallas, TX

Charles H. Christiansen, EdD, OTR, FAOTA
Executive Director
American Occupational Therapy
Foundation
Bethesda, MD

S. Blaise Chromiak, MD
Family Physician
Mobile, AL

Karen Goldrich Eskow, PhD
Professor and Chairperson
Department of Family Studies and
Community Development
Towson University
Towson, MD

Linda Fazio, PhD, OTR/L, FAOTA
Professor of Clinical Occupational
Therapy
University of Southern California
Los Angeles, CA

Georgiana Herzberg, PhD, OTR/L
Retired
Previously of Nova Southeastern
University
Jacksonville, FL

Marie F. Kuczmarski, PhD, RD, LDN
Professor of Nutrition
Department of Health, Nutrition and
Exercise Sciences
University of Delaware
Newark, DE

Kathleen Matuska, MPH, OTR/L
Associate Professor and Director
MAOT Program
St. Catherine University
St. Paul, MN

M. Beth Merryman, PhD, OTR/L
Associate Professor
Department of Occupational Therapy and
Occupational Science
Towson University
Towson, MD

Penelope Moyers, EdD, OTR, FAOTA
Professor and Chair
Department of Occupational Therapy
University of Alabama at Birmingham
Birmingham, AL

Lynne Murphy, MS, OT/L
Clinical Assistant Professor
Department of Occupational Therapy and
Occupational Science
Towson University
Towson, MD

Theresa M. Petrenchik, PhD, OTR/L
Assistant Professor
Occupational Therapy Graduate Program
University of New Mexico
Albuquerque, NM

Rebecca Renwick, PhD, OT Reg (Ont)
Professor, Department of Occupational
Science and Occupational Therapy
Graduate Department of Rehabilitation
Science
Director, Quality of Life Research Unit
University of Toronto
Toronto, Ontario, Canada

Patricia Atwell Rhynders, PhD, MPH, CHES
Associate Professor
Colleges of Health Science and
Education
TUI University
Cypress, CA

Marlene Riley, MMS, OTR/L, CHT
Clinical Associate Professor
Department of Occupational Therapy
and Occupational Science
Towson University
Towson, MD

Debra Rybski, MS, MSHCA, OTR/L
Assistant Professor
Department of Occupational Science and
Occupational Therapy
Saint Louis University
St. Louis, MO

Theresa M. Smith, PhD, OTR, CLVT
Assistant Professor
School of Occupational Therapy
Texas Woman's University
Houston, TX

Virginia C. Stoffel, PhD, OT, BCMH, FAOTA
Associate Professor and Chair
Occupational Therapy Department
University of Wisconsin
Milwaukee, WI

C. Barrett Wallis, OTR
Occupational Therapist
Mobile, AL

Ann A. Wilcock, PhD, GradDip Public
Health, BAppScOT, DipOT
Honorary Professor
Occupational Science and Occupational
Therapy
Deakin University
Geelong, Australia

Reviewers

Karen Ann V. Cameron, OTD, MEd, OTR/L
Program Director and Assistant
Professor
Occupational Therapy Department
Alvernia College
Reading, PA

Elizabeth Ciaravino, PhD, OTR/L
Assistant Professor
Occupational Therapy Department
The University of Scranton
Scranton, PA

Helen Z. Cornely, PT, MS
Associate Professor of Physical Therapy
Florida International University
Miami, FL

Janis Davis, PhD
Assistant Professor
Occupational Therapy Department
Rockhurst University
Kansas City, MO

Joanne Gallagher, EdD, OTR/L
Chair and Associate Professor
Occupational Therapy Department
Worcester State College
Worcester, MA

Lynn Gitlow, PhD, OTR/L
Director of Occupational Therapy
Husson College
Bangor, ME

Liane Hewitt, DrPH (cand), OTR/L
Assistant Professor
Occupational Therapy Department
Loma Linda University
Loma Linda, CA

Angela N. Hissong, DEd, OTR/L
Occupational Therapy Program
Director
The Pennsylvania State University
Mont Alto, PA

Kathleen Marie Kniepmann, MPH, EdM, CHES, OTR/L
Instructor
Occupational Therapy Program
Washington University in St. Louis
St. Louis, MO

Ferol Menks Ludwig, PhD, OTR, FAOTA, GCG
Professor Emeritus
Occupational Therapy Department
Nova Southeastern University
Ft. Lauderdale, FL

Patricia E. Marvin, OTD, OTR/L
Assistant Professor
Occupational Therapy Department
University of St. Augustine for Health
Professions
St. Augustine, FL

Gail F. Metzger, BS, MS, OTR/L
Assistant Professor
Occupational Therapy Department
Alvernia College
Reading, PA

Maralynne D. Mitcham, PhD, OTR/L, FAOTA
Professor and Director
Occupational Therapy Educational
Program
Department of Rehabilitation Sciences
College of Health Professions
Medical University of South Carolina
Charleston, SC

Karin J. Opacich, PhD, MHPE, OTR/L, FAOTA
EXPORT Project Director and Assistant
Director
National Center for Rural Health
Professions
University of Illinois – Rockford
Rockford, IL

Betsey C. Smith, PhD, OTR/L
Occupational Therapy Program Director
University of Hartford
West Hartford, CT

Jill Smith, MS, OTR/L
Assistant Professor of Occupational
Therapy
Milligan College
Milligan College, TN

Janet H. Watts, PhD, OTR
Retired Associate Professor
Virginia Commonwealth University
Department of Occupational Therapy
Richmond, VA
Quality Assurance and Training
Specialist
Chamberlin Edmonds Company

Acknowledgments

Although it is impossible to list every person who impacted the development and creation of this book and the ideas contained therein, we would like to acknowledge several people without whose time and talent this book would not have come to fruition. Among these are the excellent staff at F. A. Davis, specifically Christa Fratantoro, our Senior Acquisitions Editor and coach extraordinaire; Margaret M. Biblis, the Publisher for Health Professions and Medicine, who believed in the potential impact of this text before a single word was written; and Peg Waltner, our Developmental Editor, for her tireless and invaluable assistance throughout the editorial process.

We would also like to thank our visionary colleagues and contributors who shared our excitement regarding the significant role of occupational therapy in prevention and health promotion. We have learned a great deal from reading their work, and we hope you do as well.

In addition, we wish to express our gratitude to S. Blaise Chromiak and Fred Reitz for their emotional support and the countless hours they spent reviewing and editing the chapters, and to Grace Wenger for her assistance in acquiring the permissions needed for some of the figures and tables in the text. We are also grateful to the reviewers, whose helpful feedback was used to improve the content and organization of the book.

On a personal note, Maggie expresses her thanks to her family, Fred and Jess Reitz, for their tolerance during the lengthy birthing process of this book. Missed family occupational opportunities were only a part of the sacrifices they made to allow this book to come to fruition. In addition, Maggie thanks her colleagues at Towson University for their patience, and she owes a special thank-you to the following people who supported this enterprise while they were occupational therapy students at Towson University: Alex Stroup, Beth Frey, Cheryl Merritt, Gar-Wing Tsang, Grace Wenger, Sarah Biederman, and Audrey Grant.

Finally, we would like to thank our patients and clients, who have taught us so much about the power of occupation, and we thank the many students who, over the years, asked important questions and challenged us to discover and develop new explanations. We hope this book fulfills a need for occupational therapy faculty, students, and practitioners and ultimately improves the quality of care for the recipients of occupational therapy services.

Contents

Foundations and Key Concepts

Historical and Philosophical Perspectives of Occupational Therapy's Role in Health Promotion

S. Maggie Reitz

> In 1991, occupational therapy was identified as *"the only health profession that had fully embraced the concepts of: health promotion and prevention, community-based care and the individual as centre to the process"*
>
> by Steven Lewis, former leader of the national New Democratic Party in Canada as part of his remarks as the keynote speaker at the 1991 Canadian Association of Occupational Therapist (CAOT) Conference (as cited by Green, Lertvilai, & Bribrieso 2001, ¶ 2).

Learning Objectives

This chapter is designed to enable the reader to:

- Articulate humans' evolutionary, cross-cultural use of occupations to promote healing and prevent disease and disability.
- Discuss the historical development of occupational therapy as a caring health profession that has emphasized prevention, health promotion, and wellbeing since its inception.

- Describe the historical roots, documents, and literature of occupational therapy's role in health promotion and their potential use to support and enhance current health promotion interventions and innovative evidenced-based health promotion practice.

Key Terms

Client

Disability prevention

Health promotion

Moral treatment

Prevention

Shell shock

Wellness

Introduction

After a brief review of early historical views on healing, health, and the use of occupations, this chapter traces the profession's roots in the philosophy and delivery of preventive and health promotion services. Official documents and activities within the American Occupational Therapy Association (AOTA) related to health promotion and prevention will be presented. This review focuses on health-promotion activities within the United States as influenced by both domestic and international activities. This historical perspective will enable the reader to link current practice with philosophical tenets and historical interventions and policies to establish a foundation for today's health promotion interventions.

Historical and Cultural Views of Health and Healing

Many cultures around the world have developed similar beliefs regarding health, wellbeing, and occupational engagement. While historical reviews often focus on

Greek and Roman contributions, other civilizations have contributed to the development and evolution of the medical and healing arts. Travel and exploration, as well as war, have facilitated the sharing of this knowledge between cultures. Ancient beliefs have influenced health-care practices through the years and continue to inform current developments. Tai chi is an excellent example of this type of continued impact. Being knowledgeable about healing and health beliefs that span time and cultures is important as the profession of occupational therapy seeks to provide culturally competent care. The following brief review provides a glimpse into humans' rich history of engaging in healing and health-promotion occupations.

Greek mythology provides an early view of the Greeks' beliefs regarding health and healing. Asclepius, the son of Apollo, was the god of medicine (Anderson, Anderson, & Glanze, 1998). According to mythology, Asclepius was the father of Panacea, the goddess of healing, and Hygeia, the goddess of health (Lasker & The Committee on Medicine and Public Health 1997). Hygeia is depicted with her father in Figure 1-1. It is now believed the myth of Aesculapius may have arisen as a result of the efforts of one or more individuals with exceptional healing abilities. Humans attributed divine status to those abilities and the legendary Aesculapius was then worshipped throughout the ancient Mediterranean area (National Library of Medicine [NLM], 2004a).

Throughout human history, healers have been afforded a special place in society. However, in some societies those who practiced medicine were more highly respected than those interested in prevention and health promotion. This division between health promotion and healing and the overshadowing of prevention and maintenance by medicine was described by Plato (Friedland, 1998, p. 374):

> In the . . . therapeutic arts, the corrective portion is more apparent but less important, while the regulative portion is largely hidden, but far more essential. . . . [Hence] there is grave danger lest "prevention" and "maintenance," the real work of the art, be overlooked, and attention exclusively be devoted to the correction of the diseases already there.

While this division was aptly described by Plato in his world, a slightly different view was held by the indigenous people of the Americas. They had an appreciation of the link between rubbish and illness and believed prevention was of great value. The medicine of the South American Indian primarily focused on hygiene, "as such medicine ought to be, it being of greater daily importance to preserve health than to cure disease" (Spruce as cited by Vogel, 1970, p. 261).

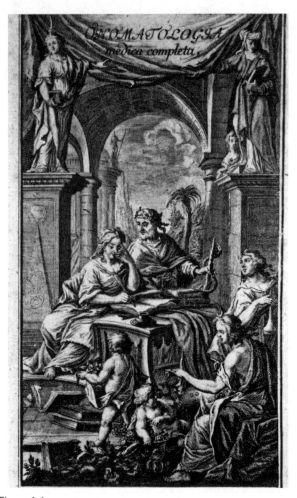

Figure 1-1 Asclepius and Hygeia in allegorical setting.
Courtesy of the National Library of Medicine.

The dichotomy between healing and prevention does not appear in early writings from Persia, China, and India. According to early Islamic writings:

> Medicine is a science from which one learns the states of the human body with respect to what is healthy and what is not, in order to preserve good health when it exists and restore it when it is lacking. (Ibn Sina, the opening to the *Qanun fi al-tibb,* cited by Savage-Smith, 1994)

In the famous Chinese medical text *Nei Chang* (*Canon of Medicine*), which dates back to 2600 BC, the Yellow Emperor, Yu Hsiung, describes both prevention and treatment (Lyons & Petrucelli, 1987). The importance of balance and the connection of humans to the physical and spiritual world were at the center of Chinese healing and prevention activities "in the last three centuries B.C." (Sivin, 1995, p. 5):

> Since ancient times [it has been understood that] penetration by [the *ch'i* of] heaven is the basis of life,

which depends on [the universal *ch'i* of] yin and yang. The *ch'i* [of everything] in the midst of heaven and earth and in the six directions, from the nine provinces and nine body orifices to the five visceral systems and the twelve joints, is penetrated by the *ch'i* of heaven. (Huang-ti nei ching t'ai su, cited by Sivin, 1995, p. 15)

The Chinese people and government are proud of their historical contributions to medicine and health. According to the Wudang Taoist Internal Alchemy (2005), recent additions to a famous temple complex that dates back to AD 140 include sculptures representing historical figures in Chinese medicine (Fig. 1-2).

Further evidence of the importance of understanding and offering acute and preventive care is found in examining long-held practices in India. Ayurveda, the science of life, originated in India about 5000 BC and was later documented by Charak:

> *Ayurveda* has been reported as one of the oldest systems of health care dealing with both the preventive and curative aspects of life in a most comprehensive way and presents a close similarity to the WHO's [World Health Organization] concept of health propounded in the modern era. (Department of Ayurveda, 2004, ¶ 1).

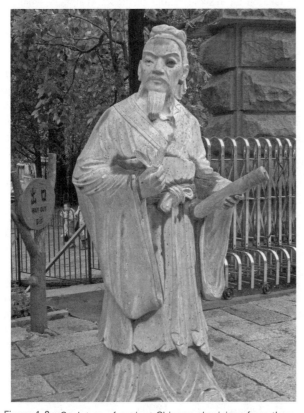

Figure 1-2 Sculpture of ancient Chinese physicians from the Taiqing Temple Complex, Laoshan Mountain, People's Republic of China.

Photography by S. Maggie Reitz.

This historical review of examples supports the continued development and evolution of health promotion as well as the need to study the effectiveness of blending preventive care with medical and rehabilitative approaches. Knowledge of history also helps practitioners better understand potential areas of tension between disciplines, as well as cultural differences in approaches to health and wellbeing.

Historical Use of Occupation to Heal and Promote Wellbeing

The historical actions, beliefs, and practices of humans through the ages also provide an important backdrop from which to view the potential to enhance health and wellbeing through engagement in occupation. The use of occupation to promote health and wellbeing through prevention of disease, injury, and social injustice has been substantially documented. Examining lessons from the past is time well spent when crafting solutions for the present, since "we cannot accurately and professionally comprehend the present or look at the future intelligently until we become acquainted with and study the past" (Stattel, 1977, p. 650). Content Box 1-1 outlines other benefits of knowing the history of one's

---

Content Box 1-1

Practical Benefits of an Awareness of Historical Influences on the Practice of Occupational Therapy in Health Promotion

- Supports the role of occupational therapy in health promotion through the realization that foundational philosophical beliefs and principles can be traced to the early 1900s.
- Enhances awareness of the unique history of occupation-based interventions for prevention and health promotion, which increases the comfort level of occupational therapists and occupational therapy assistants in this role.
- Encourages the examination of the historical influence of sociopolitical factors on the evolution of the profession and its ongoing contributions to provide solutions to societal problems.
- Strengthens society's view of occupational therapists as educated professionals through demonstration of an appreciation and synthesis of the liberal arts aspect of occupational therapy education.
- Fosters competence to facilitate interdisciplinary cooperation and respect via increased ability to articulate an understanding of the rich traditions of occupation-based service delivery.

profession and the political and sociocultural influences on that history through time.

History provides a rich description of humans' engagement in occupation for subsistence, self-expression, healing, and aesthetics (AOTA, 1979d; MacDonald, 1976; Pizzi, Scaffa, & Reitz 2006). Through the ages, many cultures have used occupations to promote healing. A variety of early philosopher-scientists as well as healers in Egypt, Rome, Greece, and Persia promoted the use of occupation as a healing agent. Pythagoras and Thales, both early Greek philosopher-scientists, used music as a treatment modality (MacDonald, 1976), as did Ibn Sina, a Persian physician, known in the west as Avicenna (Ahmed, 1990; Licht, 1948). Aristotle, the pupil of Plato, viewed praxis or "desirable and satisfying activity or action" as leading to eudaimonia, the "well-being of the soul" (Friedland, 1998, p. 374).

Physical occupations were often prescribed. The Egyptians recommended physical activity and boat trips on the Nile (Punwar, 2000) as well as music and games (Dunton, 1954). The Chinese prescribed exercise to restore wellbeing (Lyons & Petrucelli, 1987) and promote health (Levin, 1937). Gymnastics were described by Zhuangzi in fourth-century BC China as a preventive technique to ensure successful aging and longevity and became "well established as a form of therapy around the third and second centuries B.C." (Despeux, 1989, p. 241). Hippocrates recommended other physically challenging occupations, such as wrestling and riding that required linking the mind and body during treatment (MacDonald, 1976).

In addition to the use of occupations, early public health actions and the importance of occupational balance were appreciated as being linked to health and wellbeing. Hippocrates encouraged physicians to consider the influence of air and water quality in a specific geographical area as well as the occupations of the population—both healthy and unhealthy. He encouraged an examination of "the mode of life of the inhabitants, whether they were heavy drinkers, taking lunch, and inactive, or athletic, industrious, eating much, and drinking" (cited by Lasker & the Committee on Medicine and Public Health, 1997, p. 12). Pythagoras was thought to have "promoted health through a special vegetarian diet" (NLM, 2004b, ¶ 1). Other historical figures were proponents of a balanced lifestyle, including the 13th-century Byzantine writer Actuarius, also known as John the Actuary (Licht, 1948). In addition, in the fifth century, a neurologist named Caelius Aurelianus encouraged patients to become involved in their rehabilitation efforts (MacDonald, 1976).

Australian aborigines have long recognized the interdependence of human health and welfare with that of the land (Chambers, 2002). Prior to the arrival of European colonists, this society understood the importance of a lifestyle that balanced the needs of the human and nonhuman worlds. This lifestyle included a respect for earth, animals, and humans as well as a deep sense of responsibility for self and others. Ancient sacred sites, often including cave paintings and rock engravings, represent beliefs regarding origin, attachment to the land, and personal and group identity (Barunga, 1975; Edwards, 1975; Peterson, 1975). The aboriginal view of social responsibility encompassed the health and welfare of humans and animals in both the present and the future. The active process of aboriginal "Dreaming" embodies values such as prudence and social responsibility, which were practiced through spiritual, learning, and teaching occupations:

> Dreaming is the tracks you are responsible for. You grow up, then you have to maintain it spiritually. You've got to maintain it through not over-using it; you've got to do ceremonies for the different animals; you've got to do ceremonies for human beings; and as you grow and as you get older you learn your responsibilities to that area. As you grow older still, and as you marry into different families, to take on the responsibility of other people, and as your children have children you take on the responsibilities of other Dreamings—their Dreamings, the children's Dreamings, which might go on a different way from yours. (Bowden & Bunbury, 1990, p. 33)

Dreaming is consistent with the aboriginal description of knowledge as the true aboriginal currency and the belief that learning is a lifelong process (Bowden & Bunbury, 1990). To learn more about the ancient and modern culture of the Australian aboriginal people, including symbolism in aboriginal art (see Fig. 1-3), visit http://www.aboriginalart.com.au.

Indigenous people of North America share this appreciation for nature, the land, and a desire to live in harmony with the physical world (Kavasch & Baar, 1999; National Museum of American Indians [NMAI], 2005). They also have long shared a belief in the connection of dreams, visions, and rituals to health (Kavasch & Baar, 1999). Some healing practices have involved occupations such as music, drumming, and, for the Navajo, sand painting. However, sand painting that can now be purchased as art is not the same in either form or function as the sand painting that is created for healing purposes. Physically active occupations such as endurance games and footraces were believed to enhance the power of other healing practices (Kavasch & Baar, 1999).

The Wampanoag Indians have lived in eastern Massachusetts and the surrounding islands for over 12,000 years (Kavasch & Baar, 1999). This group

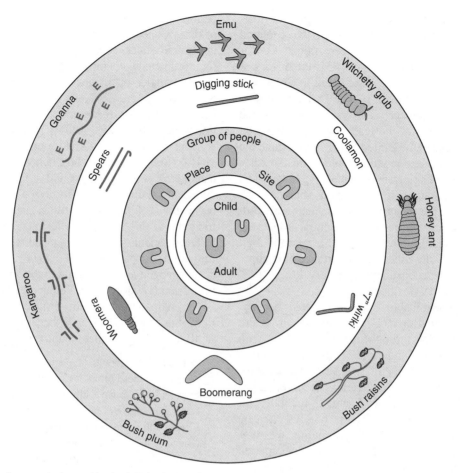

Figure 1-3 Dreamtime symbols used in aboriginal art.

Courtesy of Aboriginal Australia Art & Culture Centre, http://www.aboriginalart.com.au/site_map.html.

shared food-gathering and cultivation knowledge with the Pilgrims, thus helping the Pilgrims survive. For several hundred years, this group has played Wampanoag Fireball, a dangerous medicine game that resembles soccer with a flaming ball. In this game, men—usually young men—channel their strength to enhance the healing of a friend or a loved one. The passion and energy expended and the wounds sustained in this game are believed to minimize the impact of one's illness (Kavasch & Baar, 1999).

Other early medical writers and educators considered less dangerous occupations to be useful for both the maintenance of health and illness prevention. Cornelius Celsus, who lived from 25 BC to AD 50 (University of Texas Medical Branch, 2005), encouraged the use of occupations such as "sailing, hunting, handling of arms, ball games, running, and walking" to maintain health (MacDonald, 1976, p. 4). He also encouraged matching occupations to the needs and temperament of each person.

Bernardino Ramazzini, an 18th-century Italian physician (NLM, 2005) and a professor at Padua, "stressed the importance of prevention rather than treatment" (MacDonald, 1976, p. 5). These early proponents of occupation, the importance of client-centered care, and the influence of context planted seeds that would later take root in the era of moral treatment and the philosophy of the new discipline of occupational therapy.

Select Historical Milestones in Health Promotion and Prevention Within Occupational Therapy in the United States

The Birth of the Profession

The era of moral treatment established the foundation of ideas that would later be embraced by the founders of occupational therapy. **Moral treatment** is a "nineteenth-century humanitarian approach to treatment for individuals with mental illness that centered around productive, creative, and recreational occupations" (Spear & Crepeau, 2003, p. 1031; the history of this approach is discussed in more detail in Chapter 4, which addresses public health). The beliefs and successes of moral treatment were compatible with the visions and optimism of the leaders of various social reform movements in the United States and became the catalyst for the profession's development in the early 1900s. Educational reformers, mental hygienists, and leaders in the arts-and-crafts movement shared a philosophy stressing the importance and meaning of work and occupation and the resultant potential impact on learning and health (Breines, 1986). Harold Bell Wright eloquently described the importance of occupation by stating, "Occupation is the very life of life" (cited by Dunton, 1915, title page).

These ideas and values have supported occupational therapy practitioners' engagement in health promotion activities through the years, both with individuals and with populations. Those committed to the arts-and-crafts movement "saw activity as a means to improve society—'to socialize less accepted members of society such as the disabled, mentally ill, impoverished' " (Schemm, 1964, p. 639, as cited by Friedland, 1998, p. 375). While occupation was prescribed to ill individuals, the power of occupation to promote the overall wellbeing of society was also recognized early in the profession's development: "Although they spoke of occupation as curative, it was not in relation to medical or psychiatric conditions but rather to the human condition" and to use it as a tool to maximize human potential for the good of society (Friedland, 1998, p. 375).

In addition to those who advocated occupation to address societal problems, others wrote about the preventive qualities of occupation. Dunton proposed that occupation could be used as a preventive agent: "Another purpose of occupation may be to give the patient a hobby which may serve as a safety valve and render the recurrence of an attack less likely" (Dunton, 1915, p. 25). In addition, Dunton also believed that occupation could be a powerful tool for well individuals, and his work supports the profession's use of occupation for health maintenance (Peloquin, 1991b).

Self-Inoculation Through Occupation

MacDonald noted that "the occupational therapist of early history was the 'doctor' himself" (1976, p. 2). However, through time, it appears that individuals and communities have self-prescribed occupation both to heal and prevent illness. Sir Winston Churchill, Clifford Beers, and George Barton are examples of individuals

performing self-inoculation through occupation. The case of Barton, one of the founders of occupational therapy in the United States, is perhaps the most familiar example for occupational therapy practitioners. Isabel Newton, also a founder of occupational therapy in the United States (Licht, 1967; Neuhas, 1968) and who later became Barton's wife, described Barton's use of occupation to heal his paralysis. Physicians were so impressed with his results that referrals soon followed (Peloquin, 1991a). Beers, who was hospitalized in several mental institutions over a 5-year period at the beginning of the 20th century, credits his self-selected engagement in the occupations of drawing, writing, and reading as contributing to his recovery (Peloquin, 1991a). Dunton believed patients such as Barton and Beers, who successfully used occupations to aid in their recovery, should be acknowledged as contributing to the development of the profession (Dunton, 1915; Peloquin, 1991a).

Sir Winston Churchill, prime minister of Great Britain during World War II, began painting at the age of 40, providing another example of self-inoculation:

> Winston found hours of pleasure and occupation in painting—where problems of perspective and colour, light and shade, gave him respite from dark worries, heavy burdens, and the clatter of political strife. And I believe this compelling occupation played a part in renewing the source of the great inner strength that was his, enabling him to confront storms, ride out depression, and rise above the rough passages of his political life. (Mary Soames, Winston Churchill's daughter, Foreword, 2002, pp. vii–viii)

Pursuing a variety of occupations provided balance and perspective to his complex life of military, political, and public service. Churchill's leadership during World War II was instrumental in preventing the invasion of Britain and the expansion of Hitler's Germany, which were critical in turning the tide of the war. In recognition of his efforts, Churchill received honorary U.S. citizenship (Frenz, 1969) and was identified as one of the 100 most important people of the century (Keegan, 2003). He also received a Nobel Prize for Literature (British Broadcasting Corporation [BBC], 2005; Frenz, 1969). An excellent resource summarizing his contributions is listed in the table of website resources at the end of this chapter.

The Military and the Use of Occupation

Military leaders have long recognized the benefits of using occupation to improve their armies. These occupations primarily included physical activities for conditioning and prevention of injury (Kavasch & Baar, 1999; Levin, 1937) and included entertainment to prevent boredom and maintain morale such as has been provided by the United Service Organizations [USO] since 1941 (USO, 2005).

However, occupation does not appear to have been used for rehabilitation of soldiers until World Wars I and II. Rehabilitation is not primary prevention; it falls under the categories of secondary and tertiary prevention. The rehabilitation efforts described below were aimed at the individual needs of soldiers but were also part of a broader societal intervention through governmental policy and programs, which can be considered a form of population-based health promotion.

"During World War I, it was found in Germany, France, and England that much could be done to recondition the wounded by means of occupation" (Dunton, 1954, p. 5). Early in World War I, before the United States entered the conflict, leaders in countries already involved were concerned about the prospect of large numbers of wounded and their need for rehabilitation (Willard & Cox, 1979). The previous system of pensioning injured veterans for life was not going to be economically feasible. Thus, there was great interest in ensuring the self-sufficiency of these soldiers (Christensen, 1991).

At the onset of World War I, British physicians began to see a cluster of symptoms that became known as **shell shock.** These symptoms included "partial paralysis, convulsive movements, blindness, terrifying dreams and flashbacks, and amnesia" (NLM, 2004c, ¶ 1). At first, these symptoms were blamed on exposure to the deafening sound of shells and grenades exploding. Later it was understood that the symptoms were caused by the horrific living conditions endured during trench warfare, which included spending weeks at a time in rat-infested, corpse-laden, and flooded trenches. These conditions are detailed in an exhibit at the NLM (2004c).

In 1918, Dunton became president of the National Society for the Promotion of Occupational Therapy at the group's second annual meeting. At that meeting, he shared the Europeans' success in using occupation to treat shell shock and stressed the need for the United States to prepare well-trained occupational workers for the eventual war effort (Peloquin, 1991b). Within months, the United States entered World War I, and recruitment and education for reconstruction aids began (Dunton, 1954; Peloquin, 1991b; Willard & Cox, 1979). Recovering soldiers in World Wars I and II received instructions in basket weaving, woodwork, and other occupations to facilitate their recovery from physical injuries and from psychosocial dysfunction caused by the horrors of war (McDaniel, 1968). Figures 1-4 and 1-5 show examples of occupational therapy workshops in a U.S. Army hospital in France during World War I.

The exhibit at the NLM mentioned earlier traces shell shock from World War I to the Vietnam War, when the syndrome was "labeled Post-Traumatic Stress Disorder, a disorder now recognized by the American Psychiatric Association" (NLM, 2004c).

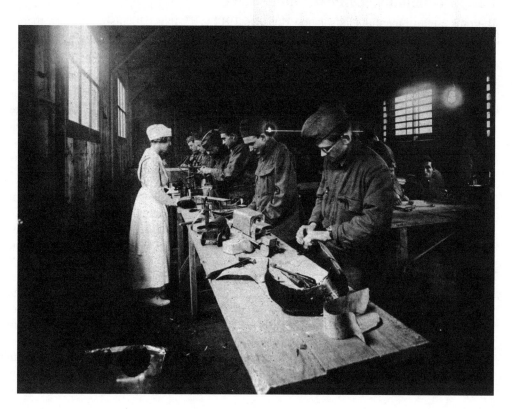

Figure 1-4 Service provision at U.S. Army Base Hospital No. 9, Chateauroux, France.

Courtesy of the National Library of Medicine (A02826).

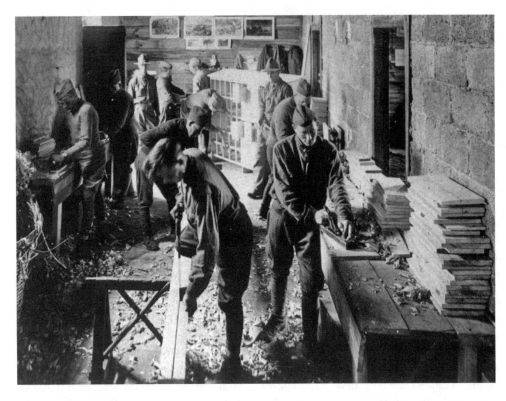

Figure 1-5   Base Hospital No. 9. Chateauroux, France, woodwork.

Courtesy of National Library of Medicine Collection. Appears as Figure 24 in "Occupational therapists before World War II (1917–40)" by M. L. McDaniel in Army Medical Specialist Corps *(pp. 69–97). Washington, DC: Office of Surgeon General, Department of the Army.*

As often happens, knowledge gained in war can later be used to favorably affect the health and wellbeing of nonmilitary populations.

Early Community and Prevention Practice

Barton's establishment of Consolation House in 1914 is the earliest example of community-based occupational therapy practice within the United States (Scaffa, 2001; Scaffa & Brownson, 2005). The doors of Consolation House opened on March 7, 1914, after extensive alterations. In an article commemorating AOTA's 50th anniversary, Barton's wife, Isabel, described the alterations and the dedication of the Consolation House (Barton, 1968). The alterations included a 6-foot tub, which Barton installed against the advice of the plumber. After many months at a sanatorium, Barton desired the opportunity to "stretch out" while bathing. The parlor of the house was turned into an office that housed books related to occupational therapy as well as a glass case exhibiting patients' craft work. The décor of Consolation House was heavily influenced by the arts-and-crafts movement of the early 1900s (Krieger, 2001).

The first floor of an old red barn on the property was converted into a workshop, and the second floor became a studio. Barton acquired a vacant lot adjacent to the house and subdivided it into three sections: a vegetable garden, a grass lawn, and an area containing flowering shrubbery and a hammock. The house provided tools for engaging in a variety of occupations,

and "experimental projects were carried out in the quest for new occupations to be offered to incapacitated individuals" (Barton, 1968, p. 342). An example of one of the many "experiments" conducted in the garden area was growing calabash with the expectation that patients could turn them into pipes. The philosophy of George Barton and Consolation House can best be expressed through his words:

> I am going to raise the cry that it is time for humanity to cease regarding the hospital as a door closing upon a life which is past, and to regard it henceforth as a door opening upon a life which is to come. I do not mean heaven. I mean a job, as better job, or a job done better than it was before. (Barton, 1968, pp. 342–43)

Consolation House was the model for the present-day University of Southern California (USC), Department of Occupational Science and Occupational Therapy's Center for Occupation and Lifestyle Redesign (Gourley, 2000; Krieger, 2001). The center was established in 1999 (USC, 2004) in a renovated 1894 Victorian mansion (Krieger, 2001) and is used for community-based practice, education, and research. Workshops modeled after Barton's program and the Hull House's work with immigrants are geared primarily for the local Latino community (Krieger, 2001).

In the United States, occupational therapy's early work in prevention focused on the prevention of infectious disease such as tuberculosis (TB). Diaz (1932) described her efforts to organize a preventorium in Puerto Rico for children of parents with TB, with the goal of decreasing the children's risk of contracting the disease. The board of directors of an association to prevent TB among children contacted Diaz to organize a new facility to house and care for 50 children between the ages of 2 and 10. Diaz performed a variety of administrative functions, including the development of a daily regimen of habit training and occupations that included "marching, sun-baths, singing, folk dancing, rest in bed, story telling, calisthenics, outdoor games, daily prayers, personal habits . . . academic classes, and some craft work" (Diaz, 1932, p. 200). Within a 1-year period, the progress of the children was reported as "remarkable. They entered the institution in very bad condition: undernourished, unhealthy, and with little or no discipline. They were returned quite different" (Diaz, 1932, p. 201).

Shaffer, a psychologist, presented a paper at the 21st annual meeting of the AOTA on recreation for prevention and therapy for social maladjustments. He argued that access to healthy play would facilitate children's development and prevent criminal habits and mental illness. He was concerned about the then-current practice of sheltering children from vigorous activity. Play, he believed, "properly engaged in, is habit training for the more serious problems of adult living" (Shaffer, 1938, p. 98). Team play was also viewed as beneficial, with the child learning how to "subordinate his desires to the common good and to develop loyalty to a purpose or a task undertaken. Thus he is learning the important secrets of a good adjustment to life" (Shaffer, 1938, p. 98).

Prevention was mentioned intermittently in the literature in the 1940s both within Canada and the United States. Dr. Howland, the first president of the Canadian Association of Occupational Therapists, identified prevention as one of five forms of occupational therapy (Friedland, 1998). In 1947, the director of the Philadelphia Committee for the Prevention of Blindness discussed the need for interdisciplinary collaboration to prevent blindness through combating its three primary causes: venereal disease, now referred to as *sexually transmitted infection*; glaucoma; and accidents (Carpenter, 1947). Carpenter believed occupational therapists, due to their interactions with families, had a key role in the early screening of visual problems in children and their parents (Reitz, 1992). Specifically, occupational therapists were encouraged to look for and intervene when symptoms of congenital syphilis or ineffective home remedies for injured eyes were present, or if they heard reports of family members or neighbors seeing colored rings around lights at night. Occupational therapists were also encouraged to take

advantage of being in the community as an opportunity to minimize adverse health conditions and prevent future illness in other family or community members, thereby joining the public health team.

The use of occupation to promote normal development was also recognized early in the profession's evolution. Manual, recreational, and musical occupations were recommended for use with children in the 1940s:

> Activities used with children should be chosen primarily for their therapeutic value, but at the same time the possibilities for a normal development of the child should be considered and activities of positive value should be chosen to encourage this development. (Gleave, 1954, p. 163)

Visionary Leaders and Modern Milestones in Health Promotion

Occupation was also seen as a preventive tool for the hospitalized patient. Fay and Kellogg (1954) described one of the roles of occupational therapy as "the prevention of the establishment of invalid habits by giving opportunity for establishing or maintaining good work habits." The benefits of engaging occupational therapy were identified as improvement in circulation, decrease in fatigue, "good sleep, good appetite, and good posture" (p. 118).

Although these were important efforts, they were falling short of the full potential that the profession of occupational therapy had to offer. This was readily apparent to visionaries such as Wiemer. Wiemer repeatedly stressed her concern (1972) that the profession was viewing its role in prevention in a too limited, "elementary" manner and that the description of the role appeared to be mere technical responses rather than professional-level problem-solving. Wiemer encouraged the profession to expand efforts across the preventive-health continuum. Figure 1-6 displays Wiemer's Preventive Health Continuum functions matched to the three levels of prevention—primary, secondary, and tertiary.

In Wiemer's view, the appropriate role of occupational therapy should encompass

> *the clear exercise of that expertise unique to occupational therapy, needed by society, and unavailable from other sources, exerting all components of occupational therapy's armamentarium impinging upon prevention rather than selected options from it,* with imaginative action to supplement and complement efforts of other disciplines [italics are original author's]. (Wiemer, 1972, p. 5)

Wiemer also noted that this role would require a change in philosophy. Occupational therapists would need to broaden their perspective regarding who they were responsible for—switching their focus from assuming responsibility for patients treated to persons they do not treat (Wiemer, 1972). This statement also holds true for current practice, as the profession largely remains reimbursement driven. The profession has renewed its commitment to improve the health and wellbeing of society, which will be demonstrated through examples and discussions of official documents in the next section of this chapter.

The 1980s saw the publication of numerous articles regarding prevention and health promotion. The director of AOTA's Practice Division presented current trends that were impacting the practice of the profession. Woven through this discussion was support for the prediction that "wellness and prevention concepts will become increasingly accepted for philosophical and economical reasons" (Bair, 1982, p. 704). Articles describing program outcome studies were published, providing data for evidence-based practice and ideas for future research. Two of these studies were conducted with children—one with preschoolers in the United States (George, Braun, & Walker, 1982) and one with infants in Israel (Parush, Lapidot, Edelstein, & Tamir, 1987). Both studies concluded that structured occupation-based programs developed by occupational therapists can enhance the development of age-appropriate skills. In addition, a study was conducted with healthy older adults to determine the effectiveness of occupational therapy intervention on self-care independence and quality of life (Kirchman, Reichenbach, & Giambalvo, 1982). Results suggest that the intervention had a positive impact on social resources, life satisfaction, and general affect.

Also in the 1980s, articles appeared in the occupational therapy literature regarding the potential role of occupational therapy in workplace injury prevention. Allen (1986) reviewed two programs addressing the impact of repetitive work injury on workers and employers. The first was a seven-session program delivered to bank employees and consisting of recommendations to modify the work environment and work habits for efficiency and effectiveness. The second was a luncheon lecture program for university employees and addressed "modifying life-style, posture, equipment, desk arrangement, and work organization" (Allen, 1986, p. 766).

Schwartz (1989) described the role of occupational therapy in industrial accident and injury prevention. Many areas of expertise required for competence in this role were identified, including knowledge of the business world (i.e., labor relations, corporate and industrial management, economics), biological science (i.e., neurosciences, kinesiology, pathology), social science, and education. Schwartz predicted "an explosive demand for prevention services. Whether called 'wellness, risk management, and cost containment,' or something else, it is going to become economically and legally imperative that employees act to prevent accidents and injuries" (1989, p. 6). This prediction was partially realized within the following decade, as the author increasingly saw retail employees wearing protective gear, though often incorrectly and inconsistently.

The AOTA's backpack awareness campaign (AOTA, 2004; Gourley, 2001a, 2001b) is another example of

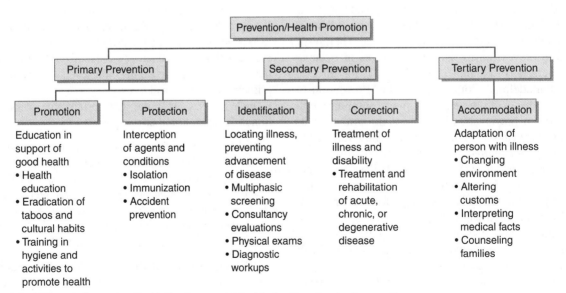

Figure 1-6 Wiemer's Preventive Health Continuum matched to the three levels of prevention.

Developed from Wiemer (1972), by Reitz (1984, 2004) with permission.

occupational therapy's potential for preventing injury. These preventive initiatives demonstrate the potential for occupational therapy to be involved in primary prevention at the level of the individual, the classroom, or the educational institution.

In the late 1990s, Wilcock and Townsend, as was earlier the case for Wiemer, articulated a vision for occupational therapy to contribute to the health and wellbeing at a societal level (Townsend, 1999; Wilcock, 1998; Wilcock & Townsend, 2000). In 2000, Wilcock described the impact of occupational science on her philosophy and work (Wilcock, 2000). The international team of Townsend and Wilcock introduced the constructs of occupational justice, occupational injustice, and other terminology to provide a language for occupational therapy assistants and occupational therapists to use as they examined broader societal and global issues through the lens of occupation. These ideas are introduced and defined in the context of population health in Chapter 6 and are also addressed during a discussion of occupational justice in Chapter 8.

Toward the end of the 1990s, a milestone in the profession's history was reached with the publication of the USC Well Elderly Study in the prestigious *Journal of the American Medical Association* (Clark et al., 1997). This study investigated the effectiveness of the USC Well Elderly program. Results indicated that "preventive occupational therapy greatly enhances the health and quality of life of independent-living adults. This landmark study reaffirmed foundational principles of occupational science and occupational therapy" (Mandel, Jackson, Nelson, & Clark, 1999, p. xi). The program was based on fundamental beliefs of the occupational therapy profession (see Content Box 1-2) as well as theoretical perspectives from the academic discipline of occupational science. A complete description is available through an AOTA publication (Mandel et al., 1999).

Content Box 1-2

Core Ideas From Occupational Therapy That Framed Lifestyle Redesign

- Occupation is life itself.
- Occupation can create new visions of possible selves.
- Occupation has a curative effect on physical and mental health and on a sense of order and routine.
- Occupation has a place in prevention.

From *Lifestyle redesign: Implementing the well elderly study* (p. 13) by D. R. Mandel, J. M. Jackson, R. Zemke, L. Nelson, & F. A. Clark, 1999, Bethesda, MD: American Occupational Therapy Association. With permission. Copyright © 1999 by American Occupational Therapy Association.

Official Documents and Activities of AOTA Related to Health Promotion and Prevention

Examples of practitioners' use of occupation in community-based practice and prevention from the profession's inception through the mid-20th century in the United States were provided above. The ability of humans to maximize their health through engagement in occupations was discussed repeatedly in the literature during this time period (Brunyate, 1967; Finn, 1972, 1977; Jaffe, 1986; Johnson, 1986a, 1986b; Reilly, 1962; West, 1967, 1969; Wiemer, 1972), including in several Eleanor Clarke Slagle lectures (Table 1-1). The discussion will now turn to an examination of official AOTA documents and activities, including the visionary leadership of Brunyate (née Wiemer) and others. A timeline of these key events appears in Table 1-2.

Report of the Task Force on Social Issues

In the 1970s, the AOTA established a task force "to identify major changes occurring within the social system and the health care systems in order to evaluate the directions and contributions of occupational therapy" (AOTA, 1972, p. 332). Ten trends (shown in Content Box 1-3) were identified as possible influencing factors on changes in health care in the next decade. Two of these trends included

1. national health insurance and legislation, and
2. new attitudes toward health care.

Echoing Plato, the task force stressed that preventive approaches were as necessary as medical approaches. The task force also described alternatives for the future of occupational therapy. Occupational therapy services were described using the five functions identified in Wiemer's (1972) preventive health care continuum (i.e., promotion, protection, identification, correction, and accommodation).

In 1979, Wiemer criticized the simplistic nature of the services described in the task force report, believing they fell short of the true potential of occupational therapy:

> My prior plea for attention to occupation regrettably resulted in action tangential to my point. In quoting my thoughts, the Task Force on Social Issues suggested: "for example,
> a. One of the highest accident rates occur in the home, therefore occupational therapists might participate in public education programs to help people become aware of the dangers of slippery rugs, slippery floors, and other hazards.

Table 1–1 Eleanor Clarke Slagle Lectures With Health Promotion Themes and Constructs

Year	Lecturer	Title	Themes
1961	Mary Reilly	Occupational Therapy Can Be One of the Greatest Ideas of 20th-Century Medicine	Humans can impact their own health and wellbeing through engagement in meaningful occupations.
1967	Wilma L. West	Professional Responsibility in Time of Change	The role of current occupational therapy should be broadened from the medical model by preparing practitioners to serve society by being health agents.
1969	Lela A. Llorens	Facilitating Growth & Development: The Promise of Occupational Therapy	Occupational therapy can promote healthy growth and development.
1971	Geraldine L. Finn	The Occupational Therapist in Prevention Programs	The need for and issues that must be addressed to develop occupational therapy's role in prevention programs.
1972	Jerry A. Johnson	Occupational Therapy: A Model for the Future	Occupation can be used to impact individual and society's need for health. Profession needs to predict changes in society so its practitioners can be prepared to make contributions to the ever-changing world.
1980	Carolyn Manville Baum	Occupational Therapists Put Care in the Health System	Practitioners need to be prepared to enter different arenas in health care, other than acute care. Examples include public health, hospital-based community outreach, and embedding prevention within curative programs.
1984	Elnora M. Gilfoyle	Transformation of a Profession	A paradigm shift is occurring with the society and the profession. The profession needs to continue to decrease its reliance on the patriarchal medical model and develop its potential to impact the wellbeing of individuals and society.
1990	Susan B. Fine	Resilience and Human Adaptability: Who Rises Above Adversity?	Occupation can be used as a tool to facilitate resilience and wellbeing in the face of traumatic life events.
1994	Ann P. Grady	Building Inclusive Community: A Challenge for Occupational Therapy	Promoting inclusion in communities of choice for individuals at the local and global level promotes adaptation, participation, and wellbeing for individuals with and without disabilities.
1996	David L. Nelson	Why the Profession of Occupational Therapy Will Flourish in the 21st Century	Engaging in meaningful occupation can promote health and quality of life.
2004	Ruth Zemke	Time, Space, and the Kaleidoscopes of Occupation	Importance of temporal rhythms, and their interactions with space, place, and culture to human health.
2006	Betty R. Hasselkus	The World of Everyday Occupation: Real People, Real Lives	Engagement in everyday occupations can promote health and wellbeing. The detrimental impact of limits to occupational engagement.

Table 1–2 Selection of Key Highlights in AOTA's Historical Involvement in Health Promotion and Disease Prevention

Year	Event	Reference
1915	Dunton proposes that occupation can be a preventative agent.	(Dunton, 1915)
1932	*American Journal of Occupational Therapy (AJOT)* publishes an article titled "Organizing a Preventorium for Children."	(Diaz, 1932)
1947	*AJOT* publishes an article on prevention of blindness.	(Carpenter, 1947)
1961	Reilly proposes that humans can impact their health through occupation: "Man, through the use of his hands as they are energized by mind and will, can influence the state of his own health."	(Reilly, 1962, p. 1)
1968	Revised AOTA definition includes the phrase "to promote and maintain health, to prevent disability."	(Willard & Spackman, 1971, p. 1)
1972	AOTA Task Force established "to delineate a model of practice for prevention and health maintenance programs."	(Jaffe, 1986, p. 11)
1977	AOTA Representative Assembly (RA) passed Resolution No. 521-77, Preventive Health Care Services.	(Jaffe, 1986)
1978	AOTA RA approved "the Philosophical Base of Occupational Therapy," which included the phrase (occupation) "may be used to prevent and mediate dysfunction."	(AOTA, 1979c, p. 785)
1978	AOTA RA convened a special session; the result was the monograph *Occupational Therapy 2001: AD.*	(AOTA, 1979b)
1986	First *AJOT* special issue on health promotion.	(AOTA, 1986)
1988	AOTA appoints first health promotion/wellness program manager.	(A. Morris, personal communication, July 1989)
1989	AOTA RA approved the position paper "Occupational Therapy in the Promotion of Health and Prevention of Disease and Disability."	(AOTA, 1989a)
1989	AOTA representatives participate in the meeting of the U.S. "Year 2000 Health Objectives Consortium."	(AOTA, 1989b)
2000	AOTA RA approved "Occupational Therapy in the Promotion of Health and the Prevention of Disease and Disability."	(Brownson Scaffa, 2001)
2007	AOTA RA approved AOTA's Statement on Stress and Stress Disorders.	(Stallings-Sahler, 2007)
2007	AOTA RA approved "Occupational Therapy Services in the Promotion of Health and the Prevention of Disease and Disability."	(Scaffa et al., 2008)

Modified from *The historical and philosophical bases for occupational therapy's role in health promotion*, presentation by S. M. Reitz at the 10th International Congress of the World Federation of Occupational Therapists, Melbourne, Australia, April 3, 1990.

b. Adolescents have a high accident rate, and parents and adolescents might be warned of the dangers of permitting or encouraging adolescents to drive high speed cars, . . ."

Any parent, spouse, sibling, or TV commercial can do that! We need to show causal relationships between various types of occupation, or lack of it, and the fact of the fall or driving accident; facts indicating, for example, the relationship between boredom, carelessness, and falling, or between fast driving and the nature of the occupational experiences of teenagers. (Wiemer, 1979, pp. 44–45)

Ten Trends Identified by AOTA Task Force That May Have an Impact on Health Care in the 1970s

- National health insurance and legislation
- Changing attitudes toward health care
- Changing educational patterns
- Change in educational consumer
- Changing patterns of work-leisure
- Changes in housing and living patterns, styles of life, and living conditions
- Technology and daily living
- The feminist movement
- Technology changes affecting career patterns and places of living
- Transmission of knowledge

From "Report of the task force on social issues," by J. A. Johnson, Chairman, Task Force, 1972, *American Journal of Occupational Therapy*, *26*, pp. 333–37. With permission. Copyright © 1972 by American Occupational Therapy Association.

The profession has begun to answer Wiemer's challenge with a return to occupation-based practice and the implementation of broader initiatives such as the USC Well Elderly program, which provides evidence for practice. Continued progress is needed in idea formation and interventions at the broader policy and population levels.

American Journal of Occupational Therapy Special Issue

This first-ever special issue on health promotion of the *American Journal of Occupational Therapy* included articles on a variety of subjects related to health promotion (AOTA, 1986). Topics included educational needs, potential role, cost and benefits of programming, and the best practice examples of that time. The guest editor of the issue defined terminology, the need for outcome measures, and other issues in health promotion.

2000 Health Consortium

In 1989, two AOTA representatives (Anne Long Morris and Evelyn Jaffe) participated in a meeting of the 2000 Health Objectives Consortium sponsored by the Institute of Medicine and U.S. Public Health Service (AOTA, 1989b). This meeting was one of many activities in the development of the health objectives for *Healthy People 2000: National Health Promotion and Disease Prevention Objectives* (U.S. Department of Health and Human Services [USDHHS], 1990). More details regarding other U.S. governmental health-promotion initiatives, including *Healthy People 2010: Understanding and Improving Health* (USDHHS, 2000), appear in Chapter 4.

AOTA Official Statements on Prevention and Health Promotion

The AOTA has published four statements on the profession's role in health promotion. The first was titled "Role of the Occupational Therapist in the Promotion of Health and Prevention of Disabilities" (AOTA, 1979a). The second, "Occupational Therapy in the Promotion of Health Care and the Prevention of Disease and Disability," followed 10 years later (AOTA, 1989a). The next most recent version was titled "Occupational Therapy in the Promotion of Health and the Prevention of Disease and Disability Statement" (Brownson & Scaffa, 2001). The most recent version is titled "Occupational Therapy Services in the Promotion of Health and the Prevention of Disease and Disability" (Scaffa, Van Slyke, Brownson, & American Occupational Therapy Association, 2008).

An evolution in the profession's knowledge and application of prevention and health promotion can be traced by reviewing the aforementioned documents. The introductory section of the first document (AOTA, 1979a) included two significant quotations. The first of these was the oft-quoted World Health Organization (WHO) definition of *health,* which is "the complete state of physical, mental, and social wellbeing, and not just the absence of disease or infirmity" (WHO, 1947, p. 29). The second is Reilly's famous statement that "man, through the use of his hands as they are energized by mind and will, can influence the state of his own health" (Reilly, 1962, p. 1). This two-page role statement was the first AOTA document to be adopted by the Representative Assembly on prevention and health promotion and thus institutionalized the vision of its leadership (Brunyate, 1967; Finn, 1972, 1977; Reilly 1962; West, 1967, 1969; Wiemer, 1972). The second version of the document was reduced to a one-page, five-paragraph document that focused on defining and differentiating between the terms *health promotion* and *wellness* (AOTA, 1989a). The term *wellness* was increasingly being used by both lay and health professionals during this time.

The third version (Brownson & Scaffa, 2001) continued to define wellness, health promotion, and three levels of prevention (i.e., primary, secondary, and tertiary), and the WHO definition of health. New terms that have emerged within the discipline, such as *lifestyle redesign,* also were defined. Readers were introduced to the U.S. national health agenda through a description of *Healthy People 2000* and *Healthy People 2010*. In addition, this version provides examples of individual-level, group-level, organizational-level, community/societal-level, and governmental/policy-level occupation-based interventions. This list of interventions was a resource for occupational therapists and occupational therapy assistants considering such work.

The current 10-page statement (Scaffa et al., 2008) continues to define health promotion and the three levels of prevention and builds on the foundation of the earlier works. The new version provides detailed examples of occupational therapy strategies at each level of prevention. In addition, it expands the discussion of the role of occupational therapy practitioners at the level of the individual, community, population, and organization as well as at the governmental and policy levels. A new feature, case studies, is used to provide details regarding the assessment and intervention process in occupational therapy health promotion practice. The current statement includes a discussion of the profession's unique contribution in this area (see Content Box 1-4).

Occupational Therapy Practice Framework: Domain and Process (Framework)

The capacity for the profession to contribute to health promotion and to disease and disability prevention is supported by the document *Framework* (AOTA, 2008). The *Framework* was developed in order to "more clearly articulate occupational therapy's unique focus on occupation and daily life activities and the application of an

intervention process that facilitates engagement in occupation to support participation in life" (AOTA, 2002, p. 609). This document provides the structure to support health promotion interventions at multiple levels, including context, performance patterns, and performance areas (i.e., education, work, play, leisure, and social participation). Although individuals are the focus of intervention approaches outlined in the tables located in the *Framework*'s appendix, the document defines the terms **client** and **prevention** more broadly than the individual level. See Table 1-3 for these and related definitions (i.e., **health promotion**, **disability prevention**, and **wellness**). The use of these definitions and language that is consistent with the World Health Organization's *International Classification of Functioning, Disability and Health (ICF)* (WHO, 2001) helps the profession make the shift to the new health system paradigm as described by Baum and Law (1997) in Table 1-4.

Centennial Vision

In 2003, the AOTA board of directors "endorsed the development of a Centennial Vision to act as a road map for the future of the profession" (Christiansen, 2004, p. 10). This effort is reminiscent of the work of the 1970 *Task Force on Social Issues* (AOTA, 1972), discussed earlier in this chapter and the long-range planning as advocated by Bair (1982). The goal of this 2-year process was to develop a plan that would

> ensure that individuals, policymakers, populations, and society value and promote occupational therapy's practice of enabling people to prevent and overcome obstacles to participation in the activities they value, to prevent health related issues, improve their physical and mental health, secure well-being, and enjoy a higher quality of life. (Christiansen, 2004, p. 10)

The first step in the development of the Centennial Vision was a scenario-building process that took place in October 2004 (Brachtesende, 2004). Various AOTA leaders and a small number of international representatives were invited to participate in this early stage of the Centennial Vision development. From this process, four possible scenarios were developed. Details regarding each scenario and the anticipated trends impacting the profession are available on the AOTA website. It is expected that the Centennial Vision effort will expand the current view of the profession's role in fostering healthier individuals, families, communities, and society.

Conclusion

The historical use of occupation by many cultures to heal, promote health, and prevent injury and disease has been well chronicled. Occupational therapy's many and varied contributions to health promotion and disease

---

Content Box 1-4

Occupational Therapy's Unique Contribution to Health Promotion and Disease/Disability Prevention

- Evaluate occupational capabilities, values, and performance
- Provide education regarding occupational role performance and balance
- Reduce risk factors and symptoms through engagement in occupation
- Provide skill development training in the context of everyday occupations
- Provide self-management training to prevent illness and manage health
- Modify environments for healthy and safe occupational performance
- Consult and collaborate with health care professionals, organizations, communities, and policymakers regarding the occupational perspective of health promotion and disease or disability prevention
- Promote the development and maintenance of mental functioning abilities through engagement in productive and meaningful activities and relationships (adapted from USDHHS, 1999, p. 4)
- Provide training in adaptation to change and in coping with adversity to promote mental health (adapted from USDHHS, 1999, p. 4)

From "Occupational therapy in the promotion of health and the prevention of disease and disability statement," by C. A. Brownson & M. E. Scaffa, 2001, *American Journal of Occupational Therapy, 55*, pp. 656–60. With permission. Copyright © 2001 by American Occupational Therapy Association.

Table 1–3 **Select Health Promotion Terms and Definitions From the AOTA Frameworks**

Term	Definition
Client	The entity that receives occupational therapy services. Clients may include (1) individuals and other persons relevant to the individual's life, including family, caregivers, teachers, employers and others who also may help or be served indirectly; (2) organizations such as business, industries, or agencies; and (3) populations within a community (Moyers & Dale, 2007 cited by AOTA, 2008, p. 669).
Disability prevention	An intervention approach designed to address clients with or without a disability who are at risk for occupational performance problems. This approach is designed to prevent the occurrence or evolution of barriers to performance in context. Interventions may be directed at client, context, or activity variables (adapted from Dunn et al., 1998 cited by AOTA, 2008, p. 659).
Health promotion	Creating the conditions necessary for health at individual, structural, social, and environmental levels through an understanding of the determinants of health: peace, shelter, education, food, income, a stable ecosystem, sustainable resources, social justice, and equity (Trentham & Cockburn 2005, cited by AOTA, 2008, p. 671).
Prevention	Promoting a healthy lifestyle at the individual, group, organizational, community (societal), governmental/policy level (adapted from Brownson & Scaffa, 2001 AOTA, 2002, p. 633 and AOTA, 2008, p.674).
Wellness	Wellness is more than a lack of disease symptoms. It is a state of mental and physical balance and fitness (adapted from *Taber's Cyclopedic Medical Dictionary*, 1997, in AOTA, 2002, p. 628 and AOTA, 2008, p. 676).

Compiled from *Occupational therapy practice framework: Domain and process*, by the American Occupational Therapy Association, 2002, Bethesda, MD: Author; *Occupational therapy practice framework: Domain and process* (2d ed.), by the American Occupational Therapy Association, 2008, Bethesda, MD: Author. Copyright © 2002, 2008 by American Occupational Therapy Association.

Table 1–4 **A Changing Health System Paradigm**

Area	Old	Medical Model
The Model	Sociopolitical (community) model	Planned or managed health
The Focus	Focus on illness	Focus on wellness
	Acute care outcomes	Wellbeing, function, and life satisfaction
	Individual	Individual within the environment
	Deficiency	Capability
	Survival	Functional ability, quality of life
	Professionally controlled	Personal responsibility, flexible choice
	Dependence	Interdependence, participation
	Treatment	Treatment, prevention
The System	Institution centered	Community centered
	Single facility	Network system
	Competitive focus	Collaborative focus
	Fragmented service	Coordinated service

From Table 1 in "Occupational therapy practice: Focusing on occupational performance," by C. M. Baum and M. Law, 1997, *American Journal of Occupational Therapy, 51*, p. 281. Copyright © 1997 by American Occupational Therapy Association.

and disability prevention are extensively documented. This historical information was reviewed as a foundation for future efforts in health promotion and prevention of disease and disability.

Interdisciplinary efforts are essential to maximize the benefits of occupational therapists and occupational therapy assistants on the health of individuals, families, communities, and populations. Health promotion is performed by a variety of trained individuals; it is not unique to a specific profession. The need for the profession to work collaboratively with other disciplines was recognized decades ago. It was believed the profession's expertise and historical concerns for health and service can best be actualized through interdisciplinary collaboration (MacDonald, 1976). These collaborative efforts can result in more efficacious outcomes that include occupation as a recognized, legitimate tool.

There is much for U.S. occupational therapy practitioners to learn through involvement with the international occupational therapy community. Knowledge can be gained through exposure to international literature (e.g., *Occupational Therapy without Borders: Learning from the Spirit of Survivors* [Kronenberg, Algado, & Pollard, 2005], *British Journal of Occupational Therapy*, *Israeli Journal of Occupational Therapy*, *Journal of Occupational Science, South African Journal of Occupational Therapy*), websites (e.g., Australian Association of Occupational Therapists, Canadian Association of Occupational Therapists, European Network of Occupational Therapy in Higher Education, World Federation of Occupational Therapists), and by attending international conferences. Although countries have differing political and economic ideologies, they share many common health promotion and prevention concerns. As a profession, occupational therapy has much to contribute to the global health and wellbeing of citizens and populations through knowledge of the healing and preventive qualities of occupation. Innovative health-promoting strategies are likely to emerge through international and interdisciplinary collaboration, maximizing the contributions of all involved.

▶ For Discussion and Review

1. As discussed in this chapter, Greek mythology had separate goddesses for healing (Panacea) and for health (Hygeia). Does this division—symbolized in ancient Greek myth—continue in occupational therapy practice today?
2. As quoted earlier, "the occupational therapist of early history was the 'doctor' himself" (MacDonald, 1976, p. 2). Will the advent of clinical doctorates enable occupational therapy to return to the role of

"prescribing" occupations for healing and health? Or might it result in further separation from the potential to serve society and eradicate occupational injustices?
3. Review AOTA's Centennial Vision home page (http://www.aota.org/nonmembers/area16/index.asp) and the four possible future scenarios. What do you see as occupational therapy's possible contributions to society's wellbeing for one of these four scenarios?

▶ Research Questions

1. By way of a document analysis, how does the frequency of articles on issues of occupational and social justice in the *American Journal of Occupational Therapy* compare to other international journals?
2. How does the development of interest in the preventive aspects of occupation in the United States compare to other countries in South America, Southeast Asia, and Europe?

▶ Occupational Engagement Assignments to Enhance Appreciation of the Historical Role of Occupational Therapy in Health Promotion

1. Select five objects that you would put in a time capsule (to be opened in 50 years) to capture the current state of occupational therapy health promotion practice. Explain your selections.
2. Develop a 15-minute skit that depicts time travelers' observations and reflections of occupational therapy interventions directed toward health and wellbeing in at least two different time periods.
3. Develop a presentation that portrays the leaders in occupational therapy from any period in time and highlights the impact of then-current political and social contexts on their professional activities.

References

Ahmed, M. (1990, November). Ibn Sina (Avicenna)—Doctor of doctors. *Muslim Technologist.*Retrieved December 4, 2004, from http://www.ummah.net/history/scholars/ibn_sina/.

Allen, V. R. (1986). Health promotion in the office. *American Journal of Occupational Therapy, 40*(11), 764–70.

American Occupational Therapy Association. (1972). Report of the Task Force on Societal Issues [J. A. Johnson, Chairman]. *American Journal of Occupational Therapy, 26*(7), 332–59.

American Occupational Therapy Association. (1979a). Association official position paper—Role of the occupational therapist in the promotion of health and the prevention of disabilities. *American Journal of Occupational Therapy, 33*(1), 50–51.

American Occupational Therapy Association. (1979b). *Occupational therapy: 2001 AD.* Rockville, MD: Author.

American Occupational Therapy Association. (1979c). Representative assembly minutes: New business—Resolutions, Resolution C, the philosophical base of occupational therapy. *American Journal of Occupational Therapy, 33*(11), 785.

American Occupational Therapy Association. (Producer; 1979d). *The early years* [video].

American Occupational Therapy Association. (1986, November). Special issue of health promotion. *American Journal of Occupational Therapy, 40.*

American Occupational Therapy Association. (1989a). Occupational therapy in the promotion of health care and the prevention of disease and disability (position paper). *American Journal of Occupational Therapy, 43*(12), 806.

American Occupational Therapy Association. (1989b, December 7). Year 2000 health consortium meets. *OT Week, 9.*

American Occupational Therapy Association. (2002). Occupational therapy practice framework: Domain and processes. *American Journal of Occupational Therapy, 56,* 609–39.

American Occupational Therapy Association. (2004). *National school backpack awareness day 2004.* Retrieved February 26, 2005, from http://www.promoteot.org/AI_Backpack Awareness.html.

American Occupational Therapy Association. (2005). *AOTA's Centennial Vision: Shaping the future of occupational therapy, planning scenarios for 2017.* Retrieved December 6, 2005, from http://www.aota.org/nonmembers/area16/links/link02.asp.

American Occupational Therapy Association. (2008). Occupational therapy practice framework: Domain and processes (2d ed.). *American Journal of Occupational Therapy, 62,* 625–88.

Anderson, K. N., Anderson, L. E., & Glanze, W. D. (1998). *Mosby's medical, nursing, allied health dictionary* (5th ed.). Baltimore: Mosby.

Bair, J. (1982). Nationally speaking: Changing trends in practice. *American Journal of Occupational Therapy, 36*(11), 704–07.

Barton, I. (1968). Consolation house, fifty years ago. *American Journal of Occupational Therapy, 22*(4), 340–45.

Barunga, A. (1975). Sacred sites and their protection. In R. Edwards (Ed.), *The preservation of Australia's aboriginal heritage* (pp. 75–76). Canberra: Australian Institute of Aboriginal Studies.

Baum, C. M., & Law, M. (1997). Occupational therapy practice: Focusing on occupational performance. *American Journal of Occupational Therapy, 51*(4), 277–88.

Bowden, R., & Bunbury, B. (1990). *Being aboriginal: Comments, observations and stories from aboriginal Australians.* Crows Nest, New South Wales: Australian Broadcasting Corporation Enterprises.

Brachtesende, A. (2004, October 20). Centennial Vision moves forward. AOTA Newsroom.

Breines, E. (1986). *Origins and adaptations: A philosophy of practice.* Lebanon, NJ: Geri-Rehab.

British Broadcasting Corporation (BBC). (2005). *Historic figures: Sir Winston Churchill (1874–1965).* Retrieved December 6, 2005, from www.bbc.co.uk/history/historic_figures/churchill_winston.shtml.

Brownson, C. A., & Scaffa, M. E. (2001). Occupational therapy in the promotion of health and the prevention of disease and disability statement. *American Journal of Occupational Therapy, 55*(6), 656–60.

Brunyate, R. W. (1967). From the president: After fifty years, what stature do we hold? *American Journal of Occupational Therapy, 21*(5), 262–67.

Carpenter, E. M. (1947). Considerations for prevention of blindness and conservation of vision. *American Journal of Occupational Therapy, 1*(6), 348–51.

Chambers, J. H. (2002). *A traveler's history of Australia* (2nd ed.). New York: Interlink.

Christensen, E. (1991). *A proud heritage: The American Occupational Therapy Association at seventy-five.* Rockville, MD: American Occupational Therapy Association.

Christiansen, C. (2004, September 20). AOTA's Centennial Vision: A map for the future. *OT Practice, 9*(17), 10.

Clark, F., Azen, S. P., Zemke, R., Jackson, J., Carlson, M., Mandela, D., Hay, J., Josephson, K., Cherry, B., Hessel, C., Palmer, J., & Lipson, L. (1997). Occupational therapy for independent-living older adults: A randomized controlled trial. *Journal of the American Medical Association, 278*(16), 1312–26.

Department of Ayurveda, Yoga Naturopathy, Unani, Siddha, and Homoeopathy, Ministry of Health & Family Welfare, Government of India. (2004). *Ayurveda—Introduction: Origin and history.* Retrieved December 20, 2004, from http://indianmedicine.nic.in/html/ayurveda/ayurveda.htm# Introduction.

Despeux, C. (1989). Gymnastics: The ancient tradition. In L. Kohn (ed.), *Taoist meditation and longevity techniques* (pp. 225–61). Ann Arbor, MI: Center for Chinese Studies, University of Michigan.

Diaz, M. P. (1932). Organizing a preventorium for children. *Occupational Therapy and Rehabilitation, 11*(3), 199–201.

Dunton, W. R. (1915). *Occupational therapy: A manual for nurses.* Philadelphia: W. B. Saunders.

Dunton, W. R. (1954). History and development of occupational therapy. In H. S. Willard & C. S. Spackman (Eds.), *Principles of occupational therapy* (2d ed., pp. 1–10). Philadelphia: Lippincott.

Edwards, R. (Ed.). (1975). *The preservation of Australia's aboriginal heritage.* Canberra: Australian Institute of Aboriginal Studies.

Fay, E. V., & Kellogg, I. M. (1954). Occupational therapy in general and surgical hospitals. In H. S. Willard & C. S. Spackman (Eds.), *Principles of occupational therapy* (2d ed., pp. 117–37). Philadelphia: Lippincott.

Finn, G. (1972). The occupational therapist in prevention programs. *American Journal of Occupational Therapy, 26*(2), 59–66.

Finn, G. (1977). Update of Eleanor Clarke Slagle Lecture: The occupational therapist in prevention programs. *American Journal of Occupational Therapy, 31*(10), 658–59.

Frenz, H. (ed.). (1969). *Nobel lectures, literature 1901–1967.* Amsterdam: Elsevier.

Friedland, J. (1998). Looking back—Occupational therapy and rehabilitation: An awkward alliance. *American Journal of Occupational Therapy, 52*(5), 373–80.

George, N. M., Braun, B. A., & Walker, J. M. (1982). A prevention and early intervention mental health program for disadvantaged pre-school children. *American Journal of Occupational Therapy, 36*(2), 99–106.

Gleave, G. M. (1954). Occupational therapy in children's hospitals and pediatric services. In H. S. Willard & C. S. Spackman (Eds.), *Principles of occupational therapy* (2d ed., pp. 138–67). Philadelphia: Lippincott.

Gourley, M. (2000, May 8). Center for occupational therapy and lifestyle redesign. *OT Practice, 5*(10), 18–19.

Gourley, M. (2001a, August 20). News: AOTA Updates: AOTA teams with L.L. Bean. *OT Practice, 6*(15), 3.

Gourley, M. (2001b, September 17). News: AOTA Updates: AOTA Spearheads backpack initiative. *OT Practice, 5*(10), 3.

Green, M. C., Lertvilai, M., & Bribrieso, K. (2001). Prospering through change: CAOT from 1991 to 2001. *Occupational Therapy Now, 3*(6) [online version]. Retrieved December 4, 2005, from http://www.caot.ca/otnow/nov01-eng/nov01.cfm.

Hasselkus, B. R. (2004). Eleanor Clarke Slagle Lecture—The world of everyday occupation: Real people, real lives. *American Journal of Occupational Therapy*, 60, 627–40.

Jaffe, E. (1986). Nationally speaking—The role of occupational therapy in the disease prevention and health promotion. *American Journal of Occupational Therapy, 40*(11), 749–52.

Johnson, J. A. (1986a). *Wellness: A context for living.* Thorofare, NJ: SLACK.

Johnson, J. A. (1986b). Wellness and occupational therapy. *American Journal of Occupational Therapy, 40*(11), 753–58.

Kavasch, E. B., & Baar, K. (1999). *American Indian healing arts.* New York: Bantam Books.

Keegan, J. (2003). *Leaders and revolutionaries: Winston Churchill. Time 100: The most important people of the century.* Retrieved December 6, 2005, from http://www.time.com/time/time100/leaders/profile/churchill4.html.

Kirchman, M. M., Reichenbach, V., & Giambalvo, B. (1982). Preventative activities and services for the well elderly. *American Journal of Occupational Therapy, 36*(4), 236–42.

Krieger, D. (2001, Winter). Something old, something new. *USC Trojan Family Magazine.* Retrieved January 2, 2005, from http://www.usc.edu/dept/pubrel/trojan_family/winter01/therapy/something.html.

Kronenberg, F., Algado, S. S., & Pollard, N. (Eds.). (2005). *Occupational therapy without borders: Learning from the spirit of survivors.* New York: Elsevier, Churchill Livingstone.

Lasker, R. D., & the Committee on Medicine and Public Health. (1997). *Medicine & public health: The power of collaboration.* New York: The New York Academy of Medicine.

Levin, H. L. (1937). Occupational and recreational therapy among the ancients. *Occupational Therapy and Rehabilitation, 17*(5), 311–16.

Licht, S. (1948). Early history of occupational therapy. In S. Licht (Ed.), *Occupational therapy sourcebook* (pp. 1–17). Baltimore: Williams and Wilkins.

Licht, S. (1967). The founding and the founders of the American Occupational Therapy Association. *American Journal of Occupational Therapy, 21*(5), 269–77.

Lyons, A., & Petrucelli, R. (1987). *Medicine: An illustrated history.* New York: Abradale Press.

MacDonald, E. M. (Ed.). (1976). *Occupational therapy in rehabilitation: A handbook for occupational therapists, students and others interested in this aspect of reablement* (4th ed.). Baltimore: Williams & Wilkins.

Mandel, D. R., Jackson, J. M., Nelson, L., & Clark, F. A. (1999). *Lifestyle redesign: Implementing the well elderly program.* Bethesda, MD: American Occupational Therapy Association.

McDaniel, M. L. (1968). Occupational therapists before World War II (1917–40). In H. S. Lee & M. L. McDaniel (Eds.), *Army Medical Specialist Corps* (pp. 69–97). Washington, DC: Office of the Surgeon General, Department of the Army. Retrieved December 4, 2005, from http://history.amedd.army.mil/booksdocs/histories/ArmyMedicalSpecialistCorps/chapter4.htm.

National Library of Medicine. (2004a). *Greek medicine: Asclepius.* Retrieved December 14, 2004, from http://www.nlm.nih.gov/hmd/greek/greek_asclepius.html.

National Library of Medicine. (2004b). *Greek medicine: Pythagoras.* Retrieved December 4, 2004, from http://www.nlm.nih.gov/hmd/greek/greek_pythagoras.html.

National Library of Medicine. (2004c). *Shell shock.* Retrieved December 5, 2004, from http://www.nlm.nih.gov/news/ww1hmdexhibit04.html.

National Library of Medicine. (2005). Untitled document. Retrieved February 24, 2005, from http://www.nlm.nih.gov/hmd/breath/breath_exhibit/FourPersp/sick/IVDb1.html.

National Museum of American Indians. (2005). *Our universes: Traditional knowledge shapes our world.* Retrieved February 24, 2005, from http://www.nmai.si.edu/subpage.cfm?subpage=dc&second=visitor&third=inside#universes.

Neuhas, B. (1968). Founder's Day at Clifton Springs. *American Journal of Occupational Therapy, 22*(4), 337–39.

Parush, S., Lapidot, G., Edelstein, P. V., & Tamir, D. (1987). Occupational therapy in mother and child health care centers. *American Journal of Occupational Therapy, 41*(9), 601–05.

Peloquin, S. M. (1991a). Looking back—Occupational therapy: Individual and collective understandings of the founders, Part 1. *American Journal of Occupational Therapy, 45*, 352–60.

Peloquin, S. M. (1991b). Looking back—Occupational therapy: Individual and collective understandings of the founders, Part 2. *American Journal of Occupational Therapy, 45*, 733–44.

Peterson, N. (1975). The ownership of sacred sites. In R. Edwards (Ed.), *The preservation of Australia's aboriginal heritage* (pp. 73–75). Canberra: Australian Institute of Aboriginal Studies.

Pizzi, M., Scaffa, M., & Reitz, S. M. (2006). Health promotion and wellness for people with physical disabilities. In H. M. Pendleton & W. Schultz-Krohn (Eds.), *Pedretti's occupational therapy for physical dysfunction* (6th ed., pp. 65–78). St. Louis, MO: Elsevier.

Punwar, A. J. (2000). The development of occupational therapy. In A. J. Punwar & S. M. Peloquin (Eds.), *Occupational therapy: Principles and practice* (3d ed.). Baltimore: Lippincott Williams & Wilkins.

Reilly, M. (1962). Occupational therapy can be one of the great ideas of 20th century medicine. *American Journal of Occupational Therapy*, 16(1), 1–9.

Reitz, S. (1984, April). *Preventive health: An essential component of occupational therapy.* Presentation at American Occupational Therapy Association Conference, Kansas City, MO.

Reitz, S. M. (1990). *The historical and philosophical bases for occupational therapy's role in health promotion.* Presentation at the 10th International Congress of the World Federation of Occupational Therapists, Melbourne, Australia.

Reitz, S. M. (1992). A historical review of occupational therapy's role in preventive health and wellness. *American Journal of Occupational Therapy, 46*, 50–55.

Reitz, S. M. (2004). *Health and wellness through: Occupation: The American Perspective* invited Open Seminar, Hospital Authority, Hong Kong.

Savage-Smith, E. (1994). *Islamic culture and the medical arts: An exhibit at the National Library of Medicine.* Bethesda, MD: National Library of Medicine [online brochure]. Retrieved December 4, 2004, from http://www.nlm.nih.gov/exhibition/islamic_medical/islamic_00.html.

Scaffa, M. E. (2001). Community-based practice: Occupation in context. In M. E. Scaffa (Ed.), *Occupational therapy in community-based practice settings* (pp. 3–18). Philadelphia: F. A. Davis.

Scaffa, M. E., & Brownson, C. (2005). Occupational therapy interventions: Community health approaches. In C. H. Christiansen, C. M. Baum, & J. Bass-Haugen (Eds.), *Occupational therapy: Performance, participation and well-being* (3d ed., pp. 477–88). Thorofare, NJ: SLACK.

Scaffa, M. E., Van Slyke, N., Brownson, C. A., & American Occupational Therapy Association Commission on Practice. (2008). Occupational therapy services in the promotion of health and the prevention of disease and disability, *American Journal of Occupational Therapy 62*(6), 694–703.

Schwartz, R. K. (1989). Cognition and learning in industrial accident injury prevention: An occupational therapy perspective. *Occupational Therapy in Health Care, 6*(1) 67–85.

Shaffer, G. W. (1938). Recreation as a preventive and therapy for social maladjustments. *Occupational Therapy and Rehabilitation, 17*(2), 97–106.

Sivin, N. (1995). State, cosmos, and body in the last three centuries B.C. *Harvard Journal of Asian Studies, 55*(1), 5–37.

Soames, M. (2002). Foreword. In W. Churchill, *Painting as a pastime* (pp. vii–viii). Delray, FL: Levinger.

Spear, P. S., & Crepeau, E. B. (2003). Glossary. In E. B. Crepeau, E. S. Cohn, & B. A. Schell, *Willard & Spackman's occupational therapy* (10th ed., pp. 1025–35). Philadelphia: Lippincott, Williams & Wilkins.

Stallings-Sahler, S. (2007). AOTA's Statement on stress and stress disorders. *American Journal of Occupational Therapy, 61,* 711.

Stattel, F. M. (1977). Occupational therapy: Sense of the past—Focus on the present. *American Journal of Occupational Therapy, 31*, 649–50.

Townsend, E. (1999). Invited comment: Enabling occupation in the 21st century: Making good intentions a reality. *Australian Occupational Therapy Journal, 46*, 147–59.

United Service Organizations (USO). (2005). *Historical timeline*. Retrieved February 26, 2005, from http://www.uso.org/pubs/8_14_34.cfm.

University of Southern California (USC), Department of Occupational Science and Occupational Therapy. (2004). *About us: Center for Occupation and Lifestyle Redesign.* Retrieved January 2, 2005, from http://www.usc.edu/schools/ihp/ot/about/center/.

University of Texas Medical Branch, Academic Resources. (2005). *Aulus Cornelius Celsus.* [Lithograph]. Retrieved February 24, 2005, from http://ar.utmb.edu/areas/informresources/collections/blocker/portraits/bios/celsus.asp.

U.S. Department of Health and Human Services. (1990). *Healthy People 2000: National health promotion and disease prevention objectives*. Washington, DC: Government Printing Office.

U.S. Department of Health and Human Services. (1999). *Mental health: A report of the Surgeon General.* Rockville, MD: Author.

U.S. Department of Health and Human Services. (2000). *Healthy People 2010: Understanding and improving health* (2d ed). Washington, DC: U.S. Government Printing Office.

Vogel, V. J. (1970). *American Indian medicine.* University of Oklahoma: University of Oklahoma Press, Norman and London.

West, W. (1967). The occupational therapist's changing responsibility to the community. *American Journal of Occupational Therapy, 21*(5), 312–16.

West, W. (1969). The growing importance of prevention. *American Journal of Occupational Therapy, 23*(3), 226–31.

Wiemer, R. (1972). Some concepts of prevention as an aspect of community health. *American Journal of Occupational Therapy, 26*(1), 1–9.

Wiemer, R. (1979). Traditional and nontraditional arenas. In *Occupational therapy: 2001 AD* (pp. 42–53). Rockville, MD: Author.

Wilcock, A. A. (1998). *An occupational perspective of health.* Thorofare, NJ: SLACK.

Wilcock, A. A. (2000). Development of a personal, professional and educational philosophy: An Australian perspective. *Occupational Therapy International, 7*(2), 79–86.

Wilcock, A. A., & Townsend, E. (2000). Occupational terminology interactive dialogue: Occupational justice. *Journal of Occupational Science, 7*(2), 84–86.

Willard, H., & Cox, B. (1979). A profile of occupational therapy and occupational therapy practice. In *Occupational Therapy: 2001* (pp. 69–70). [An interview of H. Willard by B. Cox]. Rockville, MD: American Occupational Therapy Association.

Willard, H., & Spackman, C. (1971). *Occupational therapy* (4th ed., p. 1). Philadelphia: Lippincott.

World Health Organization. (1947). Constitution of the World Health Organization. *Chronicle of the World Health Organization, 1*(1), 29–40.

World Health Organization (WHO). (2001). *The international classification of functioning, disability, and health (ICF)*. Geneva, Switzerland: Author.

Wudang Taoist Internal Alchemy. (2005). Mount Lao Shan and the temples. Retrieved December 4, 2005, from http://www.damo-qigong.net/laoshan_1.htm.

Zemke, R. (2004). The 2004 Eleanor Clarke Slagle Lecture— Time, space, and the kaleidoscopes of occupation. *American Journal of Occupational Therapy, 58,* 608–20.

Chapter 2

Occupational Therapy Conceptual Models for Health Promotion Practice

S. Maggie Reitz, Marjorie E. Scaffa, and Michael A. Pizzi

> Science is facts; just as houses are made of stones, so is science made of facts; but a pile of stones is not a house and a collection of facts is not necessarily science.
> —Henri Poincare (1854–1912)

Learning Objectives

This chapter is designed to enable the reader to:

- Describe a variety of models from within the profession of occupational therapy that could possibly support health promotion programs.
- Evaluate the advantages and disadvantages of the various models for use in occupational therapy health promotion interventions in different contexts.
- Integrate language of the American Occupational Therapy Association's (AOTA) *Occupational Therapy Practice Framework* (*Framework* [AOTA, 2008]) and the World Health Organization's (WHO) *International Classification of Functioning, Disability and Health* (*ICF* [WHO, 2001]) with the application of a theory or conceptual practice model.
- Select appropriate models that support occupational therapy health promotion intervention targeted to a specific population, health problem, or incidence of occupational apartheid.

Key Terms

Environment	Input	Occupational identity	Throughput
Environmental fit	Interests	Output	Values
Feedback	Occupational adaptation	Performance capacity	Volition
Habituation	Occupational apartheid	Personal causation	
Health promotion	Occupational	Primary energy	
Human agency	competence	Secondary energy	

Introduction

Theorists organize the building blocks of science—constructs and principles—into an organized pattern, or theory, that explains natural events. This theory construction can be guided by philosophical assumptions as depicted in Figure 2-1. The theories used by occupational therapists explain and predict human behavior in relation to health and occupational performance. This chapter reviews a selection of theories and models from occupational therapy to provide a framework for health promotion practice.

The authors believe the selected occupational therapy models are sufficiently broad to apply to the variety of populations and health behaviors addressed in this text. In addition, they are particularly well suited for use in combination with selected models from other health disciplines. Examples of models from related disciplines are presented in Chapter 3 of this text, which also provides guidance for selecting and possibly combining occupational therapy models and those from other disciplines to enhance theoretical support for health promotion programs.

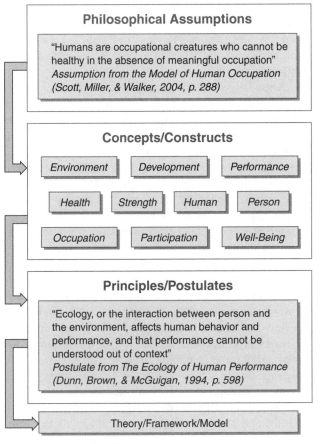

Figure 2-1   Theory construction process.

Developed by S. Maggie Reitz.

Many occupational therapy models exist that may be combined or used independently to support efforts in community-based health promotion interventions. Readers are encouraged to examine the literature for additional models—those developed within the United States and those developed in other countries—to find the model that best fits the community or health behavior of interest. This chapter reviews five recognized and widely used models, including the following:

• Ecology of Human Performance (EHP) Framework
• Model of Human Occupation (MOHO)
• Occupational Adaptation (OA) Theory
• Person-Environment-Occupation (PEO) Model
• Person-Environment-Occupation-Performance (PEOP) Model

In addition, the chapter also describes a newer model that is growing in popularity and has the potential to contribute to health promotion initiatives. Developed from an Asian perspective, this model is known as the *Kawa* ("river" in Japanese) Model (Iwama, 2005a,

2005b, 2006a; Iwama, Odawara, & Asaba, 2006; Lim & Iwama, 2006).

Prior to discussing the models, terminology used to describe the components of theory is reviewed to aid in the description of each model. In addition, schematics and health promotion practice examples are provided for each model. Through an understanding of the profession's philosophy and theories, interventions can be optimally designed. These interventions can facilitate the efforts of individuals, families, and communities as they seek to improve their health, their participation in society, and their overall quality of life through engagement in occupation.

Importance of Theory to Health Promotion Practice

Models and theories provide the foundational context for program design, implementation, and evaluation (Scaffa, 1992). However, "research and theory have little to offer society unless they are applied and used" (Royeen, 2000, p. v). When used, both occupational therapy theories and those from related disciplines can enhance the design and evaluation of health promotion programming. Thus, it is important for occupational therapists to be knowledgeable of and proficient in the use of models and theories. Many reasons exist for the limited use of theory in practice (Reitz, 1998a), including the ever-increasing pace of change, the demands placed on health-care workers that impact the art of practice (Peloquin, 1989), and the lack of available time to explore theoretical ideas in practice (Reitz, 1998a). Occupational therapists and occupational therapy assistants are not immune from significant time pressures in their work and personal lives. These pressures decrease the available time to be a competent consumer of available research and theory. Skills in time management and priority setting must be honed to acquire sufficient time to engage in theory and evidence-based practice. In addition, the use of technology and such resources as OTseeker (Bennett et al., 2003) save the occupational therapist and occupational therapy assistant time and facilitate competent, evidence-based practice supported by theory.

Additional challenges hinder proficiency in the application of theory. Few occupational therapists and occupational therapy assistants have had the opportunity to observe theory application during their fieldwork experiences. In addition, little emphasis is placed on theory in continuing-education courses. The use of inconsistent and sometimes conflicting terminology can create initial confusion and can lead to subsequent theory avoidance. However, many important reasons exist for bridging the gap between theory and practice. Miller and Schwartz (2004) identified five reasons to be knowledgeable of and competent in the use of theory (see Content Box 2-1). All five of these reasons are consistent with the AOTA *Occupational Therapy Code of Ethics* (AOTA, 2005*)*, specifically Principle 4, which addresses duties and states "occupational therapy personnel shall achieve and continually maintain high standards of competence" (p. 3).

It is imperative that occupational therapy students and occupational therapists feel comfortable when articulating the theory base of occupational therapy and when applying theory, from both occupational therapy and other related disciplines to intervention and program planning. When doing so, they blend the art of a caring practice (Peloquin, 1989, 2005) with the science of the discipline, which is supported by the occupational therapy profession's core values of justice, dignity, truth, and prudence (AOTA, 1993). The next section reviews terminology, the relationship between philosophy, theory, practice, and research to foster artful scientific practice.

Terminology and Relationships Between Philosophy, Theory, Practice, and Research

The terminology used in the discussion of theory is complex and often used in conflicting ways by theorists and writers (Miller & Schwartz, 2004). Table 2-1 was developed to help decrease confusion in this area. Frequently used terms, including *paradigm, frame of reference/conceptual model of practice, postulate/principle, concept/construct,* and *philosophical assumptions* are defined within this table. With an understanding of the "stones" that build theories and of the building blocks of knowledge, the reader is ready to organize these ideas

and systems into broader schemas that explain how the profession makes, uses, and discards ideas about people and their occupations. Reviewing Figure 2-1 will assist the reader in understanding this theory construction process.

Knowledge can be organized into systems in order to facilitate discussion of ideas and foster development of theories. These systems seek to explain the relationships between philosophy, theory, practice, and research and have been visualized and described in different ways. Disciplines organize knowledge for practical use into theories and models, and, within occupational therapy, frames of reference. These organizational structures can be viewed as parts of larger, more complex organizational systems that contain and support the knowledge used by a profession (Reitz & Scaffa, 2001).

Many schematics exist that visually represent different methods of organizing occupational therapy knowledge. Two of these methods are included for review and consideration; in one, Kielhofner employs a series of concentric circles (Fig. 2-2), while in the other, Reitz uses a comet metaphor (Fig. 2-3). These organizational schemes can be helpful tools in the study of occupational therapy knowledge. The links between the "science" of occupation and health, both within and external to the profession, and the links between theory and practice are delineated. There are similarities and differences in the way these links are displayed in the two schematics.

For example, in Figure 2-2, the paradigm is located in the center and represents Kielhofner's view that "it most directly addresses the identity and outlook of the field" (Kielhofner, 2004, p. 15). In Figure 2-3 Reitz (1998b, 2000) provides an alternate representation, which includes the recipient of care. In this view, the recipient of services appears at the comet's core in order to emphasize the importance of client-centered care. The service recipient can be an individual, family, community, or population. The paradigm is depicted as the comet's body and uses the symbolism of the comet moving through space and time to represent how the profession's past influences its current viewpoint and how the current view impacts its future trajectory. Occupational science is not included in Kielhofner's schematic. In the comet metaphor, Reitz portrays occupational science as an attractor and mediator of knowledge from other disciplines that can support the theoretical basis of occupational therapy practice. This view is consistent with the description of occupational science as "a human science that is concerned with the systematic study of the form, function, and meaning of human occupation in all contexts, including the therapeutic context" (Clark, as cited in Crist, Royeen, & Schkade, 2000, p. 49).

Content Box 2-1

Reasons for Advocating Knowledge and Competency in Theory

- To validate and guide practice
- To justify reimbursement
- To clarify specialization items
- To enhance the growth of the profession and the professionalism of its members
- To educate competent practitioners

Content from "What is theory, and why does it matter?" by R. J. Miller and K. Schwartz, 2004, in K. F. Walker and F. M. Ludwig (Eds.), *Perspectives on theory for the practice of occupational therapy* (3d ed., pp. 1–26). Austin, TX: Pro-ED.

Table 2–1   Common Theoretical Terms and Definitions

Term	Definition	Definition	Example(s)
Paradigm	Compilation of a unique set of shared ideas, values, and beliefs about a discipline, which create the foundation and vision of the profession (Kielhofner, 2004 based on the work of Kuhn, 1970).	"Typical way in which an academic discipline defines its current theoretical system, field of study, methods of research, and standards for acceptable solutions at any given time" (Mosey, 1981, p. 123).	Figures 2-2 and 2-3
Frame of Reference/ Conceptual Practice Model	Fundamental components of practice consisting of beliefs and scientific theories that are thought to be expert opinions in a discipline. Professions consist of one model and many frames of reference which are more limited and focused on one particular aspect of the profession's theory. Frames of reference include concepts, terms, and postulates that are related to specific areas of practice (Mosey, 1981).	"Presents and organizes theory used by therapists in their work . . . addresses some specific phenomena or area of human function" (Kielhofner, 2004, p. 20). Conceptual practice models give justification for specific practice methods and provide therapists with a way to understand clients' unique perspectives, occupations, experiences, and problems (Kielhofner, 2004).	Sensory Integration (Miller & Schwartz, 2004) Model of Human Occupation (Kielhofner, 2004)
Principle/Postulate	Postulates describe relationships "between two or more concepts" (Mosey, 1981, p. 36).	Principles describe the relationship between phenomena of interest (i.e., concepts/constructs).	Figure 2-1
Concept/Construct	Concepts are observable characteristics of the environment; constructs are intangible characteristics (Mosey, 1981).	Concepts identify structural features or objects (e.g., table, chair); constructs characterize observations (e.g., patience, wellbeing).	Figure 2-1
Philosophical Assumptions	"Basic beliefs about the nature of human life, the individual, society, the universe, and the relationships among these various phenomena" (Mosey, 1981, p. 17).	Beliefs that are the essence of a culture, society, discipline, or movement and which support its decision-making.	"Man is . . . an organism that maintains and balances itself in the world of reality and actuality by being in active life and active use, i.e., using and living and acting its *time* in harmony with its own nature and the nature about it" (Meyer, 1922/1977, p. 641). "Man through the use of his hands as they are energized by mind and will, can influence the state of his own health" (Reilly, 1962, p. 2).

Developed by S. Maggie Reitz.

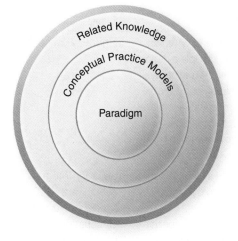

Figure 2-2   Kielhofner's view of the relationship between related knowledge, conceptual practice models, and paradigms.

From Conceptual foundations of occupational therapy *(3d ed., p. 15), by G. Kielhofner, 2004, Philadelphia: F. A. Davis. Copyright © 2004 by F. A. Davis. Reprinted with permission.*

Occupational Therapy Theories/Models

As stated above, a sampling of the occupational therapy theories and models available for use in health promotion will be described in this chapter. Determining which theories to include was a challenging task, with selection based on potential for use in support of health promotion programming. The reader is encouraged to reflect on how the presented models may be used in health promotion and to use these and other models in day-to-day practice. Of primary importance, however, is the application of the theory that best matches the population or context, rather than trying to fit the population or program to a specific model.

Although the presentation order was chosen solely on placing the selected models in alphabetical order, this sequence also has a logical flow.

- Ecology of Human Performance (EHP) Framework
- Model of Human Occupation (MOHO)
- Occupational Adaptation (OA) Theory
- Person-Environment-Occupation (PEO) Model
- Person-Environment-Occupation-Performance (PEOP) Model

The discussion starts with two of the discipline's first models to examine the human and environment interaction—the EHP Framework and the MOHO. These models are followed by the OA theory (Schultz & Schkade, 2003), which focuses on the internal process of adaptation to maximize health and participation. The discussion ends with two models having similar terminology and primary constructs, the PEO and the PEOP.

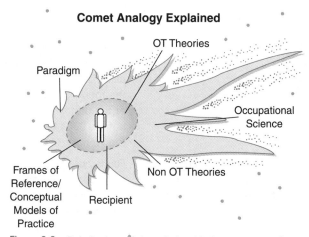

Comet Analogy Explained

Figure 2-3   Reitz's view of the relationship between paradigm, occupational science, theories, and conceptual models of practice and the recipient of the intervention.

Reproduced and adapted from S. M. Reitz in "Theoretical frameworks for community-based practice" (p. 59) by S. M. Reitz & M. Scaffa in Occupational therapy in community-based practice settings, *M. Scaffa (Ed.), 2001, Philadelphia: F. A. Davis. Copyright © 2001 by F. A. Davis. Reprinted with permission.*

An overview of the basic assumptions and constructs of each model will be presented. This overview is followed by a discussion of the model's applicability to health promotion and an example of a theory-based health promotion intervention. Theorists' responses to one or more questions posed by the authors during the preparation of this chapter appear either embedded in the text or as Content Boxes. The amount of discussion varies slightly based on the complexity of the theory or example. Prior to using any of these models in health-promotion practice, the reader is strongly encouraged to read the most recent literature both on testing of the particular model and on evidenced-based research that applies the model.

Ecology of Human Performance (EHP): Overview

The impetus for the development of this framework by the faculty at the University of Kansas was to express the complexity of context and its impact on occupational engagement. The development of the framework was influenced by the work of environmental and developmental psychologists, as well as occupational therapy theorists and occupational scientists (Dunn, Brown, & McGuigan, 1994). The primary assumptions include the following:

- To understand the occupational performance of humans, and that performance must be studied in context (Dunn, McClain, Brown, & Youngstrom, 2003)
- "People and their contexts are unique and dynamic" (Dunn et al., 2003, p. 224)

• "Contrived contexts are different from natural contexts" (Dunn et al., 2003, p. 224)

The major constructs of this conceptual practice model—the person and his or her skills, abilities, performance range, context, and habitual tasks—are displayed in Figure 2-4. Individuals' skills and abilities in combination with a perception of their context support the selection and performance of specific tasks, which are defined in the model as "objective sets of behaviors necessary to accomplish a goal" (Dunn et al., 1994, p. 599). The performance range of each individual, family, or community depends on both past experience and current resources. Limited access to resources may impact the performance range of an individual, family, community, or population, even if they have a wide repertoire of skills and abilities.

These diminished resources may be due to a temporary crisis or a more permanent situation. For example, a well-functioning community in the Sunbelt may find their ability to respond to an emergency (i.e., performance range) significantly hindered temporarily by a rare snowfall. If the same community was to experience three back-to-back hurricanes in successive hurricane seasons, resources and skills would need to be addressed, or the performance range of the community would narrow and remain constrained through the hurricane season. This situation would impact the productivity and quality of life of the individuals and the community as a whole.

The EHP model provides "five alternatives for therapeutic intervention" (Dunn et al., 1994, p. 603):

1. The *Establish/Restore* level includes traditional interventions that seek to restore function via the improvement of skills and abilities, most often

of individuals but increasingly also in families. This type of intervention also could be used at the community level.

2. At the *Adapt* level, the therapist adapts "the contextual features and task demands to support performance" (Dunn et al., 1994, p. 604), again this could be used with an individual or family in their contexts or a community.

3. At the *Alter* level, the therapist changes the actual context rather than adapting the current one. An example of such an intervention would be facilitating the move of an individual who had a series of falls in severe winter weather to a retirement community that has covered walkways so the individual will not be forced to walk outside. She can use the covered walkways to engage in occupations that she enjoys (e.g., having meals with friends) and other activities of daily living (ADLs) and instrumental activities of daily living (IADLs) such as mail retrieval.

4. The *Prevent* level of intervention seeks to "prevent the occurrence or evolution of maladaptive performance in context" (Dunn et al., 1994, p. 604). This type of intervention could be at the individual, family, or community level.

5. At the *Create* level, the goal is to create "circumstances that promote more adaptable or complex performance in context" (Dunn et al., 1994, p. 604). Policy initiatives, program development, community development, and community empowerment are all activities at this level of intervention and are examples of health-promotion activities.

In the EHP framework, intervention is always guided by the cultural context of the individual, family, community, or population. Tasks that an individual, family, community, or population pursue are influenced by skills and abilities and by personal choices, priorities, and values that are often guided by both life experience and culture. For example, a community's decision to adapt a playground to ensure it is accessible may be initiated by the work of one young (e.g., middle school) advocate with a younger disabled sibling.

Ecology of Human Performance: Applicability in Health Promotion

The relationship of the EHP to the promotion of health and wellbeing is presented in Content Box 2-2. The EHP has been identified as an appropriate framework for health promotion, as described below:

Interventions are intended to assist individuals in recognizing their health needs, acting, and gaining

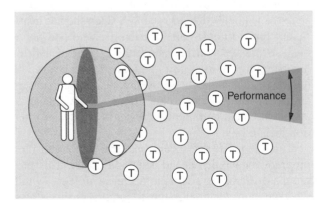

Figure 2-4 Representation of an individual with limited skills and abilities as viewed using the EHP framework. The human figure could also represent a family, a population, or a community.

From Infusing occupation into practice *(p. 109), by P. A. Crist, C. B. Royeen, & J. K. Schkade (Eds.), 2000, Bethesda, MD: American Occupational Therapy Association. Copyright 1994 by the American Occupational Therapy Association.*

competence in the performance of these behaviors. Two of the EHP's intervention alternatives relate directly to preventive health behaviors. The "Prevent" and "Create" alternatives address how therapists assess an individual's context and take steps to avoid the occurrence of negative outcomes, or formulate a new set of circumstances to encourage the individual's success. (Lutz, 1998, p. 17)

These levels of intervention can be easily matched to levels of prevention and health promotion. An intervention at the Prevent level may, for example, include the development of an interdisciplinary program to educate first-year college students about healthy eating and cooking techniques that match their limited space and available funds. This program would address both the prevention of weight gain and the enhancement of the students' performance range. Forming a community group to advocate for a walking trail that would also be accessible to wheelchair users to promote physical activity, leisure engagement, and a healthy lifestyle is an example of a Create-level intervention.

Limited EHP-related research is presently available. In one of the few existing studies, Brown, Cosgrove, and DeSelm (1997) used the EHP to examine barriers to recovery and quality of life for clients with severe and persistent mental illness. Barriers were identified through the lenses of clients and their case managers. The EHP was used to classify these barriers as relating to person or context. The study included 33 participants (20 clients and 13 case managers; some case managers were assigned to more than one participant). Results indicated that clients identified more contextual barriers while case managers most frequently identified barriers related to the person and their skills. Clients identified

lack of knowledge as a primary barrier versus lack of ability skill. Examining the potential barriers to quality of life is important to consider in health promotion intervention and program planning. Understanding the potential differences between and among community, group, family members, and service providers is important in order to maximize the intervention's overall success.

While a solid base of published research has not substantiated the EHP model, it shows promise for use in health promotion programs directed at groups, families, communities, or populations. For example, the EHP could be used to both structure a transition program within the criminal justice system and to set a direction for developing measurable outcome objectives for the program's evaluation. As with the Model of Human Occupation (MOHO), the EHP's interdisciplinary theoretical foundation makes it well suited for use in interdisciplinary health promotion programs with populations or communities. This model has been used in conjunction with a health behavior model, specifically the Health Belief Model, to design an interdisciplinary health promotion program. The Strides for Life walking program for older adults was conducted at a nutrition site in western Maryland (Stevenson, 1998) and was supported by a Health Resources and Services Administration grant (Grant #36 AH 10043-4). The decision-making or "matching" process of selecting two complementary models will be described in the next chapter.

Ecology of Human Performance: Health Promotion Example

Cindy is unknowingly used by her boyfriend to drive a getaway car after he steals a large amount of illicit drugs from an undercover police officer. After the boyfriend fires shots, they are both apprehended. She is sent to a women's detention center, since she has insufficient funds to post bail. Her family, who had previously expressed concern about the boyfriend and his habits, refuses to assist with bail. She feels betrayed by her boyfriend, abandoned by her family, and unsure about her future. Prior to her arrest, she had hoped to attend the local community college to study information technology.

Cindy requests and secures placement in a transition program for women at the detention center. This program's overarching goal is to decrease violence within the detention center through a comprehensive stress-reduction initiative. The agreement includes a commitment to participate in an 8-week group-structured interdisciplinary program. Occupational therapy is part of this program, together with yoga, physical activity, health education, and other activities. The

---

Content Box 2-2

Dr. Winnie Dunn's Reflections on the EHP

Question:
From your perspective, how do you see the EHP relating to the health and wellbeing of people?

Response:
One of our favorite things about the EHP framework is that it is NOT about disability, disease, or other "problem" focused issues . . . It is about living, how ALL of us live and thrive . . . All of us are negotiating the task, context and our own skills to conduct our daily lives, and the EHP merely illustrates these relationships. It levels the playing field, with no one standing out as the "problem." . . . We could plot anyone's life on the diagram, and all of us have challenges and successes in the interaction of task context and our own skills.

occupational therapy portion of the program is developed and delivered jointly by an occupational therapy graduate student and an occupational therapy faculty member who is also a trained health educator. This portion of the program focuses on a combination of self-assessment, occupational engagement, and education focused on the domain of occupational therapy (AOTA, 2008).

Sessions are held weekly for 1 hour (Dailey & Reitz, 2003). At the first session, each woman completes a self-assessment of occupational needs to determine which performance skills and patterns could be strengthened for enhanced ADL and IADL participation. Based on trends in the group's needs, the occupations and education units provided over the next 7 weeks are adjusted. The women participate in a variety of occupations designed to facilitate an increase in their performance range. Their performance ranges are increased by either remediating or enhancing skills through such activities as résumé writing, job interviewing, healthy low-cost leisure pursuits, parenting skills, and basic health awareness and self-screening skills. Each session concludes with a discussion of how the day's activities would enhance role performance and the women's overall health and wellbeing.

Model of Human Occupation (MOHO): Overview

From its inception, the MOHO was influenced by Reilly's work on occupational behavior (1962, 1969, 1974) and theories from other disciplines (Kielhofner, 1985a, 2004). This interdisciplinary base (Kielhofner, 2004) included theories from anthropology; sociology; psychology, including environmental and social psychology; and systems theory as described by von Bertalanffy (1968). The current version of the MOHO is based on dynamical systems theory and includes four principles upon which the rest of the model is built (Kielhofner, 2002). These principles are displayed in Content Box 2-3. Key assumptions of the MOHO that support these principles include the following:

- Humans have an innate need for occupation, and the ability to fulfill this need promotes health and wellbeing.
- Health and wellbeing depend on a constant interplay between the person and the environment.

These principles and assumptions are important to consider when applying the MOHO to health-promotion interventions.

According to Kielhofner (2004), the MOHO is a conceptual practice model. As such, it provides a framework for the therapist to investigate how people are motivated toward their occupations; how they perceive,

---

Content Box 2-3
Human Order Principles That Support the MOHO
• Humans are composed of flexible elements whose interaction with each other and with the environment depends on the situation.
• Thinking, feeling, and doing emerge out of dynamic interactions between elements within the person and those in the environment.
• Dysfunction is the result of the interaction of conditions internal and external to the person.
• Function can be enhanced through remediation of a faulty element, compensation by another element within the person, and/or by environmental modification.

Content from *A model of human occupation: Theory and application* (3d ed., p. 38), by G. Kielhofner, 2002, Baltimore: Lippincott, Williams & Wilkins. Copyright 2002 by Lippincott, Williams & Wilkins.

---

learn, and sustain performance patterns; and how the environment impacts that performance. The importance of the environment's relationship to occupational performance is a major focus (University of Illinois at Chicago [UIC], 2005a). The MOHO emphasizes that through therapy, persons are helped to engage in doing things that maintain, restore, reorganize, or develop their capacities, motives, and lifestyles.

The primary original constructs of the MOHO include feedback, input, throughput, and output. These constructs are linked in a cycle that describes how humans interact with the environment (Kielhofner, 1980a, 1980b; Kielhofner & Burke, 1980; Kielhofner & Igi, 1980). This interaction is the **output** of the system, or what was originally described as occupational behavior. **Feedback** produces information to the person regarding current behaviors and occupational performance, and the possible need for adaptation based on the feedback. **Input** refers to the information from the environment, which the person processes via throughput.

Throughput is composed of the subsystems volition, habituation, and performance capacity. **Volition** refers to the process by which persons are motivated to choose what they do. The volitional subsystem refers to one's thoughts and feelings about the process of being occupationally engaged. These thoughts and feelings reflect a person's effectiveness to act in the world (i.e., **personal causation**), what the person holds as important (i.e., **values**), and what the person finds enjoyable and satisfying (i.e., **interests**).

Habituation refers to a process whereby actions are organized into routines and patterns. This area incorporates a person's habits of daily living (i.e., learned ways of doing things that occur in an automatic way) and roles (i.e., the development of an identity and the behaviors that engage the person in that role).

Performance capacity refers to and includes the neurophysiological, cardiopulmonary, cognitive, and mental capacities of individuals that help them carry out and engage in occupations while interacting with the environment; it "refers both to the underlying objective mental and physical abilities and to the lived experience that shapes performance" (Kielhofner, 2004, p. 148). Over time, the construct of performance capacity has been increasingly viewed as blended phenomena of objective and subjective components (Kielhofner, Tham, Baz, & Hutson, 2008). The importance of mind-body unity on the lived body experience is important to truly understand occupation at the performance level. For example, physical performance and the desire to engage in physical activity can be affected by mood. In addition, the quality of physical performance can, in turn, impact mood.

The process of occupational adaptation has been added to the MOHO. The three main constructs of volition, habituation, and performance capacity are seen as continuously interacting with one another. Through this interaction, a person, family, or community chooses to engage in meaningful habits and routines that are supported by their abilities. In addition, they may choose to engage in occupations that stretch their capabilities and through the process of occupational adaptation refine their occupational identity and occupational competence:

> Occupational adaptation is dynamic and context dependent; therefore what a person does in work, play, and self-care is a function of the interaction among person, characteristics of motivation, life patterns, and performance capacity with the environment. All clients have the potential for change and to become more occupationally adaptive through occupational therapy. (Kielhofner, Forsyth, & Barrett, 2003, p. 213)

Figure 2-5 displays the process of occupational adaptation within the MOHO. In this process, **occupational identity** is the sense of self that humans or communities develop over time through reflection upon the results of their active selection and engagement in meaningful occupation. The additional construct of **occupational competence** is viewed as the sustainability of a pattern of occupation that is congruent with a person's or community's occupational identity (Kielhofner, 2002).

The environment, which includes both social and physical dimensions, is a key construct in the MOHO. Nelson's construct of occupational form (1988) has been incorporated into the language used to describe the social environment. The social environment

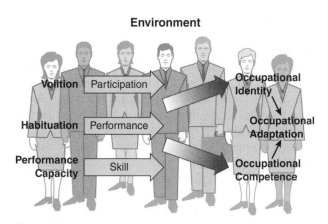

Figure 2-5 The Model of Human Occupation as a framework for use in community-based practice.

Adapted from A model of human occupation: Theory and application *(3d ed., p. 121), by G. Kielhofner, 2002, Baltimore: Lippincott, Williams & Wilkins. Copyright 2002 by Lippincott, Williams & Wilkins.*

ronment consists of groupings of humans and the expression of occupational forms those humans are socialized into, based on group membership and setting (Kielhofner, 2004); it determines what behaviors are appropriate in certain situations. For example, it may be appropriate for occupational therapy students to be flirtatious at a wedding, but this same behavior could be considered sexual harassment within the occupational form of the classroom or a fieldwork site. The physical environment includes the space (e.g., reception hall, refugee camp, prison, or office building) where occupational performance takes place and the objects within that space (e.g., tables, tents, gravel, or security portals).

The model was originally developed as a hierarchical system (Kielhofner, 1985b). Current thinking is that the process of occupational performance more closely resembles a heterarchy versus a hierarchy and that a contextually based dynamic resonance exists among phenomena. "Heterarchy is manifest throughout human occupation. When we consider any thought, emotion, or action, the parts of the human being and environment cooperate together according to local conditions created by what each element brings to the total dynamic" (Kielhofner, 2002, p. 35). Kielhofner and colleagues continue to refine the model and be influenced by changes in theory development in other disciplines and the advent of new theories.

Model of Human Occupation: Applicability in Health Promotion

Two of the three originators of the MOHO (Kielhofner, 2002) were contacted to seek their thoughts about its application to health promotion. Their responses are presented in Content Boxes 2-4 and 2-5. Research supports the belief of these theorists. For example, a health promotion study using the MOHO as the guiding theory was conducted by Aubin, Hachey, and Mercier (1999). Their study examined the relationship between subjective quality of life and meaningful daily activity in a population of people with persistent and severe mental illness. Their findings suggested positive correlations between perceived competence in daily tasks and rest, and pleasure in work and rest activities with subjective quality of life. Occupational interventions aimed at enhancing a sense of competence as defined by the MOHO were also supported.

The MOHO embraces the concept of one's participation in society and involvement in a social role. Levy (1990) suggested that multiple occupational therapy intervention principles can be used by therapists and caregivers in the physical and cognitive rehabilitation of elders to facilitate participation in valued life activities and social roles. Maintaining one's social role enables continued competence and occupational adaptation in life, which, in turn, enables optimal participation in daily living and enhances wellbeing and quality of life.

Dermody, Volkens, and Heater (1996) identified the MOHO as being compatible with efforts to assist individuals in changing their health behaviors. Specifically, they stated that as humans make choices about engaging in occupations within the environment, they can respond in a healthy way and make healthy choices, which is consistent with being in a benign or adaptive cycle. Humans also can make unhealthy choices and thus enter a vicious or maladaptive cycle. These and other research studies support the constructs of the MOHO and its application to health promotion practice.

Content Box 2-4

Dr. Janice Burke's Reflections on the MOHO

Question:
From your perspective, how do you see the MOHO relating to the health and wellbeing of people?

Response:
Health and wellbeing is a fundamental core of the model. The foundation of the model is anchored in recognition that all humans have a basic need to be engaged in activities that are meaningful. Engagement in meaningful activities serves as a catalyst to health and wellbeing in that a sense of competence, feelings of self efficacy, self-worth, and pleasure are evoked. Such feelings are hypothesized to evoke health and wellbeing.

Content Box 2-5

Dr. Gary Kielhofner's Reflections on the MOHO

Question:
From your perspective, how do you see the MOHO relating to the health and wellbeing of people?

Response:
In my view a fundamental aspect of health and wellbeing is how one participates in life occupations. This model is about the key factors that influence one's choices about, pattern of, and ability for such participation, along with the environmental support and barriers to such participation. . . . We decompose occupational health and wellbeing (referred to as occupational adaptation) into the dual components of developing an occupational identity and relying on occupational competence.

The preceding examples support the use of the MOHO in occupational therapy health promotion programming. The interdisciplinary theoretical foundation of this model also makes it well suited for use in interdisciplinary health promotion programs with populations and communities. Those addressing the global health promotion needs identified by the WHO (1986, 1997) have found the MOHO to be a useful tool, whether those efforts are interdisciplinary or solely within occupational therapy.

This model has been introduced and adopted by occupational therapists worldwide, as evidenced by MOHO assessments being translated into 13 different languages and by the scholarship cited at the MOHO Clearinghouse (UIC, 2005a, 2005b, 2005c). The MOHO has been identified as a model of choice to both understand and assist in combating occupational apartheid (Abelenda, Kielhofner, Suarez-Balcazar, & Kielhofner, 2005). **Occupational apartheid** is defined as

> the segregation of groups of people through the restriction or denial of access to dignified and meaningful participation in occupations of daily life on the basis of race, color, disability, national origin, age, gender, sexual preference, religion, political beliefs, status in society, or other characteristics. Occasioned by political forces, its systematic and pervasive social, cultural, and economic consequences jeopardize health and wellbeing as experienced by individuals, communities, and societies. (Kronenberg & Pollard, 2005, p. 67)

The MOHO also has been used as a framework to facilitate the return of displaced people to their homeland (Algado & Cardona, 2005; see Content Box 2-6), to intervene with survivors of war (Algado & Burgman, 2005), and to work with street children in Mexico and Guatemala (Kronenberg, 2005). These examples highlight the model's potential cross-cultural use to promote occupational justice by addressing occupational apartheid through enhanced health and wellbeing.

Model of Human Occupation: Health Promotion Example

The MOHO can be used to support health promotion interventions at the community level. A community can demonstrate volition through a shared history and vision expressed in a manner that supports the

---

Content Box 2-6

MOHO Influenced Goals of a Community-Based Project

- **The Volitional Subsystem**

    The objective was to prevent the loss of goals, interests, and values. We assisted community members in analyzing their new life situation in Guatemala, looking at their strengths and problems, identifying new goals, and confronting their new reality. We encouraged the recovery of the values inherent in Mayan culture, and in their cosmovision. Finally, we attempted to promote an inner locus of control through this empowerment, thus ensuring that the villagers saw themselves as the main characters in their life stories, and as survivors. This is an especially important consideration in humanitarian interventions, since traditionally such work has adopted a paternalistic position.

- **The Habituation Subsystem**

    The goals were to encourage adolescents in the role of community promoters and to return the role of "guardians of ancient wisdom" to the elders. Finally, we attempted to discourage damaging habits such as alcoholism and its consequences (such as domestic violence) by promoting healthier ways of life.

- **The Performance Subsystem**

    The goals were to develop new skills in emotional expression among the children, in community promotion and carpentry among the adolescents, and the recovery of the traditional weaving skills among the adult women.

- **The Environment**

    The goal was to develop income generating projects in order to address poverty. One of the most meaningful goals was the recovery of the cultural cycle of the community.

Reprinted from Box 25-2 "The return of the corn men: An intervention project with a Mayan community of Guatemalan *retorno*s," by S. Simó-Algado and C. E. Cardona, 2005, in F. Kronenberg, S. S. Algado, and N. Pollard (Eds.), *Occupational therapy without borders: Learning from the spirit of survivors* (pp. 336–50). New York: Elsevier, Churchill Livingstone. Copyright © 2005 by Elsevier, Churchill Livingstone. With permission.

---

wishes and concerns of its members—for example, an occupational therapist organizing a stroke club with monthly meetings at a local hospital per the request of several families who met during the rehabilitation process.

Each month, the occupational therapist and a volunteer leader open a group discussion about health and wellbeing issues affecting people coping with impairments of daily living secondary to stroke. Volitional aspects of occupational performance are raised through the identification of health and wellbeing issues critical to the group. Continued member participation is fostered through peer and professional support, as well as personal interest in discussing occupational performance areas associated with living well with stroke.

The group meets regularly, with a schedule designed to accommodate as many group members as possible. In addition, the hospital arranged for transportation in order to accommodate as many individuals as possible. With transportation provided and a schedule that fits the group's needs, there is little room for developing a maladaptive habit of not attending the group. The group also discusses the development of habits and routines that support living longer and improving quality of life, such as smoking cessation, healthy eating, and regular participation in stress-reducing occupations.

Performance capacity is addressed via the expressions of what people do in their daily lives to enact healthy habits. Barriers to health and wellbeing are discussed, and strategizing occurs through open group discussion. Group members can then call upon individual (and group) volition in order to make new choices that support health and wellness or commit further to these choices. There is constant multidirectional interaction between the individual group members, the occupational therapist, the group as a whole, and other entities, which promotes growth and change. Over time, the group and its members successfully employ strategies, and new occupational identities evolve through heightened occupational competence, demonstrating the benefits of a heterarchy.

Occupational Adaptation (OA): Overview

Occupational adaptation was originally developed as a frame of reference for linking the two primary constructs of occupational therapy: occupation and adaptation (Schkade & Schultz, 1992; Schultz, 2000; Schultz & Schkade, 1992). In later works, it was referred to as a *theory* (Schultz & Schkade, 2003). The philosophical assumptions that support this model resonate with health promotion and include the following:

- Competence in occupation is a lifelong process of adaptation to internal and external demands to perform.
- Demands to perform occur naturally as part of the person's occupational roles and the context (person-occupational-environment interactions) in which they occur.
- Dysfunction occurs because the person's ability to adapt has been challenged to the point that the demands for performance are not satisfactorily met.
- At any stage of life, the person's adaptive capacity can be overwhelmed by impairment, physical or emotional disability, and stressful life events.
- The greater the level of dysfunction, the greater the demand for changes in the person's adaptive processes.
- Success in occupational performance is a direct result of the person's ability to adapt with sufficient mastery to satisfy the self and others (Schultz & Schkade, 2003, p. 220).

The relationships between the constructs are detailed in a diagram that appears in Figure 2-6. Schultz and Schkade (2003) noted that the diagram represents the individual at a specific moment in time. The flow and interactions between the constructs at this point in time are displayed. Specifically, the diagram's left side

represents the individual's desire for mastery, and the right side represents the environment's demand for mastery, while the middle represents the interplay between these forces. The desired outcome of this process is **occupational adaptation**:

> Occupational adaptation is not about mastery per se. Rather, it is the constant presence of the desire, demand, and press for mastery in occupational contexts that provide the impetus for adaptation. . . . The person seeking to respond masterfully in occupational situations will engage in the adaptive processes. (Schultz & Schkade, 2003, p. 221)

Mastery of one's health and wellbeing can often be a difficult factor in a person's life but can be secured through occupational adaptation. For example, a poor single mother of three who works as a cashier is having a difficult time securing funds to feed her children. Based on a collaborative intervention process with an occupational therapist, the mother is able to identify less expensive, healthier, quick meals compared to the fast food she had previously relied on to feed her children. The desire to master motherhood, together with the press from the environment to feed her children, resulted in her attending, at her place of employment, a free interdisciplinary workshop on low-cost healthy food and play activities for young families.

This client-centered, occupation-focused theory can assist with organizing evaluation and intervention, where

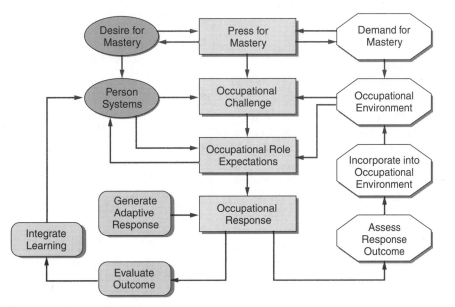

Figure 2-6 Schematic of occupational adaptation process.

Reproduced from the presentation "Theory of Occupational Adaptation: Overview" (slide # 2), by S. Schultz, n.d. Retrieved December 11, 2006, from http://www.twu.edu/ot/post_phd.htm. With permission.

the desired outcome is the ability to adapt to occupational challenges and develop occupational competence.

> The theory of occupational adaptation is intended to be used as a guide for intervention that capitalizes on the power of occupation as the primary tool to enhance the adaptive capacity of those we serve. We view the enhancement of adaptive capacity as a fundamental tool for engendering competence in occupational functioning. (S. Schultz, personal communication, February 2003)

In planning interventions, the OA model also presents two alternatives: occupational readiness and occupational activity (Schultz & Schkade, 2003). Occupational readiness works with facilitating client factors (e.g., movement functions, thought functions, mental functions of language) that are barriers to occupational performance. Working on increasing endurance through graded physical activity and instruction in energy conservation are examples of occupational readiness. Occupational activity is the use of a client-selected occupation related to the individual's occupational roles. For example, the client may choose to develop tolerance for walking in the community to complete instrumental activities of daily living (IADLs), such as home and health management and shopping. The client would then develop and execute a plan to achieve this goal (e.g., starting first with a walk to the mailbox located at the end of the driveway, increasing to a walk to the corner drugstore for a prescription, and then a walk to a strip mall that is four blocks away). In this example, the client uses the capacity and knowledge gained through occupational readiness to independently plan an approach that can lead to ongoing occupational adaptation.

Occupational Adaptation: Applicability in Health Promotion

There appears to be increasing acceptance of and research utilizing OA (Honaker, 1999; Reitz & Scaffa, 2001; Schultz & Schkade, 2003) as an occupational therapy theory. The principles of the theory are sound, as they are built upon the constructs of occupation and adaptation, which have been utilized since the profession's inception. While other models encourage the development of skills to promote adaptation, this approach supports the development of clients' adaptiveness so they can determine which skills are needed and how to gain the needed skills (Schkade, Schultz, & McClung, 2000). This approach is consistent with the goal of sustainability, which is an essential component for the long-term success of health promotion interventions. Using this theory, health promotion programming may be developed and sustained in a variety of contexts.

The development of an adaptive response is a positive way for people to develop healthy habits and promote wellbeing in their lives and in their communities. The originators of OA see a clear link between the OA theory and health promotion, as detailed in Content Box 2-7.

In this theory, the client is the agent of change (Schkade & McClung, 2001). The desired outcome as applied to health promotion is for the client to gain sufficient knowledge and skills to be able to engage in the occupational adaptation process without the presence of an occupational therapist or occupational therapy assistant. According to AOTA's *Framework* (2008), the term *client* can represent an individual, a group (e.g., a family), or a population (e.g., an organization, a community).

Adaptive energy, which includes both primary and secondary energy, is an important construct in this model when used for health promotion interventions and programming. It is particularly relevant for addressing health habits and routines. **Primary energy** describes the process of engaged, intentional focus in an occupation. The term **secondary energy** describes the phenomena of creative solutions appearing to a problem while the individual is engaged in tasks unrelated to the current occupational challenge. Schkade and McClung (2001) used a student's writer's block to describe the two types of adaptive energy. The student was spending a great deal of primary energy without

---

Content Box 2-7

Dr. Sally Schultz's Reflections on OA Theory

Question:
From your perspective, how do you see OA theory relating to the health and wellbeing of people?

Response:

- Health and wellbeing are relative. They are relative to the ability to participate in life.

- Satisfying participation in life in the presence of both facilitators and inhibitors, constitutes relative health and wellbeing.

- Satisfying participation in life is a function of competence in occupational functioning.

- Competence in occupational functioning is a function of adaptive capacity and resulting adaptiveness.

- Adaptiveness in occupational pursuits develops as a function of the development and maintenance of an innate occupational adaptation process.

- Therefore, adaptive function or adaptation is the intervening variable between occupation and participation in life or health and wellbeing.

success (i.e., trying to develop a topic and outline for a term paper). She took a break to knit a blanket for her baby, and when she returned to her schoolwork, she had both an idea and a plan for her paper. This OA strategy, labeled *shunting,* enabled her to use secondary energy to consider the problem while using primary energy to knit (Schkade & McClung, 2001). Additional examples of therapists applying this model to practice were collected and reported by Schkade and McClung. Although the majority of the examples focus on the rehabilitation process, the examples help illustrate the model's principles and process.

Research on the OA process supports its use in occupational therapy and occupational therapy in health promotion. Honaker (1999) studied patterns of adaptation in elders with rheumatoid arthritis (RA) relative to choices made when presented with occupational challenges. The author explored how elders with RA adapted in order to pursue meaningful occupation, whether a sense of mastery was experienced, and whether a perceived relationship existed between occupational participation and pain. Results of this study showed that elders with RA continued to pursue meaningful occupation despite pain but experienced a diminished sense of efficiency and mastery.

Through one's desire for mastery, OA acknowledges environmental influences on mastery and examines demands for mastery. There is a consistency in philosophy between OA and the WHO definition of **health promotion,** which is the "process of enabling people to increase control over, and to improve, their health" (WHO, 1997, p. 1). This process also can be viewed as developing mastery over one's health in order to optimize wellbeing. This theory has excellent potential for use in the creation of holistic health promotion interventions and programs, and it matches the philosophy of the profession and the principles of high-level wellness initiated by Dunn (1954), a progressive physician.

Occupational Adaptation: Health Promotion Example

Mark is a 45-year-old African American with new-onset diabetes and beginning visual impairments who was recently released from the hospital. He is single and works in a rehabilitation facility for people with substance-abuse issues. He is a former substance abuser.

The onset of visual impairments and the health issues related to diabetes have affected abilities and roles important to him as he copes with his new life situation. He wishes to return to work as soon as possible to avoid "going on welfare." He receives occupational therapy at home, limited to a small number of visits. The occupational therapy assistant, under indirect supervision of an occupational therapist, engages Mark

in learning new home-management techniques to accommodate current and probable future visual impairments. Due to Mark's new-onset diabetes, the occupational therapy assistant also helps him adapt both his eating and cooking routines and habits in order to develop a healthier lifestyle (e.g., decreasing fried foods, increasing vegetable intake), thus meeting the demand for mastery. The occupational therapy assistant recognizes that cooking is a meaningful occupation for Mark and thus helps him find large-print healthful recipes online that are within his budget to prepare.

Mark begins to develop occupational competence by meeting the occupational challenge for adaptation. The press for mastery exists for Mark, and he meets the challenge with enthusiasm. While Mark learns adaptive strategies for lifestyle enhancement in home management, the occupational therapy assistant also addresses his work situation. Together, they strategize to adapt both transportation and work areas in order for Mark to be safe with community mobility and explore areas of work in which he can still engage. Mark begins to recognize that the visual adaptive strategies learned at home can be used at work and begins to develop a level of mastery in occupational adaptation that supports a healthier lifestyle on both a physical and psychosocial level.

Person-Environment-Occupation (PEO): Overview

In the PEO model, individuals are viewed holistically with their unique combination of physical, cognitive, and affective characteristics and their life experiences. The primary assumption of the model is that the person is intrinsically motivated and continually developing. The "person" in the model can refer to an individual, a group, or an organization (Strong et al., 1999). The model has three main constructs: person, environment, and occupation.

Environment in the model is defined as the physical, social, and cultural elements of the context in which occupational performance takes place. The environment provides cues about appropriate and expected behaviors. The environment's characteristics can enable or constrain occupational performance. The environment is conceptualized on both the micro and macro levels. A micro level view of the environment focuses on the individual's context at home, work, school, and so on, and how this environment affects the person's occupational performance. The macro level view of the environment has a population-based perspective and focuses on the environmental variables that affect the occupational performance of groups of people. **Environmental fit** refers to the degree of congruence among the PEO components. A "good fit" results in optimal occupational performance for the individual (Cooper, Letts, Rigby, Stewart, & Strong, 2001), family, or community.

Adaptation is a function of environmental fit. When a person is functioning well in a new context, they can be said to have adapted well to that environment. This implies a positive and supportive relationship between the person and the environment. However, it is important to note that the person and the environment are constantly changing, and therefore adaptation is a continual process (Letts et al., 1994). The model also recognizes that problems associated with disability may not be due to the disability itself but rather are the result of a poor person-environment fit. In cases such as this, intervention may consist of changing the environment to meet the individual's needs, rather than trying to change the person to fit the environment (Law et al., 1996).

According to the PEO model, occupations are clusters of tasks and include self-care, leisure, and productive pursuits. Occupations satisfy an individual's needs for self-maintenance, self-expression, and life satisfaction. Meaningful engagement in occupations is health promoting and enhances quality of life. The model conceptualizes activities, tasks, and occupations as nested concepts. Activities are the basic units of tasks, and tasks are sets of purposeful activities that make up meaningful occupations. "Occupations are groups of self-directed, functional tasks and activities in which a person engages over a life span" (Stewart et al., 2003, p. 229).

Occupational performance is the product of the person-environment-occupation transaction. Occupational performance requires that persons mediate the sometimes conflicting demands of the environment with their view of themselves and their ever changing needs and priorities. Some elements of occupational performance can be measured objectively through observation, while subjective experiences are best measured through self-report (Law et al., 1996).

The PEO model emphasizes the physical, social, and cultural factors in the environment that hinder or facilitate occupational performance. It recognizes the developmental nature of the person-environment-occupation interaction and the individual's changing needs, roles, expectations, and goals across life stages (Law & Baum, 2001).

Traditional occupational therapy evaluation measured aspects of the person, environment, and occupation as discrete entities. The PEO model advocates measurement of the various interfaces of the PEO relationship in order to provide a more complete understanding of the variables that affect occupational

performance. In the PEO model, occupational performance is the outcome or product of the dynamic relationship between the person, the environment, and the occupation (Law, Baum, & Dunn, 2001). This is represented in Figure 2-7 as the intersection of the three spheres. A greater degree of overlap of the three spheres indicates a better fit between the person, the environment, and the occupation. The focus of intervention is on improving PEO congruence and thereby enhancing occupational performance. As a result, multiple options for change can be generated (Strong et al., 1999).

Person-Environment-Occupation: Applicability to Health Promotion

Law, one of the originators of the PEO, described the relationship between PEO and the facilitation of health and wellbeing (Content Box 2-8). Occupational therapy health promotion interventions can facilitate changes in the person, the environment, or the occupation in order to enhance occupational performance, health, and wellbeing. Interventions that address all three elements—the person, the environment, and the occupation—are more likely to be effective (Stewart et al., 2003) and have greater sustainability. Increasing access to work, school, and recreational environments and modifying/adapting occupations can facilitate improved health and occupational performance. Improving skills and

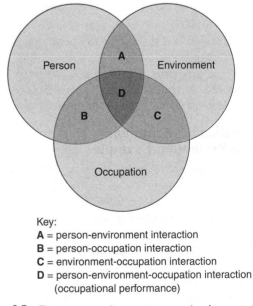

Key:

A = person-environment interaction
B = person-occupation interaction
C = environment-occupation interaction
D = person-environment-occupation interaction
(occupational performance)

Figure 2-7 The person-environment-occupation framework.

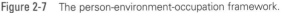

Developed from Measuring occupational performance: Supporting best practice in occupational therapy (p. 41), *by M. Law, C. Baum, & W. Dunn, 2001, Thorofare, NJ: SLACK. Courtesy of Jenny Wingrat. Copyright © 2001 by SLACK. Reprinted with permission.*

capabilities of individuals, families, and groups can enhance occupational performance and the health of communities and populations.

Applications of the PEO model have been investigated through both quantitative and qualitative research. Several studies have tested the effectiveness of the PEO model with various populations, including older adults (Cooper & Stewart, 1997) and persons in recovery (Strong, 1998). The model has been used in Canada, the United States, Russia, India, and Bosnia (Strong et al., 1999). It also was used to help create a family-centered framework for therapy with children who have cerebral palsy; although the model was not identified by name, the influence and interplay of the child (i.e., person), tasks (i.e., occupation), and environment were major components of the family-centered framework (Law et al., 1998).

The PEO model is flexible, easily understood, and can be used with people of all ages in a variety of settings. This model has the potential to facilitate a shift in practice from a narrow focus on performance components to a broader emphasis on occupational performance. The model provides occupational therapists with a framework for analyzing occupational performance problems, planning interventions, measuring outcomes, and articulating the uniqueness of occupational therapy practice (Strong et al., 1999). The model's only limitation is that it has not been extensively tested, as it is a relatively new practice model.

Content Box 2-8

Dr. Mary Law's Reflections on PEO Theory

Question:

From your perspective, how do you see PEO relating to the health and wellbeing of people?

Response:

Notions included in health and wellness . . . can be thought of in terms of person, environment and occupation. For example, health and wellness can include happiness, physical vigor, and personal safety, potentially all elements found within the person. Similarly, health and wellness can include access to meaningful activities, work, leisure or school, elements of occupation. Finally, health and wellness can include access to social networks or financial stability, two of the environments mentioned in the PEO.

The relationship between the PEO model and health and wellness can be seen throughout daily living. For example, a person cannot achieve work satisfaction if they cannot physically enter the building, nor can they experience happiness and personal safety if their environment is full of hazardous elements.

Person-Environment-Occupation: Health Promotion Example

An occupational therapist was contracted as a consultant for an existing transitional living program for homeless women and children. The program was not meeting its objectives and was in need of expert advice. The PEO model was used to evaluate the program and make recommendations for improvement.

The evaluation and intervention took place in a 15-apartment, transitional-living facility (microenvironment) in the midtown region of a southern city with a population of approximately 200,000 (macroenvironment). The "person" in this example refers to a group of 15 homeless women and their children who are residents of the transitional living apartment complex. The program's goal is to enable the 15 families to obtain and maintain their own housing in the community. Participants are allowed to remain in the transitional living apartments for a maximum of 18 months. The average length of stay over the past 5 years has been 12 months.

The occupational therapist evaluated the characteristics of the microenvironment and found that, in general, there was little social support evident among the families. They rarely interacted, except when engaged in structured program activities. All the women and children attended the same program activities. Program staff made no attempt to customize the program to individual participant needs or to change program elements over time. The families rarely participated in community events, other than to attend program-required activities in community locations, such as 12-step meetings. However, the city (macroenvironment) was abundant in resources. A community center providing after-school activities was within walking distance of the apartments. The city provided numerous no-cost or low-cost leisure opportunities, a variety of levels of educational and vocational training programs, and a diverse economic base with numerous job opportunities. However, a major barrier was the limited transportation options to these community resources.

A large percentage (70%) of the women and children were victims of domestic violence, and 50% of the women had substance-abuse problems. A few were in legal trouble and were remanded to the program by the court. Many of the women had been previously employed but had minimal work skills. None of the women were currently employed. All the women indicated a desire to work, and some wanted to return to school to further their education. Many of the women voiced a desire for parenting-skills training and nutrition education. The children ranged in age from newborn to adolescence, with most of the children of elementary school age. All the children received developmental screening, and one-third were found to be marginally delayed. The school system had identified several children as having learning disabilities, and some had obvious mental health needs. Few of the families had received any health-care services in the past year.

The range of occupations available in the microenvironment was limited. Each family had its own apartment, which facilitated participation in self-care occupations, both basic and instrumental. There was a coin-operated laundry on-site, a group meeting room, and a small playground for the children. Facility policies prohibited families from inviting visitors to their apartments. Visitors were allowed in the group meeting room, which was equipped with a kitchen, but the kitchen was off limits to residents.

A few of the problems identified by the occupational therapist included

- limited social support in both the micro (facility) and macro (community) environments;
- poor access to community resources (person-environment transaction);
- minimal opportunities for participation in work and play/leisure occupations (person-environment-occupation transactions);
- lack of customization of program activities to family needs (person-occupation transactions).

The occupational therapist recommended using the Canadian Occupational Performance Measure (COPM) to ascertain the families' occupational needs and priorities. The results would be used to customize program activities to meet the specific needs of the women and their children. This necessitated developing numerous program activities not currently provided, including parenting-skills training and nutrition education. Another recommendation was to allow the women access to the kitchen in the group meeting room to prepare snacks for visitors and to prepare food for parties for the apartment complex residents. The families began celebrating birthdays and holidays together, which facilitated the development of social-support mechanisms within the microenvironment. In addition, computers, table games, and other leisure resources were added to the group meeting room, and the name of the space was changed to the "community activities room."

Addressing the problem of transportation and access to community resources was a more challenging proposition. The bus system in this part of the city was quite limited, with few routes and minimal daytime service. The occupational therapist provided instruction on using the bus system, but this proved inadequate for many of the families' needs. Some of the women had driver's licenses, but none of them owned cars. A local car dealership was contacted, and a used car was donated for facility use. A local civic organization provided the funds for insuring the donated vehicle, and a sign-up system was initiated for the women to use the car. After a short time, the women developed a system that met the needs of all the families. In addition, a local nonprofit transportation agency offered 50% discounts on their services for the women to travel to work, school, or health-care appointments.

The PEO model continues to inform the evaluation and intervention process for these families, and new program elements are being added on a regular basis. The participants' complex needs were readily addressed by the transactional elements of the model. The COPM provided the women with a measure of control and autonomy over the intervention goals and activities, and it gave them a sense of ownership of the results. This factor emerged as a particularly important aspect of the intervention, as many of these women had lost motivation and exhibited low levels of self-efficacy.

Person-Environment-Occupation-Performance Model (PEOP): Overview

The PEOP model was initially referred to as the *person-environment-performance framework*. Originally, the model was graphically designed as a set of three nested boxes, with the person represented in the innermost box embedded in the performance component in turn, embedded in the environment (Christiansen & Baum, 1991). The subsequent version of the PEOP used a triangle, with all subcomponents (i.e., self-identity, roles, tasks, and actions) feeding into the development of occupational performance, which then reflected a state of wellbeing (Christiansen & Baum, 1997). Occupational performance was seen to be influenced by both intrinsic factors (e, g., psychological and biological) and extrinsic factors (e.g., social and cultural).

In the latest iteration of the PEOP (Fig. 2-8), the graphic representation more closely resembles the PEO model, with the use of overlapping circles, which may confuse students who are attempting to differentiate between the models. However, the PEOP is differentiated from the PEO by the clear depiction of four constructs (versus three) and by the projected outcomes. This latest version more clearly illustrates the interrelationships between the primary constructs (i.e., occupation, performance, person, and environment) and the desired outcomes of occupational performance and participation, wellbeing, and quality of life. Two basic assumptions support the PEOP:

1. "People are naturally motivated to explore their world and demonstrate mastery within it."
2. "Situations in which people experience success help them feel good about themselves. This motivates them to face new challenges with greater confidence" (Baum & Christiansen, 2005, p. 245).

The PEOP is a client-centered, top-down approach that focuses on the interaction of environment, person, and occupation—including the actual performance of an occupation.

Occupation is described as part of a hierarchy of behaviors having differing levels of "occupational complexity." Table 2-2 identifies these levels and provides examples. The model's intent is to guide intervention using occupation and to enhance occupational performance for greater participation in the community or world of meaning. It considers personal and environmental factors that enable or constrain societal participation. Baum and Law (1997) discussed the need for interventions to be contextually based in order to achieve a state of "occupational competence." When intervention is focused on context, as well as on activities and occupations that have meaning and value to the client, then health and wellbeing can be more effectively improved.

Person-Environment-Occupational-Performance Model: Applicability to Health Promotion

The PEOP views health as an enabler and not as an outcome (C. Baum and C. Christiansen, personal communication, February 2003). Health enables participation in everyday life. When people are healthy, they can optimally participate in daily occupations that promote life satisfaction and enhance quality of life. Participation may also be influenced by external factors, as noted in the model. These factors may be barriers to the promotion of health and wellbeing, thus occupational therapists can readily use the PEOP to begin identifying environmental and personal barriers to health and explore, with the client, strategies to optimize participation.

The PEOP can also be applied to community or population-based health promotion initiatives. Although the model contains four primary constructs, many additional constructs are used to describe applications of this model in the literature. One of these constructs, human agency, is of particular relevance in applying the model to health promotion. **Human agency** has been described as the natural tendency of humans to be "motivated to explore their worlds and demonstrate mastery within it. To do this, the person must effectively use the resources (personal, social, and material) available in his or her environment" (Baum & Christiansen, 2005, p. 242). This important

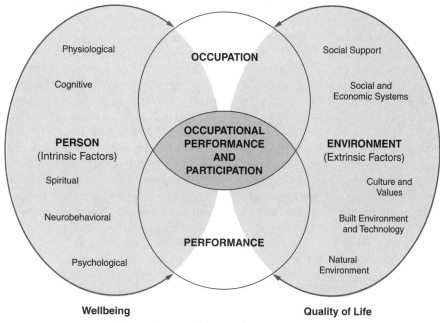

Figure 2-8 The person-environment-occupation-performance framework.

*Reproduced from Figure 11-1 in "Person-environment-occupation-performance: An occupation-based framework" (p. 246), by C. M. Baum & C. H. Christiansen, in Occupa-*tional therapy: Performance, participation, and well-being, *C. H. Christiansen, C. M. Baum, & J. Bass-Haugen (Eds.), 2005, Thorofare, NJ: SLACK. Copyright © 2005 by SLACK. Reprinted with permission.*

Table 2–2   A Hierarchy of Occupation-Related Terms and Behaviors

Term	Example
Roles: Positions in society having expected responsibilities	Adult child
	Adult grandchild
	Full-time employee
Occupations: Goal-directed pursuits that typically extend over time, have meaning to the performer, and involve multiple tasks	Shopping for self, parents, and grandparent
Tasks: Combinations of actions sharing a common purpose recognized by the performer	Making a grocery list
	Managing a grocery cart
Actions: Observable behaviors that are recognizable	Lifting
	Directing another to lift
Abilities: General traits or individual characteristics that support occupational performance	Attention, motor control, language

From "Person-environment-occupation-performance: An occupation-based framework for practice" (p. 252), by C. M. Baum & C. H. Christiansen in C. H. Christiansen, C. M. Baum, and J. Bass-Haugen (Eds.), *Occupational therapy: Performance, participation, and well-being*, 2005, Thorofare, NJ: SLACK. Copyright © 2005 by SLACK. Reprinted with permission.

construct can be broadened by replacing the word *person* with *community* or *population.*

One of the strengths of this model that makes it ideal for use in health promotion is that it provides a framework, built upon the theory, to guide intervention. Baum, Bass-Haugen, and Christiansen (2005) described a situational analysis process based on the model to assist occupational therapists in the development of theory-driven health promotion programming. This process appears to be a community version of the occupational profile described in the profession's *Framework* (AOTA, 2008). After gathering a community's occupational profile data and before initiating an intervention, it must be determined whether the community or population's needs can be best met through an occupational therapy approach. This is an important feature and is consistent with the core values of the profession (AOTA, 1993). If the community could best be served by another discipline or by working collaboratively with another discipline, it is unethical to proceed independently.

Although there has been little research on the use of the PEOP, it appears to have relevance for occupational therapy health promotion interventions. These interventions can lead to positive health behavior changes when occupational therapists examine the interactive nature of persons, occupations, environments, and the resultant occupational performance. Using the PEOP's situation analysis process can ensure that the therapist, in collaboration with the community or population, correctly and comprehensively identifies the resources and abilities available to overcome barriers to health and participation.

Person-Environment-Occupation-Performance Model: Health Promotion Example

Billy is a 12-year-old with autism. He lives with both parents and a sister in a close-knit community in a small town on the East Coast. Billy has been in inclusive school situations since he began school but has had much difficulty negotiating both the social and physical environments (contexts) of his occupational role as student.

The occupational therapist works with Billy twice a week. She focuses attention on engaging him in occupational experiences that provide the "just right challenge," which accounts for the intrinsic factors limiting participation. Billy's mother would like him to participate more actively in a sport to optimize his physical and mental health. Billy was given several choices and chose basketball, one of his father's favorite sports. The occupational therapist, in collaboration with Billy and his mother, focus on his physical and cognitive strengths (intrinsic) in order to help him develop occupational competence. They also work with the school system (extrinsic) to enable Billy to participate actively in basketball. This is achieved by exploring the possibilities for his involvement as an active participant and observer so that Billy maintains a sense of being able to participate on some level.

Billy has the support of his parents and sister at home, each of whom plays basketball with Billy to follow through with the intervention plan designed with the occupational therapist. He also plays with teammates who, over time, have accommodated for Billy's needs to catch the ball and then process which direction to run and throw the ball. The social support, directly influenced by his occupational therapy plan, assists in helping Billy attain a level of wellbeing and optimized psychosocial and physical health that supports the growth and development of any 12-year-old.

Recent Advancements and Potentially New Models

The definition of occupation, the customary focus of its use by individuals, and a growing realization that interdependence may be the best outcome of its prescription and use were discussed at the third annual conference of the Society for the Study of Occupation: USA (SSO-USA, 2004). Presentations related to interdependence, transactional approaches, and complexity science prompt the following questions: Is a broader definition of *occupation* needed that emphasizes the interdependence of humans with the environment and each other in the pursuit of occupation? Is this view of occupation more compatible with health promotion interventions and philosophy?

At first glance, the practice of tai chi displayed in Figure 2-9 may appear to be individuals independently engaging in the same occupation, but upon closer observation, the interdependent nature of the occupation becomes apparent. In time, will research find that interdependent occupations promote health and wellbeing in more powerful ways than occupational engagement in isolation? A new theoretical model that expresses the interdependence of humans and nature is the Kawa (River) Model (Iwama, 2005a, 2005b, 2006a, 2006c; Iwama et al, 2006; Lim & Iwama, 2006).

The Kawa (River) Model

A Japanese Canadian occupational therapist worked with a group of Japanese occupational therapists with the goal of designing an Eastern-influenced model for occupational therapy practice (Iwama, 2005b). Through this process, the Kawa (River) Model was developed. The model's first version appeared graphically much like other Western models, with a series of boxes imbedded in a circle, with arrows between the boxes to signify the relationships between constructs. The constructs included environmental factors, life circumstances and problems, personal assets and liabilities, and life flow and health. However, the Japanese

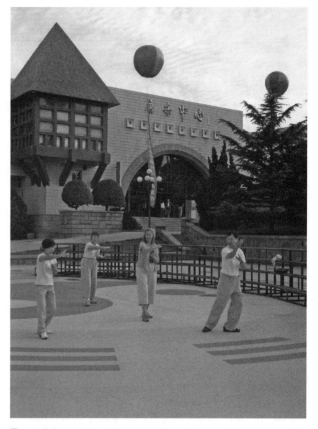

Figure 2-9   Tai chi in Qingdao, China.

occupational therapists quickly embraced one member's idea of using a river metaphor to better explain the overall value of harmony, the goal of enhanced life flow, and the relationship between the model's constructs (Fig. 2-10). The constructs were reconceptualized to support the representation of a free-flowing river as the ideal life (i.e., maximal life flow). While the final version included the original constructs, they were renamed to better reflect an East Asian philosophical perspective, including beliefs from Buddhist, Confucian, and Taoist philosophical orientations (Iwama, 2005a, 2006b, 2006c).

The Kawa Model was developed within a social structure that values interdependence and the collective more than independence and the self. Within this context, the notion of self is embedded and interconnected in a manner that precludes separation of the individual. This model is best suited for clients, families, or communities with comparable value systems. Since the model's development, its application has been primarily through case studies of individuals (Iwama, 2006a, 2006c). The three-dimensional aspects of the model can assist with visually identifying assets and liabilities through nontraditional techniques such as drawings and sculpture. Therefore, it may be particularly well

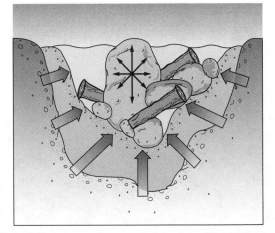

Figure 2-10 Major components of the Kawa (River) Model. Water (*mizu*) represents the individual's, family's, or community's life flow. Driftwood (*ryuboku*) represents assets and liabilities. Rocks (*iwa*) represent life circumstances and problems. Arrows represent pressures from the environment through the river's side (*kawa no soku-heki*) and the river bottom (*kawa no zoko*). Gaps represent spaces (*sukima*), which are potential areas to broaden through occupational therapy intervention and thus increase space to enhance life flow.

From Kawa River Model website: *Concepts and structures, by M. Iwama, 2006. Retrieved November 29, 2006, from http://www.kawamodel.com/. With permission.*

suited as a potential tool for community-based health-promotion programming through identification of assets and liabilities, including environmental features and problems, through the use of media or verbal techniques. Future developments of this model can be monitored through the online Kawa Model Discussion Forum: How Does Your River Flow? (Iwama, 2006b).

Conclusion

Health promotion has historically been a practice area of occupational therapy (Reitz, 1992), and the authors wish to facilitate its continued development. Contributions of occupational therapists and occupational therapy assistants to health promotion interventions have not realized their full potential. In order to do so, it is important for both occupational therapy theorists and therapists to

- reflect on the relationship between health promotion, the *Framework* (AOTA, 2008), and the core values and beliefs of the profession (AOTA, 1993), and on the beliefs of the profession's founders and current leaders;
- be knowledgeable of and able to apply theory to evidence-based health promotion program development; and
- be knowledgeable of and able to apply theory to the evaluation of the outcomes of those programs.

The end result of the above work will support the profession's continued movement toward providing health promotion services to individuals, families, groups, organizations, communities, and populations. To this end, this chapter has provided a review of several occupational therapy models and examples of their use in health promotion. In addition to occupational therapy theories and models, those from other disciplines also can be useful tools in occupational therapy health promotion. The next chapter will provide an overview of several models from health psychology, health behavior, and other areas that can further contribute to the work of occupational therapy in promoting health and wellbeing for people and their communities.

▶ For Discussion and Review

1. What are the key similarities and differences between the models described in this chapter?
2. Which model might provide guidance for developing a preventive, occupation-based intervention for military families with loved ones deployed overseas?
3. Could the occupation-based intervention for these military families be further strengthened by adding constructs from another occupational therapy model? Why or why not?
4. Which model would you select to guide an explorative study of the occupational competency of new mothers? Why did you make this selection? Which other model may also be appropriate and why?
5. How would you determine which model has been most effective for studying health and social participation of middle-aged adults in the United States?

▶ Research Questions

1. Which has more impact on the health of homeless women and children, a health promotion intervention based on the MOHO or one based on the PEO model?
2. What is the relationship between resilience and adaptation? How do these constructs impact mental health?
3. How does the environment impact a person's perception of his or her health?
4. Which occupational model(s) would support each of the above potential research questions?

Acknowledgments

The authors wish to express their appreciation to the following individuals who assisted with the preparation of this chapter: Frederick D. Reitz and Grace E. Wenger.

References

Abelenda, J., Kielhofner, G., Suarez-Balcazar, Y., & Kielhofner, K. (2005). The model of human occupation as a conceptual tool for understanding and addressing occupational apartheid. In F. Kronenberg, S. S. Algado, & N. Pollard (Eds.), *Occupational therapy without borders: Learning from the spirit of survivors* (pp. 183–96). New York: Elsevier, Churchill Livingstone.

Algado, S. S., & Burgman, I. (2005). Occupational therapy intervention with children survivors of war. In F. Kronenberg, S. S. Algado, & N. Pollard (Eds.), *Occupational therapy without borders: Learning from the spirit of survivors* (pp. 245–60). New York: Elsevier, Churchill Livingstone.

Algado, S. S., & Cardona, C. E. (2005). The return of the corn men: An intervention project with a Mayan community of Guatemalan *retornos*. In F. Kronenberg, S. S. Algado, & N. Pollard (Eds.), *Occupational therapy without borders: Learning from the spirit of survivors* (pp. 336–50). New York: Elsevier, Churchill Livingstone.

American Occupational Therapy Association. (1993). Core values statement and attitudes of occupational therapy practice. *American Journal of Occupational Therapy, 47,* 1085–86.

American Occupational Therapy Association. (2005). *Occupational therapy code of ethics (2005).* Retrieved July 5, 2005, from http://www.aota.org/general/about.asp#values.

American Occupational Therapy Association. (2008). Occupational therapy practice framework: Domain and process (2nd ed.). *American Journal of Occupational Therapy, 62,* 625–87.

American Occupational Therapy Foundation. (2005). *Collection of photographs from images of participation and health photo contest.* Retrieved December 16, 2006, from http://www.aotf.org/html/photocontestlive.shtml.

Aubin, G., Hachey, R., & Mercier, C. (1999). Meaning of daily activities and subjective quality of life in people with severe mental illness. *Scandinavian Journal of Occupational Therapy, 6,* 53–62.

Baum, C. M., Bass-Haugen, J., & Christiansen, C. H. (2005). Person-environment-occupation-performance: A model for planning interventions for individuals and organizations. In C. H. Christiansen, C. M. Baum, & J. Bass-Haugen (Eds.), *Occupational therapy: Performance, participation and well-being* (3d ed., pp. 372–92). Thorofare, NJ: SLACK.

Baum, C. M., & Christiansen, C. H. (2005). Person-environment-occupation-performance: An occupation-based framework for practice. In C. H. Christiansen, C. M. Baum, & J. Bass-Haugen (Eds.), *Occupational therapy: Performance, participation and well-being* (3d ed., pp. 242–66). Thorofare, NJ: SLACK.

Baum, C. M., & Law, M. (1997). Occupational therapy practice: Focusing on occupational performance. *American Journal of Occupational Therapy, 51*(4), 277–88.

Bennett, S., Hoffman, T., McCluskey, A., McKenna, K., Strong, J., & Tooth, L. (2003). Introducing OTseeker (occupational therapy systematic evaluation of evidence): A new evidence database for occupational therapists. [Evidence-based practice forum]. *American Journal of Occupational Therapy, 57*(3), 635–38.

Brown, C., Cosgrove, N., & DeSelm, T. (1997). Barriers interfering with life satisfaction for individuals with severe mental illness. *Psychiatric Rehabilitation Journal, 20*(3), 67–71.

Christiansen, C., & Baum, C. M. (Eds.). (1991). *Occupational therapy: Overcoming human performance and performance deficits.* Thorofare, NJ: SLACK.

Christiansen, C., & Baum, C. M. (Eds.). (1997). *Occupational therapy: Enabling function and well-being* (2d ed.). Thorofare, NJ: SLACK.

Cooper, B. A., Letts, L., Rigby, P. J., Stewart, D., & Strong, S. (2001). Measuring environmental factors. In M. Law, C. Baum, & W. Dunn (Eds.), *Measuring occupational performance: Supporting best practice in occupational therapy* (pp. 229–56). Thorofare, NJ: SLACK.

Cooper, B., & Stewart, D. (1997). The effect of a transfer device in the homes of elderly people. *Physical & Occupational Therapy in Geriatrics, 15,* 61–77.

Crist, P. A., Royeen, C. B., & Schkade, J. K. (Eds.). (2000). *Infusing occupation into practice.* Bethesda, MD: American Occupational Therapy Association.

Dailey, B., & Reitz, S. M. (2003, June). *Occupational therapy services in the criminal justice system: Healthy life skills beyond the wall.* Short course presented at the 83rd AOTA Annual Conference & Exposition, Washington, DC.

Dermody, J. L., Volkens, P. P., & Heater, S. L. (1996). Occupational therapy students' perspectives on occupations as an agent that promotes healthful lifestyles. *American Journal of Occupational Therapy, 50*(10), 835–41.

Dunn, H. (1954). *High-level wellness.* Arlington, VA: R.W. Beatty.

Dunn, W., Brown, C., & McGuigan, A. (1994). The ecology of human performance: A framework for considering the effect of context. *American Journal of Occupational Therapy, 48,* 595–607.

Dunn, W., McClain, L. H., Brown, C., & Youngstrom, M. J. (2003). The ecology of human performance. In E. B. Crepeau, E. S. Cohn, & B. A. B. Schell (Eds.), *Willard and Spackman's occupational therapy* (10th ed., pp. 223–27). Philadelphia: Lippincott, Williams & Wilkins.

Honaker, D. K. (1999). The impact of occupational activities and wellness in elders. Master's thesis, Texas Woman's University: Denton, TX.

Iwama, M. K. (2005a). Situated meaning: An issue of culture, inclusion, and occupational therapy. In F. Kronenberg, S. S. Algado, & N. Pollard (Eds.), *Occupational therapy without borders: Learning from the spirit of survivors* (pp. 127–39). New York: Elsevier, Churchill Livingstone.

Iwama, M. K. (2005b). The Kawa (river) model: Nature, life flow, and the power of culturally relevant occupational therapy. In F. Kronenberg, S. S. Algado, & N. Pollard (Eds.), *Occupational therapy without borders: Learning from the spirit of survivors* (pp. 213–27). New York: Elsevier, Churchill Livingstone .

Iwama, M. K. (2006a). *The Kawa model: Culturally relevant occupational therapy.* New York: Elsevier, Churchill Livingstone.

Iwama, M. K. (2006b). *The KAWA model discussion forum: How does your river flow?: Index.* Retrieved November 29, 2006, from http://kawamodel.phpbbnow.com/.

Iwama, M. K. (2006c). *The Kawa model website: Concepts and structures.* New York: Elsevier, Churchill Livingstone. Retrieved November 29, 2006, from http://www .kawamodel.com/.

Iwama, M., Odawara, E., & Asaba, E. (2006, October). *Cross cultural perspectives on occupation: What occupational science can gain from Japanese ways of knowing.* Paper presented at the conference of the Society for the Study of Occupation, St. Louis, MO.

Kielhofner, G. (1980a). A model of human occupation, Part 2: Ontogenesis from the perspective of temporal adaptation. *American Journal of Occupational Therapy, 34,* 657–63.

Kielhofner, G. (1980b). A model of human occupation, Part 3: Benign and vicious cycles. *American Journal of Occupational Therapy, 34,* 731–37.

Kielhofner, G. (1985a). Introduction. In G. Kielhofner (Ed.), *A model of human occupation: Theory and application* (pp. xvii–xx). Baltimore: Williams & Wilkins.

Kielhofner, G. (1985b). The open system dynamics of human occupation. In G. Kielhofner (Ed.), *A model of human occupation: Theory and application* (pp. 37–41). Baltimore: Williams & Wilkins.

Kielhofner, G. (2002). *A model of human occupation: Theory and application* (3d ed.). Baltimore: Lippincott, Williams & Wilkins.

Kielhofner, G. (2004). *Conceptual foundations of occupational therapy* (4th ed.). Philadelphia: F. A. Davis.

Kielhofner, G., & Burke, J. (1980). A model of human occupation, Part 1. Conceptual framework and content. *American Journal of Occupational Therapy, 34*(9), 572–81.

Kielhofner, G., Forsyth, K., & Barrett, L. (2003). Section II: Model of human occupation. In E. B. Crepeau, E. S. Cohn, & B. A. B. Schell (Eds.), *Willard & Spackman's occupational therapy* (10th ed., pp. 212–19). Philadelphia: Lippincott, Williams & Wilkins.

Kielhofner, G., & Igi, C. H. (1980). A model of human occupation, Part 4: Assessment and intervention. *American Journal of Occupational Therapy, 34,* 777–88.

Kielhofner, G., Tham, K , Baz, T., & Hutson, H. (2008). Performance capacity and the live body. In G. Kielhofner (Ed.), *Model of human occupation: Theory and application* (4th ed., pp. 68–48). Baltimore: Lippincott, Williams & Wilkins.

Kronenberg, F. (2005). Occupational therapy with street children. In F. Kronenberg, S. S. Algado, & N. Pollard (Eds.), *Occupational therapy without borders: Learning from the spirit of survivors* (pp. 262–76). New York: Elsevier, Churchill Livingstone.

Kronenberg, F., & Pollard, N. (2005). Overcoming occupational apartheid: A preliminary exploration of the political nature of occupational therapy. In F. Kronenberg, S. S. Algado, & N. Pollard (Eds.), *Occupational therapy without borders: Learning from the spirit of survivors* (pp. 58–86). New York: Elsevier, Churchill Livingstone.

Law, M., & Baum, C. (2001). Measurement in occupational therapy. In M. Law, C. Baum, & W. Dunn (Eds.), *Measuring occupational performance: Supporting best practice in occupational therapy.* Thorofare, NJ: SLACK.

Law, M., Baum, C., & Dunn, W. (2001). *Measuring occupational performance: Supporting best practice in occupational therapy.* Thorofare, NJ: SLACK.

Law, M., Cooper, B., Strong, S., Stewart, D., Rigby, P., & Letts, L. (1996). The person-environment-occupation model: A transactive approach to occupational performance. *Canadian Journal of Occupational Therapy, 63*(1), 9–23.

Law, M., Darrah, J., Rosenbaum, P., Pollock, N., King, G., Russell, D., Palisano, R., Harris, S., Walter, S., Armstrong, R., & Watts, J. (1998). Family-centered functional therapy for children with cerebral palsy: An emerging practice model. *Physical & Occupational Therapy in Pediatrics, 18*(1), 83–102.

Letts, L., Law, M., Rigby, P., Cooper, B., Stewart, D., & Strong, S. (1994). Person-environment assessments in occupational therapy. *American Journal of Occupational Therapy, 48*(7), 608–18.

Levy, L. L. (1990). Activity, social role retention, and the multiple disabled aged: Strategies for intervention. *Occupational Therapy in Mental Health, 10*(3), 1–30.

Lim, K. H., & Iwama, M. K. (2006, July). *The Kawa "river" model: Local to global utility.* Paper presented at the conference of the World Federation of Occupational Therapists, Sydney, Australia.

Lutz, C. S. (1998). Interdisciplinary prevention in rural communities: Outcomes evaluation of the Strides for Life walking program for older adults. Unpublished graduate project, Towson University, Towson, MD. (Supported through USDHHS, Public Health Service, Bureau of Health Professions, Health Resources and Services Administration [Grant #36 AH 10043-4] administered by the Western Maryland Area Health Education Center).

Meyer, A. (1977). The philosophy of occupation therapy. *American Journal of Occupational Therapy, 31*(10), 639–42. (Original work published 1922.)

Miller, R. J., & Schwartz, K. (2004). What is theory, and why does it matter? In K. F. Walker & F. M. Ludwig (Eds.), *Perspectives on theory for the practice of occupational therapy* (3d ed., pp. 1–26). Austin, TX: Pro-Ed.

Mosey, A. C. (1981). *Occupational therapy: Configuration of a profession.* New York: Raven Press.

Nelson, D. (1988). Occupation: Form and performance. *American Journal of Occupational Therapy, 42*(10), 633–52.

Peloquin, S. M. (1989). Sustaining the art of practice. *American Journal of Occupational Therapy, 43*(4), 219–26.

Peloquin, S. M. (2005). The 2005 Eleanor Clarke Slagle Lecture: Embracing our ethos, reclaiming our heart. *American Journal of Occupational Therapy, 59*(6), 611–25.

Ponicare, H. (n.d.). *Science is facts, ...* Retrieved October 28, 2006, from http://www.quotationspage.com/subjects/ science/.

Reilly, M. (1962). Occupational therapy can be one of the great ideas of the 20th century medicine. *American Journal of Occupational Therapy, 16*(1), 1–9.

Reilly, M. (1969). The educational process. *American Journal of Occupational Therapy, 13*(4), 299–307.

Reilly, M. (1974). *Play as exploratory learning.* Beverly Hills, CA: Sage.

Reitz, S. M. (1992). A historical review of occupational therapy's role in preventive health and wellness. *American Journal of Occupational Therapy, 46,* 50–55.

Reitz, S. M. (1998a). *Bridging the gulf between theory and practice.* Poster session presented at the 12th International

Congress of the World Federation of Occupational Therapists, Montrèal, Canada.

Reitz, S. M. (1998b). *Ways to organize OT knowledge.* Course packet, (OCTH 211). Towson, MD: Towson University.

Reitz, S. M. (2000). *Ways to organize OT knowledge.* Course packet, (OCTH 11). Towson, MD: Towson University.

Reitz, S. M., & Scaffa, M. (2001). Theoretical frameworks for community-based practice. In M. Scaffa (Ed.), *Occupational therapy in community-based practice settings* (pp. 51–84). Philadelphia: F. A. Davis.

Royeen, C. B. (2000). Foreword: The scholarship of application. In P. A. Crist, C. B. Royeen, & J. K. Schkade (Eds.), *Infusing occupation into practice* (pp. v–vi). Bethesda, MD: American Occupational Therapy Association.

Scaffa, M. (1992). *The development of comprehensive theory in health education: A feasibility study.* (Dissertation Abstracts International).

Schkade, J. K., & McClung, M. (2001). *Occupational adaptation in practice: Concepts in practice.* Thorofare, NJ: SLACK.

Schkade, J. K., & Schultz, S. (1992). Occupational adaptation: Toward a holistic approach for contemporary practice, part 1. *American Journal of Occupational Therapy, 46,* 829–37.

Schkade, J., Schultz, S., & McClung, M. (2000, March). *Occupational adaptation: Status 2000.* Paper presented at the meeting of the American Occupational Therapy Association, Seattle, WA.

Schultz, S. (2000). *Overview of theoretical models: Occupational adaptation.* In P. A. Crist, C. B. Royeen, & J. K. Schkade (Eds.), *Infusing occupation into practice* (2d ed., pp. 6–15). Bethesda, MD: American Occupational Therapy Association.

Schultz, S. (n.d.). *Theory of occupational adaptation: Overview.* Retrieved December 11, 2006, from http://www .twu.edu/ot/post_phd.htm.

Schultz, S., & Schkade, J. K. (1992). Occupational adaptation: Toward a holistic approach for contemporary practice, part 2. *American Journal of Occupational Therapy, 46,* 917–25.

Schultz, S., & Schkade, J. K. (2003). Section III: Occupational adaptation. In E. B. Crepeau, E. S. Cohn, & B. A. Schell (Eds.), *Willard & Spackman's occupational therapy* (10th ed., pp. 220–23). Philadelphia: Lippincott, Williams & Wilkins.

Scott, P., Miller, R. J., & Walker, K. F. (2004). *Gary Kielhofner.* In K. F. Walker & F. M. Ludwig (Eds.), *Perspectives on theory for the practice of occupational therapy* (3d ed., pp. 267–326). Austin, TX: Pro-Ed.

Society for the Study of Occupation: USA. (2004). *Conference abstracts: Third annual research conference.* Retrieved December 26, 2006, from http://www.sso-usa.org/prior _conference.htm#ThirdAnnual.

Stevenson, S. (1998). Interdisciplinary prevention in rural communities: Outcome evaluation of the Strides for Life walking program for older adults. Unpublished graduate project, Towson University, Towson, MD. (Supported through USDHHS, Public Health Service, Bureau of Health Professions, Health Resources and Services Administration [Grant #36 AH 10043-4] administered by the Western Maryland Area Health Education Center).

Stewart, D., Letts, L., Law, M., Cooper, B. A., Strong, S., & Rigby, P. J. (2003). Section V: The person-environment-occupation model. In E. B. Crepeau, E. S. Cohn, & B. A. Schell (Eds.), *Willard & Spackman's occupational therapy* (10th ed., pp. 227–31). Philadelphia: Lippincott, Williams & Wilkins.

Strong, S. (1998). Meaningful work in supportive environments: Experiences with the recovery process. *American Journal of Occupational Therapy, 52,* 31–38.

Strong, S., Rigby, P., Stewart, D., Law, M., Letts, L., & Cooper, B. (1999). Application of the person-environment-occupation model: A practical tool. *Canadian Journal of Occupational Therapy, 66*(3), 122–33.

University of Illinois at Chicago, MOHO Clearinghouse. (2005a). *Introduction to MOHO.* Retrieved July 23, 2005, from http://www.moho.uic.edu/intro.html.

University of Illinois at Chicago, MOHO Clearinghouse. (2005b). *Frequently asked questions.* Retrieved July 23, 2005, from http://www.moho.uic.edu/faq.html.

University of Illinois at Chicago, MOHO Clearinghouse. (2005c). *References list.* Retrieved July 23, 2005, from http://www.moho.uic.edu/referencelists.html.

von Bertalanffy, L. (1968). *General system theory: Foundations, development, applications.* New York: George Braziller.

World Health Organization. (1986). Ottawa charter for health promotion. Retrieved December 4, 2004, from http://www .who.int/hpr/NPH/docs/ottawa_charter_hp.pdf.

World Health Organization. (1997). *Jakarta declaration on leading health promotion into the 21st century.* Retrieved May 29, 2005, from http://www.who.int/hpr/NPH/docs/ jakarta_declaration_en.pdf.

World Health Organization. (2001). *International classification of functioning, disability and health.* Geneva, Switzerland: Author.

Chapter 3

Health Behavior Frameworks for Health Promotion Practice

S. Maggie Reitz, Marjorie E. Scaffa, Regina Michael Campbell, and Patricia Atwell Rhynders

Theory gives planners tools for moving beyond intuition to design and evaluate health behavior and health promotion interventions based on understanding of behavior. It helps them to step back and consider the larger picture. Like an artist, a program planner who grounds health interventions in theory creates innovative ways to address specific circumstances. He or she does not depend on a "paint-by-numbers" approach, re-hashing stale ideas, but uses a palette of behavior theories, skillfully applying them to develop unique, tailored solutions to problems.

—National Cancer Institute [NCI], 2005, pp. 4–5

Learning Objectives

This chapter is designed to enable the reader to:

- Identify theories from other disciplines for potential application to occupational therapy health promotion initiatives.
- Evaluate the advantages and disadvantages of the various models for use in occupational therapy health promotion interventions in a variety of contexts.
- Describe the potential application of a variety of models from other disciplines as theoretical support for occupation-based health promotion programs.

- Compare and contrast one occupational therapy model or theory with a model or theory from another discipline and explain how these might be combined to better address a health promotion need and develop an effective health promotion program.

Key Terms

Action stage
Bifurcations
Contemplation stage
Cues to action
Early adopters
Early majority
Enabling factors
Health-promotive environments

Innovation
Innovators
Laggards
Late majority
Macrosystem
Maintenance stage
Mesosystem
Microsystem
Ontosystem

Perceived barriers
Perceived benefits
Perceived severity
Perceived susceptibility
Precontemplation stage
Predisposing factors
Preparation stage
Reinforcing factors
Self-efficacy

Self-organization
Self-similarity
Sensitivity to initial conditions
Social climate
Social ecology
Termination stage

Introduction

While occupational therapy theories frequently focus on the adaptation and recovery of individuals, theories from other disciplines often focus on behavior change and prevention at the group, population, or societal levels. Knowledge of occupational therapy theories and those from other disciplines significantly enhances the repertoire of occupational therapists and occupational therapy assistants involved in health promotion intervention. Health promotion is described in detail in the American Occupational Therapy Association's (AOTA's) official statement on health promotion, *Occupational Therapy Services in the Promotion of Health and the Prevention of Disease and Disability* (AOTA, 2008). In this document and earlier versions of this document, health promotion is seen as a strategy to address health, wellbeing, and occupational justice with individuals and groups as well as other levels of society including, organizations, communities, and governmental agencies.

Five theories and models from a variety of health and social sciences are reviewed in this chapter as possible frameworks to supplement the use of occupational therapy conceptual practice models in health promotion practice:

- Diffusion of Innovations Theory
- Health Belief Model (HBM)
- PRECEDE-PROCEED Model
- Social Ecological Model
- Transtheoretical Model of Change (TTM)

These theories are either from or were influenced by communication studies, health education, health promotion, public health, psychology, or social psychology. Schematics and health promotion examples are included for each of these theories.

Discussion length for each theory and example varies based on the theory's maturity and complexity. In addition, the chapter also briefly introduces chaos theory, which can contribute to the manner in which occupational therapists and occupational therapy assistants view balance and change in the development of health promotion initiatives. The chapter ends with a table that provides guidance in selecting theories appropriate for supporting health promotion initiatives.

Health Behavior Theories: An Overview

The *Occupational Therapy Practice Framework* (AOTA, 2008) supports engagement in health promotion activities by occupational therapists and occupational therapy assistants. Its language and philosophy help students and practitioners describe the relationships of health promotion initiatives to both the pattern of daily life and the enhancement of health. The description of the consultation process, education process, and advocacy, as well as the examples of intervention approaches are particularly relevant. The *Framework* is an excellent starting point but is not entirely sufficient to guide practice in this area. In addition to the *Framework*'s language and occupational therapy process description, a theory-based foundation is also required to support development and implementation of evidence-based interventions.

In addition to occupational therapy theories and conceptual practice models, those from other disciplines also can be useful tools in occupational therapy health promotion. Health behavior theories are particularly relevant and can be divided into two major types: explanatory and change (NCI, 2005). Figure 3-1 shows the relationship between these types of health behavior theories. Explanatory theory, also referred to as *theory of the problem,* seeks to discover why a health condition exists and to identify modifiable factors (e.g., access to resources, attitudes, knowledge, self-efficacy). The Health Belief Model, discussed later in this chapter, is an example of explanatory theory. Change theory, also known as *theory of action,* is useful to direct decision-making around program interventions. Diffusion of Innovation, which is also described in this chapter, is an example of this type of theory.

Health behavior theories can also be classified according to their potential target: individuals, groups, or communities. Table 3-1 identifies and classifies the most prominent health behavior models currently applied in the United States (NCI, 2005). They are categorized as addressing health issues at the individual level, the interpersonal level, or the community level. A selection of these models will be described in the

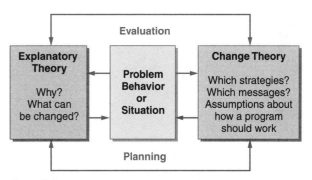

Figure 3-1 Using explanatory theory and change theory to plan and evaluate programs.

From Figure 1 in Theory at a glance *(2d ed., p. 6), by National Cancer Institute, 2005, Bethesda, MD: U.S. National Institutes of Health.*

Table 3–1   **Summary of Theories**

	Theory	Focus	Key Concepts
Individual Level	Health Belief Model	Individuals' perceptions of the threat posed by a health problem, the benefits of avoiding the threat, and factors influencing the decision to act	Perceived susceptibility Perceived severity Perceived benefits Perceived barriers Cues to action Self-efficacy
	Stages of Change Model	Individuals' motivation and readiness to change a problem behavior	Precontemplation Contemplation Decision Action Maintenance
Interpersonal Level	Social Cognitive Theory	Personal factors, environmental factors, and human behavior exert influence on each other	Reciprocal determinism Behavioral capability Expectations Self-efficacy Observational learning Reinforcements
Community Level	Community Organization	Community-driven approaches to assessing and solving health and social problems	Empowerment Community capacity Participation Relevance Issue selection Critical consciousness
	Diffusion of Innovations	How new ideas, products, and practices spread within a society or from one society to another	Relative advantage Compatibility Complexity Trialability Observability
	Communication Theory	How different types of communication affect health behavior	Media agenda setting Public agenda setting Policy agenda setting Problem identification, definition Framing

From Table 11 in *Theory at a glance* (2d ed., p. 45), by National Cancer Institute, 2005, Bethesda, MD: U.S. National Institutes of Health.

following section, which includes those addressing individual health behavior as well as group and community models of health behavior change (Glanz, Rimer, & Lewis, 2005; NCI, 2005). Those not selected are also potentially useful theories for occupational therapists. A good initial resource for the reader to acquaint themselves with these other models is the NCI publication *Theory at a Glance* (2005), available at http://www.cancer.gov/theory.pdf.

Two of the five models to be described in detail are the Health Belief Model (Rosenstock, 1974; Rosenstock, Strecher, & Becker, 1994) and Prochaska and DiClemente's Transtheoretical Model (1982, 1983, 1992). Both are examples of widely researched individual or intrapersonal health behavior models. The Health Belief Model (HBM) examines the precursors of health behavior. The Transtheoretical Model (TTM), also identified as the *Stages of Change Model* by the NCI, explains the various stages people experience as they seek to change and maintain behaviors to maximize health and wellbeing (DiClemente et al., 1991; McKenzie, Neiger, & Smeltzer, 2005). Diffusion of Innovations, identified in Table 3-1, is a community-level theory.

The remaining theoretical frameworks of health behavior change to be described include the PRECEDE-PROCEED Model (designed for program planning and evaluation) and the Social Ecology Model. These models and theories are most applicable to multilevel health promotion interventions that address the health needs of communities rather than individuals. In addition to these theories from the health and social science literature, a theory from the physical sciences that will be described, chaos theory, may prove beneficial in supporting health promotion practice. To date, this theory has not been extensively discussed in the health promotion literature; however, the authors believe it has significant potential for application in health promotion.

Diffusion of Innovations: An Overview

The Diffusion of Innovations Theory was originally developed to describe the manner in which individuals adopt new products or behaviors. The theory has been applied extensively to marketing and communications research, to public health, and to education research. Diffusion research has been supported by "an invisible college," an "informal network of researchers who form around an intellectual paradigm to study a common topic" (Rogers, 1995, p. 44).

Rogers, a communications scholar who has written a series of books on the subject, defined *diffusion* as "the process by which an innovation is communicated through certain channels over time among members of a social system" (1995, p. 5). Although some researchers consider diffusion only as the spontaneous spread of an idea or product, Rogers used the term to describe both the planned and unplanned spread of innovations. His use of the term **innovation** applies to "an idea, practice, or object that is perceived as new by an individual or other unit of adoption" (Rogers, 2003, p. 12). The actual age of the innovation is irrelevant; it is the perception of newness that characterizes an innovation. For example, health promotion has been linked with occupation and occupational therapy from the inception of the profession (Reitz, 1992) but as of yet has not been fully diffused into the profession.

Simply introducing a new construct, idea, or practice does not guarantee change. If that were the case, clients would make appropriate changes in their lives by merely being told of the value of healthy behaviors. There are characteristics of the innovation, the adopter, and the organization that combine to affect the likelihood and rate of adoption (Rogers, 1995). The four elements of the theory are detailed in Table 3-2.

Table 3–2 Concepts in Diffusion of Innovations

Concept	Definition
Innovation	An idea, object, or practice that is thought to be new by an individual, organization, or community
Communication channels	The means of transmitting the new idea from one person to another
Social system	A group of individuals who together adopt the innovation
Time	How long it takes to adopt the innovation

From *Theory at a glance* (2d ed., p. 27), by National Cancer Institute, 2005, Bethesda, MD: National Institutes of Health.

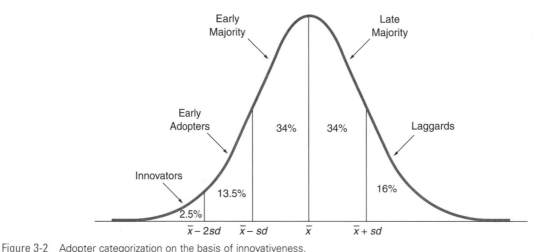

Figure 3-2 Adopter categorization on the basis of innovativeness.

From Diffusion of innovations *(p. 281), by E. M. Rogers, 2003, New York: Free Press. Copyright 2003 by E. M. Rogers. Reprinted with permission.*

Individuals, organizations, and social systems can be categorized according to their openness to adopt innovations and the communication channels they use to learn of new ideas. **Innovators,** the most daring of all adopters, usually get ideas from sources outside their communities and put those ideas into use on a local level. Because they are "ahead of their time," they are not considered to be leaders among the majority. The **early adopters** are more widely known and respected as opinion leaders. They serve as role models to those within the community and can influence adoption by raising awareness and persuading others to try the innovation. The **early majority** adopters value the opinions of the early adopters. They are likely to have a wide circle of local peers but are not seen as leaders. Because the early majority adopt just before the skeptical **late majority,** they provide an important connection in the diffusion process. The late majority are persuaded by system norms and motivated by peer pressure. **Laggards** are the last members of the social system to adopt. They are the most traditional of the adopters and can least afford the risk of trying something new (Rogers, 1995). Figure 3-2 displays the typical dispersion of a social system's members to these five categories; this dispersion resembles the normal frequency distribution.

Phases of Diffusion

The action of diffusion is phased over time, first raising awareness in the knowledge stage, then forming an opinion in the persuasion stage, moving to the decision to adopt or reject implementation of the innovation, and finally confirmation, when reinforcement for the adoption decision is needed. When enough individuals have adopted an innovation, its diffusion becomes self-sustaining (Rogers, 1995). Rogers illustrated this as the typical S-shaped curve of adoption, which was based

on the original idea of Tarde, a French social psychologist in the early 1900s (Rogers, 2003).

The curve starts slowly as innovative members of the social system adopt the innovation, then rises steeply as the early adopters spread news of the innovation's acceptance through the early majority's interpersonal networks. After the innovation has become the standard practice, the curve tapers off, as there are few individuals remaining who have not incorporated the innovation within their practice.

Figure 3-3 displays the standard S-curve of adoption for a new technology (Paulk, 1999). As mentioned earlier, while health promotion has been associated with the occupational therapy profession since its inception, it has only recently approached the level of confirmation. Figure 3-4 depicts the S-curve of adoption for

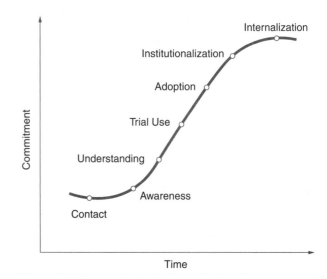

Figure 3-3 The standard technology adoption S-curve.

From Structured approaches to managing change, *by M. C. Paulk, 1999, Pittsburgh, PA: Carnegie Mellon University. Copyright © 1999 by Carnegie Mellon University. Reprinted with permission.*

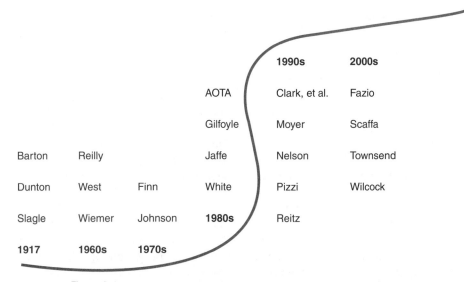

Figure 3-4   Adoption of health promotion in occupational therapy S-curve.

health promotion practice within the occupational therapy profession. Innovators and early adoptors of health promotion within the profession are identified.

Ely (1990, p. 298) described eight conditions that facilitate the adoption, implementation, and institutionalization of educational innovations:

- Dissatisfaction with the status quo
- Knowledge and skills
- Resources
- Time
- Rewards
- Participation
- Commitment
- Leadership

One of the first prompts to change comes from dissatisfaction with the current situation or the way in which things are done. It may result from a problem that cannot be solved with currently available methods. The greater the dissatisfaction, the more likely a person or organization is to implement an innovation or change. In order for an innovation to be implemented effectively, the persons involved must possess adequate knowledge and skills. If there is desire but knowledge and skills are lacking, then successful implementation is unlikely. In-services, tutorials, and formal education are all strategies that can facilitate proper implementation.

Resources, including time, are essential elements for implementation. Needed tools and materials should be readily available, and personnel resources must be adequate. Those responsible for implementing innovations must have sufficient time "to learn, adapt, integrate, and reflect on what they are doing" (Ely, 1990, p. 299). Blocks of time should be set aside and designated specifically for tasks associated with implementation.

Incentives and rewards for those who adopt an innovation facilitate successful implementation. Change is often an uncomfortable prospect, so sufficient cause for change must exist, as well as an expectation that participation in the implementation will result in positive outcomes for those involved. Individuals deem different incentives and rewards desirable, so it is important to ascertain which incentives/rewards will be most effective. Involving implementers in planning and decision-making facilitates implementation. Communication is vital to theeffort's success. It is imperative that "each person feels that he or she has had an opportunity to comment on innovations that will directly affect his or her work" (Ely, 1990, p. 300).

Stakeholder endorsement of the innovation enhances the likelihood of implementation. Opinion leaders can have a profound effect on outcomes. Commitment from superiors indicates support, which promotes confidence in those who are empowered to incorporate the innovation into practice. Easily identifiable leadership is another important element. Leaders encourage, inspire, and support others in their implementation attempts. They must ensure that the necessary materials and training are provided and are available for consultation should a problem occur (Ely, 1990).

Ely (1990) suggested that these conditions be assessed before implementation is attempted. However, he cautioned that although "most of the conditions will apply most of the time" (p. 303), cross-cultural comparisons indicate some variations; therefore, adaptation to specific situations may be necessary. Maximizing as many conditions as possible before and during the adoption process will increase implementation effectiveness: "The conditions can be used as a screening tool to identify potential problems, but they cannot be specific in determining the exact causes of the problems" (Ely, 1990, p. 303).

Diffusion of Innovations: Applicability to Health Promotion in Occupational Therapy

Although a limited amount of literature exists discussing the use of Rogers's work in health promotion, examples are available. Buller and colleagues (2005) used the Diffusion of Innovations Theory to develop and disseminate a sun-protection program for outdoor employees in ski areas. Other researchers compared tuberculosis (TB) therapy completion rates among jail inmates after their release (White et al., 2005). Compliance rates obtained through a clinical trial were compared to those achieved from repeating the innovation in the real day-to-day world of a county jail. In the clinical trial, the individuals providing the training did not have additional duties beyond providing the TB education and research. However, in the comparison group, the TB education protocol was added to the routine job duties performed by jail discharge planners. This resulted in the training being provided in a shorter timeframe and in a different setting (i.e., a private quiet room for the clinical trial versus "talking through the bars" in the real-world implementation).

Although this study highlights the difficulties in translating evidence-based practice from the clinical trial environment to the realities of real-time service delivery, it demonstrated that the Diffusion of Innovations Theory may be a helpful tool for researching the impact of dissemination approaches on health promotion programs.

The literature supports the use of the Diffusion of Innovation Theory, which has been identified as one of the few frequently used theories to support theory-driven health promotion program initiatives (Kegler, Crosby, & DiClemente, 2002). By using the characteristics of innovation, the success of programs aimed at encouraging the adoption of a new health behavior can be increased (NCI, 2005). In addition, the Diffusion of Innovations Theory has been identified as promising for use in disseminating new health promotion strategies or programs (NCI, 2005; Oldenburg & Parcel, 2002).

As with any theory discussed in this chapter, opportunities exist for further development and research to enhance strength and applicability. While descriptions of program development based on this theory are available, research comparing the efficacy and expense of various dissemination strategies remains underrepresented in the health promotion literature. This situation may be due to the need for different research strategies and measurement tools when studying the dissemination process than those traditionally used in program effectiveness studies (Oldenburg & Parcel,

2002). Another concern is that the theory provides minimal guidance on how to accomplish dissemination of innovative health promotion actions through such strategies as interpersonal influence at the community level (Kennedy & Crosby, 2002). The impact of context on the dissemination process is an additional challenge and is an area for needed research (Oldenburg & Parcel, 2002). Occupational therapists and occupational therapy assistants, with their expertise and knowledge of context and human performance, are in a position to enhance research efforts in this area.

Despite its limitations, the Diffusion of Innovation Theory has the potential to maximize success in the dissemination of broad, multilevel health promotion communitywide programming (Oldenburg & Parcel, 2002). The ultimate success of these efforts will be demonstrated in health outcomes that are linked to the achievement of national health objectives, such as *Healthy People 2010: Understanding and Improving Health* (U.S. Department of Health and Human Services [USDHHS], 2000). The Diffusion of Innovation Theory exhibits potential for use in implementing or replicating health promotion programs, including those that are occupation-based, such as that described in the following example.

Diffusion of Innovations: Health Promotion Example

An occupational therapist wanted to implement a program modeled after the Well Elderly Study, developed by University of Southern California (USC) faculty (Mandel, Jackson, Zemke, Nelson, & Clark, 1999), in the assisted-living facility in which she works. She recognized that the residents' participation in occupations was limited. As a result, their occupational performance was deteriorating (dissatisfaction with the status quo). This deterioration has impacted the residents and the other facility staff, since they are being required to provide more and more care for the residents as their abilities decline. The occupational therapist had heard of the USC program but did not know how to implement it, so she began by immersing herself in the professional literature and contacting therapists who have implemented the program (knowledge and skills).

When the occupational therapist felt comfortable with her knowledge level, she met with the facility director to present a program proposal. The director was excited about the idea and gave the occupational therapist permission to proceed. In addition, the director agreed to provide the resources needed to implement the program (commitment). The occupational therapist organized an in-service for the staff, provided information about the program (knowledge and skills), and requested input from the staff regarding implementation. Staff members asked numerous questions and provided strategies to overcome barriers to implementation (participation).

It became obvious to the occupational therapist that the staff's complete cooperation and assistance would be required. It was decided that the staff needed more training to increase the likelihood of successful implementation. The facility director agreed to pay the employees for participating in the additional training (incentives and time). The occupational therapist identified "team leaders" to participate in the training and then train the staff on their respective teams (leadership). Equipment, materials, and supplies were acquired, and the environment was modified to support the program (resources). Now the conditions are optimized to begin implementing a program tailored to maximize the wellbeing of the facility's residents.

Health Belief Model: An Overview

The Health Belief Model (HBM) was originally developed by social psychologists Hochbaum, Kegeles, Leventhal, and Rosenstock to explain preventive health behaviors (Rosenstock, 1974). Within a short time, it was adapted to study sick role (Becker, 1974) and illness behavior (Kirscht, 1974). According to Rosenstock, the model is based on Lewin's aspiration model, which is a special case of Lewin's well-known field theory (Maiman & Becker, 1974). Lewin's work provided two underlying perspectives of the model: the phenomenological orientation and the ahistorical perspective. According to Rosenstock, the founders of the HBM all agreed upon a phenomenological orientation where the individual's perceptions of self and the environment determine health behavior, not the actual environment. Their ahistorical perspective focuses attention on the current dynamics affecting an individual's behavior, not on past history or prior experiences, except if it directly relates to the current issue (Rosenstock, 1974).

The HBM describes the relationships between a person's beliefs about health and his or her health-specific behaviors. The beliefs that mediate health behavior, according to the original model, include perceived susceptibility, perceived severity, perceived benefits, and perceived barriers (Rosenstock, 1966, 1974). **Perceived susceptibility** is the individual's impression of their risk of contracting a disease or illness. Once a health condition exists, perceived susceptibility expands to include perceived resusceptibility, perceptions regarding the belief in diag-

nosis accuracy, and acceptance of the diagnosis (Becker, 1974; Rosenstock et al., 1994). **Perceived severity** refers to a person's convictions regarding the degree of seriousness of a given health problem. **Perceived benefits** are a person's beliefs regarding the availability and effectiveness of a variety of possible actions in reducing the threat of illness. **Perceived barriers** are the costs or negative aspects associated with engaging in a specific health behavior. These barriers can include fear of pain, inconvenience of seeking care, and expense (Rosenstock, 1966). Content Box 3-1 identifies a variety of barriers to health promotion, including perceived barriers and systems-level barriers to care. **Cues to action** are defined as instigating events that stimulate the initiation of behavior. These cues may be internal, such as perceptions of pain, or external, such as a famous person beginning an exercise plan or being diagnosed with breast cancer.

According to the model, in order for a person to take action to avoid illness, the positive forces must outweigh the negative forces. If an individual believes that

1. he or she is personally susceptible to the disease or illness;
2. the occurrence of the health problem is severe enough to negatively impact his or her life;
3. taking specific actions would have beneficial effects;
4. the barriers to such action do not overwhelm the benefits; and
5. the individual is exposed to cues for action, then it is likely that the health behavior will occur (Rosenstock, 1974).

Rosenstock (1966, 1974) hypothesized that the required intensity of the cue to action could vary depending upon the strength of the perceived threat. Thus, if someone already felt a high level of perceived threat when riding a bicycle without a helmet, a bike safety poster on a passing bus may be a sufficient cue to purchase and wear a bike helmet. However, for someone else with a lower degree of perceived threat, the cue to action may need to be stronger, such as their biking buddy taking a spill and receiving a mild concussion.

Perceived threat, which encompasses perceived susceptibility, has been suggested as an important first cognitive step in the health-action link described by this model (Rosenstock et al., 1994). However, in addition to perceived threat, a person needs to believe that they have the resources to address that threat before they take action. In order to maximize the likelihood of one's engagement in a health behavior, the individual must simultaneously

Content Box 3-1

Examples of Possible Barriers to Health Promotion Services or Actions

- System Barriers
  - Fragmentation of services
  - Complex systems
- Time
  - Travel time
  - Waiting time at appointment
  - Waiting interval for appointment
- Distance
- Transportation
- Cost
  - Cost of services
  - Inadequate insurance coverage
  - Transportation/parking
- Availability of Services
  - Limited office hours
  - Health-care provider shortages
- Organization of Services
  - Lack of primary providers
  - Lack of case managers
  - Lack of continuum of care
- Discrimination
  - Race
  - Sex
  - Geography (i.e., rural populations)
  - Social status
  - Age
- Stigma
- Provider-Consumer Relationships
  - Lack of expertise
  - Short encounters
- Demographic Factors
  - Education
  - Low income
  - Age
- Attitudes
  - Lack of interest in health promotion
  - Fear or anxiety
  - Skepticism
- Knowledge
- Effort
- Cultural Factors
  - Preference for folk medicine
  - Naiveté
  - Language
- Family Characteristics
  - Complexity of family
  - Family size
  - Prior negative experience

Adapted from "Barriers: A critical review of recent literature," by K. A. Melnyk, 2005, *Nursing Research, 37*(4), 196–201.

- achieve a sufficient level of motivation to examine the health issue;
- feel enough of a perceived threat to trigger action;
- decide that the health benefits outweigh the cost and efforts to overcome the perceived barriers,

which can include self-efficacy (McKenzie et al., 2005).

Figure 3-5 presents a schematic representation of the HBM with a new placement of the perceived susceptibility construct and the addition of self-efficacy. **Self-efficacy** refers to a person's beliefs about their "ability to coordinate skills and abilities to attain desired goals in particular domains and circumstances" (Maddux, 2005, p. 278). These beliefs develop through interaction with the environment during one's lifetime and are specific to particular skill sets and goals.

Health Belief Model: Applicability to Health Promotion in Occupational Therapy

The HBM is one of the most widely studied and used frameworks for health behavior change (McKenzie et al., 2005). It has been used to study and address a wide array of health topics within varied populations, including alcoholism (Bardsley & Beckman, 1988), compliance with a diabetes regimen (Becker & Janz, 1985), exercise participation following myocardial infarction (Al-Ali & Haddad, 2004), medication compliance among psychiatric outpatients (Kelly, Mamon, & Scott, 1987), and compliance with home exercise programs (Chen, Neufeld, Feely, & Skinner, 1999). As the aforementioned examples indicate, the HBM often focuses on health behaviors following the onset of a health condition. It also can be used as a tool for prevention. Examples of such use include breast self-examination (Champion, 1985), testicular self-examination (Reno, 1988), contraceptive behavior (Herold, 1983; Hester & Macrina, 1985), and, more recently, the health promotion needs of young families (Roden, 2004a, 2004b), prostate cancer detection (Kleier, 2004), osteoporosis prevention (Cline & Worley, 2006; Turner, Hunt, DiBrezzo, & Jones, 2004), and physical activity participation (Centers for Disease Control and Prevention [CDC], 1999; Juniper, Oman, Hamm, & Kerby, 2004).

Research on the model as a whole has been limited; more attention has been given to examining its various constructs in isolation. In addition, the model's predictive value is in question (Kegeles & Lund, 1982). Although the constructs are fairly well defined, the causal associations among the variables and the reasons why particular factors are more important in one population than another require further study. Also of concern is the limited research conducted to determine the validity of the HBM for use with women from nonwhite cultural backgrounds (McAllister & Farquhar, 1992).

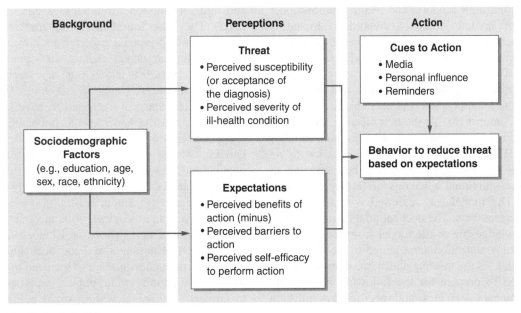

Figure 3-5   The Health Belief Model.

From Figure 1 "The Health Belief Model and HIV Risk Behavior Change" (p. 11), by I. M. Rosenstock, V. J. Strecher, & M. H. Becker, in Preventing AIDS: Theories and methods of behavioral interventions, *R. J. DiClemente & J. L. Peterson (Eds.), 1994, New York: Plenum Press. Copyright © 1994 by Plenum Press. Reprinted with permission.*

Due to concerns regarding the constructs and their failure to translate to a wellness approach for use with families, Roden revised the HBM (2004a, 2004b). Two constructs—perceived behavioral control (PBC) and behavioral intention—were added from Ajzen's theory of planned behavior (1985). In addition to including these constructs, the revised model also diminishes the influence of perceived threat, perceived seriousness, and perceived susceptibility by subsuming these constructs under PBC and the perceived notion of health. Cues to action have been reframed to assist in the model's reorientation to a health promotion perspective versus an illness-prevention focus; this reframing was accomplished through a link to the notion of perceived health instead of the previous link to the perceived threat of disease (Roden, 2004b).

The preceding concerns provide opportunities for future research. If these concerns are addressed, both the HBM and Roden's revised model for families (2004a, 2004b) have much to offer health promotion program development and can be used in conjunction with occupation-based theories. The NCI (2005) recommended this model for use with health promotion interventions or research that addresses health motivation where the individual or group has a sufficient level of perceived susceptibility. If an individual or group does not feel they are at risk, this model will not be as likely to promote health behavior change. Since the HBM has been both used and published by a variety of health disciplines (Reitz, 1990), it has good potential

for use by interdisciplinary teams. The following example describes such an approach.

Health Belief Model: Health Promotion Example

This health promotion example is hypothetical, as actual HBM examples within occupational therapy are limited (Chen et al., 1999; Kielhofner & Nelson, 1983; Reitz, 1990) and are focused primarily on compliance with rehabilitation rather than health promotion program development. In addition to this example, one of the author's real-life applications of the HBM's constructs and principles is described elsewhere in this text. This example, although fictitious, is based on knowledge of rural health issues and culture gained through participation in a series of federally supported interdisciplinary health promotion activities conducted in western Maryland (Fertman, Dotson, Mazzocco, & Reitz, 2005). These activities were part of a project supported by funds from USDHHS, Health Resources and Services Administration, Bureau of Health Professions, and the Quentin N. Burdick Program for Rural Interdisciplinary Training, and were directed by the Western Maryland Area Health Education Center in collaboration with various universities.

Recently, the dominant hand of Ashwood County's star high school football quarterback was amputated by a piece of farm machinery. This accident acted as a cue to action for the county health commissioner and the football coach (who was also the health educator at the county's lone high school). The health commissioner and coach invited various stakeholders, including farmers, school board members, and health providers, to a meeting to design a campaign to address safety on the farm. Two occupational therapists were invited to attend; one works in the school system, and the second works at the local hospital (the next closest hospital is at least a 2-hour drive). At the first meeting, the county health commissioner and coach, who are both familiar with the HBM, suggested this model be used as an organizing framework for planning the campaign to change the individual behaviors of farmers and their families. The model was reviewed with farm safety committee members. The occupational therapists, who were knowledgeable of the model from their occupational therapy education, contributed to the discussion of the model. As the meeting ended, the committee was encouraged to prepare for the following meeting by considering campaign ideas and specific ways in which they can contribute.

The two occupational therapists, both new to the county, decided they must first seek prevalence data on farm-related injuries and identify possible resources prior to the next meeting. They decided to meet in 2 days to compare notes. When they met, they discussed how farming has been identified as one of the most dangerous occupations in a variety of countries, including the United States, in terms of both death and injury (Thurston, Blundell-Gosselin, & Vollman, 2003). They also found that male farmers in Ireland had poor health-protective behaviors, "with only 18% reporting regular dental checks, 26% practicing skin protection, and 29% taking regular exercise" (Hope, Kelleher, Holmes, & Hennessy, 1999, p. 231). Farmers in the United States were found to have higher rates of suicide than the general U.S. population, whereas Canadian farmers' suicide rate, with the exception of Quebec, was at or below that of Canada's general population. The supportive tradition of farming communities in Canada was identified as possibly acting as a protective factor (Pickett et al., 2000). It was also noted that stress was an ecological problem versus a problem of individual farmers (Thurston, Blundell-Gosselin, & Rose, 2003). This supported the occupational therapists' growing understanding of the need for a comprehensive, community-wide, population-based approach to farmers' wellbeing, which would be broader than this particular event.

In addition to examining the literature, the occupational therapists also reviewed *Healthy People 2010* (USDHHS, 2000) and developed a list of health objectives that may relate to farm safety (Table 3-3). In addition, they located a free resource from the NCI (2001), *Making Health Communication Programs Work*, which they ordered by calling 1-800-4CANCER.

Table 3–3 **Examples of *Healthy People 2010* Objectives Linked to Farm-Related Injuries**

Objective Number	Objective
15-1	Reduce hospitalization for nonfatal head injuries.
15-2	Reduce hospitalization for nonfatal spinal cord injuries.
20-1	Reduce deaths from work-related injuries.
20-2	Reduce work-related injuries resulting in medical treatment, lost time from work, or restricted work injury.
20-3	Reduce the rate of injury and illness cases involving days away from work due to overexertion or repetitive motion.
20-8	Reduce occupational skin diseases or disorders among full-time workers.
20-11	(Developmental) Reduce new cases of work-related, noise-induced hearing loss.
24-3	Reduce hospital emergency department visits for asthma.
28-8	(Developmental) Reduce occupational eye injury.
28-16	(Developmental) Increase the use of appropriate ear-protection devices, equipment, and practices.
28-18	(Developmental) Reduce adult hearing loss in the noise-exposed public.

Data from *Healthy People 2010: Understanding an improving health,* by U.S. Department of Health and Human Services, 2000, Washington, DC: Government Printing Office.

In both therapists' work settings, they have seen evidence of farm injuries among parents and children that mirrored what they found in the literature, even though some of the data had been collected in Canada (Thurston, Bundell-Gosselin, & Vollman, 2003). The top three reasons for male farmers to seek medical care included eye injuries, back injuries, and skin problems. For women, the top two reasons to seek medical care were similar to the men's, but the third was general muscle and joint injuries (Thurston, Bundell-Gosselin, & Vollman, 2003). Results of a survey among Arkansas farmworkers who were still in high school indicated the most common injuries were caused by cuts, falling, lifting, and animal kicks and bites. Potentially dangerous activities this group frequently engaged in included "use of chainsaws and firearms, handling or feeding large animals, loading equipment, riding on tractors, and—perhaps most significantly—operating all-terrain vehicles" (Hogge, 2002, ¶ 10).

Based on the data gathered, the therapists brainstormed to help identify their role on the committee and arrived at three feasible contributions:

1. Create or adapt ready-to-use occupation-based activities to increase perceived threat, while increasing perceived self-efficacy of engagement in farm safety by farm families.
2. Investigate funding sources to provide seed money for the committee's work.
3. Develop outcome measures to evaluate the campaign in collaboration with the university in the next county.

The occupational therapists suggested a farm safety rodeo, modeled after bicycle safety rodeos in which they had participated during their childhood in suburban environments. At first the idea was dismissed, but after continued discussion and lack of an alternative idea, the high school coach suggested the farm safety rodeo to the homecoming parade organizers. Once the committee members could set the proposed activity within their cultural context, suggestions and modifications of the original idea ensued. Through time, the event evolved into a combined health fair and tractor rodeo. About 1 year after the original meeting, the event was kicked off, beginning with the injured football player describing his injury and rehabilitation to the crowd. According to the HBM, this part of the program could become a cue to action for the attendees and a means to increase perceived threat. Next, mini-workshops were held to help the adults address perceived susceptibility and the seriousness of farm injuries, as well as safety features, precautions, and equipment. This information was conveyed in a workshop format to enhance adults' perceptions of

self-efficacy. The *Farm Family Safety and Health Workshop Leader's Guide* (Indiana Rural Safety & Health Council, n.d.b) was a helpful resource in the workshop's development.

Meanwhile, the children who were engaged in occupation-based activities that the occupational therapists designed were assisted by high school students working as part of their required volunteer hours. Previously, barriers to participation in health fairs had been work commitments (since farming is often a 7-days-per-week job) and lack of childcare. By linking the health fair to a popular community event and removing the barrier of childcare, attendance was increased. The occupational therapists provided a variety of fun prevention-focused activities for the children, including a driving course, complete with orange cones for tricycles and bicycles, which was a miniature version of the course the adults were using for the tractors. Other activities included an obstacle course that encouraged physical activities focusing on balance and coordination. Modeling the importance of breaks when engaging in prolonged physical activity, a quiet-time coloring activity was provided, using a farm-safety coloring book available in *Careful Country: Teacher's Kit* (Indiana Rural Safety & Health Council, n.d.a).

Other committee members assisted with the rodeo and parade activities and coordinated the distribution of donations from businesses supported by the farmers and county residents. A farm equipment distributor provided safety goggles, lightweight sun-blocking shirts, and hats. Other businesses contributed food or goods, such as free samples of sunscreen and water bottles. After the health fair and driving rodeo activities, everyone participated in the homecoming parade.

One month after the successful event, the committee reconvened. From discussions with participants, including farmers, health providers, and other committee members, it was determined that a recommendation would be made for an ongoing regional project to address health behavior change both at the individual and community levels. Table 3-4 shows theories that may be of assistance to the committee as they move from the goal of changing individual farmers' health behaviors to engaging in a multicomponent, multilevel effort. The next agreed upon step was to invite the regional Area Health Education Center (AHEC) staff to seek their assistance (National AHEC Organization, 2005) in planning and seeking funding to support a community capacity building initiative (Kretzmann & McKnight, 1993). This initiative would be designed to address multiple needs of farmers and their neighbors. Community capacity building is described in detail later in this text.

Table 3-4 **Using Theory to Plan Multilevel Interventions**

Change Strategies	Examples of Strategies	Ecological Level	Useful Theories	Potential Occupational Therapy Theories
Change People's Behavior ⇕	Educational sessions	Individual	Stages of Change or TTM	EHP (Establish, Prevent, Alter)
	Interactive kiosks		Precaution Adoption Process	MOHO
	Print brochures		Health Belief Model	OA
	Social marketing campaigns		Theory of Planned Behavior	PEO PEOP
Change the Environment	Media advocacy campaigns	Community	Communication Theory	EHP (Prevent, Create)
	Advocating changes to company policy		Diffusion of Innovations	MOHO
			Community Organizing	PEO
			PRECEDE-PROCEED	PEOP
			Social Ecological Theory	

Adapted from *Theory at a glance* (2d ed., p. 46), by National Cancer Institute, 2005, Bethesda, MD: National Institutes of Health. *Note:* The last column was added by the authors.

PRECEDE-PROCEED Model: An Overview

The PRECEDE (predisposing, reinforcing, and enabling constructs in educational diagnosis and evaluation) Model was developed by Green, Kreuter, Deeds, and Partridge (1980) and is a planning model for health education and community development. The inclusion of an additional set of steps, called PROCEED (policy, regulatory, and organizational constructions in educational and environmental development), was superimposed on the original model (Green & Kreuter, 1991) to promote program evaluation. Through the years, the originators have modified the model to keep pace with trends in health promotion and public health. For example, the language has been changed to better reflect the collaborative process of working with communities in order to determine community assets. More recently, the model has emphasized the importance of genetics by adding it to Phase 2—epidemiological assessment—and reconfiguring the phases from nine to eight (Green & Kreuter, 2005). Table 3-5 identifies the theoretical underpinnings of this model.

The PRECEDE Model was designed to be readily applicable across a variety of settings. It was intended to provide structure and organization to health education program planning and evaluation. Application of this approach occurs in several phases and involves the assessment of factors in four domains: social, epidemiological, educational and ecological, and administrative and policy (Green & Kreuter, 2005). It is unique in that it begins with the desired outcome and works backward, taking into account factors that must precede a certain result.

Phase 1 of this model calls for a social assessment and situational analysis (Green & Kreuter, 2005). An analysis of the social problems that exist in a community from the inhabitants' point of view is a necessary prerequisite when assessing quality of life in a target population. The purpose of this phase is to ascertain the relationship between a given health problem and the social conditions of the community. Phase 2, the epidemiological, behavioral, and environmental assessment, evaluates health problems associated with the community's quality of life through objective measures. The first step in this process is the collection of data on vital indicators such as morbidity, mortality, fertility, and disability to determine the greatest health threats to the community (Green & Kreuter, 1999).

The second step in Phase 2 is to examine the determinants of health, specifically the genetic, behavioral, and environmental factors that impact the health problems of interest to the population or community. The ability to use genetic factors in health promotion planning is expected to improve as the field of applied genetics evolves. "Behavior" was purposely placed

Table 3–5 Diagnostic Elements of PRECEDE-PROCEED

Planning Step	Function	Example of Relevent Theory
1. Social Assessment	Assesses people's views of their own needs and quality of life	Community organization Community building
2. Epidemiological Assessment	Documents which health problems are most important for which groups in a community	Community-level theories (if the community helps to choose the health problem that will be addressed)
3. Behavioral/Environmental Assessment	Identifies factors that contribute to the health problem of interest	Interpersonal theories • Social Cognitive Theory Theories of organizational change Community organization Diffusion of innovations
4. Educational/Ecological Assessment	Identifies preceding and reinforcing factors that must be in place to initiate and sustain change	All three levels of change theories: • Individual • Interpersonal • Community
5. Administrative/Policy Assessment	Identifies policies, resources, and circumstances in the program's context that may help or hinder implementation	Community-level theories: • Community organization • Organization change

From *Theory at a glance* (2d ed., p. 42), by National Cancer Institute, 2005, Bethesda, MD: National Institutes of Health.

between "genetics" and "environment" in the model, as behaviors are needed to mitigate the influence of the other two factors (Green & Kreuter, 2005). Measures of behavioral factors can include consumption patterns, utilization rates of services, and self-care patterns. In addition, environmental factors such as access, affordability, and equity should be determined when planning a health promotion initiative. Behavioral and environmental indicators, rated high in importance and changeability, are usually selected as targets for intervention (Green & Kreuter, 1999).

In Phase 3, educational and ecological assessment, the health-related behaviors and environmental indicators identified in the previous stage, are differentiated by three categories of influence: predisposing, reinforcing, and enabling factors. **Predisposing factors** provide the motivation or rationale for the behavior—for example, knowledge, attitudes, values, and beliefs. **Enabling factors** promote motivation and include personal skills and assets as well as community resources. Predisposing and enabling factors are antecedent to the health behavior and allow for the behavior to occur. **Reinforcing factors** supply the reward or incentive of a behavior that contributes to its maintenance. Each group of factors is analyzed in terms of importance and changeability, and priorities are established for the

intervention. Based on the nature of the targets for intervention, educational methodologies are selected (Green & Kreuter, 1999).

The fourth and final phase of the PRECEDE process is administrative and policy assessment and intervention alignment (Green & Kreuter, 2005). This phase involves an assessment of policies, regulations, and organizational factors that impact the implementation of health promotion programs and the development of strategies to effectively manage these influences. Examples include assessment of budgetary implications, identification and allocation of resources, defining the nature of any cooperative agreements, and establishing a realistic intervention timetable. Omission of this important step can doom an otherwise viable intervention to failure.

The PROCEED portion of the model begins with Phase 5, implementation, and is followed by three additional phases (Green & Kreuter, 1999; 2005) that focus on evaluation. Phase 6, process evaluation, occurs as the program unfolds and allows for changes to be made to address problems before they escalate. Community reaction to the program as well as staff performance would be included in this phase of the evaluation. Impact evaluation is the focus of Phase 7 and measures the immediate effect of the program on the designated target behaviors. This includes examining the factors from Phase 3 (i.e., predisposing, enabling, and reinforcing factors). Phase 8, the final phase, focuses on outcome evaluation. In this phase, long-term changes to health status and quality of life are measured.

PRECEDE-PROCEED Model: Applicability to Health Promotion in Occupational Therapy

The PRECEDE-PROCEED Model has been used in a variety of settings with different populations, including

- planning a pedestrian injury prevention program for children (Howat, Jones, Hall, Cross, & Stevenson, 1997);
- promoting bicycle helmet use among children (Stanken, 2000);
- preventing computer work-related musculoskeletal disorders (Wilkens, 2003);
- encouraging self-management of asthma among families in Taiwan (Chiang, Huang, Yeh, & Lu, 2004);
- identifying factors related to repeat engagement in mammography in underserved women (Ahmed, Fort, Elzey, & Bailey, 2004);
- assessing fat intake of low-income mothers (Chang, Brown, Nitzke, & Baumann, 2004);
- investigating physicians' smoking-cessation counseling (Tremblay et al., 2001); among others.

This list demonstrates use of this model across a variety of populations, health problems, and geographic settings. According to Green and Kreuter (2005), 950 articles using the PRECEED-PROCEED Model have been published. The authors believe the current version of this model, with its educational and ecological approach, is compatible with the aims of a recent Institute of Medicine (2002) report on the future of public health (Green & Kreuter, 2005). Although the model has many opportunities for application, it is not theoretical, as it does not describe the relationships among the identified factors or variables (Parcel, 1984); therefore, it should be used as a planning model rather than a theory to guide research. Nevertheless, it is a potential tool for an interdisciplinary or community team, which may include an occupational therapist or an occupational therapy assistant, to use in addressing a community health concern.

PRECEDE-PROCEED Model: Health Promotion Example

In order to describe the application of the PRECEDE-PROCEED Model, we will revisit the story of the two occupational therapists working in a rural farming community. Although the health fair and tractor rodeo

were a success, the committee had identified the need to look beyond their original goal of changing individual behaviors of farmers to a broader multilevel initiative to include change directed at the environment through such processes as advocacy and policy development. The need to look beyond the individual farmers to the broader ecological system was supported by the literature (Thurston, Blundell-Gosselin, & Rose; 2003; Thurston, Blundell-Gosselin, & Vollman, 2003). After meeting with AHEC representatives, the committee transformed into a coalition and sought grant funding to complete a needs assessment using the PRECEDE-PROCEED framework as a planning tool. Working with the AHEC's university partners, funding was received to initiate the PRECEDE elements of the framework and then evaluated using the PROCEED portion.

Social Ecological Model of Health: An Overview

Ecology is a term used in the biological sciences to refer to the interrelationships and interactions between organisms and their environments. **Social ecology** refers to the "study of the influence of the social context on behavior, including institutional and cultural variables" (Sallis & Owen, 2002, p. 462). It "describes how populations fit into a physical, economical, cultural, and social environment that interacts with biological substrata" (Lemyre & Orpana, 2002, p. 1350). Organisms and their environments are made up of systems, which are organized in levels. The **ontosystem** consists of the individual with his or her unique physiological and psychological composition. Humans develop and are socialized in a **microsystem** of family and friends. This microsystem is embedded in a **mesosystem** of community, school, work, and religious organizations. The **macrosystem** creates social order through government, law, policy, and public services. Social ecology emphasizes the dynamic interaction and synergy among the various systems and their components (Lemyre & Orpana, 2002).

Ecological models of health propose that human behavior is influenced by intrapersonal, physical environment, and sociocultural factors. Ecological models focus on environmental causes of behavior and environmental interventions for health promotion. Environmental interventions occur on several levels and address intrapersonal, interpersonal, and community-level issues. Moos (1980) identified four categories of health-related environmental factors: physical settings, organizational, human aggregate, and social climate. *Physical settings* refer to features of both the natural and constructed environments. *Organizational factors* refer to the nature, size, and structure of community entities such as schools, hospitals, worksites, and places of worship, among others. The *human aggregate* refers to the demographic and sociocultural characteristics of people living in a particular area. **Social climate** refers to the norms, expectations, and support of a given social milieu. Moos believed all these factors impact health and health behaviors of individuals, families, and communities.

More recently, Stokols (1992, 1996) described four social ecological principles related to health:

- Health is influenced by physical and social environmental variables.
- Physical and social environments are multidimensional.
- Interactions between humans and their environments occur at various levels of complexity (individuals, families, worksite, community, and population levels).
- Feedback is an essential feature of human-environment interactions, with environments influencing human behavior and humans influencing the physical and social features of environments.

Stokols (1992) suggested a shift in emphasis from a focus exclusively on individual health habits and lifestyles to a person-environment-interaction (ecological) approach, combining both behavioral and environmental strategies for health promotion. He advocated for the development of health-promotive environments, which enhance the physical, mental, emotional, and social wellbeing of individuals, families, and communities. A **health-promotive environment** is a milieu (Stokols, 1992) that has the following features:

- injury-resistant, ergonomically sound design of physical spaces;
- nontoxic physical and social environments;
- adequate social support networks;
- economic stability;
- organizational flexibility and responsiveness;
- balance between environmental controllability and predictability and novelty and challenge;
- culturally meaningful aesthetic, symbolic, and spiritual elements.

Environmental influences on health behavior can occur on a small scale (e.g., in a specific situation) or a larger scale across multiple life domains. Stokols (1992) identified situations, settings, life domains, and overall life situation as four levels of environmental scale. Situations are "sequences of individual or group activities occurring at a particular time and place" (Stokols, 1992, p. 10), such as lunchtime at a middle school or the impact of food availability on students' eating patterns. Settings are "geographical locations in which various personal or interpersonal situations occur on a regular basis" (p. 10), such as worksites with excessive environmental stressors that impact the workers' physical and emotional wellbeing. Life domains are "different spheres of a person's life, such as family, education, spiritual activities, recreation, employment, and commuting" (p. 10). Family life significantly impacts health. For example, the presence of violence in the home has an extremely detrimental effect on the wellbeing of family members. Finally, *overall life situation* refers to "the major life domains in which a person is involved during a particular period of his or her life" (p. 10). This is the broadest and most complex context in which to assess the physical and social environmental determinants of health behavior.

Physical and social environments impact health in several ways. Environments can serve as mediums for disease transmission; for example, contamination of food sources, airborne diseases, and the interpersonal spread of contagions. In addition, the environment can act as a stressor; examples include overexposure to noise, interpersonal conflict, isolation, abrupt economic change, and organizational instability. The environment is also a source of danger or safety. Dangerous environmental conditions include, but are not limited to, natural disasters, pollution, crime, occupational hazards, and interpersonal violence. The environment can also function as an enabler of health behavior through the installation of safety devices, availability of health-care services, health education, and cultural practices that promote health. Finally, the environment provides health resources, such as clean air and water, sanitation services, and health insurance (Stokols, 1992).

Social Ecological Model: Applicability to Health Promotion in Occupational Therapy

Social ecological approaches to health promotion have been applied successfully to numerous health problems, including obesity prevention (Egger & Swinburn, 1997), physical activity (CDC, 1999; Sallis, Bowman, & Prat, 1998), violence prevention (Riner & Saywell, 2002), and substance abuse (Kumpfer & Turner, 1990). Social ecological approaches to health promotion have several core characteristics. They target individual and environmental aspects of health behavior and implement multiple intervention strategies across a variety of settings to address a range of

Table 3–6 **An Ecological Perspective: Levels of Influence**

Concept	Definition
Intrapersonal Level	Individual characteristics that influence behavior, such as knowledge, attitudes, beliefs, and personality traits
Interpersonal Level	Interpersonal processes and primary groups, including family, friends, and peers that provide social identity, support, and role definition
Community Level	
Institutional factors	Rules, regulations, policies, and informal structures, which may constrain or promote recommended behaviors
Community factors	Social networks and norms, or standards, which exist as formal or informal among individuals, groups, and organizations
Public policy	Local, state, and federal policies and laws that regulate or support healthy actions and practices for disease prevention, early detection, control, and management

From *Theory at a glance* (2d ed., p. 11), by National Cancer Institute, 2005, Bethesda, MD: National Institutes of Health.

community health problems. Health interventions that neglect social and physical contextual factors tend to demonstrate high levels of attrition and relapse. Programs based on social ecological principles promote healthy lifestyles by creating supportive environments (Stokols, Allen, & Bellingham, 1996). Table 3-6 identifies the key concepts of this approach.

Social Ecological Model: Health Promotion Example

The Child and Adolescent Trial for Cardiovascular Health (CATCH) project is an excellent example of a health promotion intervention based on social ecological principles. The CATCH project was developed to address risk factors for cardiovascular disease, including serum cholesterol, blood pressure, fat and sodium intake, physical activity, and tobacco use. Consistent with the social ecological principle of multilevel intervention strategies, CATCH employs approaches that target individual behavior, family involvement, classroom curricula, and school policies. The CATCH project addresses multiple life contexts and their influence on health, and it achieves its outcome of individual behavior change both directly, through increasing children's and teens' health knowledge, and indirectly, through parental influence and school policies (Grzywacz & Fuqua, 2000; Luepker et al., 1996).

The intervention was evaluated using a randomized controlled trial with 56 intervention and 400 control elementary schools. Over 5000 third graders from four states participated in the 3-year project. The CATCH intervention demonstrated efficacy in

reducing fat content of school lunches, increasing duration of physical activity in physical education classes, and improving overall nutritional intake and physical activity behaviors among children (Luepker et al., 1996).

Transtheoretical Model: An Overview

This model is also referred to as the *Stages of Change Model* (NCI, 2001, 2005). The Transtheoretical Model (TTM) was originated in the late 1970s and early 1980s. It is a complex model consisting of stages and processes of change (DiClemente et al., 1991; Prochaska & DiClemente, 1982, 1983, 1992). Prochaska, Norcross, and DiClemente (1994) identify the stages of change as: precontemplation, contemplation, preparation, action, maintenance, and termination. The **precontemplation stage** refers to the individual's inability to identify that they have a problem and as a result, they have no intention of changing their behavior. In the **contemplation stage,** the individual can identify and acknowledge a problem. They try to understand the problem and are motivated to do something to remedy the problem. The **preparation stage** is characterized by planning for change, acquiring needed resources to facilitate behavior change, and making public statements about one's intention to change. The **action stage** involves overtly changing one's behavior, and modifying the environment in such a way as to facilitate and maintain the change. The action stage requires a great deal of time, energy, and commitment. The **maintenance stage** is a long, ongoing process of recommitment to sustaining the behavior change. It is frequently the most challenging stage in the change process. The **termination stage,** the ultimate goal of the change cycle, occurs when the behavior change is so well integrated that there is minimal chance of relapse (Prochaska, Norcross, & DiClemente, 1994). Figure 3-6 displays the relationship between the various stages, while Figure 3-7 depicts the relationships between the stages and processes.

As can be seen from these figures, together with constructs from the HBM, for a young man to contemplate a testicular self-examination (TSE), he must first feel threatened by being at risk for or susceptible to testicular cancer. In addition, he would need to believe it would be a serious matter to be diagnosed with testicular cancer. Once this realization occurs,

he moves from the stage of precontemplation of action to contemplation. Cues to action can be instrumental in increasing perceived susceptibility through raising consciousness. Examples of cues to action include

- receiving information on the prevalence of testicular cancer during a health class;
- seeing a poster in the gym locker room; or
- being provided with a shower card depicting TSE.

The continued presence of a cue to action, such as a shower card, encourages self-reevaluation and facilitates movement from contemplation to preparation. In addition, increased knowledge about the benefits of early testicular cancer diagnosis through these targeted behaviors would favorably impact the man's beliefs regarding outcome expectations. More positive beliefs regarding these practices may, in turn, act as a stimulus to move from contemplation to preparation.

Continued movement toward engagement in the desired behavior will be influenced by the ongoing presence of cues to action and self-efficacy (e.g., belief in ability to successfully perform TSE) and by an ability to complete self-liberating tasks by confronting any remaining interpersonal barriers to performing TSE (e.g., dislike of touching his testicles). As an individual moves from the preparation stage to action, barriers can have a significant impact on further progress. If these barriers are removed, the individual can proceed to engagement in the behavior and realize its benefits (e.g., feeling relief from an absence of lumps and increased self-esteem for taking care of his health needs). Continued exposure to social support (i.e., helping relationships), shower cards, and mass media campaigns will facilitate maintenance of this behavior.

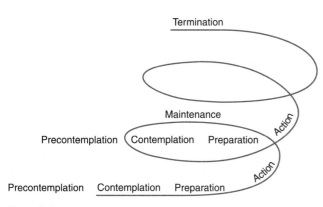

Figure 3-6   A spiral model of the the Stages of Change.

From "In search of how people change: Applications of addictive beaviors" by J. O. Prochaska, C. C. DiClemente, & J. C. Norcross, 1992, American Psychologist, *47(9), 1102–14.*

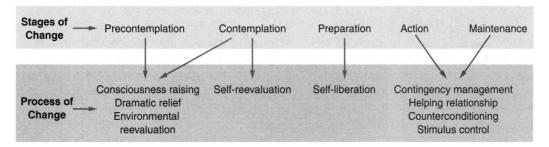

Figure 3-7   Stages of Change in which processes are most emphasized.

From "The Transtheoretical Model of behavior change," (p. 70), by J. O. Prochaska, S. Johnson, & P. Lee, in The Handbook of health behavior change *(2d ed.), S. A. Shumaker, E. B. Schron, J. K. Ockene, & W. L. McBee (Eds.), 1998, New York: Springer Publishing. Copyright © 1998 by Springer Publishing. Reprinted with permission..*

Transtheoretical Model: Applicability to Health Promotion in Occupational Therapy

Although this model has rarely been discussed in the occupational therapy health promotion literature, it recently has been discussed in terms of applicability to chronic pain management (Southam, 2005) and substance abuse (Moyers & Stoffel, 1999; Stoffel & Moyers, 2005). Beyond occupational therapy, it has been used widely in efforts to encourage and maintain health behaviors such as smoking cessation (NCI, 2005), mammography screening, dietary behaviors, medication compliance, sun exposure avoidance, unplanned pregnancy prevention, reduction or elimination of addictive behaviors (Prochaska, Redding, & Evers, 2002), and physical activity (CDC, 1999; Griffin-Blake & DeJoy, 2006). According to McKenzie and colleagues (2005), the TTM has been useful for health promotion developers in two key ways:

- It emphasizes that not all individuals are ready for change "right now," regardless if the program is available.
- It encourages the development of programs to assist individuals to prepare for change.

The NCI (2001, 2005) included this model in a list of theories to consider when addressing behavioral intentions at the individual level. The NCI identified this model's circular nature as being its strength, whereby individuals can enter the change cycle at any point and repeated attempts to change behavior or "recycle" are possible.

Prochaska and colleagues (2002) reported on the trends in the application of the model. The most frequent application is identifying the individual's stage and tailoring intervention to facilitate movement toward or readiness for the next stage: "For example, individuals in precontemplation could receive feedback designed to increase their pros of changing to help them progress to contemplation" (Prochaska et al., 2002, p. 108).

Transtheoretical Model: Health Promotion Example

This model may be employed to address the use of protective gear during leisure activities to reduce injuries and promote safe participation in physical occupations. An occupational therapist could use knowledge of this model to assist an aging female in deciding to use an assistive device during an upcoming hiking vacation after a series of falls, the most recent of which occurred during an ice storm. Movement from precontemplation to contemplation was facilitated by the granddaughter's discussion of "way cool" hiking poles she and her boyfriend saw people using when they went rock climbing the previous weekend. The operative process is one of consciousness-raising. In this case, the movement from precontemplation to contemplation could be further facilitated by a grandmother-granddaughter shopping trip to the local outdoor specialty store. (The grandmother is more willing to take suggestions from her granddaughter than her daughter.)

A few weeks later, the grandmother takes her bimonthly trip to the mall. The trip is coordinated by the staff at the retirement community where she has recently moved due to her recurring falls. During the shopping trip, the grandmother visits an outdoor specialty store and tests hiking poles without pressure from family members. She determines the poles are light enough for her to handle and sufficiently sturdy to be of assistance. Within the next few days, the hiking poles appear on her birthday wish list and are purchased, thus causing the grandmother to enter the preparation stage. The process in action is one of self-reevaluation. Action is achieved when, on her next hiking vacation, she observes younger adults using similar poles. She receives positive feedback from her fellow hikers and found she was better able to keep pace. She also found her neck to be less sore, as she felt comfortable returning to her previous hiking posture, rather than constantly trying to monitor the ground immediately in front of her feet. This served as reinforcement and began the movement from action to maintenance. It is interesting to note that this example also represents constructs from the Model of Human Occupation, in terms of volition, habits, and performance capacity.

Chaos Theory: A Brief Overview

Constructs from this theory are now used and promoted by occupational therapy practitioners (Lohman & Royeen, 2002; Royeen, 2003; Royeen & Luebben, 2002) and are considered and debated by other health, social, and medical sciences (Haigh, 2002; Hudson, 2000; Kernick, 2005; Lohman & Royeen, 2002). Particularly relevant constructs for occupational therapy health promotion include self-organization, sensitivity to initial conditions, self-similarity, bifurcations, and others.

The ultimate goal of an occupational therapy health promotion program is **self-organization,** the ability of a person, family, or community to use available resources to function independently when confronted with a challenge or a desire to self-direct evolution. The goal of self-organization can be facilitated through interventions that consider additional chaos theory constructs. **Sensitivity to initial conditions** means that small differences in input can produce large differences in output. "Small initial errors and perturbations sometimes endlessly magnify through positive feedback loops to create major changes" (Hudson, 2000, p. 218). Therefore, it is important to never underestimate the power of small inputs. For example, an appropriately timed encouraging gesture can have a major therapeutic effect, while a small, seemingly unnoticed slight can have major negative repercussions.

Another construct, **self-similarity,** is the repeated appearance of similar physical characteristics, such as structures in a snowflake or behavioral patterns (Hudson, 2000). Occupational roles and habits are behavioral patterns that evolve but follow a pattern over the life span of a human or community and are important considerations in planning health promotion initiatives. **Bifurcations** are transition points in the development or change in a system over time. "As a key parameter is increased, key thresholds are reached in which a process splits into two sub-processes or perhaps alternating rhythms" (Hudson, 2000, p. 220). At the point of a phase transition or bifurcation, the system is functioning on the border between order and disorder. It is at this "edge of chaos" where creativity, new business ventures, and dramatic change can occur (Elliott, O'Neal, & Velde, 2001). Dramatic change is often needed to promote new habits and routines to facilitate a healthy and quality life. For those instances, this theory and its constructs may provide additional guidance in the philosophical and theoretical approach to programming. Chaos theory and others discussed in this chapter may provide helpful philosophical guidance regarding the change process necessary for successful occupation-based health promotion initiatives.

Selecting and Matching Theories

Table 3-1 and Table 3-4, which appear earlier in this chapter, provide guidance in theory selection for health-promotion efforts. The rightmost column of Table 3-4 has been added to the original version of this table (NCI, 2005). This additional column includes occupational therapy theories that may be matched with the identified health behavior models for use at either the personal or community level. The five occupational therapy theories described in Chapter 2 of this text are included in this column. The intent of this table is to serve merely as a guide. Other occupational therapy and health behavior theories also may be applicable for use in combination or independently. The decision to combine theories or select only an occupational therapy or

health behavior model should be context driven and, where possible, evidence based.

Conclusion

Health promotion practice often involves an interdisciplinary team approach wherein the team membership does not conform to that of traditional hospital-based interdisciplinary teams. Community developers and organizers, community activists, spiritual and religious leaders, politicians, public health experts, nutritionists, occupational therapists, occupational therapy assistants, physical therapists, art therapists, nurses, and health educators are all examples of potential team members who may work together on a health promotion initiative. Some of the public health professionals in this group may share a common language that is represented in the health behavior models that appear in this chapter. In addition, the emerging theories not commonly associated with health promotion or occupational therapy introduced in this chapter may also provide important contributions. Hopefully, exposure to the language of these models and theories, and exposure to the models and theories themselves, will facilitate interdisciplinary work in health promotion by occupational therapists and occupational therapy assistants. Working, writing, and sharing ideas across disciplines will assist occupational therapists and occupational therapy assistants in gaining the knowledge necessary to reach their potential in the provision of health promotion services. They must possess the knowledge and skill to work together with an interdisciplinary group to effectively enhance the health capacity of diverse individuals, families, organizations, and communities.

▶ For Discussion and Review

1. What are the key similarities and differences between the models described in this chapter?
2. Which model (in conjunction with an occupational therapy model) might assist in the development of a preventive, occupation-based intervention for jail or prison inmates and their families?
3. Which model described in this chapter would you select to assist and strengthen an exploratory study of the occupational competency of new parents who have a history of domestic partner violence? Why did you make this selection? Which occupational therapy model would be appropriate to pair with this model, and why?
4. In what ways do the concepts and constructs of occupational therapy theories overlap with the

concepts of the health promotion theories described in this chapter?

5. How do the stages in the transtheoretical model impact the design of health promotion interventions?

▶ Research Questions

1. Which has more impact on the health and the healthy occupational engagement in elderly homeless men—an occupation-based health promotion intervention built on the Model of Human Occupation and HBM or one built on the Ecology of Human Performance and the Stages of Change Model?

2. What is the relationship between perceived susceptibility and adaptation? How do these constructs impact an individual's adoption of joint protection principles?

3. How does climate change impact a population's health, occupational engagement, and social participation?

4. Which theory or model best explains resiliency in children who have experienced trauma?

Acknowledgments

The authors wish to express their appreciation to the following individuals who assisted with the preparation of this chapter: Frederick D. Reitz and Grace Wenger.

References

Ahmed, N. U., Fort, J. G., Elzey, J. D., & Bailey, S. (2004). Empowering factors in repeat mammography: Insights from the stories of underserved women. *Journal of Ambulatory Care Management, 27,* 348–55.

Ajzen, I. (1985). From intentions to actions: A theory of planned behavior. In J. Kuhl & J. Beckmann (Eds.), *Action control: From cognition to behavior* (pp. 11–39). Berlin: Springer-Verlag.

Al-Ali, N., & Haddad, L. G. (2004). The effect of the health belief model in explaining exercise participation among Jordanian myocardial infarction patients. *Journal of Transcultural Nursing, 15*(2), 114–21.

American Occupational Therapy Association. (2008). Occupational therapy practice framework: Domain and processes (2d ed.). *American Journal of Occupational Therapy, 26,* 625–88.

Bardsley, P., & Beckman, L. (1988). The health belief model and entry into alcoholism treatment. *International Journal of the Addictions, 23,* 19–28.

Becker, M. H. (1974). The health belief model and sick role behavior. In M. H. Becker (Ed.), *The health belief model and personal behavior* (pp. 82–92). Thorofare, NJ: SLACK.

Becker, M., & Janz, N. (1985). The health belief model applied to understanding diabetes regimen compliance. *Diabetes Educator, 11,* 41–47.

Brownson, C. A., & Scaffa, M. E. (2001). Occupational therapy in the promotion of health and the prevention of disease and disability statement. *American Journal of Occupational Therapy, 55*(6), 656–60.

Buller, D. B., Andersen, P. A., Walkosz, B. J., Scott, M. D., Cutter, G. R., Dignan, M. B., Zarlengo, E. M., Voeks, J. H., & Giese, A. J. (2005). Randomized control testing a worksite sun protection program in an outdoor recreation industry. *Health Education and Behavior, 32*(4), 514–35.

Centers for Disease Control, National Center for Chronic Disease Prevention and Health Promotion. (1999). *Understanding and promoting physical activity.* Retrieved July 28, 2005, from http://www.cdc.gov/nccdphp/sgr/chap6.htm.

Champion, V. (1985). Use of the health belief model in determining frequency of breast self-examination. *Research in Nursing and Health, 8,* 373–79.

Chang, M., Brown, R. L., Nitzke, S., & Baumann, L. C. (2004). Development of an instrument to assess predisposing, enabling, and reinforcing constructs associated with fat intake behaviors of low-income mothers [research brief]. *Journal of Nutrition Behavior and Education, 36,* 27–34.

Chen, C-Y, Neufeld, P. S., Feely, C. A., & Skinner, C. S. (1999). Factors influencing compliance with home exercise programs among patients with upper-extremity impairment. *American Journal of Occupational Therapy, 53*(2), 171–80.

Chiang, L., Huang, J., Yeh, K., & Lu, C. (2004). Effects of a self-management asthma educational program in Taiwan based on PRECEDE-PROCEED Model for parents with asthmatic children. *Journal of Asthma, 41*(2), 205–15.

Cline, R. R., & Worley, M. M. (2006). Osteoporosis health beliefs and self-care behaviors: An exploratory investigation. *Journal of the American Pharmacists Association, 46*(3), 356–63.

DiClemente, C. C., Prochaska, J. O., Fairhurst, S. K., Velcier, W. F., Velasquez, M. M., & Rossi, J. S. (1991). The process of smoking cessation: An analysis of precontemplation, contemplation, and preparation stages of change. *Journal of Consulting and Clinical Psychology, 59,* 295–304.

Egger, G., & Swinburn, B. (1997). An ecological approach to the obesity pandemic. *British Medical Journal, 315,* 477–80.

Elliott, S., O'Neal, S. O., & Velde, B. P. (2001). Using chaos theory to understand a community-built occupational therapy practice. *Occupational Therapy in Health Care, 13*(3/4), 101–11.

Ely, D. P. (1990). Conditions that facilitate the implementation of educational technology innovations. *Journal of Research on Computing in Education, 23*(2), 298–305.

Fertman, C. I., Dotson, S., Mazzocco, G. O., & Reitz, S. M. (2005). Challenges of preparing allied health professionals for interdisciplinary practice in rural areas. *Journal of Allied Health, 34*(3), 163–68.

Glanz, K., Rimer, B. K., & Lewis, F. M. (Eds.). (2005). *Health behavior and health education* (3d ed.). San Francisco: Jossey-Bass.

Green, L. W., & Kreuter, M. W. (1991). *Health promotion planning: An educational and environmental approach* (2d ed.). Mountainview, CA: Mayfield.

Green, L. W., & Kreuter, M. W. (1999). *Health promotion planning: An educational and ecological approach* (3d ed.). Mountainview, CA: Mayfield.

Green, L. W., & Kreuter, M. W. (2005). *Health promotion planning: An educational and ecological approach* (4th ed.). New York: McGraw Hill.

Green, L. W., Kreuter, M. W., Deeds, S. G., & Partridge, K. B. (1980). *Health education planning: A diagnostic approach.* Palo Alto, CA: Mayfield.

Griffin-Blake, C. S., & DeJoy, D. M. (2006). Evaluation of social-cognitive versus stage-matched, self-help physical activity interventions at the workplace. *American Journal of Health Promotion, 20*(3), 200–09.

Grzywacz, J. G., & Fuqua, J. (2000). The social ecology of health: Leverage points and linkages. *Behavioral Medicine, 26*(3), 101–15.

Haigh, C. (2002). Using chaos theory: The implications for nursing. *Journal of Advanced Nursing, 37*(5), 462–69.

Herold, E. (1983). The health belief model: Can it help us understand contraceptive use among adolescents? *Journal of School Health, 53,* 19–21.

Hester, N., & Macrina, D. (1985). The health belief model and the contraceptive behavior of college women: Implications for health education. *Journal of American College Health, 33,* 245–52.

Hogge, A. (2002, August 16). Arkansas study shows: Young workers risk injuries on farms. *Delta Farm Press,* ¶ 10. Retrieved July 30, 2005, from http://deltafarmpress.com/mag/farming_arkansas_study_shows/.

Hope, A., Kelleher, C., Holmes, L., & Hennessy, T. (1999). Health and safety practices among farmers and other workers: A needs assessment. [Abstract]. *Occupational Medicine, 49*(4), 231–35.

Howat, P., Jones, S., Hall, M., Cross, D., & Stevenson, M. (1997). The PRECEDE-PROCEED model: Application to planning a child pedestrian injury prevention program. *Injury Prevention, 3*(4), 282–87.

Hudson, C. G. (2000). At the edge of chaos: A new paradigm for social work? *Journal of Social Work Education, 36*(2), 215–31.

Indiana Rural Safety & Health Council. (n.d.a). *Careful country: Teacher's kit.* West Lafayette, IN: Author.

Indiana Rural Safety & Health Council. (n.d.b). *Farm family safety and health workshop leader's guide.* West Lafayette, IN: Author.

Institute of Medicine. (2002). *Who will keep the public healthy? Educating public health professionals for the 21st century.* Washington, DC: National Academy of Sciences.

Juniper, K. C., Oman, R. R., Hamm. R. M., & Kerby, D. S. (2004). The relationships among constructs in the health belief model and the transtheoretical model among African-American college women for physical activity. *American Journal of Health Promotion, 3,* 354–57

Kegeles, S., & Lund, A. (1982). Adolescents' health beliefs and acceptance of a novel preventive dental activity: Replication and extension. *Health Education Quarterly, 9,* 96–112.

Kegler, M. C., Crosby, R. A., & DiClemente, R. J. (2002). Reflections on emerging theories in health promotion practice. In R. J. DiClemente, R. A. Crosby, & M. C. Kegler (Eds.), *Emerging theories in health promotion practice and research* (pp. 386–95). San Francisco: Jossey-Bass.

Kelly, G., Mamon, J., & Scott, J. (1987). Utility of the health belief model in examining medication compliance among psychiatric outpatients. *Social Science Medicine, 25,* 1205–11.

Kennedy, M. G., & Crosby, R. A. (2002). Prevention marketing: An emerging integrated framework. In R. J. DiClemente, R. A. Crosby, & M. C. Kegler (Eds.), *Emerging theories in health promotion practice and research* (pp. 255–84). San Francisco: Jossey-Bass.

Kernick, D. (2005). Migraine—New perspectives from chaos theory. *Cephalalgia, 25,* 561–66.

Kielhofner, G., & Nelson, C. (1983). A study of patient motivation and cooperation/participation in occupational therapy. *Occupational Therapy Journal of Research, 3,* 35–46.

Kirscht, J. (1974). The health belief model and illness behavior. In M. H. Becker (Ed.), *The health belief model and personal health behavior* (93–105). Thorofare, NJ: SLACK.

Kleier, J. A. (2004). Using the health belief model to reveal the perceptions of Jamaican and Haitian men regarding prostate cancer. *Journal of Multicultural Nursing & Health, 10*(3), 41–48.

Kretzmann, J. P., & McKnight, J. L. (1993). *Building communities from the inside out: A path toward finding and mobilizing a community's assets.* Evanston, IL: Northwestern University, Center for Urban Affairs and Policy Research.

Kumpfer, K. L., & Turner, C. W. (1990). The social ecology model of adolescent substance abuse: Implications for prevention. *International Journal of the Addictions, 25*(4A), 435–63.

Lemyre, L., & Orpana, H. (2002, August). Integrating population health into social ecology. *Canadian Family Physician,* 1349–51.

Lohman, H., & Royeen, C. (2002). Posttraumatic stress disorder and traumatic hand injuries: A neuro-occupational view. *American Journal of Occupational Therapy, 56,* 527–37.

Luepker, R.V., Perry, C. L., McKinlay, S. M., Nader, P. R., Parcel, G. S., Stone, E. J., Webber, L. S., Elder, J. P., Feldman, H. A., & Johnson, C. C. (1996). Outcomes of a field trial to improve children's dietary patterns and physical activity: The Child and Adolescent Trial for Cardiovascular Health (CATCH). *Journal of the American Medical Association, 275*(10), 768–76.

Maddux, J. E. (2005). Self-efficacy: The power of believing you can. In C. R. Snyder & S. J. Lopez (Eds.), *Handbook of positive psychology.* New York: Oxford University Press.

Maiman, L., & Becker, M. (1974). The health belief model: Origins and correlates in psychological theory. In M. Becker (Ed.), *The health belief model and personal health behavior.* Thorofare, NJ: SLACK.

Mandel, D., Jackson, J. M., Zemke, R., Nelson, L., & Clark, F. A. (1999). *Lifestyle redesign: Implementing the well elderly program.* Bethesda, MD: American Occupational Therapy Association.

McAllister, G., & Farquhar, M. (1992). Health beliefs: A cultural division. *Journal of Advanced Nursing, 17,* 1447–54.

McKenzie, J. F., Neiger, B. L., & Smeltzer, J. L. (2005). *Planning, implementing, and evaluating health promotion programs: A primer* (4th ed.). Needham Heights, MA: Allyn & Bacon.

Melnyk, K. A. M. (2005). Barriers: A critical review of recent literature. *Nursing Research, 37*(4), 196–201.

Moos, R. H. (1980). Social-ecological perspectives on health. In G. C. Cohen, F. Cohen, & N. E. Adler (Eds.), *Health psychology: A handbook.* San Francisco: Jossey-Bass.

Moyers, P. A., & Stoffel, V. C. (1999). Case report—Alcohol dependence in a client with a work-related injury. *American Journal of Occupational Therapy, 53*(6), 640–45.

National AHEC Organization. (2005). *Area Health Education Center (AHEC) program.* Retrieved July 30, 2005, from http://www.nationalahec.org/main/ahec.asp.

National Cancer Institute. (2001). *Making health communication programs work: A planner's guide.* Bethesda, MD: National Institutes of Health. (Reprinted 2004).

National Cancer Institute. (2005). *Theory at a glance* (2d ed.). Bethesda, MD: National Institutes of Health. Retrieved March 3, 2007, from http://www.cancer.gov/theory.pdf.

Oldenburg, B., & Parcel, G. S. (2002). Diffusion of innovations. In K. Glanz, B. K. Rimer, & F. M. Lewis (Eds.), *Health behavior and health education: Theory, research, and practice* (3d ed., pp. 312–34). San Francisco: Jossey-Bass.

Parcel, G. S. (1984). Theoretical models for application in school health education research. Special combined issue of *Journal of School Health, 54,* 39–49 and *Health Education, 15,* 39–49.

Paulk, M. C. (1999). *Structured approaches to managing change.* Retrieved March 10, 2007, from http://www.stsc.hill.af.mil/crosstalk/1999/11/paulk.asp.

Pickett, W., King, W. D., Faelker, T., Lees, R., Morrison, H. I., & Bienefeld, M. (2000). Suicides among Canadian farm operators. *Chronic Diseases in Canada, 20*(3), 1–10.

Prochaska, J. O., & DiClemente, C. C. (1982). Transtheoretical therapy: Toward a more integrative model of change. *Psychotherapy: Theory, Research and Practice, 19*(3), 276–88.

Prochaska, J. O., & DiClemente, C. C. (1983). Stages and processes of self-change of smoking: Toward an integrative model of change. *Journal of Counseling and Clinical Psychology, 51*(3), 390–95.

Prochaska, J. O., & DiClemente, C. C. (1992). Stages of change in the modification of behavior problems. In M. Hersen, R. M. Eisler, & P. M. Miller (Eds.), *Progress in behavior modification* (pp. 184–214). Sycamore, IL: Sycamore Press.

Prochaska, J. O., DiClemente, C. C., & Norcross, J. C. (1992). In search of how people change: Applications of addictive behaviors. *American Psychologist, 47*(9), 1102–14.

Prochaska, J.O., Norcross, J.C. & DiClemente, C.C. (1994). Changing for good: A revolutionary six-stage program for overcoming bad habits and moving your life positively forward. New York: HarperCollins.

Prochaska, J. O., Johnson, S., & Lee, P. (1998). The transtheoretical model of behavior change. In S. A. Shumaker, E. B. Schron, J. K. Ockene, & W. L. McBee (Eds.), *The handbook of health behavior change* (2d ed., pp. 59–84). New York: Springer Publishing.

Prochaska J. O., Redding, C. A., & Evers, K. (2002). The transtheoretical model and stages of change. In K. Glanz, B. K. Rimer, & F. M. Lewis (Eds.), *Health behavior and health education: Theory, research, and practice* (3d ed., 99–120). San Francisco: Jossey-Bass.

Reitz, S. M. (1992). A historical review of occupational therapy's role in preventive health and wellness. *American Journal of Occupational Therapy, 46,* 50–55.

Reitz, S. T. (1990). The health belief model: An overlooked tool for occupational therapy? *Physical Disabilities SIS Newsletter, 13*(11), 1–4.

Reno, D. (1988). Men's knowledge and health beliefs about testicular cancer and testicular self-examination. *Cancer Nursing, 11*(2), 112–17.

Riner, M. E., & Saywell, R. M. (2002). Development of the social ecology model of adolescent interpersonal violence prevention. *Journal of School Health, 72*(2), 65–70.

Roden, J. (2004a). Revisiting the Health Belief Model: Nurses applying it to young families and their health promotion needs. *Nursing & Health Sciences, 6*(4), 1–10.

Roden, J. (2004b). Validating the revised Health Belief Model for young families: Implications for nurses' health promotion practice. *Nursing & Health Sciences, 6*(4), 247–59.

Rogers, E. M. (1995). *Diffusion of innovations* (4th ed.). New York: Free Press.

Rogers, E. M. (2003). *Diffusion of innovations* (5th ed.). New York: Free Press.

Rosenstock, I. (1966). Why people use health services. *Milbank Quarterly, 44*(3), 94–124.

Rosenstock, I. (1974). Historical origins of the Health Belief Model. In M. Becker (Ed.), *The Health Belief Model and personal behavior.* Thorofare, NJ: SLACK.

Rosenstock, I. M., Strecher, V. J., & Becker, M. H. (1994). The Health Belief Model and HIV risk behavior change. In R. J. DiClemente & J. L. Peterson (Eds.), *Preventing AIDS: Theories and methods for behavioral interventions* (pp. 5–24). New York: Plenum Press.

Royeen, C. B. (2003). Chaotic occupational therapy: Collective wisdom for a complex profession, 2003 Eleanor Clarke Slagle Lecture. *American Journal of Occupational Therapy, 57,* 609–24.

Royeen, C. B., & Luebben, A. J. (2002). Annotated bibliography of chaos for occupational therapy. *Occupational Therapy in Health Care, 16*(1), 63–80.

Sallis, J. F., Bauman, A., & Pratt, M. (1998). Environmental and policy interventions to promote physical activity. *American Journal of Preventive Medicine, 15,* 379–97.

Sallis, J. F., & Owen, N. (2002). Ecological models of health behavior. In K. Glanz, B. K. Rimer, & F. M. Lewis (Eds.), *Health behavior and health education: Theory, research and practice.* San Francisco: Jossey-Bass.

Scaffa, M. E., Van Slyke, N., & Brownson, C. A. (2008). Occupational therapy services in the promotion of health and the prevention of disease and disability. *American Journal of Occupational Therapy 62*(6), 694–703.

Southam, M. (2005). Psychosocial aspects of chronic pain. In E. Cara & A. MacRae (Eds.), *Psychosocial occupational therapy* (2d ed., pp. 423–45). Clifton Park, NY: Thomson.

Stanken, B. A. (2000). Promoting helmet use among children. *Journal of Community Health Nursing, 17*(2), 85–92.

Stoffel, V. C., & Moyers, P. A. (2005). Occupational therapy and substance use disorders. In E. Cara & A. MacRae (Eds.), *Psychosocial occupational therapy* (2d ed., pp. 446–73). Clifton Park, NY: Thomson.

Stokols, D. (1992). Establishing and maintaining health environments: Toward a social ecology of health promotion. *American Psychologist, 47*(1), 6–22.

Stokols, D. (1996). Translating social ecological theory into guidelines for community health promotion. *American Journal of Health Promotion, 10*(4), 282–98.

Stokols, D., Allen, J, & Bellingham, R. L. (1996). The social ecology of health promotion: Implications for research and practice. *American Journal of Health Promotion, 10*(4), 247–51.

Thurston, W. E., Blundell-Gosselin, H. J., & Rose, S. (2003). Stress in male and female farmers: An ecological rather than an individual problem. *Canadian Journal of Rural Medicine, 8*(4), 247–54.

Thurston, W. E., Blundell-Gosselin, H. J., & Vollman, A. R. (2003). Health concerns of male and female farmers: Implications for health promotion. *Canadian Journal of Rural Medicine, 8*(4), 239–46.

Tremblay, M., Gervais, A., Lacroix, C., O'Loughlin, J., Makni, H., & Paradis, G. (2001). Physicians taking action against smoking: An intervention program to optimize smoking cessation counseling by Montreal general practitioners. *Canadian Medical Association Journal, 165*(5), 601–07.

Turner, L. W., Hunt, S. B., DiBrezzo, R., & Jones, C. (2004). Design and implementation of an Osteoporosis Prevention Program using the Health Belief Model. *American Journal of Health Studies, 19*(2), 115–21.

U.S. Department of Health and Human Services. (2000). *Healthy People 2010: Understanding and improving health* (2d ed.). Washington, DC: U.S. Government Printing Office.

White, M. C., Tulsky, J. P., Menendez, E., Arai, S., Goldenson, J., & Kawamura, L. M. (2005). Improving tuberculosis therapy completion after jail: Translation of research to practice. *Health Education Research, 20*(2), 163–74.

Wilkens, P. M. (2003). Preventing work-related musculoskeletal disorders in VDT users: A comprehensive health promotion program. *Work, 20,* 171–78.

Chapter 4

Public Health Principles, Approaches, and Initiatives

S. Maggie Reitz and Marjorie E. Scaffa

> Many of the improvements in personal health over the last century can be directly traced to public health efforts. While occupational and physical therapists have not traditionally performed in public health activities, the sedentary nature of American society and the increasing incidence of chronic disease and disability is challenging them to become involved in public health efforts.
>
> —Sandstrom, Lohman, & Bramble, 2003, p. 252

Learning Objectives

This chapter is designed to enable the reader to:

- Identify public health constructs and principles, policies, approaches, and initiatives that support occupation-based health promotion programs.
- Describe the relationships among U.S. public health, the new public health, community health, health promotion, prevention, wellness, and occupational therapy.
- Discuss the role of occupational therapy in public health using the language of the *Occupational Therapy Practice Framework: Domain and Processes* (referred to as the *Framework;* American Occupational Therapy Association [AOTA], 2008)
- Describe key domestic and international governmental and organizational reports and policies that support national and global health promotion.
- Utilize national and state-level documents and objectives to support occupation-based preventive programming for populations.

Key Terms

Community health

Health

Health-care disparities

Health promotion

Healthy community

New Freedom Initiative (NFI)

New public health

Occupational justice

Prevention

Preventive occupation

Public health

Wellness

World Health Organization (WHO)

Introduction

Public health is what a society does collectively to facilitate conditions that enable its members to be healthy (Institute of Medicine [IOM], 1988). "Traditionally, public health has been defined as health of populations and communities" (Tulchinsky & Varavikova, 2000, p. 2). It differs from medicine in that it focuses on facilitating health and wellbeing of populations by

assessing and monitoring health problems, informing the public and professionals about health issues, developing and enforcing health-protecting laws and regulations, implementing and evaluating population based strategies to promote health and prevent disease, and assuring the provision of essential health services. (Lasker & the Committee on Medicine and Public Health, 1997, p. 3)

In the United States, the public health system has been shaped by scientific knowledge and prevailing societal values. It also has been greatly influenced by health initiatives and policy development in Great Britain and Canada. The United States has been involved in international public health initiatives through its participation in the **World Health Organization (WHO)** since that organization's inception in 1948 (WHO, 1948). The WHO "is the United Nations' specialized agency for health." It is comprised of 192 member states that work toward "the attainment by all peoples of the highest possible level of health" (WHO, 2005a, ¶ 1). In 2000, the United Nations set eight broad goals, known as the Millennium Development Goals (MDGs), to achieve by 2015. Three of these goals—to reduce child deaths; improve maternal health; and combat HIV/AIDS, malaria, and other diseases—are directly related to health and fall under the purview of the WHO. Two other MDGs—to eradicate extreme hunger and poverty and to achieve environmental sustainability—have the potential to significantly impact health.

The WHO has four current priorities:

- Ensuring global health security by identifying emerging threats to health and managing them efficiently
- Reducing tobacco use and promoting healthy nutrition and physical activity to decrease the incidence of chronic diseases
- Increasing efforts to support the achievement of the MDGs
- Improving health-care services, including fair access for all (WHO, 2006a)

After providing a brief history of the public health in the United States, this chapter will describe the new public health; review terminology; and summarize current governmental documents and initiatives, such as *Healthy People 2010* (U.S. Department of Health and Human Services [USDHHS], 2000a). The implications of these reports for occupational therapy practice and the promotion of occupational justice will be detailed in an additional feature called **Implications for Occupational Therapy** that was added especially for this chapter. This feature was designed to assist the reader in applying various documents, principles, and approaches with a public health focus to occupational therapy interventions. The role of occupational therapy assistants and occupational therapists within interdisciplinary public health initiatives and the relationship between public health, new public health, occupational therapy, health promotion, and wellness will also be explored.

History of Public Health in the United States

"The history of public health has been one of identifying health problems, developing knowledge and expertise to solve problems, and rallying political and social support

around the solutions" (IOM, 1988, p. 70). The history of public health in the United States mirrors this description, beginning with the area's original inhabitants. The indigenous peoples of the Americas had an appreciation for hygiene and sanitation procedures, which helped maintain health and prevent disease. Early visitors from Europe noted the frequency of bathing habits and the cleanliness of homes and public areas among this population (Vogel, 1970). Appendix A identifies key historical events in public health and health care, nationally and internationally, over the last several hundred years.

In the 18th century, the solution for the public health problem of infectious disease was the institution of isolation techniques and quarantine. Hospitals were built to isolate and treat the ill. Voluntary general hospitals were established for those with physical illnesses, and public institutions for the care of the mentally ill were founded (IOM, 1988, p. 57). The first public mental health hospital in British North America was built in Williamsburg, Virginia, in 1773 (IOM, 1988; Zwelling, 1985). This Public Hospital for Persons of Insane and Disordered Minds was built in an underdeveloped area on the town's border. Before the hospital was built, individuals with mental health problems were housed in the public jail, which was a common practice in North America at that time (Zwelling, 1985).

Moral treatment, a new strategy for the care of individuals with mental illness, was initiated in the United States in the 19th century, based on the successes of Pinel in France and Tuke in England (Peloquin, 1989). In his work *Medical Philosophical Treatise on Mental Alienation* (1948), Pinel provided examples of and praise for the use of moral treatment at an asylum in Saragross, Spain, and another in Amsterdam, Netherlands.

In 1817, the Friend's Asylum, the first hospital founded in the United States to provide moral treatment, was built in Philadelphia. Peloquin presented a variety of descriptions and views of moral treatment and from them distilled an image of moral treatment as "humane treatment, a routine of work and recreation, an appeal to reason, and the development of desirable moral traits" (1989, p. 538). Documented success rates using this technique at both private asylums and public hospitals were impressive, with reported recovery rates of over 70% (Peloquin, 1989).

The Moral Management Era was eventually embraced at the Public Hospital for Persons of Insane and Disordered Minds in Williamsburg, where it flourished from 1836 to 1862 (Colonial Williamsburg Foundation, 2004) under the management of Alexander Galt and then his son John Galt II (Zwelling, 1985). John Galt instituted an extensive program of occupations, including a "carpentry shop, sewing, spinning, and weaving rooms, a shoemaking shop, patient library, a game room," and a variety of occupations performed in the hospital garden and wood yard (Zwelling, 1985, p. 32). In addition, he supplied patients with musical instruments and organized extensive social activities, such as lectures and concerts and "scheduled carriage rides about town for female patients" (Zwelling, 1985, pp. 32–33). Galt also worked to ensure the environment was as comfortable and attractive as possible. Pleasing furniture, wall hangings, table settings, and the use of flowers are examples of Galt's efforts to make hospital life less Spartan and sterile. These efforts were consistent with Galt's overall treatment strategy, which was to "emphasize the patients' sanity rather than their insanity" (Zwelling, 1985, p. 34).

The potential for moral treatment in the United States was curtailed by the Civil War (Peloquin, 1989; Zwelling, 1985) and the economic and social crises that ensued. The success of moral treatment encouraged a push for equal access to treatment by social reformers. Although the effort to gain equal access was successful, insufficient planning and funding resulted in severe overcrowding, which led to custodial care replacing curative moral treatment (Kielhofner, 2004; Peloquin, 1989). This, together with the greater emphasis on biological causes and cures of disease, reduced interest in both public health and the behavioral and environmental factors associated with mental illness. Dunton, one of the founders of occupational therapy, believed that moral treatment reemerged years later in the form of occupational therapy (Schwartz, 2003).

The problems of infectious disease and mental illness continued as a focus of public health into the 19th century, with new public health strategies evolving based on the current science of the period. An emphasis on sanitation and hygiene developed as a result of advances in bacteriology. New strategies required laboratories, which provided the impetus for the development of local and state health departments (IOM, 1988). Maps became public health tools as the impact on sanitation and public health of the physical structures within cities (e.g., streets, rivers, drains) was recognized.

The "new public health" emerged in the early 20th century when public health "increasingly focused its attention on health education, maternal and child health, and the detection of unrecognized but treatable impairments" (Lasker & the Committee on Medicine and Public Health, 1997, p. 15). The **new public health** addressed both interventions and preventive strategies to promote the health and wellbeing of populations, communities, and individuals—including equitable access to services (Goraya & Scambler, 1998; Roemer, 2000; Tulchinsky & Varavikova, 2000). The Ottawa Conference and the resultant *Ottawa Charter for Health Promotion* (WHO, 1986) have been identified as the catalyst for a paradigm shift in public health to a focus on policy (O'Connor-Fleming & Parker, 1995): "Above

all [the new public health] stresses that both society and the individual have rights and responsibilities in promoting and maintaining health through direct services and through healthy environmental and community health promotion" (Tulchinsky & Vaavikova, 2000, p. 3).

This new public health paradigm supported the continued development of local and state health departments and increased governmental involvement in public and personal health (IOM, 1988). The Centers for Disease Control and Prevention (1999) identified the top 10 achievements in public health in the 20th century: vaccinations to prevent disease, increased motor vehicle safety, safer and healthier workplaces, improved control of infectious diseases, decline in deaths from stroke and coronary heart disease, safer and healthier foods, healthier mothers and infants, advances in family planning, fluoridation of drinking water, and recognition of the health hazards of tobacco. However, near the end of the 20th century, a fiscal crisis significantly decreased available resources for problem-solving and implementing public health initiatives.

This financial crisis was one of the factors leading to the "disarray" of public health and the establishment of the Committee for the Study of the Future of Public Health. The committee was charged with developing recommendations to facilitate the mission of public health in the United States, thereby "assuring conditions in which people can be healthy" (IOM, 1988, p. 140). Although the problems addressed by U.S. public health practitioners have changed in volume and complexity since the 18th century, the focus remains on finding solutions to current population-based health problems, identifying interventions to prevent the development and spread of illness, and addressing behaviors that impact the health of society. The general goals of public health in the 21st century are to

- prevent epidemics and minimize the spread of disease;
- protect against environmental hazards;
- prevent injuries;
- promote health behaviors;
- respond to disasters and assist communities in recovery;
- assure access to health services; and
- enhance quality of life (USDHHS, 1994, ¶ 1).

Relationship Between Public Health and Medicine

At the inception of the U.S. Public Health Service in 1798 (Timmreck, 1995), there was a close relationship between leaders in public heath and medicine. This positive working relationship lasted until the early 20th century (Lasker et al., 1997). The two disciplines shared a goal of addressing the most significant health threat of the time—infectious disease. Fighting this common enemy encouraged cooperation between public health and medicine. However, advances in bacteriology and other sciences decreased the threat of infectious diseases, and a division between medicine and public heath emerged. This divide accelerated after World War II due to differences in funding and training. Limited incentives existed for collaboration in education, resulting in little to no cooperative teaching. These factors tended to facilitate "recurring tensions deriving from overlapping interests" and "the development of striking cultural differences" between the two fields (Lasker et al., 1997, p. 1).

The divide, although narrowed, continues to exist today. As in the past, opportunities to enhance the nation's health through collaboration have been missed (Lasker et al., 1997), but examples of cooperation remain. The Robert Wood Johnson Foundation commissioned a study to determine factors facilitating the division between medicine and public health and what could be done to foster positive collaboration. The New York Academy of Medicine (NYAM) was responsible for completing this study, whose timing was well matched to the growing realization of leaders in both disciplines that each could benefit from a closer working relationship. The formation of the Medicine/Public Health Initiative, a joint project between the two disciplines in 1996 (Reiser, 1997), had already begun to pave the way for success. Through the course of the NYAM's work, 414 cases of successful collaboration were gathered and reviewed.

Another example of the collaboration between public health, medicine, and other disciplines is the production of governmental reports and policies. Positive results are obtained when various practitioners, including occupational therapists and occupational therapy assistants, collaborate to provide population-based health promotion. Several key governmental reports will be described, which are significant for occupational therapists and occupational therapy assistants interested in program development and for those seeking funding and advocating for health policy. These documents are introduced after presenting relevant terminology and a description of occupational therapy's role within the new public health arena.

Terminology and the Role of Occupational Therapy in the New Public Health

While a growing trend exists in occupational therapy practice toward community-based practice and some movement has been observed toward population-based interventions, most interventions are still aimed at and delivered to individuals (Wilcock, 2003). Although some occupational therapy services may include health promotion activities at a basic level, the potential to broaden the scope of practice to address the new public health needs of the United States and the global community exists. In order for this increase in scope to occur, it is essential to understand what health promotion is and is not and its relationship to interventions at the individual, family, community, and societal level. This understanding requires familiarity with key terms.

The most often cited definition of **health** is "the complete state of physical, mental, and social wellbeing, and not just the absence of disease or infirmity" (WHO, 1947, p. 29). Although this definition has remained consistent since 1947, there has been a growing appreciation that health is "a resource for everyday life" and dependent upon other resources (WHO, 1986, p. 1). Content Box 4-1 displays the prerequisites for health identified by WHO (1986) in the *Ottawa Charter for Health Promotion.*

Unlike the definition of the term *health,* the concept of health promotion has evolved over time and setting, resulting in the existence of a variety of definitions for the term *health promotion.* The WHO (1986; 1997a, p. 1) described it broadly as the "process of enabling people to increase control over, and to improve, health." Green and Kreuter (1999) suggested that **health promotion** is "any combination of educational and ecological supports for action and conditions of living conducive to health" (p. 112). The WHO (1997a) believes health promotion has the potential for making the greatest impact on improved health status and social justice.

One way occupational therapists and occupational therapy assistants can improve health status and social justice is by maximizing the health and wellbeing of communities. A variety of definitions exist for the term **community health.** The definition that best captures the philosophy of the occupational therapy profession

---

Content Box 4-1

Prerequisites for Health

- Peace
- Shelter
- Education
- Food
- Income
- Stable eco-system
- Sustainable resources
- Social justice and equity

From *Ottawa charter for health promotion* (p. 1), by World Health Organization, 1986, Geneva, Switzerland.

has been posed by Scaffa, Desmond, and Brownson (2001): "Community health refers to the physical, emotional, social, and spiritual wellbeing of a group of people linked together in some way, possibly through geographical proximity or shared interests" (pp. 39–40). This definition is consistent with the AOTA (2008) *Framework.* Occupational therapy can assist in the promotion of health in a community of stroke survivors, small towns, college campuses, refugee camps, city boroughs, or a variety of other communities.

A primary goal of community health and health promotion is the prevention of disability, injury, and disease. **Prevention** has been defined in AOTA's *Framework* (2008, p. 674) as "promoting a healthy lifestyle at the individual, group, organizational, community (societal), governmental/policy level" (adapted from Brownson & Scaffa, 2001). Typically, prevention is classified into three levels: primary, secondary, and tertiary. These levels are defined in Table 4-1. Examples of activities for each of these prevention levels are detailed in Table 4-1 and in Figure 1-6 of Chapter 1 of this text. The WHO recognizes the increasing complexity of identifying risk factors for prevention and advocates for a broader perspective and approach, one focused on precautionary principles:

> The concepts of precaution and prevention have always been at the heart of public health practice. Public health is inherently about identifying and avoiding risk to the health of populations, as well as about identifying and implementing protective measures. In the past, public health interventions focused on removing hazards that had already been identified and "proven" (even if the etiological mechanisms were not well understood). As "modern" potential risk factors become more complex and far-reaching, the precautionary principle addresses uncertain risks and seeks to shift the ways in which science informs policy from a

strategy of "reaction" to a strategy of "precaution". Together with related approaches such as health impact assessment, precaution provides a useful means of guiding public health decisions under conditions of uncertainty, in a manner that appropriately addresses the issues of power, ownership, equity and dignity. (WHO, 2004b, p. 3)

The term *wellness* is used frequently in conjunction with *health promotion.* **Wellness** has been defined as "a dynamic way of life that involves action, values, and attitudes that support or improve health and quality of life" (Brownson & Scaffa, 2001, p. 656). Figure 4-1 depicts the role of occupational therapy in new public health, where the target of the intervention is a society as a whole or a broad population within that society. In order for occupational therapy public health interventions to realize their potential benefit to individuals, families, communities, and society, these interventions must

- be planned, delivered, and evaluated through active engagement with the population, in order to maximize ownership by the population; and must
- include participation in health-enhancing occupations by the individual, family, community, or society.

Health promotion is the primary tool used by occupational therapists and occupational therapy assistants in public health. It includes education strategies, advocacy, and other preventive interventions. Occupation-based health promotion is the process used by practitioners to assist individuals, families, communities, or society in the pursuit of occupational wellness. These efforts are supported by and consistent with the language and description of the domain of occupational therapy and the process of service delivery in the AOTA *Framework* (2008). For example, whether a health promotion intervention is

Table 4–1 Definitions of Levels of Prevention and Examples

Term	Definition	Examples
Primary prevention	Interventions with healthy individuals, communities, and populations in order to decrease risk for potential health problems	Lifestyle redesign Falls prevention
Secondary prevention	Early detection and treatment of diseases or disabilities	Developmental screenings
Tertiary prevention	Interventions with people with disabilities or traumatized communities to prevent or minimize further dysfunction	Joint protection Hurricane relief

Data from "Public health, community health, and occupational therapy" by M. E. Scaffa, S. Desmond, & C. A. Brownson in *Occupational therapy in community-based settings,* 2001, Philadelphia: F. A. Davis.

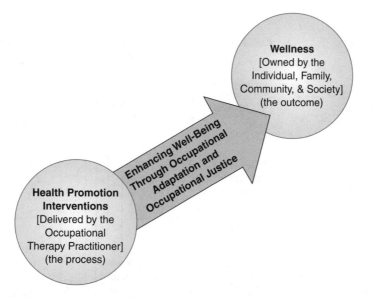

Figure 4-1   Occupational therapy's role in the new public health through occupation-based health promotion.

Courtesy of Reitz, Scaffa, & Pizzi (2004) used by S. M. Reitz in Health and wellness through occupation: The American perspective, *invited open seminar, Hospital Authority, Hong Kong, February 27, 2004.*

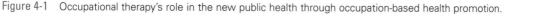

aimed at an individual, family, community, or population, the first step is to complete an occupational profile. This profile would be followed by an occupational performance analysis of the individual, family, or community population, which, with the client's feedback, would be used in the development of an occupation-based intervention. Examples of assessments that can be used to conduct an occupational profile of a community or population are described in Chapter 10. One possible type of intervention would be an interdisciplinary community-led effort to promote occupational justice through advocacy and capacity building, with the outcome being enhanced community health and occupational engagement.

The majority of occupation-based health promotion interventions in the United States are currently targeted toward the specific needs of an individual client (as is the case with most occupational therapy interventions). When efforts are aimed at a population, they are considered public health interventions. If these interventions are simultaneously aimed at decreasing occupational deprivation and occupational alienation at the societal level, they are consistent with the values of the new public health. Public health is an interdisciplinary activity; thus, occupation-based public health initiatives must be conducted as part of a broader interdisciplinary program or movement. Figure 4-2 displays three examples of the possible relationships between policy (at the local, state, and national level), governmental agencies, governmental reports, interdisciplinary public health programming, and target populations. The lines indicate the relationships for each of the three examples: America on the

Move™ (Partnership to Promote Healthy Eating and Active Living [PPHEAL], 2003), *Healthy Campus 2010: Making It Happen* (American College Health Association [ACHA], 2002), and bike helmet laws and helmet distribution programs.

International Official Health Promotion Documents and Initiatives

A variety of international documents and those from other nations provide guidance in the development of health promotion policies and interventions. Five of these documents will be described below, including

- *A New Perspective on the Health of Canadians* (Lalonde, 1974);
- *Ottawa Charter for Health Promotion* (WHO, 1986);
- *Jakarta Declaration on Leading Health Promotion into the 21st Century* (WHO, 1997a);
- *International Classification of Functioning, Disability, and Health* (WHO, 2001); and
- *Twenty Steps for Developing a Healthy Cities Project* (WHO, 1997b).

A New Perspective on the Health of Canadians

This document, often referred to as the *Lalonde Report* published in 1974, was the first definitive governmental report to outline a vision for the future

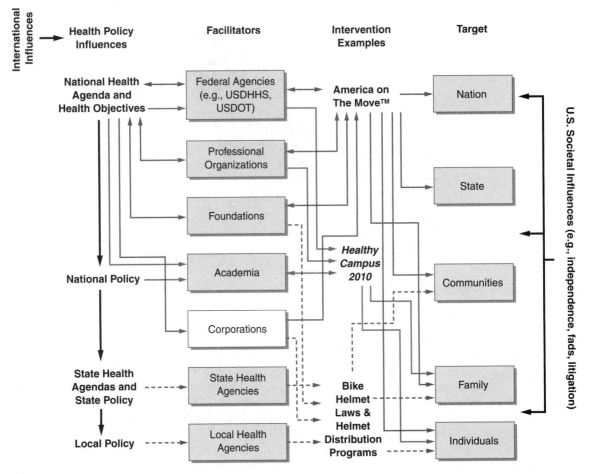

Figure 4-2   Health promotion policy in action.

Courtesy of Reitz, Scaffa, & Merryman (2004). Examples of Health Promotion Programming in the U.S. [Figure]. Used by S. M. Reitz in Occupational therapy in health promotion—Moving into a new era, *invited plenary session, Occupational Therapy Symposium 2004—Achieving Health and Wellness Through Occupation: From Theory to Practice, Hong Kong, February 28, 2004.*

health of its citizens using a "planning-by-objectives" approach. Other countries used the *Lalonde Report* and then the U.S. government's 1979 *Healthy People: The Surgeon General's Report on Health—Promotion and Disease Prevention* and the WHO's *Primary Health Care for All* initiatives as models for this approach (Green & Kreuter, 1999). *Health* was identified in the *Lalonde Report* as being dependent on the interaction of human biology, now referred to as *genetics,* the *environment, lifestyle,* and the *health-care system* (Lalonde, 1974; Tulchinsky & Varavikova, 2000). The development of health promotion policies, programs, and initiatives in the later part of the 1970s and through the 1980s was influenced by the identification of the reduction of lifestyle risk factors as a means to improve health and decrease health-care costs. However, concern was expressed that the focus on lifestyle could lead to "blaming the victim" and restriction of access to

services, which is inconsistent with public health values (Tulchinsky & Varavikova, 2000).

Ottawa Charter for Health Promotion

This document was developed in 1986 at the First International Conference on Health Promotion (Green & Kreuter, 1999; Tulchinsky & Varavikova, 2000). The preparation of this document resulted in a shift in focus from lifestyle or proximal risk factors to risk conditions and broader determinants of health (Green & Kreuter, 1999). The *Ottawa Charter* "is agreed upon by most authors as the single most important document in the history of health promotion" (Wilcock & Whiteford, 2003, p. 60). Three essential issues of concern to those involved in health were identified in the *Ottawa Charter*: caring, holism, and ecology. Figure 4-3 displays the five directions identified by the *Ottawa Charter* to reach the long-term goal of healthier communities. The figure also includes roles or actions identified by

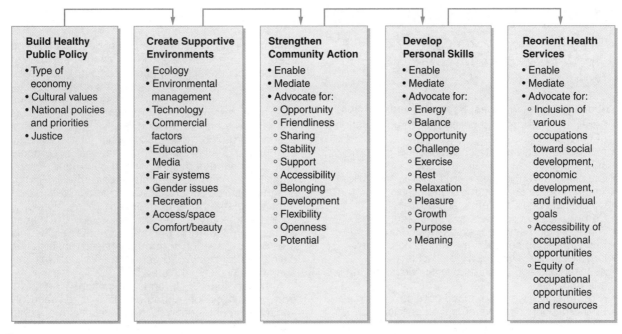

Figure 4-3   Wilcock and Whiteford's categorization of the Ottawa Charter's five directions (WHO, 1986).

From Figure 4-2 from Occupation, health promotion, and the environment (p. 61) by A. Wilcock and G. Whiteford in Using environments to enable performance, *2003, Thorofare, NJ: SLACK. Reprinted with permission from SLACK Incorporated.*

Wilcock and Whiteford (2003, p. 60) that would match the values and outcomes of occupation-based practice and research that promotes occupational justice. **Occupational justice** is "a critical perspective of social structures that promotes social, political, and economic changes to enable people to meet their occupational potential and experience well-being" (Spear & Crepeau, 2003, p. 1031). An occupationally just society promotes occupational engagement for all members through access to education, health, and recreational services that support quality of life of individuals, families, and communities through policy and public health initiatives.

Jakarta Declaration on Leading Health Promotion into the 21st Century

This document identified the critical role of the environment in health, while echoing the call of the *Ottawa Charter* to address the underlying social conditions that impact health, such as access to shelter, food, living wages, and sustainable resources (Wilcock & Whiteford, 2003). Health promotion was described as being "carried out by and with people, not on or to people" (WHO, 1997a, p. 4). Five priorities for the 21st century regarding health promotion were identified:

- Promote social responsibility for health.
- Increase investments for health development.
- Consolidate and expand partnerships for health.

- Increase community capacity and empower the individual.
- Secure an infrastructure for health promotion (WHO, 1997a, pp. 3–4).

International Classification of Functioning, Disability, and Health (ICF)

The international health community uses the *ICF* as a standard common language and framework to describe health status and factors that influence health and wellbeing (WHO, 2001). This document is one of the WHO's "family" of international classifications. The development of the *Framework* was influenced by the *ICF*. Besides providing consistent health language across nations, the *ICF* also provides a structure for advocacy for individuals with disabilities, the study of health systems, and the development and evaluation of health and social policy. Content Box 4-2 displays the services, systems, and policies defined within the classification that would be of interest in public health initiatives.

Twenty Steps for Developing a Healthy Cities Project

This is the third edition of a document that describes the ongoing work of the WHO Regional Office for Europe to improve the public health and determinants of health in the inhabitants of their cities. Eleven qualities of

Content Box 4-2

International Classification of Functioning, Disability, and Health (ICF)

Subcategories—Services, Systems, and Policies

- Services, systems, and policies for the production of consumer goods
- Architecture and construction services, systems, and policies
- Open-space planning services, systems, and policies
- Housing services, systems, and policies
- Utilities services, systems, and policies
- Communication services, systems, and policies
- Transportation services, systems, and policies
- Civil protection services, systems, and policies
- Legal services, systems, and policies
- Associations and organizational services, systems, and policies
- Media services, systems, and policies
- Economic services, systems, and policies
- Social Security services, systems, and policies
- General social support services, systems, and policies
- Health services, systems, and policies
- Education and training services, systems, and policies
- Labor and employment services, systems, and policies
- Political services, systems, and policies
- Services, systems, and policies, other specified
- Services, systems, and policies, unspecified

Data from an overview of *ICF* from *International classification of functioning, disability, and health* (p. 44) by World Health Organization (WHO), 2001, Geneva, Switzerland. Copyright © 2001 by WHO.

Implications for Occupational Therapy

The international documents briefly described can be used to inform practice and enhance the education of occupational therapy and occupational therapy assistant students. These five documents are representative of the many available international documents and have been used by occupational therapists around the world to support work in public health, health promotion, and occupational justice. Several of these and other similar international documents have been cited in descriptions of community-based rehabilitation and other occupational therapy public health initiatives directed toward marginalized people throughout the world (Kronenberg, Simó-Algado, & Pollard, 2005). In addition, the philosophy and human values represented in these documents resonate in the position paper on community-based rehabilitation developed by the World Federation of Occupational Therapists (WFOT) in June 2004.

Although the WFOT and occupational therapists from a variety of countries have been actively engaged in contributing to the public health of populations and countries in need around the world (Kronenberg et al., 2005), less has been done within the United States to promote public health and occupational justice. While innovative occupational therapy models exist, they do not reach the needs of many marginalized people within U.S. borders. Awareness of these documents is a first step in the education of students. The second step is educating students about health disparities and marginalized populations within the United States and around the world. With this knowledge, students will be better prepared to advocate for public health and occupational therapy's contribution to public health, both within their country and abroad.

a healthy city are identified in this document and appear in Content Box 4-3. Although the document and processes were designed for European cities, the document includes useful information for the design of any interdisciplinary project to impact the health of a city or community. Phase IV of the WHO Healthy Cities Network in Europe ran from 2003 through 2007. Focus areas for this phase included healthy urban planning, health impact assessment, and healthy aging. All six WHO regions have established Healthy City networks (WHO, 2005b).

U.S. Governmental Documents on Health Promotion

A variety of U.S. governmental documents are also available to provide assistance with needs assessment and health promotion program development. Six of these documents, five of which are official U.S. documents, are described below. The other document, *Unequal Treatment: Confronting Racial and Ethnic Disparities in*

Health Care (IOM, 2003), was written at the request of the U.S. Congress. These documents include

- *Healthy People 2010: Understanding and Improving Health* (USDHHS, 2000a);
- *Healthy People in Healthy Communities: A Community Planning Guide Using Healthy People 2010* (USDHHS, 2001a);
- *Unequal Treatment: Confronting Racial and Ethnic Disparities in Health Care* (IOM, 2003);
- *Healthy Campuses 2010: Making It Happen* (American College Health Association, 2002)
- *Youth Violence: A Report of the Surgeon General* (USDHHS, 2001b); and
- *Mental Health: A Report of the Surgeon General* (USDHHS, 1999).

After each document has been described, one or more implications for the profession of occupational therapy will be shared, along with thoughts regarding future directions for the specific population, health condition, or threat addressed by the report.

Content Box 4-3

Qualities of a Healthy City

A city should strive to provide

- a clean, safe physical environment of high quality (including housing quality);
- an ecosystem that is stable now and sustainable in the long-term;
- a strong, mutually supportive and nonexploitive community;
- a high degree of participation and control by the public over the decisions affecting their lives, health, and wellbeing;
- the meeting of basic needs (for food, water, shelter, income, safety, and work) for all the city's people;
- access to a wide variety of experiences and resources, with the chance for a wide variety of contact, interactions, and communication;
- a diverse, vital, and innovative city economy;
- the encouragement of connectedness with the past, with cultural and biological heritage of city dwellers, and with other groups and individuals;
- a form that is compatible with and enhances the preceding characteristics;
- an optimum level of appropriate public health and sick care services accessible to all; and
- high health status (high levels of positive health and low levels of disease).

Data from Figure 1 in *Twenty steps for developing a healthy cities project* (p. 9) by the World Health Organization (WHO), Regional Office for Europe, 1997, Copenhagen, Denmark. Copyright 1997 by WHO, Regional Office for Europe.

Healthy People 2010: Understanding and Improving Health

This document continues the tradition established with previous federal government publications, which outline proactive health goals and objectives for the United States and its citizens. These national health goals and objectives are developed through a collaborative process between governmental, professional, and nonprofit organizations, and the public. The AOTA was a member of the Healthy People Consortium, "an alliance of more than 350 national organizations and 250 State public health, mental health, substance abuse, and environmental agencies" involved in the development of *Healthy People 2010: Understanding and Improving Health* (USDHHS, 2000a, p. 2).

Healthy People 2010: Understanding and Improving Health, frequently referred to as simply *Healthy People 2010*, is comprised of a series of goals and objectives. Two overarching goals exist in *Healthy People 2010*. The first is to "increase quality and years of life," and the second is to "eliminate health disparities" (USDHHS, 2000a, p. 2). In addition to these overarching goals, the report includes 467 objectives divided into 28 focus areas. Table 4-2 lists a sampling of objectives with potential interest to occupational therapy practitioners. This list includes examples of objectives that correlate to all three levels of prevention. Achievement of these objectives will not occur through occupational therapy personnel working in isolation; progress will be made only if occupational therapy practitioners join or initiate interdisciplinary efforts to target one or more of these objectives.

Table 4–2 Examples of Healthy People 2010 Objectives Related to Health Promotion

Domain of Concern	Objective Number	Objective
Access to Quality Health Services	1-7	(Developmental) Increase the proportion of schools of medicine, schools of nursing, and other health professional training schools whose basic curriculum for health-care providers includes the core competencies in health promotion and disease prevention.
	1-8	In the health professions, the allied and associated health profession fields, and the nursing field, increase the proportion of all degrees awarded to members of underrepresented racial and ethnic groups.
Arthritis, Osteoporosis, and Chronic Back Conditions	2-1	(Developmental) Increase the mean number of days without severe pain among adults who have chronic joint symptoms.
	2-7	(Developmental) Increase the proportion of adults who have seen a health-care provider for their chronic joint symptoms.

Continued

Table 4–2   **Examples of Healthy People 2010 Objectives Related to Health Promotion—cont'd**

Domain of Concern	Objective Number	Objective
	2-8	(Developmental) Increase the proportion of persons with arthritis who have had effective, evidence-based arthritis education as an integral part of the management of their condition.
Cancer Deaths and Disabilities	3-9	Increase the proportion of persons who use at least one of the following protective measures that may reduce the risk of skin cancer: avoid sun between 10 a.m. and 4 p.m., wear sun-protective clothing when exposed to sunlight, use sunscreen with a sun-protective factor (SPF) of 15 or higher, and avoid artificial sources of ultraviolet light.
Disability and Secondary Conditions	6-3	Reduce the proportion of adults with disabilities who report feelings such as sadness, unhappiness, or depression that prevent them from being active.
	6-6	Increase the proportion of adults with disabilities reporting satisfaction with life.
	6-7	Reduce the number of people with disabilities in congregate care facilities, consistent with permanency planning programs.
Educational and Community-Based Programs	7-7	(Developmental) Increase the proportion of health-care organizations that provide patient and family education.
	7-8	(Developmental) Increase the proportion of patients who report that they are satisfied with the patient education they receive from their health-care organization.
	7-9	(Developmental) Increase the proportion of hospitals and managed care organizations that provide community disease prevention and health promotion activities that address the priority health needs identified by their community.
	7-12	Increase the proportion of older adults who have participated during the preceding year in at least one organized health promotion activity.
Heart Disease and Stroke	12-11	Increase the proportion of adults with high blood pressure who are taking action (for example, losing weight, increasing physical activity, or reducing sodium intake) to help control their blood pressure.
Injury and Violence Prevention	15-12	Increase the number of states and the District of Columbia that collect data on external causes of injury through hospital discharge data systems.
	15-33	Reduce maltreatment and maltreatment fatalities of children.
	15-39	Reduce weapon-carrying by adolescents on school property.
Mental Health and Mental Disorders	18-5	(Developmental) Reduce the relapse rates for persons with eating disorders, including anorexia nervosa and bulimia nervosa.
	18-8	(Developmental) Increase the proportion of juvenile justice facilities that screen new admissions for mental health problems.

Table 4–2   **Examples of Healthy People 2010 Objectives Related to Health Promotion—cont'd**

Domain of Concern	Objective Number	Objective
	18-9	Increase the proportion of adults with mental disorders who receive treatment.
Physical Activity and Fitness	22-1	Reduce the proportion of adults who engage in no leisure-time physical activity.
	22-7	Increase the proportion of adolescents who engage in vigorous physical activity that promotes cardiorespiratory fitness 3 or more days per week for 20 or more minutes per occasion.
	22-11	Increase the proportion of adolescents who view television 2 or fewer hours on a school day.
	22-12	(Developmental) Increase the proportion of the nation's public and private schools that provide access to their physical activity spaces and facilities for all persons outside of normal school hours (that is, before and after the school day, on weekends, and during summer and other vacations).
	22-13	Increase the proportion of worksites offering employer-sponsored physical activity and fitness programs.
Substance Abuse	26-19	(Developmental) Increase the proportion of inmates receiving substance abuse treatment in correctional institutions.

Data from *Healthy People 2010: Understanding and improving health,* by U.S. Department of Health and Human Services, 2000, Washington, DC: Government Printing Office.

Focus area 6 of *Healthy People 2010* is devoted to the promotion of wellbeing and the prevention of secondary conditions for people with disabilities. This focus area had not been included in previous versions of *Healthy People* and demonstrates a growing understanding of the health promotion needs of individuals and populations with disabilities. People with disabilities are at increased risk for secondary conditions, which include more than just physical health issues. Emotional distress prompted by barriers and lack of access to opportunities for social participation can lead to a variety of mental health issues, including sleep abnormalities and depression. Table 4-2 includes 3 of the 13 objectives related to individuals with disabilities associated with this focus area. The majority of these objectives focus on helping people with disabilities be involved in all aspects of life through improving access to education, employment, equipment, and health promotion activities. Also, three of the objectives focus directly on the mental health needs of this population.

In addition to outlining goals and objectives for the nation's health, *Healthy People 2010* provides background information regarding health determinants, data on the nation's current health status, and top health indicators. Health determinants and the relationships with health status are identified in Figure 4-4. Data such as the leading causes of death by age group are included in this report (Table 4-3 on page 83). Ten leading health priority indicators reflecting major U.S. public health concerns will be used to track the progress of *Healthy People 2010*.

> These 10 Leading Health Indicators are intended to help everyone more easily understand the importance of health promotion and disease prevention. Motivating individuals to act on just one of the indicators can have a profound effect on increasing the quality and years of healthy life and on eliminating health disparities—for the individual, as well as the community overall. (USDHHS, 2001a, p. 4)

Table 4-4 on page 84 lists the 10 leading health indicators together with corresponding public health challenges.

There are additional resources that provide updated data and information concerning the implementation of *Healthy People 2010*, which include a

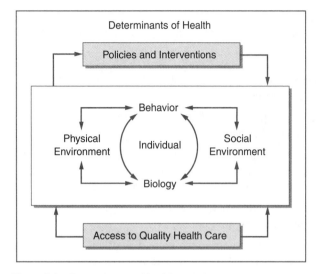

Figure 4-4 Determinants of health.

From Figure 7 in Healthy People 2010: Understanding and improving health *(p. 18), by U.S. Department of Health and Human Services, 2000, Washington, DC: Government Printing Office.*

midcourse review, tracking reports, and progress reviews. It is customary for the USDHHS to release a midcourse review of progress toward the current decade's goals and objectives. The midcourse review for *Healthy People 2010* was released in December 2006 (USDHHS, 2006) and can be found by clicking on the publications link on the *Healthy People 2010* homepage, which is accessible at http://www.healthypeople.gov/About/. A second resource is *Tracking Healthy People 2010,* a statistical companion to *Healthy People 2010,* which also can be found by clicking on the publications link on the *Healthy People 2010* homepage. This document

> is a comprehensive, authoritative guidebook on the statistics used for Healthy People—in effect the analytic framework for the program. Never before has the broad Healthy People community had this type of resource. This guidebook will assist in ensuring greater accuracy and comparability in the data produced for, and used by, Healthy People 2010 programs at the local, State, and national levels. (USDHHS, 2000b, Foreword ¶ 2)

A third type of resource is progress reviews. The first of two planned *Healthy People 2010* progress reviews began in 2002, with the goal of reviewing one of the 28 focus areas, roughly in alphabetical order, on a monthly basis (USDHHS, 2004). These progress reviews can be accessed through the *Healthy People 2010* homepage, via the implementation link.

Healthy People in Healthy Communities: A Community Planning Guide Using Healthy People 2010

In addition to *Healthy People 2010,* many parallel efforts exist, two of which are described in this chapter. The first of these efforts to be described is *Healthy People in Healthy Communities: A Community Planning Guide Using Healthy People 2010,* a guide to help citizens form and operate community coalitions (USDHHS, 2001a). A **healthy community** is described as a community that

- provides access to both preventive and clinical health services to all residents;
- has a safe and healthy atmosphere; and
- has an infrastructure (e.g., roads, schools, playgrounds, and other services) to meet the needs of community members (USDHHS, 2001a).

This guide describes the *Healthy People 2010* initiative and a step-by-step process that can be used to assess the community and to promote change. The steps—mobilize, assess, plan, implement, and track—spell out MAP-IT, which is the acronym used to identify the process. This process is briefly highlighted in Chapter 10 of this book.

While the document *Healthy People in Healthy Communities* is an excellent resource, it is not sufficient to combat the social injustices and disparities in resources that exist in communities across the United States. Funding and support for communities with the human capital to locate and use this resource are

Table 4–3   Leading Causes of Death by Age Group

Under 1 Year	Number of Deaths
Birth defects	6178
Disorders related to premature birth	3925
Sudden infant death syndrome	2991
1–4 Years	
Unintentional injuries	2005
Birth defects	589
Cancer	438
5–14 Years	
Unintentional injuries	3371
Cancer	1030
Homicide	457
15–24 Years	
Unintentional injuries	13,367
Homicide	6146
Suicide	4186
24–44 Years	
Unintentional injuries	27,129
Cancer	21,706
Heart disease	16,513
45–64 Years	
Cancer	131,743
Heart disease	101,235
Unintentional injuries	17,521
65 Years and Older	
Heart disease	606,913
Cancer	382,913
Stroke	140,366

Adapted from Figure 9 in *Healthy People 2010: Understanding and improving health* (p. 23), by U.S. Department of Health and Human Services, 2000, Washington, DC: Government Printing Office.

required. Even more critical are the efforts that must be made to ensure all communities are aware of this document and have access to the supports to realize the goal of healthy communities across the entire U.S. landscape.

Implications for Occupational Therapy

A healthy community supports optimal occupational performance as presented in the AOTA's *Framework*. However, the *Framework* does not discuss or define community but instead describes components of a community through its explanation of contexts. *Healthy People in Healthy Communities* helps occupational therapists and occupational therapy assistants begin to think in terms of a community as a potential client.

Unequal Treatment: Confronting Racial and Ethnic Disparities in Health Care

The Institute of Medicine (IOM) 2003 report *Unequal Treatment: Confronting Racial and Ethnic Disparities in Health Care* details disparities that exist in access to health care and outlines disparities that currently exist in the U.S. health-care delivery system. **Health-care disparities** are "racial or ethnic differences in the quality of healthcare that are not due to access-related factors or clinical needs, preferences, and appropriateness of intervention" (IOM, 2003, pp. 3–4). The findings of this report appear in Content Box 4-4. Evidence of health-care disparities continued with the publication of the congressionally mandated report *National Healthcare Disparities Report* (Agency for Healthcare Research and Quality, 2005). A summary of

Implications for Occupational Therapy

Occupational therapists and occupational therapy assistants take an active role in eliminating health-care disparities within the United States. Potential actions include the following:

- Participate in the AOTA and state associations and promote awareness of the IOM report.
- Require review of this and other similar reports within occupational therapy educational programs and fieldwork.
- Monitor service delivery patterns to ensure disparities do not exist.
- Advocate and be politically active to ensure necessary polices, laws, and regulations are enacted and implemented.
- Engage in evidence-based, culturally competent practice.
- Embrace and conduct research on ethical issues in service delivery.

Active involvement to eliminate health-care disparities within the United States is consistent with the *Occupational Therapy Code of Ethics* (AOTA, 2005), the *Core Values and Attitudes of Occupational Therapy Practice* (AOTA, 1993), the AOTA's statement on Health Disparities (Braveman, 2006), and the AOTA's statement *Occupational Therapy's Commitment to Nondiscrimination and Inclusion* (AOTA, 2004).

Table 4–4   **Leading Health Indicators and Corresponding Public Health Challenge**

Subject/Topic	Public Health Challenge
Physical activity	Promote regular physical activity
Overweight and obesity	Promote healthier weight and good nutrition
Tobacco use	Prevent and reduce tobacco use
Substance abuse	Prevent and reduce substance abuse
Responsible sexual behavior	Promote responsible sexual behavior
Mental health	Promote mental health and wellbeing
Injury and violence	Promote safety and reduce violence
Environmental quality	Promote healthy environments
Immunization	Prevent infectious disease through immunization
Access to health care	Increase access to quality health care

From *Healthy People in Healthy Communities 2010: Understanding and improving health* (p. 24), by U.S. Department of Health and Human Services, 2000, Washington, DC: Government Printing Office.

Content Box 4-4

Summary of Findings of Institute of Medicine (IOM) Report

- **Finding 1-1:** Racial and ethnic disparities in health care exist and, because they are associated with worse outcomes in mean cases, are unacceptable.
- **Finding 2-1:** Racial and ethnic disparities in health care occur in the context of broader historic and contemporary social and economic inequality, and evidence of persistent racial and ethnic discrimination in many sectors of American life.
- **Finding 3-1:** Many sources—including health systems, health-care providers, patients, and utilization managers—may contribute to racial and ethnic disparities in health care.
- **Finding 4-1:** Bias, stereotyping, prejudice, and clinical uncertainty on the part of health-care providers may contribute to racial and ethnic disparities in health care. While indirect evidence from several lines of research supports this statement, a greater understanding of the prevalence and influence of these processes is needed and should be sought through research.
- **Finding 4-2:** A small number of studies suggest that racial and ethnic minority patients are more likely than white patients to refuse treatment. These studies find that differences in refusal rates are generally small and that minority patient refusal does not fully explain health-care disparities.

From box in *Unequal treatment: Confronting racial and ethnic disparities in healthcare* (p. 19), by Institute of Medicine, 2003, Washington, DC: National Academies Press. Reprinted with permission from the National Academies Press. Copyright © 2003 by National Academy of Sciences.

the IOM (2003) recommendations for reducing health disparities can be found in Appendix B.

Healthy Campuses 2010: Making It Happen

This is the second document related to *Healthy People 2010* to be discussed. This document provides colleges and universities with the structure to assess the health status of their campuses and make decisions regarding priorities and interventions. In addition to this report, data collected and reported by ACHA through the National College Health Assessment (NCHA) can assist with decision-making. The NCHA collects data nationally on college and university students' health behaviors and perceptions on

- alcohol, tobacco, and other drug use;
- sexual health;
- weight, nutrition, and exercise;
- mental health; and
- injury prevention, personal safety, and violence (ACHA, 2004, NCHA ¶ 2).

Currently in the United States there are 128 accredited occupational therapy assistant education programs (AOTA, 2009). The campuses on which these programs reside may seek assistance from the Bridges to Healthy Communities 2005 program. This program is managed through the American Association of Community Colleges (AACC) in cooperation with the Centers for Disease Control and Prevention's (CDC) Division of Adolescent and School Health. Resources are available to assist with program replication and development, with an emphasis on the prevention of HIV infection.

The Bridges project is helping community colleges improve student and community health through models of integrated activities that bring together campus and community. They involve individuals, families, schools, and communities. Service learning is the primary strategy and is supplemented by a variety of specific strategies left to the creativity and imagination of the colleges. (AACC, 2004, About the project, ¶ 1)

Youth Violence: A Report of the Surgeon General

The tragic events at Columbine High School in 1999 brought the public health problem of youth violence to the forefront and were the catalyst for *Youth Violence: A Report of the Surgeon General* (USDHHS, 2001b). At the beginning of her report, the secretary of USDHHS, Dr. Donna E. Shalala, stated that "the first, most enduring responsibility of a society is to ensure the health and wellbeing of its children" (p. i). Shalala then described how President Clinton directed the Surgeon General to prepare a report summarizing the current research on the scope, causes, and possible prevention of youth violence. The Office of the Surgeon General supervised the preparation of the *Youth Violence* report, which was a collaborative effort between the USDHHS; the CDC; the National Institutes of Health, National Institute of Mental Health (NIH/NIMH); and the Substance Abuse and Mental Health Services Administration (SAMHSA).

Then Surgeon General, Dr. David Satcher, summarized the overall report findings in the preface. The following were among his comments:

- "No community is immune."
- "Intervention strategies exist today that can be tailored to the needs of youths at every stage of development, from young childhood to late adolescence."
- Strategies that are "effective for one age may be ineffective for older or younger children. Certain hastily adopted and implemented strategies may be ineffective—and even deleterious—for all children and youth" (USDHHS, 2001b, p. v).

The CDC's National Center for Injury Prevention and Control (NCIP) cooperates with other agencies to maximize collaboration and the dissemination of research, and it conducts

> research on violence-related injuries across contexts (e.g., school, family, community), roles (i.e., victim or perpetrator), and proximal causes (e.g., intoxication, bullying, robbery), combined with its emphasis on prevention strategies, complements and extends the violence-prevention activities of other federal agencies and community-based organizations. (CDC/NCIP, 2004a, The Injury Center's Niche in Preventing Youth Violence, ¶ 4)

The NCIP established research priorities for preventing youth violence. The top 7 of 15 priorities to be emphasized over the next 3 to 5 years are listed below:

- Evaluate dissemination strategies for the most effective youth violence prevention programs.
- Evaluate the effectiveness of community-wide parenting programs for youth violence prevention.
- Evaluate the effectiveness of youth violence prevention strategies.
- Identify and evaluate strategies to decrease inappropriate access to and use of firearms among youths.
- Identify modifiable sociocultural and community factors that influence youth violence.
- Identify modifiable factors that protect youths from becoming victims or perpetrators of violence.
- Clarify the relationships between youth violence and other forms of violence and determine implications for prevention. (CDC/NCIP, 2004b, *The Injury Center's Research Priorities*, ¶ 1–23)

The information gathered and disseminated from evidence-based research in these areas will inform future legislation, policies, and program development and refinement.

Implications for Occupational Therapy

The findings of the *Youth Violence* report (USDHHS, 2001b) support the need for evidence-based violence prevention practice. *Best Practices of Youth Violence Prevention: A Sourcebook for Community Action* (Thornton, Craft, Dahlberg, Lynch, & Baer, 2002) is another source for successful programs and ideas upon which to build occupational therapy's contributions to the prevention of youth violence in the community. By critically reviewing the literature for efficacious programs, the occupational therapist can more quickly be prepared to contribute to interventions that will more likely achieve desired outcomes.

The Families and Schools Together (FAST) program is another resource for occupational therapy practitioners. The original FAST program was developed by a social worker in 1988 (AOTA, 2003). The AOTA conducted a FAST violence prevention research project from September 2000 through May 2001, which was funded by the Center for Mental Health Services (CMHS), a division of the Substance Abuse and Mental Health Services Administration (SAMHSA). An occupation-based, multifamily, 10-week program was developed and implemented at two different schools, one in a Midwest city and one in a Northeast suburb. Positive program results were consistent with previous FAST initiatives, thus it was determined that occupational therapists would be appropriate FAST team leaders (AOTA, 2003).

Mental Health: A Report of the Surgeon General

Mental health is viewed as a dynamic phenomenon that reflects an individual's genetic predispositions, life experiences, and social environment. Although the physical health of the U.S. population progressively improves, mental health is often overlooked, and mental illnesses remain shrouded in stigma and misunderstanding. The report of the U.S. Surgeon General regarding mental health emphasizes the interdependent nature of physical and mental health and wellbeing, and focuses attention on the mental health needs of persons across the life span (USDHHS, 1999). Approximately 20% of individuals within the United States are affected by mental disorders in any given year; depression is a leading cause of disability in the United States, and suicide is one of the leading preventable causes of death worldwide. Yet, the availability and accessibility of mental health services lack parity with other areas of health care. Due to recent advances in neurophysiology, mental illnesses are more effectively treated than at any other point in history. However, there is a serious lack of research on efficacious strategies to prevent mental disorders and promote mental health.

Several themes are evident in the Surgeon General's report on mental health, including

- mental health and mental illness should be approached from a public health perspective;
- mental disorders are significantly disabling;
- mental health and mental illness are points on a continuum, not polar opposites;
- the mind and body are inseparable; and
- stigma is a serious barrier that reduces access to treatment, limits opportunities, interferes with full participation in society, and may result in overt discrimination (USDHHS, 1999).

The report was based on the best available scientific evidence at the time and addresses the unique mental health needs of children, adolescents, adults, and the elderly. Each stage of life is associated with specific vulnerabilities for mental illness and distinct capacities for mental health. In addition to chapters describing mental health and mental illness at each stage of the life cycle, other chapters in the report discuss issues related to the organization and financing of mental health services and issues of privacy and confidentiality.

Based on the findings of the Surgeon General's report on mental health, numerous recommendations for future action were identified, including the following:

- Continue to build the science base.
- Implement strategies to overcome stigma.
- Ensure an appropriate array of mental health services and an adequate supply of practitioners.
- Provide culturally competent care.
- Reduce barriers to evidence-based interventions. (USDHHS, 1999)

Although significant efficacy data exists to support a range of treatments for mental disorders, there is a paucity of research on preventive interventions. More attention focused on strategies for promoting mental health and facilitating resiliency is essential. The conditions necessary for developing and maintaining mental health and preventing mental illness are priorities for future research.

Implications for Occupational Therapy

The number of occupational therapists and occupational therapy assistants in mental health practice has significantly declined over the past 20 years. In 2004, only 2% of occupational therapy practitioners worked in mental health settings, down from 8.5% in 1986 (Ebb & Haiman, 1990; Gandy, 2004). It is disconcerting that occupational therapy is losing its presence in the mental health arena, where the profession first emerged and demonstrated its worth.

According to WHO, depression is the leading cause of disability in terms of years lived with disability (YLD). It is the fourth leading cause of disability as measured by DALYs (disability adjusted life years). *DALYs* refers to the sum of years of potential life lost due to premature mortality and years of productive life lost due to disability. It is expected that by the year 2020, depression will be the second leading cause of DALYs among all age groups and for both sexes (WHO, 2006c).

Since mental disorders (especially depression) are disabling, it is essential for occupational therapists to actively reinvigorate this area of practice. As "lifestyle redesign" (University of Southern California, Department of Occupational Therapy & Occupational Science, n.d.) specialists, occupational therapists can have a role in the prevention of mental disorders and the promotion of mental health. Mental health promotion can be integrated into practice regardless of the setting and population served. Genetics, life experiences, and social environment affect mental health. Occupational therapists and occupational therapy assistants can provide positive mental health promotion life experiences and can facilitate the development of social networks and thereby promote mental health. The Surgeon General's report clearly indicates that mental health is a health problem across the life span. As such, it must be addressed for all people, not just for persons with mental illness.

U.S. Government and Professional Association Public Health Initiatives

This last section will focus on initiatives sponsored by the U.S. government and U.S.-based professional organizations to impact public health in the United States and abroad. Four examples will be shared, including former President George W. Bush's New Freedom Initiative, the President's New Freedom Commission on Mental Health (Bush, 2002), the AOTA's official document on health promotion, and the American Occupational Therapy Foundation's *Occupation in Societal Crises Task Force* report.

New Freedom Initiative: Fulfilling America's Promise to Americans with Disabilities

Approximately 54 million people in the United States live with a disability. This represents nearly 20% of the population. The **New Freedom Initiative (NFI)**, announced by former President George W. Bush on February 1, 2001, is a comprehensive national framework for eliminating barriers that prevent people with disabilities from fully participating in community life. Six federal agencies are directly involved, including the Departments of Health and Human Services, Education, Labor, Housing and Urban Development, and Justice, as well as the Social Security Administration. Several other departments and agencies are involved indirectly. The NFI has six goals, which include

- increasing access to assistive and universally designed technologies;
- expanding educational opportunities;
- promoting home ownership;
- integrating Americans with disabilities into the workforce;
- expanding transportation options; and
- promoting full access to community life (USDHHS, 2003b, ¶ 3).

On June 18, 2001, as part of the NFI, former President George W. Bush issued Executive Order 13217: Community-Based Alternatives for Individuals with Disabilities:

> The Order called upon the federal government to assist states and localities to swiftly implement the decision of the United States Supreme Court in *Olmstead v. L.C.* stating: "The United States is committed to community-based alternatives for individuals with disabilities and recognizes that such services advance the best interests of the United States." (USDHHS, 2003c, ¶ 1)

The *Olmstead v. L.C.* decision, issued by the U.S. Supreme Court in July 1999, declared that unnecessary segregation of persons with disabilities in institutions violates the Americans with Disabilities Act (ADA) of 1990 and constitutes discrimination. The decision applies to all persons with physical or mental disabilities, regardless of age. It challenges local, state, and federal governments to provide accessible, cost-effective, community-based services for people with disabilities. The NFI mandates full implementation of the *Olmstead v. L.C.* decision.

In 2004, a progress report was released describing the NFI's accomplishments. Content Box 4-5 highlights some of the achievements related to each goal.

The U.S. Department of Justice (USDOJ) houses the homepage of the ADA, the forerunner of the NFI. This homepage includes links to an area that displays case studies of people whose lives and occupations have been positively impacted by the ADA (USDOJ, 2000). One of the cases pertains to a boy whose parents, with the help of the USDOJ, ensured his continued access to an after-school program operated by a national day-care chain.

Implications for Occupational Therapy

The ADA and now the NFI provide an outstanding opportunity for occupational therapists and occupational therapy assistants to become involved in a national effort to eliminate barriers to full inclusion and social participation for children, adults, and elderly persons with disabilities. Occupational therapy can positively impact all six goals of the NFI. Occupational therapy professionals have knowledge and skills in assistive technology, school-system interventions, home adaptations, work-skill development, transportation adaptations, and facilitating community integration and social participation. The U.S. Supreme Court's *Olmstead v. L.C.* decision mandates community-based services for people with disabilities. Occupational therapists are uniquely positioned to respond to the NFI and the *Olmstead* decision by developing and providing accessible, cost-effective health promotion and occupation-based interventions in the community.

President's New Freedom Commission on Mental Health

A key component of the New Freedom Initiative was the establishment of the President's New Freedom Commission on Mental Health in 2002. The commission's purpose was to conduct a comprehensive evaluation of the mental health service delivery system and provide recommendations on how the system could be improved. For nearly a year, 22 commissioners met monthly to hear testimony, analyze the mental health

Content Box 4-5

Selected Achievements of the New Freedom Initiative

Goal: Increasing Access to Assistive and Universally Designed Technologies

• Funded alternative financing programs—for example, low-interest, long-term loans to enable persons with disabilities to acquire needed technologies
• Promoted full implementation of Section 508 of the Rehabilitation Act to ensure that electronic and information technologies used by the government are fully accessible to persons with disabilities
• Developed a Web portal, DisabilityInfo.gov, that provides information about the variety of programs offered by the federal government that impact people with disabilities

Goal: Expanding Educational Opportunities for Youth With Disabilities

• Established the President's Commission on Excellence in Special Education
• Increased funding for the Individuals with Disabilities Education Act (IDEA)

Goal: Integrating Americans With Disabilities Into the Workforce

• Provided funding to purchase technology to enable telecommuting
• Implemented the Ticket to Work program
• Promoted strict enforcement of the Americans with Disabilities Act (ADA) of 1990
• Developed best practice models for hiring and retaining qualified individuals with disabilities

Goal: Promoting Full Access to Community Life

• Improved access to voting for persons with disabilities
• Provided funding for projects to reduce transportation barriers
• Trained over 1500 architects and builders in the design and construction of fully accessible housing
• Funded projects to enable older individuals and individuals with disabilities to remain in their homes
• Provided employment transportation services for individuals with disabilities
• Funded demonstration projects for the recruitment, training, and retention of direct service workers
• Established the New Freedom Commission on Mental Health

From *The President's New Freedom Initiative for People with Disabilities: The 2004 progress report, executive summary* (pp. 3–6), by the White House Domestic Policy Council Washington, DC: The White House.

system, visit innovative program models, and review research evidence (President's New Freedom Commission on Mental Health, 2003). The U.S. Department of Health and Human Services Surgeon General's 1999 report on mental health served as the scientific foundation for the commission's deliberations.

The commission was mandated to identify unmet needs, barriers to community-based services, and effective treatment approaches and to formulate policies to enhance community integration of persons with mental disorders. The ultimate goal is to create a system of services that enable persons with serious mental illnesses to live, work, learn, and participate fully in their communities.

In 2003, the final report of the commission was released. A complete transformation of the mental health service delivery system was advocated, and two principles for this transformation were outlined. First, the services must be client- and family-centered, not oriented to the needs of bureaucracies. Second, intervention should focus on building resilience and facilitating recovery, not simply on reducing symptoms. In addition, interventions should be based on the best available evidence, and the system must be convenient, accessible, and built upon client needs. According to the report, in a transformed mental health service,

• Americans understand that mental health is essential to overall health;
• mental health care is consumer and family driven;
• disparities in mental health services are eliminated;
• early mental health screening, assessment, and referral to services are common practice;
• excellent mental health care is delivered and research is accelerated; and
• technology is used to access mental health care and information (President's New Freedom Commission on Mental Health, 2003, p. 8).

The characteristics are written as goal statements in the report and serve as the framework for the commission's 19 recommendations (see Content Box 4-6).

Implications for Occupational Therapy

Two outcomes of the commission's deliberations are of special interest to occupational therapists and occupational therapy assistants. One is the provision of community-based services for persons with mental disorders. Many mental health services are provided in community settings, but few of these include occupational therapy. Occupational therapists need to promote their unique focus, abilities, and skills to these programs and advocate employment of occupational therapy professionals for the benefit of mental health clients. In addition, it is not only reasonable, but also imperative to create new occupation-based programs for mental health clients living in the community. Occupational therapists are particularly qualified to address the two broad principles of the commission's report—client- and family-centered care and building client resilience.

Content Box 4-6

Goals and Recommendations in a Transformed Mental Health System

Goal 1: Americans Understand That Mental Health Is Essential to Overall Health

Recommendations

1.1 Advance and implement a national campaign to reduce the stigma of seeking care and a national strategy for suicide prevention.
1.2 Address mental health with the same urgency as physical health.

Goal 2: Mental Health Care Is Consumer and Family Driven

Recommendations

2.1 Develop an individualized plan of care for every adult with a serious mental illness and child with a serious emotional disturbance.
2.2 Involve consumers and families fully in orienting the mental health system toward recovery.
2.3 Align relevant federal programs to improve access and accountability for mental health services.
2.4 Create a comprehensive state mental health plan.
2.5 Protect and enhance the rights of people with mental illnesses.

Goal 3: Disparities in Mental Health Services Are Eliminated

Recommendations

3.1 Improve access to quality care that is culturally competent.
3.2 Improve access to quality care in rural and geographically remote areas.

Goal 4: Early Mental Health Screening, Assessment, and Referral to Services Are Common Practice

Recommendations

4.1 Promote the mental health of young children.
4.2 Improve and expand school mental health programs.

4.3 Screen for co-occurring mental and substance use disorders and link with integrated treatment strategies.
4.4 Screen for mental disorders in primary health care, across the life span, and connect to treatment and supports.

Goal 5: Excellent Mental Health Care Is Delivered and Research Is Accelerated

Recommendations

5.1 Accelerate research to promote recovery and resilience, and ultimately to cure and prevent mental illnesses.
5.2 Advance evidence-based practices using dissemination and demonstration projects and create a public-private partnership to guide their implementation.
5.3 Improve and expand the workforce providing evidence-based mental health services and supports.
5.4 Develop the knowledge base in four understudied areas: mental health disparities, long-term effects of medications, trauma, and acute care.

Goal 6: Technology Is Used to Access Mental Health Care and Information

Recommendations

6.1 Use health technology and telehealth to improve access and coordination of mental health care, especially for Americans in remote areas or in underserved populations.
6.2 Develop and implement integrated electronic health record and personal health information systems.

From the President's New Freedom Commission on Mental Health, 2003. Retrieved May 31, 2005, from http://www.whitehouse.gov/news/releases/2002/04/20020429-2.html

Occupational Therapy in the Promotion of Health and the Prevention of Disease and Disability Statement

The AOTA supports and encourages the development of occupation-based health promotion and disease/disability prevention services and the involvement of occupational therapy practitioners in interdisciplinary health promotion efforts. The document *Occupational Therapy Services in the Promotion of Health and the Prevention of Disease and Disability* (Scaffa, Van Slyke, & Brownson, 2008) serves as the profession's official document on health promotion. This document

defines health promotion, discusses the need to address health disparities, describes levels of prevention, and details the role of occupational therapy at the community and population levels. A particularly useful aspect of this official document is the discussion of Wilcock's (1998) constructs of occupational imbalance, occupational deprivation, and occupational alienation and their relationship to health promotion.

Three critical roles for occupational therapy in health promotion are identified:

• Promoting healthy lifestyles for all clients/patients, their caregivers, and their families

- Emphasizing occupation as an essential component of prevention strategies and complementing health promotion services provided by experts in other professions through the application of occupational therapy principles
- Expanding occupational therapy interventions from a focus on individuals to include health promotion efforts with groups, organizations, communities, and policymakers (Scaffa et al., 2008)

The statement lists a variety of potential health promotion interventions at the organizational, community, population, governmental, and policy levels. In addition, the document provides case studies to illustrate the application of health promotion principles in occupational therapy practice. Occupational therapy's unique contribution to health promotion and disease/disability prevention is the profession's focus on occupational capabilities, skills, habits, roles, and routines, as well as its expertise in modifying environments for optimal, healthy, and safe occupational performance.

Occupation in Societal Crises Task Force

Shortly following the terrorist attacks of September 11, 2001, the president of the American Occupational Therapy Foundation (AOTF) appointed practitioners from across the United States and Canada to form the Task Force on Occupation in Societal Crises (Task Force). The goal of the Task Force was to delineate the influence of occupation during times of societal crisis and define the role of occupational therapists and occupational therapy assistants in disaster planning, response, and recovery.

The Task Force produced numerous publications, including McColl's (2002) article "Occupation in Stressful Times" which was published in the *American Journal of Occupational Therapy.* Other Task Force members wrote articles that were published on the AOTF website. In addition, the librarian of the Wilma West Library assembled a "Resource Note," which served as a bibliography of references on the subject. Pi Theta Epsilon, in collaboration with the Task Force, sponsored two sessions at the AOTA Annual Conference. The first, in 2003, featured a panel of experts who outlined the federal, state, and local systems responsible for responding to natural and technological disasters. Panelists urged the occupational therapy audience to become involved in disaster planning in their communities (AOTF, 2003). The second conference session, held in 2005, described the role of occupational therapy practitioners in disaster planning, response, and recovery. Over 100 practitioners attended and, in small work groups, brainstormed occupational therapy responses to several different disaster scenarios.

The AOTF Task Force collaborated with the AOTA Commission on Practice to develop an official document on the profession's role in disasters. This document is based on information gathered from focus groups, practitioners, and literature from the disaster management field. In November 2005, the Representative Assembly of the AOTA approved an official concept paper titled *Occupational Therapy's Role in Disaster Preparedness, Response and Recovery.* The Task Force's ultimate goal is to develop a network of practitioners who are trained to respond effectively to disasters. Occupational therapy professionals are uniquely prepared to address the special needs of the elderly and individuals with disabilities before, during, and after disasters. In 2004, former President George W. Bush issued the executive order Individuals with Disabilities in Emergency Preparedness. The order is designed to enhance the nation's disaster response for persons with disabilities and begins by recognizing the special needs of persons with disabilities in the planning process. The order established a coordinating council within the Department of Homeland Security to address these concerns (White House, 2004).

Implications for Occupational Therapy

Although occupational therapy can make a significant contribution to health promotion practice, it is important to acknowledge and respect the roles and contributions of other health promotion service providers, including health educators, public health personnel, nutritionists, exercise physiologists, and others. In order to demonstrate the efficacy of occupational therapy in health promotion, it is critical that energy and resources are directed at

- identifying occupational factors that impact health and wellbeing;
- developing assessment tools that measure these factors;
- evaluating occupation-based health promotion services in a variety of settings with a variety of populations; and
- documenting the effectiveness and cost benefits of occupational therapy involvement in health promotion efforts.

Many of the prevalent social problems of today have significant health components, for example, homelessness, substance abuse, mental illness, violence, and accidents. These social problems can be addressed from a prevention and health promotion perspective. Occupational therapy is uniquely positioned to provide essential and tangible responses in these areas.

Implications for Occupational Therapy

The Health Resources and Services Administration (HRSA) of the federal government funds the Bioterrorism Training & Curriculum Development Program (BTCDP). This grant program funds continuing education and curriculum development for training health professionals in bioterrorism response. Recently, HRSA expanded its focus to include all-hazards public health emergencies.

In 2005, HRSA convened a series of focus groups to discuss the role of the allied health (AH) professions in disaster planning and response. Several recommendations for action emerged from these meetings, including the need to

- develop a standardized set of basic core competencies in allied health and standardized metrics to evaluate performance;
- identify discipline-specific competencies that reflect the role of the discipline in a public health emergency—this requires role delineation and differentiation of disaster roles from traditional roles;
- create training opportunities that lead to nationally recognized certification;
- incorporate mental health issues into all aspects of training; and
- conduct research regarding the role of AH professions in disasters.

Specific ideas regarding training included the need to develop multiple layers of education, the importance of understanding chains of command, emergency response structure, and terminology. Focus group members suggested requiring that all AH professionals obtain basic disaster training in the National Incident Management System (NIMS) and participate in one training exercise/drill annually. These recommendations are all relevant for occupational therapy practitioners. Concerns were expressed regarding the lack of disaster response training requirements in AH accreditation standards, shortage of experienced instructors to teach the competencies, the difficulty of incorporating this content into already overflowing curricula, and the need for real-life experiences to evaluate student/practitioner performance of competencies. These challenges must be addressed if occupational therapy is to define its place in all-hazards public health emergency planning, response, and recovery.

Conclusion

Governmental reports and initiatives such as those described above can be instrumental in providing data and ideas to occupational therapists and occupational therapy assistants seeking funds to develop health-promotion programs. These reports summarize work and knowledge from a variety of disciplines. An additional step beyond reviewing reports on the subject of interest is to review data and evidence-based research from a variety of related fields. This review should be extensive and include sources that may at first seem unrelated to occupational therapy. For example, public health experts found information from geographic information systems and data from police reports concerning pedestrian injury rates and location of occurrence useful in studying child pedestrian injuries and developing tailored preventive strategies (Braddock et al., 1994). This type of data can assist occupational therapists employed in the school system to gain support for developing a safety program targeting needs and safety risks of students and families. Data such as this would also be important to consider in the development of school-sponsored walking programs designed to increase physical activity.

According to Wilcock, the primary impediment keeping the profession from reaching its potential contribution to population health is the "dominance of the idea of the 'individual' within the profession and the more or less exclusive focus on disability and handicap" (2003, p. 43). One way to change this thinking is to increase participation in interdisciplinary, population-based health education, research, and prevention activities. The profession remains insular and focused on its perceived ability to do it all—and to do it alone, which fails to honor its history and is a costly disservice to society. The governmental reports and other initiatives described in this chapter can provide significant guidance on the interdisciplinary, population-based health education, research, and prevention activities mentioned above. When the profession is ready to routinely seek interdisciplinary opportunities, the true potential of occupational therapy's contribution to public health and society will be realized.

This chapter encourages the involvement of occupational therapy practitioners in interdisciplinary public health initiatives and research by reviewing the history of public health, key governmental and nongovernmental reports, and national and international perspectives on health and wellbeing. This foundational knowledge, together with the data in these and future reports, will allow occupational therapists and occupational therapy assistants to advocate for the polices and programs needed to enhance public health in broader population and interdisciplinary ventures.

The belief that occupation can be health-enhancing led to the development of the concept of preventive occupation. Scaffa and colleagues (2001) defined **preventive occupation** as "the application of occupational science in the prevention of disease and disability and the promotion of health and wellbeingof individuals and communities through meaningful engagement in occupations" (p. 44). In 2006, AOTA adopted a statement on health disparities that declares, "Occupational therapy is well positioned to intervene with individuals and communities to limit the effects of health disparities on participation in meaningful occupations" (Braveman, 2006, ¶ 1). The new public health approach shares a common goal with occupational therapy—a commitment to social activism and advocacy. In addition, practitioners in these disciplines understand the impact of the social and physical environments on health. It should be easy to find willing partners with whom to join forces. "We cannot solve all problems of poverty and injustice, but we can improve survival and quality of life, step by step, one acre at a time, to achieve wondrous miracles" (Tulchinsky & Varavikova, 2000, p. 3).

▶ For Discussion and Review

1. What are the similarities and differences between occupational therapy and public health in terms of ideology, goals, and approaches?
2. How might occupational therapy provide preventive, occupation-based interventions to individuals, families, groups, and communities?
3. Briefly describe an occupational therapy health promotion intervention and the supporting U.S. and international documentation.
4. Identify and discuss aspects of the AOTA's *Framework* that support the role of occupational therapy in health promotion.
5. Read the AOTA official document on health promotion and develop three occupational therapy strategies for addressing one of the public health challenges identified in Tables 4-3 or 4-4.
6. Review one of the national health documents described in this chapter, identify a target population, and briefly outline three possible occupational therapy health promotion interventions that could be suggested to that population.

▶ Research Questions

1. Does the addition of occupational therapy interventions in health promotion programs enhance program effectiveness?
2. What are the effects of brief health promotion interventions in traditional occupational therapy settings?
3. What are the effects of brief, repeated, developmentally graded health promotion interventions in school-based occupational therapy settings?

4. What are the occupational therapy-specific competencies needed for all-hazards public health emergency planning, response, and recovery?
5. Does the addition of occupational therapy personnel to interdisciplinary health promotion programs enhance the overall effectiveness of those programs' impact on community health?

Acknowledgments

The authors wish to express their appreciation to the following individuals who assisted with the preparation of this chapter: Frederick D. Reitz, Gar Wing Tsang, and Grace E. Wenger.

References

Agency for Healthcare Research and Quality. (2005). *National healthcare disparities report.* Retrieved March 13, 2006, from http://www.ahrq.gov/qual/nhdr05/nhdr05.htm.

American Association of Community Colleges. (2004). *Bridges to healthy communities 2005.* Retrieved November 28, 2004, from http://www.aacc.nche.edu/Content/NavigationMenu/ResourceCenter/Projects_Partnerships/Current/BridgestoHealthyCommunities/AbouttheProject/AbouttheProject.htm.

American College Health Association. (2002). *Healthy Campus 2010: Making it happen.* Baltimore: Author.

American College Health Association. (2004). *ACHA-National College Health Assessment.* Retrieved November 28, 2004, from http://www.acha.org/projects_programs/assessment.cfm.

American Occupational Therapy Association. (1993). Core values and attitudes of occupational therapy practice. *American Journal of Occupational Therapy, 47,* 1085–86.

American Occupational Therapy Association. (2003). *American Occupational Therapy Association/FAST project: Role of occupational therapists in violence prevention* [Executive Summary]. Retrieved November 29, 2004, from http://www.aota.org/members/area2/limnks/link36.asp.

American Occupational Therapy Association. (2004). Occupational therapy's commitment to nondiscrimination and inclusion. *American Journal of Occupational Therapy, 58,* 668.

American Occupational Therapy Association. (2005). Occupational therapy code of ethics (2005). *American Journal Occupational Therapy, 59*(6), 639–42.

American Occupational Therapy Association. (2008). Occupational therapy practice framework: Domain and processes. *American Journal of Occupational Therapy, 56,* 609–39.

American Occupational Therapy Association. (2009, March 4). *OTA programs—Accredited.* Retrieved March 7, 2009, from http://www.aota.org/nonmembers/area13/links/link29.asp.

American Occupational Therapy Foundation. (2003). Plenary session draws attention to disaster planning. *AOTF Connection, 10*(2), 7.

American Public Health Association. (2003). *Growth of international health: An analysis and history.* Retrieved March 13, 2006, from http://www.apha.org/wfpha/pdf/ InternationalHealth Book1.pdf.

Best, J., & Cameron, R. (1986). Health behavior and health promotion. *American Journal of Health Promotion, 1,* 48–56.

Braddock, M., Lapidus, G., Cromley, E., Cromley, R., Burke, G., & Banco, L. (1994). Using a geographic information system to understand child pedestrian injury. *American Journal of Public Health, 84*(7), 1158–61.

Braveman, B. (2006). AOTA's Statement on Health Disparities. *American Journal of Occupational Therapy, 60*(6), 670.

Breines, E. (1986). *Origins and adaptations.* Lebanon, NJ: Geri-Rehab.

Brownson, C. A., & Scaffa, M. E. (2001). Occupational therapy in the promotion of health and the prevention of disease and disability statement. *American Journal of Occupational Therapy, 55*(6), 656–60.

Bush, G. (2002, April 22). Executive Order: President's New Freedom Commission on Mental Health. Retrieved May 31, 2005, from http://www.whitehouse.gov/news/ releases/2002/04/20020429-2.html.

Centers for Disease Control and Prevention. (1999). Ten great public health achievements: United States, 1900–1999. *Morbidity and Mortality Weekly Report, 48*(12), 241–43.

Centers for Disease Control and Prevention, National Center for Health Statistics. (2006). *Health, United States, 2006* (p. 29). Washington, DC: Government Printing Office.

Centers for Disease Control and Prevention, National Center for Injury Prevention and Control. (2004a). *The Injury Center's niche in preventing youth violence, CDC Injury Research agenda—Preventing youth violence.* Retrieved January 18, 2008, from http://www.cdc.gov/ncipc/ pubres/research_agenda/09_youthviolence.htm.

Centers for Disease Control and Prevention, National Center for Injury Prevention and Control. (2004b). *The Injury Center's research priorities, CDC Injury Research agenda—Preventing youth violence.* Retrieved January 18, 2008, from http://www.cdc.gov/ncipc/pubres/research_agenda/ 09_youthviolence.htm.

Colonial Williamsburg Foundation. (2004). *Public hospital exhibit.* Colonial Williamsburg, VA: Author.

Ebb, E., & Haiman, S. (1990). Enriching the fieldwork II experience: A recruitment strategy for psychosocial occupational therapy. *Occupational Therapy in Mental Health, 10,* 29–46.

Gandy, J. (2004). *Trends and issues in education* [PowerPoint presentation]. Retrieved October 3, 2005, from http:// www.aota.org.

Geller, J. L. (2000). The last half-century of psychiatric services as reflected in psychiatric services. *Psychiatric Services, 51*(1), 41–67.

Goraya, A., & Scambler, G. (1998). From old to new public health: Role tensions and contradictions. *Critical Public Health, 8*(2), 141–51.

Green, L. W., & Kreuter, M. W. (1991). *Health promotion planning: An educational and environmental approach* (2d ed.). Mountainview, CA: Mayfield.

Green, L. W., & Kreuter, M. W. (1999). *Health promotion planning: An educational and ecological approach* (3d ed.). Mountainview, CA: Mayfield.

Institute of Medicine. (1988). *The future of public health.* Washington, DC: National Academies Press.

Institute of Medicine. (2003). Unequal treatment: Confronting racial and ethnic disparities in health care. Washington, DC: National Academies Press.

Johnson, J. (1986). *Wellness: A context for living.* Thorofare, NJ: SLACK.

Kielhofner, G. (2004). The development of occupational therapy knowledge. In *Conceptual foundations of occupational therapy* (3d ed., pp. 27–63). Philadelphia: F. A. Davis.

Kronenberg, F., Simó-Algado, S., & Pollard, N. (Eds.). (2005). *Occupational therapy without borders: Learning from the spirit of survivors.* New York: ELSEVIER, Churchill Livingstone.

Lalonde, M. A. (1974). *A new perspective on the health of Canadians.* Ottawa: Ministry of National Health and Welfare.

Lasker, R. D., & the Committee on Medicine and Public Health. (1997). *Medicine & public health: The power of collaboration.* New York: The New York Academy of Medicine.

Life Online. (n.d.) *Millennium—Top 100 events, No. 6 1882 the germ theory of disease.* Retrieved November 28, 2004, from http://www.life.com/Life/millennium/events/06.html.

Lyons, A., & Petrucelli, R. (1987). *Medicine: An illustrated history.* New York: Abradale Press.

McColl, M. A. (2002). Occupation in stressful times. *American Journal of Occupational Therapy, 56*(3), 350–53.

National Library of Medicine. (2006). Map of Washington, D.C., showing projected harbor improvement and system of drainage, 1881. Retrieved September 8, 2006, from http://wwwihm.nlm.nih.gov/cgi-bin/gw_44_3/chameleon.

O'Connor-Fleming, M. L., & Parker, E. (1995). *Health promotion principles and practice in the Australian context.* New South Wales, Australia: Allen & Unwin.

Partnership to Promote Healthy Eating and Active Living. (2003). America on the Move™. Retrieved November 3, 2003, from http://www.americaonthemove.org/index.asp.

Peloquin, S. M. (1989). Looking back—Moral treatment: Contexts reconsidered. *American Journal of Occupational Therapy, 43,* 537–44.

Pinel, P. (1948). Medical philosophical treatise on mental alienation (S. Licht, Trans). In S. Licht (Ed.), *Occupational therapy sourcebook* (pp. 19–24). Baltimore: Williams and Wilkins. (Original work published 1801.)

President's New Freedom Commission on Mental Health. (2003). *Achieving the promise: Transforming mental health care in America. Executive summary* (DHHS Pub. NO SMA-0303831). Rockville, MD: DHHS.

Reiser, S. J. (1997). Topics for our times: The medicine/public health initiative. *American Journal of Public Health, 87*(7), 1098–99.

Reitz, S. M. (2003, June 22–23). *Rural interdisciplinary health promotion service learning training.* Lecture presented at the Western Maryland Area Health Education Center, Cumberland, MD.

Reitz, S., Scaffa, M., & Merryman, M. (2004). Examples of health promotion programming in the U.S. [Figure]. Used by S. M. Reitz in *Occupational therapy in health promotion—Moving into a new era,* invited plenary session,

Occupational Therapy Symposium 2004—Achieving Health and Wellness through Occupation: From Theory to Practice, Hong Kong, February 28, 2004.

Reitz, S., Scaffa, M., & Pizzi, M. (2004). Relationship between health promotion interventions & wellness from an occupational therapy perspective [Figure]. Used in *Health and wellness through occupation: The American perspective*, invited open seminar, Hospital Authority, Hong Kong, February 27, 2004.

Roemer, M. I. (2000). Foreword. In T. H. Tulchinsky & E. A.Varavikova, *The new public health: An introduction for the 21st century* (pp. xix–xxi). San Diego, CA: Academic Press.

Sandstrom, R. W., Lohman, H., & Bramble, J. D. (2003). *Health services: Policy and systems for therapists.* Upper Saddle River, NJ: Prentice Hall.

Scaffa, M. E., Desmond, S., & Brownson, C. A. (2001). Public health, community health, and occupational therapy. In M. E. Scaffa (Ed.), *Occupational therapy in community-based practice settings* (pp. 35–50). Philadelphia: F. A. Davis.

Scaffa, M. E., Van Slyke, N., & Brownson, C. A. (2008). Occupational therapy services in the promotion of health and the prevention of disease and disability, *American Journal of Occupational Therapy 62*(6), 694–703.

Schwartz, K. B. (2003). The history of occupational therapy. In E. B. Crepeau, E. S. Cohn, & B. A. Schell (Eds.), *Willard & Spackman's occupational therapy* (10th ed., pp. 5–13). Philadelphia: Lippincott, Williams & Wilkins.

Spear, P. S., & Crepeau, E. B. (2003). Glossary. In E. B. Crepeau, E. S. Cohn, & B. A. Schell (Eds.), *Willard & Spackman's occupational therapy* (10th ed., pp. 1025–35). Philadelphia: Lippincott, Williams & Wilkins.

Thornton, T. N., Craft, C. A., Dahlberg, L. L., Lynch, B. S., & Baer, K. (2002). *Best practices of youth violence prevention: A sourcebook for community action* (rev.). Atlanta: Centers for Disease Control and Prevention, National Center for Injury Prevention and Control. Retrieved November 28, 2004, from http://www.cdc.gov/ncipc/dvp/bestpractices.htm.

Timmreck, T. C. (1995). *Planning, program development, and evaluation: A handbook for health promotion, aging, and health services.* Boston: Jones and Bartlett.

Tulchinsky, T. H., & Varavikova, E. A. (2000). *The new public health: An introduction for the 21st century.* San Diego, CA: Academic Press.

University of Southern California, Department of Occupational Therapy & Occupational Science. (n.d.) *Faculty practice.* Retrieved July 23, 2008, from http://www.usc.edu/schools/ihp/ot/faculty_practice/.

U.S. Department of Health and Human Services. (1979). *Healthy People: Surgeon General's report on health promotion and disease prevention.* Washington, DC: Government Printing Office.

U.S. Department of Health and Human Services. (1980). *Promoting health/preventing disease: Objectives for the nation.* Washington, DC: Government Printing Office.

U.S. Department of Health and Human Services. (1990). *Healthy People 2000: National health promotion and disease prevention objectives.* Washington, DC: Government Printing Office.

U.S. Department of Health and Human Services. (1994). *Public health in America.* Retrieved October 1, 2006, from http://www.health.gov/phfunctions/public.htm.

U.S. Department of Health and Human Services. (1999). *Mental health: A report of the Surgeon General.* Rockville, MD: U.S. Department of Health and Human Services, Substance Abuse and Mental Health Services Administration, Center for Mental Health Services, National Institutes of Health, National Institute of Mental Health.

U.S. Department of Health and Human Services. (2000a). *Healthy People 2010: Understanding and improving health* (2d ed.). Washington, DC: Government Printing Office.

U.S. Department of Health and Human Services. (2000b). *Tracking Healthy People 2010.* Washington, DC: Government Printing Office. Retrieved November 28, 2004, from http://www.healthypeople.gov/Document/tableofcontents .htm#tracking.

U.S. Department of Health and Human Services. (2001a). *Healthy people in healthy communities: A community planning guide using Healthy People 2010.* Retrieved November 27, 2004, from http://www.healthypeople.gov/Publications/ HealthyCommunities2001/healthycom01hk.pdf.

U.S. Department of Health and Human Services. (2001b). *Youth violence: A report of the Surgeon General.* Rockville, MD: U.S. Department of Health and Human Services, Centers for Disease Control and Prevention, National Center for Injury Prevention and Control; Substance Abuse and Mental Health Services Administration, Center for Mental Health Services; and National Institutes of Health, National Institute of Mental Health. Retrieved January 18, 2008, from http://www.surgeongeneral.gov/library/youthviolence/ youvioreport.html

U.S. Department of Health and Human Services. (2003a). *Healthy People 2010: Progress reviews—Health communication.* Retrieved November 28, 2004, from http://www.healthypeople.gov/data/2010prog/focus11/.

U.S. Department of Health and Human Services. (2003b). *New Freedom Initiative.* Retrieved June 4, 2005, from http://www.hhs.gov/new freedom/init.html.

U.S. Department of Health and Human Services. (2003c). *New Freedom Initiative, Executive Order 13217.* Retrieved May 28, 2005, from http://www.hhs.gov/newfreedom/eo13217.html.

U.S. Department of Health and Human Services. (2004). *Healthy People 2010: Progress reviews.* Retrieved November 27, 2004, from http://www.hhs.gov/about/hhshist.html and http://www.healthypeople.gov/data/PROGRVW/default.htm #2010.

U.S. Department of Health and Human Services. (2005). *Historical highlights.* Retrieved September 8, 2006, from http://www.hhs.gov/about/hhshist.html.

U.S. Department of Health and Human Services. (2006). Foreword. *Healthy People 2010 midcourse review.* Retrieved January 18, 2008, from http://www.healthypeople.gov/Data/ midcourse/html/foreword.htm.

U.S. Department of Justice. (2000). *ADA tenth anniversary: Faces of the ADA.* Retrieved September 10, 2006, from http://www.usdoj.gov/crt/ada/adafaces.htm.

U.S. Department of Justice. (2006). *ADA signing ceremony.* Retrieved September 10, 2006, from http://www.usdoj.gov/ crt/ada/videogallery.htm.

Vogel, V. J. (1970). *American Indian medicine.* Norman: University of Oklahoma Press.

White House. (2004, July 22). *Executive order: Individuals with disabilities in emergency preparedness.* Press release. Retrieved June 3, 2005, from http://www.whitehouse.gov/news/releases/2004/07/print/20040722-10.html.

White House Domestic Policy Council. (2004). *The president's new freedom initiative for people with disabilities: The 2004 progress report, Executive summary.* Retrieved November 24, 2006, from http://www.whitehouse.gov/infocus/newfreedom/toc 2004.html.

Wilcock, A. A. (1998). *An occupational perspective of health.* Thorofare, NJ: SLACK.

Wilcock, A. A. (2003). Occupational therapy practice: Section II Population interventions focused on health for all. In E. B. Crepeau, E. S. Cohn, & B. A. Schell (Eds.), *Willard & Spackman's occupational therapy* (10th ed., pp. 30–45). Philadelphia: Lippincott, Williams & Wilkins.

Wilcock, A., & Whiteford, G. (2003). Occupation, health promotion, and the environment. In L. Letts, P. Rigby, & D. Stewart (Eds.), *Using environments to enable occupational performance* (pp. 55–70). Thorofare, NJ: SLACK.

World Federation of Occupational Therapists. (2004). *WFOT position paper on community based rehabilitation.* Retrieved March 6, 2006, from http://www.wfot.org/Document_Centre/default.cfm.

World Health Organization. (1947). Constitution of the World Health Organization. *Chronicle of the World Health Organization, 1*(1), 29–40.

World Health Organization. (1948, June). *Official records of the World Health Organization, No. 2. Proceedings and final acts of the International Health Conference held in New York from 19 June to 22 July 1946.* Retrieved December 4, 2004, from http://whqlibdoc.who.int/hist/official_records/2e.pdf.

World Health Organization. (1986). *Ottawa charter for health promotion.* Retrieved December 4, 2004, from http://www.who.int/hpr/NPH/docs/ottawa_charter_hp.pdf.

World Health Organization. (1997a). *Jakarta declaration on leading health promotion into the 21st century.* Retrieved May 29, 2005, from http://www.who.int/hpr/NPH/docs/jakarta_declaration_en.pdf.

World Health Organization. (1997b). *Twenty steps for developing a healthy cities project.* Retrieved February 26, 2006, from http://www.euro.who.int/healthy-cities/introducing/20050202_2.

World Health Organization. (2001). *The international classification of functioning, disability, and health (ICF).* Geneva, Switzerland: Author.

World Health Organization. (2004a). *Background for healthy cities network.* Retrieved November 27, 2004, from http://www.euro.who.int/healthy-cities/CitiesAndNetworks/20020111_1.

World Health Organization. (2004b). *The precautionary principle: Protecting public health, the environment and the future of our children.* Retrieved February 25, 2006, from http://www.euro.who.int/eprise/main/WHO/Progs/HMS/MainActs/20040129_1.

World Health Organization. (2005a). *About WHO.* Retrieved May 30, 2005, from http://www.who.int/about/en/.

World Health Organization. (2005b). *Healthy cities and urban governance.* Retrieved February 26, 2006, from http://www.euro.who.int/healthy-cities.

World Health Organization. (2006a). *Working for health: An introduction to the World Health Organization.* Geneva: Author.

World Health Organization. (2006b). *WHO regional offices.* Retrieved February 26, 2006, from http://www.who.int/about/regions/en/index.html.

World Health Organization. (2006c). *Depression.* Retrieved March 16, 2006, from http://www.who.int/mental_health/management/depression/definition/en/.

Zwelling, S. S. (1985). *Quest for a cure: The public hospital in Williamsburg, Virginia, 1773–1885.* Williamsburg, VA: Colonial Williamsburg Foundation.

Chapter 5

Cultural and Sociological Considerations in Health Promotion

Bette Bonder

> I do not want my house to be walled in on all sides and my windows to be stuffed. I want the cultures of all the lands to be blown about my house as freely as possible. But I refuse to be blown off my feet by any.
>
> —Mahatma Gandhi (1869–1948)

Learning Objectives

This chapter is designed to enable the reader to:

- Define *culture, cultural competency, race, ethnicity, socioeconomic status, enculturation, acculturation,* and *spirituality.*
- Describe the impact of culture and socioeconomic status on health and health disparities.
- Discuss reasons for addressing cultural and socioeconomic factors in designing health promotion interventions.
- Describe the ways in which culture and socioeconomic status affect behavior in terms of
  - lifestyle;
  - health behaviors;
- rates of illness and disability;
- perceptions of health, illness, and disability;
- performance areas;
- performance patterns;
- performance skills; and
- performance contexts, activity demands, and client factors.
- Discuss implications for design of culturally relevant preventive interventions in occupational therapy.

Key Terms

Acculturation

Cultural competency

Culture

Enculturation

Ethnicity

Explanatory model

External locus of control

Internal locus of control

Race

Religion

Socioeconomic status

Spirituality

Introduction

Since the inception of the occupational therapy profession, occupational therapists have been aware of the importance of culture in the occupational lives of their clients (Dunton, 1915). In the past 25 years, occupational therapy literature has increasingly addressed the centrality of culture to occupational choice and satisfaction with occupational patterns (cf. Barney, 1991; Dillard et al., 1992; Iwama, 2004; Levine, 1984). The

core values of occupational therapy practitioners are in harmony with the desire described by Alvord and Van Pelt (1999):

> Navaho healers use song to carry words of the Beauty Way; the songs provide a blueprint for how to live a healthy, harmonious, and balanced life. I would like to create such a pathway between cultures so that people can walk across and see the wonders on the other side. (p. 16)

This chapter will explore the definitions of culture and socioeconomic status, and the ways in which these affect beliefs and behaviors related to occupations, health, illness, and disability. Strategies for addressing cultural and socioeconomic factors in the occupational therapy process will also be discussed.

In the United States, socioeconomic factors are strongly associated with culture, particularly when culture is defined based on race or ethnicity. In community health and health care, there is substantial evidence that socioeconomic factors affect individual health, access to care, and outcomes of care received (cf. Bowman & Wallace, 1990; Hakansson et al., 2003); therefore, effective interventions must address both culture and socioeconomic factors.

The evidence of the impact of culture and socioeconomic status on health and wellbeing is sufficiently compelling that the professional culture of occupational therapy clearly reflects their importance. In 1999, the Representative Assembly of the American Occupational Therapy Association (AOTA, 2004) approved a statement regarding support for inclusion and nondiscrimination. That statement has been revised and is now titled *Occupational Therapy's Commitment to Nondiscrimination and Inclusion* (AOTA, 2004). These beliefs are further supported by the *Occupational Therapy Practice Framework: Domain and Process* (AOTA, 2008), which indicates "occupational therapists and occupational therapy assistants recognize that engagement in occupation occurs in a variety of contexts (cultural, physical, social, personal, temporal, spiritual, virtual)" (p. 612). In addition, the AOTA *Occupational Therapy Code of Ethics* (2005) states that occupational therapy personnel will "recognize and appreciate the cultural components of economics, geography, race, ethnicity, religious and political factors, marital status, age, sexual orientation, gender identity, and disability of all recipients of their services" (p. 639).

While it seems self-evident that culture and socioeconomic status should be considerations in care, acting on that belief is no simple matter. This chapter provides definitions and descriptions important to efforts to ensure that culture and socioeconomic status are accurately identified and addressed in designing occupation-based preventive and health-promoting interventions.

Defining Terms

Defining terms to facilitate understanding and communication is an important first step. A number of constructs require explanation before any meaningful dialogue can occur. We begin by considering **culture.** Most people probably believe they know it when they

see it but have a much more difficult time providing a concrete definition. They are not alone in this, as researchers and theorists have similar difficulty. Kuper (1999), an anthropologist, indicates "in its most general sense, culture is simply a way of talking about collective identities" (p. 3). The U.S. Department of Health and Human Services (USDHHS), indicates that "'culture' refers to integrated patterns of human behavior that include language, thoughts, communications, actions, customs, beliefs, values, and institutions of racial, ethnic, religious, or social groups" (2000, p. 80865). A variety of definitions are offered in the occupational therapy literature, a selection of which is detailed in Content Box 5-1.

While these definitions vary somewhat, they all suggest that culture is shared among members of a particular group; is learned not inherent; is localized geographically; is patterned in the sense that it describes roles, behaviors, and values; and has some element of constancy although it may change over time (Bonder, Martin, & Miracle, 2002, 2004). Thus, culture contributes strongly to beliefs and behaviors of individuals.

Another important attribute of culture is that it emerges in interaction (Bonder et al., 2004; Tedlock & Mannheim, 1995). This means that culture is not something that is concrete and fixed in the environment. Rather, it is an element of relationships among people

---

Content Box 5-1

Sample of Definitions of Culture and Cultural Context From the Occupational Therapy Literature

- "A state of manners, taste, and intellectual development at a time or place. It is the ideas, customs, arts, etc. of a given people at a given time" (Baptiste, 1988, p. 180).
- "Values, beliefs, customs and behaviors that are passed on from one generation to the next" (Christiansen & Baum, 1997, p. 61).
- "An abstract concept that refers to learned and shared patterns of perceiving and adapting to the world" (Fitzgerald, Mullavey-O'Byrne, & Clemson, 1997, p. 1).
- "Customs, beliefs, activity patterns, behavior standards, and expectations accepted by the society of which the [client] is a member. Includes ethnicity and values as well as political aspects, such as laws that affect access to resources and affirm personal rights. Also includes opportunities for education, employment, and economic support (AOTA, 1994, p. 1054)" (AOTA, 2008, p. 670).

and groups. This is why it is not possible to identify one's culture from looking at an individual. Thus, culture is not race, nor is it any other biological attribute of individuals. Rather it is socially constructed during communication.

Because race is so often used as a proxy for culture (Wang & Sue, 2005), it is important to examine this construct. The National Research Council (NRC) defines **race** as a combination of physical characteristics along with "individual, group, and social attributes" (1997, p. 2). **Ethnicity,** by the same group's definition, refers to individual, group, and social attributes in the absence of common physical features that lead to categorization of individuals into a particular group (NRC, 1997). And while some hold that race is genetic, recent scientific advances in the understanding of human heredity suggest that genetic differences among "racial" groups are tiny (Wang & Sue, 2005). Race and ethnicity are increasingly perceived as entirely social (i.e., not biological) constructs. For example, Sacks observes,

> The study of the deaf shows us that much of what is distinctively human in us—our capacities for language, for thought, for communication, and culture—do not develop automatically in us, are not just biological functions, but are, equally, social and historical in origin; that they are a gift—the most wonderful gift—from one generation to another. (1989, p. xi)

It is possible that race and ethnicity emerged as categorical markers in health care, because several health conditions, such as sickle-cell anemia and Tay-Sachs disease, are clearly clustered in particular groups (Arnason, Sigurgislason, & Benedikz, 2000). This observation has given weight to race and ethnicity as constructs, although current explanations of this clustering suggest they are found most often in particular groups because of historical proximity of groups of individuals at a time when contact between groups was limited and because they conferred some unique survival benefit in those geographic areas (Wang & Sue, 2005). For example, sickle-cell anemia, a condition found almost exclusively in African and African American groups, appears to provide some protection against malaria. Thus, race and ethnicity in health care may have become proxies for expectations about the probability that individuals might be susceptible to specific health conditions.

Race and ethnicity are also strongly correlated with access to and outcomes of health care (Smedley, Stith, & Nelson, 2003). In fact, a recently published Institute of Medicine report (Smedley et al., 2003) has focused national attention on a growing problem—that there is clear and compelling evidence that individuals from particular racial and ethnic backgrounds are at high risk of certain diseases. Diabetes, for example, occurs at a much higher incidence among individuals from some Hispanic backgrounds than for other groups. Other groups are at risk of receiving substandard care, as in the case of African Americans with heart disease. Although these associations are well documented, they are not well explained.

Racial or ethnic labels tend to obscure important differences. The label *Asian,* for example, includes such diverse groups as Japanese Americans and Hmong. The first group is relatively similar socioeconomically to the majority culture in the United States. It includes some individuals recently arrived to this country and others whose families have lived in the United States for so long that they have only a nominal affiliation with the country from which their ancestors came. The Hmong, on the other hand, have come to the United States in substantial numbers only in the last generation or so (Fadiman, 1997). Those who arrived here initially were refugees from a war-torn region in which they had been completely dispossessed. They arrived with no economic resources, no ability to speak English, and no education in the formal Western sense. This first generation settled in several communities in California and Minnesota, where they struggled to make a life for themselves and, at the same time, changed the dynamics of the communities to which they immigrated. Health and social service providers experienced new challenges as a result of this influx.

Another complicating factor in an attempt to understand how race and ethnicity (and other cultural variables) affect health is the interaction of these variables with economic considerations. **Socioeconomic status** has been defined as categorization based on education, income, wealth, and position in the social hierarchy (Krieger, Williams, & Moss, 1997). Although the United States is often presented as a classless society, differentials in power, status, and economic resources clearly exist (Mills, 1958/2005), which affects health, functional abilities, and health care (Smedley et al., 2003). Studies of child development have found that socioeconomic status affects children's hand size and strength, praxis, and other visuomotor factors (Bowman & Wallace, 1990). Culture and socioeconomic status, while clearly implicated in health status and outcomes of care, represent a complicated set of interacting considerations.

An often overlooked fact is that everyone has culture, ethnicity, and socioeconomic status. Just as clients bring cultural beliefs and values to health-care encounters, providers of care bring cultural beliefs and values to the situation. Professions are themselves cultures (Krusen, 2003). Consider the beliefs conveyed in occupational therapy education about the kinds of interventions that will restore health or prevent dysfunction. Compare those beliefs with those of surgeons. Both professions are concerned with helping clients, but their beliefs about how to do that differ dramatically.

Not only do all individuals have culture, but most also have many cultures (Bonder et al., 2002) that interact with each other. An individual might identify with all of the following: Italian American (ethnic culture), high school student (developmental-stage culture), Catholic (religious culture), hearing-impaired (physical-status culture), gay (gender-preference culture), and so on. This individual also has socioeconomic status (for a high school student, this is typically conferred by parental status) that arguably could also be considered culture; for example, middle-class suburban.

This hypothetical high school student has been enculturated into multiple cultures. The process of **enculturation** involves learning about culture through direct instruction, observation, and modeling. High school students, for example, are particularly observant about those around them and those portrayed in the media. They choose their style of dress, language, and sometimes even their gait in an attempt to be as similar as possible to their peers. This particular student has undoubtedly also learned about being an Italian American through direct instruction by his or her parents, stories told by grandparents, and so on.

This individual may have learned other cultural identities through more subtle interaction with others. Gay high school culture is somewhat hidden, and unless the student's parents are also hearing-impaired, the student may have to actively seek out others with hearing impairments to learn about this very well-established culture (for more information about the culture of individuals with hearing impairment, see Sacks, 1989).

Acculturation, by contrast, is the process by which individuals relinquish aspects of their culture to acquire those of the surrounding majority culture. So in the case of the high school student previously described, the grandparents may have been first-generation Italian Americans who immigrated to the United States from Italy. They may well have chosen to live in a largely Italian immigrant neighborhood where they could speak Italian, eat foods familiar from their country of birth, and maintain customary behaviors. Their second-generation children may have learned to speak Italian but chosen to speak primarily English, or they may have enjoyed Italian food, but also chosen to eat fast food and steak more frequently. In addition, they may have had greater opportunity for educational accomplishments that led to better paying jobs that allowed a move to the suburbs. The third-generation high school student previously described may not speak Italian at all and may equate Italian food solely with pizza. In all

these ways, acculturation, adoption of majority cultural values and behaviors, may have led the individual away from the culture of origin.

Spirituality, Religion, and Health

Recent occupational therapy literature has increasingly focused on spirituality (Belcham, 2004; Canadian Association of Occupational Therapists, 1997; 2002; Mayers, 2004; McColl, 2003; Phillips, 2003; Townsend, De Laat, Egan, Thibeault, & Wright, 1999). Spirituality appears as the central core of the Canadian Model of Occupational Performance (CMOP), as depicted in Figure 5-1 and described in more detail in Content Box 5-2.

Both religion and spirituality are important elements of culture. **Religion** is defined by hyperdictionary (2005a, ¶ 2) as "an institution to express belief in a divine power." Specific religions, depending on their particular attributes, may well be defined as cultures, since they are learned, shared, patterned, and convey values. Issues about ability to conduct religious rituals, participate in religious events, and maintain culturally prescribed religious customs (e.g., cooking particular foods, undertaking volunteer activities that are prescribed by particular religions) can be major concerns for individuals, families, and communities.

Spirituality, on the other hand, is "concern with things of the spirit" (hyperdictionary, 2005b, ¶ 1). This means that spirituality focuses on concerns about the spirit and the divine that are not necessarily associated with an established religious group or institution. According to Frey, Daaleman, and Peyton (2005), the term *nonreligious spiritual propensity* (p. 559) is sometimes found in the literature. These authors' conceptualization of spirituality focuses on two factors: life scheme and self-efficacy. They note that "spirituality may be tied to attributes of personal meaning that may or may not be tied to religious traditions" (p. 560). The focus on personal meaning is echoed by the definition proposed by the Association of Professional Chaplains (2001) that suggests that **spirituality** is "an appreciation of presence and purpose that includes a sense of meaning" (p. 81).

This focus on meaning is particularly noteworthy for occupational therapists, given the profession's emphasis on supporting the engagement of individuals and communities in meaningful occupations. For some, that meaning emerges through connection with something beyond themselves. Whether that something is identified as God, as in the case of religion, or a more generally stated "bigger purpose," as in the case of spirituality, this aspect of culture and of personal values and beliefs cannot be ignored.

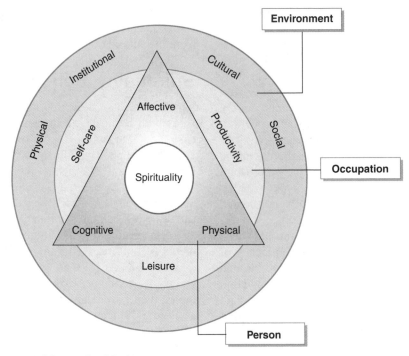

Figure 5-1 Canadian Model of Occupational Performance.

From Enabling occupation: An occupational therapy perspective, *by the Canadian Association of Occupational Therapists, 2002, Figure 1, p. 32. With permission.*

Content Box 5-2

Ideas About Spirituality From the Canadian Model of Occupational Performance

• Innate essence of self
• Quality of being uniquely and truly human
• Expression of will, drive, motivation
• Source of self-determination and personal control
• Guide for expressing self

From *Enabling occupation: An occupational therapy perspective,* by the Canadian Association of Occupational Therapists, 2002, Table 7, p. 43. With permission.

In some cultures, it could be argued that spiritual considerations guide all of life's decisions, including those about occupational choices and health behaviors (Alvord & Van Pelt, 1999). For example, many Native American cultures have a spiritual reverence for the stars. They believe that the Great Spirit gave the stars power to guide humans on Earth and impart spiritual blessings on them. The Milky Way is seen as a pathway for departed loved ones to reach the "southern star," or "abiding place of the dead." Star quilts are a manifestation of this belief and are given on the first-year anniversary of a loved one's death as a token of appreciation to those who had been especially kind to the deceased (Wicasa, 2005).

An individual can be spiritual without being religious and can be religious without being spiritual. The hypothetical high school student described earlier self-identifies as Catholic. This might imply active participation in formal religious practices (e.g., Mass) or in culturally Catholic events (e.g., discussion groups led by the parish priest), or it might mean simply having been raised in a home where Catholicism was the stated religious affiliation. Regardless of which of these is true, the student might still be highly spiritual, not at all spiritual, or (most likely) somewhere between these two poles.

In occupational therapy, both spirituality and religion have important consequences for clients' choices and for outcomes of care (Beauregard & Solomon, 2005; Schulz, 2004; Wilding, May, & Muir-Cochrane, 2005). Research suggests that spirituality or religion has implications for outcomes of care in HIV/AIDS (Beauregard & Solomon, 2005), mental health (Wilding et al., 2005), substance abuse (Rivera-Mosquera, 2005), chronic pain (Rippentrop, 2005), and many other conditions.

There is evidence that occupational therapists are somewhat reluctant to address spiritual or religious factors (Belcham, 2004; Udell & Chandler, 2000), in part because they feel unprepared or unqualified to do so. At the same time, there is growing awareness of the importance or centrality of these concerns in the occupational lives of individuals (Collins, Paul, & West-Frasier, 2001). Someone who believes that illness or disability is God's will might have very different motivation for participation in preventive interventions or remediation of dysfunction than someone who believes that "God helps those who help themselves."

Ultimately, it seems likely that in working in the community, religious and spiritual beliefs and motivations must be considered (Townsend, 1997). Without attention to these considerations, it is possible, perhaps even probable, that interventions will not address central concerns of the group. Culture, including religion and spirituality, are vital motivating factors for both individuals and groups. In order to move toward cultural competency, they must be understood and valued.

Cultural Competency

The fact that culture and the factors that fall within its sphere are so difficult to define complicates efforts to achieve cultural competency. According to the Culturally and Linguistically Appropriate Services (CLAS) standards developed by the USDHHS, Office of the Secretary (2000), **cultural competency** can be thought of as "having the capacity to function effectively as an individual and an organization within the context of the cultural beliefs, behaviors, and needs presented by consumers and their communities" (p. 80865). Unfortunately, as is the case for definitions of culture and its attributes, this is a relatively general definition, one that does not make clear the precise characteristics that allow a practitioner to say, "I am culturally competent."

The dynamic nature of culture also makes it very difficult to become and remain a culturally competent health-care provider without engaging in additional efforts to remain current. It is, perhaps, more appropriate to think of developing cultural competency as a career-long and lifelong process. It is worth the time and effort to be a culturally competent occupational therapist or occupational therapy assistant. Knowledge of and sensitivity to culture and socioeconomic status are essential to the success of the occupational therapy process in prevention and health promotion as well as rehabilitation. Furthermore, it is an expectation supported by the profession's core values and attitudes (AOTA, 1993), the Code of Ethics (AOTA, 2005), and *Nondiscrimination and Inclusion Regarding Members of the Occupational Therapy Community* (AOTA, 2004).

The Importance of Culture and Socioeconomic Status in Health and Health Care

The professional culture of occupational therapy holds that individuals should identify goals that are meaningful to them and that the therapist's interventions should be client-centered, assisting the individual to accomplish those goals (AOTA, 2008). By definition, culture influences individual and group values, beliefs, and behaviors. It is inevitable that understanding the culture of the individual or group is central to intervention. The hope is that understanding and incorporating those beliefs will improve outcomes of care. Although this remains to be validated through careful outcomes research, there is certainly a growing body of literature to suggest that it is true.

Given demographic trends in the United States, it is challenging to understand culture and incorporate it into preventive and health promotion interventions. The United States has long been a magnet for immigrants from around the world and has undergone and continues to undergo dramatic demographic change (U.S. Department of Commerce, 1999). It is estimated that by 2070, the population will be more than 50% nonwhite, with African Americans and Hispanics making up the largest proportion of the "minority" community. The population of individuals from Asia is also growing rapidly, representing a wide range of Far Eastern cultures (U.S. Census Bureau, 2000).

In the past decade, there has been growing awareness that culture and socioeconomic status have profound impact on health and health care. In its summary review of the literature about health and health care in the United States, the Institute of Medicine (Smedley et al., 2003) found repeated examples of increased health risk for individuals from minority and disadvantaged groups. Among disease differentials reported were rates of diabetes, high blood pressure and its accompanying sequelae, substance abuse, and some cancers. Similarly, access to and outcomes of care are worse for individuals from minority and socioeconomically disadvantaged communities. Such individuals received less effective pain management, fewer heart bypass procedures, fewer organ transplants, and more frequent limb amputations. All of these have consequences for subsequent occupational health, including employment, leisure activities, and ability to manage independent living.

While these data are sobering, it is important to avoid a deficit model of culture and socioeconomic status. Therapists sometimes assume deficits where none exist or inaccurately expect clients from lower socioeconomic circumstances to be less capable or more impaired than those from higher socioeconomic situations (Gajdosik & Campbell, 1991; von Zuben, Crist, & Mayberry, 1991). Given the tendency to focus on health disparities, it is important to recognize that culture often enhances aspects of function, health, and life satisfaction.

As one example, in African American communities, families feel a strong sense of obligation to care for their elderly family members (Pickett-Schenk, 2002). That care is reinforced through strong affiliation with churches, which serve as community centers, and, to some extent, social service agencies. The same is true for the influences of socioeconomic status. It is not always the case that more money equals happiness or enhanced occupational satisfaction. Several years ago, the author had a conversation with an elderly African American woman living in government-subsidized housing. After a lifetime as a housekeeper, she reported taking great pleasure in the steady (although tiny) income she received from Social Security and the opportunity to do just what she wanted to do.

Cultural and Socioeconomic Factors and Occupation

Human behavior reflects a complex interaction of cultural, socioeconomic, biological, and environmental circumstances. In many situations, this interaction is difficult to untangle. Yet the impact of this maze of factors has significant implications for engagement in occupation and for occupational therapy interventions.

An example is the emerging dilemma of Mayan families (Burns, 1993). Individuals of Mayan background tend to be of very slight stature. As a result of modest improvements in socioeconomic status, pregnant women and young children have had access to improved diets. Many Mayan children now tower over their parents. Mayan women often carry their infants in fabric slings on their backs; infants are now so much larger than a generation ago that it is exceedingly difficult for mothers to continue this for as long as was previously the case. Toddlers have become so large that their petite parents have difficulty lifting, carrying, bathing, and dressing them. In Mayan culture, respect for elders has been a central factor for generations. Now that Mayan children are taller than their parents, discipline is more difficult and respect for elders less accepted. Thus a socioeconomic change altered a biological characteristic with significant consequences for culture and for occupational performance.

An occupational therapist working with parents in this situation would have to help them find new ways to manage childcare and impose discipline. However, many Mayan mothers were raised in traditional circumstances.

One of the cultural values imposed in their childhood experiences was the importance of adhering to tradition. Thus, preventive interventions would require recognizing the challenge to traditional patterns of behavior and parents' needs for information about managing childcare and disciplinary tasks in the context of cultural beliefs.

It is important to note that increasingly, the clients for occupational therapy services are communities, not just individuals or small groups. Occupational therapists may assist in enhancing environmental characteristics of a neighborhood or providing community-focused educational interventions to enhance occupational performance. In these situations, too, understanding of the culture and socioeconomic characteristics of the community can be important to framing interventions and ensuring successful outcomes. Community ownership of programs is vital to such intervention efforts (Baker & Brownson, 1998; Bracht et al., 1994).

In examining the lives and occupational patterns of their clients, occupational therapists and occupational therapy assistants must be aware of the interaction of biological, personality, cultural, and socioeconomic status. This complex interaction means that simply learning "facts" about cultures is not sufficient to ensure culturally sensitive care. Occupational therapy practitioners must recognize the ways in which culture and socioeconomic status affect lives and behaviors, and the ways in which individual characteristics and experiences interact with culture, either to support or inhibit satisfactory accomplishment of occupations.

Lifestyle

Lifestyle choices are strongly influenced by cultural values and beliefs. Culture and socioeconomic factors affect, among many other decisions, whether or not to marry, how to raise children, vocational plans, attitudes and behaviors toward family members and the community, and engagement in religious and spiritual activities. Examples abound in the global news. In Afghanistan under the Taliban, women's roles were circumscribed such that they were not permitted to work or to be in public places unless entirely covered by a burka. The removal of the Taliban government from power meant that the laws restricting women's behaviors were liberalized; cultural expectations have lagged somewhat, such that many women still choose (for a variety of reasons) to appear in public only when clothed in a burka. This is an extreme example of cultural influence on behavior.

There are less dramatic examples in cultural groups within the United States, often defined by religious affiliation. For instance, certain groups or communities believe that women should remain in the home to raise their children, should not use birth control, and should dress in "modest" clothing. While not carrying force of law, these groups' cultural expectations hold considerable power in influencing women's lifestyle choices. In Amish communities, failure to behave as prescribed by community rules can lead to shunning by everyone in the community (Nolt, 1992). Fear of such punishment is a powerful incentive to behave in culturally appropriate ways.

Construction of Illness/Disability

Culture also influences beliefs about health, illness, and disability. Kleinman, Eisenberg, and Goode (1978) indicated that individuals and groups have **explanatory models**—that is, culturally mediated constructions of what constitutes health, what causes illness, and what would lead to cure. Western health care promotes a biological explanatory model that holds that health is the absence of disease, that disease is caused largely by microorganisms, and that pharmaceutical medicines can cure disease. It does not consider the role of optimism, spirituality, and other personal characteristics that have been shown to contribute to wellness and healing. Compare this to the "hot-cold" explanatory model prevalent in many Hispanic cultures (Loue, 1998) that suggests that health is the presence of an appropriate balance of hot and cold influences on the body, that hot and cold can be defined for various substances and occurrences, and that health can be regained by restoring balance. In this system, someone with abdominal distress might be encouraged to eat or drink substances defined as either hot or cold. Note that in this system, the labeling of substances as hot or cold is not based on the temperature but on some other aspect of the substance. So in one encounter in Guatemala, cortisone cream (a modern and unfamiliar substance) was labeled as hot when individuals using it were advised to stay out of the sun (Love, 1998).

Explanatory models also reflect beliefs about individual control over disease. Depending on cultural norms, individuals may feel that they can control their circumstances, a belief labeled **internal locus of control,** or they may feel that they are subject to uncontrollable external factors, a belief known as **external locus of control.** So in some Hispanic cultures, individuals believe that illness is the will of God and must therefore be cured by God rather than by taking medicine. Chinese individuals may believe that the patient's role is passive and dependent (Jang, 1995). Occupational therapy tends toward emphasis on individual control. This belief can lead to conflict and poor outcomes when the client is more inclined toward external locus of control. It may also understate the effects of real external forces, such as public policy and environmental constraints.

It is important to recognize that everyone has an explanatory model for illness and that Western medicine does not possess all the answers to ensuring good health. Think about your own beliefs about illness. Did your mother teach you that going outside with wet hair can cause a cold? Science has disproved this, but you may still be hesitant to go out with wet hair. In addition, there is evidence that expectations about treatment have a powerful effect on its outcome. Consider the impact of placebo surgery to treat knee problems (Bernstein & Quach, 2003), which was found to be as effective as real surgery in leading to reductions in knee pain and improvement in function.

Culturally mediated explanatory models influence health-related behaviors just as they do behaviors in other spheres of life. Beliefs about effective treatment may affect choices about seeking care. In many cultures, herbal remedies and traditional healers are perceived as the first line of intervention for illness. Only when those are unsuccessful will some individuals seek care by Western practitioners. Thus, a Chinese woman might first turn to the local herbalist, then to an acupuncturist, and only then to a Western physician.

Socioeconomic status affects choices about health care as well. Individuals living in impoverished circumstances may be unable to afford visits to physicians or the medications prescribed. They may be compelled to wait until a health condition has become an emergency before seeking care. Preventive interventions might be cheaper for society as a whole, but for individuals without financial resources, these interventions might be impossible. Even advice about diet must be tempered by the realities of poverty. Some poor neighborhoods do not have grocery stores with fresh produce. Residents who are too poor to own and maintain cars for easy transportation may be forced to purchase whatever food is available at the local convenience store, typically at prices higher than in surrounding affluent neighborhoods.

Culture and Occupation

As has already been noted, culture and socioeconomic status affect lifestyle choices. A significant characteristic of lifestyle is an individual's constellation of occupational choices. The *Framework* (AOTA, 2008) notes that occupational choice is predicated on the contexts (including culture) in which activities occur, the demands of the activity, and the characteristics of the individual. All these factors affect occupation in all areas, including activities of daily living (ADLs), instrumental activities of daily living (IADLs), education, work, play, leisure, and social participation. Further, culture and socioeconomic status influence performance patterns and performance skills.

Activity Demands

Demands of activities are mediated by socioeconomic and cultural variables. In some rural, impoverished communities (e.g., in rural Appalachia), the process of acquiring an education might be constructed to mean attending public school until age 16, when law permits withdrawal. In a middle-class suburban neighborhood, education might mean completion of an undergraduate college degree in a state-funded college or university. In an affluent suburban neighborhood, education might mean undergraduate and graduate degrees from high-status universities.

Context and Client Factors

Context for activity includes the physical and social environment. The physical environment is shaped to some extent by nature but also by humans with particular cultural values and socioeconomic resources. So, for example, a culture in which communal activities are highly valued would probably build homes conducive to easy access and in close proximity to one another. In an individualistic culture, homes might be more widely spaced, perhaps with gated access. These choices about home construction are culturally mediated and then affect a variety of interactions in the community thereafter. One elderly grandmother with whom the author is acquainted blamed the rise in youth crime to the demise of the front porch. She believed that when family outdoor activity turned to the backyard, neighborhoods lost a natural source of "neighborhood watch."

Characteristics of the individual (client factors) interact with cultural and socioeconomic factors (context) to lead to unique occupational choices. For example, in almost every culture, gender-appropriate roles are culturally defined. And yet, even when those roles are quite rigid, the personal characteristics of the individual woman will affect the way in which occupations are selected and enacted. Under the Taliban, some women in Afghanistan continued to find ways to acquire an education and to work at vocations they valued, such as health care or teaching, in spite of the possible dire consequences should their activities be discovered. In the United States, women whose cultures promote their role as homemakers and mothers may establish small businesses selling products at house parties or may demonstrate their leadership and organizational skills in their children's school organizations or in community volunteer settings.

Areas of Occupation

Activities of daily living (ADLs) are an example of performance areas of occupation that are clearly influenced by cultural and socioeconomic factors. Ability to afford skin care and grooming products, expectations about appropriate dress, access to particular food ingredients, complexity of finances and perceptions about gender roles in managing money are all examples of the ways in which self-care can differ among groups. Likewise, in making work choices, access to education and transportation, gender roles, and other culturally and socioeconomically mediated factors have substantial influence. In an excellent summary of the challenges facing young people in impoverished inner-city neighborhoods as they attempt to find work and move up the social ladder, Newman and Newman (1999) describes the ways in which cultural expectations can become an added impediment. The young people she describes lack role models who had successful careers by majority U.S. cultural standards. They battled expectations of the majority culture that they were lazy and unmotivated. Such influences affect all areas, including play, leisure, and social participation.

An often-overlooked performance area is religious observance. There is considerable evidence that for some racial or ethnic groups, religion is a central focus of life and activities (cf., Swanson, Crowther, Green, & Armstrong, 2004). Participation in religious ceremonies, attendance at worship services, and other religious activities can provide meaning to life and motivation in other areas. For some individuals, every area incorporates a religious element, so ADLs (dress in particular), work, and leisure choices all reflect religious influence.

Performance Patterns

The influence of culture and socioeconomic status on performance patterns has been well documented. In the movie *Bowling for Columbine,* Michael Moore (2002) movingly demonstrated how working individuals in impoverished neighborhoods routinely traveled several hours each way by public transportation to get their children to day care and then to their minimum-wage jobs in the suburbs. This kind of pattern is imposed by both cultural (segregation) and socioeconomic (inadequate funds to purchase and maintain a car) factors.

Performance Skills

The interaction of culture, socioeconomic status, and performance skills is perhaps more surprising. Performance skills and motor, process, and communication skills are largely characteristics of the individual. Motor and process skills are mediated largely by the central nervous system and might, therefore, be considered to be more individual than cultural or socioeconomic factors. Yet children living in poverty have high rates of lead poisoning, which causes neurological damage (Canfield et al., 2003). Consequently, such children might have impairments in both motor and process skills. There is also evidence that culture affects neurological development. Chinese individuals, whose written language is pictographic, perceive stimuli in the environment more globally than individuals from Western countries (Yoon, Hasher, Feinberg, Rahhal, & Winocur, 2000). This is believed to be a consequence of brain plasticity leading to differential development in the presence of differential environmental stimuli.

Occupational Therapy in the Promotion of Health and Wellness: Cultural and Socioeconomic Considerations

The goal of prevention in occupational therapy is avoidance of dysfunction in occupations that clients need and want to accomplish. In the case of prevention and wellness, the key question is: How can occupations of individuals and communities best be supported to avoid dysfunction and promote wellness? As with other forms of occupational therapy intervention, the process involves evaluation, intervention, and examination of outcomes (AOTA, 2008).

At each step of the process, cultural and socioeconomic factors must be addressed. In evaluation, consideration must be given to the kinds of instruments used and their applicability to individuals from various cultural or socioeconomic groups. Too often, standardized instruments ignore culture, giving an inaccurate picture of the strengths, needs, and goals of the individual (Paul, 1995). Likewise, economic resources are often overlooked. Among the relevant issues that are culturally or economically mediated, therapists should consider the following:

- What language is spoken?
- How is information conveyed and shared?
- What beliefs does the client hold about health and wellbeing? What do these constructs mean to him or her?
- In what ways are daily activities affected by cultural or economic circumstances?
- What is the nature of family and neighborhood interaction in the community?
- What is the person's gender role and age-related expectations?
- Who makes decisions for the person? A family elder? The male leader of the family? The individual?

- Are there traditional customs that influence community members' choices about interacting with Western health care?
- What are the individual's beliefs about education, work, and appropriate leisure activities?
- Does the cultural background of the individual or community include a spiritual or religious component that must be considered in promoting wellness?

The answers to these questions are all dependent on particular cultural influences. The beliefs of an individual in an inner-city Puerto Rican neighborhood will differ greatly from those of a more acculturated Mexican American individual. African Americans whose families have lived in the United States for many generations will be quite different from recent Somali refugees.

Unless the appropriate information is obtained during evaluation, intervention options cannot be appropriately identified. The emphasis on client-centered intervention in occupational therapy (AOTA, 2008) is not possible unless the client's strengths, needs, and self-identified goals are well understood.

Given the complexity of the individual, cultural, and socioeconomic factors that affect occupation and occupational choice, how can occupational therapists ensure that they gather the right information and apply it correctly to intervention? It is impossible to know everything about particular cultures and to determine all the members of that group, and even if it were possible, individual characteristics and experiences would lead each person to express cultural values and beliefs differently.

Perhaps the most helpful strategy is an inquiry-based approach to evaluation (Bonder et al., 2002). An inquiry-based approach uses ethnographic principles that encourage respectful questioning and careful observation. While it is helpful to have a fund of cultural knowledge that might guide initial and follow-up questions, genuine understanding of the individual must be based on that person's responses rather than on stereotypical descriptions of cultural groups.

Such thoughtful questioning and interpretation can yield significant benefits. As an example, one local chapter of the Alzheimer's Association developed support groups as a way to prevent excessive stress, and thereby illness, among family caregivers. However, as the service was instituted, staff noted that the majority of the families using its services were white, although the chapter was located near a large African American community. After puzzling over this for a while, one staff member read about African American culture and found that churches were described as central to community life (Swanson et al., 2004). Based on this fact, the staff person went to talk with the minister at one of the African American churches. It quickly became apparent that the church was indeed a community center for that African American community, and the minister was an important opinion leader. The staff spent time getting to know him and, through him, other community leaders. These conversations made clear to the staff that both the nature of the programs and the outreach strategies had to be changed for these communities. When the Alzheimer's Association support groups were moved to church meeting rooms and members of church leadership were present for the first several meetings, residents of the community felt much more comfortable about participating. In addition, the minister announced the groups on Sundays. These modifications made a tremendous difference in the reception of the programs in that community.

As another example, thoughtful design of environments can support cultural values and thereby provide tremendous benefits in preventing occupational dysfunction. In communities where child-raising is perceived as a community function, with close interaction among neighbors and family members, high-rise apartments with little green space can serve as a barrier to effective childcare. The resulting isolation can lead to depression for parents robbed of support networks and grandparents deprived of regular contact with grandchildren. Children lose opportunities for support from an array of adults and valuable opportunities to observe role models. Adding communal areas can support traditional values about childrearing and reduce parental stress.

Several health promotion programs that incorporate cultural elements or the social context are described in the occupational literature. Rebeiro and colleagues (2001) describe the Northern Initiative for Social Action (NISA), a consumer-run, occupation-based organization located in northeastern Ontario, Canada. Its goal is to promote participation in personally meaningful and socially valued occupations for individuals with mental illness living in the community. Thus, it is a tertiary prevention program, designed to prevent relapse and to encourage continuing health for individuals already diagnosed with a disorder. Qualitative measures of outcome suggest that the program met participants' needs for belonging.

Another example described by Frank and colleagues (2001) is a program called "New Stories/New Cultures." This is an activity-based, after-school enrichment program for students in low-income neighborhoods with large populations of African American and Hispanic American residents. The students were more likely to feel they were building skills when they were engaged in activities that were challenging and enjoyable. They term their approach a "direct cultural intervention."

Finally, DeMars (1992) describes a community health promotion intervention for Native American children and adults in Canada. The program focused on preserving the participants' ethnic heritage. Participant feedback led to modifications of the program, which was perceived as helpful in promoting wellness and life skills.

Conclusion

Effective occupational therapy intervention requires an understanding of the client's needs and wishes. Those needs and wishes are mediated by the client's personal characteristics and by his or her cultural and socioeconomic circumstances. As is true of personality and biological characteristics, the individual's cultural experiences are highly idiosyncratic, even though culture is a group phenomenon. Likewise, socioeconomic factors are interpreted differently by individuals. Thus, recommendations to incorporate cultural and socioeconomic factors into evaluation and intervention require complex skills on the part of the therapist. Acquisition of these skills is an ongoing process. Professionals who make the effort to understand their clients in the context of their cultural and socioeconomic situations are likely to find both the process and outcomes of intervention to be greatly improved.

Culture and socioeconomic status are realities of life and have significant impact on access to occupations, occupational preferences, and enactment of occupations. Thus, they are important factors in developing effective occupational therapy interventions. Occupational therapy professionals can draw upon the strengths conferred by cultural values and beliefs and can prevent occupational dysfunction by incorporating those values and beliefs in the intervention process. Townsend and Wilcock emphasize this point: "Humans are occupational beings. Their existence depends on enablement of diverse opportunities and resources for participation in culturally-defined and health-building occupations" (Townsend & Wilcock, 2004, p. 76).

▶ For Discussion and Review

1. How would you describe your own cultural influences? In what ways do they differ from your parents'?
2. What beliefs and values have you been taught as you learn to become an occupational therapist?
3. In what ways do you think your classmates and instructors share your values and beliefs? In what ways do you think they differ? How could you find out if your perceptions of their values and beliefs are accurate?

4. Reflecting on your experiences so far in working with clients or patients, what incidents have you seen in which you thought culture or socioeconomic status were factors? How did you or the therapist address them? What might you or the therapist have done differently?

5. Have you ever been misunderstood because of cultural or socioeconomic differences? What do you wish you or those with whom you were interacting might have done differently?

▶ Research Questions

Research related to occupational therapy interventions that appropriately incorporate cultural and socioeconomic factors in prevention and health promotion is sparse, with many questions yet to be answered.

1. Describe the occupational beliefs, patterns, and barriers to participation for various communities (cf., Lau, Chi, & McKenna, 1998; Piskur, Kinebanian, & Josephsson, 2002).

2. Identify effective research strategies for evaluating the success of culturally sensitive prevention efforts.

3. Describe intervention strategies for working with individuals from various cultural backgrounds.

4. Examine outcomes of intervention strategies in terms of increased self-esteem, increased participation, reduced disability, and other important health and wellness outcomes.

5. Swanson and colleagues (2004) suggest that in African American communities, churches can play a major role in providing health information and encouraging healthy behaviors. Among the many research questions they pose is: What models best describe the role of religious organizations in promoting healthy communities?

References

Alvord, L. A., & Van Pelt, E. C. (1999). *The scalpel and the silver bear.* New York: Bantam Books.

American Occupational Therapy Association. (1993). Core values statement and attitudes of occupational therapy practice. *American Journal of Occupational Therapy, 47,* 1085–86.

American Occupational Therapy Association. (2004). Occupational therapy's commitment to nondiscrimination and inclusion. *American Journal of Occupational Therapy, 58,* 668.

American Occupational Therapy Association. (2005). Occupational therapy code of ethics. *American Journal of Occupational Therapy, 59*(6), 639–42.

American Occupational Therapy Association. (2008). Occupational therapy practice framework: Domain and process

(2d ed.). *American Journal of Occupational Therapy, 62,* 625–83.

Arnason, E., Sigurgislason, H., & Benedikz, E. (2000). Genetic homogeneity of Icelanders: Fact or fiction? *Nature Genetics, 25,* 373–74.

Association of Professional Chaplains, Association for Clinical Pastoral Education, Canadian Association for Pastoral Practice and Education, National Association of Catholic Chaplains, and National Association of Jewish Chaplains. (2001). A white paper. Professional chaplaincy: Its role and importance in healthcare. *Journal of Pastoral Care, 55,* 81–97.

Baker, E. A., & Brownson, C. A. (1998). Defining characteristics of community-based health promotion programs. *Journal of Public Health Management and Practice, 4*(2), 1–9.

Baptiste, S. (1988). Murial Driver Memorial Lecture: Chronic pain, activity, and culture. *Canadian Journal of Occupational Therapy, 55,* 179–84.

Barney, K. F. (1991). From Ellis Island to assisted living: Meeting the needs of older adults from diverse cultures. *American Journal of Occupational Therapy, 45,* 586–93.

Beauregard, C., & Solomon, P. (2005). Understanding the experience of HIV/AIDS for women: Implications for occupational therapists. *Canadian Journal of Occupational Therapy, 72,* 113–20.

Belcham, C. (2004). Spirituality in occupational therapy: Theory in practice? *British Journal of Occupational Therapy, 67*(1), 39–46.

Bernstein, J., & Quach, T. (2003). Questioning the value of arthroscopic knee surgery for osteoarthritis. *Cleveland Clinic Journal of Medicine, 70,* 401–07.

Bonder, B. R., Martin, L., & Miracle, A. (2002). *Culture in clinical care.* Thorofare, NJ: SLACK.

Bonder, B. R., Martin, L., & Miracle, A. (2004). Culture emergent in occupation. *American Journal of Occupational Therapy, 58,* 159–68.

Bowman, O. J., & Wallace, B. A. (1990). The effects of socioeconomic status on hand size and strength, vestibular function, visuomotor integration, and praxis in preschool children. *American Journal of Occupational Therapy, 44,* 610–21.

Bracht, N., Finnegan, J. R., Rissel, C., Weisbrod, R., Gleason, J., Corbett, J., & Veblen-Mortenson, S. (1994). Community ownership and program continuation following a health demonstration project. *Health Education Research, 9,* 243–55.

Burns, A. F. (1993). *Maya in exile: Guatemalans in Florida.* Philadelphia: Temple University Press.

Canadian Association of Occupational Therapists (1997; 2002). *Enabling occupation: An occupational therapy perspective* (Rev. ed.). Ottawa, ON: CAOT Publications ACE.

Canfield, R. L., Henderson, C. R., Cory Slechta, D. A., Cox, C., Jusko, T. A., & Lanphear, B. P. (2003). Intellectual impairment in children with blood lead concentrations below 10μg per deciliter. *New England Journal of Medicine, 348,* 1517–26.

Christiansen, C., & Baum, C. (1997). Person-environment occupational performance: A conceptual model for practice. In C. Christiansen & C. Baum (Eds.), *Occupational therapy: Enabling function and well-being* (2d ed., pp. 47–70). Thorofare, NJ: SLACK.

Collins, J. S., Paul, S., & West-Frasier, J. (2001). The utilization of spirituality in occupational therapy: Beliefs, practices, and perceived barriers. *Occupational Therapy in Health Care, 14*(3/4), 73–92.

DeMars, P. A. (1992). An occupational therapy life skills curriculum model for a Native American tribe: A health promotion program based on ethnographic field research. *American Journal of Occupational Therapy, 46,* 727–36.

Dillard, M., Andonian, L., Flores, O., Lai, L., MacRae, A., & Shakir, M. (1992). Culturally competent occupational therapy in a diversely populated mental health setting. *American Journal of Occupational Therapy, 46,* 721–26.

Dunton, W. R. (1915). *Occupational therapy: A manual for nurses.* Philadelphia: Saunders.

Fadiman, A. (1997). *The spirit catches you and you fall down.* New York: Noonday Press.

Fitzgerald, M. H., Mullavey-O'Byrne, C., & Clemson, L. (1997). Cultural issues from practice. *Australian Journal of Occupational Therapy, 44,* 1–21.

Frank, G., Fishman, M., Crowley, C., Blair, B., Murphy, S. T., Montoya, J. A., Hickey, M. P., Brancaccio, M. V., & Bensimon, E. M. (2001). The new stories/new cultures after-school enrichment program: A direct cultural intervention. *American Journal of Occupational Therapy, 55,* 501–08.

Frey, B. B., Daaleman, T. P., & Peyton, V. (2005). Measuring a dimension of spirituality for health research: Validity of the Spirituality Index of Well-Being. *Research on Aging, 27,* 556–77.

Gajdosik, C. G., & Campbell, S. (1991). Effects of weekly review, socioeconomic status, and maternal belief on mothers' compliance with their disabled children's home exercise program. *Physical and Occupational Therapy in Pediatrics, 11*(2), 47–65.

Hakansson, C., Svartivk, L., Lidfeldt, J., Nerbrand, C., Samsioe, G., Schersten, B., & Nilsson, P. M. (2003). Self-rated health in middle-aged women: Associations with sense of coherence and socioeconomic and health-related factors. *Scandinavian Journal of Occupational Therapy, 10,* 99–106.

hyperdictionary. (2005a). *Religion.* Retrieved January 6, 2005, from http://www.hyperdictionary.com/dictionary/religion.

hyperdictionary. (2005b). *Spirituality.* Retrieved January 6, 2005, from http://www.hyperdictionary.com/dictionary/spirituality.

Iwama, M. K. (2004). Revisiting culture in occupational therapy: A meaningful endeavor. *OTJR: Occupation, Participation, and Health, 24,* 2–3.

Jang, Y. (1995). Chinese culture and occupational therapy. *British Journal of Occupational Therapy, 58,* 103–06.

Kleinman, A. M., Eisenberg, L., & Good, B. (1978). Culture, illness, and care. *Annals of Internal Medicine, 88,* 251–58.

Krieger, N., Williams, D. R., & Moss, N. E. (1997). Measuring social class in U.S. public health research: Concepts, methodologies, and guidelines. *Annual Review of Public Health, 18,* 341–78.

Krusen, N. (2003, June 5). *The occupational adaptation process during the transition from student to practitioner,* presented at AOTA Institute 05, Exploring Adaptation: An Occupational, Contextual, and Intrapersonal Process in Occupational Therapy, Texas Women's University.

Kuper, A. (1999). *Culture: The anthropologists' account.* Cambridge, MA: Harvard University Press.

Lau, A., Chi, I., & McKenna, K. (1998). Self-perceived quality of life of Chinese elderly people in Hong Kong. *Occupational Therapy International, 5,* 118–39.

Levine, R. E. (1984). The cultural aspects of home care delivery. *American Journal of Occupational Therapy, 38,* 734–38.

Loue, S. (Ed.). (1998). *Handbook of immigrant health.* New York: Plenum Press.

Mayers, C. A. (2004). Towards understanding spirituality. *British Journal of Occupational Therapy, 67,* 191.

McColl, M. A. (2003). *Spirituality and occupational therapy.* Ottawa, ON: Canadian Association of Occupational Therapists Publications, ACE.

Mills, C. W. (1958/2005). The structure of power in American society. In T. M. Shapiro (Ed.), *Great divides: Readings in social inequality in the United States* (3d ed., pp. 139–46). New York: McGraw-Hill.

Moore, M. (Writer/Director). (2002). *Bowling for Columbine* [Motion picture]. United States: Metro-Goldwyn-Mayer.

National Research Council. (1997). *Racial and ethnic differences in the health of older Americans.* Washington, DC: Author.

Newman, B. M., & Newman, P. R. (1999). *Development through life: A psychosocial approach* (7th ed.). Belmont, CA: Wadsworth.

Nolt, S. M. (1992). *A history of the Amish.* Intercourse, PA: Good Books.

Paul, S. (1995). Culture and its influence on occupational therapy evaluation. *Canadian Journal of Occupational Therapy, 62,* 154–61.

Phillips, I. (2003). Infusing spirituality into geriatric health care: Practical applications from the literature. *Topics in Geriatric Rehabilitation, 19,* 249–56.

Pickett-Schenk, S. A. (2002). Church-based support groups for African-American families coping with mental illness: Outreach and outcomes. *Psychiatric Rehabilitation Journal, 26,* 173–86.

Piskur, B., Kinebanian, A., & Josephsson, S. (2002). Occupation and well-being: A study of some Slovenian people's experiences of engagement in occupation in relation to well-being. *Scandinavian Journal of Occupational Therapy, 9*(2), 63–70.

Rebeiro, K. L., Day, D. G., Semeniuk, B., O'Brien, M. C., & Wilson, B. (2001). Northern Initiative for Social Action: An occupation-based mental health program. *American Journal of Occupational Therapy, 55,* 493–500.

Rippentrop, A. E., (2005). A review of the role of religion and spirituality in chronic pain populations. *Rehabilitation Psychology, 50,* 278–84.

Rivera-Mosquera, E. T. (2005). Differential predictors of substance abuse outcome in African American and white populations (Ohio). *Dissertation Abstracts International: Section B: The Sciences and Engineering, 65*(8-B), 3169.

Sacks, O. (1989). *Seeing voices: A journey into the world of the deaf.* Berkeley: University of California Press.

Schulz, E. K. (2004). Spirituality and disability: An analysis of select themes. *Occupational Therapy in Health Care, 18*(4), 57–83.

Smedley, B. D., Stith, A. Y., & Nelson, A. R. (Eds.) (2003). *Unequal treatment: Confronting racial and ethnic disparities in health care.* Washington, DC: Institute of Medicine.

Swanson, L., Crowther, M., Green, L., & Armstrong, T. (2004). African Americans, faith and health disparities. *African American Research Perspectives, 10*(1), 79–88.

Tedlock, D., & Mannheim, B. (1995). Introduction. In D. Tedlock & B. Mannheim (Eds.), *The dialogic emergence of culture* (pp. 1–32). Urbana, IL: University of Illinois Press.

Townsend, E. (1997). Inclusiveness: A community dimension of spirituality. *Canadian Journal of Occupational Therapy, 64,* 146–55.

Townsend, E., De Laat, D., Egan, M., Thibeault, R., & Wright, W. A. (1999). *Spirituality in enabling occupation: A learner-centered workbook.* Ottawa, ON: Canadian Association of Occupational Therapists Publications, ACE.

Townsend, E., & Wilcock, A. A. (2004). Occupational justice and client-centered practice: A dialogue in progress. *Canadian Journal of Occupational Therapy, 71*(2), 75–86.

Udell, L., & Chandler, C. (2000). The role of the occupational therapist in addressing the spiritual needs of clients. *British Journal of Occupational Therapy, 63,* 489–94.

U.S. Census Bureau. (2000). *2000 Census of Population, Public Law 94-171 Redistricting Data File.* Retrieved January 6, 2005, from http://factfinder.census.gov.

U.S. Department of Commerce. (1999). *The emerging minority marketplace.* Washington, DC: Author.

U.S. Department of Health and Human Services, Office of the Secretary. (2000). National standards on culturally and linguistically appropriate services (CLAS) in health care. *Federal Register, 65*(247), 80865–80879.

von Zuben, M. V., Crist, P. A., & Mayberry, W. (1991). A pilot study of differences in play behavior between children of low and middle socioeconomic status. *American Journal of Occupational Therapy, 45,* 113–18.

Wang, V. O., & Sue, S. (2005). In the eye of the storm: Race and genomics in research and practice. *American Psychologist, 60,* 37–45.

Wicasa, W. (2005). *Explanation of star quilt.* Retrieved March 16, 2005, from http://www.bluecloud.org/18.html.

Wilding, C., May, E., & Muir-Cochrane, E. (2005). Experience of spirituality, mental illness and occupation: A life-sustaining phenomenon. *Australian Occupational Therapy Journal, 52,* 2–9.

Yoon, C., Hasher, L., Feinberg, F., Rahhal, T. A., & Winocur, G. (2000). Cross-cultural differences in memory: The role of culture-based stereotypes about aging. *Psychology of Aging, 15,* 694–704.

Chapter 6

Population Health: An Occupational Rationale

Ann A. Wilcock

> A human being is part of the whole, called by us "Universe," a part limited in time and space. He experiences himself, his thoughts and feelings as something separated from the rest—a kind of optical delusion of his consciousness. This delusion is a kind of prison for us, restricting us to our personal desires and to affection for a few persons nearest to us. Our task must be to free ourselves from this prison by widening our circle of compassion to embrace all living creatures and the whole of nature in its beauty.
>
> —Albert Einstein

Learning Objectives

This chapter is designed to enable the reader to:

- Articulate basic concepts of population health.
- Discuss the relationship between health and occupation.
- Identify occupational determinants of health.
- Describe five approaches to population health.
- Discuss the potential role of occupational therapy in population health.
- Describe how occupational science can inform population health interventions.

Key Terms

Community

Community development

Ecological public health

Ecological sustainability

Health

Health promotion

Occupation

Occupational justice

Population health

Preventive medicine

Social epidemiology

Wellness approach

Introduction

In this chapter, the rationale for taking an occupational approach to population health will be considered. Taking this approach is an important task for occupational therapy assistants and occupational therapists because of a close association between what people do and their health status. To get some idea of the scope of the work that needs to be done in this regard, the fundamental relationship between positive or negative health and what people do or are unable to do will be examined. This will lead to tracing the possible effects of underlying occupational determinants on health. This will highlight not only the evidence of the benefits of occupation that support occupational therapy's potential contribution to population health, but also the negative consequences of occupational deprivation, alienation, and imbalance.

Occupational deprivation, alienation, and imbalance could and should also be a focus of occupational therapy research and intervention. This assertion will be justified using the framework of occupational science and population health with reference to their impact on, or potential affiliation with, occupational therapy. The exploration is begun by defining both *occupation* and *population health* in current terms and clarifying how an occupation perspective might fit within, or extend the concept of, population health.

An Occupational Perspective of Population Health

Many authors have defined *occupation* in different ways. As it is used in this chapter, **occupation** is seen as central to the human experience in that it comprises all that people do in order to fulfill basic needs and meet social and environmental challenges across the sleep–wake continuum. It can be economically, socially, or politically driven, and it can be obligatory or self-chosen to meet individual needs, pleasures, and purposes. It draws on and develops people's potential so they can do, be, and become according to their physical, social, mental, or spiritual talent, interest, and opportunity (Wilcock, 1999). Potential for, and interest in, different occupations results from what individuals learn, particularly early in life, from natural, sociocultural, and familial environments together with genetically inherited capacities. At its most basic, occupation is the means by which individuals meet their innate biological needs and is therefore essential for survival (Wilcock, 1998). All these factors link it to people's health status when the World Health Organization (WHO) definition of *health* is taken literally.

In the WHO constitution (1948), **health** was defined as a "state of complete physical, social and mental wellbeing, and not merely the absence of disease or infirmity." In later WHO strategy documents, health has also been recognized as "a resource for everyday life, not the objective of living," and as "a positive concept emphasizing social and personal resources, as well as physical capacities" (WHO, 1986, p. 5).

The term **population health** is synonymous with public health. In *Health Promotion International,* Nutbeam (1998, p. 352) defines it as "the science and art of promoting health, preventing disease, and prolonging life through the organized efforts of society." He explains that while public health has long been associated with social and political interventions to improve the health of whole populations, what is described as the "new public health" has a broader focus. This is distinguished by efforts to understand determinants of health, such as lifestyles and living conditions, so these can be maintained or improved.

Another term commonly used in the field is **ecological public health,** which emphasizes the interconnections between health and sustainable development, as well as global environmental problems and the changing nature of ill-health (Nutbeam, 1998). It can be argued that it is the occupations of people that have, in large part, altered environments and that this trend continues without thought of ecological change or the health and wellbeing of future generations. With this understanding, an occupational approach can be justified in terms of population health, the new public health, and ecological public health.

Both the new public health and ecological public health have been informed by the WHO's push for "health for all" across the globe (1978). This initiative forecasts "the attainment by all the people of the world

of a level of health that will permit them to lead a socially and economically productive life" (WHO, 1984), thereby linking occupation as an outcome of health status. Other WHO documents demonstrate appreciation of causal and outcome links between occupation and health. For example, the *Ottawa Charter for Health Promotion (OCHP)* states that

> to reach a state of complete physical, mental and social wellbeing, an individual or group must be able to identify and to realize aspirations, to satisfy needs, and to change or cope with the environment. (WHO, 1986, p. 5)

It is through engagement in occupation that people realize aspirations, satisfy needs, and change or cope with the environment. If occupational therapy assistants and occupational therapists accept that those are appropriate targets for their intervention, the *OCHP* definition of **health promotion** as "the process of enabling people to increase control over, and to improve their health" (WHO, 1986, p. 2) clearly provides a mandate for them to become involved in predisease health promotion. So, too, does the *OCHP* call for all health professionals to "move increasingly in a health promotion direction" beyond "responsibility for providing clinical and curative services" (WHO, 1986, p. 4).

As the new vision of population health has taken shape, new disciplines have emerged to conduct research or intervene according to these new ways of thinking. One of the newer disciplines is **social epidemiology**—the study of population health and ill-health informed by "social, psychological, economic, and public policy information" (Nutbeam, 1998, p. 355). This new discipline has much in common with another of similar age—occupational science. Many of its researchers study aspects of the interaction between the health consequences of the what, whys, and hows of people's occupations, which includes social, psychological, economic, physical, and spiritual factors, as well as public policies.

In the 1960s and 1970s, and over the last decade, some occupational therapists took a population health perspective and began to write about researching the links between occupation and health. Leading the earlier movement were Wilma West, Florence Cromwell, and Geraldine Finn. They argued that the way forward for the profession was via health-promoting and preventive approaches (Cromwell, 1970; Finn, 1972; West, 1969). They suggested that such approaches would address the fundamental relationship of occupation to health, thus providing an alternative to occupational therapist's "intermittent treatment of acute disease and disability" (West, 1967, p. 312). The health model West proposed was centered on a balanced regime of age-appropriate, work-play activities for all people as well as client/community-centered practice that would enrich people's physical, mental, emotional, social, and vocational abilities. In that "new mould," she envisaged that occupational therapists would consider not only the biological causes of disease and dysfunction, but also the socioeconomic and cultural (West, 1970).

Cromwell (1970), too, argued for occupational therapists to move into the arena of preventive and "Well Care" programs because of their interest in work and play behavior in ordinary environments. She described that feature of the profession's work as a universal phenomenon of great importance to health. Similarly, Finn (1972, 1977), with an interest in primary prevention, argued that this type of health care is based on an understanding of the relationship between health and the basic structural elements of society. She proposed the development of a model of practice addressing occupation's significance to human life. The directions suggested by West, Cromwell, and Finn lay dormant for at least 20 years but are relevant to today's growing interest in population health. They are also relevant to some occupational therapists' interest in the need to understand more fully the fundamental nature and purpose of occupation, and the subsequent growth of the study of people as occupational beings, which is known as *occupational science.*

Finn described *occupational science* as, fundamentally, finding out about the significance of occupation to human life. Although controversial, it is seen by some as a foundation science for occupational therapy, as well as psychology, sociology, anthropology, anatomy, and physiology. Population health research aimed at understanding aspects of the relationship between occupation as a basic structural element of society and health is consistent with occupational science's philosophy and goals. This research would provide a framework and would extend notions about life skills; lifestyles; mental, spiritual, and socioeconomic issues; humans' need to engage with and in their worlds; opportunities and justice; and sustainable development. Some such population health research has already been carried out, and studies from other fields, such as anthropology, archaeology, and human geography can also inform health professionals seeking increased understanding of the relationship between occupation and health status.

The Relationship Between Health and Occupation

Occupation calls upon and allows expression of complex human characteristics and capacities that have enabled people to survive healthily and successfully as a species throughout time. These include characteristics unique to humans, such as bipedal gait and upright posture, which allow hands to engage freely in multiple occupations. Human hand function differs from other animals mainly because of an ability to oppose the thumb to fingers, which permits unprecedented dexterity. In addition, expansion of brain function allowed increased cognitive capacity, language, creativity, and conscious awareness of self (Bronowski, 1973; Campbell, 1988; Jones, Martin, & Pilbeam, 1992). Added to posture and "handiness" characteristics, these higher cortical capacities were and are major factors in the many different ways humans meet survival needs and affect their health status through engagement in occupation. As Ornstein and Sobel (1988) claim in *The Healing Brain,* it is the integrated functioning of mind and body that maintains health as the brain makes "countless adjustments" to preserve stability between "social worlds, our mental and emotional lives, and our internal physiology" (pp. 11–12).

Because people engage in occupation as part of their daily lives, it is also part of the process of health and healing. In public health research, it is more usual to study the negative associations than the positive. Paid employment is, arguably, the central type of occupation in Western capitalist economies. As a result, many researchers, including Brenner at Johns Hopkins University, have studied the effects of unemployment on health. Brenner's research, which covered more than 30 years of the mid-20th century, indicated that health is vulnerable to subtle economic fluctuations (1977; 1979). He calculated that if a 1% increase in unemployment was sustained for 6 years, it could be linked with over 4000 admissions to mental hospitals and to an increase of 36,887 deaths. Smith (1987) reported many studies in which apparent associations were found between unemployment and physical, mental, and social ill-health. Standardized questionnaires, for example, have consistently found links between unemployment and deterioration of mental health, suicide, and self-injury. In terms of physical health, associations have been made with respiratory disorders, diabetes, ischemic heart disease, medical consultation rates, and outpatient visits to physicians.

Academics, scientists, and others in intellectual employment are frequently overwhelmed or stressed by the "chaos of information pollution" (Naisbit, 1982). Indeed, the health benefits of paid employment appear to be dependent on work quality (Warr, 1985, 1987; Winefield & Tiggerman, 1991; Winefield, Tiggerman, & Winefield, 1992; Winefield, Tiggerman, Winefield, & Goldney, 1993). When work is boring, meaningless, stressful, or alienating, for example, the incidence of mass epidemics increases (Colligan & Murphy, 1979;

Justice, 1987). This research is but a minute representation of the field, but even that small sample poses the question whether paid employment is the only form of occupation that can have health consequences. This is far from the case, as shown in Content Box 6-1. This Harvard study by Glass and colleagues (1999) is worthy of replication and promulgation by occupational therapists.

The evidence supports that there is a definite relationship between what people do or do not do and their experience of health, although it may differ from person to person. This relationship poses another question as to whether occupation-based programs can be used to counteract any potential negative effects and to promote health. To answer that question, occupational therapists from the University of Southern California researched the connection between occupational therapy preventive programs and the health risks of older adults (Clark et al., 1997). A randomized controlled study of three groups living independently in community housing in Los Angeles showed benefits across health, function, and quality-of-life domains for participants engaged in a purpose-designed occupational therapy program. The program enabled participants to successfully employ occupation-based principles of healthy living and to appreciate and talk about how occupations affect health. A nontreatment group and a third group that was engaged in only social activity tended to decline in health over the study interval.

A link between different aspects of occupation and health is recognized by the WHO and by health-promotion experts, although the concept of occupation as an entity is yet to be fully understood. An example of the links that have been made includes the *OCHP* (WHO, 1986), which lists developing personal skills as one of five strategies to improve health. The other four strategies—to build healthy public policy, to create supportive environments, to strengthen community action, and to reorient health services toward health promotion—are also calls for action. Another WHO (1993) strategic document aimed at school health programs uses the term life skills in discussing abilities and behaviors that enable people to successfully meet the challenges of daily life.

Some writers in the field of population health also recognize links between occupation and health in the way they define it. For example, Kass (1981) defined health as a state of being revealed in activity, while Greiner, Fain, and Edelman (2002) saw physical, mental, and social functioning "that realizes a person's potential" as integral to health (p. 6). In addition, as early as 1955, the medical historian Sigerist maintained that work is essential to the maintenance of health, "because an organ that does not work atrophies and the mind that does not work becomes dumb" (pp. 254–55). Addition-

ally, he wrote, work balances and determines the rhythm of life, while providing meaning and significance.

Within the general population, too, there is appreciation of a connection between what people do and their wellbeing that cries out for a better understanding of how to maintain and improve health as part of normal lifestyles. A survey of 9000 adults across the United Kingdom revealed that while people describe health in many different ways, over 30% defined it for themselves in occupational terms (Blaxter, 1990). Many described it in terms of engagement in social, family, and community activity (see Content Box 6-2). Other occupational descriptors included the notion of health as being functionally able, alert, lively, physically or psychosocially fit, full of get-up-and-go, having energy, and engaging in healthy behavior.

As ideas about health and wellbeing differ between individuals, communities, professions, societies, and cultures, so, too, does engagement in occupation. Such ideas of engagement are integral to daily life and in large part result from underlying occupational determinants. A brief look at such determinants follows so that the nature and purpose of occupation can be considered more easily as either a negative or positive agent of health.

Content Box 6-1

Psychosocial Health Benefits of Activity

A 13-year randomized controlled trial of 2761 older male and female adults in the United States found that

social and productive activities (occupations) that involve little or no enhancement of fitness lower the risk of all causes of mortality as much as fitness activities do. This suggests that in addition to increased cardiopulmonary fitness, activity may confer survival benefits through psychosocial pathways. (Glass et al., 1999, pp. 478–83)

Content Box 6-2

Common Descriptions of Health

- Being able to do what you want to when you want to
- Being able to perform physically demanding work
- Working despite an advanced age (Blaxter, 1990, pp. 28–29)
- Being keen and interested
- Doing everything easily
- Feeling like conquering the world
- *Energy* and *vitality* were terms used to describe enthusiasm about work (Blaxter, 1990, pp. 25–27).

Underlying Occupational Determinants of Health

The author's historical research (Wilcock, 1998) led to the development of a figure that charts the negative and positive effects of the occupational determinants of health and ill-health, displayed in Figure 6-1. In this figure, occupational factors that underlie people's experiences of health or ill-health are listed as the type of economy, national policies and priorities, and widely held cultural values.

Such underlying determinants led to the establishment of particular types of institutions and activities at societal levels. These include what and how technology is applied within daily life; employment opportunities; and the division of labor, legal, commercial, and materialistic influences on fiscal policies and legislation. Also included are the hows and whats of media expression and freedoms; sport and recreation opportunities; social service provisions, such as pension or welfare schemes; and the types of health-care or educational services available to different segments of communities. Particu-

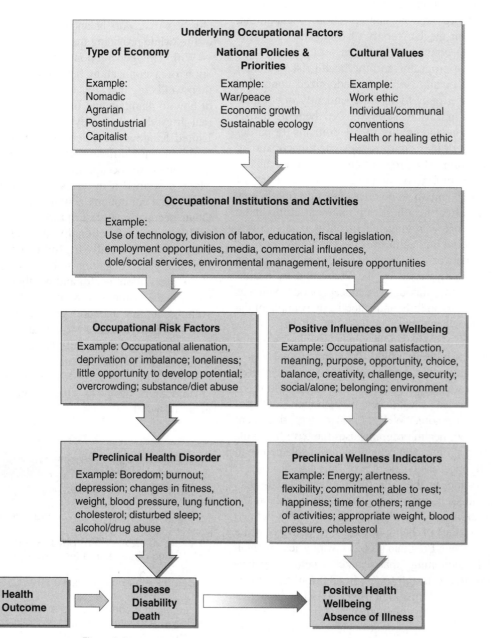

Figure 6-1 Occupational determinants of health and ill-health.

lar institutions and societal activities can result in opportunities or restrictions of occupational interests and capacities. Those, in turn, can lead to either positive influences on wellbeing or to risk factors that can negatively impact people's health in the longer term.

Risk factors might be those described as occupationally alienating or depriving (Wilcock, 1998); might result in an imbalance of, for example, too much or too little work; or might limit opportunities for social occupations and lead to loneliness. All can result in ongoing unresolved stress. As a result of such risk factors, the appearance of early preclinical health disorders can occur. These might well include changes to body weight, blood pressure, cholesterol, and levels of fitness. Additionally, liver, lung, and brain function may become disordered over a period of time, as secondary occupations involving substance abuse might be ways of coping with the stress of occupational dissatisfaction. Substance abuse occupations are common phenomena for those with illnesses such as schizophrenia when satisfaction through doing is restricted by the disease's symptoms. Substance abuse occupations are also common choices for people with too little or too much work or for those with unsatisfying jobs. In the latter case, Villarosa (1994) explained that "far too many of our people work in dangerous, unhealthy environments, enduring long hours, low pay, unfulfilling jobs, and unsanitary conditions" (p. 553). At the time Villarosa was writing, new cases of occupational disease were estimated at up to 350,000 each year in the United States. "For millions of others the toll is more subtle, but serious nonetheless: Quite literally, our jobs make us sick" (p. 566). Indeed, preclinical disorders can lead to full-blown disease, disability, and death. While the latter might appear to be an exaggeration, it is only necessary to consider the mortality statistics of unemployment studies (Smith, 1987) or the findings of the Harvard randomized-controlled trial of mortality in older people mentioned earlier (Glass, de Leon, Marottoli, & Berkman, 1999) to see that it is a hard reality.

At the other extreme are underlying factors and the institutions and activities they support that can be positive influences on health and wellbeing. These factors can provide ongoing challenges that meet the needs of individuals and communities and that provide potential opportunities for satisfaction, meaning, purpose, choice, belonging, sharing, socialness, and creativity. They can support occupations that are ecologically sustaining within environments that are accessible, beautiful, comfortable, just, and equitable. If that occurs, it is likely that so, too, will occupational indicators of wellness. These include expressions of energy and alertness, commitment and flexibility, time for others, a range of activities, openness to new challenges, and the

ability to take advantage of and enjoy adequate sleep and rest. In Western societies, the workplace can be particularly important in this regard. Stating the opposite case to the one given earlier, Villarosa explains, "For many of us, work can be profoundly rewarding and satisfying—even if we don't make a lot of money" (1994, p. 553). Individuals in rewarding employment contexts are likely to express or display happiness and contentment, to experience flow, and to have healthily appropriate height and weight ratios, blood pressure, cholesterol levels, and lung function. These by-products of a healthy work setting will further enhance the possibility of, or lead to, positive health, wellbeing, the absence of illness, and longer life expectancies (Glass et al., 1999).

Occupational Science and Population Health: Occupational Therapy Framework

Even from the limited sample of research cited above, it is possible to claim that engagement in occupation appears to benefit population health. Alternatively, it can also be claimed that occupation can be alienating or unbalanced and lead to negative health experiences. That is also the case when sociopolitical, cultural, or personal circumstances or factors result in occupational injustice or deprivation. There is a wealth of possibilities for the implementation of extensive, wide-ranging, and varied research studies. Such research would be best founded on the notion of people as occupational beings as a basic structural element of society, taking the ideas of West, Finn, and Cromwell forward into the 21st century and beyond.

Occupation-based research is necessary if occupational therapy assistants and occupational therapists are to have a legitimate role within population health. While a range of other disciplines have an interest in some aspects of occupation, and may well inform occupational science about health issues as well as population health, occupational therapy practitioners have the broadest knowledge of what occupation encompasses. For example, their concern with all that people do, why they do it, and how they feel about their experiences provides occupational therapists with the potential to consider health in terms of overall balance for communities and for individuals across the life span. This can enable positive health and occupational satisfaction as outcomes of intervention aimed at achieving a balance within daily, weekly, monthly, and yearly occupational needs and interests, across the sleep–wake continuum. It is the broad overview of what occupation encompasses that provides the particular perspective that occupational therapists can bring to population health. Beginning to show leadership in this direction in the United Kingdom, the College of Occupational Therapists adopted a definition that states, "Occupational therapy enables people to achieve health, wellbeing and life satisfaction through participation in occupation" (British College of Occupational Therapists, 2004, p. 7).

Although such definitions from national bodies are necessary to point the way forward, to become known as workers in the field of population health, at least some occupational therapists need to aim everyday practice toward positive health and wellbeing for the population at large. Others working in more traditional, medically related settings could expand wellness aspects of practice for clients with physical or mental dysfunction in line with the WHO's (2001) *International Classification of Functioning, Disability and Health (ICF)*.

The *ICF* has potential use as a tool for research, social policy, and education and is widely accepted by occupational therapists as a new way to consider disability. It also provides a strong link to population health in that it applies to everybody, not just people with medically based dysfunction. To advance a systematic discussion of occupational therapy practice in population health, the five approaches presented in *An Occupational Perspective of Health* (Wilcock, 1998)—wellness, preventive medicine, community development, occupational justice, and ecological sustainability—will be revisited (Fig. 6-2).

Wellness Approach

Within conventional medicine, the **wellness approach** is arguably closest to current occupational therapy practices. This approach is defined as "an active process through which individuals become aware of, and make choices toward a more successful existence" (Wilcock, 1998, p. 230). The wellness approach is closely aligned to the *OCHP* (WHO, 1986) call for health professionals to enable people to develop personal skills and explains that

> to reach a state of complete physical, mental, and social wellbeing, an individual or group must be able to identify and realize aspirations, to satisfy needs, and to change or cope with the environment. Health is, therefore, seen as a resource for everyday life, not the objective of living. (WHO, 1986, p. 2)

Occupational therapists are comfortable with the concept of people being enabled to identify, realize, and satisfy aspirations and needs, and in many regular

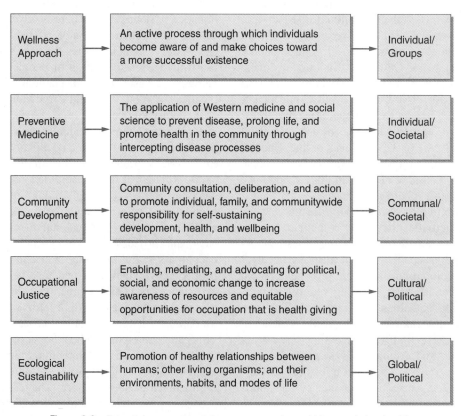

Figure 6-2 Potential occupational therapy approaches within population health.

practices, helping people with disability to change or cope with the environment is an everyday occurrence. Services based on these concepts could be extended to include the well population at large, at least in terms of consultative services and publications and the establishment of occupational health and wellness centers or clinics.

The concept of balance, too, fits the wellness approach and has been familiar within the profession's rhetoric since 1922, when Meyer advocated a balance between work, rest, play, and sleep in his seminal paper of a philosophy of occupational therapy. More recent balance rhetoric has, similarly, focused on the relationship between work (i.e., productivity), rest, and play (i.e., leisure) but has also included self-care (Canadian Association of Occupational Therapy [CAOT], 2002; Kielhofner, 2002; Reed & Sanderson, 1992; Rogers, 1984). The rhetoric reflects acceptance within occupational therapy that there is a balance of occupations that contributes to health and wellbeing (Christiansen & Baum, 1997), but a broadening of the concept of what balance may include is required for population research and practice. During the time when the notions of health promotion and wellness were gaining ground in Western societies, multidimensional aspects of balance began to emerge in which environment and culture were featured in discussion, along with work, play, and rest (Howard, 1983). These aspects of balance need studying with regard to population health. So, too, do other types of occupational balancing that might affect health, such as whether individuals or groups engage mainly in obligatory or self-chosen occupations; whether they are stressed by over- or underwork; or whether there is an imbalance between physical, mental, social, and rest occupations.

With a group of colleagues, Wilcock explored a representative sample of 146 South Australians to discover how they measured occupational balance in terms of physical, mental, social, and rest occupations against a self-rating of their health (Wilcock et al., 1997). Significantly, participants who reported their current balance to be closest to ideal balance also reported their health to be fair or excellent. The study was replicated with similar results by Lovelock and colleagues (2002) in four European countries with a sample of 200 people.

The United Kingdom's "Work-Life Balance" campaign (Department of Trade and Industry, 2002) demonstrates that there is some general awareness of the links between wellbeing and occupational balance. However, this is rare, as evident in the rise in fatigue-related disorders associated with burnout, such as chronic fatigue syndrome (Cox, 2002; Glouberman, 2002). The journey toward understanding the wellness process can be made at times when people are experiencing stress or illness.

Assisting people to reestablish an appreciation of life's purpose and meaning would fit well within traditional occupational therapy.

Occupational therapists working in medical settings may investigate whether the hospital (agency) is health-promoting. If not, they might potentially advocate for it to embrace the requirements of the *Budapest Declaration on Health Promoting Hospitals* (WHO, 1991). Such hospitals or agencies develop a corporate identity that embraces health-promoting practices and environments and actively work cooperatively with the community it serves.

Preventive Medicine

Preventive medicine was defined in 1998 as "the application of western medicine and social science to prevent disease, prolong life, and promote health in the community through intercepting disease processes" (Wilcock, 1998, p. 230). It is closely linked with the *OCHP* (WHO, 1986) call for the reorientation of health services toward the pursuit of health, in that prevention can usually be considered as workers in the health sector taking action aimed at individuals or populations at risk of illness or disease. Alternatively, prevention can be aimed at arresting the progress or reducing the consequences of ill health or disability once established. These three types of preventive strategies, known as *primary, secondary,* and *tertiary prevention,* are often thought to be synonymous with health promotion but, despite overlap, are different. Rehabilitation fits within this approach often as a form of tertiary intervention. Occupational therapists are experts in this arena, so other population health prevention possibilities that are less commonly part of everyday practice will be discussed here, namely, primary health care and health education.

Intervention within primary health care is a growing aspect of occupational therapy practice, which differs with contexts. The *Declaration of Alma Ata* (WHO, 1978) emphasized that everyone should have access to primary health care and that the whole population could be involved in its provision. It encompasses community participation and equitable distribution of and access to services, as well as costs and technology appropriate to a population. Depending on where the population is situated, primary health care may well have to address issues of food and water supplies, nutrition and activity advice, sanitation, maternal and childcare services, and job creation, as well as the more usual medical services. In the latter, occupational therapists may be involved in devising equipment such as splints, walking frames, and wheelchairs manufactured from indigenous materials by local community members. Advocacy roles concerned with overturning policies that prevent the health and wellbeing of the population are important, especially as occupation is frequently viewed as an economic rather than a health essential.

An occupational therapy preventive medicine approach should pay great attention to promulgation of the links between occupation and health with regard to risk factors. Health education is part of this approach. It concerns the immediate effects of what each person may do, as well as the social, economic, and environmental factors that may determine illness outcomes as discussed above. This may lead to occupational therapists becoming involved in feasibility studies and organizational action. Advocacy and mediation skills are essential for this, as the *OCHP* (WHO, 1986) suggests.

Community Development

The third approach to be discussed is community development. The WHO describes a **community** as

> a specific group of people, often living in a defined geographical area, who share a common culture, values and norms, are arranged in a social structure according to relationships, which the community has developed over a period of time. (WHO, 1998, p.5)

The WHO suggests that members of a community share common beliefs, values, and norms that the community has developed over time and may change in the future. These form part of each person's personal and social identity.

In 1998, the **community development** approach was defined as "community consultation, deliberation, and action to promote individual, family and community-wide responsibility for self sustaining development, health and wellbeing" (Wilcock, 1998, p. 230). This approach articulates closely with one of the five action directives of the *OCHP,* namely the strengthening of community action for health. According to the *Jakarta Declaration on Health Promotion into the 21st Century* (WHO, 1997), the actions and strategies set down by the *OCHP* remain relevant and applicable to all countries. The *Declaration* identified five priorities, all of which relate to community development in some way (see Content Box 6-3).

The *Declaration* found clear evidence that participation is essential for sustained effort toward health. In other words, with regard to health, as with other issues, people have to understand strategies and be involved in the decision-making processes for them to be effective. It follows that health literacy, and in this case occupation for health literacy, will assist participation through empowerment of communities and the individuals within them. Occupational therapists, therefore, need to put effort into making the connections between occupation and health or ill-health clear and accessible

---

Content Box 6-3

Five Priorities of the Jakarta Declaration Related to Community Development

- Promoting social responsibility for health
- Increasing investments for health development
- Expanding partnerships for health promotion
- Increasing community capacity and empowerment of individuals
- Securing an infrastructure for the promotion of health

---

to populations as a whole. They also need to be involved in extensive population education campaigns, bearing in mind the *Declaration*'s five priorities, bringing to them understanding and practical application of the relationship between occupation and health.

Occupational Justice

In 1998, Wilcock described occupational justice as social justice, although occupational justice was identified within it as occupational therapy's domain of concern (Wilcock, 1998, p. 230). Since then, written work about occupational justice has begun to emerge, and many workshops have been run on the topic in different parts of the world (Wilcock & Townsend, 2000, Townsend & Wilcock, 2004a, 2004b). Although Townsend and Wilcock are hesitant to define occupational justice at this stage of its exploration, it is done for the sake of conformity, specifically in terms of population health. From that viewpoint, **occupational justice** can be conceived as "equitable opportunity and resources to enable people's engagement in meaningful occupations" (Wilcock & Townsend, 2000, p. 85). This approach articulates well with another *OCHP* call for action, namely, to build healthy public policy and, with the *Declaration* (WHO, 1997), to empower individuals, to promote social responsibility for health, and to develop infrastructures for health promotion.

Social justice in the postmodern world envisions societies holding principles that enable freedom of expression and responsible engagement in life, without interference (Botes, 2000; Metz, 2000; Rawls, 1975). Justice in this broad sense is about the right to participate in civic governance and the right to an equitable distribution of goods, services, resources, and opportunities (Armstrong, 2000; Daniels, Kennedy, & Kawachi, 1999). However, the underlying political decisions that determine justice or health are seldom obvious in day-to-day discourse. This is also true of people's right to engage in occupations that are meaningful to them and to meet their own needs and potential.

Occupational therapists hold views that unconsciously resonate with a belief in the latter right. These embody the premise of the right to such occupations being a matter of justice, concealed within a unique concept of health and adaptation to disability. It is a premise that is only now emerging as justified with results of recent population health research. With even limited justification, not to provide opportunities for health-giving occupations can, indeed, be considered a matter of injustice and a matter of health, morbidity, or mortality. It is imperative to give consideration to what, why, and how occupations provide people with physical, mental, and social exercise while they reach toward their potential and meet unique occupational wants and needs.

It is also imperative to question why there appears to be so little emphasis in population health literature on encouraging people of any age to engage in wide-ranging occupations. Literature and funded health programs appear to focus on risk management to prevent accidents, physical occupations, or mundane hygiene tasks. This may well be because of the increasingly litigious nature of Western societies, which fails to recognize individual needs or the morbidity and mortality links between what people do or do not do, the rise in obesity as a public health concern, or economic issues about the cost of institutional care.

Sociopolitical factors determine whether occupational justice is a common experience. Occupational therapy assistants and occupational therapists have a major task ahead of them to be advocates for occupation for health interests and concerns of the population at large. In this regard, they need to brave public and political forums to advance understanding of the relationship between occupation and health or ill-health. They need to do so, because as part of a small, poorly understood or resourced profession, they, too, are victims of occupational injustices (Townsend & Wilcock, 2004b).

Ecological Sustainability

The last of the approaches to be discussed is **ecological sustainability,** which can be defined as the "promotion of healthy relationships between humans, other living organisms, their environments, habits, and modes of life" (Wilcock, 1998, p. 230). This approach fits within the newly emerging domain of ecological public health described earlier and is aimed at creating supportive environments for health as the *OCHP* mandates.

The broad scope offered by this approach is probably the most daunting for occupational therapists, who are comfortable and committed to working in medical-model

domains. Many would think it outside the scope of the profession, as it appears far from the individualistic treatment of people with a medically defined dysfunction that has been the norm for the last few decades. However, to work within population health according to WHO directives, it is important to be open to the idea that the factors influencing health are many, varied, and interactive. For example, the *OCHP* lists environmental prerequisites without which health is probably unattainable. These include a stable ecosystem and sustainable resources, as well as social justice, peace, shelter, education, food, and income (WHO, 1986, p. 2). Environmental factors are major determinants of living and working conditions, including the occupations that are required to maintain physical, mental, and social health for every person on the globe. Villarosa (1994) argues that when humans "lose respect for the earth . . . the greatest toll may be on our health" (p. 569). Yet, it is the occupations that people have engaged in throughout time that have caused the deteriorating ecological conditions that now need therapy.

With a concern for the ecosystem and sustainable resources, occupational therapists could become advocates for and advisers of the occupations suited to individuals to meet their needs yet to sustain resources and the ecology. The way forward is to be part of the economic and ecological debate, with the occupation for health needs of people at the forefront of the agenda. It is a different role, but it is the practice of occupational therapy at the global level. Once again, it calls upon knowledge of people as occupational beings combined with environmental and population health issues. The latest World Federation of Occupational Therapist's minimum standards address the relationship between people, occupation, and the environment. In the glossary of terms, it explains that this includes

> the implicit relationship between people, what they do and the context in which they do it. The essential idea is that occupational performance is both influenced by and influences personal and environmental dimensions. (Hocking & Ness, 2002, p. 33)

This concept includes understanding "how resources in the environment . . . and the local geography affect people's participation in occupation" (Hocking & Ness, 2002, p. 16).

Conclusion

Despite the development of an abstract appreciation of links between health and occupation among occupational therapy professionals and in the population generally, there remains substantial difficulty in applying occupational issues to population health. In part, this is due to people's limited understanding of themselves as occupational beings and to the fact that health-maintaining needs and functions, rather like the autonomic nervous system, are built into the organism to just go on working. It is also due to little being written in mainstream health care, which is based on the Western medical model, about the benefits of a natural lifestyle or the need for a balance of ongoing physical, mental, and social occupations as integral aspects of health. Scant information about people as occupational beings, and the inbuilt consequences of that, has led to deleterious health consequences for individuals, communities, and the global ecology. A major task for occupational therapists who wish to extend practice into the population health domain is to research and promulgate information about such links. Excitingly, that process is beginning to happen.

▶ For Discussion and Review

1. What is the impact of occupational deprivation, occupational alienation, and occupational imbalance on health?
2. Compare and contrast the five approaches to population health. What are the similarities and differences? Which approach(es) is (are) most consistent with occupational therapy philosophy?
3. How can occupational science inform population health interventions?
4. What are the positive influences on wellbeing, and how can occupational therapy enhance these factors?
5. What is the focus of social epidemiology, and how does it relate to occupation?
6. What is the relationship between occupational justice and population health?

▶ Research Questions

1. What are the impacts of occupational deprivation, occupational alienation, and occupational imbalance on the health of various populations?
2. How does occupational engagement facilitate health, healing, and wellbeing?
3. How do environmental resources and local geography affect occupational participation?

References

Armstrong, H. (2000). Reflections on the difficulty of creating and sustaining equitable communicative forums. *Canadian Journal for Studies in Adult Education, 14,* 67–85.

Blaxter, M. (1990). *Health and lifestyles.* London and New York: Tavistock/Routledge.

Botes, A. (2000). A comparison between the ethics of justice and the ethics of care. *Journal of Advanced Nursing, 20,* 55–71.

Brenner, M. H. (1977). Health costs and benefits of economic policy. *International Journal of Health Services, 7,* 581–93.

Brenner, M. H. (1979). Mortality and the national economy: A review, and the experience of England and Wales. *Lancet, 2*(8142), 568–73.

British College of Occupational Therapists. (2004). OT definition agreed. *Occupational Therapy News, 12*(2), 7.

Bronowski, J. (1973). *The Ascent of man.* London: British Broadcasting Corporation.

Campbell, B. G. (1988). *Humankind emerging* (5th ed.). New York: Harper Collins.

Canadian Association of Occupational Therapy. (2002). *Enabling occupation: An occupational therapy perspective* (Rev. ed.). Ottawa, ON: CAOT Publications ACE.

Christiansen, C., & Baum, C. (Eds.). (1997). *Occupational therapy: Enabling function and wellbeing.* Thorofare, NJ: SLACK.

Clark, F., Azen, S. P., Zemke, R., Jackson, J., Carlson, M., Mandel, D., Hay, J., Josephson, K., Cherry, B., Hessel, C., Palmer, J., & Lipson, L. (1997). Occupational therapy for independent-living older adults: A randomized controlled trial. *Journal of the American Medical Association,* 1321–26.

Colligan, M. J., & Murphy, L. R. (1979). Mass psychogenic illness in organizations: An overview. *Journal of Occupational Psychology, 52,* 77–90.

Cox, D. L. (2002). Chronic fatigue syndrome: An evaluation of occupational therapy intervention. *British Journal of Occupational Therapy, 65*(10), 461–69.

Cromwell, F. S. (1970). *Our challenges in the seventies. Occupational therapy today—Tomorrow.* Proceedings of the 5th International WFOT Congress. Zurich, Switzerland: World Federation of Occupational Therapists.

Daniels, N., Kennedy, B. P., & Kawachi, I. (1999). Why justice is good for our health: The social determinants of health inequalities. *Daedelus, 128*(4), 215–51.

Department of Trade and Industry, United Kingdom. (2002). *Work-life balance.* Retrieved September 2, 2004, from http://www.dti.gov.uk/work-lifebalance/index.html.

Finn, G. L. (1972). The occupational therapist in prevention programs. *American Journal of Occupational Therapy, 26*(2), 59–66.

Finn, G. L. (1977). Update of Eleanor Clarke Slagle Lecture: The occupational therapist in prevention programs. *American Journal of Occupational Therapy, 31*(10), 658–59.

Glass, T. A., de Leon, C. M., Marottoli, R. A., & Berkman, L. F. (1999). Population based study of social and productive activities as predictors of survival among elderly Americans. *British Medical Journal, 319,* 478–83.

Glouberman, D. (2002). *The joy of burnout.* London: Hodder & Stoughton.

Greiner, P. A., Fain, J. A., & Edelman, C. L. (2002). Health defined: Objectives for promotion and prevention. In C. L. Edelman & C. L. Mandle (Eds.), *Health promotion throughout the lifespan* (5th ed.). St Louis, MO: Mosby.

Hocking, C., & Ness, N. E. (2002). *Revised minimum standards for the education of occupational therapists 2002.* World Federation of Occupational Therapists.

Howard, R. B. (1983). Wellness: Obtainable goal or impossible dream. *Post Graduate Medicine, 73*(1), 15–19.

Jones, S., Martin, R., & Pilbeam, D. (Eds.). (1992). *The Cambridge encyclopaedia of human evolution.* Cambridge, UK: Cambridge University Press.

Justice, B. (1987). *Who gets sick: Thinking and health.* Houston, TX: Peak Press.

Kass, L. R. (1981). Regarding the end of medicine and the pursuit of health. In A. L. Caplan, H. T. Englehart, & J. J. McCartney (Eds.), *Concepts of health and disease: Interdisciplinary perspectives.* Reading, MA: Addison Wesley.

Kielhofner, G. (2002). *A model of human occupation: Theory and application* (3d ed.). Baltimore: Lippincott, Williams and Wilkins.

Lovelock, L., Bentley, J., Dunn, T., & Wallenbert, I. (2002). Occupational balance and perceived health: A study of occupational therapists. In *Conference abstracts, World Federation of Occupational Therapists Conference 2002,* Stockholm, Sweden.

Metz, T. (2000). Arbitrariness, justice, and respect. *Social Theory and Practice, 26,* 24–45.

Meyer, A. (1922). The philosophy of occupational therapy. *Archives of Occupational Therapy 1,* 1–10. (Reprinted in 1997 in *The American Journal of Occupational Therapy, 31*(10), 639–42.)

Naisbit, J. (1982). *Megatrends: Ten new directions transforming our lives.* New York: Warner Books.

Nutbeam, D. (1998). Health promotion glossary. *Health Promotion International, 13*(4), 349–64.

Ornstein, R., & Sobel, D. (1988). *The healing brain: A radical new approach to health care.* London: MacMillan.

Rawls, J. (1975). A Kantian conception of equality. *Cambridge Review,* 94–99.

Reed, K., & Sanderson, S. (1992). *Concepts of occupational therapy* (3d ed.). Baltimore: Williams & Wilkins.

Rogers, J. C. (1984). Why study human occupation? *The American Journal of Occupational Therapy, 38,* 37–49.

Sigerist, H. E. (1955). *A history of medicine, volume 1. Primitive and archaic medicine.* New York: Oxford University Press.

Smith, R. (1987). *Unemployment and health: A disaster and a challenge.* Oxford, UK: Oxford University Press.

Townsend, E., & Wilcock, A. (2004a). Occupational justice. In C. Christiansen & E. Townsend (Eds), *Introduction to occupation: The art and science of living.* Upper Saddle River, NJ: Prentice Hall.

Townsend, E., & Wilcock, A. A. (2004b). Occupational justice and client-centered practice: A dialogue in progress. *Canadian Journal of Occupational Therapy, 71*(2), 75–87.

Villarosa, L. (1994). *Body & soul: The black women's guide to physical health and emotional wellbeing.* New York: Harper Collins.

Warr, P. (1985). Twelve questions about unemployment and health. In R. Roberts, R. Finnegan, & D. Gallie (Eds.), *New approaches to economic life.* Manchester, UK: Manchester University Press.

Warr, P. (1987). *Work, unemployment and mental health.* Oxford, UK: Oxford Science Publications.

West, W. (1967). The occupational therapists changing responsibilities to the community. *American Journal of Occupational Therapy, 21,* 312.

West, W. (1969). The growing importance of prevention. *American Journal of Occupational Therapy, 23,* 223–31.

West, W. (1970). *The emerging health model of occupational therapy practice.* Proceedings of the 5th International WFOT Congress. Zurich, Switzerland: World Federation of Occupational Therapists.

Wilcock, A. A. (1998) *An occupational perspective of health.* Thorofare, NJ: SLACK.

Wilcock, A. A. (1999). Reflections on doing, being and becoming. *Australian Journal of Occupational Therapy, 46*(1), 1–11.

Wilcock, A. A., Chelin, M., Hall, M., Hamley, N., Morrison, B., Scrivener, L., Townsend, M., & Treen, K. (1997). The relationship between occupational balance and health: A pilot study. *Occupational Therapy International, 4*(1), 17–30.

Wilcock, A. A., & Townsend, E. (2000). Occupational justice: Occupational terminology interactive dialogue. *Journal of Occupational Science, 7*(2), 84–86.

Winefield, A., & Tiggerman, M. (1991). A longitudinal study of the psychological effects of unemployment and unsatisfactory employment on young adults. *Journal of Applied Psychology, 76*(3), 424–31.

Winefield, A., Tiggerman, M., & Winefield, H. (1992). Unemployment distress, reasons for job loss and causal attributions for unemployment in young people. *Journal of Occupational and Organizational Psychology, 65,* 213–18.

Winefield, A., Tiggerman, M., Winefield, H., & Goldney, R. (1993). *Growing up with unemployment.* London: Routledge.

World Health Organization. (1948). *Constitution.* Geneva, Switzerland: Author.

World Health Organization. (1978). *Declaration of Alma Ata.* Alma Ata: Reported in *World Health,* Aug./Sept. 1988.

World Health Organization. (1984). *Glossary of terms: Health for all series.* Geneva, Switzerland: Author.

World Health Organization. (1991). *The Budapest declaration on health promoting hospitals.* Geneva, Switzerland: Author.

World Health Organization. (1993). *Life skills education in schools.* Geneva, Switzerland: Author.

World Health Organization. (1997). *The Jakarta declaration on health promotion into the 21st century.* Geneva, Switzerland: Author.

World Health Organization. (1998). *Health promotion glossary.* Geneva, Switzerland: Author.

World Health Organization. (2001). *International classification of functioning, disability and health.* Geneva, Switzerland: Author.

World Health Organization, Health and Welfare, Canada, Canadian Public Health Association. (1986). *Ottawa charter for health promotion.* Geneva, Switzerland: World Health Organization.

Chapter 7

Quality of Life and Health Promotion

Michael A. Pizzi and Rebecca Renwick

> The good life is a process, not a state of being. It is a direction not a destination.
> —Carl Rogers
> The quality of life is determined by its activities.
> —Aristotle

Learning Objectives

This chapter is designed to enable the reader to:

- Define the concept of quality of life (QOL).
- Discuss the conceptual interrelationships of health promotion, wellness, and QOL.
- Describe the theoretical underpinnings of various QOL models and their applicability to occupational therapy.

- Explain the relationship between being, belonging, and becoming and QOL.
- Discuss QOL issues as they impact children, adults, and persons at the end of life.
- Apply QOL concepts in occupational therapy and health promotion practice.

Key Terms

Becoming

Being

Belonging

Good death

Happiness

Health promotion

Health-related quality of life

Quality of life

Introduction

The concept of quality of life (QOL) can be traced to Aristotle, who described happiness as a virtuous activity of the soul (Zhan, 1992). **Happiness** generally refers to shorter-term, transient feelings of wellbeing in response to day-to-day events (Horley, 1984). In the United States, QOL was introduced for political reasons, with slogans such as the "quality of American life." It was not until the late 1970s that the term was used in reference to individuals (Wolfensberger, 1994).

> The numerous attempts made to define QOL suggest that the concept includes multiple dimensions; it covers cultural, psychological, interpersonal, spiritual, financial, political, temporal and philosophical domains. Furthermore, QOL is dynamic as it reflects changes in people and the environment over time across many of its domains. (Tate, Dijkers, & Johnson-Greene, 1996, p. 2)

The World Health Organization (WHO) defines **quality of life** as

> an individual's perception of their position in life in the context of the culture and value systems in which they live and in relation to their goals, expectations, standards and concerns. It is a broad ranging concept affected in a complex way by the person's physical health, psychological state, personal beliefs, social relationships and their relationship to salient features of their environment. (WHO, 1998, p. 1569)

The first goal of *Healthy People 2010: Understanding and Improving Health* (U.S. Department of Health and Human Services [USDHHS], 2000) is to help individuals of all ages increase life expectancy and improve their QOL:

> Quality of life reflects a general sense of happiness and satisfaction with our lives and environment. General quality of life encompasses all aspects of life, including health, recreation, culture, rights, values, beliefs, aspirations, and the conditions that support a life containing these elements. *Health-related quality of life* reflects a personal sense of physical and mental health and the ability to react to factors in the physical and social environments. Health-related quality of life is more subjective than life expectancy and therefore can be more difficult to measure. (USDHHS, 2000, p. 10)

Conceptually, **health-related quality of life** supports assessments and interventions that occupational therapists and occupational therapy assistants use to determine the health and occupational performance of people in the context of their lives. Whether or not one believes health-related QOL is a client-centered concept, as QOL may depend upon who defines the concept, it still warrants further investigation for use in occupational therapy.

The *Ottawa Charter for Health Promotion* (WHO, 1986) was developed as a response to the need for a changing health-care system. The WHO was the foundation for this charter, which was one of the first documents that integrated the concepts of QOL and health promotion. QOL was described as an "important dimension" of good health, with *good health* identified as a "major resource of social, economic and personal development" (WHO, 1986, p. 1). **Health promotion** was defined as

the process of enabling people to increase control over, and to improve, their health. To reach a state of complete physical, mental and social wellbeing, an individual or group must be able to identify and to realize aspirations, to satisfy needs, and to change or cope with the environment. Health is, therefore, seen as a resource for everyday life, not the objective of living. Health is a positive concept emphasizing social and personal resources, as well as physical capacities. Therefore, health promotion is not just the responsibility of the health sector, but goes beyond healthy life-styles to wellbeing. (WHO, 1986, p. 1)

In the American Occupational Therapy Association's (AOTA's) 2008 *Occupational Therapy Practice Framework* (referred to as the *Framework*), health, wellness, and prevention are listed as outcomes of occupational therapy interventions. QOL is also noted as an outcome. It is defined as

a client's dynamic appraisal of life satisfactions (perceptions of progress toward identifiable goals), self-concept (the composite of beliefs and feelings about themselves), health and functioning (including health status, self-care capabilities), and socioeconomic factors (e.g., vocation, education, income). (adapted from Radomski, 1995; Zhan, 1992 cited by AOTA, 2008, p. 674)

This definition encompasses a person's state of being and his or her participation in the act of doing, or occupational engagement. In assessing a person's QOL, occupational therapists must be mindful of other related factors, including

- the person's spiritual being or sense of meaning within his or her current state of being, and

- environmental interactions, particularly the quality of social interactions the individual deems important.

In the *Framework,* the definition of *quality of life* fails to incorporate these other important features. Therefore, it would behoove the profession to incorporate in its definition of QOL other aspects that can influence QOL, such as spirituality.

One goal of the AOTA's vision statement emphasizes the profession's contributions in the promotion of "health, productivity, and quality of life of individuals and society (2008, innercover, ¶ 3). While the professional activities of occupational therapists and occupational therapy assistants reflect that vision in practice, health promotion language, particularly QOL, must be included so that others outside the profession clearly understand the purpose of occupational therapy interventions toward the goal of improving QOL of individuals, families, and communities.

The Canadian Association of Occupational Therapists (CAOT) has also produced formal documents that describe core principles, values, beliefs, and conceptual frameworks to guide practice. The two most recent documents include *Enabling Occupation: An Occupational Therapy Perspective* (CAOT, 2002) and *Enabling Occupation II: Advancing an Occupational Therapy Vision for Health, Well-Being, & Justice Through Occupations* (Townsend & Polatajko, 2007). The major emphasis in *Enabling Occupation I* was on client-centeredness; holism; life-span development; and the complex interplay among the person, the environment, and occupations, as well as occupational performance. In *Enabling Occupation I,* QOL is featured as a crucial overarching concept related to meaningful life occupations. The definition of QOL remains constant across both versions: "Choosing and participating in occupations that foster hope, generate motivation, offer meaning and satisfaction, create a driving vision of life, promote health, enable empowerment, and otherwise address the quality of life" (CAOT, 2002, p. 182; Townsend & Polatajko, 2007, p. 373).

These documents clearly suggest ways that occupational therapy practitioners and researchers can better understand the connections among persons, families, and populations and the impact meaningful engagement in occupations has on QOL. A deeper and richer understanding of these connections could lead to assessment, intervention, and evaluation of occupational therapy process and outcomes that are more relevant and beneficial to clients' daily lives.

Occupation and Quality of Life

Engaging in meaningful occupation is associated with a good QOL (Christiansen, Backman, Little, & Nguyen, 1999; Christiansen & Townsend, 2004). This finding is not so surprising, since occupational engagement can bolster or even transform a person's identity and sense of empowerment (Christiansen, 1999). Not engaging in meaningful occupations can result in fewer experiences that enable a person to develop competence in and mastery of occupations. Further, such limited occupational engagement can constrain a person's fulfillment of their occupational potential (Wicks, 2001). When long-standing barriers that a person cannot control hinder or prevent participation in chosen or necessary occupations that would normally provide personal meaning in life, a person is likely to experience occupational deprivation (Wilcock, 1998). The effects of occupational deprivation include a sense of isolation, emotional distance from oneself and others, perceived lack of control, and frustration (Wilcock, 1998), which can significantly detract from life quality. Consequently, the opportunity (or lack thereof) to engage in and experience meaningful occupation can significantly impact a person's subjective QOL.

Not long ago, many people with disabilities were faced with substantial barriers to participation in meaningful occupational engagement, and they had a narrow range of occupations available to them (Renwick, 2004). These restrictions to occupational engagement were due to such social forces as the stigma associated with disabilities, segregation in institutions, and public stereotypes about the capacity and potential of people with disabilities for engaging in a diverse range of occupations. Such barriers put people with disabilities at considerable risk for occupational deprivation and decrease their opportunities for developing competence and mastery and for achieving their occupational potential. In today's society, many people with disabilities still encounter some of these occupational obstacles, which can detract from their QOL. Thus, striving for a good QOL, a relevant concept for all human beings, can present additional challenges for people living with disabilities, especially within the realm of occupational engagement (Renwick, 2004). Similar occupational obstacles often confront those who are disadvantaged and marginalized in modern society (Wilcock, 1998); for example, people who live in poverty; who are unemployed, homeless, or imprisoned; or who are refugees from countries in conflict. Thus, for occupational therapists who work with clients who have disabilities or who are experiencing disadvantage and marginalization, QOL is an especially salient concept.

Quality of Life and Health Promotion

Health promotion is a multidisciplinary field that is focused on personal empowerment in that it seeks to enable "people to increase control over and to improve their health" (WHO, 1986, p. 2). This goal is broadly conceived in that it is relevant to people of all ages, whether or not they have disabilities. In these respects and in other ways, it shares some common ground with holistic approaches to QOL. For instance, the concept of personal control is inherent in numerous major holistic QOL frameworks (Renwick & Brown, 1996; Schalock, 1996a).

Health promotion also takes a broad perspective on health, including the study of socially determined influences on health; for example, poverty, housing, education, and unemployment (Evans, Barer, & Marmor, 1994). These influences are usually environmental in nature or inherent in the relationship between people and their environments, where they engage in the occupations of their daily lives (e.g., home, neighborhood and community, school, workplace, and the larger society). Thus, the concepts and principles associated with health promotion can inform occupational therapy theory and practice.

Influential Perspectives on Quality of Life

There are more than a hundred definitions for QOL (Cummins, 1995), a growing number of conceptual frameworks, and numerous instruments and measures purporting to measure the construct (Hughes, Hwang, Kim, Eisenman, & Killian, 1995). Given this vast, multidisciplinary literature on QOL, it would be very challenging to devise a categorization system that would account for all approaches. However, two major influential types of perspectives are most relevant to this discussion—the health-related approaches and the holistic approaches.

Health-related approaches typically take a biomedical view of health and focus on health status or functional abilities. These approaches may focus primarily on physical aspects of health or function (e.g., pain, mobility, fatigue) but often include attention to their psychological and social dimensions (e.g., anxiety, depression). They are frequently concerned with perceptions about a person's health or symptoms related to illness or intervention (Koot, 2001). For example, some concentrate on the impact a specific illness or disorder has on the individual's QOL, while others are concerned with how a variety of illnesses or disorders affect QOL. Some health-related QOL instruments were originally developed to assess function and health status, not QOL per se. However, biomedically oriented researchers have employed them as indicators of QOL. Bowling (1991, 1995) and McDowell and Newell (1996) review a variety of such functional health indicators of health-related QOL. Typically, health-related approaches to QOL also focus much more on measurement than on their conceptual underpinnings (Bowling, 1995; Day & Jankey, 1996). Bowling (1995) and McDowell and Newell (1996) reviewed in detail numerous measurement approaches to health-related QOL.

Holistic approaches view QOL from a broader perspective that may include health and function but go beyond these domains. Because there are different holistic approaches, it is difficult to include every model in terms of a core set of characteristics. However, most assume (but fewer explicitly indicate) that QOL arises out of the ongoing relationship that each person has with their environment. QOL is also conceptualized in terms of domains, such as the individual's emotional, physical, and material wellbeing; relationships with important others; opportunities to make personal choices and decisions or personal empowerment; social participation or inclusion; and rights and freedoms (Brown, Brown, & Bayer, 1994; Felce & Perry, 1996; Renwick & Brown, 1996; Renwick, Fudge Schormans, & Zekovic, 2003). Thus, in contrast to health-related approaches, holistic approaches are generally congruent with themes of empowerment of individuals and meaningful engagement in life occupations important to them. They are more truly measures of life goodness or quality and do not infer QOL only from the person's self-reported or assessed level of health status or functional ability.

Holistic approaches also tend to be better elaborated—that is, to have a better-developed and described conceptual basis than do health-related QOL approaches. Further, some holistic approaches are based on frameworks of QOL developed according to rigorous research methods (e.g., Lindstrom, 1994; Renwick, Fudge Schormans, et al., 2003). Some of these approaches have included the use of qualitative methods, such that the emergent conceptual frameworks and instruments based on them reflect the voices of those whose lives are being studied or assessed (e.g., Laliberte Rudman, Hoffman, Scott, & Renwick, 2004; Renwick, Nourhaghighi, Manns, & Laliberte Rudman, 2003). Grounding any measurement instrument in a clear conceptual framework is a significant step in establishing its' construct validity (Wallander, 2001).

Both health-related and holistic approaches to QOL may be relevant to occupational therapy researchers and practitioners, depending on the particular context in which they work. However, holistic approaches seem to be more clearly consistent with the core values of occupational therapy (AOTA, 2004; CAOT, 2002) and the profession's focus on the meaningful occupations people carry out in their daily lives.

Quality of Life Across the Life Span

QOL is an issue that is highly relevant at all stages of human life, from childhood to the end of life (Stark & Faulkner, 1996). Several subsequent sections provide examples of approaches that are relevant to various life stages. However, most of the attention in the literature has been focused on conceptualizations and measures of QOL for adults. There has been considerably less attention to what contributes to and detracts from a good life for children, for older adults, and for those receiving end-of-life care. The following sections focus only on holistic approaches, since they are more relevant to occupational therapy's core values.

Quality of Life for Adults

Many of the holistic conceptual frameworks of QOL for adults are found in the literature on developmental disabilities (Schalock, 1996b). However, most of these frameworks are applicable to adults with and without disabilities (Brown et al., 1994; Renwick & Brown, 1996; Felce & Perry, 1996). One model is outlined here to exemplify the holistic approaches to QOL for adults.

The Centre for Health Promotion (CHP) model (Renwick & Brown, 1996) was originally developed for adults with developmental disabilities, and measurement instruments grounded in this model were also constructed for this group. However, since then, the model has been tested for applicability with adults without disabilities, senior adults, adolescents, and adults with physical and psychiatric disabilities. Subsequently, measurement instruments based on the CHP model were developed for use with adults in each of these populations (Raphael, 1996; Renwick, Brown, & Raphael, 2000; Renwick, Nourhaghighi, et al., 2003; Laliberte Rudman et al., 2004). The CHP model was developed based on interviews and focus groups with adults with and without disabilities; a comprehensive review of the literature; and consultation with experts in the fields of disability studies, health promotion, and QOL. It assumes that individuals differ from one another and that each person is a unique human being who should be understood in a holistic way. Further, QOL has many dimensions or aspects and results from the continuous and ever-changing relationships that the person has with the environment. Thus, QOL may change over time for the individual, but these changes may differ in their extent and nature from one aspect of QOL to another. However, the basic aspects or dimensions of QOL are the same for people with and without disabilities, even though they may be experienced in different ways by each person. These basic aspects of QOL are congruent with current concepts of health, health promotion (WHO, 1986), and occupational wellbeing (Christiansen et al., 1999). The CHP model also assumes that social factors such as poverty, lack of adequate housing, lack of access to education, and unemployment can significantly affect a person's health (Evans et al., 1994) and can contribute to occupational deprivation (Wilcock, 1998).

The concept of QOL is defined as "the degree to which a person enjoys the important possibilities of his or her life" (Renwick & Brown, 1996, p. 80). The term *possibilities* refers to the significant opportunities and constraints in the various aspects of a person's life (described below) that result from the person's continuous interaction with the environment. These possibilities are associated with three major aspects of QOL (Table 7-1)—

being, belonging, and becoming—each of which has three subdimensions (Renwick & Brown, 1996).

QOL consists of both how much satisfaction a person experiences and how much importance he or she attaches to each of the nine aspects of life—physical being, psychological being, spiritual being, physical belonging, social belonging, community belonging, practical becoming, leisure becoming, and growth becoming. In addition, perceptions people have about their QOL can be positively or negatively affected by how much personal control they exert over their lives. Personal control includes

- the degree to which people make decisions and choices, within a comfortable range, and
- the spectrum of opportunities available to people as they make these choices.

For example, a person who is comfortable making most of her own decisions may perceive her life quality to be negatively affected if the range of opportunities for exercising her decisions and choices is very narrow. Similarly, a person's QOL may be diminished because he is experiencing too many demands or too

Table 7-1 Three Major Aspects of QOL With Their Subdimensions

Major Aspects of QOL	Subdimensions of QOL
Being (who the person is as an individual)	*Physical being:* concerns physical health and wellbeing
	Psychological being: focuses on mental health and wellbeing
	Spiritual being: includes important standards, values, beliefs, and experiences that guide and sustain the person (Renwick, Brown, & Raphael, 2000)
Belonging (the fit between the person and their environment)	*Physical belonging:* refers to the fit between the person and the physical environment of his or her home, school, work, neighborhood, and community
	Social belonging: includes relationships with important others and with those the person sees regularly (e.g., family, coworkers, neighbors)
	Community belonging: focuses on the person's access to community resources (e.g., employment, resources, services, public events)
Becoming (what the person does to reach their goals or hopes in life)	*Practical becoming:* includes a person's regular practical activities (e.g., paid work, participation in school or program, volunteer work, household chores, caring for self and others)
	Leisure becoming: concerns what the person does for relaxation or recreation, alone or with others (e.g., sports, hobbies, games, entertainment, socializing, and taking holidays)
	Growth becoming: encompasses what the person does to learn, change, and develop (e.g., learn new skills, cope with changes in life, take on new challenges) (Renwick, 2004; Renwick et al., 2000)

much pressure to make many decisions from too broad a spectrum of opportunities to reasonably manage (Renwick, 2004).

Since the ultimate goal of occupational therapy intervention is to enable clients to improve or maintain their QOL, the instruments based on the CHP model that were noted above can be useful to occupational therapists. These measures can be used as assessments with clients as well as in evaluation of outcomes for individual clients, groups of clients, or programs. These measures can also be used in occupational therapy research.

Quality of Life for Children

Although not as many approaches to conceptualization and measurement of QOL have been developed for children as for adults, there has certainly been attention to these issues in the literature, particularly in the area of health-related QOL (Koot & Wallander, 2001). However, there are few holistic models specifically for children. A notable exception is Lindstrom's (1994, 1995) work, which takes a public health perspective on QOL for children aged 2 to 18 years living in the five Nordic countries. Lindstrom created a model of QOL for children and an instrument consisting of several modules to assess QOL for children with and without disabilities. The scores from this measurement tool are compared with a set of basic values tied to a Nordic standard for QOL. However, the applicability of this instrument in countries with different health systems and cultural groups remains unexamined (Zekovic & Renwick, 2003).

Another QOL model focused on children with developmental disabilities (Renwick & Fudge Schormans, 2004; Renwick, Fudge Schormans, et al., 2003) will be used here as an example of holistic approaches relevant for children. This model is closely aligned with the practice of health promotion within occupational therapy. It was derived from a grounded theory analysis of in-depth personal interviews with parents of children aged 3 to 12 years who had a wide range of developmental disabilities. The conceptual framework that emerged from this qualitative analysis highlights the dynamic interplay of three elements that work together to influence QOL: the child; the child's family environment; and the larger environment beyond the family, which includes the child's neighborhood, school, day-care program, the community, and the government policies affecting this group of children and their families. The extent to which these three elements overlap, or form a good fit, has consequences for the child's life. The better the fit, the better the QOL. If the fit of these elements is poorer, QOL will be diminished for the child.

As for the CHP model for children, the conceptual framework highlights three aspects of QOL, which are shaped by the interplay among the elements previously noted:

• The child
• The family environment
• The larger environment

These major aspects have the same labels, as do those in the CHP model for adults. However, the nature of these aspects or domains of QOL for children is different and reflects the developmental issues appropriate to them. The first aspect is *being,* which refers to who the child is perceived to be in the view of others, such as family members, relatives, and people in the child's community.

Belonging is the second aspect, which refers to the connections the child has to people and places in his or her life. Included here is the extent to which family members, relatives, peers, and others in the community include the child in their activities. In addition, this domain focuses on the child's friendships and on play and other activities with friends. It also refers to the child's access to professional services and community venues, such as parks, playgrounds, pools, shopping malls, and transportation, and to the safety and security of the child's environment.

The third aspect of QOL is *becoming* and refers to the child's nurtured growth and development. It centers on the identification of the child's major needs and how well those needs are being accommodated and supported by professionals and by government policies, services, resources, and programs. In addition, this aspect of QOL is concerned with how well the expectations of others in the child's life are congruent with his or her abilities. For example, do family members, teachers, and professionals expect too much or too little from the child based on his or her abilities?

This framework treats the child's life as whole, which is consistent with core values of occupational therapy, and it focuses attention on several key occupations for this group of children:

• Play with friends
• Going to day care/nursery program or school
• Activities in the community
• Learning new things that help him or her grow or develop

A measurement instrument tapping parental perspectives on QOL for this group of children was developed based on this conceptual framework. It has been evaluated in terms of its psychometric properties and usefulness with 180 parents of children with developmental disabilities who are aged 3 to 12 years

(Renwick & Fudge Schormans, 2004). Given the connections of its conceptual foundations to core values and goals of occupational therapy and its demonstrated psychometric soundness, it has potential value for researchers and for practitioners to use in assessment and program evaluation.

The prior sections of this chapter dealt primarily with the conceptualization of QOL. An integration of QOL concepts with those of occupation and occupational participation is relevant for occupational therapy practice and has been discussed. Content Box 7-1 details some QOL assessments that can be used in occupational therapy to complement those that are traditional and contextually based. The next section focuses specifically on the elderly and those experiencing end-of-life issues.

Quality of Life Relative to End-of-Life Care and Aging

Byock (1997) contrasts the "good death" with "dying well." A good death is not necessarily a sudden, painless demise, for which most people might wish. A **good death** is often described as encompassing elements such as having family or significant others present, being without pain, being physically comfortable, and maintaining dignity through privacy and caring (Thompson & McClement, 2002). Dying well suggests that people need to prepare in order to realize this good death. This work (see Chapter 25 in this text) may be initiated by palliative and hospice care professionals using grief and bereavement as indicators on which patients or significant others might focus to realize some new meaning or identity (Field & Cassel, 1997). The process of dying well is really about living life fully while dying. If one views grief and bereavement as normal transitions of life, then the palliative and hospice practitioners can help the patient and family focus on opportunities for diminishing the suffering (Byock, 1996).

Most people wish for a long, satisfying life—that is, they value both how long they live *and* how well they live. In response, the concept of health-related QOL has emerged to emphasize health as perceived and valued by people for themselves (or, in some cases, for those close to them) rather than as seen by experts (Cohen, Mount, & Strobe, 1995; Gold, Franks, & Erickson, 1996; Patrick & Erickson, 1993). This client-centeredness is congruent with the beliefs and values of occupational therapy.

> Going well beyond traditional mortality and morbidity measures, health-related quality-of-life outcomes include physical, mental, social, and role functioning; sense of wellbeing; freedom from bodily pain; satisf-

action with health care; and an overall sense of general health. (Field & Cassel, 1997, p. 25)

Suffering and Loss of Meaning in Life

Suffering is an expansive concept and goes beyond pain. It encompasses the loss of control, anguish, terror, and hopelessness that dying patients may experience. A dying person may suffer greatly, with no evidence of physical distress, if he or she feels that life has lost any meaning. Meaning and experiencing meaning in life is often associated with the concept of QOL (Frankl, 2000) and is congruent with holistic approaches to QOL.

Cassell has suggested that a symptom or feeling becomes suffering when people perceive it as a "threat to their continued existence—not merely to their lives but their integrity as persons" (1991, p. 36). Such perceptions may have significant emotional and spiritual dimensions related to self-image, family relationships, past experiences, caregiver attitudes, and other circumstances of a patient's life (Byock, 1997). Suffering is "a personal matter—something whose presence and extent can only be known to the sufferer" but which cannot be ignored (Cassell, 1991, p. 35).

> Those caring for dying patients have a responsibility, first, to explain to people that pain and other distress can often be relieved and, second, to consider whether the patient would benefit from an exploration with a chaplain or other counselor of the nature and significance of suffering. (Field & Cassel, 1997, p. 26)

In a qualitative study of nurses involved in palliative care, Pegg and Tan (2002) discuss three emerging themes from the transcribed interviews:

- Power and showing the way of suffering through not knowing
- Being as giving by enhancing QOL
- Being as giving by sharing

The second theme is closely aligned with the core strength of occupational therapy, which focuses on optimizing participation. According to Pegg and Tan (2002),

> The participants focused [sic] on rehabilitation, symptom control and prevention of complications to enable their suffering clients to maintain their usual social roles while receiving palliative care. . . . An emphasis on participation and encouragement of a return to social activities are of primary importance in health promoting palliative care. (p. 29)

Pizzi (2004) found that QOL was a major theme that emerged from his qualitative study on narratives of hospice professionals. QOL was often discussed in conjunction with wellness and participation in living

Quality of Life Assessments for Occupational Therapy

The following is a list of several QOL assessments and related resources that may be used in occupational therapy practice and research. Both holistic and health-related QOL instruments are included here. However, the list is not all inclusive, as there are hundreds of assessments available. Where available, Web pages or reference information have been listed for ease of access.

- **Child Health Questionnaire.** A self-report and parent report survey for children and adolescents aged 5 or older. Different versions evaluate domains such as physical functioning, role/social emotional, role/social behavioral, role physical, bodily pain, general behavior, mental health, self-esteem, general health perceptions, change in health, parental impact—emotional, parental impact—time, family activities, family cohesion (Landgraf, Abetz, & John, 1966).
- **Dartmouth COOP Clinical Improvement System (Generic/General and Disease Specific).** A self-report survey for children and adolescents aged 10 and older and for adults; adult version for dialysis patients evaluates health and function, clinician attention to needs, risk/habits, preventions, bothers/concerns, diagnoses, medications, finances; user designated and provides SF-36 estimated scores (Nelson, Wasson, Johnson, & Hays, 1996).
- **Duke Health Profile.** A self-report survey evaluates functioning domains such as physical health; mental health; social health; general health; perceived health; self-esteem; and dysfunction domains of anxiety, depression, anxiety-depression, pain, disability (Parkerson, Broadhead, & Tse, 1990).
- **Kidney Disease Quality of Life.** Self-report survey measures all SF-36 domains (physical functioning, role limitations—physical, bodily pain, general health, vitality, social functioning, role limitations—emotional, mental health) plus symptoms/problems, effects of kidney disease on daily life, burden of kidney disease, cognitive function, work status, sexual function, quality of social interaction, and sleep (Hays, Kallich, Mapes, Coons, & Carter, 1994).
- **Life Satisfaction Index—Adolescents (LSI-A).** A life satisfaction measure for adolescents with long-term and progressive neurological disabilities. The instrument and supporting published scientific literature about the conceptual basis and psychometric properties are available at http://www.utoronto.ca/qol; select the publication button to order the assessment.
- **Life Satisfaction Index—Parents (LSI-P).** A life satisfaction measure for parents of adolescents with long-term and progressive neurological disabilities. The instrument and supporting published scientific literature about the conceptual basis and psychometric properties are available at http://www.utoronto.ca/qolt; select the publication button to order the assessment.
- **Quality of Life Assessment Instruments Database (QOLID).** The QOLID database is a collaborative effort of several international organizations interested in patient reported outcomes. Available at http://www.qolid.org.
- **Quality of Life Measure for Children with Developmental Disabilities: Parental Perspective.** This holistic measure of quality of life is based on a rigorously developed conceptual model. The instrument is designed for children aged 3 to 12 years who live with a wide spectrum of developmental disabilities and delays and who may also have physical disabilities. It measures quality of life on three dimensions from the perspective of the child's parent. Supporting published scientific literature on theoretical underpinnings and psychometric properties is available. To obtain this instrument and supporting materials, visit http:www.utoronto.ca/qol; select the publication button to order the assessment.
- **Quality of Life Profiles (for Several Groups and Populations, Including a Generic Version).** This family of instruments is based on the Centre for Health Promotion Model of Quality of Life. All instruments measure quality of life from a holistic perspective, and all have supporting manuals or published scientific literature. Instruments are available for the following groups and populations: adults living with developmental disabilities, adults living with physical disabilities, adults living with schizophrenia, older adults (long, short, and brief versions), generic adult version for general population, and adolescents. To obtain these instruments and supporting materials, visit http://www.utoronto.ca/qol; select the publication button to order the assessment.
- **SF-36, SF-12 (Both With Online Versions), and SF-8.** Generic self-report survey measuring domains of physical functioning, role limitations—physical, bodily pain, general health, vitality, social functioning, role limitations—emotional, mental health. Available at http://www.sf-36.org/. (Author's note: Not necessarily client-centered but is often used as the "gold standard" in medical research. To be used with that in mind.)
- **WHOGOL-100 and the WHOQOL-BREF.** Although there are generally satisfactory ways of measuring the frequency and severity of diseases, this is not the case when measuring wellbeing and quality of life. WHO, with the aid of 15 collaborating centers around the world, has therefore developed two instruments for measuring quality of life—the WHOQOL-100 and the WHOQOL-BREF. These can be used in a variety of cultural settings while allowing the results from different populations and countries to be compared. These instruments have many uses, including in medical practice, research, audit, and in policymaking. Available at http://www.who.int/mental_health/who_qol_field_trial_1995.pdf and http://www.who.int/mental_health/media/en/76.pdf.

life fully. Two of the narratives from this research are representative of themes that described QOL as an outcome of health professional end-of-life interventions. One participant commented on how rewarding it was when making a difference in the patients' QOL. This participant also commented that people often distance the end of life from the rest of the person's life continuum. Their observation was that there may be an artificial barrier due to people's discomfort with the process of death. However, the person who is in the process of dying, yet still participating in activities that enrich QOL, does not see this artificial demarcation in the life cycle. Another participant commented on the sense of fulfillment gained from assisting the family with enhancing their QOL (Pizzi, 2004). Occupational therapists and occupational therapy assistants can assist clients and caregivers in diminishing suffering and thus optimize QOL through fostering occupational participation.

An "open systems" model of care (Sulmasy, 2002) examines the interrelationships between the person's spiritual and biopsychosocial state. Either state of being can influence the other, and the "composite state" of how one is being physically, psychologically, interpersonally, and spiritually is the construct called "quality of life." Sulmasy (2002) believes that researchers should pay more attention to the importance of the relationship between the health professional and the client as a possible "context" for the patient to work out and express spiritual concerns and struggles. An example of this is the story of a patient who continued chemotherapy despite not wanting it because he enjoyed the "company" of his oncologist and feared the relationship would dissipate should chemotherapy treatments stop (Remen, 1999). Sulmasy (2002) also discusses research needs in QOL and its intimate integration with spirituality in general and with the professional's own spirituality specifically. He encourages health professionals to explore the possible impact of spiritual wellbeing and QOL on persons who are dying. In particular, he emphasizes spiritual wellbeing during the bereavement process and QOL for the survivors. To prevent caregiver burnout and to carry on the difficult but meaningful and spiritually satisfying work of supporting the dying person in life role transitions, professionals can facilitate a good death and assist the dying and their caregivers in finding meaning at the end of life and, thus, experience a QOL.

Frankl (2000) states that there are three factors that focus on meaning fulfillment:

- Doing a deed or creating a work
- Experiencing something or encountering someone (e.g., work and falling in love)
- Facing a fate that cannot be changed

He believes that humans must change themselves. No matter what unfolds in one's life, no matter the circumstance, life event, or activity, in order to create a meaningful existence, Frankl says it is the "will to meaning" that helps one through daily life. Through occupational engagement, all these areas of meaning fulfillment can be achieved, thus making meaning, or better yet, facilitating the creation of meaning by empowering one to be participatory. Participation in old age or at the end of life does not necessarily have to mean active physical engagement in occupation for one to experience QOL. It could also mean passive engagement if bed-bound or feeling spiritually connected to occupation that can be facilitated by an occupational therapy practitioner.

Pizzi (1984, 1993), Pizzi and Chromiak (2001), and Pizzi and Briggs (2004) offer many case examples of the creation of meaning and themes of care from both an occupational therapy and occupational science perspective, including meaning and QOL. Developing a sense of closure or resolution may help clients discover meaning and identity and hence an improved QOL at a time when his or her connection to the world seems to be slipping away. In these cases, patients report being at peace or even sometimes exhilarated as they experience life and others anew.

Pizzi and Chromiak (2001) cite a geriatric and a pediatric case example whereby the occupational therapy process unfolded through the discovery of things meaningful and spiritually important to each of the clients. Careful assessment of each person's life through ongoing occupational history-taking revealed the essence of each person. From there, interventions involved the making of products as well as being present with each client, which was as important as the doing process. With the older adult, named Sara, who was referred to occupational therapy because she would not complete her activities of daily living (ADLs), the meaning of occupational engagement and disengagement was much deeper and more expansive than imagined by any of the health professionals with whom she worked. It was in her cake baking that transcendence was finally achieved, giving much meaning to her and those caring for her. "From Sara, the therapist and others learned some important lessons about the power of occupation and how the mind and body, in concert with a loving environment, can work wonderful miracles, for both patient and professional" (Pizzi & Chromiak, 2001, p. 267).

In Bryan's case, a child with HIV/AIDS, the authors discussed the QOL and dignity that the therapy process preserved for him. In both cases, the therapeutic process was framed from a perspective that stressed QOL and dignity.

There is an increased likelihood that people will experience pathological aging secondary to increasing longevity. This will increase the psychosocial needs of older people near the end of their lives and pose challenges to loved ones and professional caregivers. This will also dramatically impact the QOL of the client and their caregivers (Schultz & Heckhausen, 1996). "The possibility that people will achieve a 'good death' will be significantly enhanced to the degree that we attend to the psychosocial needs of their end-of-life care and decisions" (Werth, 2002, p. 200).

Sarvimäki and Stenbock-Hult's (2000) research described QOL in old age as a sense of wellbeing, meaning, and value. A model of QOL was presented and analyzed using 300 participants aged 75 or older living in a community in Finland. They concluded that wellbeing was high in terms of being satisfied with one's living area, economic situation, and health. A Sense of Coherence test measuring meaning viewed participants as having a meaningful, intelligible, and manageable life, and participants also seemed to have a strong sense of value and self-worth. Preliminary significance was given to the model used. The researchers acknowledge that a more subjective client-centered study using the perceptions of older people about their own QOL could be valuable.

Lawton (1991) also cites the need for more subjective perspectives when exploring QOL. His conceptual model relates to QOL and older people. It consists of four major areas: perceived QOL, psychological wellbeing, behavioral competence, and objective environment (Lawton, 1991). He states that QOL is influenced by and needs evaluation from both objective and subjective perspectives. Arnold (1991) believes that there are many factors that influence QOL for the elderly and that QOL is an abstract concept that needs more specific measurement rather than simply approximating an understanding of the concept.

For occupational therapists and occupational therapy assistants working with the elderly and for those clients and caregivers involved with end-of-life issues, QOL is a very important outcome. This outcome can best be realized through interventions that are holistic in scope and that enhance the health and wellbeing of those at the end of life and their caregivers.

Conclusion

Definitions of QOL vary and are often contextually dependent. QOL, as defined by the AOTA's *Framework,* is an important possible outcome of occupational therapy health promotion approaches. When client-centered practice explores strategies to optimize participation with life and living, the result will be enhanced client health and wellbeing. The outcome of that participation, then, is an increased QOL for the individual, no matter their age or cultural, social, or medical situation (Raphael, Brown, Renwick, & Rootman, 1994). It is the responsibility of occupational therapists and occupational therapy assistants to ensure their interventions address health and medical conditions and include strategies that empower and foster community and social participation in all spheres of life, including spirituality where indicated by the client. QOL is optimized through evidence-based, client-centered, and occupation-centered focus. It is the responsibility of occupational therapy assistants and occupational therapists to be aware of QOL models, such as those described in this chapter, and to regularly review the literature for models and research that inform practice to promote QOL.

▶ For Discussion and Review

1. What makes your life good? What makes your life not so good?
2. What do you think makes life good (and not so good) for persons with a chronic disability? How would you go about determining what contributes to and detracts from their QOL?
3. How does engaging in occupation contribute to your own QOL? How does engagement in certain occupations detract from your QOL?
4. If you were at the end of life, what would contribute to fostering optimal QOL so that you could experience a good death?
5. What specific instruments can occupational therapists adapt that measure QOL from an occupation-based perspective?
6. How does the profession of occupational therapy operationalize the concept of QOL to determine the extent to which individuals, communities, and populations experience a good (or poor) QOL?

▶ Research Questions

1. How do people at the end of life or who are older community dwellers define QOL for themselves?
2. What is the nature of the relationship between experienced QOL and the engagement in occupation that is meaningful to the individual?
3. What is the nature of the relationship between health-related QOL and holistic quality of life for individuals? (For example, positively or negatively correlated? Strength or magnitude of correlation?)
4. From their own perspectives, what do people living with disabilities say about the connections between their health, function, and QOL?

5. How do disasters affect occupational participation and impact QOL for children?

Acknowledgment

The editors would like to acknowledge the assistance of Amy Wiles in the editing of this chapter.

References

American Occupational Therapy Association. (2008). Occupational therapy practice framework: Domain and processes (2d ed.). *American Journal of Occupational Therapy, 62*(6), 625–83.

American Occupational Therapy Association. (2004). *Vision statement.* Retrieved June 10, 2004, from http://www.aota.org.

Arnold, S. (1991). Measurement of quality of life in the frail elderly. In J. Birren, J. Lubben, J. Rowe, & D. Deutchman (Eds.), *The concept and measurement of quality of life in the frail elderly* (pp. 50–74). New York: Academic Press.

Bowling, A. (1991). *Measuring health: A review of quality of life measurement scales.* Milton Keynes, UK: Open University Press.

Bowling, A. (1995). *Measuring disease: A review of disease-specific quality of life measurement scales.* Buckingham, UK: Open University Press.

Brown, R. I., Brown, P. M., & Bayer, M. B. (1994). A quality of life model: New challenges arising from a six-year study. In D. Goode (Ed.), *Quality of life for persons with disabilities: International perspectives and issues* (pp. 39–56). Cambridge, MA: Brookline Books.

Byock, I. R. (1996). *Statement before the IOM Committee on Care at the End of Life on behalf of the Academy of Hospice Physicians.* Retrieved June 2004, from http://www.dyingwell.com/iomtest.htm.

Byock, I. R. (1997). *Dying well: The prospect for growth at the end of life.* New York: Riverhead Books.

Canadian Association of Occupational Therapists. (2002). *Enabling occupation: An occupational therapy perspective.* Ottawa, ON: Author.

Cassell, E. J. (1991). *The nature of suffering and the goals of medicine.* New York: Oxford University Press.

Christiansen, C. (1999). Defining lives: Occupation as identity. An essay on competence, coherence and the creation of meaning. *American Journal of Occupational Therapy, 53,* 547–58.

Christiansen, C., Backman, C., Little, B. R., & Nguyen, A. (1999). Occupations and subjective wellbeing: A study of personal projects. *American Journal of Occupational Therapy, 53,* 91–100.

Christiansen, C., & Townsend, E. (2004). An introduction to occupation. In C. Christiansen & E. Townsend (Eds.), *Introduction to occupation: The art and science of living* (pp. 1–27). Upper Saddle River, NJ: Prentice Hall.

Cohen, S. R., Mount, B. M., & Strobe, M. G. (1995). The McGill Quality of Life Questionnaire: A measure of quality of life for people with advanced disease. *Palliative Medicine, 9,* 207–19.

Cramer, J. A., & Spilker, B. (Eds.). (1996). *Quality of life and pharmacoeconomics: An introduction* (pp. 161–68). Philadelphia: Lippincott–Raven.

Cummins, R. A. (1995). Assessing quality of life. In R. I. Brown (Ed.), *Quality of life for handicapped people.* London: Chapman & Hall.

Day, H., & Jankey, S. (1996). Lessons from the literature: Toward a holistic model of quality of life. In R. Renwick, I. Brown, & M. Nagler (Eds.), *Quality of life in health promotion and rehabilitation: Conceptual approaches, issues, and applications* (pp. 39–50). Thousand Oaks, CA: Sage.

Evans, R. G., Barer, M. L., & Marmor, T. R. (1994). *Why are some people healthy and others are not? The determinants of health of populations.* Hawthorne, NY: Aldine de Gruyter.

Felce, D., & Perry, J. (1996). In R. Renwick, I. Brown, & M. Nagler (Eds.), *Quality of life in health promotion and rehabilitation: Conceptual approaches, issues, and applications* (pp. 51–62). Thousand Oaks, CA: Sage.

Field, M. J., & Cassel, C. K. (Eds.). (1997). *Approaching death: Improving care at the end of life.* Washington, DC: National Academy Press.

Frankl, V. (2000). *Man's search for ultimate meaning.* New York: MJF Books.

Gold, M., Franks, P., & Erickson, P. (1996). Assessing the health of the nation: The predictive validity of a preference-based measure and self-rated health. *Medical Care, 34*(2), 163–77.

Hays, R. D., Kallich, J. D., Mapes, D. L., Coons, S. J., & Carter, W. B. (1994). Development of the Kidney Disease Quality of Life [KDQOL] Instrument. *Quality of Life Research, 3*(5), 329–38.

Horley, J. (1984). Life satisfaction, happiness, and morale: Two problems with the use of subjective well-being indicators. *Gerontologist, 24,* 124–27.

Hughes, C., Hwang, B., Kim, J. H., Eisenman, L. T., & Killian, D. J. (1995). Quality of life in applied research: A review and analysis of empirical measures. *American Journal of Mental Retardation, 99,* 623–41.

Koot, H. M. (2001). The study of quality of life: Concepts and methods. In H. M. Koot & J. L. Wallander. *Quality of life in child and adolescent illness: Concepts, methods, and findings* (pp. 2–20). New York: Brunner-Routledge.

Koot, H. M., & Wallander. J. L. (2001). *Quality of life in child and adolescent illness: Concepts, methods, and findings.* New York: Brunner-Routledge.

Laliberte Rudman, D., Hoffman, L., Scott, E., & Renwick, R. (2004). Quality of life for people living with schizophrenia: Validating an assessment that addresses consumer concerns and occupational issues. *Occupational Therapy Journal of Research, 24,* 13–21.

Landgraf, J. M., Abetz, L., & John, E. (1966). *Child health questionnaire [CHQ]: A user's manual.* Boston: The Health Institute, New England Medical Center.

Lawton, M. P. (1991). A multidimensional view of the quality of life in frail elders. In J. Birren, J. Lubben, J. Rowe, & D. Deutchman (Eds.), *The concept and measurement of quality of life in the frail elderly* (pp. 3–27). New York: Academic Press.

Lindstrom, B. (1994). *The essence of existence: On the quality of life for children in the Nordic countries.* Goteborg, Sweden: Nordic School of Public Health.

Lindstrom, B. (1995). Measuring and improving quality of life for children. In B. Lindstrom & N. Spencer (Eds.), *Social paediatrics* (pp. 83–89). New York: Oxford University Press.

McDowell, I., & Newell, C. (1996). *Measuring health: A guide to rating scales and questionnaires.* New York: Oxford University Press.

Nelson E. C., Wasson, J. H., Johnson, D. J., & Hays, R. D. (1996). Dartmouth COOP Functional Health Assessment Charts: Brief measures for clinical practice. In J. A. Cramer & B. Spilker B. (Eds.), *Quality of life and pharmacoeconomics: An introduction* (pp. 161–68). Philadelphia: Lippincott–Raven.

Parkerson, G. R., Jr., Broadhead, W. E., & Tse, C-K. J. (1990). The Duke Health Profile: A 17-item measure of health and dysfunction. *Medical Care, 28*(11), 1056–72).

Patrick, D. L., & Erickson, P. (1993). *Health status and health policy.* New York: Oxford University Press.

Pegg, B., & Tan, L. (2002). Reducing suffering to improve quality of life through health promotion. *Contemporary Nurse, 12,* 22–30.

Pizzi, M. (1984). Occupational therapy in hospice care. *American Journal of Occupational Therapy, 38*(4), 252–57.

Pizzi, M. (1993). Environments of care: Hospice. In H. Hopkins & H. Smith (Eds.), *Willard and Spackman's occupational therapy* (8th ed., pp. 853–64). Philadelphia: Lippincott.

Pizzi, M. (2004). *Promoting a good death: Perspectives of hospice professionals.* Unpublished doctoral dissertation.

Pizzi, M., & Briggs, R. (2004). Occupational and physical therapy in hospice: The facilitation of meaning, quality of life and wellbeing. *Topics in Geriatric Rehabilitation, 20*(2), 119–29.

Pizzi, M., & Chromiak, B. (2001). Hospice: Creating meaningful environments of care. In M. Scaffa (Ed.), *Occupational therapy in community based practice settings* (pp. 253–70). Philadelphia: F. A. Davis.

Raphael, D. (1996). Quality of life of older adults: Toward the optimization of the aging process. In R. Renwick, I. Brown, & M. Nagler (Eds.), *Quality of life in health promotion and rehabilitation: Conceptual approaches, issues, and applications* (pp. 290–306). Thousand Oaks, CA: Sage.

Raphael, D., Brown, I., Renwick, R., & Rootman, I. (1994). *Quality of life theory and assessment: What are the implications for health promotion?* Toronto, ON: University of Toronto, Centre for Health Promotion and ParticipACTION.

Remen, R. (1999). Educating for mission, meaning, and compassion. In S. Glazer (Ed.), *The heart of learning: Spirituality in education* (pp. 33–49). New York: Tarcher/Putnam.

Renwick, R. (2004). Quality of life as a guiding framework for occupational intervention. In S. Bachner & M. Ross (Eds.), *Adults with developmental disabilities: Current approaches in occupational therapy* (2d ed., pp. 20–38). Bethesda, MD: American Occupational Therapy Association.

Renwick, R., & Brown, I. (1996). The Centre for Health Promotion's approach to quality of life: Being, belonging, and becoming. In R. Renwick, I. Brown, & M. Nagler (Eds.), *Quality of life in health promotion and rehabilitation: Conceptual approaches, issues, and applications* (pp. 75–86). Thousand Oaks, CA: Sage.

Renwick, R., Brown, I., & Raphael, D. (2000). Person-centered quality of life: Contributions from Canada to an international understanding. In K. D. Keith & R. L. Schalock (Eds.), *Cross-cultural perspectives on quality of life* (pp. 5–21). Washington, DC: American Association on Mental Retardation.

Renwick, R., & Fudge Schormans, A. (2004). *The children's quality of life project.* Toronto, ON: Quality of Life Research Unit, University of Toronto.

Renwick, R., Fudge Schormans, A., & Zekovic, B. (2003). Quality of life for children with developmental disabilities: A new conceptual framework. *Journal on Developmental Disabilities, 10,* 107–14.

Renwick, R., Nourhaghighi, N., Manns, P. J., & Laliberte Rudman, D. (2003). Quality of life for people with physical disabilities: A new instrument. *International Journal of Rehabilitation Research, 26,* 1–9.

Sarvimäki, A., & Stenbock-Hult B. (2000). Quality of life in old age described as a sense of well-being, meaning and value. *Journal of Advanced Nursing, 32*(4), 1025–33.

Schalock, R. L. (1996a). Reconsidering the conceptualization and measurement of quality of life. In R. L. Schalock (Ed.), *Quality of life— Volume I: Conceptualization and measurement* (pp. 123–39). Washington, DC: American Association on Mental Retardation.

Schalock, R. L. (Ed.). (1996b). *Quality of life—Volume I: Conceptualization and measurement.* Washington, DC: American Association on Mental Retardation.

Schultz, R., & Heckhausen, J. (1996). A life span model of successful aging. *American Psychologist, 51*(7), 702–14.

Stark, J., & Faulkner, E. (1996). Quality of life across the life-span. In R. L. Schalock (Ed.) *Quality of life—Volume I: Conceptualization and measurement* (pp. 23–32). Washington, DC: American Association on Mental Retardation.

Sulmasy, D. P. (2002). Psychosocial-spiritual model for the care of patients at the end of life. *Gerontologist, 42,* 24–33.

Tate, D. G., Dijkers, M., & Johnson-Greene, L. (1996). Outcome measures in quality of life. *Topics in Stroke Rehabilitation, 2*(4), 1–17.

Thompson, G., & McClement, S. (2002). Defining and determining quality in end of life care. *International Journal of Palliative Nursing, 8*(6), 288–93.

Townsend, E. A., & Polatajko, H. J. (2007). *Enabling occupation II: Advancing an occupational therapy vision for health, well-being, & justice through occupations.* Ottawa, ON: Canadian Association of Occupational Therapists.

U.S. Department of Health and Human Services. (2000). *Healthy People 2010: Understanding and improving health.* Washington, DC: U.S. Government Printing Office.

Wallander, J. L. (2001). Theoretical and developmental issues in quality of life for children and adolescents. In H. M. Koot & J. L. Wallander, *Quality of life in child and adolescent illness: Concepts, methods, and findings* (pp. 23–48). New York: Brunner-Routledge.

Werth, J. L., Jr. (2002). Behavioral science and the end of life. *American Behavioral Scientist, 46*(2), 195–203.

Wicks, A. (2001). Comment: Occupational potential: A topic worthy of exploration. *Journal of Occupational Science, 8,* 32–35.

Wilcock, A. (1998). *An occupational perspective of health.* Thorofare, NJ: SLACK.

Wolfensberger, W. (1994) Let's hang up "quality of life" as a hopeless term. In D. Goode (Ed.), *Quality of life for persons with disabilities: International perspectives and issues.* Cambridge, MA: Brookline Books.

World Health Organization. (1986). *Ottawa charter for health promotion.* Ottawa, ON: Canadian Public Health Association.

World Health Organization. (1998). The World Health Organization quality-of-life assessment (WHOQOL): Development and psychometric properties. *Social Science Medicine, 46,* 1569–85.

Zekovic, B., & Renwick, R. (2003). Quality of life for children and adolescents with developmental disabilities: Review of conceptual and methodological issues relevant to public policy. *Disability and Society, 18,* 19–34.

Zhan, L. (1992). Quality of life: Conceptual and measurement issues. *Advanced Nursing, 17,* 795–800.

Chapter 8

Occupational Justice

Melba J. Arnold and Debra Rybski

Injustice anywhere is a threat to justice everywhere.
—Dr. Martin Luther King, April 16, 1963

Learning Objectives

This chapter is designed to enable the reader to:

- Describe concepts of social justice, social injustice, and social group identity development and membership.
- Identify and define elements of oppression and explain how oppression influences social identity and its contribution to social injustice.
- Discuss concepts of occupational justice and how the interrelation between social injustice and oppression can predispose certain social groups to occupational injustice.

- Identify and define various forms of occupational injustice and apply these premises to situational examples.
- Describe how occupational justice can be incorporated in the promotion of health and wellbeing.

Key Terms

Classism
Commutative justice
Distributive justice
Injustice
Internalized oppression
Occupational alienation

Occupational
  deprivation
Occupational imbalance
Occupational injustice
Occupational justice

Occupational
  marginalization
Oppression
Participation
Participation restriction
Preventive occupation

Racism
Sexism
Social group identity
Social injustice
Social justice

Introduction

From the very beginning of the profession, occupational therapy practitioners have been concerned with justice and the wellbeing of clients. For over a decade, and through contributions of occupational therapists and occupational scientists, the profession has increased its focus on justice and its relationship to practice and occupational wellbeing. Through patient advocacy, occupational therapy has focused on the promotion of ethical and moral issues related to equal access to care for all clients, regardless of condition, illness, or station in life. Because occupational therapy concerns itself with the occupational nature of human existence, practitioners advocate for their client by addressing both the medical and nonmedical aspects of the individual's needs. Although clients may present with clinical or medical conditions, occupational therapy practitioners are concerned with how these conditions impact their clients'

ability to continue to equally participate in society and fulfill their occupational needs. Wilcock and Townsend (2000) provide a clear distinction between social justice and occupational justice by viewing the former as addressing social relations and conditions of life, while the latter deals with what people do in their relationships and conditions for living.

This chapter provides an overview of basic information that addresses the need for practitioners to further clarify the relationship between social justice and occupational justice, and the implications for practice. By developing a better understanding of the terminology and the relationship between social justice and occupational justice, occupational therapy assistants and occupational therapists can be more effective in dealing with the challenges resulting from social changes that affect human engagement in daily occupations, determine quality of life, and affect delivery of services to clients.

In order to understand the relationship between the terms *social justice* and *occupational justice,* it is important to think of social justice in both a national and international context. It is becoming exceedingly more complex to find any firm basis for a common definition of social justice across the world. Actions and behaviors that may be just in the United States might be considered unjust beyond U.S. borders. Often, decisions about social justice are based on a nation's or community's perceptions of power, influence, the allocation of limited resources, and cultural factors. Thus, it is critical to consider a multifaceted view of social justice, including how various theorists define and describe it, and to exemplify the need for a greater focus on occupational justice throughout the United States and the world.

Social Justice

The origin and use of the term *social justice* can be traced back to around 1845, but it is unknown who first coined it. However, documentation reveals that the term originated in print as early as the mid-1800s, when it was used by a Jesuit who was considered to be a political writer of that time (Shields, 1941). According to Shields (1941), because the term was recognized as having "acceptable meaning," it became more widely used among different groups in the United States and in parts of Europe. Various literature sources agree that the notion of justice has been debated as far back as the days of Socrates, Plato, and Aristotle (384–322 BC).

A literature search revealed a prevailing Judeo-Christian, philosophical, and political interconnection that contributes to the evolution of a generally recognized definition of *social justice* in modern society. An early definition recognized **social justice** as "a certain equality in society; the equality of justice, by which everyone in society gets his due from everyone else" (Shields, 1916). Current definitions reflect a similar perspective. For example, U.S. Catholic Bishops outlined three elements to further describe justice—commutative justice, distributive justice, and social justice (U.S. Catholic Bishops, 1999). The bishops agreed on these elements because they believed no single principle could govern the many possible situations society might encounter. These terms are defined as follows:

- **Commutative justice** is the fundamental fairness in agreements and relationships between individuals and social groups.
- **Distributive justice** is the allocation of income, wealth, and power in society evaluated in light of

its effect on persons whose basic material needs are not met.
- **Social justice** means that people have a right to be active, productive participants in society and that society should not hinder the ability of an individual to develop their full range of social, economic, and political participation. There is a reciprocal duty between the individual and society.

In a more comprehensive and modern approach, Wilcock and Townsend (2000) explain social justice as an experience that involves a society that is "governed justly, ethically, morally, with civil principles of fairness, [and that] promotes empowerment, provides equitable access to resources, and promotes the sharing of rights and responsibilities" (p. 84). In other words, how humans relate to each other must be the fundamental core of social justice. A social justice perspective becomes important to egalitarian societies, because it "draws attention to the ways in which we treat each other and the distribution of material wealth and the opportunities which accompany that wealth" (Wilcock & Townsend, 2000, p. 84).

Noted philosopher and social contract theorist John Rawls (2000) is known for his theoretical work on social justice. Rawls theorizes that a just system exists when there is fairness in exchange and when individual needs and potential of all who are involved are considered and treated equally in terms of distribution of resources, including civil, political, and reproductive rights, responsibilities, and opportunities. He suggests that social justice occurs when every person is treated with respect and moral equality and when the lowest member in society is afforded the same parity and fairness as all others (Rawls, 2000).

Goal of Social Justice

During the early 1900s, Italian writer. Loria saw the goal of social justice as "an order in which the prosperous and peaceable development of all will be possible" (Shields, 1941). The goal of social justice is viewed very much the same today. Adams, Bell, and Griffin (1997) consider the goal of social justice to be "full and equal participation of all groups in a society that is mutually shaped to meet their needs" (p. 3). To achieve such a goal will require individuals to engage in a participative and collaborative democratic process that is absent of domination and oppression (Gil, 1998). The concept of social justice embraces basic values that include the equal worth of all individuals, their right to have basic needs met, and their equal right to opportunities.

Given this philosophical primer on social justice one can then ask, "What is the connection between social justice and occupational therapy?" Inherent in the services provided by occupational therapy practitioners, social justice concerns must be addressed for every client. To provide quality care from a social justice perspective, it is routine to consider distinctions between clients based on age, gender, culture, ethnicity, social class, race, sexual orientation, or disability. However, also included in these criteria are a final determination of "relative deprivation" and a baseline of what qualifies as a "minimally acceptable level" of resources. Historically, occupational therapy has been in the forefront addressing issues of social justice and quality of life in order to empower clients. Emphasis on social justice is evident in the early work of Adolph Meyer and other pioneers in the occupational therapy field who provided care to institutionalized individuals who might otherwise have had little or no attention to their needs (Meyer, 1977).

Social Injustice

Social injustice cannot be discussed without addressing the role and impact of oppression. Since the core of social justice involves equal participation in society by all individuals to the extent of resources and situations, it is easy to conclude that social injustice is fortified by rules, regulations, policies, and other forms of guidance that encourage an unjust, or inequitable, disadvantage for some while greatly empowering others. The more a society strives toward the promotion of social justice, the more it is driven to understand and address the social complexities that may create inequality, difference, oppression, domination, and exploitation. Gil (1998) defines **social injustice** as "coercively established and maintained inequalities, discrimination, and dehumanizing, development-inhibiting conditions of living . . . imposed by dominant social groups, classes, and peoples upon dominated and exploited groups, classes and peoples" (p. 10). Current-day examples supporting Gil's definition include health-care inequality; discrimination based on race, age, religion, ethnicity, gender, or sexual orientation; homelessness; poverty; inadequate education; and others.

Oppression

Gil (1998) distinguishes between oppression and injustice; he defines **oppression** as human relations involving domination and exploitation. Whereas **injustice** involves coercive behavior designed to establish and maintain inequalities, discrimination, and dehumanizing situations for others. Oppression plays a major role in social injustice.

Gil (1998) describes five institutions of social life believed to shape the circumstances of living and the relative power of individuals, social groups, and classes:

(1) stewardship; (2) organization of work and production; (3) exchange of products of human work; (4) governance and legal status or authorization; and (5) biological reproduction, socialization, and social control. Gil's model not only encompasses the quality of human relationships among individuals, groups, and classes, but also the overall quality of life, whether the origin is due to relationships or economic conditions. There are other life dimensions that may be a part of oppression (e.g., psychological, social, and cultural); however, Gil (1998) believes that these five institutions are central to shaping social life in general and that the absence of these is likely to lead to oppression. Gil concludes that an oppressive society exists when people are not considered and treated as equals and therefore do not have equal rights and responsibilities concerning the key institutions of life.

Adams and colleagues (1997) offer six identifying elements of oppression. Oppression is pervasive; restrictive; hierarchical; it involves complex, multiple, crosscutting relationships; it is internalized; and it is based on "isms"—shared and distinctive characteristics. The *pervasive* nature of social inequality can be seen in social institutions and in individuals. Typically oppression is more likely to be all-encompassing and includes other elements such as bigotry, discrimination, prejudice, and personal bias. While use of the terms *oppression* or *social injustice* relative to how health care is administered to the elderly or individuals living below poverty may seem overly dramatic, these groups often face severe health-care needs and have more limits placed on their insurance and medication coverage compared to other age groups that are gainfully employed with better health-care coverage (Cummings, 2003). Oppression is *restrictive* in that it can limit self-development; for example, poor children are less likely to have the experiences, role models, and resources that might lead them to imagine themselves achieving high goals, such as becoming professionals or leaders in their country (Adams et al., 1997; Finn & Jacobson, 2003).

In the case of oppression, a *hierarchical* relationship exists when dominant groups gain a disproportionate benefit from their privileged status, as seen in the relationship between white people and people of color. In U.S. society, whites generally enjoy more positions of power and influence than other racial groups. They earn more money, hold the majority of influential positions, and make decisions about the control of hospitals, banks, lending institutions, major businesses, transportation, housing, and U.S. agriculture (Adams et al., 1997).

Power and privilege become far more complicated in situations where individuals have *complex, multiple, crosscutting group memberships* (Adams et al., 1997). The result is a continuation of hierarchical and internalized relationships that can make it difficult to determine "who is on first." For example, consider men of color who may enjoy economic opportunity not available to most women. Conversely, these same individuals may face limitations not endured by white coworkers, male or female. Despite their economic and professional status, there is greater likelihood of males of color being stopped by police while driving an upscale vehicle or having difficulty hailing a taxi than their white male counterpart (Cose, 1993; Dill & Zinn, 1990; Feagin & Sikes, 1994, all cited in Adams et al., 1997).

The element of **internalized oppression** refers to the manner in which an individual psychologically absorbs his or her role as the oppressed (Fannon, 1968; Freire, 1990; Miller, 1976, all cited in Adams et al., 1997). This form of internalization can actually impact both the oppressed and the oppressor. For example, members of minority racial, religious, or sexual orientation groups may internalize feelings of being oppressed and ultimately become their own oppressor. Paulo Freire (1970) described internalized oppression as a dual experience that occurs inside the consciousness of the oppressed. It is as if the oppressive state can ultimately consume the individual to a point of self-hatred and self-destruction and can give them a sense of no escape from their situation.

Social Identity and Oppression

Social identity plays a critical role in developing an understanding of oppression. An understanding of essential identity develops from birth and from that moment is shaped over time by the values and attitudes prevalent in the individual's context. Because identity describes who humans are, there is a strong urge to protect beliefs, values, social group affiliations, and memberships that help create a sense of self. A **social group identity** can be defined as a sense of collective similarity based on one's perception that there is a common heritage within a particular group (Bettencourt & Hume, 1999). Throughout years of development, the vast majority of people develop this within the original social group in which they are born. Humans have a tendency to strive to maintain their identity by remaining within the context of their own group. When humans move outside the boundaries of their social group, their identity begins to transform. The more individuals learn about groups outside of their own, the more likely they will feel less threatened by that group's presence.

It is very important to note that oppression cannot be understood only in terms of the individual, for people are privileged or oppressed on the basis of social group status. One of the privileges of dominant social group status is the simple luxury of having a self-image of individuality that is unique to that person. For example, a white man is rarely defined by his whiteness or maleness, regardless of his public endeavors. If he does well, he is likely to be acknowledged as a highly competent or qualified individual. By the same token, if he does poorly, the blame is attributed to him alone. The opposite is the case for subordinate group members. Under similar circumstances, the subordinate individual is considered an exception when successful but is likely to be viewed as representative of the entire social group if the person fails (Adams et al., 1997).

Paulo Freire (1970) believed that oppressive forces are not part of the natural order of things; instead, he concluded that they are the result of historical and socially constructed forces that can be changed. An example of this can be seen in the belief that oppression is manifested through the use of "isms" that are developed and sustained over time (e.g., racism, classism, heterosexism, anti-Semitism, sexism, and ableism) and are connected to other dimensions of oppressive experiences (Adams et al., 1997; Bishop, 2002; Latting, 1990). Figure 8-1 illustrates the common social identity categories in which humans are likely to be grouped. Based on the oppressive nature of the human experience, each social identity group evolves into a form of "ism." For each social identity group and each form of oppression, there is a target and an agent group. For example, Native Americans, African Americans, Latino Americans, or other individuals of color are most likely to experience racism and are considered to be the "target," or subordinate, disenfranchised group, while Caucasians are typically considered to be the "agent," or dominant, privileged group.

Understanding the various forms of "isms" inherent in oppression is important, as they contribute to the development of social identity. There are two principles that are important to understanding the impact of racism:

1. As a form of oppression, racism has a negative effect on the dominant group and the subordinate group. By using racism as a form of power, the subordinate group is stigmatized and violated, while the dominant group is encumbered with psychic and ethical cruelty.
2. There is an overt and covert level to racism in that there are conscious and unconscious forms of discriminating and prejudicial behavior that pervasively embrace the cultural norms of the dominant group (Adams et al., 1997).

The civil rights movement of the 1950s and 1960s in the United States was the catalyst for a growth in the understanding of racism. **Racism** can be defined

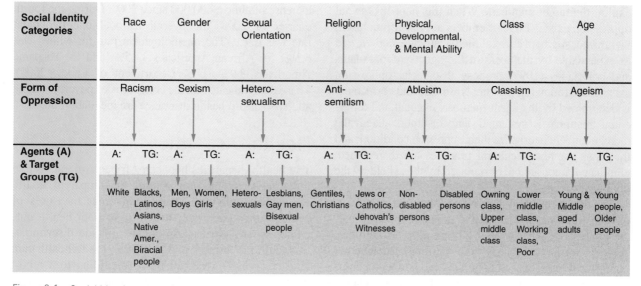

Social Identity Categories	Race		Gender		Sexual Orientation		Religion		Physical, Developmental, & Mental Ability			Class		Age	
Form of Oppression	Racism		Sexism		Hetero-sexualism		Anti-semitism		Ableism			Classism		Ageism	
Agents (A) & Target Groups (TG)	A:	TG:	A:	TG:	A:	TG:	A:	TG:	A:	TG:		A:	TG:	A:	TG:
	White	Blacks, Latinos, Asians, Native Amer., Biracial people	Men, Boys	Women, Girls	Hetero-sexuals	Lesbians, Gay men, Bisexual people	Gentiles, Christians	Jews or Catholics, Jehovah's Witnesses	Non-disabled persons	Disabled persons		Owning class, Upper middle class	Lower middle class, Working class, Poor	Young & Middle aged adults	Young people, Older people

Figure 8-1   Social identity categories.

Adapted from. Teaching for diversity and social justice by M. Adams, L. A. Bell, & P. Griffin, 1997, *New York: Routledge.*

as prejudice, discrimination, or oppression against another individual based on physical differences such as skin color or other features. According to the documentary *Race: The Power of an Illusion* (Adelman, 2003), race is a modern idea, in that ancient societies did not divide people by physical differences but by religion, status, class, or language.

Classism refers to the hierarchical nature of oppression based on economics. It evolved out of the 1960s and 1970s as an explanation of the structural factors that maintain oppressive, exploitative, economic, and social relations. When reference is made to the "upper" or "elite" class, it means individuals with power and status. The opposite is true when people are identified as "lower" class, meaning individuals without power or people who are poor. Understanding classism reveals how power, over time, can transform domination into practices that are taken as the natural order of the relationship between the oppressor and the oppressed.

Sexism refers to the social structure of patriarchy and how women internalize its existence. As a response to sexism, the feminist movement uncovered how women internalized the theory of patriarchy and became collaborators in creating and perpetuating the experience. Women ultimately challenged the traditional notions regarding human nature, sexuality, family life, and gender roles and relations (Adams et al., 1997). For over 150 years in the United States, women have worked to deconstruct the unjust relationship based on gender to gain their basic human rights and to develop their own identity as equals and individuals.

The oppressive nature of each "ism" is evident when viewed alone (see Fig. 8-1). However, consider individuals who are faced with multiple issues of "ism." Today's society is far from the clearly defined cultural groups of the past. Interracial or intercultural marriages and sexual orientation have had a major impact on how the social structure has changed and what constitutes social group membership. Although attitudes and mind-sets have changed at varying social levels, the pervasiveness of oppression of individuals based on class, race, gender, and financial status still exists (Adams et al., 1997). Imagine a homosexual individual who is also African American, Mexican, Latino, or Hispanic, with a low income and a disability. Conceivably, the degree of social injustice (oppression) experienced by such a person would be far greater than if this person was a white male or female with an elite status (Adams, et al., 1997; Bishop, 2002; Johnson, 2001). Individuals of multiple identities and diverse social group memberships, along with the complexity of their experiences resulting from oppression, will be the greatest future challenge confronting social justice and researchers in the field.

Within each "ism" category, there is a clearly identifiable dominant group (i.e., oppressor) and a subordinate group (i.e., oppressed). Social justice literature refers to the dominant group as *agents* and the subordinate group as *targets* (Adams et al., 1997). Typically, agent members are privileged at birth or may acquire their status through means of privilege. As a result of their status, agent members knowingly or unknowingly exploit the target members. When this happens, social oppression exists. Target members are disenfranchised, victimized, stigmatized, exploited, restricted, and viewed as expendable by members of the agent group. Adams and colleagues (1997) propose that social oppression exists if the following are true: Normalcy and correctness is determined by the agent member; unequal and differential treatment is systematic and institutionalized; the target members internalize their oppressed condition; and the target member's cultural practices are disregarded, eliminated, imposed on, or replaced by those held by the dominant group.

The dynamics of oppression can be found in individuals, institutions, and societal systems. Individuals create oppressive experiences by bringing their attitudes, beliefs, values, and behavior into situations, whether consciously or unconsciously. This can be seen in cases involving hate crimes or use of racial or religious slurs. Structural oppression may exist in government agencies, educational systems, and business, as manifested by the unusually high rate of imprisonment for people classed as minorities or low income or for individuals with mental illness. It is also manifested in the high rate of poverty and disenfranchised, the continuing imbalance in educational opportunities, and the existence of unfair housing and employment (Adams et al., 1997; Finn, 2003; Gil, 1998; National Alliance on Mental Illness, 2006; Thibeault, 2006).

Socioeconomical and Political Issues

Effects of oppression on social justice can be seen nationally and globally. Examples of social injustice throughout the world appear in newspapers, news magazines, and on the radio and television. Stories and data abound about the exploitation and unfair treatment of persons, typically the very young and very old, the poverty-stricken or those with low income, people with disabilities, or any combination of these characteristics. A press release by the Congressional Black Caucus (Cummings, 2004) reported economic data from the U.S. Census Bureau (USCB). The report stated that in 2003, the poverty rate for African Americans rose by 24%, bringing the ranks of poverty-stricken African Americans to 9 million. For Hispanic Americans, the poverty rate climbed by 22%, placing 9 million Hispanic Americans below the poverty line. For children in the United States, 12.9 million were living in conditions equal to that of a destitute third-world country. In 2003, the number of Hispanic Americans without health insurance rose to 13.2 million, an increase of 1.4 million since 2000. For the same year, 7.3 million African Americans were without health insurance, an

increase of almost 600,000 since 2000. During the fourth quarter of 2008, the overall national unemployment rate was 6.9%. The unemployment rate for whites was 6.3%, for African Americans 11.5%, and for Hispanic Americans 8.9% (U.S. Department of Labor, 2009). These data indicate that the conditions of poverty and the ability to afford health insurance are inevitably linked.

Health Disparities

The health disparities between African Americans and other racial groups are striking and apparent in life expectancy, infant mortality, and other measures of health status. Factors contributing to poor health outcomes among African Americans include discrimination, cultural barriers, and lack of access to health care (U.S. Census Bureau, 2000a). According to a report published in 2001 by the U.S. Department of Health and Human Services (USDHHS), the average health-related life expectancy at birth for African American males is 68.3 years, compared with 74.8 years for white males, and 75 years for African American females versus 80 years for white females. The report cited the incidence of diabetes for African Americans, a leading cause of death among this group, was twice the rate than that of white Americans. Infant mortality rates are reportedly twice as high for African Americans as Caucasians, at 14.6 and 5.8, respectively (Lukacs & Schoendorf, 2004; USDHHS, 2001).

A 2004 report from the Intercultural Cancer Council (ICC) stated that up to 80 percent of elderly women with newly diagnosed invasive cervical cancer have not had a Pap test in excess of 5 years. Older Hispanic women continue to be less likely to be screened for cancer until the later stages of the disease. Forty percent of elderly Mexican American women report never having had a mammogram. The ICC further reports that the elderly, especially among ethnic groups, get substandard care and generally have poorer mortality outcomes compared to white or more affluent patients. Within the Native American population, male elders have a greater chance of dying from malignant tumors as compared to their white or black counterparts.

Access is considered to be the primary indicator for the lack of health care for the elderly, particularly among ethnic groups. Lack of health insurance coverage, limited Medicare coverage, and political and sociocultural barriers are credited as the primary factors that limit health care for the elderly. Generally, racial and ethnic elderly minorities covered by Medicare suffer from more illnesses and are more apt to live in poverty (ICC, 2004). According to the ICC, elderly patients have expressed a physical and emotional distance from health-care systems that ultimately lead to a delay and avoidance in receiving the necessary preventive services, and this eventually leads to mortality.

An International Perspective

In addressing social injustice and oppression from a global perspective, in their 1998 conference in Rome, Catholic Bishops decreed to do whatever could be done to change international attitudes and behavior toward Africa, which is considered to be the epitome of marginalization. With 30 of the world's poorest countries, Africa houses two-thirds of the world's refugees. Throughout its history, Africa has been subjected to both internal (from its own governments) and external oppression. Throughout the world, there are over 45 million refugees and displaced persons, 80% of whom are women and children. These individuals often dwell in the poorest of countries (e.g., Eastern European countries such as Romania, the Czech Republic, Bosnia, Serbia, etc.) with no relief in sight and a growing sense of hopelessness and despair for life and culture (U.S. Catholic Bishops, 1999). Other indigenous people, as seen with the "untouchables" (Dalits or castes) in India, face an inescapable lifetime of low-level hierarchy, poverty, social exclusion, and isolation based on ancient principles of hereditary pollution (meaning once born into this social station, one cannot escape the generational cycle) and totally unrelated to any principles of race. In the hierarchical system, the Brahmans are considered to be the purest and the untouchables the most polluted. Dalits include people whose occupation in life are considered to be humiliating or unclean and involve tasks thought to have a polluting nature, such as killing or disposing of animals or working with their hides or coming into contact with human waste. Once born into this social caste, escaping the associated discrimination and stigma is nearly impossible (U.S. Catholic Bishops, 1999; Moon, Omvedt, & Zelliot, 2001).

Cases of modern-day slavery exist throughout the world, even in places such as Paris, London, New York, Los Angeles, and Zurich. According to Bales (1999), "this is the new slavery which focuses on big profits and cheap lives. It is not about owning slaves in the traditional sense of old slavery, but about controlling them completely. People become completely disposable tools for making money" (p. 4). Ruthless business owners throughout the world are benefiting from the work of modern-day slavery as reported in some sugar factories in the Caribbean or in jewelry factories and garment sweatshops in India. Workers are paid little, if anything at all, to produce goods that are shipped globally and sold to make millions of dollars for the owners. Although society will speak out against the perils of modern-day slavery, it becomes a primary economic process that keeps the cost of products low and brings high returns on investments (Bales, 1999).

In many ways, migrant workers in the United States embody modern-day slavery. Immigrants seeking to escape severely impoverished settlements arrive here willing to work under any conditions to earn wages. Employers of Mexican, Chinese, and other workers benefit from this desperation by paying below minimum-wage requirements while demanding that employees work well in excess of 40 hours per week without overtime pay. In some cases, as seen in garment factories in New York that utilize Chinese workers, it is not uncommon for employers to withhold earned wages or to make claims of having a cash flow problem to postpone payment (Goode & Maskovsky, 2001).

Vulnerable Populations

Aday's (2001) accounting of vulnerable populations gives another perspective of social injustice. She writes of how certain populations are targeted as vulnerable or at risk for poor physical, psychological, or social health. Aday concluded that the mental health and well-being of low socioeconomic status groups tend to be more adversely affected by stressful or negative events than is the case for those with higher status. Certain factors serve as predictors of populations at risk. It is already known that social status, age, gender, race, and ethnicity are significant features or predictors of vulnerable populations; individuals who fall into these vulnerable categories are at a higher risk of health disparity. Other additional contributing factors that have served as predictors of populations at risk include social capital (e.g., family structure, marital status, social networks, etc.) and human capital (e.g., schools, jobs, income, housing, etc.). Among these vulnerable groups, African Americans, Hispanics, and Asians are more likely to be in poor health than the majority of Caucasians. Health areas of concern for vulnerable populations include childbearing (e.g., low birth weight, infant mortality, prenatal care, teen births, and maternal mortality); chronic illness and disability (i.e., physical and mental); and limitations in activities of daily living and overall quality-of-life experiences. Two especially vulnerable groups—the homeless and persons with disabilities—are discussed here.

Homeless

The United States is considered to be the world's superpower, with great resources, yet hundreds of thousands of men, women, and children are classified as homeless and live on the streets each day. Homelessness is characterized by a lack of fixed, regular, and adequate nighttime residence, or the nighttime residence is a public/private shelter or institution not designed for regular sleeping or living accommodations. It is projected that by the year 2010, there will be 1.7 billion people in the United States who will have been homeless at some point in their lives. It is estimated that as many as 600,000 people reside in homeless shelters every night. Reports show there are approximately only 250,000 shelter spaces available for the homeless. Racial distribution of the homeless averages around 50% for African Americans, 35% for Caucasians, 12% for Hispanics, and 1% for Asians. Most disturbing is that at the national level, 39% of the homeless are children. Consider the impact this has on a child's ability to acquire a formal education when he or she has no permanent location or learning environment. Equally distressing are the homeless statistics for U.S. veterans. Reportedly, despite the fact that male veterans make up only 34% of the general adult male population, they comprise 40% of the homeless male population (USDHHS, 2003).

Making a case for the social injustice and oppression for the homeless is not difficult. Without medical resources, insurance, Medicare, or Medicaid, the disparity in health increases significantly in terms of chronic health problems, mental illness, and drug and alcohol addictions. Eventually, individuals arrive at the emergency room to be treated for a condition that would otherwise be cared for on an outpatient basis through routine health maintenance.

People With Disabilities

As mentioned earlier, stigma plays a major role in labeling target groups to justify the prejudice and discrimination directed toward them. In the case of persons with disabilities, those who acquire a disability from defending the country or from working are considered to be more deserving of benefits from society than individuals who sustained a disability from recklessness or other forms of behavior considered to be irresponsible. Individuals with congenital or mental disabilities experience a far greater degree of stigma as compared to individuals who may have acquired a physical disability in some other manner. Individuals with congenital disabilities are more likely to be perceived as being personally or morally responsible for the cause or onset of their disability, as if they could have prevented its onset (Smart, 2001).

Prior to the Americans with Disabilities Act (ADA), many individuals with disabilities were excluded from most social experiences, such as attending school, attaining employment, participating in recreational or leisure experiences, and shopping. The ADA evolved as a federal legislation to prevent prejudice, discrimination, and stigma (all of which are environmental limitations) against people with physical and mental disabilities. An able-bodied perspective of the ADA is that it shifts the responsibility for the disability "issues" from the individual to the U.S. population in general. Others believe that, because people with disabilities may receive certain privileges and opportunities, the ADA is a form of reverse discrimination that allows individuals to be exempted from valid employment or educational opportunities while receiving monthly disability payments. The ADA is predicated on the premise that the real issue with disabilities is the result of the prejudice that stems from the environment, and thus the U.S. Supreme Court concluded that the prevention of disadvantages associated with disability should be the responsibility of all (U.S. Department of Justice, 2005).

Smart (2001) offers three perspectives of justice relative to persons with disabilities. First, everyone receives equal treatment but not equal outcome. Prior to the ADA, individuals with a disability had the right to purchase an airline ticket, but accessibility was a problem. So, the opportunity was there, but the outcome was different secondary to the disability.

Second, everyone receives what he or she has earned, be it reward, penalty, or bad luck. Such a Darwinian perspective is based on survival of the fittest. Guiding this thought is the notion that it is a waste to provide assistance or accommodations to individuals who are considered inferior (e.g., people with disabilities), because they will not have the requisite abilities to utilize the assistance or resources in an effective (productive) manner.

Third, everyone gets what he or she needs despite individual differences. This form of justice allows for individual rights and opportunities and in doing so benefits society as a whole. The complications inherent in this perspective are in determining which needs of a person with a disability are legitimate and which ones are not. This perspective is further complicated in that many individuals in the United States believe they should be "blind" to any differences (e.g., color, ethnicity, gender, disability). However, history has shown that every group can—and have—claim to have a greater need for resources and accommodations; therefore, deciding on who should and should not receive consideration becomes very difficult. Although a goal of "everybody gets what he or she needs" is not 100% attainable, the benefits to society of striving toward this goal would be enhanced diversity and improved economic health. In this scenario, individuals gain the opportunity to be independently responsible for contributing to the growth of society. As complicated as this perspective can be, it still most effectively aligns with the original intent of the ADA.

Occupational Justice and Injustice

History of Occupational Justice

Occupational justice is a construct born out of the complexity of the 21st century. It is in its infancy of development and grew out of the call to promote "social justice by enabling development of individuals' occupational potential" (Townsend, 1993, p. 176), the driving theme in Elizabeth Townsend's 1993 Muriel Driver lectureship titled *Occupational Therapy's Social Vision* (Townsend, 1993). To raise the consciousness of the profession, she brought to the forefront issues occupational therapists face in striving to engage in client-centered practice. Townsend addressed the challenges of occupational therapists serving those individuals who not only enter traditional professional doors, but also those who hover outside in the shadows of hospitals, clinics, schools, and communities who quite frequently experience barriers to health-care services. Those most likely to be confronted are alone in the community, in adult prisons and juvenile justice centers, in Medicaid-reimbursed nursing homes, in senior community centers, and in homeless and domestic and child abuse centers. Out of this original conceptual direction arose the partnering of ideas around the concept of social justice in occupational therapy with another leader in the international occupational therapy arena, Ann Wilcock from Australia. At the time, Wilcock was studying occupation from a public health perspective as well as the evolution and development of humans as occupational beings and the human's need for occupation to establish and maintain health (Wilcock, 1993).

Townsend and Wilcock first began using the term *occupational justice* in 1997 after meeting and beginning to explore together their ideas about justice and occupation (Townsend & Wilcock, 2004a). It was in their discussions of how an occupationally just world could enhance the health of all its citizens that they began to synthesize their ideas and explore what occupational justice, and conversely what occupational injustice, meant for occupational therapists and their practice with individuals and populations. Wilcock first wrote about the concept in *An Occupational Perspective of Health* (1998a). Here her ideas regarding the profound impact of occupation on human health began to converge into a concept that related to the occupational health and wellbeing of individuals. To explore their ideas in more depth, these authors began investigating the concept of occupational justice by reviewing occupational science and occupational therapy, as well as interdisciplinary literature on social justice, and they began holding a series of conversations with therapists at occupational justice workshops around the world.

This resulted in a conceptual definition in Wilcock and Townsend's 2000 "Occupational Terminology" article in the *Journal of Occupational Science*. They initiated the discussion by referring to **occupational justice** as being "about recognizing and providing for the occupational needs of individuals and communities as part of a fair and empowering society" and that "occupational justice can be described as the equitable opportunity and resources to enable people's engagement in meaningful occupations" (Townsend & Wilcock, 2004b, p. 79). Out of these workshops also evolved the ideas, reasoning, beliefs, and principles that began the exploratory theory of occupational justice (Townsend & Wilcock, 2004a, 2004b).

Exploratory Theory of Occupational Justice

Townsend and Wilcock are reserving the right to refrain from delivering a definition of occupational justice, preferring to contemplate the concept as an exploratory theory (Townsend & Wilcock, 2004b). Discussions at the workshops around the world between 1999 and 2002 led to many contributions and the development of the possible defining features of, and linkages between, occupation and justice leading to the concept of occupational justice. As a result of asking participants three key questions—What is occupation? What is justice? and What is occupational justice?—some similar themes became apparent. Emerging key concepts referred to were enabling; equal distribution of the right and opportunities for occupations; choice in culturally and personally meaningful occupations (Townsend & Wilcock, 2004b); and equal opportunities to live, work, and play in safe and supportive environments. These were based on defining concepts of participation outlined in the 2001 World Health Organization's (WHO) *International Classification of Functioning, Disability and Health (ICF)*. Complementing the international workshops, Townsend and Wilcock (2004b) undertook an in-depth historical and interdisciplinary literature review that supported the direction and development of the exploratory theory of occupational justice.

Components of Occupational Justice

At the foundation of the exploratory theory of occupational justice emerged the ideas of equity, including those of fairness, empowerment, and civility (Wilcock & Townsend, 2000). Three interconnected pillars of knowledge were built on these foundations: the concepts of occupation, enablement, and justice. *Occupation* is the participation in one's daily life activities. *Enablement* suggests participatory and empowerment-oriented approaches to lifestyle design and practice. *Justice* was defined by discussing the underlying determinants of justice and the socially determined forms of occupational wellbeing and social inclusion that vary given individual differences and contexts (Townsend & Wilcock, 2004b).

The exploratory theory of occupational justice presents ideas, beliefs, principles, and reasoning related to the occupational nature of humans. Ideas introduced included the following: people are occupational as well as social beings; human occupational needs differ with each person; and differing forms of enablement address a variety of occupational needs, strengths, and potentials. Beliefs and principles include: humans participate in occupations as autonomous yet interdependent agents in their societal context; health depends on participation in health-building occupations; and empowerment depends on enabling choice and control in occupational participation. Reasoning that has evolved from the theory includes recognition that occupation experiences and environments are determined by economic, political, cultural, and other determinants; media, caregiving, education, and employment are examples of occupations that shape and are shaped by other occupations; and potential outcomes of occupational injustices are, for example, occupational alienation or occupational marginalization (Townsend & Wilcock, 2004b). In understanding occupational justice, it is helpful to delineate its distinguishing characteristics from those of social justice (Townsend & Wilcock, 2004a).

Distinctions Between Occupational and Social Justice

In discussions and writings about the topic of occupational justice, Townsend and Wilcock have attempted to illuminate the similarities and differences between occupational and social justice (Townsend & Wilcock, 2004a, 2004b). This effort helped provide a context for which occupational science and occupational therapy can see potential study and application of occupational justice. Some of the differences identified by the authors are highlighted in Table 8-1. These differences point out the unique contributions of occupational justice to an individual's engagement in occupation as a vehicle to occupational identity, health, and wellbeing.

Agents That Impose Occupational Injustice and Targets Who Are Predisposed to Occupational Injustice

Agent individuals, institutions, and policies that impose occupational injustice on vulnerable individuals or groups are those that supersede the individual's power to make choices in their lives about what they can and want to do. Institutions such as underfunded

Table 8–1 **Comparison of Social Justice and Occupational Justice**

Social Justice	Occupational Justice
Humans are social beings	Humans are occupational beings
Interests in social relations	Interests in health and quality of life
Same opportunities and resources	Different opportunities and resources
Possession	Enablement
Group differences	Individual differences

state systems, residential congregate living settings, educational systems, and foster care systems can eliminate opportunities for individuals' occupational potential in the guise of safety, economic changes, and guardianship. Business owners of sweatshops, for-profit organizations providing health or social services, owners who hire immigrant or migrant workers, and multinational businesses may offer work that deprives individuals of fair privileges and can be unhealthy. Occupational determinants, forms, and outcomes such as poverty, limited access to health care, and unemployment create situations where individuals can suffer the consequences of occupational injustice and can be considered agents of occupational injustice.

Occupational Injustice at Individual, Community, National, and International Levels

Occupational injustice scenarios were discussed internationally at the occupational justice workshops led by Townsend and Wilcock. They believed that sometimes it was easier to bring to participants' awareness cases where occupational injustice was observed, as opposed to where occupational justice was embraced. **Occupational injustice** was described as individuals, groups, communities, and nations experiencing a lack of meaningful occupation for its members in their daily lives. At most workshops, participants described cases of people not being allowed to fully embrace their potential as humans as occupational beings. These discussions have been carried over to clinics, classrooms, and community settings as participants have returned to their places of employment to further explore these concepts. From the ongoing dialogue, Townsend and Wilcock (2004b) illuminated four different thematic descriptions of occupational injustice: occupational alienation, occupational deprivation, occupational marginalization, and occupational imbalance.

Occupational Alienation

"Occupational alienation may occur when one's right to experience occupation as meaningful and enriching is lost" (Townsend & Wilcock, 2004b, p.80). **Occupational alienation** is associated with "prolonged experiences of disconnectedness, isolation, emptiness, lack of a sense of identity, a limited or confined expression or spirit, or a sense of meaningless" (Townsend & Wilcock, 2004b, p. 80). Individuals or groups who might experience this injustice include those enslaved (Kwong, 2001), native peoples (Aday, 2001), and confined refugees (Schisler, Conor, & Polatajko, 2002), all living or working great distances from home or loved ones. In the United States, as a result of living on reservations, Native Americans have missed opportunities for school and work that were meaningful and respectful of their culture. Consequently, they have suffered high rates of substance abuse and unemployment (Aday, 2001). Also experiencing occupational alienation are the migrant farmworkers who are illegal aliens from Mexico and Central America (Zavella, 2001), and the urban garment district workers who are illegal aliens from China (Kwong, 2001). Both groups come to work in the United States and frequently leave families and support systems behind for long periods of time. They work for very low wages and often more than 40 hours per week. They suffer greatly and may experience occupational alienation by engaging in work that is physically hard, menial, tedious, and at times dangerous to the point of injury or illness (Loh & Richardson, 2004). The injustice of this is even more severe when the workers are children robbed of opportunities to expand their occupational potential through school.

All these individuals or groups are people who should be able to have "occupational dreams" and a vision of the future that would allow occupational development through doing, being, believing, and becoming (CAOT 1999 campaign slogan adapted from Wilcock, [1998b]), as described by Fearing and Clark (2000). However, as a result of ongoing meaninglessness in the daily routines and occupations of their lives, these individuals do not reap the health-promoting benefits of occupational engagement. Children are a particularly vulnerable group to occupational injustice. Children raised in deprived orphanage environments have missed the opportunity to engage in meaningful developmental activities necessary for important integrative experiences that facilitate brain maturation (Kadlec & Cermack, 2002). In addition, abused and neglected children are particularly at risk for

occupational alienation, as exposure numbs a child's interpersonal relations and affects regulation and self-development. This prevents early childhood health co-occupations with caregiving adults and affects performance in other important occupations of participation such as school, family, and social activities (Whiting, 2001).

One group of children particularly at risk for abuse and neglect are those in the foster care system. This group has been found to have significantly more health and developmental problems than other children, particularly behavioral and emotional concerns. These are possibly a result of underlying risk factors such as abuse, chaotic family life, or interrupted attachment (Hansen, Mawjee, Barton, Metcalf, & Joye, 2004). As these children age, they become more at risk as they approach the time when they need to transition out of foster care. Results of Mech's (1994) analysis of post-placement outcomes of former foster children showed high rates of high school dropout, difficulty finding a place to live, and high public aid use known as cost-to-community. These individuals frequently suffer the effects of missing social supports, which puts them at great risk for occupational alienation.

Occupational Deprivation

"Occupational deprivation may occur when one's occupational rights to develop through participation in occupations for health and social inclusion are limited" (Townsend & Wilcock, 2004b, p. 80). **Occupational deprivation** is a term introduced by Wilcock (1998a) and elaborated on by Whiteford (2000, 2010). It is described as "a state of prolonged preclusion from engagement in occupations of necessity, and/or meaning due to factors that stand outside the control of the individual" (Whiteford, 2010, p. 305).

The individual or group does not have a choice or control over decisions in their daily lives as a result of external impositions that are beyond the realm of their influence. Whiteford sees these particular injustices as a global concern in such areas as incarceration, disability, refugeeism, sex-role stereotyping, unsatisfactory conditions of poverty, and geographic and social isolation.

Whiteford (1997) explored the deprivation of meaningful activities experienced during incarceration. Activities that were imposed or noncreative—such as meeting with prison staff, exercising, watching television, and sleeping—composed most of their day and were done mainly in social isolation. The temporal aspect of their day was extremely slow. When occupation-based activities were incorporated, the inmates saw the benefits, including "satisfaction of showing something they made to someone, letting out frustration, gaining money, and keeping hands and mind on something positive" (p. 128). It was customary to withdraw activities from inmates as a form of discipline. This exacerbated their long days of social isolation. These reflections clearly demonstrate the pain of inactivity throughout many of the inmates' days and the struggles they experienced with the meaninglessness of so much of their lives.

Disability also can be a particularly depriving experience. In the United States, people with disabilities comprise 20% of the population. Currently, 42% of individuals in the United States over age 65 have one or more disabilities (U.S. Census Bureau, 2000b). Trends indicate these numbers will continue to rise as the population ages. The ADA provided comprehensive civil rights protections to individuals with disabilities in the areas of employment, state and local government services, public accommodations, transportation, and telecommunications. Despite this landmark legislation, individuals with disabilities continue to experience occupational injustice through the inability to participate fully in everyday activities of their choice. These individuals continue to experience disparities in securing employment, with 70% being unemployed (U.S. Census Bureau, 2000b). Inaccessible transportation, public/private buildings and community facilities, and health care and social services are examples of things that hinder individuals' participation in all aspects of life. Fewer than 10% of individuals who are disabled own their own home (U.S. Census Bureau, 2000b), and those who want to live independently have difficulty finding accessible housing and are frequently forced into group living situations.

Children with disabilities comprise about 18% of the population (Newacheck et al., 1998) and are also at risk for missing the opportunity to fully participate in their communities. Under the Individuals with Disabilities Education Act (IDEA), 13% of school-age children in 2002 qualified for special education services (U.S. Department of Education, 2003). However, many children, particularly those with mild to moderate or invisible disabilities, may fail to be identified for special-needs services before entering school and may therefore miss the opportunity for early intervention or early childhood services. Disability impedes a child from full participation in school and at home.

Poverty can also lead to occupational deprivation. Poverty in the United States affects individuals in both urban and rural environments and has a limiting impact on the occupational engagement of people living in these communities. Poverty creates many challenges for families who raise children in the United States, where the official poverty rate was 12.1%. For children living below the poverty level, the rate was 16.7%, and for children under age 6, the rate was 18.5% of the population. Among black or Hispanic people, the rate of poverty was higher, with 24.1% and 21.8 %, respectively (Proctor & Dalaker, 2003). In some urban Midwestern cities affected by the economic downturn, poverty rates have increased (Proctor & Dalaker, 2003). These same communities have minority numbers that average over 60% of the population which is another risk factor for occupational deprivation (Vision for Children at Risk, 2003). Urban minority children are more likely to be poor than nonminority children. When poverty and disability converge, 28% of children living in poverty are identified as disabled (Fujiura & Yamaki, 2000), and those living in an urban community are likely to also be a minority.

This convergence may be ascribed to several risk factors. Children living in poverty often reside in housing with lead exposure (Dugbatey, Evans, Lienhop, & Stelzer, 1995), lack proper nutrition (Brown & Pollitt, 1996), and experience diminished positive family interaction due to maternal depression or parental substance abuse (Cattell, 2001). They also experience barriers to health-care access (Newacheck et al., 1998), childcare (Phillips, Voran, Kisker, Howes, & Whitebook, 1994), and social and educational services (Humphry, 1995). These poverty-related factors are associated with developmental delay in young children aged 0 to 3 years (Sonnander & Claesson, 1999) and in preschoolers (McLoyd, 1998), and are associated with academic difficulties in school-age children (Aber, Benett, Conley, & Li, 1997). These experiences deprive children of enriching occupational opportunities and limit full participation in daily living, such as going to school and playing in safe communities. This contributes to a future risk for occupational injustice when they become adults.

Poverty in rural areas poses equally devastating but different occupationally depriving conditions. Marshall (2003) investigated the effect of poor water quality due to chemical runoff from the coal industry on the lives of rural families in southeastern Kentucky. Many activities that involve using water—including hygiene, cooking, and outdoor leisure participation—were delayed or restricted. Damage to household items and clothing created an additional hardship to daily living. Occupational injustice, in the form of occupation deprivation, was noted in this population, as the interaction of context and occupation was explored.

Occupational Marginalization

"Occupational marginalization may occur when the right to benefit from fair privileges for diverse participation in occupations is deprived" (Townsend & Wilcock, 2004b, p. 80). When the right to exert individual or population autonomy through choice in occupations and the right to develop through participation in occupations for health and social inclusion is abused, there is **occupational marginalization.** This is less overt in the influence it has over people's participation in their communities. Occupational marginalization has been described as the inability of humans to exert micro, everyday choices and decision-making power as they participate in occupations. It may operate invisibly through governmental and societal policies and culture for individuals and through what they choose to do for their physical, emotional, and spiritual health (Townsend & Wilcock, 2004b). It takes on a normative expectation or standard in society for individuals to participate, as opposed to an individual's ability to participate as they wish or desire. It makes individuals relinquish self-determination and makes occupational therapists relinquish client-centered practice. Older adults in many urban impoverished communities live in fear of violence, and consequently, they feel trapped or held hostage in their homes. This self-imposed isolation sets limits on what they can and wish to do and on their health and wellbeing (Jackson, Carlson, Mandel, Zemke, & Clark, 1998).

Violence in society imposes a curse of occupational marginalization. Women who are victims of domestic violence are at risk not only for themselves but also for their children (Gallew, 2004). These women live in fear, which compromises their fragile self-determination and self-esteem, leading to occupationally marginalized lives. Children exposed to violence in the home are less likely to thrive and grow to appreciate close and nurturing relationships (Helrich, Lafata, McDonald, Aviles, & Collins, 2001). When children are occupationally marginalized through violence in their lives, severe ramifications are seen. Violence and adolescent homicide are the third leading cause of death in children aged 5 to 14 and are the second leading cause of death in 15- to 24-year-olds (USDHHS, 2000). This devastating outcome is a severe form of occupational injustice.

In for-profit health-care systems or government-subsidized school systems with strict limits on numbers of visits, therapists feel constrained when needing to practice client-enabling occupational therapy. Authentic occupational therapy requires the therapist to use well-developed clinical reasoning skills, particularly those of the narrative nature, to understand the client's occupational needs and desires and to help him or her build a new occupational future. This is very challenging in many current traditional provider environments and diminishes the opportunities for occupational therapists to enable clients who are experiencing limits on decision-making opportunities to engage in health-promoting and even therapeutic skill-building activities and occupations.

Occupational Imbalance

"Occupational imbalance may occur when the right to benefit from fair privileges for diverse participation in occupations is removed" (Townsend & Wilcock, 2004b, p. 80). Occupational imbalance is a term that emerged from Wilcock's (1998a) work on the human need for occupation and its influence on health and wellbeing. Townsend and Wilcock (2004a) discuss using **occupational imbalance** as a population-based term to identify groups of people who do not share in the labor and benefits of economic production. These people are being occupied too much or too little to experience meaning and empowerment in choosing meaningful daily occupations and establishing routines and habits. These individuals might be in both the paid and unpaid labor market. The Charter of Human Rights of the United Nations Article 23 (United Nations, 1948) states that every person has the right to work, to free choice of employment, and to equal pay for equal work. Ravaged by over 200 years of racism in the United States, black males continue to experience unequal opportunities to reach nondiscriminatory employment practices. Many black men have too little that is meaningful to do, resulting in lack of empowerment and self-determination (Darity Jr., 2003). In contrast, women working outside the home who are trying to balance family and work life are frequently quoted as stressed and overworked (Kirkby & Skues, 1998).

Certain professionals who have been traditionally underpaid for their contributions, particularly in health care, have experienced imbalance. Townsend (2002) considered this imbalance to be occupation overload. In the past decade, this was observed in the increasing patient caseload of health professionals as a result of the for-profit health-care system's economic priority in the provision of services. In a study of 10,000 nurses, Aiken, Clark, Sloane, Sochalaski and Silber (2002) found that as nursing caseloads increased above a baseline level, patient mortality increased by 7%, job dissatisfaction increased by 23%, and burnout increased by 15%. Nurses in high-caseload hospitals felt a lack of respect for what they provided to patients and planned to leave their positions within the next few years. This predicament suggests that increasing caseloads will not save money but will increase costs as nursing exits and turnovers create personnel challenges for administrators.

Occupational Justice in the Promotion of Health and Wellbeing

The World Health Organization (WHO) defines health as "a state of complete physical, mental and social well-being and not merely the absence of disease or infirmity" (1948, p.100). *Healthy People 2010,* the nationwide health agenda of promotion and disease prevention in the United States, asserts that individual health is closely linked to community health—the health of the community and environment where people live, work, and play (USDHHS, 2000). Both of these definitions allude to the individual's ability to be actively engaged in daily life. This may involve full participation in one's daily activities in one's natural environment. Participation is defined in the *ICF* as involvement in a life situation (WHO, 2001) and is about being engaged in daily life. **Participation restriction** is defined as problems an individual may experience in involvement in life situations. Participation has a positive influence on health and wellbeing. Law (2002) reflects and discusses the importance of participation in occupations of everyday life within the aggregate of a strong research evidence base illuminated by the work of the Canadian Child Center for Childhood Disability Research (Law, 2002). She defines participation more specifically from this work as "involvement in formal and informal everyday activities" (p. 641). Law also defines certain characteristics of active participation, including individual choice and control, a supportive environment, a means-rather-than-an-ends emphasis, and a challenge that matches skill and that when accomplished results in a sense of mastery (Law, 2002).

As occupational therapists have begun to recognize the importance of occupation to health, not only in its therapeutic power but also in its health promotion potential, new and creative programs have emerged. This is not a new view for occupational therapists (Reitz, 1992; Scaffa, 2001) but one that has taken on increased emphasis given national and international calls for health promotion and prevention (Kniepmann, 1997). The WHO (1986) defines health promotion as "the process of enabling people to increase control over and to improve their health" (p. iii). Fazio (2001) reflects that occupational therapists' view of health promotion emanates from the basic belief that a balance of work, rest, self-care, and leisure is necessary to optimal health and wellbeing. Occupational therapy assistants and occupational therapists know the importance of balance to the fulfillment of living in the most meaningful and healthy way. Health promotion is generally seen as operating with individuals or groups in a context without the challenges of illness, disability, or risk of such possibilities (Fazio, 2001). Health promotion provides consultations, supports, or enhancements to maximize one's health potential. Fazio comments that it is difficult to separate health promotion from prevention of illness, because if one is providing the supports for health promotion, it will translate into the prevention of illness and disability.

The Centers for Disease Control and Prevention (CDC) has shifted its focus from the prevention of mortality and morbidity to an increased emphasis on working to improve the health and wellbeing of individuals with disability (Lollar & Crews, 2003). This is an opportunity for occupational therapy to play an integral role in an interdisciplinary approach to develop new and creative health promotion programs. These new trends in practice are consistent with the American Occupational Therapy Association position paper, written by Scaffa, Van Slyke, and Brownson (2007), *Occupational Therapy in the Promotion of Health and Prevention of Disease and Disability*, in which health promotion interventions "promote healthy living practices, social participation, occupational justice, and healthy communities, with respect for cross cultural issues and concerns" (p. 2). In addition, in the *Occupational Therapy Practice Framework: Domain and Process* (referred to as the *Framework*; AOTA, 2008), health promotion is addressed as one of the key intervention approaches to support engagement in occupation for participation in society.

Occupational Justice and the Occupational Therapy Process in Health Promotion

Individuals, groups, and communities experiencing occupational injustice are at great risk for poor health. Occupational therapists who desire to focus on addressing occupational injustice will find challenges to practicing in traditional settings and with more medical-model approaches. However, those committed to client-centered and occupationally just practice will reach out to individuals, groups, and communities in new and different ways, and will naturally incorporate a health promotion approach as supported by the *Framework* (AOTA, 2002). Scaffa (2001) has led this occupational-science approach to health promotion and has defined for practitioners the concept of **preventive occupation,** which she defines as "the application of occupational science to prevent disease/disability and promote the health and wellbeing of persons and communities through meaningful engagement in occupation" (p. 44). Some examples of practice that have begun to take on this converged model address populations that are particularly vulnerable to occupational injustice.

In "The Guide to Occupational Therapy Practice," Moyers (1999) refers to the Well Elderly Study and its lifestyle-redesign program as an example of health promotion in a community of multicultural, urban-dwelling elders (Clark et al., 1996; Jackson et al., 1998). Prior to the intervention, this community of elders might have been considered as experiencing occupational injustice. Many would not leave their homes for fear of violence or other threats to safety. Many lived alone and lacked the social supports necessary to ensure healthy daily living habits and routines. Through individualized occupational therapy programs, community members were assisted in ways to improve their health and quality of life.

This evidence-based health promotion program is now being replicated across the United States in different settings, communities, and with different populations. The goal is to enhance one's health through conscious decision-making about engaging in occupations that promote healthy lifestyles and improve the quality of one's life. One population being explored is individuals at risk for ill health as a result of obesity, a national health concern. Over 60% of individuals in the United States are overweight or obese and are experiencing difficulties in managing their weight. Individualized occupational therapy that incorporates a lifestyle-restructuring program is suggested to support healthy choices, to maintain a healthy weight, and to improve the quality of one's life (F. Clark, personal communication, October 30, 2004).

In addition to the lifestyle redesign program for well elders, another example of an occupational therapy approach addressing older adults living in the community potentially at risk for occupational alienation is the occupational therapy component of a university-community partnership (Neufeld, 2004). This partnership identified the needs of and the support necessary for independence in elders living in a naturally occurring retirement community (NORC)—a community with a high population of residents over 60 years of age and that initially began as a community with a younger population. As part of the team, occupational therapists have been able to support the concept of aging in place, with recommendations and programs that support the residents' continued participation in independent living, productive activity, and leisure in their community.

In another population-based, university-community partnership serving older adults, a local Area Agency on Aging and School of Allied Health partnered to provide health promotion services to caregivers of older adults living in family homes. Caregivers can be at risk for occupational deprivation when overwhelmed by the caregiving needs of family members. The health professionals provided important information and consultations on such topics as mobility and activities of daily living (ADLs) safety, medication routines and risks, respite care, and nutrition (Saint Louis University, Doisy School of Allied Health, 2002). This caregiver-support program emphasized the important need for balance in the caregiver's life to prevent occupational overload.

Older adults living in nursing homes have been identified as being at risk of occupational deprivation (French, 2002). Wood (2003) has explored the nursing home environment for adults with Alzheimer's disease (AD) for day-to-day functioning and quality of life. Preliminary results indicate the importance of the caregivers and environmental interactions in supporting occupational engagement and quality of life for persons with AD. Health promotion programs can emphasize an ecological approach to caring for individuals with dementia that focuses on the critical features in the environment that support occupational engagement, not only for home caregivers, but also for staff and residents of institutional programs. An ecological approach would address both the social and physical features of the environment that interact with clients' capacity for occupational performance and that could be adapted to enhance their occupational potential.

Individuals with disabilities, both physical and mental, are at risk for occupational injustice and can benefit from a client-centered occupational therapy approach infused with occupational justice principles and reasoning. One population at risk for occupational injustice is adults with developmental disabilities. These individuals face issues that are problematic for reaching occupational potential. They are at risk for occupational deprivation in opportunities for participating in society in such areas as work, independent living, and leisure. The Canadian Centre for Health Promotion's approach to quality of life emphasizes the importance of participation for adults with developmental disabilities (Renwick, 2004). Occupational therapists have assisted these individuals with this model, which brings both a health promotion and a client-centered focus to intervention. The model emphasizes three domains of quality of life: (1) being, belonging, and becoming; (2) the importance and satisfaction of factors in one's life; and (3) the personal control one can have on those factors that can influence one's quality of life. The model has been used successfully in a large-scale research project and can be used to advocate for policy change to establish or enhance programs that support quality of life for adults with developmental disabilities (Renwick, 2004); this, in turn, could diminish occupational injustice.

In its decision in *Olmstead v. L. C.,* the U.S. Supreme Court recognized the role that occupational injustices can play in preventing the achievement of meaningful occupation (527 U.S. 581 1999). In the decision, it was stated that "wherever possible, people with disabilities should be provided services in the community, rather than in institutions" (p. 1). The New Freedom Initiative (Bush, 2001) brought attention to the need to assist in implementing *Olmstead* by improving the daily life experiences for people with disabilities. The New Freedom Initiative progress report has indicated areas where improvement has been made (White House Domestic Policy Council, 2004). Three examples of ways the New Freedom Initiative has helped to decrease occupational deprivation of individuals with disability are (1) increased support for individuals to purchase technology needed to telework, (2) implementation of the "Ticket to Work" program that supports training and work-related services so individuals can choose their supports needed, and (3) improved access to transportation through the "United weRide" program.

Children are another population at risk for occupational deprivation. As a result of trauma such as abuse, neglect, and violence, children experience occupational injustice and may require specialized support services. Developing best practices that focus on a transdisciplinary and family-centered approach has been shown to enhance the occupational potential in these children (Hyter, Atchinson, Henry, Sloane, & Black-Pond, 2001). Enabling families to seek support and looking at ways to continue support are health promoting and can result in breaking the cycle of trauma.

Rybski and Wilder (2004) propose that pediatric therapists can facilitate health promotion in children at risk for occupational deprivation in underserved communities. In community-based childcare centers, they have supported developmental surveillance and screening programs. This has been accomplished by empowering childcare staff, who have a keen awareness of children's abilities and challenges to participate in early identification and referral. This model utilizes a community-needs assessment approach in which health-care providers reach out to at-risk children. This approach is different from more traditional medical or educational models, where occupational therapists see children only after they have been identified by another health/education team member and then referred for early intervention or early childhood services.

Adolescents at risk are another population vulnerable to occupational injustice. Farnsworth (2000) described how young offenders, at risk for decreased social wellbeing as a result of their lifestyle and environment, spend their time. The young offenders reported that 57% of the time they were engaged in leisure occupations that were predominantly passive, and they spent 21% of their time in personal care occupations. Only 10% of the time did they report being engaged in productive occupations, such as education or employment. Leaving school and lack of financial and human resources contributed to the high percentage of engagement in passive leisure occupations. Recently immigrated adolescent male minorities are frequently at risk for gang behavior. Once an adolescent joins a gang, they often drop out of school and engage in crime and other high-risk behaviors that involve guns and drugs.

A community-based occupational therapy program to address this population was targeted in the New Occupations for Life program (Snyder, Florence, Masunaka-Noriega, & Young, 1998), an outgrowth of a Los Angeles Alternative Education program for youth. These adolescents seemed to have fallen through the cracks in society. The 6-week occupational therapy program allowed adolescent gang members to explore alternative socially acceptable and personally meaningful occupations in a safe, trusting environment. Activities that were action-oriented to meet the kinesthetic learning needs of the students were used to focus on socialization, prevocational and employment readiness, self-management, resource awareness, and community building. Program evaluation outcomes indicated a positive response and impact of the program (Snyder et al., 1998).

In a study on the occupation of leisure in adolescents and its influence on mental health, Passmore (2003) found that achievement and social leisure supported mental health while time-out leisure did not. Adolescents unable to participate in achievement and social leisure due to social or physical barriers experienced occupational injustice and a decrease in health and wellbeing. Adolescents who transition out of foster care are particularly at risk for occupational alienation as they struggle to bridge the gap between dependence and independence. Propp, Ortega, and Newhart (2003) found that when programs engage in an empowerment model called *interdependent living that fosters interdependence, connection, and collaboration,* adolescents feel a sense of power in decision-making that facilitates a move to health-promoting social participation.

Women and their children who are domestically abused may also experience occupational deprivation. Abusers may prevent women from choosing meaningful activities in which they wish to engage. Many times these women are socially isolated from support networks and are financially dependent on their abusers, interrupting any pattern of meaningful daily occupations. Gallew (2004) suggests a community-based approach emphasizing management of independent living skills while supporting a gradual reentry into community social networks. This can encourage social participation and renewed role competency as a provider and caregiver critical to the important roles in these women's lives.

Another group of individuals at risk for occupational deprivation are recently immigrated persons, some of whom are refugees or illegal immigrants. Both of these groups come into the new country with few of their home world's belongings and must start over with very little economic or social support. Sullivan, Gupta, and Spiegal (2003) investigated immigrant refugee women to better understand the changes in occupations as these women adjusted to new environments. They found that the orchestration of occupation changed in the new country, given differences of temporal and environmental factors. They also found that the functions of occupations took on varying degrees of multiplicity, such as paid employment, which provided social and cultural learning opportunities as well as subsistence. These lessons can be applied in occupational therapy population-based practices in the community and in more traditional medical settings where health promotion is advocated.

Advocacy and empowerment for occupational justice beyond practice settings and addressing sociopolitical and policy issues in health and social services takes occupational therapists clearly into the community. It requires an activist perspective that may not always be associated with contemporary occupational therapy but certainly was present in the profession's historical foundations. This activist client-centered approach for occupational therapy was further diagrammed and highlighted by Townsend and Wilcock (2004b). Steps to take in this approach included raising awareness and recognition of occupational justice and injustice, and researching and acting to change any occupational injustice they confront.

Another multistep model for social justice action, the Action Continuum, (Adams et al., 1997) can be used to address issues of occupational justice. This model is a continuum approach that has eight specific stages for practitioners to reflect upon and identify their stage of readiness to confront and take an activist approach. At one end of the continuum are actions against inclusion and social justice, and on the other end are actions for diversity and social justice. This model was taught and implemented in reflective classroom and community activities in an occupational science course that focused on occupation in a global society (Arnold & Rybski, 2003). At first students struggled to recognize themselves on the continuum, but as the course progressed and more instances of occupational injustice became apparent to them in class activities, international news discussions, and community experiences, they became more able to aspire to and act in activist ways. They were able to make recommendations for changes in ecological supports to enhance opportunities for the occupational potential of clients experiencing occupational injustice. They recognized and sought solutions to difficulties therapists face in engaging in client-centered, health-promoting practice. In addition, they sought alternative solutions to address the occupational injustice they found and, as a result of their experience, recognized in themselves the ability to take on an advocate/activist role.

Conclusion

Perhaps it is thought that social justice is "writ large," in that too much attention is attributed to its level of importance. Theorists such as Townsend (2002) challenge occupational therapy professionals and occupational scientists to explore the relationship between the profession and social justice. She encourages occupational therapy professionals to better understand the difference between what is known about social justice and what she and other occupational therapy theorists refer to as *occupational justice*. According to Townsend, there are paradigms of justice that distinguish occupational justice from social justice, yet acknowledging a relationship between the two concepts is essential in addressing a client's holistic needs. Social justice is concerned with inequality that is directed toward marginalized individuals of various target groups (e.g., social class, race, gender, disability, age, etc.). It is concerned with equitable distribution that focuses on access and opportunity. Equal opportunity and access for daily occupations such as work and education will be different for persons with disabilities and for able-bodied individuals. The role of occupational therapy is inherent in addressing the inequities of opportunity for occupational development or inequities related to lack of appropriate enablement for those living with a disability.

Vulnerable populations globally are at great risk for occupational alienation, deprivation, marginalization, and imbalance secondary to social injustice leading to occupational injustice. Occupational therapists see individuals in their daily practice who are experiencing occupational injustices and unable to engage in meaningful occupations. Occupational therapy interventions that have demonstrated ideals of occupational justice, many of which are health promotion programs, have in some cases recognized the relationship between their client-centered approaches and the concept of occupational justice, but in many cases have not gleaned a relationship. History of occupational therapy practice shows us that the roots of the profession grew out of addressing social injustices and promoting health and wellbeing through participation in valued daily activities. The newer concepts of occupational injustice can enrich occupational therapy interventions at individual, community, and population levels.

A major challenge for the profession is to delineate how to help therapists recognize the themes of occupational justice in their current practice. This could occur through continuing education case studies and research that will help therapists recognize the importance of taking an occupational justice activist role. In continuing education opportunities, stage models that instruct therapists in the continuum of recognizing and taking action to change occupational injustice can be presented.

This will allow occupational therapists to accept where they are on the action continuum in their knowledge, skill, and performance in incorporating occupational justice into their programs to enable clients to experience occupational justice. Through a collaborative enabling approach with their occupational therapists, clients will then be able to recognize the actions needed to positively impact their own occupational health and wellbeing. Lastly, advocacy for both the client and the profession of occupational therapy must include educating other health-care and community disciplines and third-party payers to develop an understanding of occupational justice relative to client needs and recovery.

Case Study 8-1

Karly is a 30-year-old obese African American woman with diabetes. She is married to a Hispanic man but has been separated for 3 years. She has two girls, ages 5 and 9, and one son, age 15. She has a GED (general equivalency diploma) and works three part-time, minimum-wage jobs to maintain her family. She receives very little, if any, financial assistance from her husband. She does not qualify for government financial assistance.

She has a history of bipolar disease and has to go for her medical checkup every 4 to 6 weeks, which occasionally affects her getting to work on time. Her bosses are not pleased and deduct from her pay for tardiness. She is not revealing the nature of her illness to her employers out of fear of being fired. She works 5 days a week and typically gets home around 10:00 to 11:30 p.m., depending on the bus system. She also has to work on rotating weekends, which she does not mind because it means a little extra money for the family. Her greatest financial difficulty is being able to afford the family needs as well as her medication, which costs $30 for each prescription. Sometimes she skips dosages to try spreading out the time between refills.

Karly has side effects from her medication, and this affects the quality and timeliness of her work, but she will not reveal her illness, as she knows the company has terminated other employees who had a mental illness. Her third job for each day is janitorial work. On this job, there is a shortage of employees, so workers have to double up on their assigned cleaning areas. This means that sometimes Karly is unable to complete her work during the regularly paid hours. Even though it takes her longer to do more work, her employer will not pay for the overtime and has threatened that anyone complaining will be terminated.

Since Karly does not have a car, she rides the bus for all transportation needs; however, she must walk several blocks from her home to catch the bus. The same applies for her children, who must ride the school bus every day.

So, she wakes up very early each day to walk with her children to catch the school bus before she goes to work. Because of her three jobs, her children are "latchkey" and are responsible for each other until their mother comes home from work, which, again, is typically very late at night.

Karly's apartment has only two bedrooms. The girls have a room and share a bed. Her son sleeps on the sofa in the living/dining area. The apartment usually does not have hot water, there are sewer problems, the locks on the doors are easily penetrated (the landlord will not upgrade the locks, and Karly cannot afford the cost of the change), the building is infested with bugs and rodents, and the only set of elevators in the building often break, so tenants are forced to use the stairs. The stairways are poorly lit, which further increases the risk for criminal behavior. Karly refuses to complain to the landlord out of fear of being evicted. She does not believe she would be able to find another apartment at a price that she could afford or that would be large enough for her three children.

Karly lives in a very large city/county area, and the crime rate for her neighborhood is dreadfully high. She constantly worries about the safety of her children. Her nearest relative lives 6 hours away, so there is no family support. The infrastructure for her community is very poor, and there are several abandoned buildings that also serve as havens for criminal acts and as shelter for homeless people. Her son has begun to verbally abuse his sisters and disregard Karly's directives on chores and safety. She had him assessed by the school and was told that he had signs of obstinate behavior disorder. Karly was not sure what this meant, and because she could not afford to pay for counseling, she decided to try and deal with it on her own.

Karly is very tired most of the time. She has little time to spend with her children. Sometimes she is so sleep deprived she becomes unable to think clearly. On occasion, she, too, has been impatient and verbally strong with her children. She loves them very much but feels that she is slowly losing control over everything that is important to her.

Questions

1. Using the scenario for Karly, identify social and occupational injustices that exist at each of the following levels: individual, institutional, and societal.
2. Explain how commutative, distributive, and social justice exists or does not exist in Karly's scenario.
3. Based on Freire's definition of "internalized oppression," does Karly's scenario indicate the presence of this experience for her?
4. List the social identity groups to which Karly belongs.
5. For each social identity group for which Karly is a member, list and describe her role as a "target" or "agent" member.
6. List the forms of oppression that Karly may experience as a result of her social identity group.
7. In what ways might Karly or her family experience each of the following?
   a. Occupational alienation
   b. Occupational deprivation
   c. Occupational marginalization
8. In what ways might Karly and her family be viewed as members of a vulnerable population prone to occupational injustice?

▶ For Discussion and Review

1. Explain Freire's concept of internalized oppression. What is the importance of understanding this concept?
2. Provide a description of the difference and relationship between social justice and occupational justice.
3. Define *occupational injustice*.
4. Identify and discuss examples of occupational injustice, including occupational alienation, occupational deprivation, occupational marginalization, and occupational imbalance.
5. Explain how occupational justice can be addressed in health promotion approaches through the occupational therapy process.

▶ Research Questions

1. Is there a direct relationship between social injustice and occupational injustice?
2. Does social group identity have a direct correlation to occupational injustice?
3. In what way does current occupational therapy practice reflect occupational justice?
4. Is there a direct relationship between occupational injustice and injustice in vulnerable populations?
5. How does occupational justice, through the occupational therapy process, influence health promotion?

References

Aber, J. L., Benett, N. G., Conley, D. C., & Li, J. (1997). The effects of poverty on child health and development. *Annual Review of Public Health, 18,* 463–83.

Adams, M., Bell, L. A., & Griffin, P. (1997). *Teaching for diversity and social justice.* New York: Routledge.

Aday, L. A. (2001). *At risk in America: The health and health care needs of vulnerable populations in the United States* (2d ed.). San Francisco: Jossey-Bass.

Adelman, L. (Executive Producer & Co-director). (2003). Race—The Power of an illusion [Film]. San Francisco: California Newsreel. (Available from California Newsreel, P.O. Box 2284, South Burlington, VT 05407.)

Aiken, L., Clarke, S., Sloane, D., Sochalaski, J., & Silber, J. (2002). Hospital nurse staffing and patient mortality, nurse burnout, and job dissatisfaction. *Journal of the American Medical Association, 288*(16), 1987–93.

American Occupational Therapy Association. (2008). *Occupational therapy practice framework: Domain and process* (2d ed.). Bethesda, MD: Author.

Arnold, M., & Rybski, D. (2003). *Broadening the concepts of community and occupation: Perspectives in a global society.* Paper presented at the Society for the Study of Occupation: USA, Park City, Utah.

Bales, K. (1999). *Disposable people: New slavery in the global economy.* Berkeley: University of California Press.

Bettencourt, B. A., & Hume, D. (1999). The cognitive contents of social group identity: Values, emotions and relationships. European Journal of Social Psychology, 29, 113–21.

Bishop, A. (2002). Understanding different oppression. In A. Bishop (Ed.). *Becoming an ally: Breaking the cycle of oppression in people* (2d ed., 78–94). London: Zed Books.

Brown, L., & Pollitt, E. (1996). Malnutrition, poverty and intellectual development. *Scientific American, 274*(2), 38–43.

Bush, G. W. (2001). *The New Freedom Initiative.* Retrieved September 12, 2004, from http://www.whitehouse.gov/news/freedominitiative/freedominitaitive.

Cattell, V. (2001). Poor people, poor places, and poor health: The mediating role of social networks and social capital. *Social Science & Medicine, 52,* 1501–16.

Clark, F., Carlson, M., Zemke, R., Frank, G., Patterson, K., Ennevor, B., Rankin-Martinez, A., Hobson, L., Crandall, J., Mandel, D., & Lipson, L. (1996). Life domains and adaptive strategies of a group of low-income, well older adults. *American Journal of Occupational Therapy, 50*(2), 99–108.

Cummings, E. E. (2003, September 3). *The August Employment Report: Job growth falls short of economic forecast.*

Retrieved September 2004, from http://www.house.gov/cummings/cbc/cbcpress.

Cummings, E. E. (2004, August 26). *Number of Americans living in poverty without health insurance.* Retrieved September 12, 2004, from http://www.house.gov/cummings/cbc/cbcpress.

Darity Jr., W. (2003). Employment discrimination, segregation and health. *American Journal of Public Health, 93*(2), 226–31.

Dugbatey, K., Evans, R. G., Lienhop, M. T., & Stelzer, M. (1995). Community partnerships in preventing childhood lead poisoning: A report on the development of a community oriented education program about childhood lead poisoning. *Journal of Environmental Health, 58*(4), 6–10.

Farnsworth, L. J. (2000). Time use and leisure occupations of young offenders. *American Journal of Occupational Therapy, 54*(3), 315–25.

Fazio, L. (2001). *Developing occupation-centered programs for the community: A workbook for students and professionals.* Upper Saddle River, NJ: Prentice Hall.

Fearing, V., & Clark, J. (2000). *Individuals in context: A practical guide to client-centered practice.* Thorofare, NJ: SLACK.

Finn, J. L., & Jacobson, M. (2003). *Just practice: A social justice approach to social work.* Peosta, IA: Eddie Bowers.

Freire, P. (1970). *Pedagogy of the oppressed* (M. B. Ramos, Trans.). New York: Seabury Press.

French, G. (2002). Occupational disfranchisement in the dependency of culture of a nursing home. *Journal of Occupational Science, 9*(1), 28–37.

Fujiura, G. T., & Yamaki, K. (2000). Trends in demography of childhood poverty and disability. *Exceptional Children, 66*(2), 187–99.

Gallew, H. A. (2004). Addressing domestic violence. *OT Practice,* 20–22.

Gil, D. G. (1998). *Confronting injustice and oppression: Concepts and strategies for social workers.* New York: Columbia University Press.

Goode, J., & Maskovsky, J. (Eds.). (2001). *The new poverty studies.* New York Columbia University Press.

Hansen, R. L., Mawjee, F. L., Barton, K., Metcalf, M. B., & Joye, N. R. (2004). Comparing the health status of low-income children in and out of foster care. *Child Welfare, 83*(4), 367–80.

Helrich, C. A., Lafata, M. L., McDonald, S. L., Aviles, A., & Collins, L. (2001). Domestic abuse across the lifespan: Definitions, identification and risk factors for occupational therapy. *Occupational Therapy in Mental Health, 16*(3/4), 5–34.

Humphry, R. (1995). Families who live in chronic poverty: Meeting the challenge of family-centered service. *American Journal of Occupational Therapy, 49*(7), 678–93.

Hyter, Y. D., Atchison, B., Henry, J., Sloane, M., & Black-Pond, C. (2001). A response to traumatized children: Developing a best practices model. *Occupational Therapy in Health Care, 15*(3/4), 113–40.

Intercultural Cancer Council. (2004). *Elderly and cancer.* Retrieved September 12, 2004, from http://www.iccnetwork.org.

Jackson, J. C., Carlson, M., Mandel, D., Zemke, R., & Clark, F. (1998). Occupation in lifestyle redesign: The Well Elderly Study occupational therapy program. *American Journal of Occupational Therapy, 52*(5), 326–36.

Johnson, A. (2001). The trouble we're in: Privilege, power and difference. In A. Johnson (Ed.), *Privilege, power and difference* (pp. 15–41). Boston: McGraw-Hill.

Kadlec, M. B., & Cermack, S. A. (2002). Activity level, organization and social-emotional behaviors in post industrialized children. *Adoption Quarterly, 6*(2), 43–57.

Kirkby, R., & Skues, J. (1998). Work stress, coping and gender. *Australian Journal of Primary Health, 4*(4), 79–88.

Kniepmann, K. (1997). Prevention of disability and maintenance of health. In C. H. Christiansen & C. M. Baum (Eds.), *Enabling function and wellbeing* (pp. 527–55). Thorofare, NJ: SLACK.

Kwong, P. (2001). Poverty despite family ties. In J. M. Goode, J. (Ed.), *The new poverty studies: The ethnography of power, politics, and impoverished people in the United States* (pp. 57–78). New York: New York University Press.

Latting, J. K. (1990). Identifying the isms: Enabling social work students to confront their biases. *Journal of Social Work Education, 26*(1), 36–39.

Law, M. (2002). Participation in the occupation of everyday life. *American Journal of Occupational Therapy, 56*(6), 640–49.

Loh, K., & Richardson, S. (2004). Foreign-born workers: Trends in fatal occupational injuries, 1996–2001. *Monthly Labor Review,* 42–53.

Lollar, D. J., & Crews, J. E. (2003). Redefining the role of public health in disability. *Annual Review of Public Health, 24,* 195–208.

Lukacs, S. L., & Schoendorf, K. C. (2004). *Racial and ethnic disparities in neonatal mortality USA.* Retrieved September 16, 2004, from http://www.nejm.org.

Marshall, A. (2003). *Water quality and the contextual nature of occupation.* Paper presented at the Society for the Study of Occupation: USA, Park City, Utah.

McLoyd, V. C. (1998). Socioeconomic disadvantage and child development. *American Psychologist, 53*(2), 185–204.

Mech, E. V. (1994). Foster youths in transition: Research perspectives on preparation for independent living. *Child Welfare, 73*(5), 603–24.

Meyer. A. (1977). The philosophy of occupational therapy. *American Journal of Occupational Therapy, 31*(10), 639–42.

Moon, V., Omvedt, G., & Zelliot, E. (2001) *Growing up untouchable in India.* Lanham, MD: Rowman & Littlefield.

Moyers, P. (1999). The guide to occupational therapy practice. *American Journal of Occupational Therapy, 53*(3), 247–322.

National Alliance on Mental Illness. (2006). *Policy topics.* Retrieved October 1, 2006, from http://www.nami.org/Template.cfm?Section=Issue_Spotlights.

Neufeld, P. (2004). Enabling participation through community and population approaches. *OT Practice, 9*(14), CE1–CE8.

Newacheck, P. W. D., Strickland, B. P., Shonkoff, J. P. M., Perrin, J. M. M., McPherson, M. M., McManus, M. M., et al. (1998). An epidemiologic profile of children with special health care needs. *Pediatrics, 102*(1), 117–23.

Olmstead v. L. C., 527 U.S. 581. (1999). Retrieved February 1, 2009, from http://supct.law.cornell.edu/supct/html/98-536.ZS.html.

Passmore, A. (2003). The occupation of leisure: Three typologies and their influence on mental health in adolescence.

Occupational Therapy Journal of Research: Occupation, Participation and Health, 23(2), 76–83.

Phillips, D. A., Voran, M., Kisker, E., Howes, C., & Whitebook, M. (1994). Child care for children in poverty: Opportunity or inequity? *Child Development, 65* (2 Spec No), 472–92.

Proctor, B. D., & Dalaker, J. (2003). *Poverty in the United States: 2002* (Current Population Reports, P60-222). Washington, DC: U.S. Census Bureau.

Propp, J., Ortega, D. M., & Newhart, F. (2003). Independence or interdependence: Rethinking the transition from "Ward of the Court" to adulthood. *Families in Society: The Journal of Contemporary Human Services, 84*(2), 259–66.

Rawls, J. (2000). *Justice as fairness: A restatement.* Cambridge, MA: Belknap Press of Harvard University Press.

Reitz, S. M. (1992). A historical review of occupational therapy's role in preventive health and wellness. *American Journal of Occupational Therapy, 46*(1), 50–55.

Renwick, R. (2004). Quality of life: A guiding framework for practice with adults with developmental disabilities. In M. Ross & S. Bachner (Eds.), *Adults with developmental disabilities: Current approaches in occupational therapy* (pp. 20–38). Bethesda, MD: AOTA Press.

Rybski, D. A., & Wilder, E. (2004). Developmental delay in children in underserved community childcare. *Manuscript submitted for publication.*

Saint Louis University, Doisy School of Allied Health. (2002). *Strengthening community support for caregivers: An interdisciplinary approach.* Training manual. St. Louis, MO.

Scaffa, M. (2001). Community-based practice: Occupation in context. In M. Scaffa (Ed.), *Occupational therapy in community based practice settings* (pp. 3–18). Philadelphia: F. A. Davis.

Scaffa, M. E., Van Slyke, N., & Brownson, C. A. (2007). *Occupational therapy in the promotion of health and the prevention of disability statement.* Retrieved July 24, 2008, from http://www .aota.org/Practitioners/OfficialStatements/41260.aspx.

Schisler, A., Conor, M., & Polatajko, H. (2002). The individual as mediator of the person-occupation-environment interaction: Learning from the experience of refugees. *Journal of Occupational Science, 9*(2), 82–92.

Shields, L. W. (1941). *The history and meaning of the term social justice.* Unpublished dissertation.

Smart, J. (2001). *Disability, society, and the individual.* Gaithersburg, MD: Aspen.

Snyder, C., Florence, C., Masunaka-Noriega, M., & Young, B. (1998). Los Angeles street kids: New occupations for life program. *Journal of Occupational Science, 5*(3), 133–39.

Sonnander, K., & Claesson, M. (1999). Predictors of developmental delay at 18 months and later school achievement problems. *Developmental Medicine and Child Neurology, 41,* 195–202.

Sullivan, C., Gupta, J., & Spiegal, J. (2003). *Occupational change in immigrant women.* Paper presented at the Society for the Study of Occupation: USA Second Annual Research Conference, Park City, Utah.

Thibeault, R. (2006). Globalisation, universities and the future of occupational therapy: Dispatches for the majority world. *Australian Occupational Therapy Journal, 53*(3), 159–65.

Townsend, E. (1993). Occupational therapy's social vision. *Canadian Journal of Occupational Therapy, 60*(4), 174–84.

Townsend, E. (2002). *Occupational justice: Is activism on occupational justice viable?* Paper presented at the Occupational Science Symposium, Los Angeles, CA, University of Southern California.

Townsend, E., & Wilcock, A. (2004a). Occupational justice. In C. Christiansen & E. Townsend (Eds.), *Introduction to occupation: The art and science of living* (pp. 243–73). Upper Saddle River, NJ: Prentice Hall.

Townsend, E., & Wilcock, A. (2004b). Occupational justice and client-centered practice: A dialogue in progress. *Canadian Journal of Occupational Therapy, 71*(2), 75–87.

United Nations. (1948). *Universal declaration of human rights.* Retrieved July 18, 2004, from http://www.un.org/rights.

U.S. Catholic Bishops. (1999). *A jubilee call for debt forgiveness.* Retrieved August 29, 2004, from http://www.nccbuscc .org/jubileepledge.

U.S. Census Bureau. (2000a). *African Americans—Health disparity.* Retrieved September 13, 2004, from http://www .cdc.gov/omhpopulation/baa.html.

U.S. Census Bureau. (2000b). *Disability.* Retrieved September 5, 2004, from http://www.census.gov/hhes/www/ disablity.html.

U.S. Department of Education, National Center for Education Statistics, Common Core of Data. (2003). *Public elementary/ secondary school universe survey* 2001–2002. Retrieved April 5, 2004, from http://www.nces.ed.gov/ccd.

U.S. Department of Health & Human Services. (2000). *Healthy People 2010: Understanding and improving health.* (2d ed.). Washington D.C.: Government Printing Office.

U.S. Department of Health & Human Services. (2001). *Closing the health gap: Reducing the health disparities affecting African-Americans.* Retrieved June 16, 2004, from http:// www.healthgapomhrc.gov/heart_disease.html.

U.S. Department of Health & Human Services. (2003). *Ending chronic homelessness: Strategies for action.* Washington, DC: Author.

U.S. Department of Justice. (2005). *A guide to disability rights laws.* Retrieved March 25, 2009, from www.ada.gov/ cguide.pdf

U.S. Department of Labor. (2009). *Employment situation summary.* Retrieved February 1, 2009, from http://www .bls.gov/news.release/empsit.nr0.htm.

Vision for Children at Risk. (2003). *Children of metropolitan St. Louis: A report to the community 2003 sixth edition* (Research report No. Sixth Edition). St. Louis, MO: Vision for Children at Risk.

White House Domestic Policy Council. (2004). *New Freedom Initiative: A progress report.* Retrieved April 2, 2004, from http://www.whitehouse.gov/news/freedominitiative.html.

Whiteford, G. (1997). Occupational deprivation and incarceration. *Journal of Occupational Sciences: Australia, 4*(3), 126–30.

Whiteford, G. (2000). Occupational deprivation: Global challenge in the new millennium. *British Journal of Occupational Therapy, 63*(5), 200–204.

Whiteford, G. (2010). Occupational deprivation: Understanding limited participation. In C. Christiansen & E. Townsend (Eds.), *Introduction to occupation: The art and science of living* (pp. 303–28). Upper Saddle River, NJ: Prentice Hall.

Whiting, C. C. (2001). School performance of children who have experienced maltreatment. *Physical and Occupational Therapy in Pediatrics, 21*(2/3), 81–89.

Wilcock, A. A. (1993). A theory of the human need for occupation. *Occupational Science: Australia, 1*(1), 17–24.

Wilcock, A. A. (1998a). *An occupational perspective of health.*Thorofare, NJ: SLACK.

Wilcock, A. A. (1998b). Reflections on doing, being and becoming. *Canadian Journal of Occupational Therapy, 65*(5), 248–56.

Wilcock, A., & Townsend, E. (2000). Occupational terminology interactive dialogue: Occupational justice. *Journal of Occupational Science, 7*(2), 84–86.

Wood, W. (2003). *Can't judge a place by its looks: Environmental dynamics, occupation and wellbeing in people with dementia.* Paper presented at the Society for the Study of Occupation: USA, Park City, Utah.

World Health Organization. (1948). *Preamble to the Constitution as adopted by the International Health Conference.* (Official Record of the World Health Organization, no. 2, p. 100).

World Health Organization. (1986). *Ottawa charter for health promotion: The first international conference on health promotion meeting in Ottawa.* Retrieved January 4, 2004, http://www.who.int/hpr/NPH/docs/ottawa_charter_hp.pdf.

World Health Organization. (2001). *International classification of functioning, disability and health.* Retrieved October 1, 2006, from http://www3.who.int/icf/icftemplate.cfm.

Zavella, P. (2001). The tables are turned: Immigration, poverty and social conflict in California communities. In J. M. Goode (Ed.), *The new poverty studies: The ethnography of power, politics and impoverished people in the United States* (pp. 102–31). New York: New York University Press.

Designing Health Promotion Interventions

Chapter 9

Evaluation Principles in Health Promotion Practice

S. Maggie Reitz, Michael A. Pizzi, and Marjorie E. Scaffa

> On my fieldwork in physical rehabilitation, I had many opportunities to observe and then eventually to evaluate patients. When I observed, I was very concerned and frankly, upset that the therapist I observed evaluated patients strictly from a "what's wrong" perspective and then, in 15 minutes proceeded to tell the patient what needed to be worked on, what their goals were and how to get their arm back in shape. The therapist never asked the patient how he was feeling, what in life was important to get back to doing and never talked about HIS goals or even anything about his social situation that he came from or where he would return. When it came time to treat, this same therapist set the patient up with a peg-board and told the patient to pick up the pegs and put them into the board and she came back 20 minutes later to see if he did it. When I asked him some questions, I found out he was a corporate lawyer who smoked two packs of cigarettes per day, had 4 children and a wife, worked 60 hours a week, and never took time for himself. He said he felt very guilty and depressed about not being the breadwinner in the future and that he missed something in life. He also said that he was pretty upset that the therapist didn't seem all that concerned about him or his health.
>
> —Occupational therapy student, 2002 (personal communication with M. Pizzi)

Learning Objectives

This chapter is designed to enable the reader to:

- Delineate the distinctions between evaluation and assessment in occupational therapy.
- Discuss philosophical issues related to evaluation while integrating the language and constructs of the *International Classification of Functioning, Disability, and Health (ICF)* developed by the World Health Organization (WHO, 2001).
- Apply the American Occupational Therapy Association's (AOTA) *Occupational Therapy Practice Framework* (AOTA, 2008) to the evaluation process.

- Implement ethical standards and guidelines in health promotion and wellness evaluation and assessment.
- Describe the concept of evidence-based assessment.
- Define the concepts of reliability, validity, and usability as they relate to standardized assessments.

Key Terms

Activity demands

Analysis of
    occupational
    performance

Assessment

Best practice

Client-centered

Client factors

Context

Cultural context

Ethics standards

Evaluation

Evidence-based
    practice

Occupational
    performance

Occupational profile

Performance patterns

Performance skills

Reliability

Standardized
    assessment

Standardized tests

Standard practice

Usability

Validity

Introduction

Occupation and client-centered practice begins with evaluating the individual's occupational participation in the context of his or her life. Evaluation and assessment are the means used to discover who people are via the creation of an occupational profile. An analysis of occupational performance determines occupational health needs and subsequent barriers. The intervention process subsequently follows, leading to eventual restoration of occupational participation in meaningful and important areas of one's life.

According to the *Standards of Practice for Occupational Therapy,* the term **evaluation** refers to "the process of obtaining and interpreting data necessary for interventions. This includes planning for and documenting the evaluation process and results" (AOTA, 2005b, p. 633). **Assessment** refers to "specific tools and instruments that are used during the evaluation process" (AOTA, 2005b, p. 663). These are the same definitions used in the *Occupational Therapy Practice Framework* (referred to as *Framework*). This chapter's goal is to provide both the knowledge and motivation to engage in evidence-based prevention and health promotion practice, specifically in terms of selecting and reporting assessment results. In addition, this chapter considers ethical issues and explores theoretical and philosophical perspectives related to the evaluation process in health promotion practice.

Best Practice and Evidence-Based Practice in Health Promotion Assessment

Leaders in occupational therapy have been encouraging practitioners to increase their use of and competence in outcome measures and to increase their engagement in best practice and evidence-based practice (Coster & Vergara, 2004; Holm, 2000, 2003; Law, 2002; Law, Baum, & Dunn, 2005). Law and Baum (2005) differentiate between the terms *standard practice* and *best practice.* **Standard practice** is the utilization of routine

approaches, which evolved from the best practices of yesterday. **Best practice** is looking beyond the current established way of delivering services and searching for new, innovative solutions that may yield better results in terms of both efficiency and effectiveness; this term is

> used in business, health, and education [and refers] to procedures which are believed to result in the most efficient provision of a product or service. Occupational therapists believe that evidence-based practice is a major element of what is now described as best practice. (Canadian Association of Occupational Therapists, Association of Canadian Occupational Therapy University Programs, Association of Canadian Occupational Therapy Regulatory Organizations, Presidents' Advisory Council, 1999, p. 268)

Best practice includes the pursuit of evidence on which to base practice and therefore must include **evidence-based practice.** Dunn defines this term as informing the client

> of what the profession knows (or does not know) about the effectiveness of the evaluations and interventions being proposed so that the recipient can make informed decisions about what services are acceptable and what he or she is willing to accept. (2005, p. 22)

While it may at first seem overwhelming to pursue evidence-based practice in any area of occupational therapy it may seem even more so in health promotion practice. This challenge, however, must be met. There are many myths about evidence-based practice that hinder its application. Law (2002) debunks key myths that relate to evidence-based practice in rehabilitation. These myths may also relate to evidence-based practice in health promotion and are presented in Table 9-1.

Law also describes the paramount role of self-directed learning in its quest and application. Law stresses that

> practitioners must maintain a humble attitude about their own practice patterns to excel at evidence-based practice. The ability to admit one's own errors and

Table 9–1 **Myths of Evidence-Based Practice in Health Promotion**

Myth	Reality
Evidence-based practice already exists.	Many practitioners take little or no time to review current research findings.
Evidence-based practice is impossible to put into place.	Even extremely busy practitioners can initiate evidence-based practice through little work.
Evidence-based practice is cookie-cutter interventions.	Evidence-based practice requires extensive expertise.
Evidence-based practice is a cost-cutting mechanism.	Evidence-based practice emphasizes the best available evidence for each client's situation.

Adapted with permission from Table 1-1 "Myths of Evidence-Based Practice," in *Evidence-based rehabilitation* (p. 7), by M. Law, 2002, Thorofare, NJ: SLACK.

oversights and to critically assess one's own prior work is crucial because knowing one's own limitations (and when to look for help) is the basis of evidence-based practice. (2002, p. 5)

This awareness of and engagement in self-directed learning, and the profession's continued movement toward the use of outcome measures, is supported by the AOTA's *Ethics Standards* (2007) and other occupational therapy codes of ethics (Canadian Association of Occupational Therapists [CAOT], 2007; Pollock & Rochon, 2002). The ethics of assessment will be discussed in more detail later in this chapter.

Bennett, Tooth, and colleagues (2003) found that although 96% of Australian occupational therapists reported believing in the importance of evidence-based research, only 56% reported using research evidence to select interventions. The most frequent sources of knowledge for decision-making were consultation with peers and participation in continuing education opportunities. Interest in and a need for education and the availability of "brief summaries of evidence" to support evidence-based decision-making was indicated from the survey results of Bennett, Tooth, and colleagues (2003, p. 13). To address the need for an evidence-based database specifically for occupational therapists, a group of Australian occupational therapists from two universities collaborated to develop a Web-accessible database called OTseeker (Bennett, Hoffman, et al., 2003). A community-based prevention example was used to describe how this database could be useful to an occupational therapist who wished to support the use of home visits and client education to reduce the risk of falls.

Professional occupational therapy associations also offer resources to assist their members to engage in evidence-based practice. For example, the AOTA provides the Evidence-Based Practice (EBP) Resource

Directory, which is an online service that links users to websites related to the evidence-based practice of the profession. "The Resource Directory is organized to connect occupational therapists, occupational therapy assistants, and students with useful Web-based resources, including

- Databases and Internet sites in occupational therapy, rehabilitation, and health outcomes
- Tutorials for acquiring basic and intermediate-level skills to search and interpret the literature relevant to occupational therapy
- National and international evidence-oriented Internet sites posted by universities, government agencies, and private organizations" (AOTA, 2009, *EBP Resource Directory*, ¶ 1).

There is also increasing emphasis on evidence-based practice in public health. According to Brownson and colleagues (2003), "Ideally, public health practitioners always incorporate scientific evidence in making management decisions, developing policies, and implementing programs" (p. 3). However, in reality, public health interventions, like those of occupational therapy, are often developed and implemented based on anecdotal evidence. Evidence-based practice in public health is defined as

the development, implementation, and evaluation of effective programs and policies in public health through application of principles of scientific reasoning, including systematic uses of data and information systems, and appropriate use of behavioral science theory and program planning models. (Brownson, Gurney, & Land, 1999, p. 86)

There are two types of evidence relevant for public health practice. The first type is data that addresses the relationship between preventable risk factors and specific diseases; for example, the link between smoking and lung cancer. This type of evidence indicates that "something should be done." The second type of evidence is data on intervention effectiveness. It delineates which interventions are most effective for what types of public health problems, and therefore it indicates specifically "what should be done" (Brownson, Baker, Leet, & Gillespie, 2003). These two types of evidence served as the foundation for the development of the national public health agenda *Healthy People 2010: Understanding and Improving Health* (U.S. Department of Health and Human Services, 2000).

Other professional associations, besides those in occupational therapy, are interested in promoting evidence-based practice among their members and other health providers. For instance, the Society for Prevention Research is "committed to the advancement of science-based prevention programs and policies through empirical research" (Flay et al., 2004, p. i). A committee was appointed by this association's board of directors to "determine the requisite criteria that must be met for preventive interventions to be judged tested and efficacious or tested and effective" (Flay et al., 2004, p. i). Efficacious prevention programs are those that do "more good than harm when delivered under optimal conditions" (Flay & last cited in Flay et al., 2004, p. 1), whereas effective programs do so under natural or "real-world" conditions.

Occupational therapists "must have the capacity to collect data to support their intervention recommendations" if they are to engage in evidence-based practice (Crepeau, Cohn, & Schell, 2003, p. 29). This is especially true when occupational therapists enter new partnerships with groups or communities. Care must be taken with the selection of both assessments and interventions.

The Language, Evolution, and Philosophical Aspects of Health Promotion Assessment

The profession has returned to its roots, with increasing interest in promoting wellbeing through building individual and community capacity. Those served may have health and occupational needs rather than medical or activities of daily living (ADLs) needs. Instead of solely identifying and focusing on problems to be worked on, strengths and potential for increased participation at the societal level are being considered. Occupational therapists and occupational therapy assistants are becoming more client-centered, which emphasizes the client as the focus of the occupational therapy process. Occupational therapy as a profession has knowledge and skills to strengthen population- and community-based program development and will need assessments to help guide intervention plans. Populations and communities are once again being viewed as potential clients by the profession, thus occupational therapy is engaged in addressing family and societal issues where people live, play, and work (AOTA, 2008).

Wilma West, Ruth Brunyate Wiemer, Geraldine Finn, and Florence Cromwell emphasized the need for occupational therapy to expand roles, responsibilities, and boundaries to explore what was possible in the community and in health promotion and disease prevention (White, 1986). Unfortunately, the occupational therapy profession did not heed their messages, which were articulated as early as 1966 (West, 1967). However, before effective interventions are developed, valid, effective, and reliable assessment and evaluative tools and processes to determine the health, occupational strengths, and needs of those to be served are required.

> Although philosophically dedicated to this concept of a healthy society, occupational therapists have not always demonstrated a commitment to match the rhetoric of their leaders. . . . It behooves all occupational therapists to accept the mandate of our professional leaders of the 1970s and to give priority to the expansion of the profession into the areas of health planning, health policy, and advocacy for disease prevention/health promotion programs. (Jaffe, 1986, p. 750)

The need for continued expansion from occupational therapy assessment and evaluation focusing on problems of individuals to those more reflective of health promotion, wellness, and prevention is especially critical in order to meet the needs of individuals and those of communities and society.

During the 1970s, occupational therapy assessments were primarily used to measure physical performance components (Mathiowetz, 1993). At that time, this was considered appropriate practice. In the 1990s, a movement within the discipline to modify the approach of assessment from bottom-up to top-down gained momentum. Articles in an *American Journal of Occupational Therapy* special issue on "critical issues in functional assessment" discussed the need to switch to a top-down approach, with primary consideration given to assessing occupational performance and secondary consideration given to assessing performance components (Fisher & Short-DeGraff, 1993; Mathiowetz, 1993; Trombly, 1993). Fisher, in her 1998 Eleanor Clarke Slagle Lecture, continued the support for a top-down approach, suggesting the use of chart reviews, life stories, or structured interviews as initial assessment tools. This top-down approach is compatible with health promotion efforts and is consistent with the *Framework* (AOTA, 2008).

Concern has been expressed that perhaps the "art of occupational therapy" has been lost or diminished (Peloquin, 1989). Instead, the profession has become more focused on the science of component occupational therapy. Increasing the knowledge and the development of ways to assess and restore performance components—such as range of motion, strength, endurance, reflexes, and self-esteem—has been an important step in the profession's development. Good work developing and refining component-based practice has enhanced the science of practice. Efforts to further refine the art of assessment need to be enhanced, especially in terms of population-based practice. A top-down approach, achieved through the completion of an occupational profile as described in the *Framework,* successfully blends the art and science of practice.

Peloquin (1989) states that

the art of practice in occupational therapy is intrinsically centered on relationships, on the qualities that make relationships meaningful, and on the meaning of occupation in a life. Demands from today's health care system make it increasingly difficult for practitioners to engage in meaningful relationships with their patients. (p. 219)

Peloquin's words continue to apply today. It is vital that these therapeutic relationships continue, as they will help sustain the art of practice and client-centered care. Holistic assessment demonstrates the willingness of the occupational therapy practitioner to discover the depths of a person's occupational health and wellness, thereby showing a caring and empathic connectedness to those served and fulfilling the requirement for evidence-based practice.

The *Framework* and the *ICF*

The *Framework* provides a blueprint for occupational therapy evaluation regardless of the population served or the setting in which the services are provided. The **occupational profile** is the first step in the evaluation process and "provides an understanding of the client's occupational history and experiences, patterns of daily living, interests, values, and needs" (AOTA, 2008, p. 646). In addition, the occupational profile allows the occupational therapist, in collaboration with the client, to identify problem areas and set priorities regarding activities of daily living, instrumental activities of daily living, education, work, play, leisure, and social participation. The term *client* as used in the *Framework* refers to the recipient of service, which may be individuals and their caregivers but may also include groups (e.g., families, classrooms), organizations, populations, and communities. The occupational profile can be

developed through a variety of ways. For individuals, structured, semistructured, or informal interviews can be appropriate tools. Focus groups, surveys, town meetings or other processes can be used when working with groups, communities, or populations.

The second step in the evaluation process is the **analysis of occupational performance,** during which the occupational therapist collects and interprets "information using assessment tools designed to observe, measure, and inquire about factors that support or hinder occupational performance" (AOTA, 2008, p. 649). This could include gathering data across the domain of occupational therapy, which includes performance skills, performance patterns, contexts, activity demands, areas of occupation, and client factors (AOTA, 2008). Descriptions of the elements of the domain of occupational therapy are presented below and are based on the *Framework*. **Performance skills** are the "abilities clients demonstrate in the actions they perform" (AOTA, 2008, p. 639). According to the *Framework,* these include motor and praxis skills, sensory-perceptual skills, emotional regulation skills, cognitive skills, and communication and social skills. **Performance patterns** include habits, routines, roles, and rituals that organize occupational behavior. These patterns may support or hinder meaningful engagement in occupations. **Context** refers to the internal and external conditions (i.e., cultural, physical, social, personal, spiritual, temporal, and virtual) that can affect the client's occupational performance. **Activity demands** refers to the required energy to perform a specific occupation. Such factors as required muscle actions, number and size of objects used, type of space, social demands among others needed for an individual, group, or community to successfully perform an occupation could dictate the activity demand of an occupation at a specific time. Areas of occupation are listed in detail within the *Framework*. **Client factors** vary greatly according to the type of client. For individuals, client factors include body structures and functions and the values and beliefs, including spirituality, within the client that may impact occupational performance At the population level, client factors would include economic, political, and social resources; values and beliefs; and other structures that the population has in common (AOTA, 2008).

During the analysis-of-occupational-performance phase of evaluation, skilled observation as well as standardized and nonstandardized assessments are used to collect data related to occupational performance (AOTA, 2008). **Standardized assessments** are defined as "assessment procedures in which processes are clearly identified, along with guidelines for interpretation of results, [and] may have established and tested normative data with which to compare results" (Spear & Crepeau, 2003, p. 1034). The occupational therapist must integrate information from the occupational profile with data from the assessments and, using clinical reasoning, must identify factors that influence performance skills and patterns and facilitate or constrain occupational performance. This analysis allows the occupational therapist to determine the client's strengths and challenges, and provides the foundation for intervention planning (AOTA, 2008).

At least two of the four aims of the *International Classification of Functioning, Disability, and Health (ICF)* relate to assessment. These two aims include establishing a common language to "describe health and health-related states" and providing "a scientific basis for understanding and studying health and health-related states, outcomes, and determinants" (World Health Organization [WHO], 2001, p. 5). The importance of a common language in the development of assessments and in reporting the results of assessments are particularly important in health promotion, which is often interdisciplinary and international in scope and potential contribution.

Although the *ICF* focuses on the functioning of the individual, components and definitions are relevant for use in population-based health promotion practice. The *ICF* provides

a conceptual framework for information that is applicable to personal health care, including prevention, health promotion, and the improvement of participation by removing mitigating societal hindrances and encouraging the provision of social supports and facilitators. It is also useful for the study of health care

systems, in terms of both evaluation and policy formation. (WHO, 2001, p. 6)

The *ICF* is divided into two parts: One addresses function and disability and the second addresses contextual factors. Each of these parts is subdivided into components. The function and disability portion is divided into "body functions and structures" and "activities and participation"; the contextual factors portion is divided into "environmental factors" and "personal factors." Table 9-2 depicts these components and the domains and constructs that are linked to each. The four components are further divided into categories. Each of the four components and many of the associated categories has relevance to the evaluation of the individual in terms of prevention and health promotion. The "activities and participation" and "environmental factors" components may have more relevance to the selection or development of assessment tools for health promotion of a group, community, or population than the "body functions and structures" and "personal factors" components. Table 9-3 displays the categories associated with the "activities and participation" and "environmental factors" components. The categories identified in this table are within the domain of occupational therapy practice and should be considered when evaluating the prevention and health promotion needs of a group or community.

The *ICF* further divides the categories of each component into subcategories, providing a detailed dissection and classification of terms related to health and health-related states. Content Boxes 9-1 and 9-2

Table 9–2 Overview of the *ICF*

Components	PART 1: FUNCTIONING AND DISABILITY		PART 2: CONTEXTUAL FACTORS	
	Body Functions and Structures	**Activities and Participation**	**Environmental Factors**	**Personal Factors**
Domains	Body functions Body structures	Life areas (i.e., tasks, actions)	External influences on functioning and disability	Internal influences on functioning and disability
Constructs	Change in body functions (physiological)	Capacity Executing tasks in a standard environment	Facilitating or hindering impact of features of the physical, social, and attitudinal world	Impact of attributes of the person
	Change in body structures (anatomical)	Performance Executing tasks in the current environment		

Adapted from portions of Table 1, in *An overview of ICF* from *International classification of functioning, disability, and health* (p. 11) by World Health Organization (WHO), 2001, Geneva, Switzerland. Copyright 2001 by WHO.

Table 9–3 *ICF* **Categories for Selected Components**

Activities and Participation	Environmental Factors
Learning and applying knowledge	Products and technology
General tasks and demands	Natural environment and human-made changes to environment
Communication	Support and relationships
Mobility	Attitudes
Self-care	Services, systems, and policies
Domestic life	
Interpersonal interactions and relationships	
Major life areas	
Community, social, and civic life	

Data from material in *An overview of ICF* from *International classification of functioning, disability, and health* (p. 30) by World Health Organization (WHO), 2001, Geneva, Switzerland. Copyright © 2001 by WHO.

identify the subcategories for a selected category from each of the components described in Table 9-3. These were selected as examples of categories that may have more relevance to prevention and health promotion efforts. The reader is encouraged to review and explore the *ICF* in its entirety at http://www3.who .int/icf/onlinebrowser/icf.cfm.

Although the *ICF* may at first appear overwhelming and cumbersome, it behooves occupational therapy practitioners to be aware of international trends in the language of health to maximize the exchange of ideas and outcome data, thus advancing both standard and evidence-based practice. The influence of this classification system can be seen in the development

Content Box 9-1

ICF *Subcategories—Community, Social, and Civic Life Category From Activities and Participation Component*

- Community life
- Recreation and leisure
- Religion and spirituality
- Human rights
- Political life and citizenship
- Community, social and civic life, other specified
- Community, social and civic life, unspecified

Data from material in *An overview of ICF* from *International classification of functioning, disability, and health* (p. 42) by World Health Organization (WHO), 2001, Geneva, Switzerland. Copyright 2001 by WHO.

Content Box 9-2

ICF *Subcategories—Services, Systems, and Policies Category From Environmental Factors Component*

- Services, systems, and policies for the production of consumer goods
- Architecture and construction services, systems, and policies
- Open-space planning services, systems, and policies
- Housing services, systems, and policies
- Utilities services, systems, and policies
- Communication services, systems, and policies
- Transportation services, systems, and policies
- Civil protection services, systems, and policies
- Legal services, systems, and policies
- Associations and organizational services, systems, and policies
- Media services, systems, and policies
- Economic services, systems, and policies
- Social security services, systems, and policies
- General social support services, systems, and policies
- Health services, systems, and policies
- Education and training services, systems, and policies
- Labor and employment services, systems, and policies
- Political services, systems, and policies
- Services, systems, and policies, other specified
- Services, systems, and policies, unspecified

Data from material in *An overview of ICF* from *International classification of functioning, disability, and health* (p. 44) by World Health Organization (WHO), 2001, Geneva, Switzerland. Copyright 2001 by WHO.

of the *Framework,* which compares the language of the *Framework* with that of the *ICF* and the *Uniform Terminology for Occupational Therapy—Third Edition* (AOTA, 1994).

Issues in Assessment

There are many issues associated with evaluation and assessment. Ethical and cultural concerns as well as the importance of and need for a client-centered approach to evaluation, assessment, and intervention are discussed in the following pages.

Client-Centered Health and Wellness Assessment

Law, Baptiste, and Mills (1995) defined **client-centered** occupational therapy as "an approach to service which embraces a philosophy of respect for, and partnership with, people receiving services" (p. 253). Partnering with those served in the evaluation process can only enhance the communication between occupational therapist and client, which will then most likely lead to increased cooperation of the client to engage in the occupational process and meet goals that are collaboratively discussed and agreed upon. There is no alternative than to collaborate with clients and their caregivers/significant others if they so choose. If clients are unable to make their needs and goals known, then goal planning should be completed in consultation with the designated significant other. Collaboration speaks to regard for others and a desire to form caring and open relationships. Outcomes will be enhanced, and quite probably improved, when the client is a part of the process from the onset. Client-centered approaches can more powerfully produce meaningful occupational therapy interventions.

Law (1998) summarized constructs of a client-centered approach and then later detailed the implications for measurement of occupational performance (as cited by Law & Baum, 2001, 2005). In this description, the construct of family can be applied to a small two-person dyad as well as a larger extended family unit.

1. Occupational performance issues/problems will be identified by the client and his or her family, not by the therapist or team; if other issues, such as safety, are not identified, the therapist will communicate these concerns directly to the client and significant others.

2. Evaluation of the success of therapy intervention will focus on change in occupational performance.

3. Our measurement techniques will enable clients to have a say in evaluating the outcomes of therapy intervention.

4. Measurement will reflect the individualized nature of people doing occupations.

5. Measurement will focus on both the subjective experience and the observable qualities of occupational performance.

6. Measurement of the environment is critical in helping therapists and clients understand the influence of the environment on occupational performance, as well as measuring the effects of changing environmental conditions during the therapy process. (Law & Baum, 2005, pp. 8–9)

In summary, in order for occupational therapy evidence-based interventions to be successful and promote health and wellbeing, effective and holistic health and wellness assessment must be utilized as a first step. With an understanding of the *ICF* and the *Framework,* previously used assessments will take on new meaning, and new assessments will be developed that will help shape and create new ways of thinking in occupational therapy. This evolving philosophy will assist the profession to more fully contribute to the health and wellbeing of individuals, communities, and society.

Cultural Issues

The context of culture is a very complex factor that needs to be negotiated with care and respect during the evaluation process. **Cultural context,** as defined in the *Framework,* is the

> customs, beliefs, activity patterns, behavior standards, and expectations accepted by the society of which the individual is a member. Includes political aspects, such as laws that affect access to resources and affirm personal rights. Also includes opportunities for education, employment and economic support. (AOTA, 2002, p. 623)

Occupational therapy assessment often focuses on an individual's **occupational performance,** which is, as defined in the *Framework,*

> the act of doing and accomplishing a selected activity or occupation that results from the dynamic transaction among the client, the context, and the activity. Improving or enabling skills and patterns in occupational performance leads to engagement in occupation or activities (adapted in part from Law et al., 1996, p. 16 as cited by AOTA, 2008, pp. 672–73)

In order for outcomes to more closely relate to a person's life and lifestyle, assessment of occupational performance must occur within context, which includes understanding and acknowledging various cultural influences. These influences may include ethnicity, family structure, sexual orientation, gender, and age.

It is important that cultural backgrounds of those served—be it a person, family system, community, or society—are accurately understood in order to individualize therapy and to develop a more collaborative experience in planning intervention and setting goals (Mattingly & Beer, 1993). McGruder (2003) believes that, besides these issues, the need "to ensure accurate assessment and to increase the likelihood of equitable treatment" (p. 85) are essential ingredients in the occupational therapy process. Evans (1992) cautioned occupational therapists to constantly review their decisions to check for possible racial bias when deciding who may or may not benefit from interventions. This self-reflection should also be conducted when decisions are made regarding access to health promotion interventions and when selecting groups for population-based programming. These efforts are supported by the *Occupational Therapy Code of Ethics (2005)* (AOTA, 2005a), specifically Principles 1A and D (Table 9-4).

The *Framework* is infused with language and terms from the *ICF* classification system. This infusion can be seen within the definitions of activity demands, areas of occupational performance, and client factors. Attempts by the profession to use internationally developed and agreed-upon terms may assist with the sharing of culturally relevant assessment and intervention successes.

Occupational therapy assessments and the entire evaluation process can be culturally influenced. For example, Pizzi recalled administering to a British homosexual man with AIDS the role checklist, an occupational therapy assessment used to determine which occupational roles a client values. He threw the assessment at the therapist and stated he wasn't filling it out, because there was no space for him to put the role of partner, and he felt the checklist was discriminatory. While this was an unexpected gesture on the client's part, it heightened the therapist's awareness about this issue.

Another patient of the same practitioner, this time in homecare, was surrounded by family members of an elderly Chinese patient, all of whom questioned the occupational therapy referral, because, culturally, the family cares for their elderly, both disabled and well members. Occupation-based recommendations were made for continued occupational performance, and occupational participation was realized within the context of the home, the family, and other cultural influences. The practitioner was very nicely shown to the door and thanked for his time. No further visits could be made, although the family was very polite about refusing help. "Cultural differences enter into the therapy process of assessment not only at the level of achieving understanding and empathy for the client but also at the level of choosing evaluation instruments and strategies and interpreting results" (McGruder, 2003, p. 87).

Health, promotion of healthy lifestyles, and prevention are culturally influenced. For example, in the North American dominant culture, there is a high value placed on independence. Many occupational therapy assessment tools are biased toward this value (Law, 1993). McGruder (2003) discusses literature in occupational therapy that "supports the need to tailor evaluation strategies carefully, particularly considering culture and racial, ethnic and class diversity" (pp. 88–89). Pizzi (2003) emphasized the need to obtain an historical account of the person as a primary strategy to assess his or her culture and diverse needs. At the very least, cultural differences should be acknowledged during assessment. Utilizing therapeutic use of self to establish the rapport needed to develop trust and maintain human dignity through the evaluation process is essential.

Ethical Issues in Health Promotion Assessment

There are many potential ethical quagmires therapists can encounter during the evaluation process. Some of these pitfalls are unique to community-based or health promotion practice, while others are more germane to the evaluation process as a whole. The AOTA *Ethics Standards* (AOTA, 2007), which includes the *Occupational Therapy Code of Ethics (2005)* (AOTA, 2005a), the *Guidelines to the Occupational Therapy Code of Ethics* (Slater, 2006), and the *Core Values and Attitudes of Occupational Therapy Practice* (AOTA, 1993), provide guidance regarding behavior to aspire to during evaluation and intervention. The *Ethics Standards* are a set of documents that can assist the occupational therapist and occupational therapy assistant in fulfilling their commitment to provide the best possible evaluation and intervention services to their clients. They can be particularly helpful in self-reflection of health promotion service provision, as these services are often provided in contexts with no or limited supervisory assistance. Awareness and commitment to the *Ethics Standards* prevents unintentional harm to clients and encourages the delivery of services that reflect well upon the practitioner and the profession.

Examples follow of potentially unethical behaviors and the rationale supporting why these behaviors are unethical or illegal. This list of unethical behaviors is not exhaustive but is illustrative to provoke the reader's thinking. Many resources, including the AOTA, the National Board for Certification in Occupational Therapy (NBCOT), and state regulatory bodies are available to consult if the reader has questions or concerns about these or other issues.

Table 9–4 Selection of Principles That Influence Assessment in Health Promotion

1. Occupational therapy personnel shall demonstrate a concern for the safety and well-being of the recipients of their services. (BENEFICENCE)	Occupational therapy personnel shall: 1A. Provide services in a fair and equitable manner. They shall recognize and appreciate the cultural components of economics, geography, race, ethnicity, religious and political factors, marital status, age, sexual orientation, gender identity and disability of all recipients of their services. 1D. Recognize the responsibility to promote public health and the safety and well-being of individuals, groups, and/or communities.
2. Occupational therapy personnel shall take measures to ensure a recipient's safety and avoid imposing or inflicting harm. (NONMALEFICENCE)	Occupational therapy personnel shall: 2A. Maintain therapeutic relationships that shall not exploit the recipient of services sexually, physically, emotionally, psychologically, financially, socially, or in any other manner.
4. Occupational therapy personnel practitioners shall achieve and continually maintain high standards of competence. (DUTY)	Occupational therapy personnel shall: 4B. Conform to AOTA standards of practice and official documents. 4D. Be competent in all topic areas in which they provide instruction to consumers, peers, and/or students. 4E. Critically examine available evidence so they may perform their duties on the basis of current information. 4H. Refer to or consult with other service providers whenever such a referral or consultation would be helpful to the care of the recipient of service. The referral or consultation process should be done in collaboration with the recipient of service.
5. Occupational therapy personnel shall comply with laws and Association policies guiding the profession of occupational therapy. (PROCEDURAL JUSTICE)	Occupational therapy personnel shall: 5D. Take reasonable steps to ensure employers are aware of occupational therapy's ethical obligations, as set forth in this Code, and of the implications of those obligations for occupational therapy practice, education, and research.
6. Occupational therapy personnel shall provide accurate information when representing the profession. (VERACITY)	Occupational therapy personnel shall: 6B. Disclose any professional, personal, financial, business, or volunteer affiliations that may pose a conflict of interest to those with whom they may establish a professional, contractual, or other working relationship. 6D. Identify and fully disclose to all appropriate persons errors that compromise recipients' safety. 6E. Accept responsibility for their professional actions that reduce the public's trust in occupational therapy services and those that perform those services.

From *Reference guide to the Occupational Therapy Code of Ethics* (pp. 6–8), D. Y. Slater (Ed.), 2006, Bethesda, MD: American Occupational Therapy Association. Copyright 2006 by American Occupational Therapy Association. With permission.

Five of the many potential issues therapists may face during the evaluation process include (1) competence to select and perform assessments, (2) conflict of interest, (3) copyright infringement, (4) failure to perform due diligence, and (5) misrepresentation of results. Each are described below and are linked to one or more principles of the *Occupational Therapy Code of Ethics (2005)* (AOTA, 2005a), the *Guidelines to the Code,* or *Core Values and Attitudes* that direct and define appropriate behavior.

Competence

A competent, ethical occupational therapist would complete a thorough literature review and a needs assessment prior to developing a health promotion program for a group, community, institution, or organization. This behavior is supported by Principles 4B, 4D, and 4E of the *Occupational Therapy Code of Ethics (2005)* as are the core values of truth and prudence. These principles appear in Table 9-4. If the occupational therapist has had no previous experience in this type of work, seeking a mentor or obtaining additional training or education would be appropriate first steps. Principle 4H (see Table 9-4) and *Guideline* 4.1, which states, "Occupational therapy personnel developing new areas of competence (skills, techniques, approaches) must engage in appropriate study and training, under appropriate supervision, before incorporating new areas into their practice" (Slater, 2006, p. 17), are relevant to this issue. Tickle-Degnen (2002) encourages occupational therapists to be guided by evidence when selecting assessments.

Conflict of Interest

A multitude of possible situations exist where conflicts of interest may arise. One example would be if a supervisor directs his or her employees to routinely use an assessment and/or a canned health promotion program from which they receive royalties with no efforts to individualize choice for the client's needs. This is a conflict of interest in that financial gain may be influencing assessment and practice decisions. This behavior would be in violation of the value of truth and Principles 2A and 6B (see Table 9-4) and *Guidelines* 6.1 and 6.2 (Slater, 2006), which caution occupational therapy practitioners to avoid any situation that has the potential to inappropriately influence their judgment or result in the exploitation of a client.

Another example would be if two coworkers opened a private health promotion practice that competes for business with their primary employer. Their behavior would be even more problematic if, without permission, they used materials for their private practice that were developed while they were employees and were owned by the primary employer. This behavior would be in violation of Principle 5 (see Table 9-4) and *Guideline* 3.2, which states, "Occupational therapy personnel shall be diligent stewards of human, financial, and material resources of their employers. They shall refrain from exploiting these resources for personal gain" (Slater, 2006, p. 17). In addition, the behavior would violate *Guideline* 6.4 and, to a lesser degree, 6.5. *Guideline* 6.4 states, "Occupational therapy personnel shall not accept obligations or duties that may compete with or be in conflict with their duties to their employers" (Slater, 2006, p. 19), whereas *Guideline* 6.5 cautions occupational therapy personnel not to "use their position or the knowledge gained from their position in such a way that knowingly gives rise to real or perceived conflict of interest between themselves and their employers, other association members or bodies, and/or other organizations" (Slater, 2006, p. 19).

Copyright Infringement

Although individuals can attempt to justify "borrowing" and "copying" a copyrighted assessment instead of purchasing it, this behavior is both illegal and unethical. Depending on the purpose, asking local academic institutions to borrow assessments can also be unethical. If the purpose of the loan is to review the assessment for possible use and purchase, this would be both prudent and fiscally responsible. However, if the purpose was to make a copy for their use, it would be both unethical and illegal. Employees are duty bound to educate their employers of the necessity for access to the appropriate assessments to provide competent service to recipients. This duty is supported by the values of justice and truth and by *Guideline* 3.1, which states, "Occupational therapy practitioners take steps to make sure that employers are aware of the ethical principles of the profession and occupational therapy personnel's obligation to adhere to those ethical principles" (Slater, 2006, p. 17).

Failure to Perform Due Diligence

Working expediently can be a positive attribute, but it can also lead to unethical behavior if sufficient care is not taken to select the best available assessment, to properly administer the assessment, and to properly report results. If the person knows the best assessment and is able to perform it but does not do so, this behavior is inappropriate and has the potential to harm the object of the assessment, be it an individual, a family, or a community. This behavior would thus violate Principles 1 and 2 (see Table 9-4). Another concern is this behavior's potential to negatively impact society's view of the profession and the reputation of the profession's members, which would be in violation of Principle 6E.

There are numerous resources available for occupational therapists to become knowledgeable about both standard practice and best practice in assessment (Hyner, et al., 1999; Law, 2002; Law, Baum, & Dunn, 2005). Besides these and other texts, additional resources are available. The AOTA provides information on evidence-based practice through its website and continuing-education opportunities. Other professional organizations and state associations also provide resources and educational opportunities. It is essential that occupational therapists use these resources to maintain their competence in selecting the best available assessment to use in health promotion interventions with the individual, family, community, or population. If occupational therapists conduct assessments they are not competent to perform, they fail to uphold the value of truth and are in violation of Principles 1, 2, 4, and 5 (see Table 9-4). It is important for occupational therapy personnel to know their strengths and weaknesses and to be honest with themselves and the recipients of their care.

Misrepresentation of Results

Modifying assessment data for financial gain is obviously an unethical and illegal behavior. For example, it is unethical to misrepresent the outcome of a community-needs assessment to create the illusion that a health-promotion program you can provide is required when the assessment actually indicates that the community is in greater need of other services that are more appropriately provided by another occupational therapist or discipline. This behavior is in conflict with the core value of truth, Principle 2A (see Table 9-4), and *Guidelines* 6.1 and 6.2 as described above. *Guideline* 1.3 states, "Occupational therapy practitioners must be truthful about their individual competencies. . . . In some cases the therapist may need to refer the client to another professional to assure that the most appropriate services are provided" (Slater, 2006, p. 15), and it provides helpful guidance as to appropriate behavior.

A second example of misrepresentation of results occurs when results are manipulated in an attempt to be helpful to an individual, family, or community. Although it may be tempting to falsify data to ensure that a community or individual receives needed health promotion services, it is still fraudulent and unethical. This behavior is also not supported by the *Ethics Standards*.

Assessment Selection

Completing an occupational profile (AOTA, 2008) provides the occupational therapist with the background information necessary to assist in selecting appropriate assessment tools, including standardized tests. **Standardized tests** are administered and scored following a prescribed system and are either norm-referenced or criterion referenced (Imel, 1990). More specifically, according to Surrey and colleagues (2003), the prevailing criteria indicate that a standardized test is an instrument that must meet the following six conditions:

- Establishment of reliability
- Verified validity
- Specific and clear administration instructions
- Appropriate instructions for interpretation of the results
- Well established equipment standards
- Normative data based on large population samples (pp. 97–98)

Many factors must be considered prior to selecting assessment tools or tests. Windsor (2002, 2003) developed a test critique assignment for a graduate research class at Towson University. This assignment required students to answer questions regarding the ease of a test's administration, cost, and psychometric properties (e.g., reliability, validity, standard error of measurement). A modified version of selected questions from this assignment appears in Content Box 9-3.

Content Box 9-3

Considerations for the Selection of a Test or Standardized Assessment

1. What is the purpose or function of the test?
2. Is the purpose compatible with the client's goals?
3. Will the test provide data about the client's occupational performance?
4. What is the validity of the test?
5. What is the reliability of the test?
6. What is the appropriate test population (e.g., age, diagnostic group)?
7. What is the test's cost to the client?
8. What is the cost to the institution or agency?
9. Does this cost include test materials/manual/answer sheets?
10. Are the test materials easy to manipulate, use, clean?
11. Is the test administered in a group or individually?
12. How long does the test administration take?
13. How easy is it to administer/score?
14. Does fatigue affect the result?
15. Do you have the required skill/training to administer the test?
16. Do you have the required skill/training to interpret the test results?

Adapted from *Test critique assignment* by M. M. Windsor, 2002 & 2003, for OCTH 613 Advanced Research Methods in Occupation-Based Practice, Towson, MD: Towson University. Adapted with permission.

The questions included in Content Box 9-3 address the three primary attributes requiring scrutiny when selecting a test: **validity, reliability,** and **usability** (Lyman, 1998). These three attributes are defined and described in Table 9-5. A clear link between the constructs to be measured in an assessment and an accepted theory is necessary to enhance the assessment's validity. The presence of this link should be considered when selecting an assessment tool. Also, care must be taken prior to selecting an assessment designed for a specific population (e.g., individuals with physical disabilities in the United States) if using it with a different population (e.g., new immigrant families from the Sudan who are experiencing stress from war and resettlement). Usability, or practical factors, must always be considered when selecting health promotion assessments, whether the client is an individual, a family or group, or a community.

Polgar (2003) reported varying recommendations or guidelines for a minimum level of reliability depending on a test's purpose. In general, the purposes of assessment in health promotion (e.g., screening, assessment of attitudes) do not require the same level of reliability as a test to determine an individual's discharge placement. Whereas a 0.90 minimum level of reliability is recommended for placement decisions, it may be appropriate for health promotion screenings to require a reliability coefficient of only 0.80. Although a reliability coefficient of 0.60 is often considered too low for use in a clinical context, it has been proposed as an acceptable minimum level of reliability for group attitude tests, if the results are reported for the group as a whole (Polgar, 2003). Detailed information regarding critiquing standardized assessments (Polgar, 2003) and interpreting test scores (Lyman, 1998; Silverlake, 1999) are available.

It is more challenging to locate standardized health-promotion occupation-based assessments than assessments for other areas of occupational therapy practice. However, even if standardized assessments are unavailable, both usability and alignment with client needs and preferences must be considered when selecting a non-standardized assessment tool. A variety of resources (AOTA, 1996; Boop, 2003; Christiansen & Baum, 1997; Hyner et al., 1999; Law et al., 2005; Letts, Baum, & Perlmutter, 2003 [assessments specific for older adults]; Paul & Orchanian, 2003) are available to assist the occupational therapist in identifying, locating, and selecting appropriate assessments for health promotion interventions.

Component Versus Holistic Assessment and Objective Versus Subjective Assessment

It has been difficult to find holistic prevention/health promotion and wellness assessments specific for occupational therapy that have some level of validity and reliability, though these assessments exist in other disciplines. Development of such assessments has been limited in occupational therapy, with the majority of assessment tools being component-driven, emphasizing a person's deficits and problems and being objective in nature (versus client-centered and coming from, or at least including, the client's subjective experiences). This appears to be an area for further development and growth in occupational therapy.

While the profession's official documents value diversity; the promotion of healthy lifestyles; the prevention of disease; and the principles of being client-centered, occupation-based, and holistic, the assessment tools and the overall evaluation process simply do not reflect many of these factors. Using only component-based assessments with interventions that focus only on improving the performance of that function or structure does not speak to the possibilities that occupational therapy can afford a client. The *Framework,* while acknowledging these as client factors, emphasizes participation. The overarching goal of occupational therapy, according

Table 9–5 **Necessary Attributes to Consider in the Selection of Assessments**

Term	Definition/Description	Source
Reliability	The consistency of measurements when the testing procedure is repeated on a population of individuals or groups (American Educational Research Association [AERA], 1999, p. 25)	Polgar, 2003
Validity	The degree to which evidence and theory support interpretations of test scores or assessment results (AERA, 1999, p. 9)	Polgar, 2003
Usability	All such practical factors such as cost, ease of scoring, time required, and the like (AERA, 1999, p. 9)	Lyman, 1998

to the *Framework*, is "supporting health and participation in life through engagement in occupation" (AOTA, 2008, p. 660). If the *Framework* is used as intended, it is vital that assessments take on a more global and holistic perspective. Practitioners, including those working in a more component-driven and often reimbursement-driven environment, are focused on function. *Function* is often used to describe occupational performance, because occupational therapy enhances and facilitates both function and occupational performance. However, in order for the profession to move forward and to continue developing its unique identity, practitioners need to continually reflect on the following questions:

- Is this really occupational therapy?
- Is the client's uniqueness being considered in the assessment process?
- Is the focus on the client's needs, goals, aspirations, and hopes?
- Will the intervention help to facilitate a level of occupational engagement that is satisfactory to the client?

One strategy to address these questions is to ensure clients have as much input as they wish during the evaluation process.

No one knows the client better than the client. The occupational therapist's ability to clinically reason through a situation to assist a client to optimize their health and wellbeing is crucial. However, occupational therapy knowledge and application of that knowledge can result in an objective bias toward what the practitioner deems is important in the client's life. The practitioner may then make decisions regarding assessment and intervention that are unduly influenced by what the practitioner believes is right and good. When occupational therapists add to the assessment process the dimension of a client's subjective responses, such as their narrative, story, or occupational history, then intervention that follows will more likely automatically include an integration of both the client's perceptions of their life story and the practitioner's clinical reasoning skills. The astute, expert therapist effectively uses conditional reasoning. This enables him or her to evaluate the client within the social contexts of home and community and thereby identify the client's current and future needs more appropriately (Benamy, 1996).

Lund, Tamm, and Branholm (2001) explored and compared patients' and professionals' perceptions about participation in care. First they examined how patients perceived their participation in the planning of their rehabilitation. They next described the nurses' and occupational therapists' view of the strategies used to encourage patients' participation, and then they compared the perceptions of the two groups (i.e.,

patients and health-care providers). Data were collected through semistructured interviews with 57 hospitalized patients, 39 nurses, and 11 occupational therapists. On the basis of the data, patients were categorized as

- relinquishers,
- participants, and
- occasional participants.

Professionals were categorized as information providers and rehabilitation practitioners. Approximately the same strategies used by the professionals to encourage patient participation were provided regardless of patient category. It was suggested that professionals needed to be sensitive to the patient's desire to participate in the planning of a rehabilitation program. Further research was recommended to investigate which circumstances affected patients' participation and which strategies professionals could use to encourage their participation.

Conclusion

Measurement of occupational performance includes the use of both quantitative and qualitative assessment approaches, from the perspective of the client, his or her family or caregiver, and the occupational therapist.

> As occupational therapists develop an evidence-based practice, a valid measurement process is essential in providing evidence of the effectiveness and efficiency of our services. Our measurement practices need to fit within a client-centered practice where persons, their families and therapists work in partnership to enhance occupational performance. Our clients expect, and have a right to know and receive, evidence of the outcomes of occupational therapy service provision. (Law & Baum, 2001, p. 15)

The likelihood of a client following up with health-promotion or prevention interventions will be greater when the client values the occupational therapy process through being a part of the process. In addition, the client is more likely to feel included and respected. The next chapter will describe several health promotion assessments that foster the collaborative relationship.

▶ For Discussion and Review

1. A professor copies an assessment for educational purposes, because the department states it does not have enough money budgeted to purchase one for each student. Describe how this is or is not an ethical problem, and defend your position.

2. What does the *Framework* say about assessment and evaluation? Is there a distinction? Should components of occupational performance be included? Why or why not?
3. Describe how validity and reliability of assessments is related to best practice and evidence-based practice.

▶ Research Questions

1. Develop a qualitative study to examine practitioners' understanding and application of ethical reasoning when selecting and using assessments to determine the needs of individuals, families, or communities.
2. Design a quantitative or mixed-method research study to determine (a) the most frequently used assessments in occupational therapy health promotion and (b) the rationale for their selection.

Acknowledgments

The authors would like to acknowledge the assistance of Alexander J. Stroup and Grace E. Wenger in the preparation of this chapter.

References

American Occupational Therapy Association. (1993). Core values and attitudes of occupational therapy practice. *American Journal of Occupational Therapy, 47,* 1085–86.

American Occupational Therapy Association. (1994). Uniform terminology for occupational therapy—Third edition. *American Journal of Occupational Therapy, 48,* 1047–54.

American Occupational Therapy Association. (1995). Clarification of the use of terms assessment and evaluation. *American Journal of Occupational Therapy, 49,* 1072–73.

American Occupational Therapy Association. (1996). *Occupational therapy assessment tools: An annotated index* (2d ed.). Bethesda, MD: Author.

American Occupational Therapy Association. (2005a). Occupational therapy code of ethics (2005). *American Journal Occupational Therapy, 59,* 639–42.

American Occupational Therapy Association. (2005b). Standards of occupational therapy practice. *American Journal Occupational Therapy, 59,* 663–65.

American Occupational Therapy Association. (2007). Enforcement procedures for the *Occupational Therapy Code of Ethics* (edited 2007). *American Journal of Occupational Therapy, 61,* 679–85.

American Occupational Therapy Association. (2008). Occupational therapy practice framework: Domain and process (2d ed.). *American Journal of Occupational Therapy, 62,* 625–83.

American Occupational Therapy Association. (2009). *Evidence-based practice resource directory.* Retrieved January 19, 2009, from http://aota.org/Educate/Research/Evidence Directory.aspx.

Benamy, B. C. (1996). *Developing clinical reasoning skills: Strategies for the occupational therapist.* San Antonio, TX: Therapy Skill Builders.

Bennett, S., Hoffman, T., McCluskey, A., McKenna, K., Strong, J., & Tooth, L. (2003). Introducing OTseeker (occupational therapy systematic evaluation of evidence): A new evidence database for occupational therapists. *American Journal of Occupational Therapy, 57*(3), 635–38. [Evidence-based practice forum.]

Bennett, S., Tooth, L., McKenna, K., Rodger, S., Strong, J., Ziviani, J., et al. (2003). Perceptions of evidence-based practice: A survey of Australian occupational therapists. *Australian Journal of Occupational Therapy, 50,* 13–22.

Boop, C. (2003). Appendix A—Assessments: Listed alphabetically by title. In E. B. Crepeau, E. S. Cohn, & B. A. Schell (Eds.), *Willard & Spackman's occupational therapy* (10th ed., pp. 981–1004). Philadelphia: Lippincott, Williams & Wilkins.

Brownson, R. C., Baker, E. A., Leet, T. L., & Gillespie, K. N. (2003). *Evidence-based public health.* New York: Oxford University Press.

Brownson, R. C., Gurney, J. G., & Land, G. (1999). Evidence-based decision-making in public health. *Journal of Public Health Management and Practice, 5,* 86–97.

Canadian Association of Occupational Therapists. (2007). *Canadian Association of Occupational Therapists code of ethics.* Retrieved April 16, 2007, from http://.caot.ca/default.asp?pageid=35.

Canadian Association of Occupational Therapists, Association of Canadian Occupational Therapy University Programs, Association of Canadian Occupational Therapy Regulatory Organizations, & Presidents' Advisory Council. (1999). Joint position statement on evidence-based occupational therapy. *Canadian Journal of Occupational Therapy, 66*(5), 267–69.

Christiansen, C., & Baum, C. (Eds.) (1997). Index of assessments. In *Occupational therapy: Enabling function and well-being* (2d ed., pp. 607–608). Thorofare, NJ: SLACK.

Coster, W., & Vergara, E. (2004). Finding the resources to support EBP: What to do when the university library isn't next door. *OT Practice, 9*(50), 10–15.

Crepeau, E. B., Cohn, E. S., & Schell, B. B. (2003). Occupational therapy practice, Section I Occupational therapy practice today. In E. B. Crepeau, E. S. Cohn, & B. B. Schell (Eds.), *Willard and Spackman's occupational therapy* (10th ed., pp. 27–30). Philadelphia: Lippincott, Williams & Wilkins.

Dunn, W. (2005). Measurement issues and practice. In M. Law, C. Baum, & W. Dunn, (Eds.), *Measuring occupational performance: Supporting best practice* (2d ed., pp. 21–32). Philadelphia: SLACK.

Evans J. (1992). What occupational therapists can do to eliminate racial barriers to health care access. *American Journal of Occupational Therapy, 46*(8), 679.

Fisher, A. G. (1998). Uniting practice and theory in an occupational framework—1998 Eleanor Clark Slagle Lecture. *American Journal of Occupational Therapy, 52*(7), 509–21.

Fisher, A. G., & Short-DeGraff, M. (1993). Nationally speaking—Improving functional assessment in occupational therapy: Recommendations and philosophy for change. *American Journal of Occupational Therapy, 47*(3), 199–201.

Flay, B. R., Biglan, A., Boruch, R. F., Castro, F. G., Gottfredson, D., Kellam, S., et al. (2004). *Standards of evidence: Criteria for efficacy, effectiveness and dissemination.* Falls Church, VA: Society for Prevention Research.

Holm, M. B. (2000). The 2000 Eleanor Clarke Slagle Lecture—Our mandate for the new millennium: Evidence-based practice. *American Journal of Occupational Therapy, 54*(6), 575–85.

Holm, M. B. (2003). Top ten reasons for becoming an evidence-based practitioner. *OT Practice, 8*(3), 9–11.

Hyner, G. C., Peterson, K. W., Travis, J. W., Dewey. J. E., Foerster, J. J., & Framer, E. M. (Eds.). (1999). *SPM handbook of health assessment tools.* Pittsburgh, PA: The Society of Prospective Medicine & the Institute for Health & Productivity Management.

Imel, S. (1990). *Adult literacy learner assessment* (ERIC Digest No. 103). Retrieved October 31, 2005, from http://www.ericdigests.org/pre-9217/adult.htm (ERIC Document Reproduction Service No. ED325658).

Jaffe, E. (1986). The role of occupational therapy in disease prevention and health promotion. *American Journal of Occupational Therapy, 40*(11), 749–52.

Law, M. (1993). Evaluating activities of daily living: Directions for the future. *American Journal of Occupational Therapy, 47,* 233–37.

Law, M. (1998). *Client centered occupational therapy.* Thorofare, NJ: SLACK

Law, M. (2002). *Evidence-based rehabilitation*: A guide to practice Thorofare, NJ: SLACK.

Law, M., Baptiste, S., & Mills, J. (1995). Client-centered practice: What does it mean and does it make a difference? *Canadian Journal of Occupational Therapy, 62,* 250–57.

Law, M., & Baum, C. (2001). Measurement in occupational therapy. In M. Law, C. Baum, & W. Dunn (Eds.), *Measuring occupational performance: Supporting best practice in occupational therapy* (pp. 3–19). Thorofare, NJ: SLACK

Law, M., & Baum, C. (2005). Measurement in occupational therapy. In M. Law, C. Baum, & W. Dunn (Eds.), *Measuring occupational performance: Supporting best practice in occupational therapy* (2d ed., pp. 3–20). Thorofare, NJ: SLACK

Law, M., Baum, C., & Dunn, W. (Eds.) (2005). *Measuring occupational performance: Supporting best practice in occupational therapy* (2d ed.). Thorofare, NJ: SLACK

Letts, L., Baum, C., & Perlmutter, M. (2003). Person-environment-occupation assessments with older adults. *OT Practice, 8*(10), 8–9.

Lund, M. L., Tamm, M., & Branholm, I. B. (2001). Patients' perceptions of their participation in rehabilitation planning and professionals' view of their strategies to encourage it. *Occupational Therapy International, 8,* 151–67.

Lyman, H. B. (1998). *Test scores and what they mean* (6th ed.). Boston: Allyn & Bacon

Mathiowetz, V. (1993). Role of physical performance components evaluations in occupational therapy functional assessment. *America Journal of Occupational Therapy, 47*(3), 233–37.

Mattingly, C., & Beer, D. (1993). Interpreting culture in a therapeutic context. In H. Hopkins & H. D. Smith (Eds.), *Willard and Spackman's occupational therapy* (8th ed., pp. 154–161). Philadelphia: Lippincott.

McGruder, J. (2003). Culture, race, ethnicity and other forms of human diversity in occupational therapy. In E. B. Crepeau, E. S. Cohn, & B. A. Boyt Schell (Eds.), *Willard and Spackman's occupational therapy* (10th ed., pp. 81–95). Philadelphia: Lippincott, Williams & Wilkins.

Paul, S., & Orchanian, D. P. (2003). *Pocket guide to assessment in occupational therapy.* London: Thomson, DelarLearning.

Peloquin, S. (1989). Sustaining the art of practice in occupational therapy. *American Journal of Occupational Therapy, 43*(4), 219–26.

Pizzi, M. (2003). Diversity lecture presented to occupational therapy students, University of Florida, Gainesville, FL, March 2003.

Polgar, J. M. (2003). Critiquing assessments. In E. B. Crepeau, E. S. Cohn, & B. B. Schell (Eds.), *Willard and Spackman's occupational therapy* (10th ed., pp. 299–313). Philadelphia: Lippincott, Williams & Wilkins.

Pollock. N., & Rochon, S. (2002). Becoming an evidenced-based practitioner. In M. Law (Ed.), *Evidence-based rehabilitation: A guide to practice* (pp. 31–46). Thorofare, NJ: SLACK.

Silverlake, A. C. (1999). *Comprehending test manuals: A guide and workbook.* Los Angeles: Pyrczak.

Slater, D. Y. (Ed.). (2006). *Reference guide to the Occupational Therapy Code of Ethics.* Bethesda, MD: American Occupational Therapy Association.

Spear, P. S., & Crepeau, E. B. (2003). Glossary. In E. B. Crepeau, E. S. Cohn, & B. A. Boyt Schell, *Willard & Spackman's occupational therapy* (10th ed., pp. 1025–1035). Philadelphia: Lippincott, Williams & Wilkins.

Surrey, L. R., Nelson, K., Delelio, C., Mathie-Majors, D., Omel-Edwards, N., Shumaker, J., & Thurber, G. (2003). A comparison of performance outcomes between the Minnesota Rate of Manipulation test and the Minnesota Manual Dexterity Test. *Work, 20,* 97–102.

Tickle-Degnen, L. (2002). Communication evidence to clients, managers, and funders. In M. Law (Ed.), *Evidence-based rehabilitation: A guide to practice* (pp. 221–54). Thorofare, NJ: SLACK.

Trombly, C. (1993). The issue is—Anticipating the future: Assessment of occupational function. *American Journal of Occupational Therapy, 47*(3), 253–57.

U.S. Department of Health and Human Services. (2000). *Healthy People 2010: Understanding and improving health* (2d ed.). Washington, DC: Government Printing Office.

West, W. (1967). The occupational therapist's changing responsibility to the community. *American Journal of Occupational Therapy, 21*(5), 312–16.

White, V. (1986). Promoting health and wellness: A theme for the eighties. *American Journal of Occupational Therapy, 40*(11), 743–48.

Windsor, M. M. (2002). *Test critique assignment.* OCTH 613 Advanced Research Methods in Occupation-Based Practice. Towson, MD: Towson University.

Windsor, M. M. (2003). *Test critique assignment.* OCTH 613 Advanced Research Methods in Occupation-Based Practice. Towson, MD: Towson University.

World Health Organization. (2001). *The international classification of functioning, disability, and health (ICF).* Geneva, Switzerland: Author.

Chapter 10

Assessments for Health Promotion Practice

Michael A. Pizzi, S. Maggie Reitz, and Marjorie E. Scaffa

> The assessment offers therapists using a client-centered approach the opportunity to communicate to clients that they care about the client's view of the situation, that they want to understand the context of the person's life, that they are committed to helping, that they have some expertise that may be of assistance, and that they can be trusted to do what the client has said he or she wants.
> —Pollock & McColl, 1998, p. 90

Learning Objectives

This chapter is designed to enable the reader to:

- Select appropriate occupational therapy assessments for health promotion and prevention practice.
- Identify assessments from other disciplines specific to the prevention of injury and disability and to the promotion of health and wellness that can be utilized or adapted for occupational therapy practice.
- Describe the variety of quality-of-life (QOL) assessments available, and discuss their usefulness in occupational therapy health promotion practice.

- Describe and implement an occupation-based wellness screening tool that can be used with people of all life stages and from a variety of populations.
- Identify assessment approaches and tools appropriate for evaluating the health promotion needs of communities.

Key Terms

Achievable risk

Appraised risk

Capacity assessment

Client

Community assessment

Family systems theory

Health risk appraisals (HRA)

Macro level

Meso level

Micro level

Occupational wellness

Relative risk

Introduction

In a health-care environment that is becoming more focused on health promotion and prevention, occupational therapy has an opportunity to contribute to and lead the movement to create healthy individuals, communities, and wellness-oriented societies. This chapter describes currently available occupational therapy assessments that may be appropriate for health promotion practice and discusses health promotion and quality-of-life assessments that can be utilized by occupational therapists.

These assessments can be used specifically to prevent injury and disability and to promote health and wellbeing. Community assessment is discussed, and a health promotion occupational therapy screening tool designed for adults or caregivers is introduced to incorporate into the occupational therapy evaluation process.

Occupational Therapy Assessments

Many of the well-known assessments in occupational therapy measure components or portions of a person's occupational performance. The areas of occupation measured may include "activities of daily living (ADLs), instrumental activities of daily living (IADLs), rest and sleep, education, work, play, leisure, social participation" (American Occupational Therapy Association [AOTA], 2008, p. 628). Many assessments used in occupational therapy come from other disciplines or are informal assessments created to suit the practitioner's particular work environment. This ad hoc approach is often a source of great frustration among occupation-centered practitioners who are attempting to engage in best practice. While some of these assessments may be holistic and may focus on health and wellbeing, their validity and reliability can be questioned.

In the current economic and health-care climate, it is essential that assessments provide the foundation for evidence-based and best practice, as defined in the previous chapter. Client-centered, occupation-focused occupational therapy assessments exist that are relevant for health promotion practice. Several of these will be discussed in this chapter, including the Canadian Occupational Performance Measure (COPM); three assessments based on the Model of Human Occupation, including the Occupational Circumstances Assessment Interview and Rating Scale (OCAIRS, Version 4.0), the Occupational Self Assessment (OSA), and the Family Assessment of Occupational Functioning (FAOF); and the Assessment of Motor and Process Skills (AMPS). A listing of additional occupational therapy assessments that may be useful in health promotion practice can be found in Content Box 10-1. While these are not specifically designed for health promotion practice, many are closely aligned with the principles and practice of health promotion.

Content Box 10-1

Potentially Useful Assessments for Health Promotion Practice

Occupational Performance
- Canadian Occupational Performance Measure (COPM)
- Model of Human Occupation Screening Tool (MOHOST)
- Occupational Circumstances Assessment Interview Rating Scale (OCAIRS)
- Occupational Performance History Interview—second version (OPHI-II)
- Occupational Questionnaire
- Occupational Self-Assessment (OSA)—adult and child versions
- Perceived Efficacy and Goal Setting System for Children
- School Function Assessment
- Self-Assessment of Occupational Functioning (SAOF)
- Volitional Questionnaire—adult and child versions

Play
- Child Behaviors Inventory for Playfulness
- Children's Playfulness Scale
- ChIPPA (Child-Initiated Pretend Play Assessment)
- Pediatric Interest Profiles (PIPs)
- Play History
- Preferences for Activities of Children (PAC)
- Preschool Play Scale, Revised
- Test of Playfulness (ToP)

Leisure
- Activity Index & Meaningfulness of Activity Scale
- The Experience of Leisure Scale (TELS)
- Idyll Arbor Leisure Battery includes
  - Leisure Assessment Inventory
  - Leisure Attitude Measure
  - Leisure Interest Measure
  - Leisure Motivation Scale
  - Leisure Satisfaction Measure

- Knowdell Leisure & Retirement Activities Card Sort
- Leisure Interest Profile for Adults
- Leisure Interest Profile for Seniors
- Modified Interest Checklist
- NPI Interest Checklist

Work
- COP System Career Guidance Program
- Geist Picture Interest Inventory—Revised
- Hall Occupational Orientation Inventory
- Transition Planning Inventory
- Transition to Work Inventory
- Work Adjustment Inventory
- Work Environment Impact Scale (WEIS)
- WorkPlace Mentor
- Workplace Skills Survey

ADLs and IADLs
- Assessment of Motor and Process Skills
- Kohlman Evaluation of Living Skills
- Psychosocial Impact of Assistive Devices Scale
- Task Management Strategies for Caregivers

Social Participation
- CASP-19 (Control, Autonomy, Self-Realization, and Pleasure)
- Children's Assessment of Participation & Enjoyment (CAPE)
- Community Integration Measure
- Community Integration Questionnaire
- Health-Related Quality of Life
- Participation Scale
- RAND Social Health Battery
- Satisfaction With Performance Scaled Questionnaire

Roles, Habits, and Routines
- Adolescent Role Assessment
- National Institutes of Health Activity Record

Content Box 10-1
Potentially Useful Assessments for Health Promotion Practice—cont'd

- Role Change Assessment
- Role Checklist
- Routine Task Inventory
- Self-Discovery Tapestry
- Worker Role Interview

Context

- Accessibility Checklist
- Americans With Disabilities Act Guidelines Checklist for Buildings & Facilities
- Environmental Rating Scales
- Home Assessment Profile
- Home Observation & Measurement of the Environment (HOME)
- Life Stressor and Social Resources Inventory
- Readily Achievable Checklist
- Safety Assessment of Function and the Environment for Rehabilitation (SAFER)
- School Setting Interview (SSI)
- Social Climate Scale: Community-Oriented Programs Environment Scale
- Social Climate Scale: Family Environment Scale
- Test of Environmental Supportiveness
- Westmead Home Safety Assessment

Developmental Assessments

- Denver Developmental Screening Test II
- Evaluation Tool of Children's Handwriting (ETCH)
- First STEP Developmental Screening Tool for Evaluating Preschoolers
- Hawaii Early Learning Profile (HELP)
- Miller Assessment for Preschoolers

Social and Interaction Skills

- Aggression Questionnaire
- Burks Behavior Rating Scales
- Infant Toddler Social and Emotional Assessment

- Interpersonal Style Inventory
- Mother–Child Interaction Checklist
- OT PAL (Psychosocial Assessment of Learning)
- Parent–Child Relationship Inventory
- Social Adjustment Scale—Self Report
- Social Interaction Scale (SIS)
- Student Behavior Survey

Coping and Adaptation

- Adolescent Coping Orientation for Problem Experiences
- Caregiver Strain Index
- Carer's Checklist
- COPE/ Brief COPE
- Coping Health Inventory for Parents
- Coping Inventory/Early Coping Inventory
- Holmes-Rahe Life Change Index
- OT-Quest
- Parenting Stress Index
- Resiliency Scales for Adolescents
- Rhode Island Stress & Coping Inventory
- Sickness Impact Profile
- Spiritual Wellbeing Scale
- Student Adaptation to College Questionnaire
- Ways of Coping Questionnaire

Psychological Processes

- Adult Self-Perception Profile
- Children's Nowicki-Strickland Internal-External Locus of Control
- Color-A-Person Body Dissatisfaction Test
- Culture Free Self-Esteem Inventories
- Depression and Anxiety in Youth Scale
- General Self-Efficacy Scale
- Multidimensional Self-Concept Scale
- Piers-Harris Children's Self-Concept Scale

Note: Many of these assessments are described in Asher (2007).

Canadian Occupational Performance Measure (COPM)

The Canadian Occupational Performance Measure (COPM), developed by Law and colleagues (1998), is an occupational therapy assessment that can be very useful as a health promotion and wellness tool. The COPM is a semistructured interview divided into three areas: self-care, productivity, and leisure. The occupational therapist interviews clients to determine their perceived occupational performance and their satisfaction with that performance. Clients rate their perceived performance and satisfaction on a scale of 1 to 10. It is client-centered; uses the Canadian Model of Occupational Performance as a theoretical basis; and has been used as a measurement tool in practice, education, and research (McColl, Paterson, Davies, Doubt, & Law, 2000).

The major strength of this assessment is that it is truly client-centered. In addition, the COPM has demonstrated validity and reliability. Criterion validity and construct validity have been supported (Law, Baum, & Dunn, 2005; McColl et al., 2000), and test-retest reliability has been reported from 0.75 to .89 (Law et al., 2005). The primary weaknesses of the COPM are that the therapist must be a skilled interviewer (McColl & Pollock, 2005), it is time-consuming (McColl et al., 2000), and clients must be willing and able to participate. This is an excellent tool to assess a client's perceptions, if he or she can participate; otherwise, it may need to be used in conjunction with other tools or education in order to assess potential areas of occupational engagement. McColl and colleagues (2000) have demonstrated the utility of the COPM in community practice. The global use of this assessment, which has been translated into 22 languages (McColl & Pollock, 2005), speaks to its ability to put the value of client-centered care into action.

Model of Human Occupation (MOHO) Assessments

When the Model of Human Occupation (MOHO) was developed (Kielhofner & Burke, 1980), it was a different and exciting theoretical model from which to develop practice, especially on the individual level. The MOHO has much to offer health promotion practice, not only at the individual level but also at the family and community level (see Chapter 2 in this text). Although many assessments based on the MOHO have been developed (University of Illinois at Chicago, Department of Occupational Therapy, 2005), two assessments are deemed particularly useful in health promotion: the Occupational Circumstances Assessment Interview and Rating Scale and the Occupational Self Assessment (Kielhofner, personal communication, 2004). A third potential assessment in health promotion practice is the Family Assessment of Occupational Functioning (FAOF), which is currently being revised and tested to improve reliability and validity. These three assessments are described here.

Occupational Circumstances Assessment Interview and Rating Scale (OCAIRS)

The Occupational Circumstances Assessment Interview and Rating Scale (OCAIRS) is a modification of the original Occupational Case Analysis Interview and Rating Scale. The acronym remains the same even though the assessment's title has been updated to better reflect the current theoretical constructs and principles of the MOHO, specifically the 2002 published version of the MOHO (Kielhofner, 2002). The latest version of the OCAIRS is available from the MOHO Clearinghouse (Forsyth et al., 2005). This assessment is classified as a semistructured interview that guides the gathering of information in 12 areas (Content Box 10-2) based on the MOHO. These areas include constructs from the original MOHO, as well as the client's interpretation of past experience and their readiness for change. The OCAIRS can be used with adolescents, adults, and older persons who have sufficient emotional and cognition functional abilities. The purpose of this assessment is to determine a person's occupational participation and occupational adaptation process as a precursor to developing an intervention plan with the client to maximize his or her successful community adjustment (Forsyth et al., 2005).

Content Box 10-2

OCAIRS Assessment Areas

- Roles
- Habits
- Personal causation
- Values
- Interests
- Skills
- Short-term goals
- Long-term goals
- Interpretation of past experiences
- Physical environment
- Social environment
- Readiness for change

Data from *A user's manual for the Occupational Circumstances Assessment Interview and Rating Scale (OCAIRS, Version 4.0)* (p. 3), by K. Forsyth, S. Deshpande, G. Kielhofner, C. Henriksson, L. Haglund, L. Olson, S. Skinner, & S. R. J. Kulkarni, 2005, Chicago: Model of Human Occupation Clearinghouse, University of Illinois at Chicago.

There are three versions of the OCAIRS; they are designed specifically for use with individuals in a mental health setting, a forensics mental health setting, and a physical disability setting. All three versions use the same rating scale and criteria. Four forms are available for each setting. These forms are similar in structure but are modified to the contextual features of the setting. Table 10-1 describes the forms' general structure. In order to use this assessment, the occupational therapist should be familiar with current MOHO terminology, should be skilled in the interview process, and should have experience in psychosocial practice (Forsyth et al., 2005). Novice users of the OCAIRS should use the full questions in the recommended sequence. Experienced users who use Form 1 may modify both the questions and their order to enhance the interview process and outcome.

Upon interview completion, the therapist must rate each item using specific criteria to assign a score based on how well the measured item influences the client's participation. This scale includes four possible ratings, described by the acronym FAIR:

F: the item "facilitates participation in occupation";
A: the item "allows participation in occupation";
 I: the item "inhibits participation in occupation"; and
R: the item "restricts participation in occupation." (Forsyth et al., 2005, p. 11).

With experience, the assessment can be administered in 20 to 30 minutes, with an additional 5 to 10 minutes for interpretation and recording of results. Studies on both a Swedish version of the original instrument and the second version of the OCAIRS provided evidence

Table 10–1 Structure of Forms for OCAIRS

Form Interview	Description
Form 1	Full questions
Form 2	Abbreviated questions
	Full rating scale
Form 3	Note section
	Abbreviated questions
	Full rating scale
Form 4	Keyword list for use during administration of any of the other forms.

Data from *A user's manual for the Occupational Circumstances Assessment Interview and Rating Scale (OCAIRS, Version 4.0)* (p. 28), by K. Forsyth, S. Deshpande, G. Kielhofner, C. Henriksson, L. Haglund, L. Olson, S. Skinner, & S. R. J. Kulkarni, 2005, Chicago: Model of Human Occupation Clearinghouse, University of Illinois at Chicago.

of excellent inter-rater reliability and adequate internal consistency (Haglund, Thorell, & Walinder, 1998; Henry, 2003). In addition, when compared to the Global Assessment Scale, the OCAIRS was found to have satisfactory concurrent validity (Brollier, Watts, Bauer, & Schmidt, 1989). No studies on the reliability and validity of the current version have been published.

A strength of the OCAIRS is that it assesses several areas that are relevant for health promotion practice. Therapists in health promotion practice need information on a person's habits and daily routines, personal challenges, goals and plans to accomplish those goals, social support, sense of self-efficacy, ability to adapt to change, and readiness for change. This instrument provides this information and rates these areas in terms of their impact on occupational participation. The focus on occupational participation and its impact on health is particularly salient for health promotion practice. Other strengths of the OCAIRS includes the ability of the interviewer to adjust the questions as needed, the obtainment of both quantitative and qualitative data, and the relatively short time frame needed for administration and interpretation. A weakness of the assessment is that it can be lengthy, particularly if the client and therapist explore the scope of problems rather than solely identifying the problems (McColl & Pollock, 2005). The weakness for health promotion practice is that it does not necessarily measure health issues directly but rather addresses occupational areas of participation that impact health and wellbeing.

Occupational Self Assessment (OSA)

The Occupational Self Assessment (OSA) is a client-centered, self-report assessment designed to "capture clients' perceptions of their own occupational competence and of the impact of their environments on their occupational adaptation" (Kielhofner, 2002, p. 221). The second version of the OSA was copyrighted in 1998 and revised in 2006. Care was taken to translate constructs from the MOHO into everyday language that is not culture-bound. In addition to the MOHO, the OSA is also based on principles of a client-centered approach. The OSA is most useful with higher-level-functioning individuals who are able to be reflective and plan, who have the capacity for realistic self-appraisal, and who wish to collaborate in goal-setting (Baron, Kielhofner, Iyenger, Goldhammer, & Wolenski, 2006).

The OSA was designed to measure competence and values for everyday tasks. Clients are given a list of 21 items and asked to rate their perceived level of competence regarding a particular task and the importance of each task. (Table 10-2 identifies these items and their relationship to the MOHO constructs.) Clients rate their occupational competence by circling one of the four possible responses (Baron et al., 2006, p. 14), which include the following:

- "I have a lot of problems doing this."
- "I have some difficulty doing this."
- "I do this very well"
- "I do this extremely well."

Clients rate their occupational identity (i.e., values) from the following possible four responses (Baron et al., 2006, p. 14):

- "This is not so important to me."
- "This is important to me."
- "This is more important to me."
- "This is most important to me."

After clients rate their occupational competence and their occupational identity for each item, they determine a maximum of four priority areas for change. The areas are then rank-ordered to distinguish which is of highest priority. The identified areas of potential change become the foundation for collaborative intervention planning (Baron et al., 2006).

The occupational therapist can examine the gap between clients' rated value of a particular item and their rating of their occupational competence for that same item. The gap can be considered a measure of satisfaction with their competence. A small gap indicates more satisfaction, while a large gap indicates less satisfaction and greater potential for an area to be identified

Table 10–2 **MOHO Constructs and Related OSA Items**

Constructs	Items
Skills/Occupational Performance	• Concentrating on my tasks
	• Physically doing what I need to do
	• Taking care of the place where I live
	• Taking care of myself
	• Taking care of others for whom I am responsible
	• Getting where I need to go
	• Managing my finances
	• Managing my basic needs (food, medicine)
	• Expressing myself to others
	• Getting along with others
	• Identifying and solving problems
Habituation • Habits • Roles	• Relaxing and enjoying myself • Getting done what I need to do • Having a satisfying routine • Handling my responsibilities • Being involved as a student, worker, volunteer, and/or family member
Volition • Personal Causation • Values • Interests	• Doing activities I like • Working toward my goals • Making decisions based on what I think is important • Accomplishing what I set out to do • Effectively using my abilities

Adapted from *A user's manual for the Occupational Self Assessment* by K. Baron, G. Kielhofner, A. Iyenger, V. Goldhammer, & J. Wolenski, 2006, p. 63. Copyright © 1998 by University of Illinois at Chicago. With permission.

as a priority for change. However, some clients may prefer to first address goals that seem easier or more reachable. In client-centered practice, it is important to understand why clients select their particular goals, especially if they do not match the items with the greatest gap between competence and value.

As with the administration of any assessment, it is important to consider the comfort and selection of the environment. When the OSA is used in health promotion with an individual, family, or group, the assessment could be completed at home in between sessions or as part of an initial session. Clients usually take between 10 and 20 minutes to complete this pencil-and-paper self-assessment. Afterward, the occupational therapist should allot an additional 15 minutes for joint intervention planning, if

an intervention is indicated. The OSA can be used for reevaluation purposes as a postintervention outcome measure to assess changes in occupational competence by following the specific guidelines as outlined in the user's manual (Baron et al., 2006).

The OSA has numerous strengths. It measures several areas of occupational participation, practitioners can collaborate with the client to make intervention decisions, and studies have provided evidence of its psychometric properties (Baron et al., 2006). Two international studies using the OSA have demonstrated preliminary construct validity and the usefulness of the tool across language, cultural, and diagnostic groups (Kielhofner, 2002). As mentioned previously, it also can be used for reevaluation purposes to measure outcomes. Another strength is that the OSA is linked to theory and can be used to help explain this theory to clients. As it is a self-report, other assessments may need to be used in conjunction with the OSA to determine occupational function and the impact of impairments on one's health and occupational participation. Reliability measures, such as internal consistency and test-retest, have not been reported (McColl & Pollock, 2005).

Users of any MOHO-based assessment should routinely monitor the MOHO Clearinghouse at http://www.moho.uic.edu/ for information on the latest versions, the status of translations, and the reliability and validity studies. The current version of the OSA no longer includes items on the environment; an environmental scale is currently being revised. A version of the OSA for children, the Child Occupational Self Assessment (COSA), has been developed (Kielhofner, 2002). Results of preliminary studies on psychometric properties are available through the MOHO Clearinghouse website. Both the OSA and COSA instruments show promise for use in health promotion programs to enable client-centered interventions and to address enhancing occupational competence for improved wellbeing and quality of life.

Family Assessment of Occupational Functioning (FAOF)

The Family Assessment of Occupational Functioning (FAOF) was designed to evaluate the occupational function of family units using the MOHO and family systems theory as a framework (Shepherd, Scaffa, & Pizzi, 1989). Occupational therapists often include caregivers and family members in the evaluation process but rarely evaluate the occupational function of the family as a whole. In contrast, family assessments are plentiful in the family therapy literature but do not include occupation-focused assessment items.

Family systems theory describes a family system as open and having a complex organizational structure that maintains a steady, stable state through interactions with its environment. Family systems have the capacity to grow, develop, and change over time. Family members are interdependent, engaging in complex interactions. A change in one family member's function can affect all others in the family system. Therefore, an individual cannot be completely understood outside the context of his or her family (Caskie, 1998). Families are more than the sum of their parts, and describing individual family members explains little about family functioning. In order to obtain an accurate understanding of family dynamics, the family system must be evaluated as a unit.

Although the MOHO was originally conceptualized for individuals, it shares much in common with family

systems theory. Families can be thought to consist of the same three interrelated elements (i.e., volition, habituation, and performance capacity) as described in the MOHO (Kielhofner, 2002, 2004). Family volition (i.e., personal, or in this case family, causation; values; and goals) is strongly influenced by cultural background and socioeconomic status. Family habituation reflects family habits and roles. The family's performance capacity consists of the combined abilities and skills of family members that are available for the performance of family functions. Family functions are the occupations that families engage in to meet the needs of individual members, portions of the family, and the family as a whole. The needs addressed by families include daily care, affection, socialization, self-definition, educational/vocational, economic, and recreation (Turnbull & Turnbull, 1990). In addition, families make a significant contribution to the physical and mental health of their members. Family interactions can facilitate or hinder health promotion, disease prevention, and recuperation or rehabilitation efforts of individual family members (Turk & Kerns, 1985).

The FAOF was developed to identify areas of family occupational behavior that facilitate or constrain family adaptation. The assessment was originally conceptualized as a way to evaluate a family's adjustment to disability, but it has much wider applicability. It can be used to assess any family in need of occupational intervention, including families affected by substance abuse, domestic violence, or disaster. The FAOF consists of 42 items addressing the three elements of the MOHO and the environmental context of the family. In the current version, there are 6 items in each of the following categories: values, interests, personal causation, roles, habits, skills, and environment. Scores are calculated for each category, with the overall sum used as the total score for the instrument. High scores are indicative of adaptive occupational functioning, or the ability of family members to meet the family's needs and to fulfill social expectations for productive participation. The assessment items have a "we" orientation and are designed to describe various aspects of family occupational behavior. All items are rated on a 5-point Likert scale from "very true about our family" (5) to "not at all true" (0). The assessment is a self-reported measure that can be given to multiple family members to determine the degree of congruence of perceptions of family functioning.

Content validity of the instrument was established using a panel of 14 experts—occupational therapists who used the MOHO in their practice or research. The FAOF items were rated for clarity, relevance to the MOHO and to family systems theory, and appropriateness for occupational therapy practice. Approximately

94% of the assessment items were rated 3.5 or higher (on a 5-point Likert scale) in all areas. Sixty-eight percent of the items demonstrated 80% or greater agreement among the raters regarding the MOHO component being evaluated. In addition, 94% of the items were rated 3.5 or higher for clarity, 97% were rated 3.5 or higher for relevance to the MOHO, 98% were rated 3.5 or higher for relevance to family systems theory, and 98% were rated 3.5 or higher for relevance to occupational therapy practice (Pledger, 1990). The results of the content validity study were used to revise the assessment.

Chessler (1992) tested the concurrent validity of the FAOF, comparing scores on the FAOF to those on the Family Hardiness Index (FHI), which was developed by family therapists McCubbin, McCubbin, and Thompson (1986). The FHI was designed to measure family resiliency and adaptability. One member of each of 25 families completed both instruments. Approximately 75% of the respondents were female. The correlation coefficients by category and overall were low, ranging from .012 to .342, indicating that these instruments are not measuring comparable constructs. Continued research is needed to further establish reliability and validity of the FAOF.

A significant strength of the FAOF is that it is a family-oriented occupational therapy assessment based on occupational therapy theory and focused on family systems rather than on individuals. It was tested both with families affected by a physically challenged family member and by those without a physically challenged individual. The FAOF may be further strengthened by reviewing the MOHO's evolution and considering additional items based on new constructs; for example, it may be appropriate to add an item based on the use of occupational adaptation, which is now incorporated into the latest version of the MOHO (Kielhofner, 2002, 2004). Further studies are needed to strengthen the psychometric properties, but this tool can be a much needed and welcome addition for practitioners concerned about the impact of occupational impairments on the health and wellbeing of families.

The Assessment of Motor and Process Skills (AMPS)

The Assessment of Motor and Process Skills (AMPS) is an observational assessment used to measure the quality of an individual's performance of instrumental activities of daily living (IADL) in context by occupational therapists who have been trained and calibrated in administration of this tool (AMPS Project International [AMPS PI], n.d.b). This client-centered assessment is conducted during the performance of client-selected relevant tasks. It

was developed by Fisher and published in 1995 (Gitlin, 2005) and remains one of the few standardized measures of performance in occupational therapy (Fisher, 2006). Originally, the AMPS was developed to measure solely IADL performance and included 56 possible tasks (Gitlin, 2005). However, based on feedback from raters, simpler personal activities of daily living (PADL) were added to the AMPS (Fisher, 2006). Currently, the AMPS includes 85 tasks that range from easy to difficult (AMPS PI, n.d.a) and that fall within the ADL and IADL categories of the *Occupational Therapy Practice Framework* (referred to as *Framework;* AOTA, 2008). To use this assessment, the therapist, in collaboration with the client, selects 2 of the 85 tasks to perform, based on cultural appropriateness and level of challenge. The quality of occupational performance in the two tasks "is assessed by rating the effort, efficiency, safety, and independence of 16 ADL motor and 20 ADL process skill items" (AMPS PI, n.d.d, ¶ 1). The ADL motor and process skills are similar to those defined under the activities and participation domains of the *International Classification of Functioning, Disability and Health (ICF)*, published by the World Health Organization (WHO) in 2001 (AMPS PI, n.d.d).

The ADL motor skills items are used to rate the client's ability to move his or her body and required objects, while the ADL process skills are used to rate the client's level at choosing and manipulating tools and materials, completing each step, and adapting to problems that arise (AMPS PI, n.d.d; Bray, Fisher, & Duran, 2001). Client performance is rated on a 4-point scale, where 1 is assigned for "markedly deficient performance," 2 for "ineffective performance," 3 for "questionable performance," and 4 for "competent performance" (Fisher, 2006, p. 389). The AMPS is appropriate to use with individuals who are interested and participate in ADL or IADL tasks and who are developmentally at or above age 3 (Fisher, 1999).

The strengths of the AMPS are more numerous than its limitations. Reliability and validity have been well established. In terms of reliability, internal consistency (r = .74 to r = .93) and test-retest (r = .74 to r = .91) have been reported across studies (Gitlin, 2005; Law et al., 2005). Validity, including content and construct validity, has also been reported (Gitlin, 2005; Law et al., 2005). The AMPS has been internationally recognized as an excellent tool and has been translated into several languages and found to be culturally relevant. The major limitations are the mandatory rigorous training and calibration required of practitioners and the necessity for using computer scoring to report results for use in research and efficacy studies (AMPS PI, n.d.c).

It must be noted that the authors of this chapter do not support the idea that ADL or IADL assessments are health promotion or wellness assessments; rather, its believed these measures provide data that, taken with the results of other assessments, contributes to a broad understanding of an individual's performance in life and the identification of potential areas to address through health promotion interventions. A version of the AMPS, the School AMPS, has been developed for use in classrooms and has been the subject of validity and reliability investigations (Atchison, Fisher, & Bryze, 1998; Fingerhut, Madill, Darrah, Hodge, & Warren, 2002; Fisher, Bryze, & Atchison, 2000). As with any assessment, continued research on validity and reliability is required. In terms of health promotion practice, this version of the AMPS may be an excellent resource for occupational therapists working in schools. It could be used as part of a process to maximize a student's health and wellbeing through enhancing performance at school. This enhanced performance then has the potential to positively impact occupational performance at home, further contributing to participation and quality of life.

Wellness and Health Promotion–Specific Assessments

This section covers a selection of assessments developed specifically for health promotion activities. Included is information on health-risk appraisals, occupation-focused assessments, and quality-of-life assessments.

Health Risk Appraisals (HRAs)

Health risk appraisals (HRAs), or health hazard appraisals (HHA), are self-assessments (pencil-and-paper or computerized) designed to determine the health risks of an individual or population. "The HRA/HHA is an instrument that requires people to answer a number of questions about their health behavior, health history, and the results of a few clinical screenings (height, weight, blood pressure, and cholesterol)" (McKenzie & Smeltzer, 1997, p. 45). The data from the individual respondent is compared to a computerized database to determine the person's risk of dying from a variety of causes as compared to others of the same race, age, and gender. Many HRA/HHAs provide information on life expectancy, risk of developing various diseases, risk-reduction strategies, and associated increases in life expectancy for each prevention strategy (Breckon, Harvey, & Lancaster, 1998).

Originally, HRA/HHAs were developed by physicians to use in patient education, but now they are also used to motivate people to change their health behaviors and provide data for needs assessment and program evaluation. Currently, HRA/HHAs are used as a component of health education programs in a variety of settings, including worksites, schools, community centers, health fairs, and health-care organizations (Alexander, 1999; Strecher & Kreuter, 1999). There are a plethora of HRA/HHA instruments available (Table 10-3). Most have been designed to determine the overall risk of a variety of diseases, but some are available to measure the risk of a single disease. These instruments provide not only individual results, but also aggregate data that can be used for health promotion program planning and evaluation.

HRA/HHAs have three basic components: a questionnaire, a risk estimate, and health education messages and reports. The questionnaire is designed to elicit information regarding lifestyle factors and health history. The risk estimate calculates the individual's relative risk of morbidity and mortality in comparison to the population average. The health education messages and reports are designed to educate individuals about their risks and recommended health behavior changes (Alexander, 1999).

There are numerous benefits of HRA/HHAs. Typically, these assessments are individualized, confidential, comprehensive, inexpensive, easy to use, and require little time to administer. They emphasize modifiable risk factors and have the potential to motivate health behavior change by providing preventive health information in an organized, accessible manner. HRA/HHAs also have significant limitations. They are not a substitute for medical advice, they do not diagnose disease, and they do not predict an individual's future cause of death. In addition, these assessments do not address social or environmental risk factors, have limited impact in terms of health behavior change, and are not an appropriate single modality health promotion approach (Alexander, 1999).

It is important to recognize that the reliability of HRA/HHAs varies among instruments and that self-scoring (in contrast to computer scoring) reduces reliability. In addition, there is significant variation in the self-reporting of specific risk factors and clinical screening measurements (McKenzie & Smeltzer, 1997). Data from white, middle-class adults were typically used to develop HRA/HHAs. Therefore, these may not be appropriate for use with children, the elderly, and minority populations (Alexander, 1999). However, there is little controversy over their use as a health-education tool, and they are deemed to have a high degree of face validity. Validity of the instruments focuses on the precision of the algorithms that predict morbidity and mortality. The accuracy of the algorithms

Table 10–3 Health Risk Appraisals

Name of HRA	Source	Paper Format	Computer Format	Target Ages	Special Features
ASAP! Adult Health Survey	Institute for Corporate Health A McLaughlin Young Company PO Box 29191 Dallas, TX 75229 Asap-survey.com/science.htm	Yes	Online version	Adults	Based on stages of change theory
CPM Customized Health Risk Assessment	CPM Marketing Group, Inc. 1200 John Q Hammons Dr., Suite 300 Madison, WI 53717 http://www.cpm.com	Yes	Online version	Adults	Specifically targets African American and Latino/Hispanic populations
Health Risk Appraisal	University of Michigan Health Management Research Center 1015 East Huron Street Ann Arbor, MI 48104-1688 http://www.hmrc.umich.edu/services/hra.html	Yes	Online version and touch-screen version	Adults	Based on Centers for Disease Control and Prevention (CDC) questionnaire
The Healthier People Network HRA	The Healthier People Network, Inc. 3114 Mercer University Dr., Suite 200 Atlanta, GA 30341 http://www.thehealthierpeoplenetwork.org	Yes	Keyboard offline	Adults	Originally established by the CDC and the Carter Center of Emory University
HealthStep Health Assessment	StayWell Health Management 2700 Blue Water Rd., Suite 850 St. Paul, MN 55121 marketing@staywell.com http://www.staywellhealthmanagement.com	Yes	None	Adults	Comprehensive assessment focusing on increasing employee health and decreasing health-care costs
Maternal Health Risk Assessment	Slabaugh Morgan White & Associates 7204 Glen Forest Dr., Suite 304 Richmond, VA 23226	No	Touch-screen version	Adults	Specifically designed for pregnant women

MedAppraise Adult Health Survey	Total Health Management 602 Courtland Street, Suite 300 Orlando, FL 32804	Yes	Online version	Adults	Identifies individuals at risk for near-term hospitalization
Senior Health Profiles	National Research Corporation Payer Solutions Division 1245 Q St. Lincoln, NE 68508 http://payersolutions.nationalresearch.com	Yes	None	Adults under 65	Specifically designed for older adults and adults of all ages with disabilities
Stanford Educational Assessment of Risk & Readiness for Change (SEARCH)	Stanford Health Improvement Program Stanford Prevention Research Center Hoover Pavilion 211 Quarry Rd., Suite N049 Stanford, CA 94305	Yes	None	Adults	Based on social cognitive theory and stages of change theory
Well Check— Adolescent Wellness Assessment	LifeQuest 2620 Thousand Oaks Blvd, S-2300 Memphis, TN 38118 dhogan@bellsouth.net	Yes	None	Children aged 13–17	Designed specifically for adolescents
Youfirst Senior Health Risk Assessment	Greenstone Healthcare Solutions 7000 Portage Rd., MS 9682-203-40 Kalamazoo, MI 49001 arthur.n.gerth@am.pnu.com http://www.ghsnet.com	Yes	None	Adults 55+	Allows individuals to see how daily lifestyle decisions impact present and future health status along with how positive health choices influence healthy behavior.

is only as good as the source data used in the calculations (Edington, Yen, & Braustein, 1999).

Risk assessment involves identifying precursors and calculating relative risk, appraised risk, and achievable risk. Precursors are health-risk behaviors, family history of certain diseases, and physiological measures of body function, such as blood pressure. **Relative risk** indicates the person's risk of dying from specific causes relative to the population average. **Appraised risk** refers to the total risk of dying from all causes within a specified time frame. **Achievable risk** demonstrates the benefits of reducing all unhealthy precursors to specified target levels and is a measure of the reduced risk associated with health behavior change (Alexander, 1999). HRAs are typically accurate in categorizing individuals by risk level but are not good predictors of an individual's risk of dying from specific causes. Combining HRAs with clinical screening of blood pressure, weight, cholesterol, and other physiological parameters increases their validity and usefulness (Edington et al., 1999).

Occupation-Focused Health Assessments

In occupational therapy, there are few published assessments for health promotion practice available. However, a few have been recently developed that are more focused on health and wellness related directly to occupational performance and participation. These are the Healthy Living Screening Tool, the Pizzi Holistic Wellness Assessment, and the Occupational Wellness Assessment.

Healthy Living Screening Tool

Pizzi, Scaffa, and Reitz developed a health promotion screening tool that specifically addresses areas of the AOTA's *Framework*, occupational performance, and participation. This screening tool is intended to obtain general information regarding health status from adult clients or caregivers. It is a self-assessment checklist, which is reviewed in collaboration with the occupational therapist.

The rating assigned to each category is the individual's perception of importance or meaning to one's life. A section titled "Wanting to Change" provides the practitioner with information on the clients' readiness for change based on the Stages of Change Model (see Chapter 3 in this text). Another section "What One Can Do" allows the immediate inclusion of clients in their own intervention plan and shows respect for their own solutions to their daily living issues (client-centered versus expert-centered). The "Comments" section was provided for practitioners to make observations (e.g., tone of voice, eye contact, affect) that may be indications to perceived susceptibility (Health Belief Model) or

readiness for change (Stages of Change Model). Things verbalized (e.g., "I don't like that I get sad when I can't do something") could also be an indication of perceived susceptibility or severity (e.g., of depression). Since this is a new tool, data on its validity and reliability are not yet available. As the tool is used more widely, performance in these areas will be determined, along with its strengths and limitations. The assessment is not yet published.

The Pizzi Holistic Wellness Assessment

The Pizzi Holistic Wellness Assessment (PHWA) emphasizes that clients' subjective perspectives of their health can guide occupational therapists in developing interventions best suited to people's goals, desires, needs, and occupational lifestyles (Pizzi, 2001). Individuals are generally more motivated to participate in the intervention process when provided with occupational choices that are important and meaningful to them. The PHWA is designed to assess clients' self-perceptions of health and identify strategies to involve individuals in problem-solving solutions to enhance or restore their own health.

The PHWA is a self-assessment designed to help people become aware of their most important health issues and how they affect daily occupational performance. Developing awareness and perceiving health risks and issues related to occupational performance are critical areas for occupational therapists to address. (For an overview of health behavior models potentially helpful in occupational therapy health promotion efforts, see Chapter 3 in this text.)

Eight specific areas of health were identified through an interdisciplinary literature review. This highly individualized and qualitative assessment uses a scale of 1 to 10 for each health area, in which individuals can rate their perceived levels of health. In the qualitative sections, clients strategize, in collaboration with the occupational therapist, ways to improve specific health areas that affect occupational participation and performance; for example, being in an abusive relationship, experiencing unresolved grief, having rheumatoid arthritis, or being overweight or too thin.

The strengths of the assessment are that it is client-centered; focused on barriers to occupational participation, both perceived and real; and includes the individual in developing health promotion strategies toward optimizing health in areas of interest to the person. This approach helps demystify the perceived power of the occupational therapist and places greater emphasis on empowering the individual to take responsibility for her or his own health. A basic foundational concept of the assessment is that occupational therapists and occupational therapy assistants are but facilitators of health.

True health restoration can only be achieved through the client's healthy occupational participation.

Another strength of the PHWA is that it is the first self-assessment of health and wellbeing relative to one's occupational participation in numerous occupational areas. In addition, the tool can be administered to loved ones of the person being assessed to obtain other perceptions of occupational participation, which is not found in other assessments. The weakness of this approach is that results of self-assessment often require further explanation. This additional information can be obtained through the use of the occupational questions in each area and through a one-on-one discussion with the client about the results. The PHWA has been successfully used with a number of populations and has great practical utility. Good beginning face validity and content validity have been demonstrated. The tool has been used with occupational therapy students, clients with various mental health and physical impairments, and with well elders in the community (Pizzi, 2001). The PHWA has been found to be useful clinically, additional research on its psychometrics is required. This tool has potential to contribute to occupational therapy health promotion efforts by assisting clients in self-identifying barriers to occupations, the removal of which may promote quality and participation in life. The PHWA can be obtained at www.michaelpizzi.com.

Occupational Wellness Assessment (OWA)

Another health promotion–specific tool is the Occupational Wellness Assessment (OWA) developed by White, Davidson, and Reed (2004). This assessment, currently in a research version only, was developed through a collaborative research project between Texas Woman's University and the Veteran's Affairs Medical Center (VAMC) in Houston, Texas. The project objectives were to (1) develop an occupational wellness profile of older veterans with disabilities based on the findings from interviews and quality-of-life assessment, and (2) design an OWA to reflect the uniqueness of veterans with disabilities. For the purposes of this assessment, **occupational wellness** was defined as "daily patterns of meaningful, purposeful and satisfying occupations of individuals that contribute to maintaining health and wellness" (White, Davidson, Reed, & Garber, 2000, p. 59).

Assessment development was facilitated by data collection from nine veterans over 50 years of age and eight family members and was implemented in two phases. Phase 1 was profile development using a qualitative methods approach, and Phase 2 was instrument development. After thematic analysis in Phase 1, themes were compared with the literature and a panel of experts was engaged in oversight review. The occupational wellness model provided additional support for assessment development (White et al., 2000). Three major themes for assessment were determined: occupation, values, and sense of control.

The research edition of the OWA is comprised of these three themes, with 12 questions in each theme. Each question has multiple answers that clients can check if they apply to their life situation. After each question, the client indicates if there were 0 to 4 or more answers. According to the authors, the assessment takes 30 to 45 minutes to complete. "Ultimately, a longitudinal study will determine the OWA's potential for changing individual's occupational wellness or problems encountered over time" (White et al. 2004, p. 11). There are no current published results of outcomes from the OWA, but further research on the effectiveness beyond the population of veterans will be worthwhile.

Quality-of-Life Assessments

The President's Commission for the Study of Ethical Problems in Medicine and Biomedical and Behavioral Research noted that

> quality of life [is] an ethically essential concept that focuses on the good of the individual, what kind of life is possible given the person's condition, and whether that condition will allow the individual to have a life that he or she views as worth living. (LaPuma & Lawlor, 1990, p. 2919)

According to the *Framework,* an aspect of quality of life (QOL) is an individual's appraisal of life satisfaction and progress toward his or her goals. Although quality of life is considered a potential outcome of occupational therapy intervention, it is important to consider that not all people who experience an improved QOL will perceive progress toward their goals. One reason for this might be that perhaps these goals are not self-determined but are determined by others (for example, family, significant others, or health professionals). Another possibility, in the case of a person who is terminally ill (see Chapter 25 in this text), is where the goal, not determined or spoken by the individual, is only to achieve a pain-free physical state. If clients do not perceive progress toward their goals, then the *Framework* definition of QOL has not been enhanced. (The term **client** can refer to individuals, groups, communities, or society.) In situations like these, then, it is vital to include patient and caregiver education and client-centered care when assessing for and intervening to achieve optimal QOL as an occupational therapy outcome. Occupational therapists can collect client-centered information that helps create individualized QOL interventions, with QOL being determined and measured from the perspective of the client being served.

QOL definitions in the literature emphasize various aspects of the construct. For instance, some highlight physical or psychological or social functioning (or some combination of these), life satisfaction, or psychological wellbeing (Bowling, 1991; McDowell & Newell, 1987; Schalock, Keith, Hoffman, & Karan, 1989). The definition developed as part of the Centre for Health Promotion (CHP) conceptual approach is concise yet holistic. It views QOL as "the degree to which the person enjoys the important possibilities of his or her life" (Rootman et al., 1992, p. 23), which expands the concept of QOL. More broadly defined,

> Possibilities refer to the opportunities and constraints in people's lives as well as the balance between these. They result from the ongoing interaction between persons and their environments and thus depend on characteristics of both persons and environments. There are two types of possibilities that operate in concert. Some possibilities occur "by chance," in that they are not primarily under a person's own control. An individual's gender, genetic endowment (including inherited physical disorders), historical time of birth, and socioeconomic status of the person's birth parents are exemplars of this kind of possibility. Other possibilities occur "by choice"; that is, they are, to a great extent, amenable to much more control by individuals. Individuals' decisions and choices about a whole range of life events exemplify this second kind of possibility. These include decisions about how to spend one's discretionary savings, selection of friends, joining groups and organizations, and choice of occupation. (Renwick, Brown, Rootman, & Nagler, 1996, p. 80)

Osoba (2002) discusses health related quality of life (HRQOL) assessments used at various levels of care: the micro, meso, and macro levels. At the **micro level** of care, the individual is key and the goal is to effect a health benefit for that person. The **meso level** targets groups of individuals with commonalities like diagnosis, age, or gender. The **macro level** involves health decision-making aimed at effecting health outcomes for communities, cities, states, or a country. Osoba (2002) discusses several HRQOL assessments, both generic and condition-specific, especially those related to working with people with cancer. Osoba makes a strong argument for the inclusion of QOL assessment and discusses strategies for increasing clinical meaningfulness of the outcomes so that practice can be strengthened and made more evidence-based.

In her work on QOL and people with developmental disabilities, Brown (1996) stated that

> quality of life measurement can not only provide reliable and valid data but also identify effective goals within specified domains and suggest intervention strategies. Through this approach, the social and educational environment of the individual can be modified. As a result, behavior, performance, and perception can change for the individual and for those around the individual. In this sense, quality of life measurement is highly innovative and can be directed to program needs rather than simply comparing individuals with others. Rather than regarding quality of life measures as normative, it might be more satisfactory to describe them as idiosyncratic scales, which look for specific interests, needs, concerns, and perceived changes of individuals within specific contexts. (p. 255)

QOL is an essential aspect of assessment and intervention in order to promote health and enhance wellbeing. It is vital that occupational therapists, occupational therapy assistants, and occupational scientists who study occupational engagement include the important construct of QOL in their work. This perspective could enhance the profession's already well-established reputation for being a holistic and client-centered profession. Three generic QOL assessments—the Quality of Life Index for Adults, the WHO Quality of Life Assessment, and the KINDL-R—will be discussed here briefly. Chapter 7 in this text further elaborates on the construct of QOL and includes a list of potentially useful QOL assessments.

The Quality of Life Index for Adults (A-QLI) is a comprehensive, multidimensional assessment of QOL for older adults that examines physical health, self-care, pain, social relations/support, psychological wellbeing, spirituality, meaning and purpose in life, and personal values. The questionnaire can be self-administered or administered by phone or in a face-to-face interview. A second questionnaire format is for providers to fill out when clients are aphasic or otherwise unable to respond reliably to the assessment. These tools were developed and tested by Becker and Diamond, at the University of Wisconsin–Madison and are available for use royalty-free by contacting the developers (Becker, Shaw, & Reib, n.d.).

In 1991, the WHO initiated a project to develop a cross-culturally appropriate QOL assessment tool. An international team of researchers collaboratively developed a variety of instruments that assess individuals' perceptions within their cultural context and values. These assessments have been widely field-tested around the world and are available in 29 languages. The WHO Quality of Life Assessment-BREF (WHOQOL-BREF) instrument, a shorter version of the 100-item original, is made up of 26 items that measure physical and psychological health, social relationships, and the environment (WHO, 2007). The WHOQOL-BREF can be self-administered or administered by interview. The BREF version achieved a .89 or higher correlation on subscores with the original longer version and demonstrated good content validity, discriminant validity, internal consistency, and test-retest reliability (Frank-Stromberg & Olsen, 2004).

The KINDL-R Questionnaire for Measuring Health-Related Quality of Life in Children and Adolescents was originally developed in Germany in 1994 by Bullinger and was revised by Ravens-Sieberer and Bullinger (1998a, 1998b) for use with healthy children and adolescents as well as clinical populations. The tool measures QOL aspects of physical wellbeing, emotional wellbeing, self-esteem, family, friends, and school. The KINDL-R is actually a flexible set of instruments for different age groups of children that can be completed by both the child or adolescent and their parents. The questionnaire has been tested with 3000 healthy and chronically ill children and their parents and demonstrates a high degree of reliability (.70) and satisfactory convergent validity. Currently, there are three age-related versions for children (aged 4–7, 8–12, and 13–16) and two for parents (based on the child's age) available. In addition, a short, 12-item form is available as are several disease-specific forms for children with obesity, asthma, and diabetes. The assessment is available in numerous languages, including English, German, French, Italian, Spanish, and Russian (Ravens-Sieberer & Bullinger, 2000).

Community Assessment

Community assessment can be defined in two distinct ways. First, it can refer to the assessment of individuals in order to prepare them for community reintegration (e.g., discharge from the hospital, release from prison) or to facilitate their transition to a new community (e.g., downsizing and moving to a retirement community). Second, it can refer to the assessment of the community as the client. Referring to a community as a patient or client is consistent with the definition of the term *client* in the *Framework* (AOTA, 2008).

According to Jimenez, occupational therapists "can look at communities on the macro level and treat them as patients, too" (cited in Brachlescende, 2003, p. 8). Jimenez and the Omaha Nation Community Response Team conducted a community needs assessment with the Omaha Reservation in Macy, Nebraska, "to find

out what people in the community wanted and what was culturally relevant" (cited in Brachlescende, 2003, p. 8). The outcome of this collaborative effort was the development of a community-based program called Strengthening Family Partnerships. This program provides a variety of services, including individual assessment and culturally meaningful prevention activities.

Assessment of Individuals for Integration and Transition

If community integration and the prevention of secondary or new health issues (i.e., primary prevention) are the goal of intervention, a variety of assessment options are available from which to choose. Many of these have already been discussed above and in the previous chapter. Additional examples include the Interest Checklist, developed by Matsutsuyu (1969) and revised by Rogers, Weinstein, and Figone (1978), and the Modified Interest Checklist available through the Model of Human Occupation Clearinghouse (Asher, 2007; University of Illinois at Chicago, Department of Occupational Therapy, 2005).

In the case of an older adult coping with a new disability or hospitalized for an exacerbation of a chronic disease, assessments that are both occupation-based and that address prevention can be useful tools. The Community Adaptive Planning Assessment (Spencer & Davidson, 1998), the COPM (Letts, Baum, & Perlmutter, 2003; McColl et al., 2000), the Activity Card Sort (Baum, 1995; Sachs & Josman, 2003), and SAFER (Letts et al., 2003) are examples of assessments that may be useful for older adults who wish to review their living arrangements or who are planning their transition to new living contexts.

Assessment of the Community

There are two general types of scenarios where an occupational therapist may implement a community assessment. The first type occurs when a community has already identified its problem or need and the occupational therapist, in collaboration with the client (i.e., the community), further explores the issue and then plans an intervention. Whenever possible, the project should include selecting and using an appropriate outcomes assessment to measure the intervention's effectiveness. The second type of scenario would be when the occupational therapist, individually or within an interdisciplinary team, is contracted to perform a community needs assessment. This type of opportunity is described next.

When the community is the client, it may be more appropriate to conduct a **capacity assessment,** which focuses on assets and possibilities (Dudgeon, 2003) rather than a needs assessment, which often focuses on diagnoses and deficiencies:

> Capacity assessment is based upon the capacities, skills, and assets of community members, agencies, and organizations. . . . Community members at all levels need to be involved in decisions that affect them; they should help plan programs where they are expected to be participants. (Nieto, Scaffner, & Henderson, 1997, ¶ 2)

Capacity assessment is consistent with social and occupational justice as well as health promotion and prevention. Wilcock believes the contribution of occupational therapy to community development extends beyond rehabilitation to include prevention by "helping the socially and occupationally disadvantaged who are at-risk of ill-health in the future" (2003, p. 40). Occupational therapists who engage in community development "could enable people to recognize the occupational needs of others, as well as their own, and to take action to meet such needs more effectively" (Wilcock, 2003, p. 40). The capacity inventory, as described by Kretzmann and McKnight (1993), can be used in community capacity assessment and development. Another example of such an assessment is the Individual Capacity Inventory (Foundation for Community Health, 2004).

Examples of other community-wide assessments that may be appropriate, especially for interdisciplinary efforts, include the Planned Approach to Community Health (PATCH; U.S. Department of Health and Human Services [USDHHS], Centers for Disease Control and Prevention [CDC], n.d.) and the MAP-IT strategy. The PATCH program was an application of the PRECEED portion of the PRECEED-PROCEED Model and served as the catalyst for the development of the PROCEED portion of that model (Green & Kreuter, 1992). "The goal of PATCH is to increase the capacity of communities to plan, implement, and evaluate comprehensive, community-based health promotion programs" (USDHHS, CDC, n.d., p. CG1-1). The PATCH process, which includes five phases, is illustrated in Figure 10-1 (USDHHS, CDC, n.d., p. I-O-1).

One key to the PATCH system is the coordination of resources at the local, state, regional, and national levels. Figure 10-2 details this coordination process (Kreuter, 1992). PATCH was developed with the goal of facilitating the abilities of local and state health agencies to develop community-based health promotion initiatives directed toward the health priorities of that community. Therefore, another important aspect of the PATCH system is the focus on providing community guidance and receiving community direction through the consensus process (McKenzie & Smeltzer, 2001). The small-group-dynamics expertise of occupational

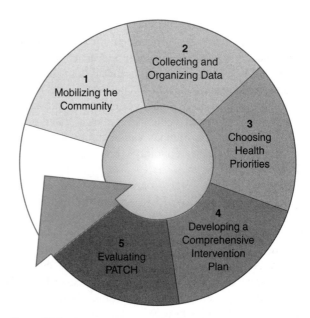

Figure 10-1 Five phases of the PATCH process.

From Planned approach to community health: Guide for the local coordinator, *by U.S. Department of Health and Human Services, Centers for Disease Control and Prevention, (n.d.), Atlanta: National Center for Chronic Disease Prevention and Health Promotion. p. I-0-1.*

therapists can be instrumental in the process of building a community's capacity to promote health.

PATCH materials are available in PDF format on the CDC website to assist in navigating through the five-phase process. These materials include a large file titled *Planned Approach to Community Health: Guide for the Local Coordinator* (USDHHS, CDC, n.d.), which contains three documents. These three documents include the *Concept Guide,* which explains the five phases of the process; the *Meeting Guide,* which provides a series of tools to engage the community in each phase of the process; and the "Visual Aids" section, which provides camera-ready materials.

The MAP-IT (Mobilize, Assess, Plan, Implement, and Track) strategy was developed as part of the *Healthy People in Healthy Communities* (USDHHS, 2001) program to facilitate community success in making changes that impact their health. Examples of community-developed and targeted health goals included

- reduction in the number of assaults;
- reduction of child endangerment as a result of methamphetamine use by parents;
- de-escalation of school tension prior to the use of deadly force.

The MAP-IT process is well detailed in Chapter 2 of *Healthy People in Healthy Communities,* which is available online at http://www.healthypeople.gov/Publications/HealthyCommunities2001/Chapter_2.htm.

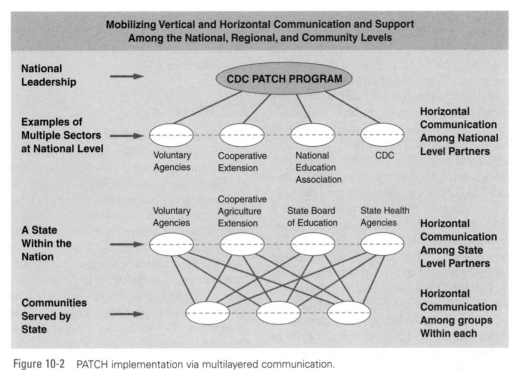

Figure 10-2 PATCH implementation via multilayered communication.

From "PATCH: Its origin, basic concepts, and links to contemporary public health policy," by M. W. Kreuter, 1992, Journal of Health Education, *23(3), p. 137. Copyright © 1992 by American Alliance for Health, Physical Education, Recreation, & Dance. With permission.*

The MAP-IT process is well matched with the philosophy of occupational therapy, as it is client-centered, is focused on facilitating healthy occupational engagement at the community-level, and is concerned with tracking outcomes.

Assessments from other disciplines may be useful for specific areas or types of community assessment and development. These additional assessments can be found by exploring the health education, health-promotion, health behavior, and environmental health literature. For example, Moudon and Lee (2003) reviewed 31 environmental instruments that evaluated walking and biking environments. Two of these instruments were identified for possible use by lay communities. The first instrument is the Walkability Checklist (National Highway Traffic Safety Administration, U.S. Department of Transportation [NHTSA, USDOT], 2004a), which could be used by an individual or a group to assess either a portion of a community or the entire community. This checklist is available online and addresses sidewalk safety, pedestrian-automobile interface, other safety factors, and aesthetics. By using this checklist with a local community organization, an occupational therapist could achieve the overarching goal of "supporting health and participation in life through engagement in occupation" (AOTA, 2008, p. 626), for that community.

Also available with the Walkability Checklist is a list of possible immediate actions and community actions to address the identified problems (NHTSA, USDOT, 2004b). An occupational therapist could assist an interested group in planning and conducting the survey and in displaying the results to maximize their impact when communicating with local stakeholders and policymakers. For example, local youth organizations could be contacted to clear undergrowth growing too close to paths used by small children and replace it with flowering bulbs, donated by a local garden supplier or purchased with grant money. These efforts could both enhance the safety and attractiveness of the paths, thereby increasing their usage. Governmental agencies also could be contacted regarding the safety hazards of tree roots disrupting paths and sidewalks. Elected officials could be contacted regarding proposals to provide paths or lighting for existing paths. The second instrument, the Bikeability Checklist, is also available online and addresses ease of use and safety (Pedestrian and Bicycle Information Center, USDOT, 2004).

Equally important to developing an ideal intervention is a plan to assess the program to be developed. The PRECEDE-PROCEED Model, discussed in-depth in Chapter 3 of this text, provides guidance for simultaneous health promotion program development and outcome evaluation planning (Green & Kreuter, 1999). Although the model provides overall guidance, specific tools must be identified to measure outcomes in the community. An example of such a tool is the Stanford Health Assessment Questionnaire (HAQ), a well-recognized and internationally used tool to measure health outcomes of people with chronic conditions (Bruce & Fries, 2003) and well individuals (Bruce & Fries, 2003; Lubeck & Fries, 1992). The HAQ is one of the oldest self-report outcome assessments and is available in over 60 languages (Bruce & Fries, 2003). This tool was modified (Lubeck & Fries, 1992) to measure health outcomes specifically for people with HIV symptoms and was named the AIDS Health Assessment Questionnaire (AIDS-HAQ).

Two other assessment options include the SF-12 Health Survey (SF-12) and the Health Impact Assessment (HIA). The SF-12 has been used to measure the health of individuals within the medical model. Work by Burdine, Felix, Abel, Wiltraut, and Musselman (2000) indicates that the SF-12 has potential for use as a population health measure. A copy of this tool and directions for requesting permission to reproduce are provided by Hyner and others (1999). The HIA is a program and policy assessment that should be conducted prior to implementing a program or policy. The HIA process is defined as "a combination of procedures, methods and tools by which a policy, program or project may be judged as to its potential effects on the health of a population, and the distribution of those effects within the population" (European Centre for Health Policy [ECHP], 1999, p. 4). Beyond maximum health of the target population, the HIA must ensure that the policy or program is consistent with the following values: democracy, equity, sustainable development, and the ethical use of evidence. Governments in Europe and global organizations such as the WHO are encouraging the use of this process in order to ensure the protection of communities before the implementation of programs or policies (ECHP, 1999).

Another role for an occupational therapist in health promotion assessment is the adaptation of the tool to the cultural or special needs of the community of interest. The use of preexisting assessments in this type of service delivery can be extremely helpful and can strengthen the intervention. However, they also may be problematic due to issues of cultural relevance or distinctive needs of the target population. For example, a U.S.-based company wanting to provide a health-risk assessment for their community (i.e., employees) as part of a health promotion program should proceed cautiously before using any assessments developed for U.S. workers to evaluate employees of other nationalities, especially those located overseas. If an appropriate, culturally relevant and accurate assessment cannot be identified, then a decision will need to be made as to whether an existing assessment can be modified or a culturally relevant assessment must be developed.

Conclusion

This chapter provided an overview of select assessments both from within the occupational therapy profession and from other disciplines and entities. To be evidence-based practitioners, occupational therapy assistants and occupational therapists must keep pace with the literature within occupational therapy and must review literature from related health and social sciences. It requires an investment of time to identify and wisely select assessments for health promotion interventions. The proper selection of a health promotion assessment, as well as its effective administration, adaptation, and data interpretation, is replete with challenges. However, the resulting contribution to improved social participation and community health warrant this investment of time and energy to address these challenges. The promotion of occupational justice and the resultant wellbeing of individuals and communities will be best achieved using scientific methods, including the application of reliable and valid health-promotion assessments.

▶ For Discussion and Review

1. Since the 1960s, health promotion and wellness have been discussed in the profession's literature, yet there are few assessments that specifically address these areas. What may have been the reason for this, and what can be done presently and in the future to better address health promotion and improve the health of individuals, communities, populations, and society?

2. Select one assessment that could be used in occupational therapy health promotion and investigate the most current research on its reliability, validity, and usefulness in occupational therapy practice.

3. What skills and knowledge can occupational therapists and occupational therapy assistants bring to interdisciplinary community assessment and intervention efforts?

4. Search the literature for a recent research study on
   a. an occupational therapy health promotion assessment,
   b. a health promotion assessment from a different discipline, or
   c. a community assessment.

Which of these studies would you replicate? Why and how?

5. Compare and contrast two health promotion assessments. How relevant might they be to occupational therapy practice? Can they be adapted for practice? In what type of setting can they be used?

▶ Research Questions

1. What is the reliability and validity of the COPM with military service personnel returning from active duty?
2. What is the reliability and validity of the PHWA with recent immigrants?
3. What factors impact rural, suburban, and urban park utilization by families?
4. What are the outcomes of an occupation-based acquaintance rape-prevention program?
5. What is the relationship between health risks as identified by HRAs and occupational participation?
6. How does occupational function in families with disabled members differ from occupational function in families with no disabled members?

Acknowledgments

The authors wish to express their appreciation to the following individuals who assisted with the preparation of this chapter: Frederick D. Reitz and Grace E. Wenger.

References

Alexander, G. (1999). Heath risk appraisal. In G. C. Hyner, K. W. Peterson, J. W. Travis, J. E. Dewey, J. J. Foerster, & E. M. Framer (Eds.), *SPM handbook of health assessment tools* (pp. 5–8). Pittsburgh, PA: The Society of Prospective Medicine & The Institute for Health & Productivity Management.

American Occupational Therapy Association. (2008). Occupational therapy practice framework: Domain and process (2d ed). *American Journal of Occupational Therapy, 62,* 625–83.

AMPS Project International. (n.d.a.) *AMPS Inservice.* Retrieved April 30, 2007, from http://www.ampsintl.com/AMPSinservice.htm.

AMPS Project International. (n.d.b.) *AMPS Training Courses.* Retrieved April 28, 2007, from http://www.ampsintl.com/training.htm.

AMPS Project International. (n.d.c.) *How is the AMPS unique?* Retrieved April 28, 2007, from http://www.ampsintl.com/benefits.htm.

AMPS Project International. (n.d.d.) *What is the AMPS?* Retrieved April 28, 2007, from http://www.ampsintl.com/overview.htm.

Asher, I. E. (2007). *Occupational therapy assessment tools: An annotated index* (3d ed.). Bethesda, MD: American Occupational Therapy Association.

Atchison, B. T., Fisher, A. G., & Bryze, K. (1998). Rater reliability and internal scale and person response validity of the School Assessment and Process Skills. *American Journal of Occupational Therapy, 52*(10), 609–639.

Baron, K., Kielhofner, G., Iyenger, A., Goldhammer, V., & Wolenski, J. (2006). *A user's manual for the Occupational Self Assessment (OSA) (Version 2.2).* Chicago: Model of Human Occupational Clearinghouse, Department of Occupational Therapy, College of Applied Health Sciences, University of Illinois at Chicago.

Baum, C. M. (1995). The contributions of occupation to function in persons with Alzheimer's disease. *Journal of Occupational Science, 2*(2), 59–67.

Becker, M. A., Shaw, B. R., & Reib, L. M. (n.d.) *Quality of life assessment manual.* Retrieved July 30, 2007, from http://www.fmhi.usf.edu/institute/pubs/pdf/mhlp/qol.pdf.

Bowling, A. (1991). *Measuring health: A review of quality of life measurement scales.* Philadelphia: Open University Press.

Brachlescende, A. (2003, June 23). Strengthening family partnerships. *OT Practice, 8*(11), 8–9.

Bray, K., Fisher, A. G., & Duran, L. (2001). The validity of adding new tasks to the Assessment of Motor and Process Skills. *American Journal of Occupational Therapy, 55*(4), 409–15.

Breckon, D. J., Harvey, J. R., & Lancaster, R. B. (1998). *Community health education: Settings, roles and skills for the 21st century* (4th ed.). Gaithersburg, MD: Aspen.

Brollier, C., Watts, J. H., Bauer, D., & Schmidt, W. (1989). A concurrent validity study of two occupational therapy evaluation instruments: The AOF and OCAIRS. *Occupational Therapy in Mental Health, 8*(4), 49–59.

Brown, R. I. (1996). People with developmental disabilities: Applying quality of life to assessment and intervention. In L. E. Young & V. Hayes (Eds.), *Transforming health promotion practice* (pp. 253–67). Philadelphia: F. A. Davis.

Bruce, B., & Fries, J. F. (2003). *The Stanford Health Assessment Questionnaire: Dimensions and practical applications.* Retrieved December 20, 2004, from http://www.hqlo.com/content/1/1/20.

Burdine, J. N., Felix, M. R., Abel, A. L., Wiltraut, C. J., & Musselman, Y. J. (2000). The SF-12 as a population health measure: An exploratory examination of potential for application. *HSR: Health Services Research, 35*(4), 885–904.

Caskie, P. D. (1998). What kind of system is the family? *Family Systems, 1*(1), 7–19.

Chessler, B. (1992). *Concurrent validity of the assessment of family functioning with the family hardiness index.* Unpublished master's research project, Virginia Commonwealth University, Richmond.

Dudgeon, B. J. (2003). Section IV community integration. In E. B. Crepeau, E. S. Cohn, & B. B. Schell (Eds.), *Willard and Spackman's occupational therapy* (10th ed., pp. 570–578). Philadelphia: Lippincott, Williams & Wilkins.

Edington, D. W., Yen, L., & Braunstein, A. (1999). The reliability and validity of HRAs. In G. C. Hyner, K. W. Peterson, J. W. Travis, J. E. Dewey, J. J. Foerster, & E. M. Framer (Eds.), *SPM handbook of health assessment tools* (pp. 135–141). Pittsburgh, PA: The Society of Prospective Medicine & The Institute for Health & Productivity Management.

European Centre for Health Policy. (1999). *Gothenburg consensus paper—Health impact assessment: Main concepts and suggested approaches.* Retrieved November 27, 2004, from http://www.euro.who.int/document/PAE/Gothenburgpaper.pdf.

Fingerhut, P., Madill, H., Darrah, J., Hodge, M., & Warren, S. (2002). Classroom-based assessment: Validation for the School AMPS. *American Journal of Occupational Therapy, 56*(2), 210–13.

Fisher, A. (2006). *Overview of performance skills and client factors.* In H. M. Pendleton, & W. Schultz-Krohn (Eds.), *Pedretti's occupational therapy for physical dysfunction* (6th ed., pp. 372–402). New York: Elsevier.

Fisher, A. G. (1999). *Assessment of motor and process skills* (3d ed.). Fort Collins, CO: Three Star Press.

Fisher, A. G., Bryze, K., & Atchison, B. T. (2000). Naturalistic assessment of functional performance in school settings: Reliability and validity of the School AMPS scales. *Journal of Outcome Measurement, 4*(1), 491–512.

Forsyth, K., Deshpande, S., Kielhofner, G., Henriksson, C., Haglund, L., Olson, L., Skinner, S., & Kulkarni, S. (2005). *A user's manual for the Occupational Circumstances Assessment Interview and Rating Scale (OCAIRS, Version 4.0).* Chicago: Model of Human Occupation Clearinghouse, University of Illinois at Chicago.

Foundation for Community Health. (2004). *United Way Needs Assessment, Individual Capacity Inventory.* Retrieved November 7, 2004, from http://fch.evansville.net/capinv.html.

Frank-Stromberg, M., & Olsen, S. J. (2004). *Instruments for clinical health care research* (3d ed.). Boston: Jones & Bartlett.

Gitlin, L. N. (2005). Measuring performance in instrumental activities of daily living. In M. Law, C. Baum, & W. Dunn (Eds.), *Measuring occupational performance: Supporting best practice* (2d ed., pp. 227–47). Philadelphia: SLACK.

Green, L. W., & Kreuter, M. W. (1992). CDC's planned approach to community health as an application of PRECEED and an inspiration for PROCEED. *Journal of Health Education, 23,* 140–47.

Green, L. W., & Kreuter, M. W. (1999). *Health promotion planning: An educational and environmental approach* (3d ed.). Mountainview, CA: Mayfield.

Haglund, L., Thorell, L., & Walinder, J. (1998). Assessment of occupational functioning for screening of patients to occupational therapy in general psychiatric care. *Occupational Therapy Journal of Research, 4,* 193–206.

Henry, A. D. (2003). Section II The interview process. In E. B. Crepeau, E. S. Cohn, & B. B. Schell (Eds.), *Willard and Spackman's occupational therapy* (10th ed., pp. 297). Philadelphia: Lippincott, Williams & Wilkins.

Hyner, G. C., Peterson, K. W., Travis, J. W., Dewey, J. E., Foerster, J. J., & Framer, E. M. (Eds.) (1999). *SPM handbook of health assessment tools.* Pittsburgh, PA: The Society of Prospective Medicine & The Institute for Health & Productivity Management.

Kielhofner, G. (2002). *Model of human occupation: Theory and application* (3d ed.). Baltimore: Lippincott, Williams & Wilkins.

Kielhofner, G. (2004). The model of human occupation. In *Conceptual foundations of occupational therapy* (3d ed., pp. 147–70). Philadelphia: F. A. Davis.

Kielhofner, G., & Burke, J. (1980). A model of human occupation, part 1: Conceptual framework and content. *American Journal of Occupational Therapy, 9,* 572–81.

Kretzmann, J. P., & McKnight, J. L. (1993). *Building communities from the inside out: A path toward finding and mobilizing a community's assets.* Evanston, IL: Northwestern University, Center for Urban Affairs and Policy Research.

Kreuter, M. W. (1992). PATCH: Its origin, basic concepts, and links to contemporary public health policy. *Journal of Health Education, 23*(3), 135–39. Retrieved March 25, 2006, from http://wonder.cdc.gov/wonder/prevguid/p0000064/p0000064.asp.

LaPuma, J., & Lawlor, E. F. (1990). Quality-adjusted life years: Ethical implications for physicians and policy makers. *Journal of the American Medical Association, 263,* 2917–21.

Law, M., Baptiste, S., Carswell, A., McColl, M., Polatjko, H., & Pollock, N. (1998). *Canadian occupational performance measure manual* (3d ed.). Ottawa, Ontario: CAOT Publications ACE.

Law, M., Baum, C. M., & Dunn, W. (2005). Occupational performance assessment. In C. H. Christiansen, C. M. Baum, & J. Bass-Haugen (Eds.), *Occupational therapy: Performance, participation, and wellbeing* (3d ed., pp. 339–70). Thorofare, NJ: SLACK.

Letts, L., Baum, C., &. Perlmutter, M. (2003). Person-environment-occupation assessments with older adults. *OT Practice, 8*(10), 8–9.

Lubeck, D. P., & Fries, J. F. (1992). Changes in quality of life among persons with HIV infection. *Quality of Life Research, 1,* 359–66.

Matsutsuyu, J. (1969). The Interest Checklist. *American Journal of Occupational Therapy, 23,* 323–28.

McColl, M. A., Paterson, M. N., Davies, D., Doubt, L., & Law, M. (2000). Validity and community utility of the Canadian Occupational Performance Measure. *Canadian Journal of Occupational Therapy, 67,* 22–30.

McColl, M. A., & Pollock, N. (2005). Measuring occupational performance using a client-centered perspective. In M. Law, C. Baum, & W. Dunn (Eds.), *Measuring occupational performance: Supporting best practice in occupational therapy* (2d ed., pp. 81–91). Thorofare, NJ: SLACK.

McCubbin, H., McCubbin, M., & Thompson, A. (1986). Family Hardiness Index. In H. McCubbin & A. Thompson (Eds.), *Family assessment for research and practice* (pp. 125–30). Madison, WI: University of Wisconsin Press.

McDowell, I., & Newell, C. (1987). *Measuring health: A guide to rating scales and questionnaires.* New York: Oxford University Press.

McKenzie, J. F., & Smeltzer, J. L. (1997). *Planning, implementing and evaluating health promotion programs: A primer* (2d ed.). Boston: Allyn & Bacon.

McKenzie, J. F., & Smeltzer, J. L. (2001). *Planning, implementing, and evaluating health promotion programs: A primer* (3d ed.). Boston: Allyn & Bacon.

Moudon, A. V., & Lee, C. (2003). Walking and bicycling: An evaluation of environmental audit instruments. *American Journal of Health Promotion, 18*(1), 21–37.

National Highway Traffic Safety Administration, U.S. Department of Transportation. (2004a). *How walkable is your community? Walkability checklist.* Retrieved November 7, 2004, from http://www.nhtsa.dot.gov/people/injury/pedbimot/ped/walk1.html.

National Highway Traffic Safety Administration, U.S. Department of Transportation. (2004b). *Making your community more walkable.* Retrieved November 7, 2004, from http://www.nhtsa.dot.gov/people/injury/pedbimot/ped/walk2.html.

Nieto, R. B., Scaffner, D., & Henderson, J. L. (1997). Examining community needs through a capacity assessment. *Journal of Extension 35*(3). Retrieved November 7, 2004, from http://www.joe.org/joe/1997june/a1.html.

Osoba, D. (2002). A taxonomy of the uses of health-related quality-of-life instruments in cancer care and the clinical meaningfulness of the results. *Medical Care, 40*(6), pp. III-31–III-38.

Pedestrian and Bicycle Information Center, U.S. Department of Transportation. (2004). *Bikeability checklist. How bikeable is your community?* Retrieved November 7, 2004, from http://www.bicyclinginfo.org/pdf/bikabilitychecklist.pdf.

Pizzi, M. (2001). The Pizzi Holistic Wellness Assessment. *Occupational Therapy in Health Care, 13*(3/4), 51–66.

Pledger, K. C. (1990). *Pilot study of comparison between the family assessment of occupational functioning and the family hardiness index.* Unpublished master's research project, Virginia Commonwealth University, Richmond.

Pollock, N., & McColl, M. A. (1998). Assessment in client-centered occupational therapy. In M. Law (Ed.), *Client-centered occupational therapy* (pp. 89–105). Thorofare, NJ: SLACK.

Ravens-Sieberer, U., & Bullinger, M. (1998a). Assessing the health related quality of life in chronically ill children with the German KINDL: First psychometric and content-analytical results. *Quality of Life Research, 7*(5), 399–407.

Ravens-Sieberer, U., & Bullinger, M. (1998b). News from the KINDL-Questionnaire—A new version for adolescents. *Quality of Life Research, 7,* 653.

Ravens-Sieberer, U. & Bullinger, N. (2000). *KINDL-R Questionnaire for measuring health-related quality of life in children and adolescents, revised version: Manual.* Retrieved July 30, 2007, from http://www.kindl.org/daten/pdf/ManEnglish.pdf.

Renwick, R., Brown, I., Rootman, I., & Nagler, M. (1996). Conceptualization, research and application: Future directions. In R. Renwick, I. Brown, & M. Nagler (Eds.), *Quality of life in health promotion and rehabilitation: Conceptual approaches, issues and applications* (pp. 357–67). Thousand Oaks, CA: Sage.

Rogers, J., Weinstein, J., & Figone, J. (1978). The Interest Checklist: An empirical assessment. *American Journal of Occupational Therapy, 32,* 628–30.

Rootman, I., Raphael, D., Shewchuk, D., Renwick, R., Friefeld, S., Garber, M., Talbot, Y., & Woodill, G. (1992). *Development of an approach and instrument package to measure quality of life of persons with developmental disabilities.* Toronto: University of Toronto, Centre for Health Promotion.

Sachs, D., & Josman, N. (2003). The Activity Card Sort: A factor analysis. *Occupation, Participation, and Health, 23*(4), 165–74.

Schalock, R. L., Keith, K. D., Hoffman, K., & Karan, O. C. (1989). Quality of life: Its measurement and use. *Mental Retardation, 27,* 25–31.

Shepherd, J., Scaffa, M., & Pizzi, M. (1989). *Family assessment of occupational functioning.* Unpublished assessment, Virginia Commonwealth University, Richmond.

Spencer, J., & Davidson, J. (1998). The Community Adaptive Planning Assessment: A clinical tool for documenting future planning with clients. *American Journal of Occupational Therapy, 52*(1), 19–30.

Strecher, V. J., & Kreuter, M. W. (1999). Health risk appraisal from a behavioral perspective: Present and future. In G. C. Hyner, K. W. Peterson, J. W. Travis, J. E. Dewey, J. J. Foerster, & E. M. Framer (Eds.), *SPM handbook of health assessment tools* (pp. 75–82). Pittsburgh, PA: The Society of Prospective Medicine & The Institute for Health & Productivity Management.

Turk, D. C., & Kerns, R. D. (1985). *Health, illness and families.* New York: John Wiley & Sons.

Turnbull, A. P., & Turnbull, H. R. (1990). *Families, professionals and exceptionality: A special partnership.* Columbus, OH: Merrill.

University of Illinois at Chicago Department of Occupational Therapy. (2005). *Model of Human Occupation Clearinghouse, MOHO related resources.* Retrieved February 5, 2005, from http://www.moho.uic.edu/mohorelatedrsrcs.html#OtherInstrumentsBasedonMOHO.

U.S. Department of Health and Human Services, Centers for Disease Control and Prevention. (n.d.). *Planned approach to community health: Guide for the local coordinator.* Atlanta: National Center for Chronic Disease Prevention and Health Promotion. Retrieved March 25, 2006, from http://www.cdc.gov/search.do?action=search&queryText=PATCH&x=17&y=9.

U.S. Department of Health and Human Services. (2001). *Healthy people in healthy communities: A community planning guide using healthy people 2010.* Retrieved November 27, 2004, from http://www.healthypeople.gov/Publications/HealthyCommunities2001/toc.htm.

White, V., Davidson, H., & Reed, K. (2004). *Occupational wellness and the occupational wellness assessment instrument.* Houston, TX: Texas Women's University. Unpublished paper.

White, V., Davidson, H., Reed, K., & Garber, S. (2000). Enhancing quality of life through occupational wellness. *Proceedings of the second national Department of Veterans Affairs rehabilitation research and development conference.*

Retrieved August 1, 2007, from http://www.rehab.research .va.gov.

Wilcock, A. A. (2003). Occupational therapy practice, Section 2, Population interventions focused on health for all. In E. B. Crepeau, E. S. Cohn, & B. B. Schell (Eds.), *Willard and Spackman's occupational therapy* (10th ed., pp. 30–45). Philadelphia: Lippincott, Williams & Wilkins.

World Health Organization. (2001). *International classification of functioning, disability and health.* Geneva, Switzerland: World Health Organization.

World Health Organization. (2007). *WHOQOL-BREF.* Retrieved July 31, 2007, from http://www.who.int/ substance_abuse/research_tools/whoqolbref/en/index.html.

Chapter 11

Health Promotion Program Development

Linda S. Fazio

> Preventive care programs cannot be viewed as replacing the already valued contributions of occupational therapy. But if we fail to use our professional knowledge to contradict those forces which create poor health, we are, in fact, guilty of contributing to the poor health of our communities and their citizens. A creative way of lessening the critical shortage of occupational therapists is to prevent the conditions which require occupational therapy. Occupational therapy belongs in the community.
>
> —Gillette, 1973, p. 130

Learning Objectives

This chapter is designed to enable the reader to:

- Describe the process of developing an occupation-centered community program.
- Understand the process of assessing the need for community services.
- Discuss the importance of community program planning to enhance achieving program goals and objectives.
- Recognize the importance of a thorough investigation of population, condition, and context in the development of a community profile.

- Describe the relationships between program goals, objectives, and programming activities.
- Appreciate the importance of theory and evidence-based research to guide programming and evaluation.
- Describe the types of program evaluation and their uses.

Key Terms

Community
Community profile
Evidence-based practice
Formative evaluation

Goal
Objectives
Outcome evaluation
Primary prevention

Program evaluation
Secondary prevention
Stakeholder

Theory
Volition

Introduction

Occupational therapists and occupational therapy assistants frequently engage in program development in common practice settings such as hospitals and schools. On occasion, these efforts include other disciplines in program planning and execution. In addition to these familiar settings, the community is becoming an increasingly popular site for program development. Occupational therapy programs anchored in the community can engage in prevention, restoration, maintenance, and health promotion, singly or in any combination. This chapter will describe the steps an occupation-centered practitioner may follow during the conception, development, implementation, and evaluation of a community program directed toward prevention of illness and disability and the promotion of health and wellbeing. Interwoven with the descriptions of this process are small vignettes of actual program development experiences. The chapter will conclude with a case example of the creation of an occupation-based community program.

Definitions of Community

A variety of definitions exist in the literature for the term community. For the purposes of this chapter, **community** refers to a group of people related by a characteristic such as age, gender, disability, culture, or social similarities. In practice, the concept of community is not necessarily limited to a geographic location. The label community "can be affixed to a place (locale) in combination with a spirit of sharing, membership, and commitment or it can simply *be* a spirit of sharing, membership, and commitment" (Fazio, 2001, p. 2).

Practitioners in the community must make a commitment to the broad context encompassed by this term, and they have an ethical obligation to serve the needs of community members (American Occupational Therapy Association [AOTA], 2005) within the scope of practice defined by the *Occupational Therapy Practice Framework* (referred to as *Framework;* AOTA, 2008). Regardless of whether the occupational therapist or occupational therapy assistant resides in or is a member of the community, in order to properly serve a community, one must understand the community and share in its problems and victories. There is an implicit expectation that occupational therapy practitioners be responsive to the needs of the community and of individual clients. This responsiveness requires an awareness of what might be described as the "greater good" and a concern for social justice (Wilcock, 1998). Certainly not all community-based programs are charitable in structure, but an expectation of charity in spirit exists.

Levels of Prevention in the Community

Sultz and Young (2004) described the work of epidemiologists and health service planners in their use of a matrix for placing known facts about a particular disease or condition in the sequence of its origin and progression when untreated: "This schema is called the natural history of disease" (Sultz & Young, 2004, p. 6) and describes three levels of prevention: primary, secondary, and tertiary. The first, or primary, level is the period during which the individual is at risk for a disease, disorder, or injury and is of particular significance to occupational therapy providers developing community programs. It is within this period that behavioral, genetic, environmental, and other factors that increase the individual's likelihood of developing or acquiring the particular condition are identified. Primary prevention is key during this phase.

Kniepmann (1997) and Pope and Tarlov (1991) used the same prevention terminology previously described but did so only in response to the prevention of illness and disabling conditions. According to these authors, **primary prevention** refers to actions and strategies directed toward the greater society; minimizing environmental risk factors would be an example. Occupational therapy addresses health promotion and disability prevention as components of primary prevention (Brownson & Scaffa, 2001).

The next level is **secondary prevention,** which includes efforts to target specific at-risk groups in the community. Occupational therapists and occupational therapy assistants are instrumental at this level of prevention, as they provide interventions along the developmental continuum. These interventions may include prenatal and parenting classes for teens as well as home and community safety programs for the well elderly. Another example of secondary prevention is teaching healthy seniors how to access public transportation in an effort to widen their options for meaningful occupation, thus maintaining health (Fazio, 2001).

Occupational therapists currently target what is described as the tertiary prevention phase of disability limitation and rehabilitation as a major arena for intervention. Although a role exists for occupational therapy after onset of disease and diagnosis, it is in the first phase when health promotion and protection are most needed and effective.

Developing the Idea for Programming

Program development starts with the formation of an idea or the identification of a need. Content Box 11-1 outlines this and other general steps in program development. A program idea is most often borne of interest and a strong desire to do something to address a community need or problem. Ideally, the community itself identifies the need. There may be no better example of what Kielhofner (2002) has described as volition as when a community joins together to meet a common goal. **Volition** has been defined

> as a pattern of thoughts and feelings about oneself as an actor in one's world which occurs as one anticipates, chooses, experiences, and interprets what one does. Volitional thoughts and feelings pertain to what one holds important (values), perceives as personal capacity and effectiveness (personal causation), and finds enjoyable (interests). (Kielhofner, 2002, p. 44)

This measure of efficacy, the ability to achieve desired results, is driven by a "boundless enthusiasm," or what the American Heritage Dictionary (2008, ¶ 1) defines as passion. Passion for an idea may carry both the community and the program developer through long hours of hard work, disappointments, and resulting changes in trajectories. It is not uncommon that while designing a program, the scope of an intervention may evolve. In addition, the original target population may be expanded to other groups in ways not originally considered.

Programs are designed to clearly focus effort and activity in meeting the needs of an identified group (Fazio, 2001). Even when driven by passion for a place, an activity, a group of people, or a particular illness or condition, a program seldom is developed without an

Steps in Community Program Development

1. Investigate personal attributes the programmer(s) bring to the project (e.g., knowledge, skills, experience, and passion).
2. Explore ideas for occupation-centered programs; consider a population; identify the potential purpose of the program.
3. Develop a community profile. Investigate archival data (e.g., demographic, epidemiologic studies, census data) and collect face-to-face data in the community. Using multiple means to research the potential population, thoroughly investigate condition and context.
4. Conduct Phase I and Phase II of the needs assessment.
5. Review the results of the needs assessments and identify what has been accomplished:
   a. Is more information needed? For whom—the community? The service population?
   b. Does the programmer(s) have the skills and knowledge base to meet the expressed need? Will others with more experience or specialized knowledge be required?
   c. Do earlier ideas regarding the tentative purpose and outcomes of the program still fit? How will the passion be mobilized?

Note: Steps 3 and 4 may be reversed or conducted simultaneously. Adapted from *Developing occupation-centered programs for the community: A workbook for students and professionals* (p. 101), by L. S. Fazio, 2001, Upper Saddle River, NJ: Prentice Hall. Copyright © 2001 by Prentice Hall.

identified need. Occupation-centered program developers may not always find an immediate match between need and their passion; however, this gap prompts further examination. Perhaps redefining purpose toward finding another environment/context for the program is warranted. Passion must not be used to create a need when one does not exist.

In program development, occupational therapists and occupational therapy assistants share core values and attitudes regarding practice and subscribe to the *Occupational Therapy Code of Ethics* (AOTA, 2005). These values include altruism, equality, freedom, justice, dignity, truth, and prudence (AOTA, 1993). Together with the *Code of Ethics* and related documents, these values are as binding for the practitioner in the community as they are for other occupational therapy contexts and provide for the client's protection as the highest priority.

Opportunities for program development can arise in current employment settings to build upon programs previously developed by other occupational therapists or related health-care providers. Occupational therapy practitioners may be encouraged to replicate a success-ful program. For example, a manager may request that a therapist design a program to extend existing services to a new location or to expand present rehabilitation/intervention services to include prevention measures. Generally, therapists engaged in program development are intrigued by the challenge of solving a puzzle or problem and become impassioned by the process as well as the idea.

Opportunities also exist to develop innovative, occupation-centered program ideas based on observed needs of a community or population. For example, an occupational therapist with a grand passion for kayaking and ocean sports was convinced that differently abled children and their families would desire to engage in these challenging sports, which would build confidence and personal efficacy (as it had done for him). Other program ideas based on knowledge of a community or observation may be less innovative but worthy of action. For instance, an occupational therapy assistant may identify the need to develop a safe biking program after observing unsafe practices in the community.

Assessing the Need for Services

There are many ways to discover or assess the needs of a group or a community. Often advocates for themselves, community members may identify a need and have strong ideas about programming. They may find a program developer who has already demonstrated expertise through the design, development, and evaluation of other programs. Physicians, teachers, city officials, religious or spiritual leaders, other therapists, and health-care providers may also present a need and ideas for programming to a community, as in the following example.

A team of cardiothoracic surgeons wants to add prevention programming to their practice. These practitioners have long counseled their patients about diet and exercise, but in these times of rising costs, both financial and in terms of quality of life, prevention with results is becoming an increasing priority. The need seems apparent. However, a first step would be to further verify need by investigating trends to support prevention programming for this population (Fazio, 2001).

Supportive information, such as the following from the *New York Times,* may be found for the desired program:

> The number of hospitals offering alternative therapies nearly doubled from 1998 to 2000, according to a survey by the American Hospital Association, to 15.5 percent of all hospitals, and the association says hospitals of all sizes are continuing to open alternative or complementary medicine centers where patients or local residents can drop in for a few hours for treatments. (Abelson & Brown, 2002, ¶ 3)

After an idea is conceived, the next step is to ascertain if perceived need is not only present, but also a priority among the community or population. It has been estimated that over $10 billion per year is spent on alternative forms of health care, including supplements (Eisenberg et al., 1993). In addition, 572 U.S. physicians who responded to a mailed survey that included a list of 16 examples of "unconventional medicine" reported being most amenable to referring their patients for "relaxation techniques, biofeedback, therapeutic massage, hypnosis, and acupuncture" (Blumberg, Grant, Hendricks, Kamps, and Dewan, 1995, p. 32). The list also included spiritual healing, herbal remedies, energy healing, megavitamin therapy, chiropractic care, rolfing, yoga, and others (Blumberg et al.,1995). The public's willingness to spend so much time and money on unconventional therapies and physicians being agreeable to referring patients for at least a portion of these techniques suggests a need among the community for the proposed program.

To continue with this example, the cardiothoracic team may already have space and funding for the proposed expansion. They now need a plan to assess the target population holistically. An occupational therapist can develop a needs assessment plan, together with clients and other practitioners with shared interests and potential contributions (e.g., health educators, nutritionists, physical therapists, nurse practitioners). It is likely that the physician group may have identified this need based on their perceptions of what is best for their clients/patients, but they may not have verified their perceptions with the potential participants. This verification would be the work of the programmer(s).

Phase I and II Needs Assessment

Thus, the physicians have provided what Fazio (2001) describes as Phase I of the needs assessment: identifying the need(s) of the targeted population as articulated by the care provider, practitioner, community leaders, or, on rare occasions, the community as a whole. It is then necessary for the programmer to conduct Phase II to assess specific perceived needs of the target population or the broader community. From the combined results of Phase I and Phase II, the information needed to develop both the program and the outcome research questions is identified. This development is done through constructing a series of profiles, which include demographics of the participant population (e.g., ethnicity, age range, gender, professions), the condition (in this example it may be those at risk for coronary heart disease or those who may be postsurgical or posttrauma), and the context (e.g., residence, income levels).

This information is combined to form the service profile, which the programmer will use to determine the degree of fit with the needs of those involved at all levels. This exemplifies how a potential program may find the programmer. The converse case involves the programmer with a passion of his or her own. It is common for an idea to develop so firmly that potential programmers search for those who may need the programming they have in mind.

The Phase I and II experiences of the earlier example regarding the potential programmer with a passion for water sports and ocean kayaking is now described. One of the first steps taken was to investigate occupational therapy facilities that provided services to children with developmental delay, autism, and cerebral palsy. The programmer narrowed the profile for Phase I of the needs assessment to a geographic area within approximately 10 to 15 miles from the ocean. In such a community, it was likely residents would have an appreciation for water sports, and many might already be participants.

After developing a brief introduction of his programming idea and an interview protocol, several therapists were interviewed to determine if they would support the programming idea (Phase I of the needs assessment). Generally, in this case they did not. Although some of the therapists interviewed enjoyed ocean sports (e.g., surfing, swimming, kayaking), they believed the parents would consider these activities to be far too unsafe and potentially dangerous for their children to engage in at any level.

Discouraged but undaunted, the programmer, with the cooperation of the therapists, conducted Phase II of the needs assessment via a focus group with parents of the children seen at the facilities. Prior to this visit, he investigated statistics regarding safety (as an ocean lifeguard, he could have made assumptions regarding safety, but as a programmer, he could not), he interviewed instructors in existing water programming for individuals who were differently abled (utilizing expert and experienced practitioners), he conducted a task analysis of riding a body board, and he performed a self-analysis regarding the characteristics of his passion.

The programmer came to the parents' focus group far better prepared and grounded than when initiating Phase I of the needs assessment. The parent group exhibited a mixed response to the potential programming, but their concerns regarding safety were addressed early on via a skillful and motivating introduction that included videos of a young surfer with a spinal injury returning to his favored occupation. Another video was shown of a differently abled child being introduced to a surfboard and the same child later riding the board with her instructor. The proposed gains of efficacy, achievement, confidence, and joy were evident in the video.

Phase II was expanded to the children themselves in an ocean orientation. This is an example of how Phase II can become a marketing venue for a programmer who initiates an idea and then seeks a need. It also demonstrates the effectiveness of a careful Phase I followed by research that permits the programmer to target the Phase II presentation to the concerns identified in Phase I. This type of programming is not for everyone, and there are potential dangers involved. The programmer must be fully prepared and credentialed to ensure safety in this or any other type of programming. Adventure programming is captivating, but one child's adventure may be another's nightmare. It does not mean that ocean programming cannot be utilized for a wide range of children; this is where an occupational therapist's knowledge of occupation, task analysis, grading of activities, and goal setting is essential. Ocean programming can include relaxation exercises, appreciating the sound of the surf (Fig. 11-1), making sand castles, and surfing.

Developing Community Profiles

The creation of a community profile can sometimes be done simultaneously with establishing a need. The **community profile** includes a description of the population, their condition, and their context. AOTA's (2008) *Framework* is the central work to guide the practice of occupational therapy. Its intent is to help the practitioner understand engagement in areas of occupation as they are translated through performance skills; performance patterns, with consideration for context;

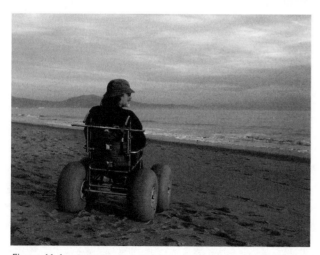

Figure 11-1   Ocean programming can provide access to the sounds of the sea.

Photo courtesy of the American Occupational Therapy Foundation, Bethesda, MD.

the demands of the selected activity; and the client factors that influence performance. Of particular interest to the practitioner in the community is the description of context that includes cultural, physical, social, personal, spiritual, temporal, and virtual factors (AOTA, 2008). These contextual elements are important considerations for any practice, but even more so for those programs in the community, where an awareness of the intricacies of context is experienced firsthand.

Spencer (2003) described contextual domains, suggesting that each of these environmental domains be examined at different levels, or contextual scales. These scales move from those closest to the individual to those that are more remote. According to Spencer,

> the concept of environmental scale is important not only because it draws attention to different kinds of influences on occupational engagement, but also because it has important implications for who controls the environment and, therefore, the processes by which environmental change might occur. (2003, p. 429)

Observing the individual from the perspective of contexts, moving from the immediate scale to a proximal scale, to a community scale, and to a societal scale, is a useful marker for the community-centered practitioner to maintain attention on the individual as he or she is influenced by, and influences, these contexts. Awareness of the complexity of context is important to understanding all aspects of programming, from the parameters of the community to assessing the need for programming, establishing appropriate and targeted programming, and evaluating outcomes. In describing the process of profiling the community in order to achieve a better understanding of the factors that must be considered in building programs, Fazio (2001) suggested sorting the community by layers (Fig. 11-2). Her description of the development of programming for a homeless runaway teenage population is compatible with Spencer's description of "scales."

Developing Community Programming Goals, Objectives, and Activities

When preparing to write goals and specific objectives for developing a program, it is important to connect the programming plan, implementation plan, and evaluation plan. In program development, a **goal** is what is aimed for, what is hoped to be achieved; **objectives** are attached to each goal to ensure the desired result is accomplished. Within occupation-centered program development for a community, the use of the term *goal*

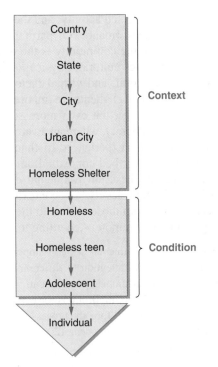

Figure 11-2   Layers of community.

Adapted from Developing occupation-centered programs for the community: A workbook for students and professionals *(p. 81), by L. S. Fazio, 2001, Upper Saddle River, NJ: Prentice Hall. Copyright © 2001 by Prentice Hall.*

should reflect the needs of the community of clients/ patients/members, and the use of the term *objective* should consider the profiles of individual participants.

When goals and objectives are well connected and when objectives are measurable, the program's effectiveness can be demonstrated. Program goals should benefit all participants, but if not all participants meet their personal objectives, this does not mean the program has failed. However, writing and achieving goals that capture the program's essence is important for future program marketing and to engage others who might wish to offer support (e.g., funding, time, in-kind donations). For instance, in a gang-prevention program, research suggests that the focus should be on strengthening the relationship between parent and child through a project or programming that requires a joint effort for the common good.

Goals for such a program might be

- to empower children to create change for positive global futures and
- to encourage parent–child teamwork.

Of course, these goals are not measurable as written, so objectives must accompany them that, collectively, will meet the conditions of the goal. The above two goals may be combined and enhanced to form the

following goal and associated objective:

> Goal: Building a better community together through parent–child teamwork
> Objective: Each parent–child team will participate in one neighborhood graffiti cleanup day by the end of the 8-week program.

DiLima and Schust (1997) provided a list of criteria for community-programming objectives. They recommended that objectives be performance-, behavior-, or action-oriented. Content Box 11-2 identifies additional criteria for writing program objectives.

When writing objectives, programmers need to be descriptive and specific in order to clarify the outcome measures and to determine if the desired outcome has been achieved. Well-written objectives enhance the programmer's ability to evaluate the program's effectiveness. Verb choice indicates the action that will be performed and may include such words as *identify, learn, cooperate, demonstrate, explore, promote,* or *support.* A noun that identifies the expected outcome should follow the verb. The objective is completed by providing the expected level or condition and the time frame for objective attainment. For example, an objective for a potential community bike safety program might be parents learning and demonstrating the safe use of bike helmets for their child prior to a joint child–parent bike ride by the program's second week.

A program may have only one goal, but several objectives may be required for participants to achieve that goal. Everyone involved in staffing the program must be able to observe and recognize when the objectives have been accomplished. A tracking method for progress and objective attainment must be readily accessible to the various staff members throughout the program.

Content Box 11-2

Criteria for Well-Written Program Objectives

- Objectives must be precise in their language (do not use general or vague verbs).
- Objectives must be measurable.
- Objectives must be clear and state the level, condition, or standard of performance.
- Objectives must be results oriented and have stated outcomes.
- Objectives must have clear descriptions of the content and performance.
- Objectives must have a specific time for completion.

From *Community health education and promotion: A guide to program design and evaluation* (p. 209), by S. N. DiLima & C. S. Schust (Eds.), 1997, Gaithersburg, MD: Aspen. Copyright © 1997 by Aspen.

Many planners begin with the idea for a program and the intervention mode or modality, and then seek to position and justify it through the steps of program development. Hippotherapy, arts and crafts, play, and computers are examples of modalities that may be selected, around which goals and objectives are written. There are many options for programming design and more for occupation-based community program activities. Table 11-1 identifies sources for programming materials/interventions.

There are many ways to meet program objectives and goals. The established program should reflect the community's culture and the philosophy and experience of both the community and the programmer or program team. The occupational therapist's expertise must include the ability to properly select a conceptual model or theory that guides development of the intervention.

Use of Theory to Guide Programming

Practitioners think about what they see, what they do, and how these elements are interrelated. Reed (1998) described this "organized way of thinking about given phenomena" (p. 521) as **theory.** According to Reed, the focus of the profession is "occupational endeavors" that are studied through four major constructs: "person, environment, health, and occupation" (p. 521). Since these constructs are multilayered and complex, many theories have been developed (Reed, 1998). This variety of theories provides community-based practitioners with options to frame discussions of target phenomena and to guide program design and development.

In addressing questions stimulated by the interweaving of community, occupation, and intervention, the need emerges for meaningful ways to integrate these

Table 11–1 **Sources for Occupation-Centered Programming Supplies and Materials**

Company and Contact Information	Products
Attainment Company, Inc. (800-327-4269)	Multiple options/supplies for children and adults with special needs
Childswork/Childsplay (800-962-1141); e-mail: care@GenesisDirect.com	Social and emotional needs of children and adolescents
Communication Skill Builders (602-323-7500)	Communication supplies/activities for children and adults
Communication/Therapy Skill Builders (a Division of the Psychological Corporation; 800-211-8378)	Child and adult assessment and intervention tools
Dick Blick Art Materials (800-828-4548); website: http://www.dickblick.com	Arts and crafts supplies
Imaginart (800-828-1376); e-mail: imaginart@aol.com	Therapy supplies for children, physical rehabilitation, and mental health
PCI Educational Publishing (800-594-4263)	Supplies for cognitive and emotional independence
S & S Healthcare (800-243-9232); website: http://www.snswwide.com	Arts, crafts, games, and exercise for education, therapy, and rehabilitation
S & S Opportunities (800-937-3482)	Child and adult rehabilitation equipment, supplies, and furnishings
Tandy Leather and Crafts/TLC Direct (888-890-1611); website: http://www.tandyleatherfactory.com	Leathercraft, Indian lore
Wellness Reproductions, Inc. (800-669-9208)	Supplies and resources for mental health facilitators, educators, and therapists
Whole Person Associates (800-247-6789); website: http://www.wholeperson.com	Stress management, wellness/health promotion, and emotional self-care resources

constructs into a practice discipline appropriate for today and the future. Theories and conceptual models provide the foundation for program design and implementation, and help set parameters for program evaluation (Scaffa, 1992). Practitioners and programmers can use one or more models to provide structure for the comprehensive services that are offered to a community or population.

The following is an example of how more than one conceptual model may need to be used. The stage of human development must be taken into account when developing prevention or health maintenance programs geared to the needs of children and adolescents. In particular, when programming goals suggest the encouragement of moral decision-making, an awareness of developmental theory regarding social, moral, and ethical development is critical. In selecting meaningful and effective learning/teaching strategies and venues, developmental responsiveness must be considered as well. Developmental theory may be combined with a theory or model from health psychology or another health-related discipline to support a community-based health promotion program. Several possible options for these types of theories are described in Chapter 3 in this text.

For many occupational therapists practicing in the field of pediatrics, developmental theory guides goal and objective selection in all settings—a clinic, a hospital, a school, or the wider community. Pediatric occupational therapists should also be aware of other models and theories from related disciplines that may be used in community-based health promotion programming. When constructing programming for children and adolescents, it may also be appropriate to combine behavioral or other approaches or models already in use at a facility with developmental approaches. If the facility is not currently using a specific approach or model, the programmer must be mindful of suggesting and using models that are compatible with the facility's mission and philosophy.

Some practitioners may neglect theory as they develop population-based or community programs by incorrectly assuming, perhaps, that when an intervention is used for prevention, models to guide such work are not necessary. In fact, in the development and execution of prevention programs, theories and models are particularly important. As in all practices, models are utilized to identify what is important and to guide the development of goals and objectives and to guide choices of assessments, programming, and measurement of outcomes. Many theories and models contain diagrammatic representations of constructs and their interrelationships. These schematics, along with written descriptions can assist the program developer in ascertaining relationships and dynamics and in anticipating reactions and responses.

These health promotion theories may move occupational therapists and occupational therapy assistants beyond the individual practice models they typically employ by adding more holistic ways to view the individual within the community.

For example, in trying to understand and articulate the placement of occupation-centered programs in the community, work conducted by occupational scientists may assist the process (Clark, 1993; Clark et al., 1991; Clark, Wood, & Larson, 1998; Yerxa et al., 1990). There are also useful theoretical orientations and models from occupational therapy that can be employed in community programming. Reitz and Scaffa (2001) reviewed four occupational therapy models suited for community health program planning: the Model of Human Occupation, Ecology of Human Performance, Occupational Adaptation, and the Person-Environment Occupational Performance Model. A preliminary selection of a theory or model should occur in Phase I. The choice may be revisited and changed as additional information is gathered through the community profile and as Phase II unfolds.

Searching for Evidence That Programming Will Be Effective

In addition to selecting a theory or model during Phase I, a search of current research on evidence-based outcomes from previous programming efforts directed at the same or a similar population should be conducted. This process is commonly referred to as **evidence-based practice**—searching for evidence that the programming will be effective based on the work of other practitioners and researchers. An awareness of the most recent literature may benefit even the most experienced practitioner and may contribute to improved programming. Lou (2002) proposed that although textbooks cannot keep pace with the evidence required by practitioners, recent advances do make it possible to be an evidence-based practitioner. These advancements include the availability of improved research, enhanced information resources, and more accessible and reliable information technology. While there will always be the benefit of receiving an expert opinion from an experienced practitioner, today's occupation-centered community program developer must be a highly competent information technology user. Content Box 11-3 describes Lou's (2002) steps for collecting evidence.

Formulating a clear, focused question is crucial for conducting evidence-based research. There are a variety of choices of where to search for the answer to

Content Box 11-3

Steps for Acquiring Evidence

1. Define your question by using the three elements: situation, intervention and comparison, and outcome.
2. Select appropriate information sources.
3. Choose the best databases or printed sources.
4. Apply a search strategy using subject terms, keywords, and/or index entries.
5. Modify your strategy to achieve a more efficient search.

From *Evidence-based rehabilitation: A guide to practice* (p. 73), by J. Q. Lou, 2002, Thorofare, NJ: SLACK. Copyright © 2002 by SLACK with permission.

a specific research question. Scholarly publications may include books, journals (peer- and non-peer-reviewed), and professional magazines. A search of electronic bibliographic databases—compilations of published research, scholarly articles, books, newspaper articles, and other such sources—and the Internet may also be helpful. Numerous databases, each with a particular focus, are available. However, the user is cautioned that the content of websites is not always evaluated for scientific rigor. For many conventional occupational therapy practices, MEDLINE is a reliable database offering medically and biomedically related sources.

However, for community programs, where the goal involves maintaining emotional and social health and preventing related dysfunction, answers may not be easily found in the medical and biomedical literature. More suitable databases may include Ovid (AARP, AgeLine), CINAHL (nursing and allied health), HAPI (health and psychosocial instruments), PsychLit, and SocioFile. OTseeker, an online database, provides information on randomized clinical trials that would be of interest to occupational therapists and occupational therapy assistants gathering evidence to direct program development. OT Search, which is an occupational therapy bibliographic system of the American Occupational Therapy Foundation and the AOTA, may also be of assistance.

Evidence for the Potential Effectiveness of the Program: Program Evaluation

A program's ultimate goal is to achieve its desired outcomes. Measuring outcomes is one aspect of program evaluation. At some point during program implementation, programmers must be prepared to answer the following questions:

- Is the program effective?
- Is it doing what it was planned to do?
- Were program goals met?
- Were the stated objectives met?
- Was the program implemented as planned?

Occupation-based programmers must be able to answer these additional questions:

- Were occupation-based methods used?
- Did they enhance the program?
- If so, how?

The evaluation process should begin in earnest when the program objectives are established to meet the identified goal. If the objectives are measurable and accurate in their expression of the goal, it is less likely that problems will be encountered in the evaluation phase. The first measures are most often quantitative. It is necessary to determine who received the services and how often. Without first knowing that everyone has received the programming specified in the objectives, further steps cannot be taken to evaluate whether the services met expectations and were effective.

Qualitative measures of outcome are helpful to measure the quality of the program and may include focus groups or interviews to gain perceptions and opinions from participants regarding the program. These measures may be useful in helping maintain a program participant's enthusiasm and often enhance marketing efforts; however, such methods may not necessarily help ensure objectives are being achieved. Greene (1994) discussed social program evaluation and suggested it may be a unique form of social inquiry. Additional qualitative measures may include observation, ethnography, narrative/storytelling, and numerous other designs and techniques.

According to Greene, and appropriate to many communities, "qualitative methods can give voice to the normally silenced" (1994, p. 541). Since many developing community programs fall into the category of social programming and the populations served may not necessarily advocate for themselves, a comprehensive evaluation that includes both quantitative and qualitative measures is warranted. Evaluation is a continuous process of asking questions and collecting data of all kinds. It is a critical part of all successful programming efforts. There must be a systematic and organized process of collecting, analyzing, and storing data, and this process must be considered when developing the overall program plan.

Methods of Evaluation

There are many ways to evaluate program effectiveness. Forer (1996) described **outcome evaluation** as the method of evaluation that "concentrates on the *results* of services, programs, treatments, or intervention strategies generally following termination of services or during a predetermined follow-up period" (p. ix). The primary goal in all program evaluation efforts is, of course, evaluating the effectiveness of the entire program, including the full array of services. Weiss (1972) emphasized that **program evaluation** is a broader concept than outcome evaluation and suggested that the components of program evaluation be expanded to include not only evaluation of outcomes, but also needs assessment, process evaluation, and program efficiency and effectiveness. It is essential to create congruence between needs, goals and objectives, programming, and outcomes from the beginning of the program-development process.

While programming centers on a community or population, it would be shortsighted to neglect the reality that programs are designed to benefit individuals—members of groups within a community or a population. Therefore, the needs of each individual must be considered, and these needs collectively provide the basis for the program. For most programs, monitoring individual process and progress provides incremental measures that ultimately aid in the evaluation of the full program's effectiveness. Formative measures allow the programmer to know how participants are responding to the program and to see their progress toward goals and objectives. These measures contribute to the **formative evaluation** process described by McKenzie and Smeltzer (1997) as gathering "immediate feedback during program planning and implementation to improve and refine the program" (p. 225).

When occupation-based community-centered programs are evaluated, the following two questions should be asked:

- How will it be determined that the desired occupational behaviors occurred?
- When and how will the occupational behaviors be measured?

All programs must be able to demonstrate effectiveness in order to justify their continued existence. Such evaluation also provides the information that is needed to continue improving the congruence between the goal, objectives, and programming. This is the function of formative evaluation.

Formative evaluation can also include staff and stakeholders. **Stakeholders** are persons who may or may not benefit directly by being involved in the potential program (McKenzie & Smeltzer, 1997) but who have a stake in the program's outcome and often the ability to influence that outcome. Focus groups may be used to gather input from stakeholders and staff. It is generally through a combination of formative measures

that necessary changes can be identified. Day-to-day programming facilitates the achievement of the program objectives and, ultimately, its goal(s). If objectives are not being met, then alterations, adjustments, and fine-tuning may be made in daily programming. If the goal is not satisfied, adjustments of the objectives may be required as well. The results of formative measures are then coupled with those from summative measures that occur at the end of a programming cycle to determine program effectiveness.

Programmers often develop their own assessment instrument(s) based on program goals and objectives. In some cases, they may purchase instruments for individual participants that are designed to accompany the theoretical models selected to guide program development. Some assessments may be copied from texts or articles, while others are copyright protected. Hinojosa and Kramer (1998) have provided an excellent resource for client evaluation. Additional excellent resources by Asher (2007) and Cohn, Schell, and Neistadt (2003) offer comprehensive overviews of evaluation and introduce the reader to detailed chapters describing the evaluation process and specific assessments appropriate to selected areas of practice. Assessment selection should be based on the tool's potential contribution to determine program effectiveness. The program evaluation is linked to the progress individual clients make, so a consistent baseline measure of performance must be included. In some instances, that measure will be made by agencies or practitioners other than the programmer, so efforts are required to access that information when setting objectives.

Other Measurement Considerations

In some programs, neither individual measurement of progress nor traditional models of evaluation and intervention are used. However, an awareness of the progress of individuals and the match between their goals and objectives with those of the program should still be considered. An example of this would be a program targeting the development of moral judgment in adolescents as they prepare to transition into the roles of young adulthood (Fazio, 2001). The goal may specifically target the development of skills to decrease teens breaking the law in the community (e.g., graffiti). Accompanying objectives may focus on skills to find work and a residence or perhaps the provision of opportunity to explore and engage in alternative meaningful occupations. These objectives are measurable and related to outcomes. Not all adolescents participating in such a program may be successful in attaining each objective, and they may not all accomplish the goal; however, it is important to remember that programs may still be successful even if all participants are not (Fazio, 2001).

Case Examples of Program Development and Evaluation

In some cases, new services are developed and implemented within existing programs. In other situations, newly developed programs are free-standing and autonomous. Two examples are provided here, one new service is embedded within an existing school program, and the other is a new program developed in response to an identified community problem.

A New Service Within an Existing Program

An ocean therapy program might be a good fit with the work of school-based therapists by providing a summer program to assist children in maintaining end-of-term achievements in skill and behavior development noted in their Individualized Educational Plans (IEPs). Certainly it would be important to collaborate with both the therapist, who sees the child during the school year, and the parent. The programmer would initiate the evaluation process for the program with the needs assessment, which in turn would guide the selection of the population and the best model to ensure success of the participants and the program. For such a program to be successful, it is assumed that the goals of individuals would be similar enough so that each child would benefit from the group experience.

For example, the ocean therapy camp model could provide intervention to enhance the intervention the child is receiving from the school-based occupational therapist and to assist in meeting the goals of the child. In addition to maintaining existing therapeutic gains and goals, the camp experience might supplement the child's individual therapy with opportunities to learn socialization through structured group experiences, provide opportunities to build confidence and efficacy, as well as other benefits. If this is the case, the programmer might consider establishing baseline measures and continuing formative and summative measures around the goals of socialization, self-confidence, and efficacy. Marketing efforts for such a camp would be enhanced if indicators of success could be demonstrated, in addition to what the child's primary therapist might identify.

A New Program Developed in Response to an Identified Problem

At the request of city health authorities, a Phase I assessment of need was initiated at a mission serving homeless teenagers. The primary identified concern was for the control of sexually transmitted infections (STIs) in the teen population. The solution was initially thought to be condom use, and although condoms were distributed on a regular basis, the rate of STIs had not declined. Following the Phase II focus groups and individual interviews, it was determined that the solution would not be found by focusing on the perceived problem (STIs). Substantial brainstorming, research, and investigation of appropriate theoretical models—including those related to the development of moral judgment, volition, habituation, adaptation, and engagement in occupation—were conducted. As a result, the following goal, objective, and programming were established to respond to the need(s) and to guide program development:

> *Goal:* To advocate for oneself in dating and other relationships, by effecting positive change in one's relationship with the environment (efficacy).
>
> *Objective:* Adolescents participating in the program will be provided with developmentally appropriate information and skills via weekly modules, which they can use to make informed choices about practiced sexual behaviors.
>
> *Programming:* Modules developed to include the acquisition of information and the development of skills structured around the subsystems of volition, habituation, and performance capacity.

Clearly, this brief scenario omits some significant work; however, it depicts how the goal of encouraging self-efficacy was enabled through an objective of providing developmentally appropriate information and skills with which to make informed choices about practiced sexual behaviors. This is very different from distributing condoms. The linkages among efficacy, cognitive and moral development, and sexual-health habits guided the development of a program that provided information and enhanced skills appropriate to adolescents' occupational and developmental needs.

It may appear simplistic to suggest that the first line of program evaluation, the objective measurement of outcome, is identified by the words *be provided with developmentally appropriate information and skills*. A simple attendance/participation grid can be used to evaluate this measure, and data regarding the number of participants who received the information can be obtained. However, little more than this is known from just this measure.

To make the objective measure stronger, pre- and post-tests can be used to determine practiced sexual behaviors, but this still does not really provide the information that will support the merit of continued programming. A traditional research paradigm can be used to track participants to determine how many remain free of STIs over time or how many become established in a transition facility and are no longer homeless. Those who have worked with similar populations know this to be extremely difficult; however, it would likely be an effective measurement of the program's effectiveness and the measure to ensure continued funding for such a program.

Managing numerous outcome measures, particularly over time, will require an effective data-management system and must be considered in the programmer's time and cost planning. Focusing on the development of efficacy, a stronger pre- and post-measure that would provide compelling evidence that the programming had, in fact, helped to achieve this larger goal would be essential. Such instruments as Rotter's (1966) Internal/External Scale would offer a measure of participants' perception of internal versus external locus of control. Rosenberg's (1965) Self-Esteem Scale was initially developed for use with adolescents and would offer a pre- and post-test measurement of positive and negative attitudes toward one's abilities and accomplishments.

Conclusion

This chapter has offered a brief general overview of the process of developing community-based, health-promotion programs that enhance and encourage the practice of meaningful occupations by children, adolescents, and adults of all ages. The role of theory and evidence-based research in program development was presented. Scenarios were used to demonstrate what it means to develop one's idea and how to proceed with needs assessment, including the need to develop goals, objectives, and outcome measures. Resources for the selection of program activities to meet objectives and program goal(s) were identified. A discussion of program evaluation offered suggestions to determine program effectiveness. There are several dimensions, or tiers, of measurement needed to fully evaluate a program. Program evaluation begins with determining the dimensions within which program success will be measured. Staffing, space consideration, funding, development of marketing strategies, and timelines have received only cursory inclusion through examples but are all critical pieces of the program development process.

▶ For Discussion and Review

1. What are you passionate about? From this passion, formulate a program idea and identify a potential community or population who may benefit from an occupation-based program.
2. Is there an unmet health need on your college or university campus? What students from which other disciplines may have a shared interest or potential skills to assist in developing a program to meet this health need?
3. Identify a community or population of interest and develop a needs assessment strategy to determine their health promotion needs.
4. What are the roles of theory and research evidence in the development of health promotion programs?
5. Describe several strategies for formative and summative evaluation of community-based programs.

▶ Research Questions

1. Does an education program contribute to the improved wellbeing of first-time parents?
2. Does a parenting/coping-skill-building program contribute to the improved wellbeing of first-time parents of a child with special needs?
3. Does a community support group contribute to the improved wellbeing of caregivers of spouses who have dementia? Does it increase the amount of time that they can live together in the community?
4. Is the Canadian Occupational Performance Measure (COPM) an effective outcome measure for community-based health promotion programs?

References

Abelson, R., & Brown, P. L. (2002, April, 13). Alternative medicine is finding its niche in nation's hospitals. *New York Times*. Retrieved October 16, 2006, from http://proquest .umi.com.

American Heritage Dictionary of the English Language. Fourth Edition. Retrieved April 26, 2008, from http://dictionary .reference.com/browse/passion.

American Occupational Therapy Association. (1993). Core values statement and attitudes of occupational therapy practice. *American Journal of Occupational Therapy, 47,* 1085–86.

American Occupational Therapy Association. (2008). *Occupational therapy practice framework: Domain and process.* Bethesda, MD: Author.

American Occupational Therapy Association. (2005). American Occupational Therapy Code of Ethics. In *The reference manual of the official documents of the American Occupational Therapy Association, Inc.* (pp. 121–25). Bethesda, MD: Author.

Asher, E. (2007). *Occupational therapy assessment tools: An annotated index* (3d ed.). Bethesda, MD: American Occupational Therapy Association.

Blumberg, D. I., Grant, W. D., Hendricks, S. R., Kamps, C. A., & Dewan, M. J. (1995). The physician and unconventional medicine. *Alternative Therapies, 1*(3), 31–35.

Brownson, C., & Scaffa, M. (2001). Occupational therapy in the promotion of health and the prevention of disease and disability statement. *American Journal of Occupational Therapy, 55*(6), 656–60.

Clark, F. (1993). Occupation embedded in a real life: Interweaving occupational science and occupational therapy. *American Journal of Occupational Therapy, 47,* 1067–78.

Clark, F., Parham, D., Carlson, M., Frank, G., Jackson, J., Pierce, D., Wolfe, R. J., & Zemke, R. (1991). Occupational science: Academic innovation in the service of occupational therapy's future. *American Journal of Occupational Therapy, 45,* 300–10.

Clark, F., Wood, W., & Larson, E. (1998). Occupational science: Occupational therapy's legacy for the 21st century. In M. Neistadt & E. Crepeau (Eds.), *Willard and Spackman's occupational therapy* (9th ed., pp. 13–21). Philadelphia: Lippincott-Raven.

Cohn, E., Schell, B., & Neistadt, M. (2003). Occupational therapy evaluation. In E. Crepeau, E. Cohn, & B. Schell (Eds.), *Willard and Spackman's occupational therapy* (10th ed., pp. 277–447). Philadelphia: Lippincott, Williams & Wilkins.

DiLima, S. N., & Schust, C. (1997). *Community health education and promotion: A guide to program design and evaluation.* Gaithersburg, MD: Aspen.

Eisenberg, D. M., Kessler, R. C., Foster, C., Norlock, F. E., Calkins, D. R., & Delbanco, T. L. (1993). Unconventional medicine in the United States—Prevalence, costs, and patterns of use. *New England Journal of Medicine, 328*(4), 246–52.

Fazio, L. (2001). *Developing occupation-centered programs for the community: A workbook for students and professionals.* Englewood Cliffs, NJ: Prentice Hall.

Forer, S. (1996). *Outcome management and program evaluation made easy: A toolkit for occupational therapy practitioners.* Bethesda, MD: American Occupational Therapy Association.

Gillette, N. P. (1973). Occupational therapy belongs in the community. In L. A. Llorens (Ed.), *Consultation in the community: Occupational therapy in child health* (pp. 127–30). Dubuque, IA: Kendall/Hunt.

Greene, J. C. (1994). Qualitative program evaluation. In N. Denzin & Y. Lincoln (Eds.), *Handbook of qualitative research* (pp. 530–44). Thousand Oaks, CA: Sage.

Hinojosa, J., & Kramer, P. (1998). *Occupational therapy evaluation: Obtaining and interpreting data.* Bethesda, MD: American Occupational Therapy Association.

Kielhofner, G. (2002). *A model of human occupation: Theory and application* (3d. ed.). Philadelphia, PA: Lippincott, Williams & Wilkins.

Kniepmann, K. (1997). Prevention of disability and maintenance of health. In C. Christiansen & C. Baum (Eds.), *Occupational therapy: Enabling function and wellbeing* (pp. 531–53). Thorofare, NJ: SLACK.

Lou, J. Q. (2002). Searching for evidence. In M. Law (Ed.), *Evidence-based rehabilitation* (pp. 71–94). Thorofare, NJ: SLACK.

McKenzie, J. F., & Smeltzer, J. L. (Eds.). (1997). *Planning, implementing, and evaluating health promotion programs: A primer.* Needham Heights, MA: Allyn & Bacon.

Pope, A., & Tarlov, A. (Eds.). (1991). *Disability in America: Toward a national agenda for prevention.* Washington, DC: Institute of Medicine, National Academy Press.

Reed, K. (1998). Theory and frame of reference. In M. Neistadt & E. Crepeau (Eds.), *Willard and Spackman's occupational therapy* (9th ed., pp. 521–24). Philadelphia: Lippincott-Raven.

Reitz, S. M., & Scaffa, M. (2001). Theoretical frameworks for community-based practice. In M. Scaffa (Ed.), *Occupational therapy in community-based practice settings* (pp. 51–84). Philadelphia: F. A. Davis.

Rosenberg, M. (1965). *Society and the adolescent self-image.* Princeton, NJ: Princeton University Press.

Rotter, J. B. (1966). Generalized expectancies for internal versus external control of reinforcement. *Psychological Monographs: General and Applied, 80,* 1–28.

Scaffa, M. (1992). *The development of comprehensive theory in health education: A feasibility study.* Dissertation Abstracts International.

Spencer, J. C. (2003). Evaluation of performance contexts. In E. Crepeau, E. Cohn, & B. Schell (Eds.), *Willard and Spackman's occupational therapy* (10th ed., pp. 427–48). Philadelphia: Lippincott, Williams & Wilkins.

Sultz, H., & Young, K. (2004). *Health care USA: Understanding its organization and delivery.* Sudbury, MA: Jones and Bartlett.

Weiss, C. (1972). *Evaluation research: Methods for assessing program effectiveness.* Englewood Cliffs, NJ: Prentice Hall.

Wilcock, A. A. (1998). *An occupational perspective of health.* Thorofare, NJ: SLACK.

Yerxa, E., Clark, F., Frank, G., Jackson, J., Parham, D., Pierce, D., Stein, C., & Zemke, R. (1990). An introduction to occupational science: A foundation for occupational therapy in the 21st century. *Occupational Therapy in Health Care, 6,* 1–17.

Chapter 12

Enhancing Community Health Through Community Partnerships

Patricia Atwell Rhynders and Marjorie E. Scaffa

The ultimate goal of community health is to enable every member of a community to experience a level of wellbeing that allows participation in, and enjoyment of, his or her chosen daily activities.

—Scaffa & Brownson, 2005, p. 482.

Learning Objectives

This chapter is designed to enable the reader to:

- Describe the characteristics of a healthy community.
- Identify threats to community health.
- Define basic concepts of epidemiology.
- Discuss the principles of community health intervention.

- Identify components of effective community health interventions.
- Apply occupational therapy concepts to the development of community health initiatives.
- Describe the RE-AIM model and how it applies to program evaluation.

Key Terms

Capacity building
Coalition
Collaboration
Community
Community action partnership
Community-based intervention
Community-centered intervention

Community development
Community development partnership
Community health
Community health initiatives
Community-level intervention
Community organization partnership

Comprehensive health promotion
Epidemiology
Health disparities
Health promotion
Health protection
Incidence
Lifestyle
Lifestyle practices
Occupational profile

Prevalence
Prevention
Reciprocal determinism
Resiliency factors
Risk factors
Situational analysis
Social capital
Sustainability
Synergy

Introduction

The increased interest in health promotion and community health in recent decades represents a rebirth of historical beliefs and practices, framed in new terminology and contexts. Despite successes in increasing immunization rates, self-care, and patient education, health education alone to facilitate behavior change is no longer sufficient to address complex health issues. As health educators and other health professionals realized the need to make it easier for people to make healthy choices, they also realized the need for complementary social, political, organizational, regulatory, and economic supports. **Comprehensive health promotion,** defined as the "combination of educational and environmental supports for action and conditions of living conducive to health" (Green & Kreuter, 1991, p. 14), takes place in communities and is a challenging enterprise that requires interdisciplinary expertise.

Traditionally, each discipline is prepared to address a certain aspect of community health. But collaboration among health professionals, in concert with community members, is critical to the success of communit health interventions. Community health merges science (human biology, epidemiology), lifestyle (health education, social and behavioral sciences), and health care (economics, political science); therefore, a continuum of services is necessary to facilitate and support health and wellness (Green & Ottoson, 1999). Occupational therapy is uniquely poised to impact community health, as it encompasses aspects of science, lifestyle, and health care organization. Madill, Townsend, and Schultz suggested that occupational therapists can promote health in the community by playing a role in "improving access to health care, developing an environment conducive to health, strengthening social networks and social supports, promoting positive health behaviour [sic] and coping, and increasing knowledge about health" (1989, p. 79).

Occupational therapists are acutely aware of the need to anticipate trends and develop action plans accordingly (Fazio, 2001; Finn, 1972; Johnson, 1973). Trends in health-care financing have resulted in more acutely and chronically ill persons being treated at home and in community settings. In the 1980s, collaboration was trendy; now it is required by many funding organizations. As the trend toward collaboration with opinion leaders, community members, and other stakeholders gains prominence as best practice in health promotion, occupational therapists will benefit from learning skills in planning, educating, empowering, and advocating broad-based social supports for health-promoting environments (Madill et al., 1989). Occupational therapists are not only important members of the community health team, but also they can play a leadership role in promoting the health of the community. This chapter describes the characteristics of a healthy community, identifies threats to community health, discusses principles and components of effective community health interventions, and examines the role of occupational therapy in the promotion of community health.

sense of purpose. Communities in this sense may be religious, professional, cultural, political, recreational, and myriad others based on groups of people's common bonds.

Another definition of *community,* used in *Healthy People 2010* and more practical for this chapter, is "a specific group of people, often living in a defined geographical area, who share a common culture, values, and norms and who are arranged in a social structure according to relationships the community has developed over a period of time" (U.S. Department of Health & Human Services [USDHHS], 2000, p. 7-27). Even this definition acknowledges that community is more than just a place. It is a dynamic entity that changes and evolves as its people, norms, and values change. This concept of an ever-changing community in which people influence their environment and in which the environment, in turn, influences the people is called **reciprocal determinism,** as depicted in Figure 12-1.

The interaction among people and their environments is an especially important concept in **community health,** which refers to "the extent to which people in a community are able to realize their aspirations, satisfy their needs, and cope with their environment" (Lasker & Weiss, 2003, p. 35). The concept of reciprocal determinism complements the early epidemiological triangle that depicts the interaction among the host, the agent, and the environment in causing and spreading infectious diseases. Many studies have shown the link between community quality, health behaviors, and health outcomes (Molinari, Ahern, & Hendrix, 1998).

According to the American Occupational Therapy Association (AOTA), occupational therapy enables individuals to accomplish the activities of daily living

Community Health

When we think of "community," perhaps we think of our hometown, a cultural group to which we belong, or even the community of scholars and students with whom we associate. Freie (1998) describes it as follows:

> **Community** is an interlocking pattern of just human relationships in which people have at least a minimal sense of consensus within a definable territory. People within a community actively participate and cooperate with others to create their own self-worth, a sense of caring about others, and a feeling for the spirit of connectedness. (p. 23)

This definition characterizes the essence of community not necessarily as a physical place but as a connection that people have formed and a shared

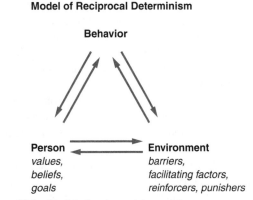

Figure 12-1 Model of reciprocal determinism.

Adapted from "The new causal principle of cognitive learning theory: Perspectives on Bandura's 'Reciprocal Determinism'" by D. C. Phillips & R. Orton, 1983, Psychological Review, 90(2), 158–65.

that have importance to them, specifically those related to the primary occupations of humankind: work, play, education, social participation, and self-care (AOTA, 2008a). These are the very activities that take place within a community; they affect and are affected by the physical, temporal, and cultural environment of that community. By recognizing the dynamic relationships between people and their environments—reciprocal determinism—the range of factors that contribute to or impede health and wellness can be identified. Those insights can then be used to develop appropriate community health promotion interventions.

Because the health of individuals is linked with that of their communities, healthy people in healthy communities is an aim of *Healthy People 2010.* The *Healthy People 2010* document describes a healthy community as one that "embraces the belief that health is more than merely an absence of disease; a healthy community includes those elements that enable people to maintain a high quality of life and productivity" (USDHHS, 2001a, p. 1). The World Health Organization's (WHO) description of a healthy community considers the environmental, social, and economic resources of a community, along with the emotional and physical abilities that allow people to realize their aspirations and satisfy their needs (World Health Organization [WHO], 1986).

Health Disparities

In general, the health of Americans has improved during the past decade, yet in some groups, health indicators have remained stable or have declined. A disproportionate number of Americans in ethnic and racial minority groups lack access to preventive health services and therefore have higher rates of morbidity and mortality than whites. The health status of individuals and populations is affected by several variables, including biological endowment, lifestyle behaviors, and social and environmental circumstances. The diversity in biological, social, ethnic, racial, and economic characteristics among people can result in health disparities. *Healthy People 2010* defines **health disparities** as "differences in health status among distinct segments of the population including differences that occur by gender, race or ethnicity, education or income, disability, and geographic location" (p. 11). Health disparities are well documented. A few examples are provided in Content Box 12-1.

Healthy People 2010 has two broad goals: (1) to increase the quality and years of healthy life and (2) to eliminate health disparities. In seeking to achieve these goals, several of *Healthy People 2010*'s objectives call for "an increase in access to quality health care, an increase in community-based programs that are culturally

and linguistically appropriate, an increase in minority health professional graduates, and improved data gathering to better understand health disparities and service needs" (Wilson, 2006, p. 21). The Centers for Disease Control and Prevention (CDC) initiated REACH 2010 (Racial and Ethnic Approaches to Community Health 2010) to eliminate health disparities among minorities. REACH 2010 identified six priority areas to target: cardiovascular disease, immunizations, breast and cervical cancer, diabetes, HIV/AIDS, and infant mortality.

In addition, racial and ethnic minorities experience greater disability from mental illness than do whites. Minorities do not have higher rates of mental illness than whites, but they do have less access to mental health care. As a result, these populations have a greater frequency of lost workdays and more significant limitations in daily activities than their white counterparts. The social and economic environment of inequality that persons of color experience has a significant negative impact on mental health (USDHHS, 2001b). For more information, see http://www.mentalhealth.org/cre/.

The causes of these disparities are being investigated, but most researchers agree that the etiology is multifactorial and includes biological, socioeconomic, and cultural influences. Cultural norms, beliefs, and practices regarding diet, hygiene, sexual behavior, and illness can significantly impact health

---

Content Box 12-1

Documented Health Disparities

- African Americans have higher infant mortality than whites (MacDorman, Minion, Strobino, & Guyer, 2002)
- African American children living in poverty have higher rates of asthma than white children living in poverty and than black or white children not living in poverty (Akinbami, LaFleur, & Schoendorf, 2002).
- White adolescents have higher rates of death due to unintentional injury than African American adolescents (Anderson, 2002).
- Native Hawaiians are more than two times more likely to develop diabetes than non-Hispanic whites (National Diabetes Information Clearinghouse, 2003).
- African American women are more likely to die of breast cancer than are women of any other racial or ethnic group (Centers for Disease Control and Prevention [CDC], 2008).
- Although African Americans and Hispanics combined represented only 25% of the U.S. population in 1999, they accounted for approximately 55% of adult AIDS cases and 82% of pediatric AIDS cases of the total prevalence reported in that same year (CDC, 2008).

status. Consequently, culture should be considered in the development of community health interventions. In addition, lower socioeconomic status, regardless of other racial or ethnic characteristics, has a negative impact on health and therefore should be targeted specifically (Issel, 2004).

Threats to Community Health

Environmental, social, organizational, and political factors can interfere with the physical and mental health of individuals and families in a community. These threats to community health may include poverty, pollution, crime, violence, and discrimination, among others. One of the functions of **epidemiology** is to identify the health threats in any particular community or population, including the distribution, frequencies, and determinants of disease, injury, and disability in human populations. It serves as the scientific foundation for community health interventions (MacMahon & Trichopoulos, 1996). Epidemiology uses measures of incidence and prevalence to analyze patterns of disease, injury, and disability distribution in communities; identify health trends; develop population health interventions; and make informed health policy decisions (Scaffa, 2001). **Incidence** is a measure of the number of new cases of disease, injury, or disability within a specified time frame. Incidence rates are typically reported in terms of the number of new cases per year per 1000 population (Green & Ottoson, 1999; Pickett & Hanlon, 1990). **Prevalence** is a measure of the total number of cases of disease, injury, or disability that exist in a community at one point in time (Pickett & Hanlon, 1990). Knowing the incidence and prevalence of disease, injury, disability, and death in a population helps to target community health efforts in areas where they can have the greatest impact on health (Green & Ottoson, 1999).

Population Health Strategies

Population health strategies are designed to reduce the incidence rate through prevention activities and reduce the duration of the disease through early detection and effective treatment. Combining the two strategies of prevention and early detection is the most effective approach to reducing overall prevalence. **Prevention** is defined as

> actions and interventions designed to identify risks, and reduce susceptibility or exposure to health threats prior to disease onset (primary prevention), detect and treat disease in early stages to prevent progress or recurrence (secondary prevention), and alleviate the effects of disease and injury (tertiary prevention).

(Joint Committee on Health Education and Promotion Terminology, 2001, p. 101)

Additional population health strategies include health services, health promotion, and health protection. Health services are interventions typically provided by health-care and medical professionals after symptoms are present or a diagnosis is evident. **Health promotion** refers to interventions directed at lifestyle and involves any planned combination of educational, political, regulatory, environmental, and organizational supports for actions and conditions of living conducive to the health of individuals, groups, or communities (Green & Kreuter, 1991). **Health protection** refers to "any planned intervention or services designed to provide individuals and communities with resistance to health threats, often by modifying policy or the environment to decrease potentially harmful interactions" (Green & Ottoson, 1999; Joint Committee on Health Education and Promotion Terminology, 2001, p. 101). The combination of health promotion, health protection, prevention, and early detection strategies provides the most comprehensive approach to community and population health.

Population health interventions often focus on reducing **risk factors,** those lifestyle behaviors or environmental conditions that, on the basis of scientific evidence or theory, are thought to influence susceptibility to a specific health problem (Turnock, 2001). In addition to reducing risk factors, health promotion interventions attempt to increase resiliency or protective factors that contribute to overall health and wellbeing. **Resiliency factors** are those characteristics that appear to increase an individual's or population's ability to avoid the development of disease or disability (Scaffa, 1998).

Community health initiatives are one type of population health intervention. **Community health initiatives** are defined as the public and private efforts of individuals, groups, and organizations to promote, protect, and preserve the physical, psychological, social, and spiritual health of those in the community (McKenzie & Smeltzer, 1997; Scaffa, 2001). Effective community health promotion programs integrate educational, social, and environmental interventions. Educational interventions regarding health can be delivered through schools, workplaces, community organizations, medical care settings, and the media. Social interventions are economic, political, legal, and organizational activities designed to improve the health of the community. Environmental interventions involve physical, chemical, or biological modifications that reduce the risk of acquiring a disease, disability, or injury (Green & Anderson, 1982).

Community Health Interventions

Community-health interventions can be viewed on a continuum, from community-based through community-level to community-centered (Scaffa & Brownson, 2005). **Community-based interventions** refer to providing health services in community settings where people live, work, play, and go to school. These interventions are typically targeted at individuals to encourage health behavior change; however, the family may also be a focus of intervention. In this approach, the professional is the expert and "visits" the community. Services may be provided in a variety of venues, including homes, schools, churches, clinics, libraries, and recreation centers. Examples of this type of intervention are services for home health, community mental health, and assisted living.

Community-level interventions, also sometimes referred to as *community-focused interventions,* are population-based approaches that are designed to facilitate health outcomes through sociocultural, economic, political, and environmental changes. These programs may seek to modify the norms or behaviors of a population in an effort to improve health (e.g., smoking). Community-level interventions are usually based on loose partnerships, and decisions are made by the funding source. In this process, the professional is the expert and leads the community. Examples of this type of intervention are public health programs to reduce smoking, drinking and driving, and sexually transmitted infections.

Community-centered interventions, sometimes referred to as *community-driven,* are also population-based; however, they are initiated by the community itself, using existing resources and seeking additional support as needed. Typically, coalitions are formed to identify common concerns and address community problems. Program planning and evaluation are participatory, and community members develop the intervention strategies. In this model, community members are the experts and the professional serves as a facilitator, consultant, mentor, and educator. An example might be communities along the Gulf Coast after Hurricane Katrina organizing and initiating medical and mental health services for those residents remaining in the region. Each of these types of interventions has appropriate uses depending on the nature of the health problem and the optimal strategies for addressing it (Issel, 2004; Scaffa & Brownson, 2005).

Principles of Community Health Intervention

Research has identified three main principles upon which community health promotion efforts should center:

1. The manner in which social and community institutions are organized and resources distributed is the most important determinant of health in Western societies.
2. The information that community members have as to health determinants and communication channels is as valid as that of the "experts."
3. Identifying and responding to community health needs requires a multilevel, multisectoral, inclusive, participatory, empowering, holistic approach (Raphael, 2003).

The ability of the individual to achieve and maintain health depends upon access to health information and services, choices about health behaviors, and the environmental and social conditions in which they live. Social indicators such as socioeconomic status; education levels; safety; civic involvement; crime rates; family stability; and availability of culture, recreation, and adequate housing are all important influences on the health of a community. In short, these social indicators are the elements that promote a good quality of life.

Therefore, when looking at community health, there is more to consider than simply the medical indicators, such as rates of infant mortality, incidence of diabetes and hypertension, and other medical-model measures. Although those are important concerns, community health also depends on organizations and systems such as public and private health services, schools, faith groups, nonprofit organizations, transportation systems, and economic and political systems. The environment, in terms of availability of and effectiveness of these systems, affects the health of the community, and the health of the community affects the environment. This reciprocal determinism is a cycle that can be influenced by interventions directed toward the people or the systems, but ideally the interventions should be directed toward both. Because this is a daunting task, collaboration is the key to successful comprehensive community health promotion. In fact, Gilfoyle (1986) and Jaffe (1986) identified creative partnerships as opportunities for occupational therapists to assume collaborative leadership roles in designing a healthy society.

Successful health interventions for communities and effective occupational therapy services for individuals share some characteristics in common. Both are client-centered, tailored to specific needs, build on existing resources and strengths, and prepare participants to

Content Box 12-2

Characteristics of Effective Community Interventions

Effective community health interventions

- are tailored to a specific population within a particular setting;
- involve participants in planning, implementation, and evaluation;
- integrate efforts aimed at changing individuals, social and physical environments, communities, and policies;
- link participants' concerns about health to broader life concerns and to a vision of a better society;
- use existing resources within the environment;
- build on strengths found among participants and their social networks and communities;
- advocate for the resources and policy changes needed to achieve the desired health objectives;
- prepare participants to become self-managers and self-advocates;
- support the diffusion of innovation to a wider population;
- seek to "institutionalize" successful components and to replicate them in other settings.

Reproduced with permission from *Occupational therapy in community-based practice settings* by M. Scaffa, 2001, Philadelphia: F. A. Davis.

become self-sufficient. Collaboration is essential for either of these approaches to be efficacious. Other characteristics of effective community health interventions are listed in Content Box 12-2.

Collaboration, Partnerships, and Coalition-Building

Collaboration is a word that is often misused, even with good intentions, to describe the process of people working together toward a common goal. But, more than that, collaboration is part of a continuum that starts with cooperation and builds to a more lasting relationship, or **coalition,** in which people or organizations create a new structure to serve a common purpose while retaining their own identities. Each member brings certain strengths that, when synergistically combined, are greater than the sum of the individual members. **Collaboration** can be defined as "a mutually beneficial and well-defined relationship entered into by two or more organizations to achieve results they are more likely to achieve together than alone" (Winer & Ray, 1994, p. 24). It requires a balance among differing individual and organizational philosophies, modes of service delivery, and sources of power. For individuals and organizations accustomed to the medical model, collaboration involves moving from managing stakeholders—"people

who have a vested interest in the issues"—to viewing stakeholders as equal partners (Brownson, 2001, p. 97).

There are three types of community partnerships: (1) **Community action partnerships** are those that form to address a specific community issue or problem, or to take advantage of a unique opportunity. (2) **Community organization partnerships** are made up of agencies and organizations that provide a similar service or share a common mission. This type of partnership is formed in order to collaborate toward some mutually agreed-upon goals. (3) **Community development partnerships** are designed to encourage participation and collaboration by people, organizations, and agencies to increase community assets and improve the quality of life of the community as a whole (Gamm, 1998).

Because the collaborative approach can accomplish more than an individual one, it makes sense that the greater the diversity of a collaboration's members, the greater their capacity to view issues from different perspectives and to bring different expertise and resources. Broad representation from the community is foremost, but a variety of disciplines, including health professions, sociology, community psychology, political science, public administration, social work, education, law enforcement, urban planning, business, and local government, can also bring unique resources.

Healthy People 2010 is a collaborative effort among federal, state, and territorial governments, in conjunction with private, public, and nonprofit organizations. This is reflected in *Healthy People 2010*'s MAP-IT method of creating a healthy community (USDHHS, 2001a). The *Healthy People in Healthy Communities: A Community Planning Guide Using Healthy People 2010* (USDHHS, 2001a) offers a step-by-step guide for using a collaborative approach to address community health (Content Box 12-3). Effective collaboration for community health requires the professional to build trust, identify community leaders, collect surveillance data, map community assets, and build coalitions. Each of these steps will be described in some detail.

Building Trust

Perhaps the most vital component of community health promotion is trust. Health professionals are accustomed to being recognized as experts, leaders, and resources. In community health, the role of professionals in the community differs from their roles in secondary and tertiary settings, moving from that entails expert to that of equal partner and collaborator. Collaboration entails both costs and benefits. Many organizations are unaccustomed to making collaborative decisions, sharing information, functioning as partners rather than leaders, and recognizing community members as equals. Establishing and maintaining trust includes mutual recognition of the

---

Content Box 12-3

MAP-IT

The *Healthy People in Healthy Communities: A Community Planning Guide Using Healthy People 2010* (USDHHS, 2001a) offers a step-by-step guide for a collaborative approach to address community health as follows:

- **M**obilize individuals and organizations that care about the health of your community into a coalition.
- **A**ssess the areas of greatest need in your community, as well as the resources and other strengths that you can tap into to address those areas.
- **P**lan your approach: Start with a vision of where you want to be as a community, then add strategies and action steps to help you achieve that vision.
- **I**mplement your plan using concrete action steps that can be monitored and will make a difference.
- **T**rack your progress over time.

---

costs and benefits, realistic expectations, and clear goals for the partnership.

Reliability, respect, roles, and rituals are important in establishing trust with community members and other collaborative partners. Reliability demonstrates to the community that a person or agency can be depended upon, honors their word, and is committed to the community's wellbeing. An example is a person or agency maintaining a regular presence in the community by attending and volunteering at events that are important to the community, even if they are not directly related to one's project.

Respect for each member of the coalition is essential. Community residents and informal leaders play as important a role in community health as professionals do. Without their involvement, community health programs will fail. Each member of the coalition should be shown equal consideration.

Roles and expectations should be based on members' special interests and expertise, and must be clarified in order to avoid conflict. Rituals can help solidify the group's identity as a unit by personalizing collaborative work and reminding members of the vision they are trying to achieve. A ritual can be as abstract as beginning each meeting with an inspirational quote or as simple as serving an ethnic snack at each meeting. Create a symbolic custom and make it a tradition.

Identifying Community Leaders

When asked to identify community leaders, many people will list mayors, city council members, police chiefs, and other people who hold similar positions.

These people certainly play a role in creating community environments conducive to health. In reality, though, people are most influenced by peers. In many communities, it is the grandmother who sits on her stoop and watches children play, the shop owner who extends credit to regular customers, or an elder in the church who are recognized as informal community leaders. Faith groups, Neighborhood Watch clubs, parent-teacher associations, and other such groups are comprised of informal community leaders and can help identify other leaders who have broad-based respect. As reliability is demonstrated—for instance, by attending meetings and events in the community, visiting with parents as they bring their children to school, and visiting senior centers and community centers—you will begin to see familiar faces. Recognize these people as community leaders and opinion leaders, and observe the influence they have on their peers.

Collecting Surveillance Data

A good way to approach community health is to identify priorities based on a combination of community interest and data collection. This approach incorporates both support and participation as the means to establish baseline data against which subsequent outcomes can be measured. As recommended in the MAP-IT model, *Healthy People 2010* can provide insight into the leading indicators of health and the issues that may be of concern in a community. Other sources of data are local, county, and state health departments; school records; senior centers; Head Start programs; nonprofit organizations; crime reports; major employers; chambers of commerce; and faith community leaders. In addition to the formal collection of secondary data, collection of primary data via surveys, observations, focus groups, and conversations with people in the community can help assemble a comprehensive picture of the community. These interactions also offer an ideal opportunity to discuss previous community development endeavors and to learn how the community views those programs. Learning about what community members liked and disliked about other programs can help guide program development.

Mapping Assets

Professionals tend to focus on the needs and problems that affect community health, while ignoring the strengths of the community. Deficiency, or needs-oriented, programs create a cycle of client-centered programs that serve people rather than empower them. (Interestingly, the word client is derived from the Greek for "one who is controlled;" McKnight, 1996.)

Yet, communities also possess strengths—assets—that can facilitate community health promotion. Asset-based methods recognize that communities are comprised of people who have competencies and talents and the power of social norms and values. Fulfillment in life depends on whether those gifts can be applied and appreciated (McKnight, 1996). This concept is directly related to the goal of occupational therapy—empowering individuals to accomplish daily life activities that are meaningful to them.

The assets of a community give the community its identity. These assets can be categorized into natural, built, social, economic, and service components (Content Box 12-4) [Canadian Rural Partnership, 2002]). Even the bleakest of neighborhoods has assets in the form of individuals, associations, and institutions. Identifying and mapping them will provide a balanced perspective in an analysis of the community. Recognition of community assets can form the foundation of sustainable community health promotion.

Mapping can begin by simply walking through a neighborhood with a local resident; counting the homes that are well cared for; observing the residents who sit on their porches; noting parks, schools, police and fire stations, shops, churches, childcare providers, employers, bus stops, community gardens, banks, cultural organizations, natural landmarks; and so on. It includes noting which assets are within the control of the community and which are not. For example, individual capacities, churches, and cultural practices are within the control of the community. Hospitals, transportation systems, and public services are not. During the mapping process, also note community needs, such as neglected or abandoned homes, liquor stores, places where litter accumulates, unsafe or inaccessible locations, and graffiti. Some of these needs may become the community's desired focus of their efforts.

Emphasizing assets to overcome needs involves more than making a list of positive aspects of a community.

It is essential to find out what residents value about their community and why. Informal conversations, focus groups, or community meetings are good ways to develop a community profile and to learn about what the residents would like to change. Reflecting on the community's assets while considering ways to effect change is crucial to promoting community engagement in a way that actually strengthens the community's capacity to sustain a health-promoting environment and enjoy a satisfying quality of life.

Building Coalitions

Coalitions bring together members of the community to work for the common good. Coalition partners may include government agencies, advocacy groups, healthcare organizations, educational institutions, and local businesses, among others (Aspen Reference Group, 2000). Each partner brings unique perspectives, skills, and resources to the effort, and the coalition provides a mechanism for community empowerment and capacity development. In addition, coalitions have the potential to use existing resources more efficiently and coordinate services more effectively (Scaffa & Brownson, 2005).

Coalitions are more likely to be sustainable and effective if they are made up of established community organizations rather than temporary, ad hoc task forces. The steps in coalition building are fairly simple and begin with identifying potential coalition members, both individual stakeholders and community agencies. The coalition membership should represent the diversity that exists in the community, and cultural issues should be addressed throughout the process. The next step is for the coalition members to identify and articulate a shared vision for the health of their community. Without a realistic, common goal with defined tasks, the coalition is likely to disband quickly. Credibility and trust, as described earlier, are critical to building relationships among coalition members; without them, effective action is nearly impossible (Issel, 2004).

Coalitions and partnerships can exist at different levels. According to Alter and Hage (1992), the lowest level of partnership, an obligational network, is characterized by simple information exchange across groups and organizations that are members of the coalition. The next level of partnership, the promotional network, collaborates in identifying common problems, solutions, and goals. Each organization retains its autonomy and fulfills a specified role in the coalition. The highest level of partnership, the systemic network, is capable of addressing complex community problems through resource sharing, joint decision-making, and a focus on the greater good rather than on organizational priorities. Each of these partnership levels can be effective, depending on the nature of the community health

---

Content Box 12-4

Categories of Community Assets

- Natural—such as environment, waterways, forests
- Built—physical, such as a community center, church, park, evidence of new construction
- Social—social aspect of living in the community, such as local opinion leaders, youth, and elders with wisdom to share, cultural traditions, history
- Economic—jobs and a varied economy, stores, banks
- Service—such as health, educational, and social services

From *Asset mapping: A handbook* by Canadian Rural Partnership, 2002. Retrieved February 7, 2009, from http://rural.gc.ca/conference/documents/mapping_e.phtml#1.

problem being addressed and the capacity of existing resources to respond.

Coalition building is facilitated by active participation of coalition members; opportunities for formal and informal communication; and establishing roles, division of labor, procedures, and processes early in the coalition's development. In addition, determining mechanisms for conflict resolution, identifying training needs of coalition members, and acquiring needed technical assistance will positively affect coalition function (Parker et al., 1998).

Community Health and Occupational Therapy

Although many models in occupational therapy focus on designing interventions for individuals, Baum, Bass-Haugen, and Christiansen (2005) describe applying the Person-Environment-Occupation-Performance Model to organization- and community-centered interventions. In this model, the person represents intrinsic factors—internal capabilities or constraints on occupation, including physiological, cognitive, spiritual, neurobehavioral, and psychological factors. The environment represents extrinsic factors—environmental enablers or barriers to occupational performance, such as the natural and built environments, culture and values, social support, and social and economic systems. The extrinsic factors impact quality of life, while the intrinsic factors affect wellbeing.

Baum and colleagues (2005) use the term **situational analysis** to capture the multifaceted nature of assessment used in the model. This term is defined as "a process that involves the collection of information and the analysis of factors intrinsic and extrinsic to the individual, the organization or the population to determine the occupational performance issues that will impact the ability to reach client-centered goals" (p. 372). A situational analysis for the purpose of designing community-health interventions would include the following:

- A general description of the population, including health behaviors, disease, injury, and disability incidence and prevalence statistics
- An environmental scan to identify environmental enablers and barriers
- Interviews with stakeholders to ascertain community goals related to health and occupation
- Measures of health status and intrinsic factors to determine the constraints and capabilities for occupational performance
- Measures of occupational participation and community engagement (Baum et al., 2005)

In essence, this is the process of developing an occupational profile and completing an analysis of the occupational performance of a community. According to the *Occupational Therapy Practice Framework: Domain and Process* (referred to as *Framework*; AOTA, 2008a), an **occupational profile** is defined as "information that describes the client's occupational history and experiences, patterns of daily living, interests, values, and needs. Because the profile is designed to gain an understanding of the client's perspective and background, its format varies depending on whether the client is a person, organization, or population" (p. 647). An analysis of occupational performance includes the identification of intrinsic and extrinsic factors that impact occupational participation and community engagement.

After the situational analysis, or client evaluation, has been conducted, an intervention plan can be created in collaboration with community members. The plan should address community priorities and utilize existing resources and community strengths. Intervention approaches may include any combination of the following: create, promote, prevent, educate, consult, compensate, adapt, modify, maintain, remediate, restore, and establish (AOTA, 2008a; Baum et al., 2005). The desired outcomes of community health interventions are consistent with the outcomes of occupational therapy outlined in the *Framework*. These include, but are not limited to, health and wellness, prevention of injury, disease and disability, occupational performance, role competence, adaptation, client satisfaction, and quality of life (AOTA, 2008a). From this discussion, it is clear that the constructs, processes, and outcomes of occupational therapy can be applied to community-health initiatives.

Quality of Life

Quality of life is a goal of *Healthy People 2010* and an aspiration for us all. Quality of life can be defined as "the degree to which a person enjoys the important possibilities of his or her life" (University of Toronto, Centre for Health Promotion, n.d., p. 1). There are social, community, organizational, physical, spiritual, and emotional dimensions to quality of life. These dimensions are interrelated with community assets and with the domains of occupational therapy. According to Johnson (1986), before the mid-19th century, "health was an aspiration of life itself, rather than an outcome" (p. 755). She proposed an expanded description of quality of life as including purpose and meaning, spanning the stages of health over a lifetime. See Chapter 7 for a detailed discussion of quality of life

The Quality of Life Research Unit at the University of Toronto's Centre for Health Promotion has developed a multidimensional, holistic model that applies to persons with and without disabilities. The Quality of Life Model has three life domains: (1) Being, (2) Belonging, and (3) Becoming. These domains complement those of occupational therapy and are applicable across the life stages:

- *Being* includes the physical, psychological, and spiritual dimensions of life. This domain is concerned with physical health, self-esteem, values, and spiritual beliefs.
- *Belonging* describes a sense of connectedness with the physical, social, and community environments. Belonging is assessed within the contexts of home, work, neighborhood, and community. Social belonging (in terms of personal relationships) and community belonging (in terms of access to and availability of leisure, recreation, education, health, and income) are addressed within this domain.
- *Becoming* exemplifies the process of achieving goals and ambitions, of realizing hopes and dreams. There are practical, leisure, and growth facets to becoming that include school, work, or volunteer activities, leisure and stress reduction, self-improvement, and adaptability to change.

A basic tenet of this model is that quality of life results from the meaningfulness the person places upon each domain and the sense of satisfaction the individual has with each dimension. Because it is so personalized, the Quality of Life Model is applicable to the development and fulfillment of participation for all people, regardless of life stage or health status. Just as with the client-centered approach in clinical practice, quality of life must be defined and measured from the client's perspective—in the case of community health, the community is the client.

Promoting Quality of Life Through Occupation

Johnson (1986) engaged the concept of dynamic wellness to enhance therapists' roles in not only assisting clients to adapt to limitations but also to support them in fulfilling their dreams and goals—in other words, quality of life. She tied together the dynamics of occupation with those of wellness and pointed out the key concept that both health and illness are variable states that respond to life and lifestyle modifications. She advocated the compatibility of occupational behavior, knowledge, and skills in assessing clients' habits and lifestyle, with the holistic goal of wellness as a context for living.

In health promotion practice, **lifestyle** refers to the choices individuals make regarding health behaviors.

These behaviors become habits that can be positive or negative. The *Framework* addresses habits as an important aspect of occupational therapy in reestablishing clients' occupational performance after an illness or injury (Youngstrom, 2002a). One strategy employed in health promotion is to support adoption of healthful behaviors. Successful maintenance of such behaviors requires habituation of the practices (Green & Kreuter, 1999). Whether on an individual or community level, occupational therapists' expertise in habitual performance patterns has the potential to enrich health-promotion programs.

Lifestyle practices are no longer viewed as individual behaviors but as "socially conditioned, culturally imbedded, economically constrained patterns of living" (Green & Kreuter, 1991, p. 17). Therefore, lifestyle modification offers the potential for promoting community health. The Well Elderly program (Clark et al., 1997), a landmark study of community-dwelling well elderly, confirmed the value of occupation-based lifestyle redesign in promoting health and improving quality of life. Occupational therapists assumed a role as collaborator rather than as medical-model expert and helped participants habituate healthy occupations. A follow-up study found the effects were sustained without ongoing intervention (Clark et al., 2001). Furthermore, the intervention has been evaluated using health economics research methodologies to calculate the cost-benefits and the quality-of-life value of preventive occupation (Clark, Carlson, Jackson, & Mandel, 2003). The findings were very positive; the average health-care savings exceeded the cost of occupational therapy intervention.

Active learning, or learning by doing, is a component of occupational therapy that can be used to advance quality of life in community health promotion. For instance, occupation can form the basis of community-based nutrition education by incorporating cooking activities to complement didactic lessons. In addition, occupation-based parenting education can be expanded to include health promotion messages that address *Healthy People 2010* indicators such as injury prevention, nutrition, and the impact of environmental tobacco smoke on children and other family members (USDHHS, 2000). Occupation can contribute to the reduction of health disparities, a focus of *Healthy People 2010,* as shown by an interdisciplinary health promotion education program for elders living in public housing communities (Cornely, Elfenbein, & Macias-Moriarty, 2001). Occupation in the form of community volunteerism can use existing communication networks to promote interpersonal relationships and the sharing of health messages.

Promoting Community Health

If there is one overarching theme in community health, it is the notion that professionals and community members must work side by side to achieve the goal of promoting health. As mentioned earlier, the role of equal partner is unfamiliar to many professionals, but it is essential to the success of community health promotion. Community health promotion is most successful when the strategies of capacity building, leadership development, and shared visioning are incorporated. The rich resources of intrinsic knowledge, skills, and abilities held by individuals can enhance the community's capacity to promote health.

Capacity Building

Capacity building in community health is the mobilization of community assets identified during the mapping process—most notably, human and cultural assets—in combination with organizational assets to make the community a healthier place to live. The community's ability to solve problems and strengthen assets must be increased and must be internally focused. The Center for the Advancement of Collaborative Strategies in Health (Lasker & Weiss, 2003, p. 21) has identified three short-term outcomes that must be achieved in order to build the capacity needed for successful collaborative community health efforts: individual empowerment, bridging social ties, and synergy. Individual empowerment and bridging social ties relate directly to improving community health and to building the community's capacity to solve problems. Lasker and Weiss (2003) refer to **synergy** as the breakthrough in thinking and action that occurs when individuals and groups pool their knowledge, skills, and resources in a way that offers an advantage over those of the individual contributors. Synergy promotes creativity; holistic thinking; realistic, pragmatic decision-making; and transformation. The capacity for comprehensive responses to community needs is a highly valued aspect of the synergy of effective partnerships (Lasker, Weiss, & Miller, 2001).

Rather than project-specific activities, community capacity building calls for long-term systemic changes in ways that engage organizations and individuals to participate in identifying and influencing the community's determinants of health. The inclusion of citizens along with both health- and nonhealth-sector participants is a fundamental concept of capacity building. Some of the strategies that make participation easy for diverse groups of stakeholders are holding meetings at times when community members can participate, avoiding technical and medical jargon, and including all participants as full partners with decision-making responsibilities rather than as only advisors. Using existing social networks and their natural communication channels is the most effective way to spread messages among community members.

Health promotion literature (Hawe, Noort, King, & Jordens, 1997) includes descriptions of capacity building in three major categories:

1. Infrastructure to facilitate health service delivery
2. Sustainability of community-based programs after outside funding resources have retreated
3. Problem-solving abilities of communities that help members identify health needs and potential solutions

In other words, occupational therapists can act as catalysts to engage community members as they move from dependency to self-reliance, self-confidence, and self-fulfillment. Occupation, engagement, and participation are as critical to building community capacity as they are to building individual fulfillment.

Leadership Development

Building capacity requires building leadership skills. When building leadership skills, the occupational therapist plays a role strikingly similar to that of the therapeutic relationship in the traditional medical model. Just as the therapist cannot perform rehabilitation exercises for a client, the therapist cannot empower a client or a community. Rather, the therapist facilitates the empowerment process by encouraging the individual (or community) to define the problem, teaching concepts, modeling behaviors and supporting their practice, suggesting adaptations as needed, encouraging continual development, and celebrating achievements.

Empowered people possess adequate knowledge and skills to feel a sense of control over their lives, to make decisions, and to take positive action. Empowerment and leadership development are the desired products of capacity building. More tangible results such as coalition meetings, community cleanup events, community-built playgrounds, and so on, are not the end product in themselves; they are evidence of the community's capacity to mobilize their assets and address local issues. The natural community leaders identified during the early stages of community assessment should play a primary role in any formal training sessions. Basing the training upon the occupational therapy principle of active learning allows community members to demonstrate and practice their new skills.

Leadership development in community health is an ongoing process that requires time and patience. Many of the people in the community are interested in improving the community but have no experience in social action, community change, public speaking, conflict resolution, or bringing their ideas to fruition. The goal of training is to help them adapt to leadership as a new occupation. The occupational therapist can act as a facilitator, guiding self-assessment, self-awareness, and self-advocacy, and encouraging increased social participation. Doing so in the context of leadership training increases both individual and collective capacity to promote change by raising participants' awareness that they can individually and collectively set and achieve goals.

Shared Visioning

Even in the best of circumstances, after having mapped community assets, recruited participants, and empowered leaders, it is not likely that everyone will agree as to what constitutes community health. Bringing the group together to create a shared vision for community health offers an opportunity to reflect on the group's history and its future. Celebrating accomplishments can promote a sense of collective pride and can set the stage for collective visioning.

Storytelling is one strategy to promote visioning. People may not have a list of community health concepts in mind, but they may be able to tell a story of the life they wish to lead in a healthy community. If storytelling is not comfortable for the group, start with a list of questions to guide the discussion. For example, in 5 years, what health-promoting hobbies will people engage in? What opportunities will there be for children, youth, adults, and elders to participate in meaningful recreation? What features of the community will promote physical activity for all? Where will people gather to socialize? What health services will be available? How will people learn about the services? What will we be most proud of in our community? What will visitors notice about our community?

Prioritizing and building consensus are slow processes; hosting a series of community dialogues allows participants to demonstrate their leadership skills in these areas. The fact that people believe they can help shape the future of their community is the benefit of visioning. What the vision *is* isn't the primary concern; it's what the vision *does* that matters (Senge, 1990). Harness the energy of the visioning process by launching small action teams that will work toward specific aspects of the vision. Having results visible to the community will reaffirm the idea that change is possible and will promote more participation.

The study circle is another strategy for bringing people of diverse backgrounds together to develop a vision for community health. Multiple small groups meet regularly throughout the community to share ideas and propose resolutions. The intention of the study circle is not necessarily to reach agreement but to give equal voice to all members. Study circles are facilitated by someone who is neutral and able to promote understanding of differing perspectives. The format usually progresses from a personal experience to sharing different viewpoints to considering strategies for change. Each study circle's ideas are compiled and shared at larger forums as part of the visioning process. Because they concentrate on nonjudgmental dialogue as opposed to judgment-laden discussion, study circles offer participants an opportunity to learn tolerance and communication skills.

Study circles may be issue-specific and time-limited or may adapt to new issues and remain ongoing. Successful study circles have centered on celebrating diversity, creating community for every generation, race relations, education, school improvement, and a host of other issues (Everyday Democracy, 2008). Occupational therapists can facilitate study circles that promote health and help break down barriers to independence through social participation and community-level occupational adaptation.

Opportunities and Challenges

The opportunities for community health promotion are endless, yet challenges are a reality as well. Most significant community health problems are complex and multidimensional and require complex, multidimensional solutions. Most sources of grant funding for community health, including private and public funds, now encourage or require collaboration. The type of professional culture redefinition that is necessary for collaborative action is difficult because of historical roles as "experts," territorialism, competition for funding, and lack of shared terminology. Many agencies "talk the talk but don't walk the walk" of collaboration and community empowerment. Building community trust can be difficult because of underrepresentation of minorities in health professions, historical exploitation of disadvantaged communities, and feelings of helplessness and hopelessness among disenfranchised communities. Furthermore, evaluation of collaborative programs as a shared process is foreign to most disciplines.

Real engagement in community health requires equal participation at all levels—the community members may be unable to do it without help, but professionals cannot do it without the active participation of community members. Everyone who will be affected by the decisions should be included in making them. The diversity of communities challenges practitioners to learn the cultural nuances of health.

As a profession, occupational therapy has adapted to cultural, historical, and technological change (Youngstrom, 2002b). The profession's adoption of the World Health Organization's *International Classification of Functioning, Disability and Health* (WHO, 2001) terminology was one step toward a shared language that positions occupational therapy as a partner among other health-care disciplines. The profession's rich history of holistic assessment and intervention to address the work, play, and self-care habits of individuals within the context of their environments provides a substantive platform for occupational therapists' involvement in community health promotion practice. Identifying issues, problems, and goals that have personal meaning to clients, mobilizing resources and developing, prioritizing, and implementing strategies for reaching those goals are all occupational therapy's role whether working with individuals or communities. Like engagement at the individual level, community engagement depends upon subjective characteristics such as the psychological and emotional aspects of being part of a community and the objective aspects of the community in terms of its physical characteristics. Occupational therapy's focus on participation and engagement as ways to *build skills for the job of living* applies to communities as well as to individuals.

Sustaining Engagement: The Value of Occupation

Sustainability refers to the ability to maintain programs or initiatives long-term. The goal of sustainability is to holistically integrate programs that improve health and quality of life into the fabric of the community. The analogy of a three-legged stool is often used (Lachman, 1997). The legs of the stool represent economic, social, and environmental components, and the seat is sustainability. Without balance among the three legs, the seat falls and sustainability cannot be achieved.

The matter of sustainability is included in Wilcock's explanation of **community development,** which she describes from an occupational therapy point of view as

> community consultation, deliberation, and action to promote individual, family, and community-wide responsibility for self-sustaining development, health, and wellbeing. It is a holistic, participatory model aimed at facilitating a community's social and economic development, based on community analysis, use of local resources, and self-sustaining programs. (Wilcock, 1998, p. 238)

Sustainability is built systematically. Celebrating successes is one way to motivate commitment, which in turn promotes sustainability. Sustainability is an especially acute problem in situations in which a program has been funded and planned by an outside organization and launched in a community without the type of community participation and capacity building discussed throughout this chapter. Once the funding stream changes, these programs often dissolve.

Occupational therapists can offer community partners a unique perspective on sustaining programs and community development. If community health efforts are geared toward *Healthy People 2010* indicators, occupational therapists can frame that goal in terms that are meaningful and have value to community members. For example, promoting physical activity can be difficult with people who do not value exercise programs as part of their activities of daily living or self-care. Framed in context as occupation, though, physical activity may take form as dancing or gardening classes at the community center. Occupational deprivation can be addressed through community development and capacity building by increasing access to public transportation or creating safe places to play, walk, and socialize. Occupational alienation may be at the core of substance abuse and crime issues in a community; promoting occupational balance is an important contribution to building the community's capacity for health. Promoting social participation and use of leisure time can foster neighborliness and trusting relationships.

By now, it should be obvious that community health is a collaborative effort. It cannot be achieved without building and sustaining partnerships. Partnerships at individual and organizational levels depend upon **social capital,** which is defined as "the features of social organization, such as networks, norms and trust, that facilitate coordination and cooperation for mutual benefit" (Putnam, 1993, ¶ 4). Putnam has found that social capital is vital for economic development, effective government, coordination, and communication. Social capital, trust, norms, and networks play a role in reciprocal determinism of the community. Trust and cooperation foster trust and cooperation; success in one partnership reinforces the value of partnerships in general. As social capital is used, it builds upon itself, creating more social capital and strengthening the fabric of the community.

Examples of Community Health Initiatives

Organization-Based

An example of a partnership for community health is the AOTA relationship with Rebuilding Together (AOTA, 2008b). Rebuilding Together is a nonprofit organization whose goal is to preserve and revitalize houses and communities, assuring that low-income homeowners, particularly those who are elderly and disabled and families with children, live in warmth, safety, and independence (Rebuilding Together, 2008). They are neighbors helping neighbors, building social capital and creating an environment conducive to health. Successful partnerships benefit all involved. In addition to the benefit to the community, this particular partnership benefits occupational therapy. The AOTA lists the following as benefits: broadening public awareness of the need for home modification and occupational therapy's role in doing so, building stronger foundations for other community partnerships, and increasing options for expanded practice opportunities.

Community-Based

The "Wellness in Tillery" project undertaken by East Carolina University's occupational therapy faculty and students presents an excellent model of capacity building using occupation-based health promotion in a community of African American elders (Barnard et al., 2004). Community members were included as full partners throughout the needs assessment, program design and implementation, and evaluation phases. The ultimate goal was for the community to maintain the program after the initial project concluded. In order to build the project team members' capacity, participants assumed responsibility for documenting sessions' activities, and students compiled scrapbooks that would later serve as a leaders' guide for replicating the program. Additionally, a "wellness toolkit" including all materials, games, and music used throughout the program was donated to the community center where the program was held.

Evaluation of Community Health Interventions

Community-based health promotion efforts have demonstrated varying degrees of success. More research is needed to identify the factors that make these programs effective. Historically, the most effective outcomes have been achieved by HIV-prevention programs. The characteristics of these programs that seem to influence their success are:

- an emphasis on changing social norms regarding risky behaviors;
- engaging community peers as health educators;
- tailoring the intervention to specific subpopulations and local contexts;
- extensive formative evaluation throughout the needs assessment, intervention development, and implementation process in order to make mid-course corrections as needed (Merzel & D'Afflitti, 2003).

One framework for evaluating the processes, impacts, and outcomes of community health partnerships is RE-AIM (Content Box 12-5). According to Glasgow, Vogt, and Boles (1999), "the ultimate impact of an intervention is due to its combined effects on [these] 5 evaluative dimensions" (p. 1323).

Reach indicates the degree to which the intervention reaches those in need; it is measured by the number and characteristics of people who participate in or who are affected by a program or policy. The number and characteristics of the participants are then compared with the demographics of the target population to determine the program's reach.

Efficacy refers to the positive consequences or benefits of participating in the program. It is calculated by subtracting the unanticipated negative consequences of the intervention from its positive outcomes. Typically, efficacy measures include physiological markers of health, evidence of behavioral and lifestyle modification, quality-of-life indicators, and participant satisfaction ratings.

Adoption refers to the percentage and representativeness of settings, organizations, and agencies that implement the program or policy. Adoption of any innovation follows a predictable pattern. Assessing the reasons for failure to adopt is critical for future program modification (Glasgow et al., 1999).

Implementation is a measure of the degree to which a program or policy was provided, delivered, or implemented as intended. Assessment of implementation answers the questions of who, what, where, when, and how the intervention took place. Implementation indicates the level of fidelity to the program plan.

The final aspect to program evaluation is *maintenance,* or the extent to which the program or policy is routinized, adhered to, or sustained over time. It also "measures the extent to which innovations become a relatively stable, enduring part of the behavioral repertoire of an individual or organization or community" (Glasgow et al., 1999, p. 3).

The purpose of the RE-AIM Model is to broaden the evaluation of interventions from an exclusive focus on efficacy to identifying the characteristics that make a

---

Content Box 12-5

The RE-AIM Model

R Reach
E Efficacy
A Adoption
I Implementation
M Maintenance

program effective in real-world environments. This approach is compatible with social ecological and systems theories. A program may be highly efficacious but have very limited reach, a low level of adoption (possibly due to cost), and an inability to sustain itself. The RE-AIM framework provides decision-makers with more comprehensive information on the overall effectiveness and impact of community health interventions.

Conclusion

It can be asserted that the greatest resource of any society is a healthy population. Unfortunately, many of the prevalent social problems of today have significant negative consequences on health—for example, homelessness, substance abuse, mental illness, violence, and accidents. These social problems can be addressed from a community health promotion perspective. However, no one discipline, organization, or agency can effect community change alone. Real, lasting change requires partnerships. Kickbusch (1997) emphasizes the importance of community partnerships and the impact of social issues on health outcomes:

> In my view, health promotion outcomes are measures that show that the determinants of positive health have been strengthened within a given nation, community and/or setting. They are those elements which contribute to the health, quality of life, and social capital of a society. And they can only be "produced" by an organized, partnership-based community effort. This is a significant shift that looks not only at how other sectors produce health, but also at the wider societal contribution of the health sector. The concern of societies will increasingly be social not physical health. (p. 267)

One of the goals outlined in the official AOTA (2007) document *Occupational Therapy in the Promotion of Health and the Prevention of Disease and Disability Statement* is to promote "healthy living practices, social participation, occupational justice, and healthy communities" (p. 2). Three major roles for occupational therapy in health promotion were also identified. These include

- promoting healthy lifestyles for all clients, patients, their caregivers, and families;
- incorporating occupation as an essential feature of health promotion programs; and
- providing health promotion interventions with individuals and populations.

Clearly, it is within occupational therapy's purview to plan, develop, and participate in community health interventions.

Following the guiding principles of the profession, occupational therapy practitioners can help people create habits that promote health in a community context; they can help people establish roles as community leaders and advocates; and they can help people come together to develop community performance patterns that sustain health. Ultimately, the sustainability of community health must be under the control of the community. This, too, is in keeping with occupational therapy's foundations, as the goal is to release control to the client/community and to be flexible and responsive in meeting their changing needs. Demonstrating the efficacy of occupational therapy in community health promotion will require identifying occupational factors that impact health and wellbeing, developing assessment tools that measure these factors, and evaluating occupation-based health promotion services in a variety of settings with a variety of populations.

▶ For Discussion and Review

1. What does *community* mean to you? What communities do you belong to? Do you know who the leaders are in those communities?
2. How does the *Framework*'s alignment of occupation with the *International Classification of Functioning*'s focus on functional engagement in life relate to reciprocal determinism?
3. Discuss ways to demonstrate reliability, respect, roles, and rituals when establishing trust with community members and other collaborative partners.
4. What does *quality of life* mean to you? How do you achieve it? As an individual, how do you contribute to the quality of life in your community? As an occupational therapist, how will you contribute to the quality of life in your community?
5. Describe your vision for a healthy community. Use the following questions to guide your discussion: What health-promoting hobbies will people engage in? What opportunities will there be for children, youth, adults, and elders to participate in meaningful recreation? What features of the community will promote physical activity for all? Where will people gather to socialize? What health services will be available? How will people learn about the services? What will you be most proud of in your community? What will visitors notice about your community?
6. How can occupational therapists help communities meet the *Healthy People 2010* objectives? Have you been involved in any activities related to the *Healthy People 2010* objectives?

▶ Research Questions

1. How do health disparities impact occupational performance?
2. What is the relationship between occupational deprivation and quality of life?
3. Which occupational therapy assessments are most useful in developing occupational profiles of communities?
4. Are occupation-based community health interventions more effective than interventions without an occupation-based component?
5. What are the occupational factors that impact community health and wellbeing?

References

Akinbami, L. J., LaFleur, B. J., & Schoendorf, K. C. (2002). Racial and income disparities in children with asthma in the United States. *Ambulatory Pediatrics, 2,* 382–87.

Alter, C., & Hage, J. (1992). *Organizations working together: Coordination in interorganizational networks.* Newbury Park, CA: Sage.

American Occupational Therapy Association. (2007). *Occupational therapy in the promotion of health and the prevention of disease and disability statement.* Retrieved February 20, 2008, from http://www.aota.org/Practitioners/Resources/Docs/Official.aspx.

American Occupational Therapy Association. (2008a). Occupational therapy practice framework: Domain and process (2d ed.). *American Journal of Occupational Therapy, 62*(6) 625–83.

American Occupational Therapy Association. (2008b). *AOTA & Rebuilding Together.* Retrieved February 7, 2009, from http://www.promoteot.org/AI_BGInfo.html.

Anderson, R. (2002). Deaths: Leading causes for 2000. *National Vital Statistics Report, 50*(16), 7–17.

Aspen Reference Group. (2000). *Community health: Education and promotion manual.* Gaithersburg, MD: Aspen.

Barnard, S., Dunn, S., Reddic, E., Rhodes, K., et al. (2004). Wellness in Tillery: A community-built program. *Family and Community Health, 27*(2), 151–57.

Baum, C. M., Bass-Haugen, J., & Christiansen, C. H. (2005). Person-environment-occupation-performance: A model for planning interventions for individuals and organizations. In C. H. Christiansen, C. M. Baum, & J. Bass-Haugen (Eds.), *Occupational therapy: Performance, participation and wellbeing* (3d ed.). Thorofare, NJ: SLACK.

Brownson, C. A. (2001). Program development for community health: Planning, implementation and evaluation strategies. In M. Scaffa (Ed.), *Occupational therapy in community-based practice settings.* Philadelphia: F. A. Davis.

Canadian Rural Partnership. (2002). *Asset mapping: A handbook.* Retrieved February 7, 2009, from http://rural.gc.ca/conference/documents/mapping_e.phtml#1.

Centers for Disease Control and Prevention. (2008). *Racial and ethnic approaches to community health.* Retrieved February 7, 2009, from http://www.cdc.gov/reach/.

Clark, F., Azen, S., Carlson, M., Mandel, D., et al. (2001). Embedding health-promoting changes into the daily lives of independent-living older adults: Long-term follow-up of occupational therapy intervention. *Journal of Gerontology, 56B*(1), 60–63.

Clark, F., Azen, S. P., Zemke, R., Jackson, J., Carlson, M., Mandel, D., et al. (1997). Occupational therapy for independent-living older adults: A randomized controlled trial. *Journal of the American Medical Association, 278,* 1321–26.

Clark, F. A., Carlson, M., Jackson, J., & Mandel, D. (2003). Lifestyle redesign improves health and is cost-effective. *OT Practice, 8*(2), 9–13.

Cornely, H., Elfenbein, P., & Macias-Moriarity, L. (2001). Interdisciplinary health promotion education for low income older adults. *Journal of Physical Therapy Education, 15,* 37–41.

Everyday Democracy. (2008). *Profiles of successful study circle programs strengthening neighborhoods.* Retrieved February 7, 2009, from http://www.everyday-democracy.org//en/Article.295.aspx.

Fazio, L. (2001). *Developing occupation-centered programs for the community: A workbook for students and professionals.* Upper Saddle River, NJ: Prentice-Hall.

Finn, G. (1972). The occupational therapist in prevention programs. *American Journal of Occupational Therapy, 26,* 59–66.

Freie, J. F. (1998). *Counterfeit community: The exploitation of our longings for connectedness.* Lanham, MD: Rowman & Littlefield.

Gamm, L. D. (1998). Advancing community health through community health partnerships. *Journal of Healthcare Management, 43*(1), 51–66.

Gilfoyle, E. M. (1986). Professional directions: Management in action (presidential address). *American Journal of Occupational Therapy, 40,* 593–96.

Glasgow, R. E., Vogt, T. M., & Boles, S. M. (1999). Evaluating the public health impact of health promotion interventions: The RE-AIM framework. *American Journal of Public Health, 89*(9), 1322–27.

Green, L. W., & Anderson, C. L. (1982). *Community health.* St. Louis, MO: Mosby.

Green, L. W., & Kreuter, M. (1991). *Health promotion planning: An educational and environmental approach* (2d ed.). Mountain View, CA: Mayfield.

Green, L. W., & Kreuter, M. (1999). *Health promotion planning: An educational and ecological approach* (3d ed.). Mountain View, CA: Mayfield.

Green, L. W., & Ottoson, J. M. (1999). *Community and population health* (8th ed.). Boston: WCB/McGraw-Hill.

Hawe, P., Noort, M., King, L., & Jordens, C. (1997). Multiplying health gains: The critical role of capacity-building within health promotion programs. *Health Policy 39,* 29–42.

Issel, L. M. (2004). *Health program planning and evaluation: A practical, systematic approach for community health.* Boston: Jones and Bartlett.

Jaffe, E. (1986). The role of occupational therapy in disease prevention and health promotion. *American Journal of Occupational Therapy, 40,* 749–52.

Johnson, J. (1973). Occupational therapy: A model for the future. *American Journal of Occupational Therapy, 27,* 229–45.

Johnson, J. (1986). Wellness and occupational therapy. *American Journal of Occupational Therapy, 40,* 753–58.

Joint Committee on Health Education and Promotion Terminology. (2001). Report of the 2000 joint committee on health education and promotion terminology. *American Journal of Health Education, 32*(2), 90–103.

Kickbusch, I. (1997). Think health: What makes the difference? *Health Promotion International, 12*(4), 265–72.

Lachman, B. (1997). *Linking sustainable community activities to pollution prevention: A sourcebook.* MR-855-OSTP, Santa Monica, CA: RAND Corporation.

Lasker, R., & Weiss, E. (2003). Broadening participation in community problem solving: A multidisciplinary model to support collaborative practice and research. *Journal of Urban Health, 80,* 14–47.

Lasker, R., Weiss, E., & Miller, R. (2001). Partnership synergy: A practical framework for studying and strengthening the collaborative advantage. *Millbank Quarterly, 79*(2), 179–205.

MacDorman, M. F., Minion, A. M., Strobino, D. M., & Guyer, B. (2002). Annual summary of vital statistics: 2001. *Pediatrics, 110,* 1037–52.

MacMahon, B., & Trichopoulos, D. (1996). *Epidemiology principles and methods.* Boston: Little, Brown.

Madill, H., Townsend, E., & Schultz, P. (1989). Implementing a health promotion strategy in occupational therapy education and practice. *Canadian Journal of Occupational Therapy, 56,* 67–72.

McKenzie, J. F., & Smeltzer, J. L. (1997). *Planning, implementing and evaluating health promotion programs: A primer* (2d ed.). Boston: Allyn & Bacon.

McKnight, J. L. (1996). *A twenty-first century map for healthy communities and families.* Institute for Policy Research: Author.

Merzel, C., & D'Afflitti, J. (2003). Reconsidering community-based health promotion: Promise, performance and potential. *American Journal of Public Health, 93*(4), 557–74.

Molinari, C., Ahern, M., & Hendrix, M. (1998). Gains from public-private collaborations to improve community health. *Journal of Healthcare Management, 43,* 498–511.

National Diabetes Information Clearinghouse. (2003). *National diabetes statistics.* Retrieved October 30, 2006, from http://diabetes.niddk.nih.gov/dm/pubs/statistics/index.htm.

Parker, E. A., Eng, E., Laraia, B., Ammerman, A., Dodds, J., Margolis, L., et al. (1998). Coalition building for prevention. *Journal of Public Health Management Practice, 4*(20), 25–36.

Phillips, D. C., & Orton, R. (1983). The new causal principle of cognitive learning theory: Perspectives on Bandura's "Reciprocal Determinism." *Psychological Review, 90*(2), 158–65.

Pickett, G., & Hanlon, J. J. (1990). *Public health: Administration and practice.* St. Louis, MO: Times Mirror/Mosby.

Putnam, R. D. (1993). The prosperous community: Social capital and public life. *American Prospect, 4*(13). Retrieved September 10, 2006, from http://www.prospect.org/archives.

Raphael, D. (2003). Toward the future: Policy and community actions to promote population health. In R. Hofrichter (Ed.), *Health and social justice* (pp. 453–68). San Francisco: Jossey-Bass.

Rebuilding Together. (2008). *About us.* Retrieved February 7, 2009, from http://www.rebuildingtogether.org/section/about/.

Scaffa. M. (1998). Adolescents and alcohol use. In A. Henderson, S. Champlin, & W. Evashwick (Eds.), *Promoting teen health: Linking schools, health organizations and community.* Thousand Oaks, CA: Sage.

Scaffa, M. (2001). *Occupational therapy in community-based practice settings.* Philadelphia: F. A. Davis.

Scaffa, M. E., & Brownson, C. (2005). Occupational therapy interventions: Community health approaches. In C. H. Christiansen, C. M. Baum, & J. Bass-Haugen (Eds.), *Occupational therapy: Performance, participation and wellbeing* (3d ed.). Thorofare, NJ: SLACK.

Senge, P. (1990). *The fifth discipline: The art & practice of the learning organization.* New York: Doubleday.

Turnock, B. J. (2001). *Public health: What it is and how it works.* Gaithersburg, MD: Aspen.

University of Toronto, Centre for Health Promotion. (n.d.). *The quality of life model.* Retrieved February 7, 2009 from http://www.utoronto.ca/qol/concepts.htm

U.S. Department of Health & Human Services. (2000). *Healthy People 2010* (2d ed.). 2 vols. Washington, DC: U.S. Government Printing Office.

U.S. Department of Health & Human Services. (2001a). Healthy people in healthy communities: A community planning guide using *Healthy People 2010.* Retrieved August 21, 2004, from http://healthypeople.gov/Publications/HealthyCommunities2001/toc.htm.

U.S. Department of Health and Human Services. (2001b). *Mental health: Culture, race, and ethnicity—A supplement to mental health: A report of the Surgeon General.* Rockville, MD: U.S. Department of Health and Human Services, Substance Abuse and Mental Health Services Administration, Center for Mental Health Services.

Wilcock, A. (1998). *An occupational perspective of health.* Thorofare, NJ: SLACK.

Wilson, L. S. (2006). A call for diversity awareness and cultural competency. *OT Practice, 11*(19), 21, 24.

Winer, M., & Ray, K. (1994). *Collaboration handbook: Creating, sustaining and enjoying the journey.* St. Paul, MN: Amherst H. Wilder Foundation. ERIC document #ED390759, retrieved August 1, 2007, from http://www.eric.ed.gov.

World Health Organization. (1986). A discussion document on the concept and principles of health promotion. *Health Promotion, 1,* 73–78.

World Health Organization. (2001). *International classification of functioning, disability and health.* Geneva, Switzerland: Author.

Youngstrom, M. J. (2002a, September). Introduction to the occupational therapy practice framework: Domain and process. *OT Practice,* CE1–CE7.

Youngstrom, M. J. (2002b). The occupational therapy practice framework: The evolution of our professional language. *American Journal of Occupational Therapy, 56,* 607–608.

Occupational Therapy's Contributions to Health Behavior Interventions

Chapter 13

Promoting Exercise and Physical Activity

S. Maggie Reitz

Physical inactivity is estimated to cause 2 million deaths worldwide annually. Globally, it is estimated to cause about 10–16% of cases each of breast cancer, colon cancers, and diabetes, and about 22% of ischaemic heart disease. Estimated attributable fractions are similar in men and women. Opportunities for people to be physically active exist in the four major domains of their day.

These are:

• At work (whether or not the work involves manual labour)
• For transport (walking or cycling to work, to shop etc)
• During domestic duties (housework, gathering fuel etc)
• In leisure time (sports and recreational activities)

—World Health Organization (WHO), 2006b, ¶ 3

Learning Objectives

This chapter is designed to enable the reader to:

• Discuss the history of organizations and international events promoting engagement in exercise and physical activity.
• Detail health risks associated with physical inactivity and health benefits of engaging in physical activity across the life span.
• Use national physical activity level data to foster support for occupational therapy interventions geared toward increasing physical activity levels among individuals with and without disabilities, families, and communities.

• Discuss the historical role and research within occupational therapy regarding engagement in physical activity as a healthy occupation.
• Discuss assessment and intervention approaches.
• Identify the benefits of interdisciplinary programming to facilitate engagement in occupations that promote physical activity.

Key Terms

Active Community
  Environments
  Initiative (ACES)

Barriers

Fitness ethic

Physical activity

Self-presentational
  concerns

Introduction

In this chapter, methods to facilitate a fitness ethic and engagement in physically active occupations among individuals, families, communities, and populations are

described. The discussion begins with a review of the Olympics and the historical use of organized physical activity within and between nations. The establishment of a governmental organization in the United States to promote health and wellbeing through exercise and physical activity is then reviewed. Next, current terminology connected with physical activity, and national health objectives related to physical activity levels included in *Healthy People 2010: Understanding and Improving Health* (U.S. Department of Health and Human Services [USDHHS], 2000) are identified. Prevalence rates of physical activity in various countries, including the United States, also will be presented. This will be followed by a brief review of barriers to participation and threats to health resulting from physical inactivity.

After introducing the recommended levels of physical activity to promote health, a variety of programs to facilitate achieving these recommended levels are described. This review will include interventions for individuals with and without disabilities, families, and communities. A brief historical examination of the role of occupational therapy in promoting exercise and physical activity follows. The discussion of the current and future possible role of occupational therapy in this area will incorporate the language detailed in the *International Classification of Functioning, Disability, and Health (ICF),* developed by the World Health Organization (WHO) in 2001, and the *Occupational Therapy Practice Framework* (referred to as *Framework)* (American Occupational Therapy Association [AOTA], 2008). An example of an interdisciplinary grant-supported health promotion program to increase physical activity among older adults also is described.

Historical Trends

In this section, the development of events and governmental actions to promote physical activity and fitness will be traced through time. The term **fitness ethic** was specifically developed for this chapter to convey a perspective that highly values physical fitness and activity. The importance of a fitness ethic in the prevention of disease and injury has been promoted since the time of Hippocrates (460–377 BC):

> All parts of the body which have a function, if used in moderation and exercised in labours in which each is accustomed, become thereby healthy, well-developed and age more slowly, but if unused and left idle they become liable to disease, defective in growth, and age quickly. (Jones as cited by Levin, 2001, p. 28)

The three examples that follow include the Olympics, the evolution of the U.S. President's Council on Youth Fitness, and U.S. National Health Objectives.

Olympics

The first Olympiad was held in 776 BC on the Olympia plains in Greece and, as with those that followed, was dedicated to the Olympian gods. The games were also held for a variety of nonreligious reasons, including promoting a fitness ethic, showcasing the physical qualities and performances of youth, and encouraging civil relationships among the cities of Greece. Beginning around the 9th century BC, a formal truce between disputing factions was instituted as part of the ancient games and has been reintroduced to the modern games. The ancient games continued for nearly 12 centuries until banned by Emperor Theodosius in AD 393 due to their connection to pagan cults (International Olympic Committee [IOC], 2005b).

In 1896, the Olympic Games were reintroduced as an international event. During the late 1800s, several factors converged to revive interest in a fitness ethic and international competition, including improved transportation and communication between countries, the growing number of international literary and scientific congresses, and a determination to transform rivalry into "noble competition" (Foundation of the Hellenic World, 2005, ¶ 2). The United States and 13 other countries participated in the 1896 Olympic Games in Athens, Greece, with the greatest number of athletes coming from Greece, Germany, France, and the United Kingdom (IOC, 2005c). Women first competed in the modern games in Paris, France, in 1900, in which the number of competing countries had increased to 24 (IOC, 2005d).

The games have continued to grow over the years, with the Winter Olympics being added in 1924 (IOC, 2005a) and the Paralympic Games added in 1952 (IOC, 2006). The most recent Winter and Paralympic Games were held in Italy. Over 35,000 spectators were present for the opening ceremonies of the XX Torino 2006 Olympic Winter Games. An estimated 2 billion people around the globe viewed broadcasts of the ceremony (Torino, 2006b). A total of 252 medals were awarded to 26 different countries at these games, which were held in several venues in Italy (Torino, 2006a). The 84 gold medals awarded were conferred upon athletes from 18 nations. During the 2008 Summer Games in Beijing, China, athletes from 81 countries received a total of 958 medals, 302 of them gold (Beijing Organizing Committee, n.d.).

The Olympics have not always been positive events that promote global wellbeing. They have been used as an opportunity for terrorist attacks, as seen in the brutal murder of Israeli athletes at the Munich Games in 1972 and the Atlanta Games bombing in 1996. The games also have been used for political leverage, such as when the United States chose to boycott the Olympics hosted by the former Soviet Union after the Soviet invasion of Afghanistan (Kindersley, 1996). While these unfortunate events were attempts to misuse the Olympics, the games remain the most recognized form of global goodwill. They remain a prime example of a macro-level occupation that promotes a fitness ethic as well as global cooperation and communication.

The President's Council on Physical Fitness and Sports (PCPFS)

Since the mid-1950s, U.S. presidents have been committed to enhancing a fitness ethic and thereby increasing the physical activity level of U.S. citizens (PCPFS, USDHHS, 2004). In 1956, concerned about research findings that showed U.S. youth falling behind their European counterparts in terms of fitness, President Eisenhower established the President's Council on Youth Fitness. In 1963, President Kennedy broadened the scope of the council to address U.S. citizens of all ages; to reflect this increased scope, its name was changed to the President's Council on Physical Fitness. The word *sports* was added to the council's name in 1966 by President Lyndon B. Johnson "to emphasize the importance of sports participation throughout life" (PCPFS, USDHHS, 2004, ¶ 2).

Through the years, the PCPFS has worked with the president to support and develop a variety of resources and activities to promote a fitness ethic and civil sports competition. On June 20, 2002, President Bush announced a new initiative called *HealthierUS*. The event, which was held on the White House lawn, included many examples of and opportunities for physical activity, including a climbing wall, batting cage, and aerobics (PCPFS, USDHHS, 2002). Content Box 13-1 displays the "four pillars" of the Healthier US program. (Details regarding progress toward the objectives of this public health initiative are provided at http://wonder.cdc.gov/data 2010/HU.HTM [Centers for Disease Control and Prevention {CDC}, 2006d].) Another initiative to use technology as a tool to promote physical activity was launched in 2003 with the unveiling of the PCPFS interactive website in Dallas, Texas). Other recent and long-standing initiatives of the PCPFS include the President's Challenge Physical Activity and Fitness Award Program, the Presidential Active Lifestyle Award (PALA), the State Champion Award, the National Student Demonstration Program, Steps to a HealthierUS, "May Month"—National Physical Fitness and Sports Month, the PCPFS Research Digest, and partnerships with various businesses and organizations to promote physical activity (PCPFS, USDHHS, 2004). The President's Challenge Physical Activity and Fitness Award Program provides incentives for people of all ages and abilities to become physically active. The corresponding website provides teachers guidance on providing accommodations to students with disabilities (Content Box 13-2).

Content Box 13-1

Four Pillars of HealthierUS

- Be physically active every day
- Eat a nutritious diet
- Get preventive screenings
- Make healthy choices/avoid risky behavior

From *About the President's Council on Physical Fitness and Sports,* by the President's Council on Physical Fitness and Sports, U.S. Department of Health and Human Services, 2004, p. 11.

Content Box 13-2

Suggested Accommodations for the President's Challenge Programs

With a little consideration and flexibility, any student can qualify for any of the President's Challenge programs. Making accommodations is consistent with the goal of motivating students for lifelong physical activity by recognizing their achievements. Using their professional judgment, trained instructors may qualify students who do not reach PCPFS standards in a given program. We recommend the following guidelines:

1. Review the individual's records to identify medical, orthopedic, or other health problems that should be considered prior to participation in physical activities, including physical fitness testing.
2. Determine whether the individual has a disability or other problem that adversely affects performance on one or more test items.
3. Consider whether the individual has been participating in an appropriate physical fitness program that develops and maintains cardiorespiratory endurance, muscular strength and endurance, flexibility, and body composition.
4. Administer the President's Challenge program, making modifications as needed or substituting alternate events or activities.
5. After completing the program, decide if the individual has performed at a level equivalent to a President's Challenge award.

If you have questions about these guidelines, you can call us toll-free at 800-258-8146.

From *The President's Challenge: Accommodating students with disabilities* by the President's Council on Physical Fitness and Sports, U.S. Department of Health and Human Services, 2006.

Terminology

As the preceding historical discussion indicates, the terminology used to describe physical activity and health has evolved over time and was influenced by scientific advances and policy initiatives. The general term **physical activity** has been defined as "bodily movement produced by the contraction of skeletal muscle and that substantially increases energy expenditure above the basic level. Physical activity can be categorized in various ways including type, intensity, and purpose" (CDC, National Center for Chronic Disease Prevention and Health Promotion [NCCDPHP], 1999, p. 20). Various national governmental health organizations have published lists of physical activity–related terms that are helpful for interdisciplinary teams working on

program intervention and evaluation (CDC 2006c, 2006e; CDC, NCCDPHP, 1999). Portions of these lists are consolidated in Content Box 13-3, which includes a description of the activity intensity and duration requirements to meet the current recommended levels of physical activity. The use of a common terminology facilitates the dissemination and replication of programs and research between disciplines.

Content Box 13-3

Physical Activity Terminology

Cardiorespiratory Fitness[1] (also called *aerobic endurance* or *aerobic fitness*)
- Cardiorespiratory endurance is the ability of the body's circulatory and respiratory systems to supply fuel and oxygen during sustained physical activity.

Exercise[1]
- Exercise is physical activity that is planned or structured. It involves repetitive bodily movement done to improve or maintain one or more of the components of physical fitness—cardiorespiratory endurance (aerobic fitness), muscular strength, muscular endurance, flexibility, and body composition.

Household Physical Activity[1]
- Household physical activity includes (but is not limited to) activities such as sweeping floors, scrubbing, washing windows, and raking the lawn.

Inactivity[2]
- Less than 10 minutes total per week of moderate- or vigorous-intensity lifestyle activities (i.e., household, transportation, or leisure-time activity).

Insufficient Physical Activity[2]
- Doing more than 10 minutes total per week of moderate- or vigorous-intensity lifestyle activities (i.e., household, transportation, or leisure-time activity), but less than the recommended level of activity.

Kilocalorie[1]
- The amount of heat required to raise the temperature of 1 kg of water 1°C. Kilocalorie is the ordinary calorie discussed in food or exercise energy-expenditure tables and food labels.

Leisure-Time Inactivity[2]
- No reported leisure-time physical activities (i.e., any physical activities or exercises such as running, calisthenics, golf, gardening, or walking) in the previous month.

Leisure-Time Physical Activity[1]
- Leisure-time physical activity is exercise, sports, recreation, or hobbies that are not associated with activities as part of one's regular job duties, household, or transportation.

Metabolic Equivalent (MET)[1]
- The standard metabolic equivalent, or MET, level. This unit is used to estimate the amount of oxygen used by the body during physical activity.
- 1 MET = the energy (oxygen) used by the body as you sit quietly, perhaps while talking on the phone or reading a book. The harder your body works during the activity, the higher the MET. Any activity that burns 3 to 6 METs is considered moderate-intensity physical activity.
- Any activity that burns >6 METs is considered vigorous-intensity physical activity.

Moderate Physical Activity[2]
- Reported moderate-intensity activities in a usual week (i.e., brisk walking, bicycling, vacuuming, gardening, or anything else that causes small increases in breathing or heart rate) for greater than or equal to 30 minutes per day, greater than or equal to 5 days per week; or vigorous-intensity activities in a usual week (i.e., running, aerobics, heavy yard work, or anything else that causes large increases in breathing or heart rate) for greater than or equal to 20 minutes per day, greater than or equal to 3 days per week or both. This can be accomplished through lifestyle activities (i.e., household, transportation, or leisure-time activities).

Content Box 13-3

Physical Activity Terminology—cont'd

Occupational Physical Activity[1]

- Occupational physical activity is completed regularly as part of one's job. It includes activities such as walking, hauling, lifting, pushing, carpentry, shoveling, and packing boxes.

Physical Activity[3]

- Bodily movement produced by the contraction of skeletal muscle and that substantially increases energy expenditure.

Physical Fitness[1]

- Physical fitness is a set of attributes a person has in regards to a person's ability to perform physical activities that require aerobic fitness, endurance, strength, or flexibility and is determined by a combination of regular activity and genetically inherited ability.

Regular Physical Activity[1]

- A pattern of physical activity is regular if activities are performed:
  - most days of the week, preferably daily;
  - 5 or more days of the week if moderate-intensity activities (in bouts of at least 10 minutes for a total of at least 30 minutes per day); or
  - 3 or more days of the week if vigorous-intensity activities (for at least 20-60 minutes per session).

Transportation Physical Activity[1]

- Transportation physical activity is walking, biking or wheeling (for wheelchair users), or similar activities to and from places such as work, school, place of worship, and stores.

Vigorous-Intensity Physical Activity[1]

- Vigorous-intensity physical activity may be intense enough to represent a substantial challenge to an individual and refers to a level of effort in which a person should experience
  - large increase in breathing or heart rate (conversation is difficult or "broken");
  - a "perceived exertion" of 15 or greater on the Borg Scale (the effort a healthy individual might expend while jogging, mowing the lawn with a nonmotorized pushmower, participating in high-impact aerobic dancing, swimming continuous laps, or bicycling uphill, carrying more than 25 lb up a flight of stairs, standing or walking with more than 50 lb for example);
  - greater than 6 metabolic equivalents (METs); or
  - any activity that burns more than 7 kcal/ min.

Weight-Bearing Physical Activity[1]

- Any physical activity that imparts a load or impact (such as jumping or skipping) on the skeleton.

From the sources identified below.
[1]From *Physical activity for everyone: Physical activity terms,* by Centers for Disease Control and Prevention, 2006c, pp. 1–3.
[2]From *U.S. physical activity statistics: Definitions,* by Centers for Disease Control and Prevention, 2006e, p. 1.
[3]From *Physical activity and health: A Report of the Surgeon General—Chapter 2. Historical background, terminology, evolution of recommendations, and measurement,* by National Center for Chronic Disease Prevention and Health Promotion, 1999, p. 21.

U.S. National Health Objectives Related to Physical Activity

As described in Chapter 4 of this text, *Healthy People 2010* (USDHHS, 2000) outlines the U.S. Health Objectives for the decade between 2000 and 2010. The current document and its predecessors focus on increasing rates of physical activity as a means to enhance the nation's health agenda. The process of establishing goals for the nation's health was first documented in the publication *Healthy People: Surgeon General's Report on Health Promotion and Disease Prevention,* which focused specifically on the health needs of older adults (USDHHS, 1979). This report mentioned exercise and fitness primarily as it related to the prevention of cardiovascular disease. The *Healthy People* reports that followed increasingly stressed the importance of physical activity. Physical activity and fitness was included as one of five health promotion focus areas for the decade between 1980 and1990 (USDHHS, 1980). In later versions of *Healthy People,* physical activity continued to be included as a focus area (USDHHS, 1990; 2000).

Table 13-1 lists current national health objectives related to increasing physical activity in adolescents, college students, and adults (USDHHS, 2000). It also includes objectives related to individuals with disabilities;

Table 13–1 *Healthy People 2010* **Objectives Related to Physical Activity and Fitness**

Objective Number	Objective
Adults	
22-1	Reduce the proportion of adults who engage in no leisure-time physical activity.
22-2	Increase the proportion of adults who engage regularly, preferably daily, in moderate physical activity for at least 30 minutes per day.
22-3	Increase the proportion of adults who engage in vigorous physical activity that promotes the development and maintenance of cardiorespiratory fitness 3 or more days per week for 20 or more minutes per occasion.
2-9	Reduce the proportion of adults with osteoporosis.
Muscular Strength/Endurance and Flexibility	
22-4	Increase the proportion of adults who perform physical activities that enhance and maintain muscular strength and endurance.
22-5	Increase the proportion of adults who perform physical activities that enhance and maintain flexibility.
Children and Adolescents	
22-6	Increase the proportion of adolescents who engage in moderate physical activity for at least 30 minutes on 5 or more of the previous 7 days.
22-7	Increase the proportion of adolescents who engage in vigorous physical activity that promotes cardiorespiratory fitness 3 or more days per week for 20 or more minutes per occasion.
22-8	Increase the proportion of the Nation's public and private schools that require daily physical education for all students.
	22-8a Middle school and junior high school (target 25%)
	22-8b Senior high schools (target 5%)
22-9	Increase the proportion of adolescents who participate in daily school physical education.
22-10	Increase the proportion of adolescents who spend at least 50 percent of school physical education class time being physically active.
22-11	Increase the proportion of adolescents who view television 2 or fewer hours on a school day.
7-2	Increase the proportion of middle, junior high, and senior high schools that provide school health education to prevent health problems in the following areas: unintentional injury; violence; suicide; tobacco use and addiction; alcohol and other drug use; unintended pregnancy, HIV/AIDS, and STD infection; unhealthy dietary patterns; inadequate physical activity; and environmental health.
Access	
22-12	(Developmental) Increase the proportion of the Nation's public and private schools that provide access to their physical activity spaces and facilities for all persons outside of normal school hours (that is, before and after the school day, on weekends, and during summer and other vacations).
22-13	Increase the proportion of worksites offering employer-sponsored physical activity and fitness programs.
22-14	Increase the proportion of trips made by walking.
	22-14a Adults aged 18 years and older (target 1 mile or less)
	22-14b Children and adolescents aged 5 to 15 years (target trip to school 1 mile or less)

Table 13–1   *Healthy People 2010* **Objectives Related to Physical Activity and Fitness—cont'd**

Objective Number	Objective
22-15	Increase the proportion of trips made by bicycling.
	22-15a Adults aged 18 years and older (target 5 miles or less)
	22-15b Children and adolescents aged 5 to 15 years (target trip to school 2 miles or less)
2-6	(Developmental) Eliminate racial disparities in the rate of total knee replacements.
3-10	Increase the proportion of physicians and dentists who counsel their at-risk patients about tobacco use cessation, physical activity, and cancer screening.
Young Adults	
7-3	Increase the proportion of college and university students who receive information from their institution on each of the six priority health-risk behavior areas.
People With Disabilities	
2-2	Reduce the proportion of adults with chronic joint symptoms who experience a limitation in activity due to arthritis.
6-10	(Developmental) Increase the proportion of health and wellness and treatment programs and facilities that provide full access for people with disabilities.
6-12	(Developmental) Reduce the proportion of people with disabilities reporting environmental barriers to participation in home, school, work, or community activities.
24-4	Reduce activity limitations among persons with asthma.
24-9	Reduce the proportion of adults whose activity is limited due to chronic lung and breathing problems.

From *Healthy People 2010 Understanding and improving health,* by U.S. Department of Health and Human Services, 2000, Washington, DC: Government Printing Office.

however, these objectives address only barriers to physical activity or the basic level of physical activity required for activities of daily living (ADLs) and instrumental activities of daily living (IADLs). No specific objectives for moderate or vigorous physical activity could be located for people with disabilities, children, families, older adults, or other populations.

Children and Adolescents

While nine *Healthy People 2010* national health objectives relate directly to adolescents, only four (i.e., 7-2, 22-8a, 22-14b, and 22-15b) directly pertain to younger children. Two of these objectives address modes of transportation (i.e., walking and bicycle use). Although these are important methods of increasing physical activity, corresponding safety issues need to be addressed though injury prevention (e.g., availability, use of bicycle helmets) and efforts to reduce barriers (e.g., access to safe pathways). The limited emphasis on increasing physical activity among children seen in *Healthy People 2010* may change in future editions as a result of accelerating childhood obesity rates and the sedentary lifestyle epidemic.

Trend data indicate that the proportion of students biking and walking to school in the United States dropped by 40% within a 20-year period (Killingsworth & Lamming, 2001). Research is being conducted to look at the barriers and factors related to these methods of commuting to school. For example, Sisson, Lee, Burns, and Tudor-Lock (2006) investigated the prevalence and suitability of bicycle commuting to a subset of elementary schools in Arizona. The prevalence was similar to other studies with the median prevalence ranging between 3.1% and 1.3%. The presence of and type of biking polices varied. The researchers reported the presence of methods to decrease thefts and promote safety. Although fears of injuries are a common barrier, none were reported by the schools in the study sample.

Ries and colleagues (2008) explored patterns of physical activity among urban adolescents, specifically focusing on environmental features. Their findings indicate that urban adolescents prefer to attend facilities that are clean and comfortable, safe, close to home, inexpensive, and frequented by other physically active adolescents. Young men were more likely than women to use outdoor spaces, and both tended to limit their use to daylight hours. When indoor and outdoor facilities were unavailable, the adolescents turned to less desirable places, such as streets and vacant lots, but tried to avoid areas with known criminal activity. The findings also suggest that occupational therapy program developers should recognize the importance of offering urban youth a variety of age-appropriate activities on a flexible schedule in a safe place.

Adults and Older Adults

Eleven *Healthy People 2010* objectives are directed toward adults as a group, but none directly address the need to increase physical activity among older adults. As will be seen in Chapters 23 and 24, levels of physical activity have been associated with successful aging and decreased risk of falls. The *Healthy People 2010* objectives that address physical activity do so in a tangential manner. These include objectives that can be achieved through physical activity, such as decreasing osteoporosis through weight-bearing exercise. Of the remaining objectives, one directly focuses on college-aged adults, one addresses a racial disparity, and five are related to the needs of individuals with disabilities.

Prevalence Rates

Low rates of participation in physical activity are of concern across age, ethnic, and racial groups in the United States. This concern is also experienced internationally in both Western countries (De Bourdeaudhuij, Sallis, & Saelens, 2003) and those that are becoming increasingly industrialized (Rastogi et al., 2004). The following sections cover prevalence rates of engagement in physical activity by various age groups. These sections also include an examination of rates based on cultural and geographic categories, and a review of differences in prevalence rates between individuals with and without disabilities.

Prevalence Rates by Age Groups: Children

According to results from a 2002 telephone survey of over 3000 households, patterns of engagement in physical activity by children aged 9 to 13 in the United States vary by gender, ethnicity, and socioeconomic class. This survey was the first administration of the Youth Media Campaign Longitudinal Survey (YMCLS) and supports the need for the development of tailored, culturally competent, age-appropriate interventions to promote physical activity levels in children while simultaneously decreasing barriers reported by parents. While most children, regardless of ethnicity, participated in unstructured physical activity (75% to 79%), only 47% of white, 26% of black, and 24% of Hispanic children participated in organized physical activity. The three most frequently reported organized physical activities children engaged in, regardless of gender, age, or ethnicity, were baseball/softball, soccer, and basketball. In addition, basketball and riding a bicycle were the two most frequently reported free-time physical activities (Duke, Huhman, & Heitlzle, 2003).

Prevalence Rates by Age Groups: Adolescents

Although many adolescents in the United States engage in sufficient physical activity to meet long-term health benefits, others do not, according to national data gathered as part of the Youth Risk Behavior Surveillance System (Grunbaum et al., 2004). Rates vary by gender, ethnicity, and grade level. Table 13-2 displays exertion-level differences in high school students by gender. Boys demonstrate greater engagement in all levels of exertion. In 2003, only about 50% of high school girls reported participating in a team sport or engaging in the recommended level of vigorous physical activity. In addition, whites generally have the highest participation rates in vigorous and moderate physical activity, followed by Hispanics, and then blacks. Less than half of black females engage in sufficient physical activity to positively impact health. Engaging in physical activity is most prevalent among students in the first years of high school and least among students in the 12th grade. Also, participation in daily physical education varies by state. The state with the highest participation in physical education is North Dakota (37.2%) and the lowest is Maine (8.2%).

Table 13–2 **Percentage of High School Students Participating in Physical Activity, by Gender, 2003**

	Female	Male
Insufficient amount of physical activity	40.1%	26.9%
No moderate or vigorous physical activity	13.1%	10.0%
Participated in strengthening exercises	43.4%	60.1%
Played on one or more sports teams	51.0%	64.0%
Watched 3 or more hours of television a day	37.0%	39.3%

Data from Tables 52 and 56 of "Youth risk behavior surveillance—United States, 2003" by J. A. Grunbaum et al., 2004, *Mortality and Morbidity Report,* pp. 81, 85.

Prevalence Rates by Age Groups: Adults

According to the results of the 2000 and 2001 Behavioral Risk Factor Surveillance System (BRFSS), most adults in the United States failed to reach physical activity levels that would promote health (Macera et al., 2003). Data for 2004 indicated that only 30% of U.S. adults participated in the recommended levels of physical activity, with the 2010 target goal being 50% participation (CDC, 2006c). There are also regional differences in engagement in physical activity (Macera et al., 2003). In some states, including Georgia, Kentucky, Louisiana, Mississippi, Missouri, Oklahoma, and Tennessee, less than 40% of the adult population met physical activity recommendations. These states also had higher reported rates of no participation in leisure-time physical activities. Tracking data such as these is helpful for both policy advocacy and tailoring program development.

Prevalence Rates by Age Groups: Older Adults

The CDC (2006c) tracking data for 2004 indicated that only 27% of U.S. adults aged 65 to 74 and 16% of those aged 75 and older met the recommended level of physical activity. Participation rates in leisure-time physical activities also fall below target levels. Almost half (44%) of U.S. adults aged 65 to 74 and roughly two-thirds (61%) of those aged 75 and older reported no leisure-time physical activity. The data for older adults were not reported by gender, ethnicity, or geographic location.

Gender, Cultural, and Socioeconomic Differences

Levels of physical activity participation differ by gender, ethnicity, and socioeconomic class. In general, men are more physically active than women. By age 75, approximately 50% of women and 33% of men engage in no physical activity. African Americans and Hispanics have lower rates of physical activity than whites. In addition, people with less education and lower incomes tend to engage in less physical activities than those from higher levels of education and income (USDHHS, 2000).

Disability Status Differences

Participation rates and patterns differ between individuals with and without disabilities (CDC, 2006c). Individuals with disabilities have lower participation rates in regular, moderate, or vigorous physical activity and in leisure-time physical activity. While 33% of U.S. nondisabled adults reported participating in moderate or vigorous physical activity, only approximately one in five (18%) people with disabilities reported participation in this level of physical activity. Interestingly, people with symptoms of arthritis reported about the same degree of participation at this level (31%) as those without arthritis symptoms (30%).

Geographic/Regional Differences

In general, adults in the North Central and Western states have higher rates of participation in physical activities than adults in the Northeast and Southern states (USDHHS, 2000). According to the 2001 BRFSS, the percentage of adults who met the physical activity recommendations ranged by state from 28.9% in Kentucky to 54.6% in Alaska (Macera et al., 2003). Physical activity–level data are available in map form from BRFSS, at http://apps.nccd.cdc.gov/gisbrfss/default.aspx. Figure 13-1 also displays exercise data from BRFSS for 2004—specifically, the percentage of adults by state who reported participating in exercise during the prior month. Data for 2003 are available by state in a similar map format, displaying the percentage of adults who participated in more than 20 minutes of vigorous physical activity 3 or more days per week. Also available at this site are data on the number of adults who participated in 30 or more minutes of moderate physical activity 5 or more days per week and in vigorous physical activity for more than 20 minutes 3 or more days per week. This site and the data it tracks have implications for occupational therapy practitioners in terms of program development, policy advocacy, and personal health habits.

Prevalence of Physical Activity in Other Countries

In general, health promotion advocates and professionals in other Western countries have encountered similar difficulties in increasing the levels of physical activity among their fellow citizens. However, researchers in Australia report not only a similar lack of success (e.g., Pate et al., 2003), but also an increasing trend in levels of physical inactivity (Marshall et al., 2004). Groups of researchers in Australia have been conducting efficacy studies to determine the best population-based methods to address the Australians' growing trend toward sedentary lifestyles (Marshall, Bauman, Patch, Wilson, & Chen, 2002). Findings support the influence of access to a safe and adequate physical environment (Giles-Corti, Macintyre, Clarkson, Pikora, & Donovan, 2003), which can vary regionally on the success of population-based intervention to encourage the development of habitual physical activity engagement (Marshall et al., 2004). An Australian initiative to increase physical activity that can be tailored to the individual is available at http://www.10000steps.cqu.edu.au/. A comparable program, Shape Up America! (2005–2006), exists in the United States and will be described later in this chapter.

2004 Percentage of Respondents Reporting YES

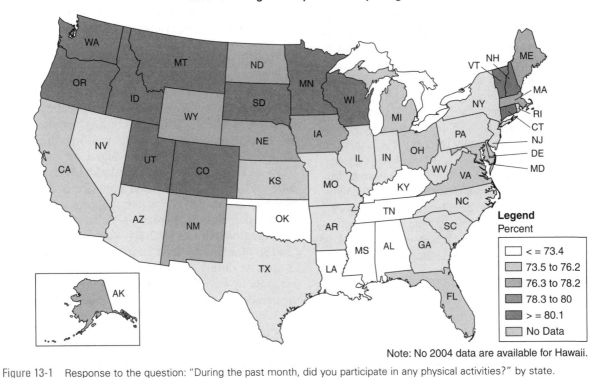

Note: No 2004 data are available for Hawaii.

Figure 13-1   Response to the question: "During the past month, did you participate in any physical activities?" by state.

From National Center for Chronic Disease Prevention and Health Promotion, Behavioral Risk Factor Surveillance System (BRFSS), BFRSS Maps, 2004, Atlanta: U.S. Department of Health and Human Services, Centers for Disease Control and Prevention.

Physical activity–level changes are occurring in large portions of non-Western countries. For example, in India, increased industrialization, the development of the computer industry, and other positive economic development results have all caused physical activity levels in urban areas to decrease (Rastogi et al., 2004). This trend will most likely occur in other nations, such as the People's Republic of China, where similar economic changes seem to be occurring at an even faster pace. Given China's tremendous population, which numbered 1.3 billion in 2005 (WHO, 2006a), attention should be focused on encouraging the continuation of traditional values and activities that promote physical activity, especially among urban and suburban populations. Otherwise, the health risks and sequela that follow a major shift to physical inactivity will dramatically impact the health and economy of China.

Barriers to Physical Activity Engagement

Although various cultural, gender, and individual differences exist regarding the strength and applicability of **barriers** to engagement in exercise and physical activity, those most frequently discussed in the literature include time, place, access, and self-esteem-related constructs. These barriers will be briefly discussed below. In addition, the impact of the occupational role of care giving on engagement in physical activity and disability status will also be addressed.

Time

Lack of time is a barrier to engagement in physical activity (Anderson, 2003; Reynolds, 2001). One of the five barriers reported in another study was "lack of parents' time" (Duke, Huhman, & Heitlzler 2003, p. 787). After expense and transportation issues, this was the third most frequently reported barrier. Data from a study of 743 10th-grade students in the United States were analyzed to determine psychosocial predictors of physical activity habits. Stress was identified as a possible barrier to adolescent females' physical activity habit patterns (Reynolds et al., 1990). It was theorized that stress may act as a barrier through the perception of time pressure (Reynolds et al., 1990). Lack of time was also found to be a barrier among sedentary older adults (Dergance et al., 2003).

Place

Research findings indicate that environment can be a barrier to engagement in physical activity. Specifically, the convenience of destinations (King et al., 2003); the design of communities, including street design; housing density; public transport; and facilities for walking, bicycling, and other active leisure pursuits impact levels of physical activity either positively or negatively (CDC, NCCDPHP, 2003; De Bourdeaudhuij et al., 2003). Walking, the least expensive and seemingly most available mode of physical activity, is not always easy or safe. In the United States, "facilities for pedestrians are often inconvenient or nonexistent, leading to fatality rates per mile traveled 36 times higher than for occupants of cars and light trucks" (Pucher & Dijkstra, 2000, cited by Pucher & Renne, 2003, p. 73).

Environmentall barriers are even more of a problem for individuals with disabilities. A series of on-site surveys conducted at 50 physical activity facilities in western Oregon found none of the sites (e.g., parks, gymnasiums) in full compliance with the Americans with Disabilities Act (Cardinal & Spaziani, 2003). Little research has been conducted on barriers to physical activity for adults with developmental disabilities. In a study of adults with developmental disabilities in the north of England, it was found that environmental and policy barriers prevented 92% of the sample from meeting recommended levels of physical activity sufficient to decrease health risks (Messent, Cooke, & Long, 1999).

A study of Dutch adolescents (aged 12 to 18) indicated that the aesthetics of the community positively impacted whether the adolescents engaged in more physical activity (de Bruijn et al., 2006). Results from the same study showed that adolescents who lived farther away from facilities were more physically active. The authors feel this may be because these adolescents valued physical activity to such a level that they were more resourceful in locating facilities and overcoming barriers of distance. These varying results indicate the need for continued research and a degree of caution before making assumptions about what is and is not a barrier to physical activity performance.

Access

Insufficient financial resources (Henderson & Bialescki, 1991, Messent et al., 1999), lack of transportation, and unavailability of recreation environments or local opportunities are examples of access issues that can act as barriers to physical activity participation. The YMCLS (Duke et al., 2003), discussed earlier, reported the barriers that parents perceived limited their children's participation in physical activity. The most frequently reported barrier was expense; 47.5% of girls' parents and 45.8% of boys' parents indicated this as a barrier. Transportation, resources, and safety of community were also reported as barriers. Transportation was the primary barrier reported by adolescent girls and their parents in a

pilot study of an intervention to reduce television watching and to increase physical activity among African American girls from low-income neighborhoods (Robinson et al., 2003). Participation rates were higher among girls with ready access to bus transportation to the program site.

Weekend and evening school use has been identified as a potential method to enhance access to physical activity space and resources. Most schools have both indoor and outdoor facilities suitable for use by the public. A telephone survey was conducted to determine the barriers and benefits of allowing access to school facilities for physical activity (Evenson & McGinn, 2004). More public schools had facilities to share than private schools. Public schools also shared those facilities more often. Outdoor facilities were available, whether at public schools, private schools, or the college level more often than indoor facilities. Barriers to sharing facilities included concerns over using student-designated space, supervision, personnel limitations, and safety and liability issues.

Self-Esteem, Self-Presentational Concerns, Self-Concept, and Body Image

Self-esteem, self-concept, self-efficacy, body image, and self-presentational concerns can affect engagement in physical activity throughout the life span. Pedersen and Seidman (2004) found a positive relationship between achievement in team sports and self-esteem among poor urban youth from diverse cultural backgrounds. Data from another study of adolescents found that for both girls and boys, self-efficacy was linked to engagement in physical activity (Reynolds et al., 1990); therefore, increasing self-efficacy is an important factor to address. Ziviani and colleagues (2006) found that young children (i.e., 7 to 8 years old) whose parents perceived them as being teased by peers engaged in less physical activity during weekends than their peers, as measured by a pedometer. There was no difference in physical activity levels during school days. In addition, cultural differences in body image should be considered during program development. For example, Robinson and others (2003) reported that African American women and girls are less concerned about achieving a slender body, experience fewer symptoms of eating disorders, and report less body dissatisfaction.

Research findings (Anderson, 2003; Focht & Hausenblas, 2004) indicate that many women choose to exercise or not exercise due to **self-presentational concerns.** While some women may exercise to promote their perceived physical attractiveness, others may avoid or discontinue exercise due to concerns about their appearance during the activity (Anderson,

2003; Dergance et al., 2003; Focht & Hausenblas, 2004). The presence of mirrors and other people exercising are common in fitness settings. These contextual features may serve as barriers for women with social physique anxiety, especially when beginning an exercise program (Focht & Hausenblas, 2004).

Pedersen and Seidman (2004) investigated the influence of team-sport participation and achievement on self-esteem in a group of poor urban adolescent girls. Based on this study and related literature, they recommend that young girls be afforded the opportunity to participate in team sports. They also identified early adolescence as a critical time period to foster this participation, in order to maximize impact on self-esteem. During this time, many young women drop out of school or sports activities due to limited opportunities and societal pressure to engage in more traditional gender-role activities.

In addition, ethnic differences regarding self-consciousness as a barrier were examined in a study of 210 community-dwelling older sedentary adults in South Texas. While 18.9% of the European Americans reported self-consciousness as a barrier, none of the Mexican Americans reported this factor as a deterrent (Dergance et al., 2003).

Occupational Roles: Child and Adult Caregiving

Although the impact of the caregiving role could have been included in the previous discussion regarding insufficient time, this topic merits a separate examination. This is especially warranted given the importance of occupational role in the occupational therapy and occupational science literature. When caring for an ill child, spouse, or aging relative, previous exercise habits may no longer be performed. In addition, women with multiple roles may experience chronic strain, which can be a barrier to exercise (Anderson, 2003; Verhoef & Love, 1992). Women caregivers report feeling guilty when taking the necessary time to perform health occupations such as exercise. Similarly, it is reported that women fail to engage in such occupations because they do not feel entitled to such pursuits (Reynolds, 2001) or view physical activity as a low priority; thus, time is rarely, if ever, allotted (Henderson & Bialeschki, 1991). In women, parenthood (i.e., cohabitating with any child aged 17 or younger) was negatively associated both with engagement in physical activity and the quantity of activity engagement. In addition, self-reported role overload and the presence of time barriers were predictive of quantity of physical activity engagement (Verhoef & Love, 1992), regardless of parental status.

This research further supports the need to tailor physical activity health promotion messages and programs (Verhoef & Love, 1992) to the individual needs of caregivers, whether they are women or men. In addition, there also is a need to promote increased amounts of physical activity engagement in those who are caregivers or who perceive themselves in role overload but are already engaging in some limited amount of physical activity. This population may benefit from a different approach and resources.

Health Benefits of Physical Activity and the Health Risks of Physical Inactivity

The health benefits of participating in regular physical activity and the related health risks of physical inactivity have been well documented. The WHO (2006b) presents facts regarding the impact of physical inactivity on the health and financial wellbeing of citizens and nations (Content Box 13-4). Physical inactivity can adversely impact body function and structures (e.g., bones, muscles, heart) in many ways, ultimately increasing risk for disease and impacting long-term health and survival (Content Box 13-5). While tobacco use is currently the leading cause of death within the United States, unhealthy diets and inactivity may soon surpass tobacco use for that dubious distinction (Mokdad, Marks, Stroup, & Gerberding, 2004).

Regular physical activity reduces people's risk for heart attack, colon cancer, diabetes, and high blood pressure and may reduce their risk for stroke. It also helps to control weight; contributes to healthy bones, muscles, and joints; reduces falls among older adults; helps to relieve the pain of arthritis; reduces symptoms of anxiety and

---

Content Box 13-4

WHO Physical Activity Facts

- "Appropriate regular physical activity is a major component in preventing the growing global burden of chronic disease."
- "At least 60% of the global population fails to achieve the minimum recommendation of 30 minutes moderate intensity physical activity daily."
- "The risk of getting a cardiovascular disease increases by 1.5 times in people who do not follow minimum physical activity recommendations."
- Inactivity increases medical costs—by an estimated $75 billion in the U.S. in 2000.
- "Increasing physical activity is a societal, not just an individual problem, and demands a population-based, multi-sectoral, multi-disciplinary, and culturally relevant approach."

From *Global strategy on diet, physical activity and health: Physical activity* by, World Health Organization, 2006b, ¶ 1. Copyright © 2006 by World Health Organization. With permission.

Content Box 13-5

Health Benefits of Regular Physical Activity

1. Improves glucose metabolism
2. Reduces body fat
3. Lowers blood pressure
4. Reduces risk and impact of diabetes due to benefits 1–3
5. Reduces risk and impact of cardiovascular disease due to benefits 1–3
6. Reduces risk of breast and colon cancer
7. Improves and maintains health of muscles, bones, and joints
8. Controls weight
9. Decreases anxiety and symptoms of depression
10. Decreases risk of early death

Data from *Global strategy on diet, physical activity and health: Physical activity* by World Health Organization, 2006b, and *Physical activity and health: A Report of the Surgeon General,* by the USDHHS, 1996.

depression; and is associated with fewer hospitalizations, physician visits, and medications. (CDC, 2006b, ¶ 6)

Regular moderate physical activity also has been associated with increased longevity compared to individuals who are less active. Higher levels of physical activity have even greater favorable impact on mortality (CDC, NCCDPHP, 1999).

The evidence linking breast and colon cancer to physical inactivity is compelling. At this time, the connection between physical inactivity and prostate cancer is inconsistent; however, physical activity has been identified as a possible protective agent for lung and endometrial cancers (Hardman, 2005). The importance of establishing healthy physical activity habits early in life as a way to decrease risk factors is increasingly stressed in the literature. However, physical activity can and should also be promoted within older populations. Engagement in even limited (i.e., once a week) moderate physical activity among postmenopausal women has been shown to decrease risk of premature death (Kushi et al., 1997). In addition, routine physical activity has been shown to decrease the frequency of hot flashes, osteoporosis, and hip fractures in postmenopausal women (Reynolds, 2001).

While links between diabetes, obesity, heart disease (Reynolds, 2001), and longevity (Glass, de Leon, Martolli, & Berlma, 1999) seem logical, research is also showing a connection between overall psychological wellbeing and cognitive function and physical activity. Time spent participating in physical education also has been found to be related to academic achievement in elementary school-aged girls (Carlson et al., 2008). In

addition, walking was found to reduce the risk of dementia among men in the Honolulu-Asia Aging Study (Abbott et al., 2004). Menec and Chipperfield (1997) found a strong relationship between subjective wellbeing and active engagement in leisure pursuits and physical activity among a group of older Canadian adults. The authors propose that older adults may exercise not to prevent health conditions but rather to experience the positive psychological benefits of physical activity. Enhanced self-esteem and personal identity has also been reported for adults with disabilities who continued to engage in physical activities (Sherril as cited by Reynolds, 2001). Remaining active also helps prevent secondary complications such as weight gain. Other studies report that physical activity decreases depressed mood and levels of anxiety and stress, and increases self-esteem and feelings of competence and mastery. The social components of leisure-related physical activity can be a factor in reducing loneliness and depressed mood (Reynolds, 2001). In addition, social and productive occupations have been linked to decreased mortality among older U.S. adults (Glass et al., 1999).

Research continues to explore the links and linking mechanisms between other diseases and physical inactivity as well as those between other types of cancer and physical inactivity. Smith and colleagues (2004) reported that increased physical activity, weight loss, or a combination of the two can reduce visceral fat and abdominal diameter, thereby decreasing the development of insulin resistance syndrome. This reduction is particularly noteworthy based on the increased understanding of the link between insulin resistance syndrome and cardiac vascular disease, diabetes, and hypertension (Rao, 2001).

The growing understanding of physical inactivity's financial impact and the impact on longevity and quality of life is enhancing efforts among U.S. public and private organizations to increase exercise among U.S. residents to recommended levels. A report of the Surgeon General (CDC, NCCD, 1999) encouraged efforts to afford all U.S. citizens, including special populations, opportunities to reap the health benefits of physical activity. These efforts will be described in the following section.

Governmental and National Organizations and Documents That Promote Physical Activity

This section describes additional current national and governmental initiatives promoting physical activity. The President's Council on Physical Fitness and Sports was described earlier in this chapter. The selection of additional governmental and national efforts to promote physical activity and overall health includes the following:

- Active Community Environments Initiative
- MyPyramid
- Rescuing Recess
- Shape Up America!
- We Can!™ (Ways to Enhance Children's Activity & Nutrition)

Active Community Environments Initiative (ACES)

The Division of Nutrition and Physical Activity of the CDC, NCCDPHP (2003), established the **Active Community Environments Initiative (ACES).** This initiative's primary goal is developing accessible leisure facilities that promote the use of bicycles and walking. The ACES includes program development and partnerships. Programs include walk-to-school day, KidsWalk-to-School program, and a variety of other activities to encourage bicycling and walking. Two examples of collaborative ACES partners include the National Park Services Rivers, Trails, and Conservation Assistance Program and the Environmental Protection Agency. The development of an active community environments guidebook is under way to assist public health practitioners to partner with transportation and city planners in promoting the ACES goals (CDC, NCCDPHP, 2003).

MyPyramid

The federal government's food pyramid was first published in 1992 (Dixon et al., 2001). The revised food pyramid, called MyPyramid, includes a recommendation for incorporating physical activity in order to achieve a healthy lifestyle (U.S. Department of Agriculture, n.d.). (This initiative will be discussed in more detail in Chapter 14, which covers weight management and obesity reduction.) Versions of this new pyramid for adults and children are available online. The graphic of the new pyramid includes a person ascending steps, emphasizing the importance of physical activity engagement (Fig. 13-2). Adults can use a Web-based program to calculate nutritional needs based on physical activity level (see http://www.mypyramid.gov/mypyramid/index.aspx). A game targeted toward children between the ages of 6 and 11 is also available to encourage healthy eating and exercise (see http://www.mypyramid.gov/kids/index.html).

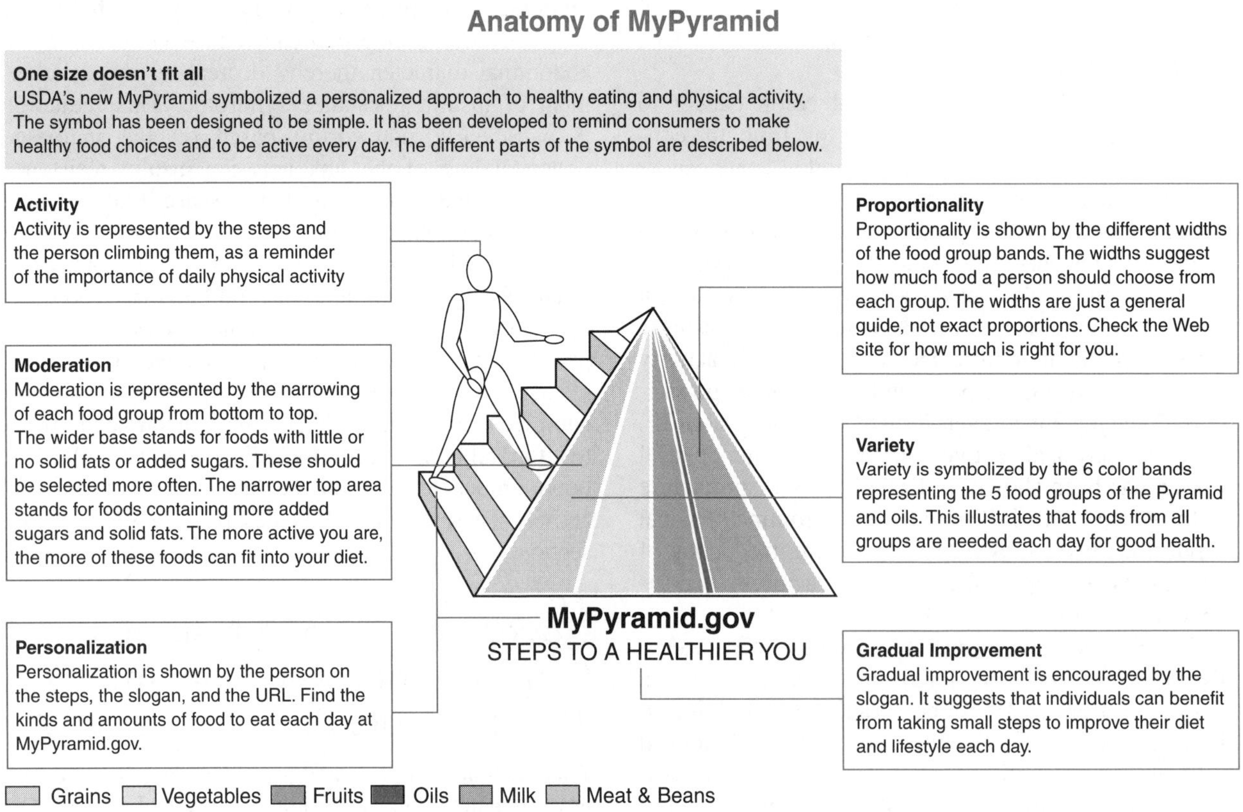

Anatomy of MyPyramid

One size doesn't fit all
USDA's new MyPyramid symbolized a personalized approach to healthy eating and physical activity. The symbol has been designed to be simple. It has been developed to remind consumers to make healthy food choices and to be active every day. The different parts of the symbol are described below.

Activity
Activity is represented by the steps and the person climbing them, as a reminder of the importance of daily physical activity

Moderation
Moderation is represented by the narrowing of each food group from bottom to top. The wider base stands for foods with little or no solid fats or added sugars. These should be selected more often. The narrower top area stands for foods containing more added sugars and solid fats. The more active you are, the more of these foods can fit into your diet.

Personalization
Personalization is shown by the person on the steps, the slogan, and the URL. Find the kinds and amounts of food to eat each day at MyPyramid.gov.

Proportionality
Proportionality is shown by the different widths of the food group bands. The widths suggest how much food a person should choose from each group. The widths are just a general guide, not exact proportions. Check the Web site for how much is right for you.

Variety
Variety is symbolized by the 6 color bands representing the 5 food groups of the Pyramid and oils. This illustrates that foods from all groups are needed each day for good health.

Gradual Improvement
Gradual improvement is encouraged by the slogan. It suggests that individuals can benefit from taking small steps to improve their diet and lifestyle each day.

MyPyramid.gov
STEPS TO A HEALTHIER YOU

☐ Grains ☐ Vegetables ☐ Fruits ■ Oils ☐ Milk ☐ Meat & Beans

Figure 13-2 New food pyramid that includes physical activity recommendation.

From MyPyramid, 2005, U.S. Department of Agriculture.

Rescuing Recess

A coalition of organizations, including the National Parent Teacher Association (PTA), the Cartoon Network, and others established the Rescuing Recess campaign. The centerpiece of this campaign is a very youth-centric Web page, which suggests fun physical activities for children. For adults, encouraging, supportive statements are available from a variety of experts and advocates, including CNN's Dr. Sanjay Gupta, the president of the Education Association, and the lead CDC epidemiologist. In addition, useful tools and facts are provided to assist individuals in being effective advocates for the inclusion of recess in the school day.

USA TODAY reported data from the National Center for Education Statistics that may initially seem to discount the need for this campaign. However, a closer looks reveals issues of unequal access. While 83% to 88% of elementary school students receive at least 30 minutes of recess each school day, the length of recess varies by socioeconomic status. Schools attended by children from wealthier families offer about 50% more recess time than those attended by students from low-income families (Toppo, 2006).

Shape Up America!

This national not-for-profit organization was developed through a collaboration between the U.S. government, businesses, and organizations concerned about health, physical activity, or nutrition. The two primary objectives of this initiative are to

- promote maintaining a healthy weight through healthy eating and increased physical activity and
- disseminate information regarding evidence-based methods to reach and maintain a healthy body weight.

The website associated with this organization provides an introduction to the 10,000 Steps Program, a meal and snack calculator, and other interactive online tools, such as a body fat lab and a cyberkitchen (Shape Up America!, 2005–2006).

We Can!™ (Ways to Enhance Children's Activity & Nutrition)

This national project (National Heart, Lung, and Blood Institute, n.d.) was launched on June 1, 2005, and involves four organizations within the National Institutes of Health NIH):

- National Heart, Lung, and Blood Institute (NHLBI)
- National Institute of Diabetes and Digestive and Kidney Diseases (NIDDK)
- National Institute of Child Health and Human Development (NICHD)
- National Cancer Institute (NCI)

The goal of the We Can!™ project is to provide parents of 8- to 13-year-old children easy access to information that can change behaviors linked to improving long-term health outcomes through the maintenance of a healthy weight. The three behavior changes identified as instrumental to achieving this goal include

- improving choices of food,
- increasing physical activity, and
- decreasing time spent in front of screens.

The project's website provides data on such topics as the amount of time youth spend viewing various screens (e.g., televisions, DVDs, video games, homework, Internet chatting), eating habits, and other health data. A variety of activities and strategies are provided to help reach each of the three goals. The suggestions are communicated by using simple, captivating language, such as "energy IN," "energy OUT," and "wean the screen."

Theoretical Models and Research

Any population- or individual-based intervention, including those previously described, must be based on well-supported theory and be evaluated to determine its effectiveness in order to warrant replication. Chapters 2 and 3 discuss the importance of theory-driven programs. A variety of theoretical models reviewed in those chapters have been used to frame physical activity intervention programs and evaluation of those programs, as well as to investigate physical activity patterns. The following section will describe a selection of theories that appear promising for physical activity program development and evaluation. Particular emphasis will be placed on the Transtheoretical Model (TTM). This section will also cover family-focused research undertaken by disciplines other than occupational therapy and occupational science. Occupation-based models are addressed later in this chapter as they relate to the role of occupational therapy in promoting physical activity. A brief review of potential evaluation measures also is included.

Stages of Change

A study compared three models—the Stages of Change Model, also known as the TTM; the self-efficacy theory; and the Decisional Balance Model (Marcus, Pinto, Simkin, Audrain, & Taylor, 1994)—in order to examine exercise patterns among women in three Rhode Island workplaces. Results were consistent with those reported in the literature at the time: Most employed women did not participate in regular physical activity. While components of the three models were found to explain some of the poor exercise behaviors, none measured roles, which was the most striking finding. Women with children under the age of 18 at home were less likely (p <.05) to be in the highest stages of exercise participation (i.e., either action or maintenance). Unmarried women were most likely (p <.05) to engage in vigorous activity and to be runners (p <.05). These results support the need for using occupation-based models to investigate physical activity patterns among working women.

The TTM seems to be one of the most frequently used theories in physical activity research (Marshall & Biddle, 2001). For example, Renger, Steinfelt, and Lazarus (2002) used this model as the basis for developing a media campaign to increase physical activity by targeting self-efficacy through a discussion of the benefits and barriers to physical activity. The campaign was more successful than expected; similar to the study of Robinson and colleagues (2003), the key action appeared to be cognizance and sensitivity to local community culture and dynamics. Other researchers have used the model to study stages of change in Belgian adolescents (De Bourdeaudhuij et al., 2005), Hong Kong Chinese university students (Callaghan, Eves, Norman, Chang, & Lung, 2002), Scottish university students (Woods, Mutrie, & Scott, 2002), urban undergraduate university students in the United States (Sallis, Calfas, Alcaraz, Gehrman, & Johnson, 1999), and older adults in Rhode Island (Riebe et al., 2005).

Resnick and Nigg (2003) tested the TTM and components of the theory of self-efficacy in a study of exercise patterns among 179 white women residing in a continuing care community. Data supported the influence of social support and health status on both self-efficacy and outcome expectations, which in turn influenced exercise stage of change placement and exercise behavior. Implications for program development included

- enhancing self-efficacy in individuals with perceived poor health as a necessary precursor of willingness to engage in physical activity and
- using the stages of change to tailor interventions.

Since the TTM views change as a dynamic process, it is well-suited for investigation of physical activity. A meta-analysis of 71 published research studies that included at least one of the primary TTM constructs supported the use of this model for physical activity research (Marshall & Biddle, 2001). The authors of this meta-analysis offered recommendations for future research, including

- explore the "moderators and mediators of stage transition" (p. 229) and
- avoid replicating studies that merely examine participants' stage and core constructs.

This model has potential for use in conjunction with occupational therapy models as well as interventions based on occupational science. It also has potential to be adapted for use with families, as families are increasingly seen as contextual features that can impact the development and retention of healthy habits.

Families

Limited research exists regarding family-based interventions for enhancing physical activity participation. The American Heart Association (n.d.) suggested that a helpful exercise strategy is to perform physical activity with family or friends. They also suggested recording family fitness activities and celebrating via rewards when a milestone is achieved. While this recommendation makes sense and is consistent with health promotion and occupational therapy theories, additional research is needed to provide supporting evidence.

The Child and Adolescent Trial for Cardiovascular Health (CATCH) was a 5-year study (1991 to 1994) at 96 U.S. schools located in four different geographical regions. The goal of this randomized controlled field trial was to reduce cardiovascular risk among third- through fifth-grade students (Kelder et al., 2003). The CATCH trial included multiple components, which are displayed in Content Box 13-6. The family and home-based components supplemented school-based components. The program focused on health behaviors in relation to tobacco use, food choices, and physical activity (Osganian, Parcel, & Stone, 2003).

Lytle, Ward, Nader, Pedersen, and Williston (2003) completed one of many studies that examined the institutionalization of CATCH. Their qualitative study addressed the family and other program components. Findings indicated that the physical education component had the highest level of institutionalization, while the family and classroom components had the lowest. These findings are not surprising, since the family component did not appear to be a main focus of the program.

The family has been suggested as an important resource in educating and supporting pregnant women to engage in moderate physical activity (Weallens, Clark, MacIntrye, & Gaudoin, 2003). A study of first-time mothers in Scotland indicated that 40% of pregnant women did not receive any advice from health-care professionals regarding the benefits of exercise for themselves or their fetuses (Weallens et al., 2003). Women

Content Box 13-6

CATCH Components

School-Based Interventions

- Classroom component
- Nutrition curricula
  - Smoking curricula
  - Physical activity curricula
  - School environment component
  - Meal preparation changes (e.g., decrease total fat)
  - Physical education curricula to emphasize moderate to vigorous physical activity levels
  - School policy initiatives to support not smoking

Home-Based Interventions

- Family component
  - Take-home activities
  - Family fun nights stressing healthy foods and physical activities

Data from *Institutionalization of a school health promotion program: Background and rationale of the CATCH-ON Study,* by S. K. Osganian, G. S. Parcel, & E. J. Stone, 2003.

from lower socioeconomic backgrounds received less advice at all stages of pregnancy ($p < 0.01$). Interdisciplinary approaches that include an occupational therapy intervention that highlights the importance of physical activity habits during and after pregnancy should be available for this underserved population. In addition, general role preparation for motherhood should be included in occupational therapy interventions where appropriate.

Although recruiting families to participate in research is more challenging than recruiting individuals, Robinson and colleagues (2003) were very successful in a pilot study of an intervention to reduce television watching and promote physical activity among adolescent African American girls. This success appears to be linked to cultural awareness, cultural competence, and close adherence to the use of Bandura's social cognitive model. These findings highlight the importance of the use of culturally relevant and accurate assessment measures in occupational therapy evidence-based research. The next section will include several promising examples of such instruments for use in research with families and other populations.

Assessment Measures

Many outcome measures are available for use in physical activity research. This section includes a brief presentation of five such measures selected on the basis of being closely related to occupations, ease of use, or frequency of citations in the literature. These measures

include the use of an activity diary, the Borg scale, the International Physical Activity Questionnaires (IPAQ), a pedometer, and two community surveys. Resnick and Nigg (2003) describe a variety of other measures and provide an excellent resource for research in this area. Another source for physical activity measures can be found on a portion of the Active Living Research website, which is located online at http://www.activelivingresearch .org/index.php/Measuring_Physical_Activity/184. Other measures, such as the Behavioral Risk Factor Surveillance System, were discussed earlier in this chapter (CDC, 2006a).

Activity Diary

The use of an activity diary was found to be a potentially effective method for collecting information on the frequency of physical activity among a group of school-aged children in a region of England (Wormald et al., 2003). A total of 91% of the requested activity diaries were submitted. Of those, 11% were invalid and were therefore not coded. Suggested strategies to maximize the likelihood of diary completion included the following:

- Provide age-appropriate incentives
- Embed diary completion into a part of the school curriculum
- Reduce data-collection period from 5 days to 4 days per week (i.e., 2 school days and 2 weekend days)
- Clarify repeatedly that students are not being tested or graded on activity diary completion
- Instruct teachers and parents on ways to assist with diary completion
- Provide reminders to participants, teachers, and parents

Although this research utilized written activity diaries as a tool for the population studied, Zhu and Hasegawa-Johnson (2002–2003) identified three concerns about using written diaries to study physical activity:

- Expense of scoring
- Accuracy of scoring
- Burden on participants

To address these concerns, they developed and validated the Portable E-diary System for assessing physical activity. Determining the appropriate type of activity diary requires analysis of various factors, including participant preference, age, education level, and experience with technology.

Borg Scale

One method for measuring physical activity is the Borg Rating of Perceived Exertion (RPE). This self-report instrument "is based on the physical sensations a person experiences during physical activity, including increased heart rate, increased respiration or breathing rate, increased sweating, and muscle fatigue" (CDC, 2007, ¶1). When multiplied by 10, this rating is thought to provide a close estimate of a person's actual heart rate during physical activity. Ratings between 12 and 14 appear to match the definitions of moderate to vigorous levels of physical activity.

International Physical Activity Questionnaires (IPAQ)

An international consensus group of experts on physical activity assessment developed two instruments to gather data on the prevalence of physical activity for international comparison. The short version of this questionnaire was designed for national and regional surveillance. The longer version was constructed to facilitate more detailed data-gathering on daily sedentary and physical activity, which is needed for program evaluation and other research. The instruments have been tested for reliability and validity and have been translated into a variety of languages, including Arabic, Italian, Korean, Malay, Polish, and three versions of Spanish (International Physical Activity Questionnaires, n.d.).

Pedometer

Pedometers are a common tool for measuring physical activity and can easily be clipped to a belt or waistband. Croteau (2004) found pedometers useful for measuring physical activity engagement as well as for increasing participation levels. A variety of types and styles of pedometers are available. Crouter, who researches pedometer accuracy, reviewed five pedometer models for members of the National Education Association (Wallace, 2008). The models ranged in price from $16.99 to $59.95 and varied in features and accuracy. Although additional features are interesting and intriguing, step counting accuracy is of primary importance.

Population-Based Surveys of the Environment

Two examples of population-based surveys that can be undertaken in the community are described below: Walkability Checklist: How walkable is your community? (U.S. Department of Transportation [USDOT], 1997) and the Bikeability Checklist: How bikeable is your community? (Pedestrian and Bicycle Information Center, n.d.). These are two of many available tools that range from measures for use by community members to more sophisticated research instruments such as the Systematic Pedestrian and Cycling Environmental Scan (SPACES), an environmental assessment instrument developed in Australia (Pikora et al., 2002) to investigate suitability for both occupations.

Both the Walkability and Bikeability checklists are easy-to-use tools that are available online and use a six-point Likert scale to access community suitability for these occupations. These tools may also be used as an initial step for either an independent occupation-based intervention or an occupation-based intervention embedded into a broader interdisciplinary effort. Both checklists include a survey of conditions, a list of strategies to seek improvements, and a contact list for additional resources. The Bikeability checklist and supporting components are accessible in one file, while the Walkability checklist separates the components into individual files. The Walkability checklist may be reproduced courtesy of the USDOT.

The literature addressing the impact of the built environment on health is growing (Frumkin, 2003; Jackson, 2003; Pollard, 2003). Design features reported to be important for parks that relate to physical activity engagement include signage and safe, pleasant, meandering pathways. The public health literature is beginning to discuss the link between access to drinking water, toilets, safety features such as good lighting and well-maintained trails (Frumkin, 2003), existence of walking and bike paths, street design, public transit (Librett, Yore, & Schmid 2003), proximity of place (Powell, Martin, & Chowdhury, 2003), and physical activity. Organizations such as Active Living Research, a program of the Robert Wood Johnson Foundation, provide grants and resources for research on physical activity in order to advocate for policy changes supportive of healthy lifestyles.

Additional instruments are under development and show promise. One such instrument is the Stanford Brief Activity Survey (Taylor-Piliae et al., 2006). It is important to review the literature to consider both recently developed and existing methods and instruments to measure physical activity participation for evaluating an occupation-based program to increase physical activity.

Occupational Therapy's Role in Promoting Physical Activity

Historical Involvement

The opportunity to participate in physical activity has been of concern to occupational therapy practitioners since the profession's inception. Occupational therapists' use of a variety of manual and physical activities, including calisthenics, with individuals with psychosocial and physical dysfunction is well documented (Dunton, 1915; MacDonald, 1976; Tracy, 1910). However, the potential broader use of these activities to promote a healthy lifestyle and prevent illness or secondary complications was also understood (Dunton, 1915; Tracy, 1910).

As was the case with other areas of occupational therapy, the preceding type of practice all but disappeared due to the allure of working within the medical model during later decades. The profession's dismissal of exercise as a therapeutic tool within the legitimate domain of occupational therapy is exemplified by the introduction of one of the first theory-based research studies on physical activity using an occupational therapy perspective. Rust, Barris, and Hooper (1987) conducted a study on exercise participation among 140 U.S. women. In the introduction to this study, it seems the authors believe they need to acknowledge possible controversy surrounding the study and justify the role of occupational therapy both in the study and in the use of exercise. This perspective may have been due to the then-prevailing thought that exercise was a therapeutic tool for physical therapy and was not viewed to be of sufficient value as an activity worthy of study as an occupation. The authors address this possible criticism by countering that for many regular participants, exercise is a discretionary leisure pursuit and thus is justified to be studied, used, and understood by occupational therapists (Rust et al., 1987).

The Model of Human Occupation (MOHO) was used as the theoretical framework for this study (Rust et al., 1987). Specifically, the researchers were interested in exploring the impact of personal causation, values, interests, habits, and roles on exercising. Results indicated a link between those who were identified as having "internalized the role of exerciser," to perceived competence in that role and to the development of a routine that supported their engagement in physical activity (Rust et al., 1987, p. 32). Interestingly, results did not support the assumption of the MOHO, which purports a link between values and interests and specific occupations. Although the participants valued and knew the importance of exercise as a health habit, this did not carry over to engagement patterns. This finding was consistent with other research findings at the time of the study; the challenge was to have interested people who valued exercise to actually engage in regular exercise. Rust and colleagues recommended that future research address environmental press and the following factors to assist in getting people to actively engage in exercise:

- The influence of peers and significant others who regularly exercise
- The availability of a group with which to participate
- The proximity of setting
- The flexibility of schedules that allow time for exercise

Current Occupational Therapy Research and Literature

Ziviani currently appears to be the occupational therapist most actively involved in disseminating research on physical activity engagement. Ziviani and colleagues (2004, 2006; 2008) have published in a variety of occupational therapy journals the results of their research on physical activity engagement in Australia. The title of the 2004 article "Walking to School: Incidental Physical Activity in the Daily Occupations of Australian Children," exudes occupation. Results of this study underscore the strong influence of parental and generational health habit patterns on their offspring. In addition, Reynolds (2001) has published a review of the literature in physical activity research, within occupational therapy and other disciplines, that provides a basis for health promotion program development. This literature influenced the development of the potential role of occupational therapy in the use of physical activity to promote health.

Potential Role

Four primary areas of expertise that support the role of occupational therapists and occupational therapy assistants in the promotion of physical activity have been identified. These areas of expertise are based on literature cited in this chapter; direct service delivery experience with individuals and groups; and the study and teaching of occupational therapy history, philosophy, and theory. While there are many other skills and areas of expertise that occupational therapists and occupational therapy assistants may use to increase physical activity levels, these were seen as the primary areas of unique expertise:

- Human development through the life span and facilitating developmental transitions
- Occupation-based assessment and intervention
- Intersection of person, environment, and occupation
- Advocating for equal assess to physical activity environments and occupations for individuals with disabilities

A variety of current and potential interventions that utilize these four areas and others are described next in more detail.

Developmentally Based Interventions

The literature describes the progressive decline in physical activity as children become adolescents, particularly for young girls (Garcia et al., 1995; Weallens et al., 2003), then as they become young adults, adults, and on into older adulthood. In addition, periods of transition of place and the resulting stress can generate a retreat to a more sedentary lifestyle (Calfas et al., 2000). Also, new mothers were asked to recall physical activity patterns since childhood (Weallens et al., 2003). Results of a survey of 42 Scottish women indicated a steady decline in physical activity since childhood, including during pregnancy. The type of activities also changed as the women aged. Team sports were most prevalent during childhood and adolescence. These activities were replaced by aerobics and exercising at gymnasiums in adulthood. During pregnancy, vigorous activities were avoided and replaced by yoga, walking, and swimming.

The more physical activity that can be embedded into lifelong occupations that individuals, groups, and communities value, the more likely results of improved health will be seen. Populations may need greater attention at times of transition from one developmental stage to another, as this is often when physical activity declines. In addition, programs should be tailored to reflect the developmental needs of distinct age groups. Perceived control has been linked to activity level, including preventive actions such as exercise in older adults.

Researchers have theorized that older adults may be more likely to participate in physical activity if the message is consistent with an internal locus of control. Older adults' physical activity levels may increase (Menec & Chipperfield, 1997) by enhancing their perception of control over their physical activity engagement through messages that emphasize personal choice in options to manage health and health issues. Targeting all older adults with similar programming and strategies should be avoided, as research indicates that physical activity performance and intention to participate in physical activity vary in subgroups of older adults (Riebe et al., 2005).

It is important that occupational therapists and occupational therapy assistants promote programs and policies for people through the lifespan, targeted to the needs of each age group. It is most critical to start when individuals are young and can develop life long healthy habits. Thus the list below focuses heavily on children and adolescents:

- developmentally appropriate resources to encourage physical activity at recess;
- availability of adaptive physical education and resources at recess for students with disabilities;
- providing education to students, parents, and families as to the health benefits of physical activity (Reynolds, 2001);
- physical education for students from kindergarten through college;

- sports and other physical activities programming (e.g., culturally relevant dance) in middle school to assist with the transition and continuation of activities in high school;
- safe bike and walking paths to school;
- less parking permits in high school;
- safe bike and walking paths from retirement communities to local shopping; and
- interdisciplinary, longitudinal studies of physical activity engagement and outcomes.

In addition to advocating for these resources, occupational therapists can develop and evaluate programs that teach skills for life-stage transitions in order to include physical activity as an important health maintenance occupation. Examples of such initiatives include

- occupation-based retirement planning;
- occupation-based assessment and prescription, to include physical activities for
  - first-year high school students,
  - first-year college students,
  - graduating college students,
  - new parents,
  - returning military service personnel and their families, and
  - new widows and widowers.

Occupation-Based Interventions

Robinson and colleagues (2003) described a culturally relevant intervention that used an occupation—dance—to increase interest in physical activity and decrease television watching. None of the researchers were occupational therapists, but the results support the power and potential of an occupation-based intervention. Programs like Shape Up America!'s 10,000 steps and other initiatives are increasingly encouraging embedding physical activity into routine task and role performance to promote health. The energy expenditure for a variety of occupations is displayed in Figure 13-3. The profession's expertise in work simplification and energy conservation can be adapted to help individuals, families, and communities to reexamine their work and IADL performance to increase levels of physical activity. In addition, occupational scientists can develop studies to determine whether

- increasing the use of embedded occupations with physical activity features increases health outcomes, and whether
- increasing targeting multiple health-promoting occupations simultaneously enhances health outcomes and addresses the current discrepancy in the research literature (Akamatsu, Nakamura, & Shirakawa, 2005).

Examples of Moderate Amounts of Physical Activities		
Common Chores	**Less Vigorous More Time** ↑	**Sporting Activities**
Washing and waxing a car for 45–60 minutes		Playing volleyball for 45–60 minutes
Washing windows or floors for 45–60 minutes		Playing touch football for 45 minutes
Gardening for 30–45 minutes		Walking $1\frac{3}{4}$ miles in 35 minutes (20 minutes/mile)
Wheeling self in wheelchair for 30–40 minutes		Basketball (shooting baskets) for 30 minutes
Pushing a stroller $1\frac{1}{2}$ miles in 30 minutes		Bicycling 5 miles in 30 minutes
Raking leaves for 30 minutes		Dancing fast (social) for 30 minutes
Walking 2 miles in 30 minutes (15 minutes/mile)		Water aerobics for 30 minutes
Shoveling snow for 15 minutes		Swimming laps for 20 minutes
Stair walking for 15 minutes		Basketball (playing game) for 15–20 minutes
		Bicycling 4 miles in 15 minutes
		Jumping rope for 15 minutes
	More Vigorous Less Time ↓	Running $1\frac{1}{2}$ miles in 15 minutes (10 minutes/mile)

Source: www.surgeongeneral.gov/topics/obesity/calltoaction/fact_whatcanyoudo.htm

Activity	Calories Burned per 30 minutes
Walking (leisurely), 2 miles per hour	85
Walking (brisk), 4 miles per hour	170
Gardening	135
Raking leaves	145
Dancing	190
Bicycling (leisurely), 10 miles per hour	205
Swimming laps, medium level	240
Jogging, 5 miles per hour	275

Figure 13-3 ENERGY OUT activities.

Reproduced from We Can!™ Ways to Enhance Children's Activity & Nutrition: ENERGY OUT Activities, *by the National Heart, Lung, and Blood Institute (n.d.).*

Intersection of the Person, Environment, and Occupation

Chapter 2 described several models and theories that have as their main constructs the person, environment, and occupation:

- Ecology of Human Performance Model
- Model of Human Occupation
- Occupational Adaptation
- Person-Environment-Occupation-Performance Model
- Person-Environment-Occupation Model

These theoretical frameworks can be used to support the activities described below or other interventions that focus on the interaction between humans, their environment, and occupations that require moderate physical activity.

The emphasis of this chapter is on program initiatives targeted toward groups and populations. However, occupational therapists also have much to offer individuals preparing or wishing to continue participating in physically active populations. This consultation should supplement rather than supplant medical clearance from their primary health-care provider.

While additional adaptations may need to be individually tailored, there are health risks that must be addressed to maximize the safety of physical activity engagement. Many of these risks are evident at the intersection of the person, occupation, and environment and can be identified with a quick environmental scan. For instance, when an environment is selected for a walking program, thought must be given to such physical features as lighting, surface, grade of inclines and altitude, weather patterns, presence of physical barriers (e.g., locked gates, unrestrained dogs), proximity to emergency assistance, and access to restrooms and water. Other considerations include frequency of use of the path or trail and the level of seclusion, as well as proximity to and patterns of criminal activity in the area.

In addition to environmental features, person and occupation features should be examined for potential health risks. In terms of person factors, the need to prepare for the activity is important by selecting appropriate clothing and equipment. Sunscreen, including for the lips; head gear; appropriate footwear; sunglasses; clothing for layering, depending on the altitude, season, and weather; walking stick; medicines; water bottle(s); map; cell phone; and a healthy snack are all important considerations. The length of the walk and the terrain will dictate the need for items from the preceding list. In terms of the occupation of walking, health risks can be minimized by grading the length of walk, the rate of pace, the place, and the inclusion of one or more other participants.

Communities, including schools, are excellent sites for collaboration to increase physical activity at the individual and group level. Many of these opportunities can involve improving access and modifying contextual factors or barriers as well as program development. A number of these potential interventions address what is referred to in the literature as *bikeability, walkability,* and the *impact of the built environment.* Governmental and nonprofit organizations can work together to communicate the availability of easy access to short to moderate walkways. A pamphlet produced by such a coalition includes maps and directions for five easy-access circular walks close to public transportation in the Chilterns area of Buckinghamshire in the United Kingdom. The free pamphlet, which is available at rail stations, also reviews the benefits of walking and other resources for walks, and encourages walkers to visit and support the local shops and other businesses after a walk (Chilterns Conservation Board, n.d.). By typing the word "walks" in the search box of the corresponding website, http://www.chiltern-saonb.org/default.asp, additional information on short (1 to 3 miles), medium (4 to 6 miles), and long (over 7 miles) walks, as well as stroller and wheelchair routes

and other activities can be obtained. Occupational therapists, with their knowledge and appreciation of built and natural environments, can be valuable assets to these and other initiatives in research, policy advocacy, and program development (Ziviani, Scott, & Wadley, 2004).

Completing the Bikeability or Walkability checklist for a community is an excellent example of the potential to examine and improve the interactions of the person, environment, and occupation to facilitate physical activity. Using six items from the 2001 BRFFS on moderate and vigorous physical activity levels, Sharpe, Granner, Hutto, and Ainsworth (2004) found a link between engaging in physical activity and the presence of supportive policies. By becoming knowledgeable about local zoning laws and ordinances (Librett et al., 2003) and the relationship between zoning and health (Hirschhorn, 2004), occupational therapists and occupational therapy assistants can be prepared to advocate for local ordinances or state legislation to promote physical activity and overall health.

Inclusion of Individuals and Families With Disabilities

The potential impact of increased physical activity on the long-term health and wellbeing of individuals with physical disabilities can be dramatic. Although the overall prevalence rate for spinal cord injury is lower than other disabilities—given the young average age of the people involved and the potential for many secondary conditions that can be decreased by physical activity—this should be an area of emphasis for occupational therapy interventions. It is possible to increase physical activity through targeted programming. Warms, Belza, Whitney, Mitchell, and Stiens (2004) conducted a pilot study of 16 volunteers who had sustained a spinal cord injury and who were not currently exercising. The vast majority of participants (81%) advanced to the next stage within the stages of change theory, indicating more readiness to embark and maintain an exercise regimen, and 60% actually increased their level of physical activity. The researchers were from a School of Nursing and a Rehabilitation Medicine Department; none were from occupational therapy. While research has been conducted among individuals with physical disabilities and their engagement in physical activity, less attention has been paid to individuals with mental illness and developmental disabilities (Messent et al., 1999).

Possible actions to be taken by occupational therapists and occupational therapy assistants to enhance the engagement of people with disabilities include

- conducting community assessments;
- developing programs in all settings, including mental health settings (Reynolds, 2001);

- evaluating programs;
- advocating for "equity in access" for those with limited income (Ziviani et al., 2008);
- using resources such as the National Center on Physical Activity and Disability to advocate for accessible parks and playgrounds;
- communicating access issues and information to the media;
- participating in urban planning to ensure the design encourages physical activity engagement (Ziviani et al., 2008);
- making sure school teachers and administrators are aware that occupational therapists have the expertise to assist with providing accommodations for students with disabilities to meet the President's Challenge;
- educating staff of sheltered housing regarding the importance of physical activity for adults with developmental disabilities (Reynolds, 2001); and
- engaging in interdisciplinary efforts that address individual and population-based health promotion programs.

For more information on health promotion for individuals with disabilities, see Chapter 19 of this book.

Conclusion

This chapter has reviewed the need for interventions, barriers to interventions, and the promise of occupational therapy's contributions to individual and population-based interventions to increase physical activity within the U.S. population. The need to facilitate a fitness ethic for people at all developmental stages and ability levels is essential for health. Occupational therapy's philosophy and theory have much to offer international, national, state, regional, and local efforts to tailor physical activity programs to interest, ability, gender, geographical region, and culture. The influence of physical activity habits on the continuation of exercise over time has been demonstrated (de Bruijn et al., 2006). Additional research is needed on constructs that are well supported by occupational therapy philosophy and theory, such as habit and competency, as well as their impact on physical activity engagement across cultures, genders, ability levels, and age groups. The outcomes from such research are needed to promote policy changes, which is the first step in achieving measurable gains in long-term health indicators in individuals, families, and communities.

Case Study 13-1

From the author's experience, interventions aimed at improving physical activity or other healthy habits within a community are enhanced by working with an interdisciplinary team. Expertise in small group dynamics and activity analysis allows occupational therapists and occupational therapy assistants to effectively function as contributing members of interdisciplinary health promotion teams.

An interdisciplinary team of students was provided the opportunity to develop an intervention to increase physical activity for a rural senior center within a condensed summer educational experience. The experience was supported by a federal grant (i.e., Quentin N. Burdick program) and included four different educational institutions from two neighboring states. A team of one occupational therapy student, one social work student, and two nursing students developed the Strides for Life: A Walking Program for Older Adults program (Stevenson, 1998). The program consisted of a preparatory education program and a walking program with an incentive component, and it was based on a combination of the Health Belief Model and the Ecology of Human Performance. One unique feature of the program was the construction and use of bead bracelets to track walking distance. Participants were encouraged to count steps performed during the course of their daily routines. A total of 18 individuals participated in the program, with the first three to walk a total of 20 miles receiving incentives (i.e., gift certificates from local grocery stores and restaurants).

A separate interdisciplinary team, consisting of two occupational therapy students and two social work students, conducted an evaluation of the program in the following fall. Of the original 18 participants, 12 were included in the follow-up survey. In addition to the participant survey, interviews were conducted with the nutrition site manager and the director of Planning and Human Resources for the county's Commission on Aging. Although the data were insufficient to draw conclusions, the results are helpful to consider for future program development. Of the 12 participants, 7 continued their involvement with the program. This result was consistent with the data displayed on the chart used at the senior center to track participants' mileage. Both administrators indicted that the program development and implementation had been enhanced due to its interdisciplinary composition. In addition, it was suggested that the use of additional visual aids (e.g., pictures of cross-sections of arteries of those who exercise versus those who don't) and case studies would strengthen the initial introduction of the program (Stevenson, 1998).

Continued

Questions

1. What additional incentives would be age and culturally appropriate for program participants?
2. What other disciplines might have been able to contribute to the program's development?

3. Would you utilize the administrators' suggestions? Why or why not?

▶ For Discussion and Review

1. How much physical activity do you engage in during the average week of your semester? During exam week?
2. Identify barriers to engagement in physical activity. How did, or could, you overcome these barriers?
3. Review the Rescuing Recess website at http://www.rescuingrecess.com. How could you as an occupational therapist in an elementary or middle school use this website and your skills as an occupational therapist to increase access to physical activity for all students?

▶ Research Questions

1. What is the impact of occupational role performance on engagement of physical activity throughout the life span?
2. What is the influence of care of pets on engagement in physical activity?
3. Do choices of leisure-oriented physical activity differ by gender, cultural background, or geographical location?

References

Abbott, R. D., White, L. R., Ross, G. W., Masaki, K. H., Curb, J. D., & Petrovitch, H. (2004). Walking and dementia in physically capable elderly men. *Journal of the American Medical Association, 292*(12), 1447–53.

Akamatsu, R., Nakamura, M., & Shirakawa, T. (2005). Relationships between smoking behavior and readiness to change physical activity patterns in a community in Japan. *American Journal of Health Promotion, 19*(6), 406–409.

American Heart Association. (n.d.). *Get fit with family & friends* [Brochure]. Glen Allen, VA: Mid-Atlantic Affiliate.

American Occupational Therapy Association. (2008). Occupational therapy practice framework: Domain and processes (2d ed.). *American Journal of Occupational Therapy, 56,* 625–683.

Anderson, C. B. (2003). When more is better: Number of motives and reasons for quitting as correlates of physical activity in women. *Health Education Research, 18*(5), 525–37.

Beijing Organizing Committee for the Games of the XXIX Olympiad. (n.d.). *Home.* Retrieved January 25, 2008, from http://en.beijing2008.cn/en.shtml.

Calfas, K. J., Sallis, J. F., Nichols, J. F., Sarkin, J. A., Johnson, M. F., Caparosa, S., et al. (2000). Project GRAD: Two-year outcomes of a randomized controlled physical activity intervention among young adults. *American Journal of Preventive Medicine, 18*(1), 28–37.

Callaghan, P., Eves, F. F., Norman, P., Chang, A. M., & Lung, C. Y. (2002). Applying the transtheoretical model of change to exercise in young Chinese people. *British Journal of Health Psychology, 7,* 267–82.

Cardinal, B. J., & Spaziani, M. D. (2003). ADA compliance and the accessibility of physical activity facilities in western Oregon. *American Journal of Health Promotion, 17*(3), 197–201.

Carlson, S. A., Fulton, J. E., Lee, S. M., Maynard, L. M., Brown, D. R., Kohl, III, H. W., & Dietz, W. H. (2008). Physical education and academic achievement in elementary school: Data from the early childhood longitudinal study. *American Journal of Public Health, 98*(4), 721–27.

Centers for Disease Control and Prevention. (2006a, May). *Behavioral Risk Factor Surveillance System.* Retrieved June 4, 2006, from http://www.cdc.gov/BRFSS/.

Centers for Disease Control and Prevention. (2006b, May). *Physical activity and good nutrition: Essential elements to prevent chronic diseases and obesity.* Retrieved June 8, 2006, from http://www.cdc.gov/nccdphp/publications/aag/dnpa.htm.

Centers for Disease Control and Prevention. (2006c, March 22). *Physical activity for everyone: Physical activity terms.* Retrieved July 4, 2006, from http://www.cdc.gov/nccdphp/dnpa/physical/terms/index.htm.

Centers for Disease Control and Prevention. (2006d, April). *Steps to a HealthierUS (measures).* Retrieved June 1, 2006, from http://wonder.cdc.gov/data2010/HU.HTM.

Centers for Disease Control and Prevention. (2006e, March). *U.S. physical activity statistics: Definitions.* Retrieved July 1, 2006, from http://www.cdc.gov/nccdphp/dnpa/physical/stats/definitions.htm.

Centers for Disease Control and Prevention. (2007, May). *Physical activity for everyone: Measuring physical activity intensity: Perceived exertion (Borg Rating of Perceived Exertion Scale).* Retrieved August 9, 2008, from http://www.cdc.gov/nccdphp/dnpa/physical/measuring/perceived_exertion.htm.

Centers for Disease Control and Prevention, National Center for Chronic Disease Prevention and Health Promotion. (1999). *Physical activity and health: A report of the surgeon general.* Retrieved May 29, 2006, from http://www.cdc.gov/nccdphp/sgr/prerep.htm.

Centers for Disease Control and Prevention, National Center for Chronic Disease Prevention and Health Promotion. (2003). *ACES: Active Community Environments Initiative.* Retrieved January 25, 2005, from http://www.cdc.gov/nccdphp/dnpa/aces.htm.

Chilterns Conservation Board. (n.d.). *Simply walk . . . Stile free: Access just got easier!* [Pamphlet]. Buckinghamshire County Council, United Kingdom: Author.

Croteau, K. A. (2004). A preliminary study on the impact of a pedometer-based intervention on daily steps. *American Journal of Health Promotion, 18*(3), 217–20.

De Bourdeaudhuij, I., Philippaerts, R., Crombez, G., Matton, L., Wijndaele, K., Balduck, A. L., & Lefevre, J. (2005). Stages of change for physical activity in a community sample of adolescents. *Health Education Research, 20*(3), 357–66.

De Bourdeaudhuij, I., Sallis, J. F., & Saelens, B. E. (2003). Environmental correlates of physical activity in a sample of Belgian adults. *American Journal of Health Promotion, 18*(1), 83–92.

de Bruijn, G-J., Kremers, S. P. J., Lensvelt-Mulders, G., de Vries, H., van Mechelen, W., & Brug, J. (2006). Modeling individual and physical environmental factors with adolescent physical activity. *American Journal of Preventive Medicine, 30*(6), 507–12.

Dergance, J. M., Calmbach, W. L., Dhanda, R., Miles, T. P., Hazuda, H. P., & Mouton, C. P. (2003). Barriers to benefits of leisure time physical activity in the elderly: Differences across cultures. *Journal of the American Geriatrics Society, 51*(6), 863–68.

Dixon, L. B., Cronin, F. J., & Krebs-Smith, S. M. (2001). Let the pyramid guide your food choices: Capturing the total diet concept. *Journal of Nutrition, 131*(suppl.), 461S–472S.

Duke, J., Huhman, M., & Heitlzler, C. (2003, August 22). Physical activity levels among children aged 9–13 years—United States, 2002. *Morbidity and Mortality Weekly Report, 52*(33) 785–88.

Dunton, W. R. (1915). *Occupational therapy: A manual for nurses.* Philadelphia: W. B. Saunders.

Evenson, K. R., & McGinn, A. P. (2004). Availability of school physical activity facilities to the public in four U.S. communities. *American Journal of Health Promotion, 18*(3), 243–50.

Focht, B. C., & Hausenblas, H. A. (2004). Research note: Perceived evaluative threat and state anxiety during exercise in women with social physique anxiety. *Journal of Applied Sport Psychology, 16,* 361–68.

Foundation of the Hellenic World. (2005). *The revival of the ancient Olympic Games.* Retrieved October 8, 2005, from http://www.fhw.gr/olympics/ancient/en/300.html.

Frumkin, H. (2003). Healthy places: Exploring the evidence. *American Journal of Public Health, 93*(9), 1451–56.

Garcia, A. W., Broda, M. A. N., Frenn, M., Coviak, C., Pender, N. J., & Ronis, D. L. (1995). Gender and developmental differences in exercise beliefs among youth and prediction of their exercise behavior. *Journal of School Health, 65*(6), 213–19.

Giles-Corti, B., Macintyre, S., Clarkson, J. P., Pikora, T., & Donovan, R. J. (2003). Environmental and lifestyle factors associated with overweight and obesity in Perth, Australia. *American Journal of Health Promotion, 18*(1), 93–102.

Glass, T. A., de Leon, C. M., Martolli, R. A., & Berlman, L. F. (1999). Population based study of social and productive activities as predictors of survival among elderly Americans. *British Medical Journal, 319,* 478–83.

Grunbaum, J. A., Kann, L., Kinchen, S., Ross, J., Hawkins, J., Lowry, R., et al. (2004). Youth risk behavior surveillance—United States, 2003. *Morbidity and Mortality Weekly Report, 53*(SS-2), 1–95. Available from http://www.cdc.gov/HealthyYouth/yrbs/index.htm.

Hardman, A. E. (2005). *Physical activity, obesity and cancer: A review of current knowledge on epidemiology and recommendations.* Nordic Symposium: Cancer and Physical Activity, Copenhagen, November 29–30.

Henderson, K. A., & Bialeschki, M. D. (1991). A sense of entitlement to leisure as constraint and empowerment for women. *Leisure Sciences, 13,* 51–65.

Hirschhorn, J. S. (2004). Zoning should promote public health. *American Journal of Health Promotion, 18*(3), 258–60.

International Olympic Committee. (2005a). *Olympic Games: All the games since 1896.* Retrieved October 8, 2005, from http://www.olympic.org/uk/games/index_uk.asp.

International Olympic Committee. (2005b). *Olympic Games: Ancient Olympic Games.* Retrieved October 8, 2005, from http://www.olympic.org/uk/games/ancient/index_uk.asp.

International Olympic Committee. (2005c). *Olympic Games: Athens 1896, Games of the I Olympiad.* Retrieved October 8, 2005, from http://www.olympic.org/uk/games/past/index_uk.asp?OLGT=1&OLGY=1896.

International Olympic Committee. (2005d). *Olympic Games: Paris 1900, Games of the II Olympiad.* Retrieved October 8, 2005, from http://www.olympic.org/uk/games/past/index_uk.asp?OLGT=1&OLGY=1900.

International Olympic Committee. (2006). *Paralympics.* Retrieved April 15, 2006, from http://www.olympic.org/uk/games/paralympic/index_uk.asp.

International Physical Activity Questionnaires. (n.d.). *Background.* Retrieved January 24, 2009, from http://www.ipaq.ki.se/index.htm.

Jackson, R. J. (2003). The impact of the built environment on health: An emerging field. *American Journal of Public Health, 93*(9), 1382–84. [Editorial].

Kelder, S. H., Mitchell, P. D., McKenzie, T. L., Derby, C., Strikmiller, P. K., Luepker, R. V., et al. (2003). Long-term implementation of the CATCH physical education program. *Health Education and Behavior, 30*(4), 463–75.

Killingsworth, R. E., & Lamming, J. (2001, July). Development and public health. *Urban Land,* 12–17.

Kindersley, D. (1996). *Chronicle of the Olympics.* New York: DK Publishing.

King, W. C., Brach, J. S., Belle, S., Killingsworth, R., Fenton, M., & Kriska, A. M. (2003). The relationship between convenience of destinations and walking levels in older women. *American Journal of Health Promotion, 18*(1), 74–82.

Kushi, L. H., Fee, R. M., Folsom, A. R., Mink, P. J., Anderson, K. E., & Sellers, T. A. (1997). Physical activity and mortality in postmenopausal women. *Journal of the American Medical Association, 277*(16), 1287–92.

Levin, S. (2001, October). *Approaching physical activity from a policy perspective.* Presented at the national conference of State Legislatures: NCSL's New England Health Promotion Institute, Nashua, NH.

Librett, J. J., Yore, M. M., & Schmid, T. L. (2003). Local ordinances that promote physical activity: A survey of municipal policies. *American Journal of Public Health, 93*(9), 1399–1403.

Lytle, A. L., Ward, J., Nader, P. R., Pedersen, S., & Williston, B. J. (2003). Maintenance of a health promotion program in elementary schools: Results from the CATCH-ON study key informant interviews. *Health Education & Behavior, 30*(4), 503–18.

MacDonald, E. M. (Ed.). (1976). Occupational therapy in rehabilitation: Its history and place in health and social services of today. In *Occupational therapy in rehabilitation: A handbook for occupational therapists, students and others interested in this aspect of reablement* (4th ed., pp. 1–14). Baltimore: Williams & Wilkins.

Macera, C. A., Jones, D. A., Yore, M. M., Ham, S. A., Kohl, H. W., Kimsey, C. D., Jr., & Buchner, D. (2003, August 13). Prevalence of physical activity, including lifestyle activities among adults—United States, 2000–2001. *Mortality and Morbidity Weekly Report, 52*(32), 764–69. Retrieved October 9, 2005, from http://www.cdc.gov/mmwr/preview/mmwrhtml/mm5232a2.htm.

Marcus, B. H., Pinto, B. M., Simkin, L. R., Audrain, J. E., & Taylor, E. R. (1994). Application of theoretical models to exercise behavior among employed women. *The Science of Health Promotion, 9*(1), 49–55.

Marshall, A. L., Bauman, A. E., Owen, N., Booth, M. L., Crawford, D., & Marcus, B. H. (2004). Reaching out to promote physical activity in Australia: A statewide randomized controlled trial of a stage-targeted intervention. *American Journal of Health Promotion, 18*(4), 283–87.

Marshall, A. L., Bauman, A. E., Patch, C., Wilson, J., & Chen, J. (2002). Can motivational signs prompt increases in incidental physical activity in an Australian health-care facility? *Health Education Research, 17,* 743–49.

Marshall, S. J., & Biddle, S. J. (2001). The transtheoretical model of behavior change: A meta-analysis of applications to physical activity and exercise. *Annals of Behavioral Medicine, 23*(4), 229–46.

Menec, V. H., & Chipperfield, J. G. (1997). Remaining active in later life: The role of locus of control in senior's leisure activity participation, health, and life satisfaction. *Journal of Aging and Health, 9*(1), 105–25.

Messent, P. R., Cooke, C. B., & Long, J. (1999). Primary and secondary barriers to physically active healthy lifestyles for adults with learning disabilities. *Disability and Rehabilitation, 21*(9), 409–19.

Mokdad, A. H., Marks, J. S., Stroup, D. F., & Gerberding, J. L. (2004). Actual causes of death in the United States, 2000. *Journal of the American Medical Association, 291*(10), 1238–45.

National Heart, Lung, and Blood Institute. (n.d.). *Live It: ENERGY OUT activities.* Retrieved May 18, 2008, from http://www.nhlbi.nih.gov/health/public/heart/obesity/wecan/live-it/energy-out.htm.

Osganian, S. K., Parcel, G. S., & Stone, E. J. (2003). Institutionalization of a school health promotion program: Background and rationale of the CATCH-ON study. *Health Education & Behavior, 30*(4), 410–17.

Pate, R. R., Saunders, R. P., Ward, D. S., Felton, G., Trost, S. G., & Dowda, M. (2003). Evaluation of a community-based intervention to promote physical activity in youth: Lessons from active winners. *American Journal of Health Promotion, 17,* 171–82.

Pedersen, S., & Seidman, E. (2004). Team sports achievement and self-esteem development among urban adolescent girls. *Psychology of Women Quarterly, 28,* 412–22.

Pedestrian and Bicycle Information Center. (n.d.). *Bikeability checklist: How bikeable is your community?* Retrieved November 7, 2004, from http://www.bicyclinginfo.org/pdf/bikabilitychecklist.pdf.

Pikora, T. J., Bull, F. C. L., Jamrozik, K., Knuiman, M., Giles-Corti, B., & Donovan, R. J. (2002). Developing a reliable audit instrument for physical activity. *American Journal of Preventative Medicine, 23*(3), 187–94.

Pollard, T. (2003). Policy prescriptions for healthier communities. *American Journal of Health Promotion, 18*(1), 109–13.

Powell, K. E., Martin, L. M., & Chowdhury, P. P. (2003). Places to walk: Convenience and regular physical activity. *American Journal of Public Health, 93*(9), 1519–21.

President's Council on Physical Fitness and Sports, U.S. Department of Health and Human Services. (2002). *News, speeches, & photos: Photos from the kick-off of the President's HealthierUS initiative—Council member Denise Austin leads a workout at the White House.* Retrieved April 22, 2006, from, http://www.fitness.gov/photos-healthieruswhitehouseevent06.20.02.htm.

President's Council on Physical Fitness and Sports, U.S. Department of Health and Human Services. (2004). *About the President's Council on Physical Fitness and Sports.* Retrieved October 8, 2005, from http://www.fitness.gov/about_overview.htm.

President's Council on Physical Fitness and Sports, U.S. Department of Health and Human Services. (2006). *The President's Challenge: Accommodating students with disabilities.* Retrieved May 29, 2006, from http://www.presidentschallenge.org/educators/disabilities.aspx.

Pucher, J., & Renne, J. L. (2003). Socioeconomic of urban travel: Evidence from the 2001 NHTS. *Transportation Quarterly, 57*(3), 49–77.

Rao, G. (2001). Insulin resistance syndrome. *American Family Physician, 65*(11), 1165–66.

Rastogi, T., Splegelman, D., Reddy, K. S., Bharathi, A. V., Stampfer, M. J., Willett, W. C., & Ascherio, A. (2004). Physical activity and risk of coronary heart disease in India. *International Journal of Epidemiology, 33*(4), 759–67.

Renger, R., Steinfelt, V., & Lazarus, S. (2002). Assessing the effectiveness of a community-based media campaign targeting physical activity. *Family and Community Health, 25*(3), 18–30.

Resnick, B., & Nigg, C. (2003). Testing a theoretical model of exercise behavior for older adults. *Nursing Research, 52*(2), 80–88.

Reynolds, F. (2001). Strategies for facilitating physical activity and wellbeing: A health promotion perspective. *British Journal of Occupational Therapy, 64*(7), 330–36.

Reynolds, K. D., Killen, J. D., Bryson, S. W., Maron, D. J., Taylor, C. B., Maccoby, N., et al. (1990). Psychosocial predictors of physical activity in adolescents. *Preventive Medicine, 19,* 541–51.

Riebe, D., Garber, C. E., Rossi, J. S., Greaney, M. L., Nigg, C. R., Lees, F. D., Burbank, P. M., & Clark, P. G. (2005). Physical activity, physical function, and stages of change in older adults. *American Journal of Health Behavior, 29*(1), 70–80.

Ries, A. V., Gittelson, J., Voorhees, C. C., Roche, K. M., Clifton, K. J., & Astone, N. M. (2008). The environment and urban adolescents' use of recreational facilities for physical activity: A Qualitative study. *American Journal of Health Promotion, 23*(1), 43–50.

Robinson, T. N., Killen, J. D., Kraemer, H. C., Wilson, D. M., Matheson, D. M., Haskell, W. L., et al. (2003). Dance and reducing television viewing to prevent weight gain in African-American girls: The Stanford GEMS pilot study. *Ethnicity and Disease, 13,* S1-65–S1-77.

Rust, K. M., Barris, R., & Hooper, F. H. (1987). Use of the model of human occupation to predict women's exercise behavior. *Occupational Therapy Journal of Research, 7*(1), 23–35.

Sallis, J. F., Calfas, K. J., Alcaraz, J. E. Gehrman C., & Johnson, M. F. (1999). Potential mediators of change in a physical activity promotion course for university students: Project GRAD. *Annals of Behavorial Medicine, 21*(2), 149–58.

Shape Up America! (2005–2006). *Shape Up America!: Healthy weight for life.* Retrieved July 5, 2006, from http://www.shapeup.org/.

Sharpe, P. A., Granner, M. L., Hutto, B., & Ainsworth, B. E. (2004). Association of environmental factors to meeting physical activity recommendations in two South Carolina counties. *American Journal of Health Promotion, 18*(3), 251–57.

Sisson, S. B., Lee, S. M., Burns, E. K., & Tudor-Locke, C. (2006). Suitability of commuting by bicycle to Arizona elementary schools. *American Journal of Health Promotion, 20*(3), 210–13.

Smith, D. A., Ness, E. M., Herbert, R., Schechter, C. B., Phillips, R. A., Diamond, J. A., & Landrigan, P. J. (2004). Abdominal diameter index: A more powerful anthropometric measure for prevalent coronary heart disease risk in adult males. *Diabetes, Obesity and Metabolism, 7,* 370–80.

Stevenson, S. (1998). *Interdisciplinary prevention in rural communities: Outcomes of the Strides for Life Walking Program for Older Adults.* Unpublished graduate project, Towson University, Towson, MD.

Taylor-Piliae, R. E., Norton, L. C., Haskell, W. L., Mahbouda, M. H., Fair, J. M., Iribarren, C., et al. (2006). Validation of a new brief physical activity survey among men and women aged 60–69 years. *American Journal of Epidemiology, 164*(6), 598–606.

Toppo, G. (2006). School recess isn't exactly on the run. *USA TODAY.* Retrieved on May 17, 2006, from http://www.usatoday.com/news/health/2006-05-16-school-exercise_x.htm.

Torino 2006. (2006a). *Medals.* Retrieved April 15, 2006, from http://www.torino2006.org/ENG/IDF/MDL/MDL_Big.html.

Torino 2006. (2006b). *The Olympic emption of the opening ceremony.* Retrieved April 15, 2006, from http://www.torino2006.org/ENG/OlympicGames/gare_e_programma/cerimonie.html.

Tracy, S. E. (1910). *Studies in invalid occupation.* Boston: Whitcomb & Barrows.

U.S. Department of Agriculture. (n.d.). *Steps to a healthier you.* Retrieved July 2, 2006, from http://www.mypyramid.gov/index.html.

U.S. Department of Health and Human Services. (1979). *Healthy People: Surgeon General's report on health promotion and disease prevention.* Washington, DC: Government Printing Office.

U.S. Department of Health and Human Services. (1980). *Promoting health/preventing disease: Objectives for the nation.* Washington, DC: Government Printing Office.

U.S. Department of Health and Human Services. (1990). *Healthy People 2000: National health promotion and disease prevention objectives.* Washington, DC: Government Printing Office.

U.S. Department of Health and Human Services. (2000). *Healthy People 2010: Understanding and improving health* (2d ed.). Washington, DC: Government Printing Office.

U.S. Department of Health and Human Services, National Institutes of Health. (n.d.). *We Can!™ (Ways to Enhance Children's Activity & Nutrition).* Retrieved June 3, 2006, from http://www.nhlbi.nih.gov/health/public/heart/obesity/wecan/whats-we-can/.

U.S. Department of Transportation, National Highway Traffic Safety Administration. (1997). *Walkability checklist: How walkable is your community?* Retrieved November 7, 2004, from http://www.nhtsa.dot.gov/people/injury/pedbimot/ped/walk1.html.

Verhoef, M. J., & Love, E. J. (1992). Women's exercise participation: The relevance of social roles compared to non-role-related determinants. *Canadian Journal of Public Health, 83*(5), 367–70.

Wallace, G. K. (2008, January). *Staying fit and eating healthy at any age.* Retrieved May 18, 2008, from http://www.nea.org/neatoday/0801/theguide.html.

Warms, C. A., Belza, B. L., Whitney, J. D., Mitchell, P. H., & Stiens, S. A. (2004). Lifestyle physical activity for individuals with spinal cord injury: A pilot study. *American Journal of Health Promotion, 18*(1), 14–20.

Weallens, E., Clark, A., MacIntyre, P., & Gaudoin, M. (2003). A survey of exercise patterns in primigravidae at a Scottish NHS Trust: More consistent support and advice required for women and their families. *Health Education Journal, 62*(3), 234–45.

Woods, C., Mutrie, N., & Scott, M. (2002). Physical activity intervention: A transtheoretical model-based intervention designed to help sedentary young adults become active. *Health Education Research, 17*(4), 451–60.

World Health Organization. (2001). *International classification of functioning, disability and health.* Geneva, Switzerland: Author.

World Health Organization. (2006a) *Core health indicators, country compare: China population.* Retrieved May 21, 2006, from http://www3.who.int/whosis/country/compare.cfm?country=CHN&indicator=TotalPop&language=english.

World Health Organization. (2006b). *Global strategy on diet, physical activity and health: Physical activity.* Retrieved May 21, 2006, from http://www.who.int/dietphysicalactivity/publications/facts/pa/en/index.html.

Wormald, H., Sleap, M., Brunton, J., Hayes, L., Warburton, P., Waring, M., & White, M. (2003). Methodological issues in piloting a physical activity diary with young people. *Health Education Journal, 62*(3), 220–33.

Zhu, W., & Hasegawa-Johnson, M. (2002–2003). *A portable E-diary system for assessing physical activity and travel.* Retrieved May 18, 2008, from http://www.isle.uiuc.edu/ research/ediary.html.

Ziviani, J., Macdonald, D., Jenkins D., Rodger, S., Batch, J., & Cerin, E. (2006). Physical activity of young children. *Occupational, Participation and Health, 26*(1), 4–14.

Ziviani, J., Scott, J., & Wadley, D. (2004). Walking to school: Incidental physical activity in the daily occupations of Australian children. *Occupational Therapy International, 11*(1), 1–11.

Ziviani, J., Wadley, D., Ward, H., Macdonald, D., Jenkins D., & Rodger, S. (2008). Physical activity of young children. *Australian Occupational Therapy Journal, 55*(2), 2–11.

Chapter 14

Weight Management and Obesity Reduction

Marie Kuczmarski, S. Maggie Reitz, and Michael A. Pizzi

> Obesity has reached epidemic proportions globally, with more than 1 billion adults overweight—at least 300 million of them clinically obese—and is a major contributor to the global burden of chronic disease and disability. Often coexisting in developing countries with under-nutrition, obesity is a complex condition, with serious social and psychological dimensions, affecting virtually all ages and socioeconomic groups.
>
> —World Health Organization (WHO), 2005, ¶ 2

Learning Objectives

This chapter is designed to enable the reader to:

- Discuss the prevalence and associated health and mortality risks of obesity.
- Describe obesity prevention and intervention guidelines across the life span.
- Explain the role of occupational therapy in weight regulation and obesity reduction.
- Discover possible personal biases against overweight individuals.
- Describe the benefits of partnering with a nutritionist when addressing weight regulation for program planning and implementation.
- Identify and access resources to plan weight-regulation interventions for individuals, families, or communities.

Key Terms

Abdominal diameter index

Basal metabolic rate

Body mass index (BMI)

Energy-dense foods

Energy imbalance

Healthy body weight

Moderate physical activity

Obesity

Overweight or pre-obese

Thermic effect of food

Vigorous physical activity

Introduction

Maintaining a healthy body weight across the life span can reduce the risk for developing certain chronic conditions and subsequently promote healthy aging. This requires a lifelong commitment to healthy living. Lifestyle behaviors emphasizing moderation and variety in eating practices, regular physical activity, adequate sleep, abstinence from tobacco, and moderate consumption of alcohol promote overall health and wellbeing. Greater food availability, especially of tasty **energy-dense foods,** encourages overeating and makes it difficult to eat healthy. Energy density is determined by the fat, fiber, and water content of foods. Energy-dense foods have a high fat content. Frequent consumption of these types of foods without adequate physical activity can lead to obesity.

Being overweight or obese can restrict or possibly severely limit people's engagement in occupations, their level of participation in society, and their overall wellbeing. Thus, health-care practitioners, including occupational therapists and occupational therapy assistants, have a responsibility to educate the public about weight management and to evaluate and assist their clients to achieve and maintain healthy body weights. Evaluation can entail examining occupational performance, including performance skill and patterns as well as contexts, activity demands, and client factors as defined in the *Occupational Therapy Practice Framework* (referred to as the *Framework*; American Occupational

Therapy Association [AOTA], 2008). Occupational therapists and occupational therapy assistants must be unbiased in their interactions and must be proficient at suggesting and assisting with adaptations that provide larger individuals with options regarding occupational engagement.

This chapter provides an overview of weight regulation; prevalence of overweight and obesity; health risks, including psychosocial and physical risks; mortality risks; the economic burden of obesity; prevention and treatment recommendations and guidelines for overweight and obesity throughout the life span; and weight bias. The chapter also includes a discussion of registered dietitian and physician roles as well as that of occupational therapy in weight management, weight regulation, and the reduction of obesity. A registered dietician served as lead author for this chapter; the remaining authors are occupational therapists. Together, they provide an interdisciplinary perspective on this content.

Weight Regulation

It is thought that the body exerts a stronger defense against undernutrition and weight loss than it does against weight gain. Weight gain can be described in three phases. The first is the pre-obese static phase, when the individual is in long-term energy balance and body weight is constant. The second phase is termed *dynamic* and occurs when the individual gains weight as a result of energy intake exceeding energy expenditure over a prolonged period. The obese static phase is the last phase and is when energy balance is regained but weight is now higher than during the pre-obese static phase. Once the obese state is established, the physiological processes tend to defend the new weight (WHO, 2000).

Weight gain is the result of **energy imbalance,** where energy intake has exceeded energy expenditure over a considerable period of time. This imbalance can result from increased energy intake, decreased energy expenditure, or a combination of both factors. The food and beverages an individual consumes determine energy intake. The macronutrients—protein, carbohydrates, and fats—provide energy. Protein and carbohydrates provide 4 kcal/g while fats provide 9 kcal/g.

The components of energy expenditure include basal metabolic rate, the effect of physical activity, and the thermic effect of food. **Basal metabolic rate,** which is energy expenditure at rest, 12 hours or more after eating, and in a thermally neutral environment, is the largest component. It represents approximately 50% to 70% of daily total energy expenditure. Physical activity represents the most variable component, at approximately 20% to 40% of total energy expenditure.

The energy expenditure of activity is influenced by the intensity, the duration, the frequency with which the activity is performed, the individual's body mass, and the individual's efficiency of performance. The smallest component is the **thermic effect of food**—the energy expenditure associated with the digestion, absorption, transport, metabolism, and storage of energy from ingested food and beverages—which averages 10% of energy intake (Gropper, Smith, & Groff, 2009).

Genetic, environmental, and behavioral factors all contribute to weight status (U.S. Department of Health and Human Services [USDHHS], 2000). The conditions of overweight and obesity develop from an interaction of these factors, rather than from any single factor alone. **Overweight** or **pre-obese** is described as an excess of body weight compared to set standards, while **obesity** is categorized by an excessive accumulation of body fat. Obesity, a complex multifactorial chronic disease, can result from a minor energy imbalance that leads to a persistent weight gain over time. Cutler, Glaeser, and Shapiro (2003) noted that the increase in median weight observed in U.S. adults over the past two decades requires a net energy imbalance of only about 100 to 150 kcal per day.

Although the physiological mechanisms are not fully understood, there is evidence of a genetic contribution to human obesity. The human OB gene (i.e., leptin gene) has been mapped to chromosome 7 (Escott-Stump, 2002). The hormone leptin is thought to act as a lipostat. It is secreted by adipocytes in proportion to triglyceride stores and binds to hypothalamic receptors. Leptin has multiple functions: inhibiting food intake, stimulating and maintaining energy expenditure, and influencing metabolism. Defects in the cortical, hypothalamic, endocrine, or metabolic components of the weight-regulatory system can also result in energy imbalances.

Cultural and physical contexts contribute to the development of obesity. There is agreement among some experts that the environment, rather than biology, is driving this epidemic (Hill, Wyam, Reed, & Peters, 2003). The increase in energy-dense, readily available foods coupled with aggressive and sophisticated food marketing by the mass media (Cummings, Parham, & Strain, 2002; Joint FAO/WHO Expert Consultation, 2003) and the increase in the portion size of food sold and served (Young & Nestle, 2002) promote higher energy consumption by the U.S. population. The WHO (2000) recognized the likelihood that behavioral aspects of eating were impacting the rise in obesity but stressed that additional research must be conducted before drawing specific conclusions.

Home, school, or workplace environments may either support or impede healthy weight. School lunch and snack programs have traditionally served high-fat and high-calorie foods. However, there has been a recent move toward healthier lunches in schools, which has been highly supported across the country (Frazao, 1999). Beside not offering healthy meal choices, many schools also impede healthy weight by restricting opportunities for physical activity. In 2003, daily participation in high school physical education classes was 28%, a drop from 42% in 1991. More than one-third of young people in grades 9 through 12 do not regularly engage in vigorous physical activity (Chronic Disease Prevention, 2003).

Physical and social contexts can greatly influence levels and types of food intake. The workplace can be a food trap, as coworkers will go out to lunch, which may lead to eating high-fat and carbohydrate-laden meals. When dining out, people tend to eat more or eat higher-calorie foods. The fat density of these meals exceeds that of food eaten at home (Frazao, 1999). However, in people's homes and communities, positive role models for weight control may influence childhood patterns of eating and can be a support to healthier eating, physical activity, and overall lifestyle management.

The technological advances in U.S. society have reduced the energy cost of engaging in occupations. Cutler and colleagues (2003) calculated that a 40-minute change from light household activity like food preparation and meal cleanup to sedentary activity like television watching would lead to a 4-pound increase in approximately 6 months in steady state weight for the average male. According to 2007 data, nearly 4 in 10 adults (37.7%) in the United States engaged in insufficient amounts of physical activity; slightly more than 1 in 10 (13.5%) were described as inactive (Centers for Disease Control and Prevention [CDC], 2007). Also, adults with lower incomes and education levels are more likely to be physically inactive (Barnes & Schoenborn, 2003). In 2007, approximately 22% of U.S. men and 26% of U.S. women reported no leisure-time physical activity. Only 47% of women and 51% of men engaged in recommended physical activity levels (CDC, 2007). Conditions have been established in the United States whereby genetic predispositions for increases in body weight are more likely to be expressed.

Psychological factors and prescription drugs can also influence weight status. Depressive symptoms can lead to binge eating, resulting in weight gain (Malhotra & McElroy, 2002). Other behaviors such as compulsivity, impulsivity, and neuroticism can also lead to excessive food intake (Camarena et al., 2004). As early as 1985, Gopalaswamy and Morgan reported that the rate of obesity is "2–5 times more prevalent" among psychiatric patients receiving drug treatment than the general population (cited by Camarena et al., 2004,

p. 127). Several classes of psychotropic medications, including antidepressants, mood stabilizers, and, "to a lesser degree, anxiolytics" (Devlin, Yanovski, & Wilson, 2000, p. 858), are associated with unwanted weight gain (Malhi, Mitchell, & Caterson, 2001; Malhotra & McElroy, 2002). There is evidence of "marked weight gain" with the use of monoamine oxidase inhibitors for depression (Camarena et al., 2004, p. 128). In fact, weight gain is one of the most frequent reasons for noncompliance with prescribed psychotropics (Devlin et al., 2000).

Prevalence of Overweight and Obesity

According to the WHO (2000), obesity is a global epidemic. The prevalence of overweight and obesity in the United States has been continually rising in both genders, in all age groups, and in all racial/ethnic groups since the 1980s and has reached epidemic proportions. Obesity is also on the rise in the United Kingdom and "has become one of the most serious health problems in Western society" (Warren, Brennan, & Akehurs, 2004, p. 9). In a study of 13 European countries, the United States, and Israel (Lissau et al., 2004), adolescents in the United States were found to have the highest prevalence of being overweight. Adolescents in Ireland, Greece, and Portugal were found to have the next highest prevalence rates.

The **body mass index (BMI),** the ratio of weight (with minimal clothing) in kilograms to height (without shoes) in meters squared, is a useful clinical tool to classify individuals as normal, underweight, or overweight. Content Box 14-1 provides the formula to calculate BMI. A weakness of the BMI is that some muscular individuals may be classified as obese when they are not. For children, *overweight* is defined as a BMI at or above the 95th percentile of gender-specific BMI for age growth charts. For adults, *overweight* or *pre-obese* is defined as a BMI of 25 to 29.9 kg/m^2. Class I obesity is a BMI of 30 to 34.9 kg/m^2, Class II obesity is a BMI of 35 to 40 kg/m^2, and extreme obesity is a BMI higher than 40 kg/m^2 (WHO, 2000).

Measured heights and weights from the National Health and Nutrition Examination Survey (NHANES) conducted from 2003 to 2004 in the United States have been used to estimate the current prevalence of overweight and obesity. The NHANES is a nationally representative cross-sectional survey of the total civilian noninstitutionalized population in the United States, conducted by the National Center for Health Statistics, an arm of the CDC.

From 2003 to 2004, approximately 13.9% of 2- to 5-year-old children, 18.8% of 6- to 11-year-old

Content Box 14-1

BMI Formulas (USDHHS, 2001)

$$BMI = \frac{weight\ is\ kilograms}{height\ in\ meters\ squared}$$

Example: A person with a weight of 170 pounds and a height of 5 feet 9 inches would have a BMI of about 25, calculated as follows.

First convert 170 pounds into kilograms (2.2 pounds equals 1 kilogram):

$$\frac{170\ lb}{2.2\ lb} = 77.27\ kg$$

Next convert 5 feet 9 inches (5.75 feet) into meters (3.28 feet equals 1 meter):

$$\frac{5.78\ ft}{3.28\ ft} = 1.75\ m$$

Finally, insert your conversions into the BMI equation:

$$\frac{77.2\ kg}{1.75^2\ m} = \frac{77.2\ kg}{3.06\ m^2} = 25$$

The following formula for BMI uses weight in pounds and height in inches.

$$BMI = \frac{weight\ in\ pounds}{height\ in\ inches\ squared} \times 703$$

children, and 17.4% of 12- to 19-year-old individuals were overweight (Ogden et al., 2006). The prevalence of overweight among Mexican American male children and adolescents was significantly greater than in non-Hispanic white male children and adolescents. Female Mexican American and non-Hispanic black children and adolescents were significantly more likely to be overweight compared with non-Hispanic white female children and adolescents. About two out of three adults (66.3%) aged 20 years or older are overweight, and one out of three (32.2%) is obese (Ogden et al., 2006). Non-Hispanic black and Mexican American women were more likely to be obese compared with non-Hispanic white women.

Health Risks

There are many well-documented health risks associated with being overweight or obese. According to Sturm, "obesity has roughly the same association with chronic health problems as does twenty years' aging; this greatly exceeds the associations of smoking or problem drinking" (2002, p. 245). While the physical health risks are more apparent and often are more frequently the subject of research and publications, increasing attention is being focused on how being overweight impacts psychosocial health. A discussion

of these psychosocial risks as well as physical health and mortality risks follows.

Psychosocial Risk Factors

There are psychosocial and health risks associated with being overweight in childhood. Overweight children often experience psychological stress from being teased, bullied, and ostracized (Janssen, Craig, Boyce, & Pickett, 2004). In addition, being overweight in the critical developmental stage of adolescence can result in "psychosocial burdens" (Lissau et al., 2004, p. 27). Researchers in Canada examined the relationship between obesity and bullying behaviors that were identified as "physical, verbal, relational, and sexual harassment" (Janssen et al., 2004, p. 1187). Results indicate that children who are overweight or obese are at increased risk for being the targets of bullies and for developing into bullies than children of average size. Being a victim, perpetrator, or both may have long-term negative ramifications for healthy psychosocial development.

The impact of obesity on psychological wellbeing was identified by Sarlio-Lahteenkorva, Stunkard, and Rissanen as "impaired quality of life, body image disparagement, low self-esteem, stigmatization, and binge eating" (as cited by Rapoport, Clark, & Wardle, 2000, p. 1726). The lack of attention to these psychosocial aspects of obesity together with recognized limitations of traditional dietary and behavioral obesity treatments were the catalyst for the development of a "nondieting" approach. This new approach included both size acceptance and nondieting. Healthy lifestyle choices (e.g., healthy eating and engaging in physical activity) are emphasized, with the goal of enhancing overall wellbeing and quality of life. Modest weight loss may result from this approach but is not a primary goal (Rapoport et al., 2000).

Physical Risk Factors

The association between obesity and insulin resistance and the link between insulin resistance, hypertension, and abnormal lipid profile have been reported in childhood and adolescence. Obesity in childhood and adolescence has also been associated with type 2 diabetes mellitus, asthma, sleep apnea, gallbladder disease, and orthopedic problems (Barlow & Dietz, 1998; Wang & Dietz, 2002). The integrity of lower-limb joints is put at risk with excessive weight (Jenkins, 2003), which can lead to limitations in mobility and social participation and can thus cause additional weight gain. Among children older than 3 years, obesity is a strong predictor of adult obesity. Parental obesity more than doubles the risk of adult obesity among both nonobese and obese children aged 10 and younger (Escott-Stump, 2002).

Being overweight during childhood and adolescence is significantly associated with insulin resistance, abnormal lipid profile, and elevated blood pressure in young adulthood (Steinberger & Daniels, 2003). Breastfeeding has been identified as having a protective effect against obesity in childhood and adolescence (Jenkins, 2003) and should be promoted for this and other health benefits. Once obesity is established in childhood or adolescence, vigorous efforts should be directed at intervention. Lifestyle modifications and weight management in childhood could reduce the risk of developing insulin resistance syndrome, type 2 diabetes mellitus, and cardiovascular disease. Weight loss by obese youth results in a decrease in insulin concentration and improvement in insulin sensitivity (Steinberger & Daniels, 2003).

An excessive amount of abdominal fat that is out of proportion to total body fat is an independent predictor of risk for developing type 2 diabetes, hypertension, cardiovascular disease, and morbidity. Waist circumference is positively correlated with abdominal fat. In most adults with a BMI of 25 to 34.9 kg/m², there is an increased relative risk for developing obesity-associated risk factors if waist circumference exceeds 40 inches (102 cm) in men and 35 inches (88 cm) in women. These waist circumference cutpoints lose their incremental predictive power in clients with a BMI >35 kg/m², because these clients will exceed the cutpoints (National Institutes of Health [NIH], National Heart, Lung, and Blood Institute [NHLBI], 1998a, 1998b). The term *apple-shaped* has been used in health education and health promotion literature to describe body types with increased waist circumferences, and the term *pear-shaped* is used to describe people whose hips and thighs are larger than their waists (NIH, NHLBI, 2001). Apple-shaped individuals, with waists as large as or larger than their hips, may have a higher risk for coronary heart disease (NIH, NHLBI, 2001).

Smith and colleagues (2004) compared various anthropometric measures to determine the one that best predicted coronary heart disease in adult men. The **abdominal diameter index** was calculated by dividing the abdomen's diameter by the thigh circumference, as measured with a caliper while the client was in a supine position. This measurement was found to be more predictive than the waist and hip circumference measurements routinely used by health promotion practitioners. Smith and colleagues (2004) suggested that this measure was particularly predictive because it more closely measured the influence of the insulin resistance syndrome (i.e., metabolic syndrome; see Content Box 14-2) on the development of coronary heart disease. Although the researchers did not believe the abdominal diameter index would replace the circumference measurements by health providers, they recommend its use in research on how body shape impacts coronary heart disease.

Content Box 14-2

Definition of Metabolic Syndrome (Also Referred to as Insulin Resistance Syndrome)

Metabolic syndrome is defined by the National Cholesterol Education Program as the presence of any three of the following conditions:

- Excess weight around the waist (waist measurement of more than 40 inches for men and more than 35 inches for women)
- High levels of triglycerides (150 mg/dL or higher)
- Low levels of HDL, or "good," cholesterol (below 40 mg/dL for men and below 50 mg/dL for women)
- High blood pressure (130/85 mm Hg or higher)
- High fasting blood glucose levels (110 mg/dL or higher)

From *Insulin resistance and pre-diabetes,* by National Diabetes Information Clearinghouse, National Institute of Diabetes and Digestive and Kidney Diseases, National Institutes of Health, 2005; National Cholesterol Education Program, Third Report of the Expert Panel on Detection, Evaluation, and Treatment of High Blood Cholesterol in Adults (Adult Treatment Panel III), National Heart, Lung, and Blood Institute, National Institutes of Health, May 2001. With permission.
Note: Other definitions of similar conditions have been developed by the World Health Organization and the Association of Clinical Endocrinologists.

Mortality Risks

Obese adults, persons with a BMI >30 kg/m², have a 50% to 100% higher risk of death from all causes compared to adults with a BMI from 20 to 25 kg/m². For both men and women, hypertension was the most common overweight and obesity-related health condition. The prevalence of hypertension among adults who have Class 1 obesity is about 49% and 34% for men and women, respectively. The prevalence of type 2 diabetes mellitus, gallbladder disease, and osteoarthritis increased sharply among both overweight and obese men and women with increasing obesity class. The prevalence of high blood cholesterol (i.e., >240 mg/dL) in obese adults was higher than normal-weight persons but did not increase with increasing weight category. For men and women with Class 1 obesity, the prevalence of hypercholesterolemia was approximately 39% and 40%, respectively (Must et al., 1999).

Obesity is strongly associated with insulin resistance in normoglycemic individuals and in persons with type 2 diabetes mellitus (Steinberger & Daniels, 2003). Insulin resistance syndrome includes hyperinsulinemia, obesity, hypertension, dyslipemia, and type 2 diabetes mellitus (Rao, 2001). An increase in the risk for cancer is also a consequence of obesity (Bianchini, Kaaks, & Vainio, 2002; Bray, 2002).

Obesity is significantly associated with higher rates of death due to cancer of the esophagus, stomach, colon and rectum, liver, gallbladder, pancreas, kidney, prostate, breast, uterus, ovary, and cervix (Calle, Rodriguez, Walker-Thurmond, & Thun, 2003). Calle and colleagues (2003) estimated that the current patterns of overweight and obesity in the United States could account for 14% of all deaths in men and 20% in women.

Weight Bias

Rand and Macgregor (1991) studied 47 obese individuals who had gastric restrictive surgery and successfully maintained a 45 kg (22 lb) weight loss for greater than 3 years. The participants were asked if they would rather be obese or have other disabilities. All these patients would prefer to be deaf or dyslexic, or have diabetes or heart disease than be obese. In addition, 92% also preferred leg amputation over obesity, and 89% would rather be legally blind than obese. These data exemplify the tremendous social stigma attached to obesity and the intense psychological burden imposed on large persons living in a culture that glorifies thinness.

Modern culture idealizes thinness and disparages obesity. There has been documented weight bias in many aspects of work (e.g., employment, salary, and promotion practices), and societal bias (e.g., media representation) has played a major role in the development of negative images and stereotypes (Greenberg, Eastin, Hofschire, Lachlan, & Brownell, 2003; Puhl & Brownell, 2001). A study by Schwartz, Chambliss, Brownell, Blair, and Billington (2003) on weight bias among health professionals, especially those specializing in obesity, concluded that there was significant implicit weight bias. Characteristics such as lazy, stupid, and worthless were indicated on both implicit and explicit measures of weight bias among those health professionals studied. Despite working with obese persons, weight bias still existed.

Weight biases could adversely affect the care obese people receive. Because of bias, perceived or real, preventive care could be compromised. Two studies found decreased likelihood of obtaining preventive health services among obese women, after controlling for the effect of other known barriers to care. Fontaine, Faith, Allison, and Cheskin (1998) surveyed nearly 7000 women and found that obese women were less likely than normal-weight women to obtain preventive services (i.e., clinical breast examinations, gynecological examinations, and Pap smears) but had a greater number of overall physician visits (Fontaine et al., 1998). In a similar study, Wee, McCarthy, Davis, and Phillips (2000) examined the relationship between

obesity and screening with Pap smears and mammograms among 11,435 women and found that overweight and obese women were less likely than normal-weight women to be screened for cervical and breast cancer.

If individuals are uncomfortable in health-care settings, it would not be surprising if they avoided care (Schwartz et al., 2003): "Weight related bias or stigma contribute to the physical and psychosocial consequences of obesity. The strength of social bias against obese individuals is evident from the fact that even health professionals . . . are not immune" (Schwartz et al., 2003, p. 1039). Although there is no evidence that occupational therapy practitioners engage in this type of discrimination, it is important to monitor behavior to ensure that it does not occur. The AOTA's *Occupational Therapy Code of Ethics* (2005), the AOTA's *Statement on Obesity* (Blanchard, 2006) and the AOTA's *Occupational Therapy's Commitment to Nondiscrimination and Inclusion* (Hansen & Hinojosa, 2004) assert that all recipients of care should be treated with dignity and respect, regardless of their physical characteristics.

Foti (2005) encouraged occupational therapists and occupational therapy assistants to be cognizant of language and to avoid potentially offensive terms such as *obese* and *morbidly obese*. The current trend is to use terms such as *clinically severe obesity* or *extreme obesity* in an effort to avoid judgmental language. Foti advocated for even less judgmental terms such as *persons of size* or *exceptionally large individuals or persons* (2005, p. 9).

Economic Burden of Obesity

Wang and Dietz (2002) calculated the economic cost of obesity in persons aged 6 to 17 years using multiyear data from the National Hospital Discharge Survey, 1979–1999. Obesity-associated annual hospital costs, after adjusting for inflation, increased more than threefold from the years 1979 to 1981 to the years 1997 to 1999. Based on 2001 U.S. dollar value, the cost was $127 million during 1997 through 1999.

Compared to adults with normal body weights, obese individuals have 38% more physician visits and 48% more inpatient days per year (Finkelstein, Ruhm, & Kosa, 2005). Based on 1998 data, Finkelstein, Fiebelkorn, and Wang (2003) estimated that obesity-attributable medical expenditures account for 5.3% of U.S. annual health expenditures. Two years later, Finkelstein, Ruhm, and Kosa (2005) reported that it ranged from 5% to 7%, for a total of $75 billion per year. The increase in medical expenditures is not the only cost of obesity. The expense of decreased productivity, missed days at work, and premature deaths related to obesity also must be considered. The estimated annual cost of obesity for a company with 1000 employees is $285,000 (Finkelstein, Fiebelkorn, & Wang, 2005). It has been estimated that the annual indirect costs of obesity was $64 billion and that the total direct and indirect costs of obesity may be as high as $139 billion per year (Finkelstein, Ruhm, & Kosa, 2005).

In adults, mortality increases with BMI greater than 25 kg/m². Life expectancy of obese individuals may be shortened by 2 to 5 years. Weight loss can result in substantial health and economic benefits. For example, in a large proportion of overweight adults, a 10-pound weight loss can reduce or prevent hypertension. This can result in reductions in stroke incidence, myocardial infarctions, and heart failure, thus enhancing length of life and quality of life and decreasing the economic burden on society (Chobanian et al., 2003).

Healthy Lifestyle Behaviors: Dietary and Physical Activity Recommendations

Food choices, physical activity, lifestyle, environment, and genes all affect an individual's wellbeing and overall health status. The *Dietary Guidelines for Americans (Dietary Guidelines),* a joint publication by the U.S. Department of Agriculture (USDA) and the USDHHS (2005), provides science-based advice to promote health and reduce risk for chronic disease through diet and physical activity in healthy children aged 2 and older and adults of any age. The key recommendations of the 2005 *Dietary Guidelines* are grouped into nine interrelated focus areas. The integrated messages encourage U.S. citizens to eat fewer calories, be more physically active, and make wiser food choices.

A key recommendation is to maintain body weight in a healthy range, balancing calories from foods and beverages with calories expended. A **healthy body weight** is defined as having a BMI from 18.5 to 24.9 kg/m² for adults and having a BMI from the 5th to the 85th percentile of gender-specific BMI for age growth charts for ages 2 through 20 years. To reduce the risk of chronic disease, the *Dietary Guidelines* recommend that adults engage in at least 30 minutes of moderate-intensity physical activity most days of the week. Children should engage in at least 60 minutes of physical activity most, preferably all, days of the week (Institute of Medicine [IOM], 2002; USDA & USDHHS, 2005). The *Dietary Guidelines* and the IOM (2002) recommend 60 minutes of daily moderate- to vigorous-intensity physical activity on most days of the week to prevent weight gain in adulthood and to accrue the weight-independent health benefits of exercise. **Moderate physical activity** is defined as any activity

that burns 3.5 to 7 kcal/min and results in achieving 60% to 73% of peak heart rate. Examples of moderate physical activity include walking briskly (4 to 5 mph), mowing the lawn, dancing, swimming, or bicycling on level terrain. **Vigorous physical activity** is defined as any activity that burns more than 7 kcal/min and results in achieving 74% to 88% of peak heart rate. Examples of vigorous physical activity include jogging, participating in high-impact aerobic dancing, swimming continuous laps, or bicycling uphill. A combination of aerobic, strength, and flexibility activities are beneficial to health. Physical activity increases energy expenditure and is essential to weight loss and maintenance. In addition, weight-bearing activities are beneficial for bone health.

The *Dietary Guidelines* encourage increased intake of fruits, vegetables, whole grains, and fat-free or low-fat milk products. Grains, especially whole grains, form the foundation of a nutritious diet. Whole grains include whole wheat, whole oats/oatmeal, popcorn, brown rice, whole rye, whole grain barley, wild rice, buckwheat, bulgur, millet, and sorghum. They provide energy and fiber, and enriched products provide selected B vitamins, iron, and folate. A nutrient-dense diet also includes a variety of five to nine fruits and vegetables daily. These foods are significant contributors of vitamins A and C, potassium, magnesium, folate, carotenoids, and other phytochemicals that reduce risk for chronic disease. Diets rich in milk and milk products can reduce the risk of low bone mass. In addition, some randomized clinical trials have shown that obese people consuming a balanced, reduced-calorie diet that included three servings of dairy a day lost significantly more weight, more body fat, and more trunk fat compared to obese participants who simply reduced calories and consumed little or no dairy products (Zemel, Thompson, Milstead, Morris, & Campbell, 2004; Zemel et al., 2005).

Balance and moderation in eating practices is essential for a healthful diet. Consuming a diet low in saturated fat, trans-fatty acids, and cholesterol and moderate in total fat; limiting sugar and sodium intake; and moderating consumption of alcoholic beverages to one drink per day for women and two drinks per day for men is recommended. A drink is considered 12 oz of regular beer, 5 oz of wine, or 1.5 oz of 80-proof distilled spirits.

The acceptable macronutrient distribution ranges (AMDR) for adults, recommended by the IOM in 2002, was 20% to 35% of total energy from fats, 45% to 65% from carbohydrates, 25% (maximum) from sugar, and 10% to 35% of total energy from protein. For children, AMDR for fat is 30% to 40% of total energy for ages 1 to 3 years and 25% to 35% for ages 4 to 18 years, while the AMDR for carbohydrates is

45% to 65% of total energy. The AMDR for protein is 5% to 20% for young children and 10% to 30% for older children. The IOM (2002) published formulas to calculate daily energy needs of individuals based on their physical activity levels. Although no upper tolerable level was recommended by the IOM (2002) for dietary cholesterol, the *Dietary Guidelines* and the American Heart Association (2008) recommend that daily dietary cholesterol intake be less than 300 mg per day, saturated fat intake be less than 7%, and trans fat intake be less than 1% of total daily energy intake.

The *Dietary Guidelines* recommends using the updated food pyramid, MyPyramid (USDA, 2005a), which is described in Chapter 13, and the Dietary Approaches to Stop Hypertension (DASH) eating plan to guide healthy food choices. Grains form the foundation of both eating plans (NIH, NHLBI, 2003). The DASH diet was introduced in 1997 to prevent and treat high blood pressure without medications. It was designed intentionally to be higher in potassium, magnesium, calcium, fiber, and protein and lower in sodium, saturated and total fats, and cholesterol than the typical U.S. consumption (National Dairy Council [NDC], 2003).

A nutrient comparison of the DASH diet to an isocaloric diet similar to what U.S. residents eat found that the total fat content of the diets differed substantially, 26% versus 36%, respectively (Lin et al., 2003). Although the DASH diet contains less red meat, poultry, and fish than the control diet, the total protein content of this diet is higher due to the daily consumption of two to three dairy products and whole grains. It is effective in decreasing blood pressure and reduces heart disease risk by lowering homocysteine levels. The DASH diet is consistent with current dietary recommendations to prevent and treat other disorders such as osteoporosis, heart disease, and colon cancer. If the U.S. population as a whole adopted the DASH diet, it is estimated that it would reduce deaths from cardiovascular disease by approximately 15% and from stroke by about 27%. It has been demonstrated to reduce all causes of mortality (NDC, 2003).

Lichtenstein, Russell, and Russeman collaborated to adapt the food guide pyramid to portray the special diet needs of older adults (as cited in Amersbach, 1999). Then, Tufts University researchers updated their Food Pyramid to correspond to the USDA's MyPyramid. The Modified MyPyramid for Older Adults still emphasizes nutrient dense food choices and the importance of fluid balance (Lichtenstein, Rasmussen, Yu, Epstein, & Russell, 2008; Tufts Univeristy, 2007). The modified pyramid, can be viewed at http://nutrition .tufts.edu/docs/pdf/releases/ModifiedMyPyramid.pdf. One of the two key differences is the inclusion of an additional base of eight glasses of water/fluids to remind the elderly of the importance of drinking water and other liquids to decrease their risk of constipation and dehydration. These fluids are required even if thirst is absent (Amersbach, 1999). It is also important for older adults to understand that beer, wine, and other alcoholic beverages do not count toward the recommended daily allowance of liquids. The other difference is the inclusion of physical activities characteristic of older adults, such as walking, yard work, and swimming, as a foundation to the pyramid (Lichtenstein et al., 2008; Tufts University, 2007).

Emphasized in the Modified MyPyramid for Older Adults are icons depicting packaged fruits and vegetables, which are forms that may be more appropriate for older adults than fresh items. For example, bags of frozen pre-cut vegetables can be resealed and single-serve portions of canned fruit are easier to prepare and have a longer shelf life, minimizing waste. Such factors are important to consider as older adults may experience a flare-ups of arthritis or other mobility issue or be less likely to go out to replenish their food supply when the weather turns either very cold or very hot. Another integral part of the Modified MyPyramid for Older Adults is a flag at the top of the pyramid suggesting that some older adults may need supplements. Since some people find it difficult to consume adequate amounts of calcium, and Vitamins D and B_{12} from food alone, especially when calorie intake decreases, the needs for these supplemental nutrients increase with age (Lichtenstein et al., 2008).

Weight Management

Successful weight management is essential to the overall health of children, adolescents, and adults of all ages (American Dietetic Association, 2002, 2006). It requires a lifelong commitment to such lifestyle behaviors as healthful and enjoyable eating practices and daily physical activity. Therefore, lifestyle modifications in food intake and physical activity are the hallmarks of both effective weight loss and management interventions. Any changes in dietary intake and physical activity patterns that decrease energy intake below energy expenditure will result in weight loss. The key to managing weight throughout life is a positive attitude and the right motivation. Internal motivators such as improved health, increased energy, self-esteem, and personal control increase an individual's chances for lifelong weight-management success.

Even the most effective therapy prescribed by the most careful health professional team will manage weight successfully only if clients are fully engaged. Compliance with recommendations improves when clients have positive experiences with and trust in their care providers. Professionals should encourage and empathize, not criticize, and they should communicate the health benefits of weight loss, not just the pounds lost. Empathy builds trust and is a potent motivator. Barlow, Trowbridge, Klish, and Dietz (2002) found that many health-care providers need guidance in motivating individuals and families. Barlow and Dietz (2002) recommend that future research identify strategies that motivate families to make and maintain recommended behavioral changes. This will be helpful and might improve outcomes of obesity interventions.

Guidelines for Treatment of Overweight and Obesity in Children

In 2005, the American Medical Association in collaboration with the Health Resources and Services Administration and CDC revised the 1998 recommendations on childhood obesity (Barlow & the Expert Committee, 2007). This Expert Committee noted that a good outcome was the establishment of permanent healthy lifestyle habits, regardless of weight change, because of the long-term health benefits of these behaviors. A long-term health benefit is sustained improvement in medical conditions. The BMI percentile should be used to assess outcomes. The target is generally to be below the 85th percentile, although some children are healthy in the overweight category (85th–94th percentile). The committee proposed a four-stage systematic approach. Stage 1 is prevention plus; Stage 2, structured weight management; Stage 3, comprehensive multidisciplinary intervention; and Stage 4, tertiary care intervention. The outcome of Stage 1 would be improved BMI status through the adoption of healthy eating and activity habits. After 3 to 6 months if a child has not made improvements, Stage 2 would be implemented. Stage 2 involves more targeted structured behaviors with the support of a registered dietitian and other health counselors. Stage 3 increases the intensity of behavior changes, the frequency of visits, and the specialists involved to maximize support for behavior modifications. Stage 4 involves intensive inventions geared to more severely obese youths. Health professionals should recommend changes in eating and activity to achieve a weight loss of up to 1 pound per month for children 2 to 5 years if BMI is >21 or 22 kg/m^2 and a maximum weight loss of 2 lb per week for persons 6 to 18 years of age.

An appropriate weight goal for all obese children is to achieve a BMI below the 85th percentile. This goal should be secondary to the primary goal of healthy eating and physical activity. To increase physical activity, several approaches may be used, ranging from limiting inactivity, such as television watching, to adding vigorous activity to their leisure pursuits. The Expert Committee recommended limiting television and video time to a maximum of 2 hours per day and no television viewing if the child is less than 2 years of age (Barlow & the Expert Committee, 2007). The best form of activity is any that is sustainable. For prepubertal children, simply increasing time spent in free play, especially outdoors, is beneficial. Team sports, individualized sports such as dance, and family activities like bike riding are all options with appeal to different children. Behavioral research emphasizes that people are more likely to exercise and prefer physical activity when they have a choice of the type of activity (Baker et al., 2005).

The Expert Committee acknowledged that childhood obesity programs can lead to sustained weight loss when treatment focuses on behavior changes and is family based. Families need to learn the skills necessary to change behavior and to maintain those changes. These skills include developing awareness of current eating habits, activity patterns, and parenting behaviors, and identifying and modifying problem behaviors. Interventions should be started early, and families must be ready for changes (Barlow & the Expert Committee, 2007).

Guidelines for Obesity Prevention for Youth

Prevention and early identification of overweight and obesity in children is critical, because long-term outcome data for successful treatment approaches of overweight are limited. Throughout childhood and adolescence, there should be routine assessments of eating and physical activity patterns and recognition of excessive weight gain relative to linear growth. The American Academy of Pediatrics recommends that the BMI of all children and adolescents be calculated and plotted on the CDC growth charts once a year (Krebs & Jacobson, 2003). If there are significant changes in growth patterns (i.e., an upward crossing of BMI percentiles), discussions with parents/caregivers to raise their awareness should be conducted in a nonjudgmental, blame-free manner. This approach should prevent an unintended negative impact on the child's self-esteem (Krebs & Jacobson, 2003).

Guidelines for obesity-prevention programs for children should encourage a health-centered approach that focuses on the whole child, physically, mentally, and socially. A nurturing environment should be created that helps children recognize their own worth and respects cultural food practices and family traditions.

A comprehensive, successful program should develop and implement activities that create a supportive environment, provide education on healthful eating, and promote and facilitate opportunities for meaningful and enjoyable physical activity. It is important to remember that what is meaningful and enjoyable physical activity will vary with each child and will be impacted by family context and resources. For example, for a middle-class child who really wants a dog and whose family can afford the expense, securing the dog may better promote healthy habits than purchasing a bicycle. While bicycle riding may not be performed on a daily basis, omitting any of the twice-daily dog walks could lead to various undesirable consequences a child would want to avoid. The child and dog would both also expend calories during shared play. In addition, reviewing and instituting healthy eating habits for the dog may also reinforce healthy eating habits for the child.

Good nutrition focuses on the *Dietary Guidelines.* Understanding portion sizes and energy density, and regularly eating from all five food groups of the food guide pyramid are of prime importance (Johnson & Nicklas, 1999; Weight Realities Division of the Society for Nutrition Education [WRDSNE], 2003). The MyPyramid for Kids (USDA, 2005b), depicted in Figure 14-1, together with the catchphrase "Eat right. Exercise. Have fun." will help to convey the information needed to properly balance diet and exercise to parents, children, and teachers alike. Several occupation-based resources based on MyPyramid for Kids are available from http://www.mypyramid.gov/kids/index.html. These resources include an interactive computer game, which is available via download; a coloring page; and a worksheet—all are geared for children between the ages of 6 and 11. The computer game, MyPyramid Blast Off Game, encourages players to eat healthy by keeping track of their fuel choices.

Healthy eating patterns include consuming a variety of foods, having regular meals and snacks, responding to body signals of hunger and fullness, and eating meals as a family whenever possible. The American Academy of Pediatrics encourages parents and all caregivers to promote healthy eating patterns by offering nutritious snacks such as vegetables, fruits, low-fat dairy products, and whole grains; encouraging children's autonomy in self-regulation of food intake; setting appropriate limits on choices; and modeling healthy food choices (Krebs & Jacobson, 2003). The Joint FAO/WHO Expert Consultation (2003) also recommended limiting the intake of sugar-sweetened soft drinks, because it has been estimated that each can or glass of these beverages consumed on a daily basis increases the risk of becoming obese by 60%. In addition, all children should aim to achieve at least 1 hour of daily activity; reduce sedentary activities; limit television watching; increase strength, endurance, and fitness; and learn skills for sports and activities that can continue throughout life (WRDSNE, 2003).

Safe and effective programs should include measures to prevent related problems such as eating disorders, hazardous weight loss, nutrient deficiencies, size discrimination, and body hatred (WRDSNE, 2003). During childhood and adolescence, there are several windows of opportunity to influence changes in lifestyle behaviors. Educating youth early on the importance of healthy habits and patterns is critical, because behaviors, particularly food practices, established in childhood and adolescence are often continued into adulthood (Birch & Fisher, 1998; Housman, 2003). Jenkins (2003) identified adolescence as the most opportune time to provide primary and secondary obesity-prevention programs, because this is when youths begin to make their own food choices and when chronic eating conditions develop.

Preventing Childhood Obesity

The Institute of Medicine's *Preventing Childhood Obesity: Health in the Balance* consists of goals and recommendations for a national effort to prevent obesity and to promote healthy weight in children and youth from different segments of society (IOM, 2004). Implementing the IOM actions will require the involvement of multiple stakeholders—the federal government, state and local governments, industry and the media, state and local education authorities and schools, parents and families, and health-care professionals. Health-care professionals such as dietitians, occupational therapists, and occupational therapy assistants should serve as role models for healthful eating and regular physical activity. They should take leadership roles in advocating childhood obesity prevention in local schools and communities. Health-care providers should routinely measure their young clients' height and weight and calculate their BMI during every health-supervised visit. This action would indicate to parents and families that BMI is just as important as routine immunizations or screening tests in protecting children and adolescent health.

For many young adults in the United States, beginning university life is a major transition. Young adults who go to college must negotiate a new environment and learn new habits and routines. This transition period can trigger the development of either healthy or unhealthy dominating habits. Decisions and choices made at this transition period regarding eating, drinking alcohol, and physical activity may lay down behaviors that will remain for a lifetime (Cason & Wenrich, 2002; Housman, 2003; Jenkins, 2003). Thus, college is an excellent opportunity (Housman, 2003, p. 12) to

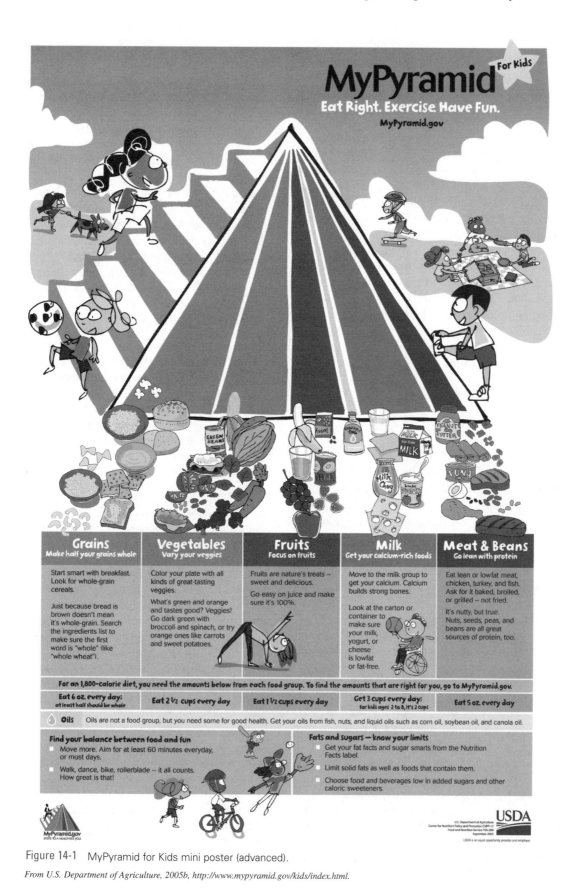

Figure 14-1   MyPyramid for Kids mini poster (advanced).

From U.S. Department of Agriculture, 2005b, http://www.mypyramid.gov/kids/index.html.

instill healthy habits for life. Cason and Wenrich found that among college students, "males eat more fast food than females ($p = .001$) and the majority of females considered themselves to be overweight and on weight-loss diets ($p = .048$)" (cited by Housman, 2003, p. 13).

Although students know that they and their peers are not making wise food and activity choices, most are unaware of the relationship between their nutrition and activity practices and their current and future health status. Students did not anticipate changing their behavior unless they gained weight, had greater access to healthy food choices and better workout equipment, or had a friend who was pursuing healthier behaviors (Cason & Wenrich, 2002; Housman, 2003). These are important considerations when developing program interventions for this age group. If interventions are to be effective, more extensive research assessing the needs of college students and influences on their behaviors is required (Cason & Wenrich, 2002; Housman, 2003). Investigating whether peers can be catalysts for changing and maintaining healthy eating habits would be one example of this type of research.

Guidelines for Treatment of Overweight and Obesity in Adults

Before initiating an intervention, the client should be evaluated for readiness to lose weight. This evaluation should include reasons for weight loss, previous attempts at weight loss, support expected from family and friends, understanding of the risks and benefits, attitudes toward physical activity, time and resource availability, and potential barriers to change. Weight-loss therapy is inappropriate for most pregnant and lactating women, individuals with major depression, and those with illnesses for whom caloric restriction might exacerbate their condition. Management involves weight loss; maintenance of body weight; and approaches to control other health risks of obesity factors such as hypertension, type 2 diabetes, coronary heart disease, cigarette smoking, and sleep apnea.

Weight-loss therapy is recommended for adults with a BMI of 30 kg/m² or greater and a BMI between 25 and 29.9 kg/m² with two or more risk factors (North American Association for the Study of Obesity [NAASO] & NHLBI, 2000). Obesity-associated disease and risk factors include hypertension, cigarette smoking, high low-density lipoprotein cholesterol, low high-density lipoprotein cholesterol, impaired fasting glucose, family history of cardiovascular disease, and age (i.e., males 45 years or older, females 55 years or older). The three goals defined by the NIH, NHLBI (1998a, 1998b) are

- to prevent further weight gain,
- to reduce body weight, and
- to maintain a lower body weight over time.

The American Dietetic Association also includes improvements in eating, exercise, and physical and emotional health, apart from weight loss, as goals of weight-management interventions (Cummings et al., 2002). A safe and effective weight-management plan is one that combines diet modification, increased physical activity, and behavior therapy.

For individuals wanting to prevent further weight gain, America on the Move—a program of the Partnership to Promote Healthy Eating and Active Living (PPHEAL), a national nonprofit organization of public and private organizations—is a possible intervention option. This program advocates increasing physical activity by taking an additional 2000 steps per day over current walking habits and decreasing energy intake by 100 kcal per day (PPHEAL, 2003).

> The Partnership's mission is to promote healthy eating and physical activity lifestyle behaviors through a public/private partnership grounded on consumer understanding. The Partnership is a 501 (c) 3 nonprofit organization with national reach. We conduct and support best practice research that focuses on healthy eating and active living. We then bring these best practices to communities across the United States. (PPHEAL, 2004b, ¶ 1–2)

The PPHEAL (2004a) is directed by leaders from prestigious academic institutions (e.g., Yale University), large food manufacturing companies (e.g., Kraft Foods), and consumer organizations (e.g., the Consumer Federation of America). This appears to be an excellent resource for individuals, families, and health professionals interested in weight management.

Weight-Reduction Strategies

For individuals desiring to lose weight, there are a variety of programs and services, ranging from community-based classes to commercial weight-loss centers and treatment by individual health-care professionals. The IOM (1995) derived sets of criteria to evaluate programs and approaches for the treatment and prevention of obesity. Three criteria—the match between the program and consumer, program soundness and safety, and program outcomes—were recommended for individuals to select a program and then periodically evaluate whether the program meets their changing needs.

There is growing realization that interventions to promote weight-reduction maintenance may need to be different from those that facilitate weight loss. Some success with delaying weight regain has been achieved through the use of longer treatment periods and greater emphasis on physical activity (Jeffery et al., 2000). However, additional cost-effective, long-term, or continuous care interventions that promote and support long-term weight maintenance (Jeffery et al., 2000; WHO, 2000) are required. Research is needed to examine the behavioral factors associated with eating (WHO, 2000), the mechanisms involved with the higher long-term success rate in preadolescents who had behavior interventions (Jeffery et al., 2000), the potential for meaningful occupations to facilitate continued engagement in physical activity, and other possible innovative strategies. In addition, new theories from the behavioral sciences should be examined for applicability (Jeffery et al., 2000).

Dietary Therapy

The initial goal of weight-loss therapy is to decrease body weight by 10% from baseline. A reasonable time frame for this goal is 6 months of therapy. For overweight individuals with a BMI from 27 to 35 kg/m^2, a reduction of 300 to 500 kcal per day from the current level will result in a loss of approximately 0.5 to 1 lb per week. For individuals with a BMI >35 kg/m^2, deficits of 500 to 1000 kcal per week from the current level will lead to an average weight loss of about 1 to 2 lb per week. Overall, the diet should be low in calories; however, it should not be less than 800 kcal per day, since very-low-calorie diets may reduce resting energy expenditure by 20%. They can also result in nutrient inadequacies if not supplemented with vitamins and minerals. In general, diets containing between 1000 to 1200 kcal/day for women and between 1200 to 1600 kcal/day for men should be selected. In addition to reduction in total energy intake, dietary fat intake needs to be reduced.

Controversy exists regarding the macronutrient (i.e., protein, lipid, and carbohydrate) composition of weight-reduction diets. However, lifestyle intervention programs utilizing a high-carbohydrate, low-fat diet combined with physical activity are effective for weight reduction (Diabetes Prevention Program Research Group, 2002; Tuomilehto et al., 2001). Diets based on MyPyramid or the DASH eating plan provide at least half the grains as whole grains and are rich in fiber. Low-glycemic index foods such as oatmeal, all-bran cereals, fruits, and legumes lower the blood glucose response to a meal. This appears to result in better management of diabetes mellitus and lowers the risk of developing chronic disease and obesity (Gropper et al., 2009).

The American Dietetic Association recommends a "total diet approach," where the overall food pattern is more important than one food or meal (Freeland-Graves & Nitzke, 2002). The eating plan should include a variety of foods from the major food groups. Appealing foods that a person can enjoy eating in moderation for the rest of his or her life can include readily available food and favorite foods (Freeland-Graves & Nitzke, 2002).

Practitioners should acknowledge that overeating, which can lead to obesity, and physical inactivity can both be related to psychosocial issues. Client-centered evaluation and interventions that promote healthy changes in eating behaviors need to address these issues. This can be done by targeting three interacting spheres of influence:

- The environment, which influences the likelihood that healthy eating behaviors will be adopted through social norms, influential role models, cues to action, reinforcements, and opportunities for action
- Personal characteristics, including knowledge, attitudes, beliefs, values, confidence in one's ability to change eating behaviors, and expectations about the consequences of making those changes
- Behavioral skills and experience, which are related to selecting or preparing specific foods, dietary self-assessment, and decision-making

Psychosocial and contextual factors that support and encourage overeating must be addressed in occupational therapy interventions.

Physical Activity

Walking and swimming are recommended as initial activities, but a wide variety of occupations such as gardening, household chores, and team or individual sports are also appropriate. Table 14-1 displays the calorie expenditure for a variety of activities. Physical activities should initially be performed for 30 minutes per day for 3 days a week, progressing to 45 minutes per day for 5 days a week. The goal is to expend between 100 to 200 kcal per day. For most obese individuals, exercise should be initiated slowly, with care taken to avoid injury, and the intensity should be gradually increased. All adults should set a long-term goal to accumulate at least 30 minutes or more of moderate-intensity physical activity on most, preferably all, days of the week. Examples of moderate amounts of activity, occupation-based interventions, and additional information regarding physical activity and health promotion are provided in Chapter 13.

Behavior Therapy

Behavior therapy helps with initial compliance to eating and physical activity changes and has the potential to also assist with long-term weight-loss maintenance.

Table 14–1 **Energy Cost of Physical Activities**

Moderate Physical Activity	Approximate Calories/hr for a 154-lb Person*
Hiking	370
Light gardening/yard work	330
Dancing	330
Golf (walking and carrying clubs)	330
Bicycling (<10 mph)	290
Walking (3.5 mph)	280
Weight lifting (general light workout)	220
Stretching	180
Vigorous Physical Activity	**Approximate Calories/hr for a 154-lb Person***
Running/jogging (5 mph)	590
Bicycling (>10 mph)	590
Swimming (slow freestyle laps)	510
Aerobics	480
Walking (4.5 mph)	460
Heavy yard work (chopping wood)	440
Weight lifting (vigorous effort)	440
Basketball (vigorous)	440

* Calories burned per hour will be higher for persons who weigh more than 154 lb (70 kg) and lower for persons who weigh less. From Dietary Guidelines for Americans, 2005 (6th ed.) by USDA and USDHHS, 2005, Washington, DC: U.S. Government Printing Office, p. 17.

Specific strategies that are helpful in achieving and maintaining weight loss include self-monitoring of eating practices and physical activity, stress management, stimulus control, problem-solving, contingency management, cognitive restructuring, and social support (NIH, NHLBI, 1998a, 1998b).

The Transtheoretical Model of Change (described in Chapter 3), social cognitive theory, and relapse prevention were identified by Chambliss (2004) as models that have provided useful constructs for weight-management lifestyle initiatives, including "readiness to change, decisional balance, self-monitoring, goal setting, social support, stimulus control, and relapse prevention" (p. 145). Figure 14-2 provides a flowchart that details the four phases of behavioral weight management, from assessment to maintenance. Research indicates that behavior techniques that focus on changing eating and physical activity levels are effective for initial weight loss but are not as effective for long-term maintenance of weight loss (Jeffery et al., 2000).

Drohan (2002) describes a behavior-modification approach for primary-care nurses to use with families with preschool-aged children, which can be equally applicable to other health professions. This approach includes using a red, yellow, green light method to categorize and monitor age-appropriate food choices and consumption levels. In addition, several practical tips are provided for parents to use in support of self-monitoring, social reinforcement, stimulus control, and modeling, which have been identified as the most appropriate family-based behavioral treatment strategies. Examples of each of these strategies appear in Content Box 14-3.

There has been limited research on the effectiveness of various behavioral therapy techniques. With the growing realization and interest in the global obesity epidemic, additional outcome research should be available in the future. Although limited in number, some promising results, especially in the international literature, are being described. For example, the effectiveness of cognitive-behavioral therapy (CBT) on health-related quality of life (HRQL) in Italian individuals with obesity—with and without binge eating—was studied (Marchesini et al., 2002). Results of this study indicated that structured sessions of CBT had a positive impact on HRQL and on weight loss. The CBT intervention was adapted for those individuals with binge-eating

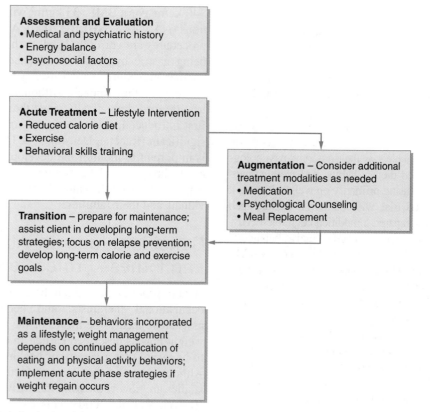

Figure 14-2 Steps in behavioral weight-management interventions.

Redrawn from Figure 1, Phases of behavioral weight management intervention. In "Behavioral approaches to obesity treatment," by H. O. Chambliss, 2004, National Association for Physical Education in Higher Education, *56, p. 144.*

Content Box 14-3

Practical Behavior Modification Techniques for Parents

1. Self-Monitoring

- Keep habit logs of foods and amounts eaten. Physical activity type and duration is important to record as well.

2. Social Reinforcement

- Remember to praise your child for good habits as soon as you notice them, like not eating while watching television.
- Contracting with your child is often useful in encouraging behavior change.
- The reward should not be food, money, or gifts. It is best if the reward is a special privilege or activity, like going to the zoo or staying up a half hour past bedtime.

3. Stimulus Control

- All eating should be done in only one place (e.g., like in the kitchen or at the dining room table).
- Children should not eat while doing another activity, especially not while watching television.
- Give your child a special dish to eat from. They should use this dish whenever they eat, even for just a snack. This will give them more control over their eating.
- Try not to serve meals family style. Give small, individual portions instead. If your child wants more, have them wait 5 to 10 minutes before serving and ask if they are still hungry.
- Remember the 5 "onlys":
  - Only in the dining room
  - Only while sitting
  - Only from a proper plate
  - Only when not doing anything else
  - Only when hungry

4. Modeling

- Do not eat things in front of your child that you do not want them to eat. Do not do things in front of your child that you do not want them to do. Children look up to their parents and will copy your actions.
- Call attention to your good health behaviors whenever possible.

From entries selected from Table 3 in "Managing early childhood obesity in the primary care setting: A behavior modification approach," S. M. Drohan, 2002, *Pediatric Nursing, 28*(6), 609. With permission.

behavior. These people had higher average changes in HRQL than participants without binge-eating habits, but they experienced less success with weight loss. When developing behavioral weight loss and management interventions, consideration should be given to tailoring the interventions based on whether the individual has an associated binge-eating disorder.

A study conducted in the United Kingdom provides encouragement for developing approaches that focus on psychosocial issues and have as their outcome psychological wellbeing, changed dietary habits, and weight management—without focusing primarily on weight loss. In a randomized controlled trial with 63 obese middle-aged women, researchers compared a modified cognitive-behavioral treatment (M-CBT) with standard cognitive-behavioral treatment (S-CBT). Both the S-CBT and M-CBT approaches focused on self-acceptance, along with healthy eating and activity patterns. The M-CBT also focused on psychological wellbeing and long-term weight management versus weight loss. Both groups experienced improvement in emotional wellbeing, physical health, and modest weight loss. These results were maintained over the following year (Rapoport et al., 2000). The literature should be reviewed frequently to identify research results to further enhance program development and to tailor interventions.

Pharmacotherapy and Weight-Loss Surgery

Pharmacotherapy should be considered after intervention with diet, physical activity change, and behavior therapy has proven ineffective to promote weight loss after 6 months. It is currently limited to individuals in the United States who have a BMI >30 kg/m² or those with a BMI >27 kg/m² with obesity-related risk factors or disease. The U.S. Federal Drug Administration (USFDA) has approved the use of sibutramine (e.g., Meridia) and orlistat (e.g., Xenical) for long-term use in weight loss. Sibutramine is an appetite suppressant that affects the norepinephrine and serotonergic mechanisms in the brain. An increase in blood pressure and tachycardia are the known side effects of this drug. Constipation and dry mouth were also reported as common side effects (Smith & Goulder, 2001, as cited by Warren, Brennan, & Akehurst, 2004), as were headache, anorexia, rhinitis, and pharyngitis (Abbott Laboratories, 2003). In the United Kingdom, continued use of sibutramine is limited to those individuals who are found to be responders—those "who lose 2 kg after 1 month and 5% of their initial weight after 3 months" (Warren et al., 2004, p. 9). Orlistat inhibits fat absorption and thus may reduce the absorption of fat-soluble vitamins and nutrients (NAASO & NHLBI, 2000). Common side effects include changes in bowel habits such as urgency, gas, and oily discharge or spotting (Roche Pharmaceuticals, 2000; USFDA, 2000).

Surgery is an option for well-informed and motivated clients who have clinically extreme obesity (BMI >40 kg/m²) or a BMI >35 kg/m² with comorbid conditions (NAASO & NHLBI, 2000). A variety of surgical procedures are currently used, with the most common being gastric bypass. Vertical banded gastroplasty is another procedure, which uses a band to restrict the capacity of the stomach. Although the mortality rate has dropped dramatically since these procedures were first introduced, side effects and complications can be significant (Racette, Deusinger, & Deusinger, 2003). It is important to monitor the development of new surgical techniques and be cognizant of the impact such surgeries have on the eating habits and patterns of individuals and their families.

Considerations for All Health and Fitness Professionals

Health professionals, including registered dietitians, occupational therapists, and occupational therapy assistants, need to be aware of the potential to harbor weight bias as described earlier. In addition, they need to be aware that a variety of healthy body types exist. Although most of the literature focuses on weight loss, studies are now addressing the "new weight paradigm" (Rapoport et al., 2000). This paradigm includes both "size acceptance" and nondieting approaches to weight management (Rapoport et al., 2000).

Health and fitness professionals often approach health care for large people with the belief that health improvement can be attained only through weight loss.

> Unequivocal acceptance of the notion that thinness equals health and fitness presents an obstacle for large people who want to improve their health through lifestyle changes in eating and activity patterns. This belief when held by health professionals can weaken the working relationship between the professional and the large client. Since the health benefits of exercise and sound nutrition are significant for people of all sizes, the strategy for health care professionals should be to assist people of all sizes in eating healthier and becoming more active. (Lyons & Miller, 1999, p. 1141)

Role of Registered Dietitians and Others in Weight Management and Obesity Prevention

As the primary nutrition practice professionals, registered dietitians are responsible for assessment and recommendations related to food behavior. They can help individuals formulate reasonable, healthy eating approaches tailored to their needs. They can also assist adults and families with overweight children by teaching skills to effectively monitor and change eating behaviors. The registered dietitian's attention to the client's concerns, feelings, values, and lifestyle behaviors beyond food behaviors helps the client assume an active role in communicating these issues to other care providers (Cummings et al., 2002).

A variety of other experienced health professionals also can participate in many aspects of weight-management programs. They can contribute to obesity prevention among their own clients and among the general population by creating awareness of obesity-related health risks while being sensitive to psychosocial issues and the negative impact of weight bias. Physicians can determine the appropriate type of weight-management plan. Registered dietitians, occupational therapists, occupational therapy assistants, nurses (Tod & Lacey, 2004), and physical therapists can play pivotal roles in modifying weight status. Racette and colleagues (2003) encouraged physical therapists "to recognize individuals who are obese and . . . address obesity-related issues with their patients" (p. 283). Mental health providers must monitor the literature about the latest research findings regarding the relationship between prescribed psychotropic medications and weight gain and must be aware of how a "hostile cultural climate" impacts the self-esteem of obese individuals (Devlin et al., 2000, p. 854).

A recent interdisciplinary study examined strategies to improve the reliability of 24-hour dietary recalls in the elderly. The interdisciplinary team included faculty from health sciences, communication sciences and disorders, and psychiatry as well as a speech-language pathologist (Shumaker et al., 2003). Understanding the impact of memory and memory aids on the level of participation in 24-hour dietary recalls is important, because recalls are a time- and cost-effective method for examining diet habits. Although the use of an encoding strategy was not found to enhance memory in this particular study, Shumaker and colleagues concluded that additional research was required. They also determined that "allied health professionals can develop improved encoding strategies and visual aids" to facilitate improved reporting of types of foods consumed as well as portion sizes (2003, p. 200).

Role of Occupational Therapy in Weight Management and Obesity Prevention[1]

Occupational therapists and occupational therapy assistants support "health and participation in life through engagement in occupation" (AOTA, 2008, p. 626).

Within the domain of occupational therapy, the practitioner considers the client's performance in the areas of occupation, performance skills, performance patterns, context and environment, activity demands, as well as client factors (AOTA, 2008). A client-centered approach is essential during both the evaluation and intervention processes. A description of one possible approach for obesity prevention using the *Framework* (AOTA, 2008) is briefly summarized below. This summary is followed by other examples of possible interventions.

During the evaluation process, the occupational therapist conducts an occupational profile, emphasizing the client's priorities and goals. The Lifestyle Performance Interview is one possible method for collecting this type of data (Velde & Fidler, 2002). Items and probes suggested for obtaining information of food and eating patterns (Content Box 14-4) may be modified to explore the meaning of food and whether eating is an unhealthy dominating habit.

An appropriate intervention might be to assist in the selection and adaptation of occupations that would increase physical activity demands and energy expenditure across areas of occupation (e.g., work, leisure, instrumental activities of daily living). Examples of these strategies include parking further from stores and the work place to increase the number of steps taken in a day and doing one's own housework versus using a

---

Content Box 14-4

Lifestyle Performance Interview: Food and Eating Pattern Probes

- To what extent do you engage in meal preparation?
- How frequently do you eat out? Eat alone? With others?
- Do you share cooking, meal planning, eating with another/others? Describe.
- How important is food to you?
- Do you shop for food? What is that experience like for you?
- Are there tasks related to obtaining, planning, and eating food that you find enjoyable? Describe. Are there some you find a chore or not enjoyable? Describe.
- Who did the cooking, shopping, and related tasks in your family?
- How would you describe your mealtime routines and behaviors? For example, regularity, casual, sit-down, family style?
- What are the most difficult or problematic parts of your present meal preparation or eating? How do you manage these?

Reprinted from "Data gathering: Conducting the lifestyle performance interview" by B. P. Velde & G. S. Fidler, 2002, in *Lifestyle Performance: A Model for Engaging the Power,* p. 63. Thorofare, NJ: SLACK. With permission from SLACK Incorporated.

---

[1] Portions of this segment were adapted from material developed by Reitz (n.d.) for the Western Maryland Area Health Education Center.

cleaning service. Through the use of an interest checklist (Henry, 2003), such as the Neuro Psychiatric Institute Interest Checklist (Matsutsuyu, 1969) or the Occupational Questionnaire (Smith, Kielfhofner, & Watts, 1986), the client identifies and prioritizes possible new or familiar occupations. If indicated, the therapist provides consultation regarding body mechanics or methods to grade participation based on evaluation and knowledge of client factors (i.e., body functions and structures) and activity demands.

Another avenue for intervention is through the analysis of the client's performance patterns (i.e., habits, routines, and roles) that may contribute to physical inactivity, overweight, or obesity. The client can also be a group or population, and interventions can be targeted toward occupational performance patterns (i.e., habits and roles) of a particular community or population. Dominating unhealthy habits, routines, and roles are the focus of this type of analysis. Recommendations to facilitate behavior change can then be provided based on a variety of conceptual models of practice. Interventions could include maintaining a weekly eating habit log (Drohan, 2002) to monitor food choices, having the client explore new pleasure or "comfort" occupations that may be substituted for feelings associated with current unhealthy food consumption or other unhealthy but pleasurable occupations, or changing their routine in order to take a healthy lunch. Perceived risks and barriers to changes in occupations, occupational routines, roles, and contexts also should be identified during the intervention.

The Lifestyle Redesign® Weight Management Program is a potentially beneficial approach for individuals. Obesity intervention is one of the most frequently provided lifestyle-redesign services at the Faculty Practice of the University of Southern California's (USC) Department of Occupational Science and Occupational Therapy (USC, 2004). The Lifestyle Redesign® program includes five key elements:

- Participating in an intensive 6-month lifestyle-modification program
- Implementing a radical reorganization of lifestyle, not just dieting
- Losing weight while eating nutritionally dense, healthy foods
- Developing healthy habits of eating and daily activity
- Enabling prospective bariatric clients to lose enough weight to improve surgical outcomes or eliminate the need for surgery entirely (USC, 2004, ¶ 8)

Approximately 160 individuals have already participated in this weight-loss lifestyle-redesign program.

Any intervention must also include an analysis of the client's context for possible supports or barriers to behavior change. The cultural context should be analyzed for possible modification to facilitate healthy behavior change, such as a cooking activity with culturally relevant healthy food alternatives or with supportive family and friends. Tod and Lacey (2004) reported public weighing and the fear of being the largest person in a group as potential barriers to participation in weight-loss programs. However, the popularity of television shows, such as the *The Biggest Loser* that publicly help obese individuals may be a positive health support for people coping with weight issues. Use of an online support group is a potential intervention option, especially for those who may find more public options embarrassing. In addition, programs or supports offered through the client's place of worship may be seen as less threatening.

The client's pattern of time usage and its link to unhealthy and healthy habits also should be evaluated. For example, one may examine the relationship of food consumption to engagement in occupational roles and occupations in terms of the rhythms of the day, week, month, or year. A values-clarification exercise may be conducted to assess whether the individual is internally or externally motivated to change behaviors and which behaviors/occupations are of primary importance.

Contexts that promote overeating should also be addressed in prevention efforts and interventions. An awareness of family influences and an appreciation of the relationship between eating behaviors and social contexts can be important in the development of early healthy eating habits. Food preferences are a learned behavior with the exception of "innate" preferences for foods that taste sweet or salty. Both infants and children are "biased to reject new foods," preferring familiar foods such as that eaten by family members and friends (Drohan, 2002).

The impact of changing contexts on weight and weight management should also be considered. The fear of gaining the "freshman 15" has been receiving media attention each fall (Lang, 2003; Sommers, 1999). However, research indicates that the actual average weight gain among college freshmen appears closer to 4 lb (Graham & Jones, 2002; Lang, 2003). While this figure is considerably less than the feared 15 lb, it still has the potential for promoting unhealthy habits (e.g., setting up an expectation that it may be fine to gain that weight) and resulting in health consequences later in life. Families can assist in preventing unhealthy weight gain in the first semester of college by sending "care packages" containing fruit rather than cookies and by discouraging all-you-can-eat meal plans.

Academic occupational therapy programs can promote healthy eating and weight through their varied roles on campus. Faculty can initiate or participate in interdisciplinary efforts to address selected objectives from *Healthy Campus 2010: Making It Happen* (American College Health Association [ACHA], 2002). Advocating for increased availability of a variety of healthy food choices for students, faculty, and staff could be one of many recommendations made by such a group. In addition, students can be encouraged to examine their own health habits and establish goals for healthier living. One of the assignments for first-year occupational therapy students at Towson University is a personal problem-solving project based on the work of Carkhuff (1985). The goal of the assignment is to use a real-life problem to develop or refine problem-solving skills. Students have selected a variety of topics, including time management, smoking cessation, and healthy eating (S. Lawson, personal communication, June 17, 2004).

College students are not the only group in which a change in context can result in weight gain. An older adult with a history of healthy eating and physical activity routines reported the difficulty she and peers were having with weight gain since moving to a continuum of care retirement community campus. Peers reported gaining 3 to 70 lb since relocating to the facility. Perceived contributing factors included the popularity of the all-you-can-eat dining option and easy access to high-quality desserts (P. Thomson, personal communication, March 30, 2004). As with college students, sending flowers or fruit/vegetable baskets versus high-calorie cookie and candy gifts may be appreciated by older relatives who are trying to avoid the Retirement 25.

There are many occupational therapy theoretical models available to assist in the development and support of interventions. Content Box 14-5 details possible interventions based on the Ecology of Human Performance (Dunn, Brown, & McGuigan, 1994). The occupational adaptation (OA) theory (Schkade & McClung, 2001; Schultz & Schkade, 2003) can be used to support interventions aimed at facilitating the individual's internal adaptation process to select healthy foods and occupations that enable weight loss or maintenance without external reinforcement or assistance. Using principles and constructs from OA, the therapist can employ both occupational readiness (e.g., teaching how to read labels for nutrition information) and occupational activity (e.g., locating and testing possible comfortable venues for walking in preparation of the self-selected new role of "walker"). The therapist may assist the client in identifying factors that could impact the perceived comfort of a possible venue, such as climate-controlled conditions; crowding; and the likelihood to experience threatening, harassing, or embarrassing social situations. The potential

---

Content Box 14-5

Possible Interventions Using the Ecology of Human Performance Framework

Establish/Restore
- Healthy occupations that promote energy expenditure
- Healthy choice-making during grocery shopping
- Healthy food preparation
- Use of Internet for behavior change support

Alter
- Alter work context if necessary (e.g., from food service to other service provision).
- Alter social supports (e.g., identify and confront potential saboteurs of new lifestyle plans).
- Alter eating context from all-you-can eat settings to restaurants that use portion control.

Adapt
- If uncomfortable with face-to-face group or individual counseling, investigate options of e-counseling or support.
- Adapt family vacation plans from a theme park tradition to a national park tradition.
- Adapt family outings to include bringing along snacks versus going to fast-food restaurants.
- Adapt summertime family activity from attending movies to going to "pick your own fruit" farms.

Prevent
- Prevent enabling by avoiding displaying unhealthy snacks in intervention areas even during holidays.
- Provide nutrition newsletters and health promotion reading materials in waiting rooms.

Create
- Advocacy group for removal of soda machines from health service venues and have them replaced with water and healthy snack alternatives
- Collaborate with local registered dietitians to design healthy cooking night at local elementary school.
- Advocacy group for removal of soda machines from high schools and have them replaced with water and healthy snack alternatives
- A worksite wellness program, including an area for a Healthy Lunch Bunch to meet and eat

Headings from "The ecology of human performance: A framework for considering the effect of context" by W. Dunn, C. Brown, & A. McGuigan, 1994, *American Journal of Occupational Therapy, 48,* 595–607.

---

for the occupational activity to be pleasurable and repeated will be enhanced by selecting the most comfortable context in which to engage in the activity.

Occupational therapy practitioners often act as health advocates and resources for their families. While this may be most common following a traumatic event such as a heart attack, stroke, car accident, or diagnosis of depression, the role can expand to providing guidance to prevent disease and disability or secondary conditions. Modeling healthy, tasty, and fun family meal selection, preparation, and consumption can make the occupation of eating both an instrumental activity of daily living and a healthy, family bonding experience. In addition, occupation-based strategies like those described above and others described in the case study that follows may be unique alternatives for overweight clients who are seeking healthier eating choices.

Role of Interdisciplinary Interventions in Weight Management and Obesity Prevention

Models from disciplines other than occupational therapy can also be helpful. For example, many of the health promotion and education models address barriers to engaging in health behaviors and may assist the client-therapist team in examining all potential barriers when selecting a venue for engagement in physical activity. Clients could also be evaluated to determine their placement in the Stages of Change or Transtheoretical Model, and recommendations can be provided for occupations/activities that promote movement to the next stage of change (Prochaska & DiClemente, 1983; Werch & DiClemente, 1994). These models are described in detail in Chapter 3.

Individuals from many disciplines can make contributions to a client's, family's, community's, or nation's efforts in weight management. Interventions are strengthened by interdisciplinary collaboration. A case study called "Mrs. P." was developed by an interdisciplinary group of faculty from five different universities and colleges representing the fields of occupational therapy, medical technology, nursing, physical therapy, public health, respiratory therapy, and social work. This case study can be helpful for students from each of the represented disciplines working together or alone to examine the contributions of each to the client and family who desire to reduce weight for health. The case study and corresponding learning materials can be found via the obesity prevention module located on the Rural Interdisciplinary Health Promotion (RIHP) website (http://ahec.allconet.org/newrihp/modules-op-over.html), which is supported by the Western Maryland Area Health Education Center and funded by the Quentin N. Burdick Program, USDHHS, Bureau of Health Professions.

Policy Advocacy

In addition to providing direct services, registered dietitians, occupational therapists, and occupational therapy assistants are encouraged to play key roles in supporting national and local initiatives that promote healthy eating and regular physical activity. The AOTA (2007) released a document on obesity to articulate to the public and to policymakers the potential role of occupational therapy in the prevention and management of obesity. This advocacy effort is further strengthened when performed in a coordinated and collaborative manner in support of public policies that increase opportunities for healthy eating, exercise, and research to improve intervention and prevention strategies.

Legislators are increasingly becoming aware of and concerned about the impact of obesity on the nations' health and budget. Faircloth (2004), who serves in the Maine legislature, describes a legislative proposal developed by the citizens of Maine. The proposal includes the following initiatives:

- Dedicate one percent of gas taxes to human-powered transportation so that all citizens (not just those who can afford treadmill and gyms) enjoy healthy options such as well-maintained trails and sidewalks.
- Guarantee every citizen freedom of information to see calories listed on major chain restaurants (costing big chains nothing as they always have this information) and empowering citizens to take personal responsibility for themselves and their children.
- Guarantee freedom from exploitation with public schools offering healthy choices in vending machines.
- Guarantee freedom from exploitation of our children, prohibiting use of public schools as corporate advertising tools. (Faircloth, 2004, pp. 47–48)

The media, consumer advocacy groups, and nonprofit health advocacy groups such as the Center for Science in the Public Interest (CSPI) can be important partners in efforts to encourage policy development and disseminate research to assist in facilitating healthy weight. Careful monitoring of policy decisions is essential. Recently, the USDA amended its rules to label frozen French fries, including batter-coated fries, as a fresh vegetable (Martin, 2004). The change was made at the request of the Frozen Potato Products Institute, who considered "rolling potato slices in a starch coating, frying them, and freezing them is the equivalent of waxing a cucumber or sweetening a strawberry" (Martin, 2004, p. 3A).

The approval of the Safe Routes to School program is a recent example of a positive policy initiative. On February 12, 2004, the U.S. Senate approved legislation "to fund transportation projects throughout the country, including initiatives to promote physical activity. Included in the bill is $420 million for the Safe Routes to School program, a program designed to promote walking and biking to school" (American Heart Association, 2004).

Conclusion

Overweight and obesity have reached nationwide epidemic proportions in the United States. Both *Healthy People 2010* (USDHHS, 2000) and *Healthy Campus 2010* (ACHA, 2002) "have developed major goals to promote health in relation to diet and weight" (Housman, 2003, p. 18). In addition, *The Surgeon General's Call to Action to Prevent and Decrease Overweight and Obesity* (USDHHS, 2001) outlines strategies for activities and interventions in five settings: (1) families and communities, (2) schools, (3) health care, (4) media and communication, and (5) worksites. The IOM's *Preventing Childhood Obesity: Health in the Balance* (2004) also describes a prevention-focused action plan for families, schools, industry, communities, and government to decrease the number of obese children and youth in the United States. As part of an interdisciplinary healthcare team, registered dietitians, occupational therapists, and occupational therapy assistants can be instrumental in helping to improve the nation's health through healthy weight management. In order to remain current in evidence-based strategies and at-risk groups and populations, continued review of recent research and governmental reports is required. At the time this book went to press, the *Clinical Guidelines on the Identification, Evaluation, and Treatment of Overweight and Obesity in Adults* (NIH, NHLBI, 1998a) were under revision (NIH, NHLBI, n.d.). The reader is encouraged to visit http://www.nhlbi.nih.gov/guidelines/obesity/index.htm to remain abreast of these changes.

Case Study 14-1

This case study is based on a real-life example provided by an occupational therapist promoting weight reduction and healthy eating choices among her extended family. The Stevensons, an African American family of six, were leading the typical hectic life of a blended U.S. family. The two younger children, a daughter aged 8 and a son aged 14, were involved in a variety of after-school activities, and both parents were employed full-time. Two older twin children from a previous marriage, aged 17, visited every other weekend. All four children spent a great amount of time performing sedentary school and leisure-related computer activities.

The entire family was overweight and rarely participated in group physical activities or other healthy habits, with the exception of the 14-year-old son, who participated in football during the fall. Although the two younger children participated in a variety of after-school activities, each child had only one with a physical activity component. The family's eating habits relied heavily on fast food and family quick-serve restaurants. Meals were often high in calories, fat, and salt. The father had a history of diabetes. The 14-year-old son, a lineman on the junior varsity high school football team, was beginning to have knee problems, which were exacerbated by his weight.

While on vacation, the father experienced a heart attack. After this event, a cousin named Sadie, who was an occupational therapist and who had already been concerned about the family's health, saw this as an opportunity to provide guidance on healthy eating choices. For the first time, the family was open to listening to and enacting Sadie's suggestions, which were occupation-based interventions that focused both on healthy eating and increasing physical activity. Since Sadie lived in a different state, the interventions tended to occur during different holidays and other family events when the families traveled to spend time together. At first, the interventions were just a series of spontaneous suggestions based on many years of using activity analysis and occupation-based intervention. Sadie eventually designed an intervention plan centered on her one-on-one time with the family during holidays, with phone calls and e-mail reinforcement between family gatherings. The primary interventions included

1. modeling and teaching healthy food shopping, storage, and cooking;
2. educating parents on the benefits of time-deepening (e.g., multitasking) strategies to maximize the parents' ability to have time to engage in physical activity while also having time to shop and cook healthy meals;
3. reinforcing and clarifying messages and directions from other health providers;
4. using computer-based learning activities and health-monitoring activities; and
5. selecting holiday and birthday gifts that encouraged fun food exploration, food knowledge, or physical activity.

When her cousin's family visited, Sadie involved the children in selecting the weekend menu, preparing the shopping list from a recipe book, purchasing the food, and helping prepare the food. Emphasis was placed on time-efficient, fun, and creative meals. Desserts were always included but were focused on in-season, locally grown fruit, when possible. The parents were surprised about how quick, simple, healthy, and satisfying many of the meals were. They also enjoyed dining in a relatively quiet, relaxing environment. The added benefits of eating at home, where the children could be excused from the table while the adults lingered over decaffeinated tea and coffee

Continued

instead of having to fight traffic, find parking, and wait in line to eat also became apparent.

The children enjoyed being in the kitchen and engaging in a fun activity with their favorite adult cousin. One of the resources that provided menu ideas was the *Heart-Healthy Home Cooking African American Style* (NHI, NHLBI, 1997) cookbook. This cookbook includes 20 culturally relevant, healthy recipes, where the food is prepared in a manner that reduces saturated fat, cholesterol, and sodium but does not adversely impact flavor. This activity helped dispel the myth that "soul food" could not be healthy. (A new cookbook is now available: *Heart Healthy Home Cooking African American Style—With Every Heartbeat Is Life* [NHI, NHLBI, 2008].)

After the menu was decided on and the food selected, Sadie had the children find the food pyramids online and analyze their diet for the day. The older children enjoyed impressing their cousin with how fast they could locate the pyramids, including the special pyramid and associated coloring book they discovered for the youngest sibling. Sadie introduced the older children to the NHLBI website and showed them how to access the BMI calculator (http://www.nhlbisupport.com/bmi/), encouraging them to read the associated section on the limitations of the BMI. The adolescents quickly found additional educational materials for their parents, and soon the entire family was gathered around the computer looking at the online interactive meal planner (http://hin.nhlbi.nih.gov/menuplanner/menu.cgi).

The second intervention focused on the parents and their schedule. Through a time and activity analysis of a typical week, Sadie was able to help the mother develop a plan to walk at the high school track while waiting to take her son home from football practice. Instead of sitting in the car being bored and snacking, she began to walk on the track. The mother found that she did not notice the craving to snack as much while she walked and sipped from a water bottle. Much to Sadie's amazement, the mother expanded the original plan and started walking at the track during halftime of her son's football games instead of sitting in the bleachers eating nachos.

After a while, the father joined his wife during her halftime routine. He found it less stressful than sitting and waiting for the second half of the game to begin. The couple soon realized they enjoyed the walks and could do a lot of planning for the remainder of the weekend and upcoming week during this time. In addition, as they began to reconfigure their lives and priorities, they became very aware of the unhealthy snack and food options available to them and their children at school events. The parents encouraged the high school booster club to provide healthier alternatives at the snack shack during games and other school functions.

Meanwhile, Sadie reviewed the hospital dietician's diet suggestions and provided additional clarification to the father. She encouraged him to take advantage of a follow-up appointment and helped him develop questions about eating choices, including the frequency with which he could eat some of his favorite, less healthy foods. Later, she served as a resource as he weighed the pros and cons of two job offers. The job he finally selected involved significantly more physical activity than a desk job (e.g., daily walk of a few miles). The job decision was partially based on his appreciation of the benefits gained from walking with his wife and the time-deepening nature of being able to perform his recommended walking as part of his work routine.

Sadie found her skills as an occupational therapist helpful in selecting age-appropriate gifts that encouraged healthy eating and physical activities to reinforce her relatives' transition to a healthier lifestyle. Over the next year, gifts for the parents included *The Volumetrics Eating Plan: Techniques and Recipes for Feeling Full on Fewer Calories* (Rolls, 2005), which was written by a leading nutrition researcher, and a subscription to the *Nutrition Action Healthletter,* published by the CSPI. Unusual and age-appropriate cookbooks were purchased for the children. An additional gift to help enforce healthy occupation engagement by the entire family was the interactive dance game, *Dance Dance Revolution* (DDR). The family already owned the necessary television and game console, so the only additional purchase was the game software and floor mats (additional information is available at http://www.ddrgame.com/info.html).

Questions

1. Review AOTA's *Framework* and Sadie's interventions. Which areas of performance, performance skills, activity demands, contexts, and client factors were impacted for individual family members or for the family as a whole?

2. What occupational therapy theoretical model would support Sadie's interventions? After considering the model and its components and principles, can you identify additional interventions?

3. The Parent Teacher Association became energized after the parents drew attention to the long-term health impact of the types of food sold at after-school events. They contacted you and a local dietician. What model(s) described in Chapters 2 and 3 may be helpful to organize this project?

▶ For Discussion and Review

1. What occupational therapy model or frame of reference would you use to support the profession's involvement in weight management?
2. Have you ever observed weight bias in a healthcare setting? Have you ever observed weight bias in other contexts? What can be done to reduce the occurrences of weight bias?
3. Locate a Web resource on weight management and obesity reduction. Identify the strengths of the site. Do you have any suggestions for improving this site?
4. Were you surprised by any of the prevalence rates reported in this chapter? Why or why not?
5. Can you identify psychosocial factors in a person's life that influence weight gain?
6. What may be some occupation-based interventions to empower people to strive toward healthy weight management?

▶ Research Questions

1. Does the use of occupation-based interventions enhance the ability to maintain or decrease weight?
2. What are the predictors of successful weight maintenance after weight reduction?
3. Do individuals who have an occupational therapy intervention prior to gastric bypass surgery have a smoother postoperative recovery period?

References

Abbott Laboratories. (2003). *Meridia®: U.S. prescribing information.* Retrieved June 22, 2004, from http://www.rxabbott.com/pdf/meridia.pdf.

American College Health Association. (2002). *Healthy Campus 2010: Making it happen.* Baltimore: American College Health Association.

American Dietetic Association. (2002). Weight management. *Journal of the American Dietetic Association, 102,* 1145–55.

American Dietetic Association. (2006). Position of the American Dietetic Association: Individual-, family-, school- and community-based interventions for pediatric overweight. *Journal of the American Dietetic Association, 106*(6), 925–45.

American Heart Association. (2004, February 17). Safe routes to school funding passes U.S. Senate. *Advocacy Pulse: News from the Hill.*

American Heart Association. (2008). *Eating a heart-healthy diet.* Retrieved January 27,, 2009, from http://www.americanheart.org/presenter.jhtml?identifier=1510.

American Occupational Therapy Association. (2000). Occupational therapy code of ethics (2000). *American Journal Occupational Therapy, 54,* 614–16.

American Occupational Therapy Association. (2005). Occupational therapy code of ethics (2005). *American Journal of Occupational Therapy, 59*(6), 639–42.

American Occupational Therapy Association. (2007). Obesity and occupational therapy position paper. *American Journal of Occupational Therapy, 61*(6), 701–03.

American Occupational Therapy Association. (2008). Occupational therapy practice framework: Domain and processes (2d ed.). *American Journal of Occupational Therapy, 62,* 625–83.

Amersbach, G. (1999). *More water, more fiber, fewer calories: Reinventing the food pyramid for older adults.* Retrieved March 28, 2004, from http://www.nutrition.tufts.edu/magazine/1999fall/pyramid.html.

Baker, S., Barlow, S., Cochran W., Fuchs, G., Klish, W., Krebs, N., Strauss, R., Tershakovec, A., & Udall, J. (2005). Overweight children and adolescents: A clinical report of the North America Society for Pediatric Gastroenterology, Hepatology and Nutrition. *Journal of Pediatric Gastroenterology and Nutrition, 40,* 533–43.

Barlow, S. E., & Dietz, W. H. (1998). Obesity evaluation and treatment: Expert Committee recommendations [Electronic version]. *Pediatrics, 102*(3). Retrieved June 11, 2003, from http://www.pediatrics.org/cgi/content/full/102/3/e29.

Barlow, S. E., & Dietz, W. H. (2002). Management of childhood and adolescent obesity: Summary and recommendations based on reports from pediatricians, pediatric nurse practitioners, and registered dietitians. *Pediatrics, 110*(1), 236–38.

Barlow S. E. and the Expert Committee. (2007). Expert Committee recommendations regarding the prevention, assessment, and treatment of child and adolescent overweight and obesity: Summary report *Pediatrics, 120,* S164–S192.

Barlow, S. E., Trowbridge, F. L., Klish, W. J., & Dietz, W. H. (2002). Treatment of child and adolescent obesity: Reports from pediatricians, pediatric nurse practitioners, and registered dietitians. *Pediatrics, 111*(1), 229–35.

Barnes, P. M., & Schoenborn, C. A. (2003). Physical activity among adults: United States, 2000. *Advance data from vital and health statistics,* No. 333, 1-24, Hyattsville, MD: National Center for Health Statistics.

Bianchini, F., Kaaks, R., & Vainio, H. (2002). Overweight, obesity, and cancer risk. *The Lancet Oncology, 3*(9), 565–74.

Birch, L. L., & Fisher J. O. (1998). Development of eating behaviors among children and adolescents. *Pediatrics, 101*(3), 539–49.

Blanchard, S. A. (2006). AOTA's statement on obesity. *American Journal of Occupational Therapy, 60*(6), 680.

Brachtesende, A. (2004, May 31). Clark receives university's top honor. *OT Practice,* 9–10.

Bray, G. A. (2002). The underlying basis for obesity: Relationship to cancer. *Journal of Nutrition, 132*(11 suppl), 3451S–3455S.

Calle, E. E., Rodriguez, C., Walker-Thurmond, K., & Thun, M. J. (2003). Overweight, obesity, and mortality from cancer in a prospectively studied cohort of U.S. adults. *New England Journal of Medicine, 348*(17), 1623–24.

Camarena, B., Santiago, H., Aguilar, A., Ruvinskis, González-Barranco, J., & Nicolini, H. (2004). Family-based association study between the Monoamine

Oxidase A Gene and obesity: Implications for psychopharmacogenetic studies. *Neuropsychobiology, 49,* 126–29.

Carkhuff, R. (1985). *PPS, productive problem solving.* Amherst, MA: Human Resource Development Press.

Cason, K., & Wenrich, T. (2002). Health and nutrition beliefs, attitudes, and practices of undergraduate college students: A needs assessment. *Clinical Nutrition, 17*(3), 52–70.

Centers for Disease Control and Prevention. (2007). *U.S. Physical Activity Statistics.* Retrieved January 27, 2009, from http://apps.nccd.cdc.gov/PASurveillance/DemoCompare ResultV.asp?State=0&Cat=3&Year=2007&Go=GO#result.

Chambliss, H. O. (2004). Behavioral approaches to obesity treatment. *QUEST, 56,* 142–49.

Chobanian, A. V., Bakris, G. L., Black, H. R., Cushman, W. W. C., Green, L. A., Izzo, J. L., et al. (2003). The seventh report of the Joint National Committee on prevention, detection, evaluation, and treatment of high blood pressure. *Hypertension, 42*(16), 1206–52.

Chronic Disease Prevention. (2003). *Physical activity and good nutrition: Essential elements to prevent chronic diseases and obesity: At a glance.* Retrieved June 16, 2003, from http://www.cdc.gov/nccdphp/aag/aag_dnpa.htm.

Cummings, S., Parham, E. S., & Strain, G. W. (2002). Weight management: Position of the American Dietetic Association. *Journal of the American Dietetic Association, 102,* 1145–55.

Cutler, D. M., Glaeser, E. L., & Shapiro, J. M. (2003, January). *Why have Americans become more obese?* Presented at the Economics of Obesity conference. Washington, DC.

Devlin, M. J., Yanovski, S. Z., & Wilson, G. T. (2000). Obesity: What mental health professionals need to know. *American Journal of Psychiatry, 157,* 854–66.

Diabetes Prevention Program Research Group. (2002). Reduction in the incidence of type 2 diabetes with lifestyle intervention or metformin. *New England Journal of Medicine, 346,* 393–403.

Drohan, S. H. (2002). Managing early childhood obesity in the primary care setting: A behavior modification approach. *Pediatric Nursing, 28*(6), 599–610.

Dunn, W., Brown, C., & McGuigan, A. (1994). The ecology of human performance: A framework for considering the effect of context. *American Journal of Occupational Therapy, 48,* 595–607.

Escott-Stump, S. (2002). Chapter 10: Weight management, undernutrition, and malnutrition. In *Nutrition and diagnosis-related care* (5th ed., pp. 431–43). Philadelphia: Lippincott, Williams & Wilkins.

Faircloth, S. (2004, Fall). Six ways government promotes obesity & what to do about it. *Diversity: Allied Health Careers, 3*(2), 47–48.

Finkelstein, E. A., Fiebelkorn, I. C., & Wang, G. (2003). National medical spending attributable to overweight and obesity: How much, and who's paying? *Health affairs.* Retrieved June 11, 2003, from http://www.healthaffairs .org/free content/v22n4/s2.pdf.

Finkelstein, E. A., Fiebelkorn, I. C., & Wang, G. (2005). The costs of obesity among full-time employees. *American Journal of Health Promotion, 20*(1), 45–51.

Finkelstein, E. A., Ruhm, C. J., & Kosa, K. M. (2005). Economic causes and consequences of obesity. *Annual Review of Public Health, 26,* 239–57.

Fontaine, K. R., Faith, M. S., Allison, D. B., & Cheskin, L. J. (1998). Body weight and health care among women in the general population. *Archives of Family Medicine, 7,* 381–84.

Foti, D. (2005). Caring for the person of size. *OT Practice, 10*(2), 9–14.

Frazao, E. (1999). *American's eating habits: Changes and consequences.* Agricultural Information Bulletin No 750. Washington DC: U.S. Government Printing.

Freeland-Graves, J., & Nitzke, S. (2002). Total diet approach to communicating food and nutrition information: Position of the American Dietetic Association. *Journal of the American Dietetic Association, 102,* 100–08.

Graham, M. A., & Jones, A. L. (2002). Freshman 15: Valid theory or harmful myth? *Journal of American College Health, 50*(4), 171–73.

Greenberg, B. S., Eastin, M., Hofschire, L., Lachlan, K., & Brownell, K. D. (2003). Portrayals of overweight and obese individuals on commercial television. *American Journal of Public Health, 93,* 1342–48.

Gropper, S. S., Smith J. L., & Groff, J. L. (2009). Chapter 8: Body composition, energy expenditure, and energy balance. In *Advanced nutrition and human metabolism* (5th ed., pp. 279–300). Belmont, CA: Wadsworth Cengage Learning.

Hansen, R. H., & Hinojosa, J. (2004). Occupational therapy's commitment to nondiscrimination and inclusion (edited 2004). *American Journal of Occupational Therapy, 58*(6), 668.

Henry, A. D. (2003). Section II: The interview process in occupational therapy. In E. B. Crepeau, E. S. Cohn, & B. A. B. Schell (Eds.), *Willard and Spackman's occupational therapy* (10th ed., pp. 285–97). Philadelphia: Lippincott, Williams & Wilkins.

Hill, J. O., Wyam, H. R., Reed, G. W., & Peters, J. C. (2003). Obesity and the environment: Where do we go from here? *Science, 299,* 853–55.

Housman, C. (2003). *Identification of engagement in healthy and unhealthy occupations in Towson University undergraduate students: Eating behaviors and substance use and abuse.* Unpublished graduate project, Towson University, Towson, MD.

Institute of Medicine. (1995). *Weighing the options: Criteria for evaluating weight-management programs.* Washington, DC: National Academy Press.

Institute of Medicine. (2002). *Dietary reference intakes for energy, carbohydrate, fiber, fat, fatty acids, cholesterol, protein, and amino acids.* Washington, DC: National Academies Press.

Institute of Medicine. (2004). *Preventing childhood obesity: Health in the balance.* Washington, DC: National Academies Press.

Janssen, I., Craig, W. M., Boyce, W. F., & Pickett, W. (2004). Associations between overweight and obesity with bullying behaviors in school-aged children. *Pediatrics, 113*(5), 1187–94.

Jeffery, R. W., Drewnowski, A., Epstein, L. H., Stunkard, A. J., Wilson, G. T., Wing, R. R., & Hill, D. R. (2000). Long-term maintenance of weight loss: Current status. *Health Psychology, 19,* 5–16.

Jenkins, C. D. (2003). *Building better health: A handbook of behavioral change.* Washington, DC: Pan American Health Organization.

Johnson, R. K., & Nicklas, T. A. (1999). Dietary guidance for healthy children aged 2 to 11 years: Position of American Dietetic Association. *Journal of the American Dietetic Association, 99,* 93–101.

Joint FAO/WHO Expert Consultation. (2003). *Diet, nutrition and the prevention of chronic diseases.* Geneva, Switzerland: World Health Organization.

Krebs, N. F., & Jacobson, M. S. (2003). Prevention of pediatric overweight and obesity. *Pediatrics, 112*(2), 424–30.

Lang, S. (2003, August 28). *CU nutritionists: Junk food, all-you-can-eat make "freshman 15" a reality.* Retrieved June, 15, 2004, from http://news.cornell.edu/Chronicle/03/8.28.03/frershman-15.html.

Lichtenstein, A. H., Rasmussen, H., Yu, W. W., Epstein, S. R., & Russell, R. M. (2008). Modified MyPyramid for Older Adults. *Journal of Nutrition,138,* 5–11.

Lin, P. H., Aickin, M., Champagne, C., Craddick S., Sacks, F. M., McCarron, P., et al. (2003). Food group sources of nutrients in the dietary patterns of the DASH-sodium trail. *Journal of the American Dietetic Association, 103*(4), 488–96.

Lissau, I., Overpeck, M. D., Ruan, W. J., Due, P., Holstein, B. E., & Hediger, M. L. (2004), and the Health Behavior in School-aged Children Obesity Working Group. Body mass index and overweight in adolescents in 13 European countries, Israel and the United States. *Archives of Pediatric Adolescent Medicine, 158,* 27–33.

Lyons, P., & Miller, W. (1999). Effective clinical care and health promotion for large people. *Medicine and Science in Sports Exercise, 31*(8), 1141–46.

Malhi, G. S., Mitchell, P. B., & Caterson, I. (2001). "Why getting fat, Doc?" Weight gain and psychotropic medications. *Australian and New Zealand Journal of Psychiatry, 35,* 315–21.

Malhotra, S., & McElroy, S. L. (2002). Medical management of obesity associated with mental disorders. *Journal of Clinical Psychiatry, 63*(Suppl 4), 24–32.

Marchesini, G., Natale, S., Chierici, S., Manini, R., Besteghi, L., Di Domizio, S., Sartini, A., Pasqui, F., Baraldi, L., Forlani, G., & Melchionda, N. (2002). Effects of cognitive-behavioral therapy on health-related quality of life in obese subjects with and without binge eating disorder. *International Journal of Obesity, 26,* 1261–67.

Martin, A. (2004, June 15). French fries are legally a vegetable. *Baltimore Sun,* 3A. [Chicago Tribune]

Matsutsuyu, J. (1969). The interest checklist. *American Journal of Occupational Therapy, 23,* 323–28.

Must, A., Spadano, J., Coakley, E. H., Field, A. E., Colditz, G., & Dietz, W. H. (1999). The disease burden associated with overweight and obesity. *Journal of the American Medical Association, 282*(16), 1523–29.

National Dairy Council. (2003). A new look at dietary patterns and hypertension. *Dairy Council Digest.* Retrieved June 11, 2003, from http://www.nationaldairycouncil.org.

National Diabetes Information Clearinghouse. (2005). *Insulin resistance and pre-diabetes.* Retrieved on November 27, 2005, from http://diabetes.niddk.nih.gov/dm/pubs/insulinresistance/.

National Institutes of Health, National Heart, Lung, and Blood Institute. (1997). *Heart-healthy home cooking African American style* (NIH Publication No. 97-3792). Bethesda, MD: U.S. Department of Health and Human Services.

National Institutes of Health, National Heart, Lung, and Blood Institute. (1998a). *Clinical guidelines on the identification, evaluation, and treatment of overweight and obesity in adults.* Bethesda, MD: U.S. Department of Health and Human Services.

National Institutes of Health, National Heart, Lung, and Blood Institute. (1998b). *Current clinical practice guidelines and reports.* Retrieved February 1, 2009, from http://www.nhlbi.nih.gov/guidelines/current.htm.

National Institutes of Health, National Heart, Lung, and Blood Institute. (2001). *Healthy heart handbook for women* (NIH Publication No. 00-2720). Bethesda, MD: U.S. Department of Health and Human Services.

National Institutes of Health, National Heart, Lung, and Blood Institute. (2003). *The DASH diet.* Retrieved June 13, 2003, from http://www.nhlbi.nih.gov.

National Institutes of Health, National Heart, Lung, and Blood Institute. (2008). *Heart healthy home cooking African American style—With every heartbeat is life.* Available from http://emall.nhlbihin.net/product2.asp?sku=08-3792&p=2&h=3&g=23&r=1.

North American Association for the Study of Obesity (NAASO), and National Heart, Lung, and Blood Institute. (2000). *Practical guide to the identification, evaluation, and treatment of obesity and overweight in adults.* (NIH Publication No. 00-4084).

Ogden, C. L., Carroll, M. D., Curtin, L. R., McDowell, M. A., Tabak, C. J., & Flegal, K. M. (2006). Prevalence of overweight and obesity in the United States, 1999–2004. *Journal of the American Medical Association, 295,* 1549–55.

Partnership to Promote Healthy Eating and Active Living. (2003). *America on the move.* Retrieved November 3, 2003, from http://www.americaonthemove.org/index.asp.

Partnership to Promote Healthy Eating and Active Living. (2004a). *About us.* Retrieved February 7, 2004, from http://www.ppheal.org/about_us.html.

Partnership to Promote Healthy Eating and Active Living. (2004b). *Welcome to the partnership to promote healthy eating and active living.* Retrieved February 7, 2004, from http://www.ppheal.org/index.html.

Price J. H. (October 11, 2005). America gets more physical. *Washington Times.* Retrieved October 14, 2005, from http://washingtontimes.com.

Prochaska, J. O., & DiClemente, C. C. (1983). Stages and processes of self-change of smoking: Toward an integrative model of change. *Journal of Counseling and Clinical Psychology, 51*(3), 390–95.

Puhl, R., & Brownell, K. D. (2001). Bias, discrimination and obesity. *Obesity Research, 9,* 788–805.

Racette, S. B., Deusinger, S. S., & Deusinger, R. H. (2003). Obesity: Overview of prevalence, etiology, and treatment. *Physical Therapy, 83*(3), 276–88.

Rand, C. S. W., & Macgregor, A. M. C. (1991). Successful weight loss following obesity surgery and the perceived liability of morbid obesity. *International Journal of Obesity, 15,* 577–79.

Rao, G. (2001). Insulin resistance syndrome. *American Family Physician, 65*(11), 1165–66.

Rapoport, L., Clark, M., & Wardle, J. (2000). Evaluation of a modified cognitive-behavioural programme for weight management. *International Journal of Obesity, 24,* 1726–37.

Reitz, S. M. (n.d.). Discipline roles in obesity prevention and weight management: Health promotion; role of occupational therapy in obesity prevention. In *Rural interdisciplinary health promotion, module three—Obesity prevention.* Available at http://www.allconet.org/ahec/rihp.

Roche Pharmaceuticals. (2000). *Patient information about XENICAL® (orlistat) capules.* Nutley, NJ: Roche Laboratories.

Rolls, B. J. (2005). *The volumetrics eating plan: Techniques and recipes for feeling full on fewer calories.* New York: HarperCollins.

Rural Interdisciplinary Health Promotion. (n.d.). *Module three—Obesity prevention.* Available at http://www.allconet.org/ahec/rihp.

Schkade, J., & McClung, M. (2001). *Occupational adaptation in practice: Concepts and cases.* Thorofare, NJ: SLACK.

Schultz, S., & Schkade, J. K. (2003). Section III: Occupational adaptation. In E. B. Crepeau, E. S. Cohn, & B. A. B. Schell (Eds.), *Willard and Spackman's occupational therapy* (10th ed., pp. 220–24). Philadelphia: Lippincott, Williams & Wilkins.

Schwartz, M. B., Chambliss, H. O., Brownell, K. D., Blair, S. N., & Billington, C. (2003). Weight bias among health professionals specializing in obesity. *Obesity Research, 11*(9), 1033–39.

Shumaker, N. L., Ball, A. L., Neils-Strunjas, J., Smith, R., Weiler, E., & Krikorian, R. (2003). Using memory strategies to improve 24-hour dietary recalls among older adults. *Journal of Allied Health, 32*(3), 196–201.

Smith, D. A., Ness, E. M., Herbert, R., Schechter, C. B., Phillips, R. A., Diamond, J. A., & Landrigan, P. J. (2004). Abdominal diameter index: A more powerful anthropometric measure for prevalent coronary heart disease risk in adult males. *Diabetes, Obesity and Metabolism, 7,* 370–80.

Smith, N. R., Kielhofner, G., & Watts, J. H. (1986). The relationship between volition, activity pattern, and life satisfaction in the elderly. *American Journal of Occupational Therapy, 40,* 278–83.

Sommers, E. (1999, August). *College freshmen can avoid the "Freshman 15."* Web MD. Retrieved June 15, 2004, from http://cnn.com/HEALTH/diet.fitness/9908/19/freshmane.fifteen.

Steinberger, J., & Daniels, S. R. (2003). Obesity, insulin resistance, diabetes, and cardiovascular risk in children. *Circulation, 107,* 1448–53.

Sturm, R. (2002). The effects of obesity, smoking, and drinking on medical problems and costs. *Health Affairs, 21*(2), 245–53.

Tod, A. M., & Lacey, A. (2004). Overweight and obesity: Helping clients to take action. *British Journal of Community Nursing, 9*(2), 59–66.

Tufts University. (2007). *Modified MyPyramid for Older Adults.* Retrieved January 30, 2009, from http://nutrition.tufts.edu/1197972031385/Nutrition-Page-nl2w_1198058402614.html.

Tuomilehto, J., Lindstrom, J., Eriksson, J. G., Valle, T. T., Hamalainen, H., Ilanne-Parikka, P., Kiukaanniemi, S. K.,

Laakso, M., Louheranta, A., Rastas, K. M., Salminen, V., & Uusitupa, M. (2001). Prevention of type 2 diabetes mellitus by changes in lifestyle among subjects with impaired glucose tolerance. *New England Journal of Medicine, 344,* 1343–50.

University of Southern California, Department of Occupational Science and Occupational Therapy. (2004). *About us.* Retrieved June 15, 2004, from http://www.usc.edu/schools/ihp/ot/about/faculty_practice/index.html.

U.S. Department of Agriculture. (2005a). *MyPyramid mini poster.* Retrieved November 27, 2005, from http://www.mypyramid.gov/professionals/index.html.

U.S. Department of Agriculture. (2005b). *MyPyramid for Kids mini poster (advanced).* Retrieved November 27, 2005, from http://www.mypyramid.gov/kids/index.html.

U.S. Department of Agriculture and U.S. Department of Health and Human Services. (2005). *Dietary guidelines for Americans, 2005* (6th ed.). Washington, DC: U.S. Government Printing Office. Available at http://www.healthierus.gov/dietaryguidelines.

U.S. Department of Health and Human Services. (2000). *Healthy People 2010: Understanding and Improving Health* (2d ed.). Washington, DC: U.S. Government Printing Office.

U.S. Department of Health and Human Services. (2001). *The Surgeon General's call to action to prevent and decrease overweight and obesity.* Washington, DC: U.S. Government Printing Office.

U.S. Food and Drug Administration, Center for Drug Evaluation and Research, Consumer Drug Information. (2000). *Xenical consumer information.* Retrieved June 13, 2004, from http://www.fda.gov/cder/consumerinfo/xenical.htm.

Velde, B., & Fidler, G. (2002). *Lifestyle performance: A model for engaging the power of occupation.* Thorofare, NJ: SLACK.

Wang, G., & Dietz, W. H. (2002). Economic burden of obesity in youths aged 6 to 17 years: 1979–1999 [Electronic version]. *Pediatrics, 109*(5), e81. Retrieved April 2, 2008, from http://www.pediatrics.org/cgi/content/full/109/5/e81.

Warren, E., Brennan, A., & Akehurst, R. (2004). Cost-effectiveness of sibutramine in the treatment of obesity. *Medical Decision Making, 24*(1), 9–19.

Wee, C. C., McCarthy, E. P., Davis, R. B., & Phillips, R. S. (2000). Screening for cervical and breast cancer: Is obesity an unrecognized barrier to preventive care? *Annals of Internal Medicine, 132,* 697–704.

Weight Realities Division of the Society for Nutrition Education. (2003). Guidelines for childhood obesity prevention programs: Promoting healthy weight in children. *Journal of Nutrition, Education & Behavior, 35*(1), 1–4.

Werch, C. E., & DiClemente, C. C. (1994). A multi-stage model for matching prevention strategies and messages to youth stage of use. *Health Education Research, 9*(1), 37–46.

World Health Organization. (2000). *Obesity: Preventing and managing the global epidemic.* Geneva, Switzerland: Author.

World Health Organization. (2005). *Global strategy on diet, physical activity and health: Obesity and overweight.*

Retrieved November 27, 2005, from http://www.who.int/ dietphysicalactivity/publications/facts/obesity/en/.

Young, L. R., & Nestle, M. (2002). The contribution of expanding portion size to the U.S. obesity epidemic. *American Journal of Public Health, 92,* 246–49.

Zemel, M. B., Richards, J., Russel, J., Milstead, A., Gehardt, L., & Silva, E. (2005). Dairy augmentation of total and central fat loss in obese subjects. *International Journal of Obesity, 29*(4), 341–47.

Zemel, M. B., Thompson, W., Milstead, A., Morris, K., & Campbell, P. (2004). Calcium and dairy acceleration of weight and fat loss during energy restriction in obese adults. *Obesity Research, 12*(4), 582–90.

Chapter 15

Preventing Substance Abuse in Adolescents and Adults

Penelope Moyers and Virginia C. Stoffel

> I only wish we would spend a fraction of the money on prevention. . . . We know prevention is the biggest bang for our buck.
> —Rhode Island Representative Patrick Kennedy, in an address to the National Mental Health Association Annual meeting, June 8, 2006, Washington, DC.

Learning Objectives

This chapter is designed to enable the reader to:

- Discuss the need for and the importance of prevention of substance-use disorders.
- Describe the Transtheoretical Model of Behavior Change and demonstrate its application in designing prevention strategies for persons with substance-use disorders.
- Augment the Transtheoretical Model with an occupational perspective in order to understand and differentiate the role of occupational therapy in the prevention of substance-use disorders.

- Identify prevention strategies and programs assessed in the literature and understand the conditions under which the evidence-based strategy prevents substance-use disorders.
- Develop and implement occupational therapy prevention strategies targeted to persons at risk for substance-use disorders.

Key Terms

Brief interventions

Downstream interventions

Midstream interventions

Motivational interviewing

Social competence

Upstream interventions

Introduction

Occupational therapists and occupational therapy assistants need to be educated about how substance use affects the communities in which they live, work, and play. Whether they are researchers, educators, practitioners, or a blend of these roles, they need to know incidence rates for illicit drug and alcohol use. While the cost of treatment for persons with substance-use disorders rises, restrictions in insurance coverage remain and the number of persons who are uninsured is growing. With limited treatment options available, substance use has devastating effects on families and communities (Oggins, 2003). The information presented in this chapter breaks from the traditional approach of imparting intervention strategies to treat persons with substance-use disorders. Instead, it encourages occupational ther-

apists and occupational therapy assistants in all areas of practice to consider ways to prevent problems related to substance use from occurring, particularly focusing on how the promotion of participation in life activities and occupations may play a role.

In this chapter, the authors review prevalence data of substance abuse to demonstrate the need for and the importance of prevention. Next, the Transtheoretical Model of Behavior Change (TMBC) is used to select prevention strategies and programs as well as the timing of intervention to enhance program effectiveness. This application of the TMBC is augmented with an occupational perspective in order to foster understanding and differentiation of the role of occupational therapy in the prevention of substance-use disorders. Next, based on a review of evidence-based literature, successful prevention strategies are shared and areas where additional research is needed are identified. The last section of the chapter delineates how occupational therapists and occupational therapy assistants might develop and implement prevention strategies targeted to a range of age groups in a variety of settings.

Prevalence of Substance-Use Disorders

In 2001, an estimated 16.6 million people were classified with dependence on or abuse of either alcohol or illicit drugs, of which 2.4 million were classified as abusing both, 3.2 million were abusing only illicit drugs, and 11.0 million were abusing only alcohol (Substance Abuse and Mental Health Services Administration [SAMHSA], 2002). In comparing the rates of dependence on and abuse of alcohol among adults aged 18 and older, those with serious mental illness (SMI) had a 20.3% rate, which is much higher than adults without SMI who had a rate of 6.3%.

There were statistically significant increases between 2000 and 2001 of those who used marijuana, cocaine, pain relievers, tranquilizers, and hallucinogens (SAMHSA, 2002). In 2002, 6.5 million people used ecstasy at least once in their lifetime, but by 2001, this number rose to an estimated 8.1 million. Similarly, in 1999, the number of people aged 12 and older who had used OxyContin for nonmedical purposes at least once in their lifetime was 221,000, rising to approximately 975,000 persons by 2001. The highest rate of illicit drug use was for 18- to 20-year-olds.

These statistics about prevalence of use do not portray a comprehensive picture about the impact of substance use on society. However, per capita use is certainly important to monitor, because there is a relationship between population use and the prevalence of societal problems—for example, driving while intoxicated, domestic violence, and homicide (Babor, Aguirre-Molin, Marlatt, & Clayton, 1999; Gutman & Clayton, 1999). Habitual users of alcohol and drugs are more likely to experience unintentional injuries (Smith, Branas, & Miller, 1999) and motor vehicle crashes (Zador, Krawchuk, & Voas, 2000) and are more likely to demonstrate violent aggressive behavior and to become a victim of violence (Reiss & Roth, 1993–94). When compared to those who do not use substances, persons who use and abuse substances have a greater likelihood of dying or becoming injured from falls, drownings, burns, exposure to cold, and unintended shootings (Hingson, Heeren, Jamanka, & Howland, 2000).

Family members of the substance user are typically affected by the way their loved one is behaving.

Domestic violence and unemployment of the primary breadwinner are two of the disabling consequences of substance use that family members experience. The impact of parental substance abuse on young children, not only before birth but also across the child's lifetime, has been documented. Young children may have different patterns of cognitive development when compared with children from families with no history of alcoholism (Corral, Holguin, & Cadaveira, 2003). Recent meta-analytical studies indicate that cognitive effects of illicit drugs taken by the mother in utero may be subtle in their impact (Lester, LaGasse, & Seifer, 1998). Additionally, children with prenatal exposure to alcohol abuse are reported to demonstrate mood disorders as they age (O'Connor et al., 2002).

Prevention Approaches

These statistics suggest that the occupational performance (impoverished and dominating habits) patterns of many individuals with substance-use disorders affect themselves and their families, as well as "the health of towns, nations, cities, neighborhoods, and communities" (Clark, Wood, & Larson, 1998, p. 18). In addition, targeting the ill effects of substance abuse is a focus area for *Healthy People 2010* (U.S. Department of Health and Human Services [USDHHS], 2000). The goal is to "reduce substance abuse to protect the health, safety, and quality of life for all, especially children" (p. 9).

While the need for prevention is clear, determining which preventative approaches are effective remains problematic. *Healthy People 2010* identifies opportunities for preventing substance-use disorders (USDHHS, 2000, p. 6), including the development of research-supported programs for diverse racial and ethnic populations. These programs must be studied using high-quality process and outcome evaluations. In terms of other opportunities for prevention, there may be particular policies that could be adopted, such as administrative revocation of driver's licenses for lower legal blood alcohol limits or higher prices and taxes for alcoholic beverages. In addition, targeting college students, high school, middle school, and elementary school-aged children is important for raising awareness. Strengthening families by supporting the parental role in providing alternative activities, in engaging in meaningful occupations, and in building the skills and confidence of children may be successful as well. According to *Healthy People 2010* (USDHHS, 2000), "government, employers, the faith community, and other organizations in the private and nonprofit sectors must increase their level of cooperation and coordination to ensure that multiple service needs are met" (p. 8).

Determining effectiveness of prevention programs depends upon the target of the intervention, often differentiated in the public health literature as downstream, midstream, and upstream interventions (Babor et al., 1999; Gutman & Clayton, 1999). **Downstream interventions** target the individual and focus on treating an existing substance-use disorder and on preventing a reoccurrence of that disorder. **Midstream interventions** are those strategies that incorporate into primary health care and into work-, community-, school-, and university-based programs the identification of persons at risk for substance-use disorders and the provision of intervention to reduce these risks. National, state, and local policies and broad population-based programs aimed at the prevention of substance abuse, such as national media campaigns, comprise what are considered **upstream interventions.**

Both Babor and colleagues (1999) and Gutman and Clayton (1999) have indicated that the effectiveness of downstream interventions range from 30% to 50% of clients remaining abstinent after 1 year of formal alcohol and drug abuse treatment, thus grading the performance of downstream interventions as "half full." Midstream and upstream interventions were both graded as "one-third full" for alcohol abuse (Babor et al., 1999) and "one-quarter full" for drug prevention (Gutman & Clayton, 1999). Prevention efforts at midstream typically have stronger effects subsequent to the intervention but actually may have a minimal effect over time. In some cases, these midstream prevention programs have had little apparent effect, as in the case of the widely disseminated Drug Abuse Resistance Education (DARE) informational program used in many U.S. school districts (Clayton, Cattarello, & Johnstone, 1996). Some midstream programs have actually facilitated substance use because of the unintended consequence of exposing young people to information and role models that enable them to pick and choose the drugs they would like to experience (Palinkas, Atkins, Miller, & Ferreira, 1996).

The lesson learned is that prevention is not just a single program or method but is effective only when multiple strategies are incorporated in a variety of environments within upstream, midstream, and downstream programs. This wide scope for intervention is directed at many relevant audiences, such as children, adolescents, college students, employers and employees, parents and other family members, teachers, community and business leaders, the media, the criminal justice system, and legislators and other policymakers. Of importance is the need for theoretical development and research to understand the complex factors and interactions that more than likely determine whether prevention strategies will work as planned.

The Occupational Perspective on Substance Abuse Prevention

The report card of the success of current prevention programs would suggest that additional components are needed. Perhaps a missing component of existing prevention strategies is the occupational therapy perspective of occupational justice, where occupational therapists and occupational therapy assistants believe that the health of the community and its members is partially dependent upon the availability of healthy occupations for everyone (Wilcock, 2003). According to Wilcock (1993), availability of occupations is extremely important, because "occupations help individuals meet their bodily needs of sustenance, self-care, shelter, and safety; occupations develop skills, social structures and technology aimed at superiority over predators and the environment." In addition, occupations "exercise and develop personal capacities enabling the organism to be maintained and to flourish" (p. 20).

Communities that do not implement strategies to reduce access to alcohol and illicit drugs and provide opportunities for participation in meaningful activities are inadvertently facilitating the isolation or estrangement of people from their healthy occupations. Substance abuse perpetuates a cycle of occupational alienation (Wilcock, 1998), where meaning is no longer derived from usual occupations but instead is transferred to substance-using activities and occupations, such as raising money for the drugs or spending time using (Moyers & Stoffel, 2001). Eventually, as withdrawal from customary occupations continues, occupational deprivation (Wilcock, 1998) may occur. The community context in which the person lives may be such that the interaction between the person and the environment limits occupational choices, thereby resulting in occupational deprivation. For instance, the person may no longer be able to (or is deprived of) work due to the strong drive to spend time exclusively on maintaining the addiction, while the context maintains the negative cycle of addiction through easy access to the drugs of choice and through restriction of access to the treatment interventions needed in order to disrupt this cycle of addiction.

The Transtheoretical Model of Behavior Change (TMBC), described in Chapter 3, outlines five stages of positive change and recovery, including precontemplation, contemplation, preparation, action, and maintenance (DiClemente & Prochaska, 1998). Goals related to each of these five stages of change can be developed and incorporated within downstream, midstream, and upstream substance-use prevention programs. Examples of goals related to the stages of change are provided in Table 15-1 (see Moyers & Stoffel, 2001, p. 329).

Table 15–1 **The Stages of Change**

Stage	Focus of Prevention	Occupational Therapy Strategy
Precontemplation: Not aware of any need for change, not aware of any risks for substance use, and is unlikely to take action soon.	Bring the risky environments, occupational performances, and activities and occupations to awareness. Move to contemplation.	• Educate about risks and their consequences to occupational performance. • Facilitate self-evaluation of current occupational performance to note mismatch between performance and values. • Promote evaluation of environments in terms of barriers and facilitators to healthy engagement in activities and occupations. • Use decisional balance exercises to articulate pros and cons for making changes in occupational performance and to explore pros and cons for not making a change.
Contemplation: Feels ambivalent about change, has not yet decided to change but is thinking that there may be a need to change.	Tip the balance of pros and cons to the pro side of making a change. Move to preparation.	• Facilitate self-evaluation of current occupational performance to note mismatch between performance and values. • Promote evaluation of environments in terms of barriers and facilitators to healthy engagement in activities and occupations. • Use decisional balance exercises to articulate pros and cons for making changes in occupational performance. • Foster self-efficacy or belief in ability to change through experience of success in key activities and occupations.
Preparation: Has decided to change and is planning steps toward achieving the change goal.	Finalize the plan for change and facilitate commitment for implementation. Move to action.	• Foster self-efficacy or belief in ability to change through experience of success in key activities and occupations. • Identify resources to facilitate and support change. • Determine alternative occupations and activities. • Avoid unhealthy environments or alter environment to support health. • Substitute healthy occupations and activities for current unhealthy ones. Use activity sampling if not aware of possible new activities • Replace unhealthy occupational performance with healthy performance.

Continued

Table 15–1   **The Stages of Change—cont'd**

Stage	Focus of Prevention	Occupational Therapy Strategy
Action: Tries out new behaviors. Behaviors are unstable.	Support the new behaviors and encourage further action as needed. Move to maintenance.	• Foster self-efficacy or belief in ability to change through experience of success in key activities and occupations. • Identify resources to facilitate and support change. • Determine alternative occupations and activities by sampling activities. • Avoid unhealthy environments or alter environment to support health. • Substitute healthy occupations and activities for current unhealthy ones. • Replace unhealthy occupational performance with healthy performance. • Reward new occupational performance. • Teach how to self-reward. • Introduce support networks for modeling and facilitating further change.
Maintenance: Establishes new behaviors on a long-term basis.	Provide periodic booster sessions to maintain healthy behaviors. Help stay in maintenance, or if relapses into old risky behaviors, move to contemplation and begin again.	• Foster self-efficacy or belief in ability to change through experience of success in key activities and occupations. • Reward new occupational performance. • Teach how to self-reward. • Introduce support networks for modeling and facilitating further change. • Promote incorporation of new occupational performances into habits, routines, and roles. • Encourage continual self-monitoring to identify emerging risky environments, occupational performances, and activities and occupations.

Adapted from *Brief interventions and brief therapies for substance abuse* by K. L. Barry, 1999, Rockville, MD: Center for Substance Abuse Treatment, Substance Abuse and Mental Health Services Administration; and *Group treatment for substance abuse: A stages-of-change therapy manual* by M. M. Velasquez, G. G. Maurer, C. Crouch, & C. C. DiClemente, 2001, New York: Guilford Press.

Similar to the process of occupational therapy interventions—where there is continual reassessment and interaction between evaluation, intervention, and outcomes—these stages of change are not linear, because individuals may move back and forth between them. Reoccurrence of the risky or addictive behavior may indicate the need for individuals to revert back to earlier stages and to progress through them again. Table 15-1 provides further clarification of how to apply these stages to prevention and outlines possible occupational therapy strategies. These strategies are guides for designing downstream, midstream, and upstream types of programming.

The goal of prevention strategies, whether delivered through downstream, midstream, or upstream programs, is to decrease the likelihood of the population's engagement in risky activities and behaviors, or if already engaged in risky activities, to prevent the escalation of risk to the point of addiction. Optimally, the outcome of prevention is the development of a personal value system and public norms that promote personal responsibility for one's own health and for contributing to the health of the community. Healthy communities depend on, and are sustained through development of supportive contexts, the engagement of the population in constructive occupations such as activities of daily living, instrumental activities of daily living, education, work, leisure, and social participation. If reduced engagement in healthy occupations and increased engagement in unhealthy occupations (e.g., activities associated with using alcohol and drugs) occurs and is widespread within a population, communities may experience increased crime and escalating economic and social decline. Values important for promoting personal responsibility for health include the following (modified from Moyers & Stoffel, 2001, p. 330):

- Using substances is not essential for occupational performance unless prescribed for specific medical reasons or unless involving the appropriate use of over-the-counter medications (e.g., for fever reduction and treatment of headache or colds, or to enhance nutrition with vitamins, etc.).
- Using substances uncontrollably leads to health, social, and possibly legal problems and interferes with occupational performance and engagement in activities and occupations.
- Using substances as performance enhancers (e.g., anabolic steroids, creatinine, ephedra, blood doping) for sports is dangerous and may lead to liver cancer, cerebrovascular accident (CVA), myocardial infarction, a weakened immune system, mania, delusions, and homicidal rage (National Institute on Drug Abuse, 2007).

- Using substances to solve emotional problems is dangerous and may lead to permanent impairments in body structures and body functions, performance skill erosion (motor, process, and communication/interaction), performance pattern disruption (habits, routines, and roles), and occupational alienation and deprivation.
- Achieving an artificially altered emotional and cognitive state is not acceptable and interferes with occupational performance and engagement in activities and occupations.
- Learning coping strategies is important for managing life problems and for facilitating occupational performance and engagement in activities and occupations within a community.
- Enhancing protective factors and reversing/reducing known risk factors to alcohol and illicit drug use is helpful when choosing occupations and when selecting contexts within a community for engagement in healthy occupations.
- Developing social competencies is necessary for articulating needs related to engagement in occupations and activities necessary for a wholesome lifestyle supported within a healthy community.

Evidence-Based Prevention Programs

In order to understand the potential role of occupational therapy in promoting health and reducing risk for substance use, it is helpful to review the literature for evidence-based prevention and health promotion programs. Most of the identified programs targeted midstream interventions, but downstream and upstream programs were also included. See Table 15-2 to examine the evidence-based prevention programs discussed in this chapter; the vast majority are provided as group interventions. Four common models of group work include the

- group education model, in which participants are taught health-related information;
- skills training model, in which participants are taught behavioral and cognitive-behavioral skills, such as anger management;
- group process model, where participants gain therapeutic benefits from their interactions with other group members and the group leader; and
- check-in group model, where brief individual interventions are provided in a group setting (Weiss, Jaffee, de Menil, & Cogley, 2004).

Family Programs

Spoth, Redmond, and Lepper (1999) studied a prevention program based on a biopsychosocial model called the Iowa Strengthening Families Program (ISFP), which was conducted with 446 families from 22 rural school districts in the Midwest. The programmatic goals were to enhance the protective and resiliency processes of the family and to decrease the family-based risk factors that may contribute to the adolescent's potential for developing a substance-use disorder. The program consisted of six separate but concurrent youth and parent sessions designed to build skills in risk reduction. There was also a joint family curriculum where skills learned in the separate sessions were practiced. These joint sessions occurred immediately after the individual sessions. Program content examples are listed in Table 15-3.

The ISFP was compared to another family program called Preparing for the Drug-Free Years (PDFY), which arose from a social development model (Spoth, Reyes, Redmond, & Shin, 1999). The goal of the PDFY program was similar to the ISFP and was designed to enhance the protective parent-child interactions. Another goal was to reduce family-based risk factors that could contribute to an adolescent's early substance use. The difference in this program from the ISFP was that there were only five sessions, each lasting 2 hours. The parents attended all five sessions while the child was required to attend only one session. Content for both programs was similar (see Table 15-3).

The results of these studies (Spoth, Redmond, & Lepper, 1999; Spoth, Reyes, et al., 1999), as indicated in Table 15-2, showed that both family programs were effective in reducing the initiation of use, frequency of use, and composite use of adolescents over a 3-year period. However, the ISFP, which involved the adolescent more than the PDFY program, demonstrated a greater number of significant effects on the outcome measures. However, both programs were effective in reducing the adolescent's reported use, and a cost-benefit analysis (Spoth, Guyll, & Day, 2002) reported significant benefit for every dollar invested in the two family-focused prevention programs, with the ISFP having a greater benefit per investment dollar.

School Programs

School programs have been effective in reducing current alcohol and drug use, intention to use, and alcohol behavior, and they have been effective in improving social adjustment and self-efficacy around alcohol and drug refusal skills. In addition to preventing alcohol use, several of the programs effectively targeted illicit drug, tobacco, marijuana, and polydrug use. Most of these programs gave minimal coverage to teaching knowledge about drugs and alcohol and their long-term physical and emotional effects. Instead, information was provided about the more immediate negative consequences of alcohol and drug use, particularly highlighting the decreasing social acceptability of use. Norms related to actual adult and adolescent drug and alcohol use were provided to illustrate any discrepancy between the adolescent's current use and that of most individuals their age.

The emphasis of these school-based programs was on general interpersonal skills and on social competence. **Social competence** refers to personal and interpersonal effectiveness in stress management, self-esteem, health knowledge, problem-solving, assertiveness, and social support (Caplan et al., 1992). Methods for teaching in these programs typically involved cognitive-behavioral strategies, such as demonstration, behavioral rehearsal, feedback and reinforcement, and behavioral homework assignments for further practice. Research generally indicated that to sustain effectiveness over time, booster sessions were helpful in maximizing any preventative effect of these school-based programs (see Tables 15-3 and 15-4).

Epstein, Griffin, and Botvin (2000) used statistical modeling to show that the adolescent's general competence was linked directly to refusal assertiveness 1 year after the prevention program and was indirectly related to less alcohol use 2 years after the prevention program. *General competence training* refers to embedding refusal-assertiveness skills within a context of broader personal and social skills training. Thus, it seems that the most promising school-based prevention programs are comprehensive in nature, incorporating a broad set of skills training. This wider focus is justified when considering that the lack of skills needed for coping with daily life hassles increases vulnerability to interpersonal and intrapersonal pressures to use alcohol and drugs (Epstein et al., 2000).

Prevention programming for college students that involved a downstream program incorporating a type of brief intervention strategy was included in Table 15-2. **Brief interventions** may include a 5-minute to 1-hour session (sometimes several short sessions over time) in which the focus is to investigate a potential problem and to motivate the person to do something about his or her substance abuse (Barry, 1999). Brief interventions do not require a face-to-face visit with a therapist, as phone calls, mailings, and workbooks may substitute.

At-risk college students were mailed personalized normative feedback about their responses to self-report items assessing their drinking habits, alcohol-related problems, and perceptions of drinking norms. Students could use this mailing to determine how their drinking

Text continues on page 294

Table 15–2 Evidence-Based Prevention

Author	Aim	Design	Participants	Intervention(s)	Outcome
			FAMILY INTERVENTION		
Midstream Intervention Spoth, Reyes, et al. (1999); Spoth, Redmond, & Lepper (1999); Spoth, Redmond, & Shin (2001)	To determine the difference in efficacy of two brief interventions on three measures: initiation of use, frequency of use, and composite use over time	Randomized design with pretest data collected when participant's in 6th grade and follow-up data collected in the 7th, 8th, and 10th grades. Schools were unit of assignment.	Included 667 sixth graders and their families from 33 rural schools in 19 contiguous counties in the Midwest	Preparing for Drug Free Years Program (PDFY) (five sessions); Iowa Strengthening Families Program (ISFP) (seven sessions); a minimal contact condition	Significant detectable effects 4 years past baseline in all three outcome measures for both interventions over the minimal contact condition, with ISFP demonstrating a greater number of significant effects. Effect sizes were small to medium.
Midstream Intervention Spoth, Guyll, & Day (2001)	To determine the cost-effectiveness of the two interventions described above	Benefits = savings from avoidance of costs that would have occurred as result of substance use disorder. Costs = direct and indirect costs spent per participant and adjusted for inflation	Same as above	Same as above	PDFY = $5.85 benefit per $1 invested ISFP = $9.60 benefit per $1 invested
			SCHOOLS AND COLLEGES		
Midstream Intervention Botvin, Schinke, et al. (1995)	Determine efficacy of two skills-based substance-abuse prevention programs compared to a control condition on a self-report questionnaire assessing current substance use and intentions for future use.	Schools were unit of assignment. Pairs of matched schools were randomly assigned. Pretest was given in 7th grade and follow-up in 9th grade.	Six junior and intermediate high schools in New York City with a total of 757 seventh-grade students.	Fifteen sessions in 7th grade and booster sessions in 8th grade of eight sessions in the following: generic skills intervention (GSI), culturally focused intervention (CFI), and information-only control	Both GSI and CFI were better than control group in significantly decreasing intent to drink beer, wine, or liquor; how often drank alcohol; how often got drunk; and amount of alcohol consumed per drinking occasion at 2-year follow-up. The CFI was more effective than the GSI.

Continued

Table 15–2 Evidence-Based Prevention—cont'd

Author	**Aim**	**Design**	**Participants**	**Intervention(s)**	**Outcome**
SCHOOLS AND COLLEGES					
Midstream Intervention Botvin, Baker, et al. (1995); Botvin, Baker, et al. (1990)	Determine long-term efficacy of a school-based broad-spectrum multicomponent approached prevention program compared to a control condition on nine drug-use outcome variables and eight poly-drug use variables.	Schools were unit of assignment. Groups of schools with high, medium, and low cigarette smoking prevalence rates. Like prevalence schools in same geographic area were matched and then randomly assigned. Pretest immediately prior to program with 6 years of follow-up.	Fifty-six public schools in New York state with 18 schools assigned to E1 condition, 16 schools assigned to E2 condition, and 22 schools were assigned to control condition. There were a total of 3597 adolescents.	Fifteen sessions in 7th grade with booster sessions in 8th and 9th grades. Curriculum involving teaching of information and skills for resisting social influences to use drugs and for improving generic personal and social skills. E1 group teachers received formal 1-day training and feedback during implementation. E2 group teachers were trained via videotape and no implementation feedback.	Both E1 and E2 groups had similar significant reductions over controls in both drug and polydrug use. Those in the sample who received at least 60% of the required program had stronger effects from the prevention (i.e., 44% fewer drug users and 66% fewer polydrug users).
Midstream Intervention Eisen et al. (2002); Eisen et al. (2003)	Determine effectiveness of commercially available skill-based substance abuse prevention program compared to usual alcohol and drug education curriculum on reducing tobacco, alcohol, and illegal drug use prevalence rates.	Schools were unit of assignment. Pairs of matched schools were randomly assigned. Pretest (6th grade)–posttest (7th grade) with 1-year follow-up (8th grade).	Thirty-four schools in multiple cities throughout United States for a total of 7426 sixth-grade students. Seventeen schools received usual curriculum and 17 received intervention.	Forty-session curriculum with eight key sessions of Lion-Quest Skills for Adolescence (SFA) was offered in the 7th grade. Control—usual education, including school assemblies, teacher-devised curricula, or DARE exposure.	SFA helped reduce the prevalence of lifetime and monthly occurrence of marijuana use and binge drinking for both genders and across all racial/ethnic groups.

Study	Purpose	Design	Sample	Intervention	Results
Midstream Intervention Caplan et al. (1992)	Assess impact of school-based social competence training on skills, social adjustment, and self-reported substance use.	Classes were unit of assignment. Classes were stratified within ability groupings and randomly assigned to program and control conditions. Pretest–posttest design.	Involved 282 sixth and seventh graders in inner-city and suburban middle schools in south-central Connecticut. Six classes received the program and nine classes were assigned to the control.	Twenty-session curriculum of Positive Youth Development Program (PYDP) involving six units, including stress management, self-esteem, problem-solving, substances and health, assertiveness, and social networks. Control group received a series of lessons pertaining to the physical effects of drug use.	Intervention promoted the self- and teacher-reported skills, social, and interpersonal effectiveness in diverse settings. Program students remained stable in their self-reported intentions to use substances. Control students became more inclined to use. Program did not affect self-reported experimental use but did affect self-reported excessive use.
Midstream Intervention Bagnall (1990)	Effectiveness of a school-based alcohol education program on alcohol-related knowledge, attitudes, and behavior	Pretest–posttest design with posttest occurring 10 months after intervention. Schools were unit of assignment. Three schools in each region were assigned (method unknown) to two intervention groups and one control group.	Involved 1560 students (12 to 13 years old) in three schools per region located in England, Wales, and Scotland.	Group S1 had teachers who participated in the development of the program and then administered it to their students. Group S2 teachers implemented the program after a 30-minute briefing. Control group had no exposure to alcohol education.	Both intervention groups equally showed increased alcohol-related knowledge. There was no impact on positive attitudes toward alcohol. There was an increase in alcohol consumption and associated consequences; however, the proportional increase over time was greater for the control group. Education groups exhibited more restrained behavior in maximum consumption.

Continued

Table 15–2 Evidence-Based Prevention—cont'd

Author	Aim	Design	Participants	Intervention(s)	Outcome
SCHOOLS AND COLLEGES					
Downstream Intervention Collins et al. (2002)	Efficacy of mailed informative feedback for at-risk college drinkers on drinking quantity and frequency, peak blood alcohol concentration, and number of alcohol-related problems.	Random assignment separately by gender. Pretest-posttest (at 6 weeks post) and follow-up at 6 months.	One hundred at-risk college drinkers (reported at least two heavy drinking episodes in the previous month) enrolled in introductory psychology classes at Syracuse University. Mailed brief intervention = 49 and control group = 50.	Intervention group received personalized normative feedback (PNF) or summaries of responses to self-report items along with normative data for Syracuse students and nationally and didactic material. Control group received a standard psychoeducational brochure about alcohol use.	PNF group noted a greater discrepancy between self and others' drinking, consumed significantly fewer drinks per heaviest drinking week, and engaged in heavy episodic drinking less frequently than controls at the 6-week posttest. No difference was found at the 6-month follow-up.
COMMUNITY					
Downstream Intervention Monti et al. (1999)	Efficacy of brief motivational interviewing to reduce alcohol-related consequences and alcohol use among adolescents treated in emergency rooms.	A randomized two-group design. Pretest-posttest (3 month) with 6-month follow-up.	A sample of 18- to 19-year-olds (n = 94) who presented at the ER with a positive blood alcohol concentration or a report of drinking alcohol prior to the event that precipitated treatment (e.g., motor vehicle accident, assault, fall, intoxication only).	Standard care (SC) control group of 5-minute session, including handout on avoiding drinking and driving and a list of local treatment agencies. Motivational interviewing (MI) session for 30 to 40 minutes as well as materials received by SC participants.	MI resulted in significant reductions in alcohol-involved injury, alcohol-related problems, and motor vehicle moving violations (harm-related effects). At 6-month follow-up, the MI group showed a 32% reduction in drinking and driving and had half the occurrence of alcohol-related injuries of the SC group. Both groups reduced drinking.

| **Midstream Intervention** Pierre et al. (1992) | Effectiveness of America's Stay SMART Program, a social competence and drug prevention program offered in Boys & Girls Clubs, on alcohol, marijuana, and cigarette behavior and knowledge and attitudes regarding these drugs. | Nonequivalent groups. Clubs were the unit of assignment with five clubs in Stay SMART only, five clubs in Stay SMART with boosters, and four clubs in the control group. Pretest-posttest (3 months) with 15-month and 27-month follow-up. | Fourteen Boys & Girls Clubs with similar demographics located in cities with populations ranging from 17,000 to 630,000 across a range of states in the East, South, Midwest, and West; 161 13-year-old members of Boys & Girls Clubs with 52 youths in Stay SMART only group, 54 youths in Stay SMART with boosters, and 55 youths in control group. | Stay SMART program was adapted from Botvin's Life Skills Training Program (Botvin, Eng, & Williams, 1980) and is based on the personal and social competence skills approach to prevention by helping members identify and resist, through nine sessions, peer and other social pressure to use alcohol, cigarettes, and marijuana or to engage in early sexual activity. The 2-year booster program, SMART Leaders, included five sessions in year one and three sessions in year two, trained club members to become drug-free role models. | Over the 24 months following the program, members in Stay SMART had decreased marijuana-related and cigarette-related behavior and overall drug-related behavior. Members in the program groups had increased knowledge concerning drugs. The members in the booster groups only showed fewer positive attitudes toward marijuana and alcohol. Booster session results did not give strong support for including a booster program due to the similar effects as the Stay SMART only program. |

Continued

Table 15–2 Evidence-Based Prevention—cont'd

COMMUNITY

Author	Aim	Design	Participants	Intervention(s)	Outcome
Upstream Intervention Holder et al. (1997); Voas et al. (1997)	Evaluation of the drinking and driving component of a five-element Community Trial Project involving a Community Mobilization component to develop organization support, a Responsible Beverage Service component to establish standards for servers, a Drinking and Driving component, an Underage Drinking component, and an Alcohol Access component to control outlet and density.	Analysis of three experimental communities implementing three enforcement techniques targeting the effects on perceived risk of arrest, drinking and driving, and alcohol-involved traffic accidents. Experimental communities were matched to comparison communities. Baseline for control and experimental communities consisted of five observation periods. The experimental community then received the Drinking and Driving component with observation while the comparison community was only observed.	Three communities, one in Northern California, one in Southern California, and the third one in South Carolina.	Media advocacy training to increase news attention to DUI enforcement, special DUI police patrols, DUI sobriety checkpoints, and special breath testing.	Media advocacy resulted in increased DUI coverage. Additional police officer hours for DUI enforcement, greater use of Breathalyzer equipment, increased officer training, and more checkpoints produced increased DUI enforcement. The combined effects of increased DUI news coverage and DUI enforcement led to an increase in perceived risk of arrest and decreased drinking and driving. Alcohol-involved traffic crashes were reduced in comparison to control communities.

Upstream Intervention Wagenaar et al. (2000)	Analysis of a trial of Communities Mobilizing for Change on Alcohol to determine the effect on reducing the accessibility of alcoholic beverages to youths under the legal drinking age.	Fifteen communities with an average population of 20,836 were matched and then randomly assigned.	Random assignment of communities to intervention or control condition. Pretest–posttest (3 years) with multiple time-series design involving multiple baselines and posttest observations.	One-to-one meetings with community leaders, and development of a local strategy team to create base of active citizen involvement; to advocate for media coverage; and to promote change in policies, procedures, and practices in the community.	Significantly and positively changed the behavior of 18- to 20-year-olds in propensity to provide alcohol to younger teens (effect size = 0.76) and changed the practices of on-sale alcohol establishments (effect size = 1.18), making them less likely to sell to minors. May have had limited effect on the drinking of younger adolescents.
Upstream Intervention Pentz et al. (1989)	Effectiveness of community trial for primary prevention of adolescent drug abuse of cigarette smoking, and alcohol and marijuana use, as measured by reduction of use and prevalence, reduction of drug use morbidity, and promotion of nondrug use social norms.	Forty-two schools in 15 communities of Kansas City (Kansas and Missouri) for a total of 5065 students. Eight schools were randomly assigned to program or control condition, 20 schools could reschedule existing programming and were assigned to program, and 14 could not reschedule existing program and were assigned to control condition.	Quasi-experimental design initiated in Kansas City, Kansas, and Kansas City, Missouri. Within each Standard Metropolitan Statistical Area, cohorts of adolescents were assigned by school to intervention or delayed intervention. Pretest–posttest (1-year follow-up). Baseline assessments occurred at 6th or 7th grade.	Introductory training of community leaders, establishment of community coordinating structure, training of program implementers (mass media representatives, teachers, student peer leaders, parents, principals, community agency leaders, and school and local government administrators), and implementation of program components of mass media campaign, educational programs for youths, parent education and organization, community organization, and policy change.	Prevalence rates of use for all three drugs were significantly lower at 1-year follow-up in the intervention condition compared to the delayed intervention condition (17% vs. 24% for cigarette smoking, 11% vs. 16% for alcohol use, and 7% vs. 10% for marijuana use in last month). Net increase in drug use prevalence was half of the prevalence in delayed intervention schools.

Table 15–3 **Key Components of Prevention Programs**

CONTENT OF PREVENTION PROGRAMS		
Family Programs	**School Programs**	**Community Members**
Learning about risk factors for substance use	Stress management and reduction of anxiety; management of emotions	Affordable downstream programs to provide treatment
Providing guidelines for substance-related behaviors and monitoring compliance with guidelines	Self-esteem, self-confidence, and personal responsibility	Community mobilization of leaders and key organizations
Promoting parent–child bonding	Cognitive-behavioral skills for problem-solving and decision-making	Responsible beverage service and sales practices
Providing consequences for substance-related behaviors	Substances and health, negative consequences of use, prevalence rates among adults and adolescents, and skills to resist advertising pressure promoting alcohol and tobacco use	Strategies to reduce drinking and driving
Managing anger, family conflict, and other strong emotions	Assertiveness and effective communication	Reduction of retail availability of alcohol and access to illicit drugs; local regulation of alcohol to decrease density and hours of sale; reduction of alcohol availability to minors
Enhancing positive child involvement in family tasks	Social networks and developing positive personal relationships	Law enforcement to increase risk of arrest; to enforce drinking-while-intoxicated laws
Developing effective family communication	Skills for coping with social influence to drink alcohol and use drugs	Local news media to increase public awareness and concern about alcohol and drug use
Using activities to increase family cohesiveness	Knowledge related to alcohol and drugs and education to modify normative expectations	Policy changes in schools and local government
	Peer leaders and role models	
Teaching the adolescent family member how to cope with negative peer influence		Availability of leisure activities to support engagement in healthy occupations
	Living a healthy and drug-free life	
Improving peer relationships		Economic promotion to increase access to jobs

compared to the norms of drinking in the general population (Collins, Carey, & Sliwinski, 2002). As noted in Table 15-2, the mailed feedback brief intervention at the 6-week posttest period was effective in reducing the consumption of drinks per heaviest drinking week and the frequency of engagement in heavy episodic drinking. Unfortunately, the impact of this social norms intervention approach was not maintained at the 6-month follow-up. This study illustrates the value of interventions that enhance recognition of the discrep-ancy between one's own behaviors and that of others who do not have a problem with alcohol, as well as highlights the need for brief booster interventions to further decrease use of alcohol and drugs.

Community Programs

Community programs identified in Table 15-2 included downstream, midstream, and upstream interventions. Monti and colleagues (1999) determined the efficacy of a harm-reduction brief intervention to reduce the

Table 15–4 **Occupational Therapy Prevention Programs**

Target Audience	Prevention Process	Occupational Therapy Prevention Focus	Prevention Delivery Site
Families	**Promoting Resiliency** Enhance protective factors: • Create strong bonds among family members • Implement clear parental rules for conduct • Celebrate family successes • Develop clear communication Reduce risk factors: • Rid routines of chaos • Improve nurturance of children • Reduce incidence of unpredictable aggressive or overemotional behavior • Increase open and honest communication	• Developing a shared value system • Establishing preventative family rituals, traditions, and daily routines • Building shared occupations • Facilitating healthy occupational performance of individual family members	**Downstream** • In family homes • Family outpatient treatment **Midstream** • Schools • Employment sites • Community sites **Upstream** • Policy supporting healthy families
Schools	Providing healthy environments for learning Building substance-free learning environment • Drug and alcohol policies • Smoke-free environment • Make available school counselors and health-care personnel • Become a site for Students Against Destructive Decisions (SADD) (previously known as Students Against Driving Drunk) or other self-help groups such as Alcoholics Anonymous if needed • Provide well-supervised extracurricular activities, field trips, dances, and so on • Investigate patterns of tardiness or absenteeism • Provide alternative punishments to expulsion when possible	• Facilitating the adoption of conventional norms about substance abuse • Creating role models • Promoting full involvement of all students in learning and in extracurricular activities • Assessing impact of family use of substances on learner and provide resources • Rewarding success and motivating positive change behaviors • Promoting replacement rituals for drinking as a right of passage	**Midstream** • Elementary • Middle school • High school • Community colleges • Universities and colleges **Upstream** • Policy supporting drug and alcohol programs in schools and universities • Development of broad population programs targeting schools and universities

Continued

Table 15–4 **Occupational Therapy Prevention Programs—cont'd**

Target Audience	Prevention Process	Occupational Therapy Prevention Focus	Prevention Delivery Site
Employers	Building substance-free workplace Focusing on creating a healthy work environment that values principles of wellness • Drug and alcohol policies • Smoke-free environment • Employee assistance programs (EAPs) • Reasonable productivity requirements and expectations • Adequate rewards for performance • Provide company outings or activities that are substance free	• Providing stress-reduction programs • Encouraging use of breaks and time off • Promoting healthy nutrition and physical fitness • Enriching jobs to increase employee autonomy and professional development • Preventing excessive absenteeism and monitoring accidents and injuries • Making available information on substance use	**Downstream** • Employee assistance programs • Occupational health programs • Referral process to treatment programs **Midstream** • The main employers in the community • Human resource departments **Upstream** • Policy development through Occupational Safety and Health Administration • Inclusion of intervention for substance use in employer health-care insurance programs
Communities	Building caring, responsible, and safe communities • Use a public health model • Advocate for appropriate legislation • Obtain funding for prevention programs • Launch national media campaigns • Introduce and enforce laws favorable to decreased substance use	• Work with media to publish or air stories about successful prevention activities and programs • Work with community leaders to fund prevention programming that is easily accessible • Work with local governments to sponsor alcohol-free or family-friendly activities • Work with groups to offer prevention programming • Keep libraries stocked with prevention and healthy lifestyle information	**Midstream** • Places of worship • Fitness clubs • Community centers • Clubs, philanthropic, and civic organizations • Senior citizen centers • Libraries • Public parks and recreation centers • Community courts **Upstream** • Local and state government • Criminal justice system • Media

alcohol consumption of older adolescents who were treated in the emergency room. The brief intervention in this study involved **motivational interviewing** (Miller & Rollnick, 2002), a type of therapeutic style with a focus on providing empathy, avoiding arguments, developing discrepancy between one's drinking and that of the general public, promoting self-efficacy, and facilitating personal choice. In the emergency room setting, the motivational interview involved five components:

1. Reviewing the event and circumstances leading to the emergency room visit
2. Exploring the motivation to continue drinking and to quit drinking
3. Providing personalized feedback regarding current drinking problem
4. Imagining the future if continuing to drink and if quitting or cutting down on drinking
5. Establishing drinking reduction goals for the future

Motivational interviewing was found effective in decreasing alcohol consumption, incidence of drinking and driving, traffic violations, and alcohol-related injuries and problems (Monti et al., 1999).

The midstream program in Table 15-2 was similar to the school-based programs previously described, except that the prevention program was implemented within Boys and Girls Club programming (Pierre, Kaltreider, Mark, & Aikin, 1992). The prevention program included both life skills training (e.g., decision making and independent thinking) and specifics about alcohol and drugs (e.g., alcohol and drug myths and realities and gateway drugs). This program was different from most of the school programs by including 2 years of booster sessions. In the first year of the booster sessions, attendees were encouraged to become peer leaders and role models in their ability to cope with peer pressure to use alcohol or drugs and to engage in sexual activity. The second-year booster sessions focused on personal and social competence. After the second-year booster sessions, prevention activities were incorporated within the general activities of the Boys and Girls Club so that skills were continually developed and enhanced.

The remaining prevention studies were targeted to the upstream program level and were broad-based population interventions (see Tables 15-3 and 15-4). After reviewing these community population prevention programs, the authors developed a community influence model that incorporated the main aspects of the programs found in the literature and included the occupational perspective that is missing from current programs. This model is graphically displayed in Figure 15-1. According to our community model, a healthy community depends on its citizens collectively engaging in positive activities and occupations. In turn, this healthy community provides the supportive contexts to continually encourage engagement in health-producing activity, especially providing economic opportunities to maintain one's livelihood and community safety and various learning opportunities important for raising children.

Examine Figure 15-1, starting at the bottom box labeled "M, Community Health." The figure's overall message is that a community remains healthier by preventing problems related to alcohol and drug abuse. Community health is negatively affected when the community does not engage in prevention of alcohol and drug abuse. Examine the top of Figure 15-1 and note that prevention depends upon the enactment of local government and organizational policies on alcohol and drug use, alcohol sales and service policies, and level of local regulation of alcohol (Holder et al., 1997). When policies are in place, this leads to the arrow labeled "C" at the figure's top right. Local communities can enforce regulations restricting the types of alcoholic beverages sold, raising the minimum age for purchase, rezoning outlets to control density, and implementing cost controls such that economic availability is reduced. Enforcement results in community access to alcohol and drugs eventually being decreased (as indicated under label "D") because of consistent law enforcement. The alternative would mean that community access to drugs and alcohol would either remain the same or could actually increase because of failure to enforce policies that restrict access to alcohol.

Strictly enforcing licensing requirements for serving alcohol is another important method for limiting access to drugs and alcohol. Encouraging establishments that serve alcoholic beverages to modify their alcohol serving and sales practices by training servers how to refuse service to intoxicated patrons and underage persons is a component of restricting access. The goal is for the establishment to also reduce a customer's likelihood of driving while intoxicated. Enforcing criminal laws for serving minors and holding intoxicated individuals liable for any damage and injury caused while drinking is useful for controlling access and is essential for reducing social acceptability of drunken behavior (label "F").

There should be community efforts to raise awareness of socially acceptable levels of alcohol use. Awareness should also be raised regarding the ways in which drinking patterns can be modified through severing the relationship between drinking and community events (arrow G). The community could limit the serving of alcohol and could improve law enforcement to prevent the unlawful use of alcohol and drugs during community-sponsored activities. Community leaders should also explore ways to

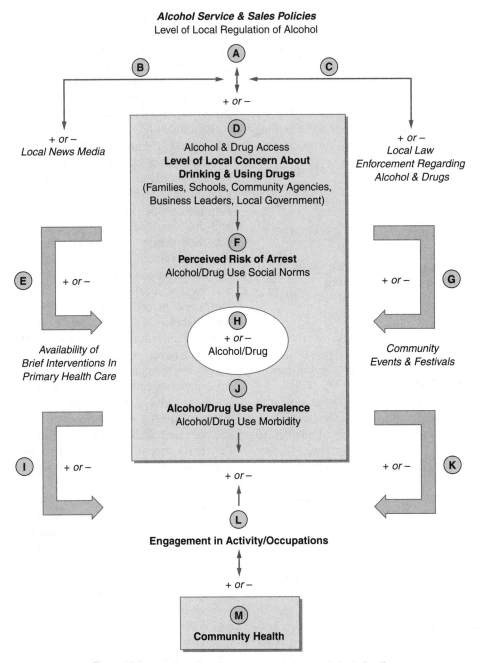

Figure 15-1   Community Influence Model, drug and alcohol policy.

decrease access to alcohol, especially for minors, through the provision of better control and of adult supervision during parties and school activities such as dances and sporting events. Communities allowing alcohol at festivals and events create access to alcohol and may be decreasing the ability to enforce existing laws and policies.

In this model (arrow B), the local media plays a role in creating community awareness and works with the police (arrow C) to publicize enforcement of laws related to drinking and driving, drug trafficking and purchasing of illegal substances, public intoxication, and disorderly conduct. When the public is aware of potential for arrest (arrows E and G), there is deterrence to driving after drinking, an effective way to reduce alcohol-involved injury and death (label "F"). It is important for the local media to educate the public about nontraffic risk activity as well, such as boating; stair-climbing; or operating machinery, equipment, or power tools at home or at work when drinking or when intoxicated. Another nontraffic risk activity is drinking and smoking in a potentially flammable environment.

Presence of these prevention factors within a community determines the rate at which citizens initiate alcohol and drug use (label "H"). Once intake is initiated, the availability of brief intervention in primary care and of treatment when indicated (arrow I) is a factor in determining whether alcohol and drug use escalates to the point of high rates of morbidity or death (label "J"). High rates of addiction in a community may lead to occupational alienation and deprivation (arrow K) such that portions of the population are deprived of work opportunities (label "L") and may become homeless or may become involved in crime to support an expensive drug habit (label "M").

Role of Occupational Therapy

Table 15-4 displays prevention programs in terms of the target audience, the prevention process, the focus of the occupational therapy program, and the site of program delivery divided according to downstream, midstream, and upstream interventions. The TMBC, combined with an occupational perspective, is used to guide the development of programming.

Recall that the goal of any prevention program targeting precontemplation or contemplation is to bring the risky behaviors to the person's or the target population's attention and to motivate a decision to make a change in these behaviors. As they embrace community-based practice in multiple settings, occupational therapists and occupational therapy assistants are in a position to identify and intervene with persons whose alcohol or drug use may be hazardous or harmful to their health and occupational performance, or with persons who are at risk for developing more serious alcohol- and drug-related behaviors. Unfortunately, occupational therapy practitioners and primary healthcare providers often seem reluctant to tackle this goal of moving the target population from precontemplation to contemplation or from contemplation to preparation. Reasons for avoiding this responsibility may include the following:

• Perceived lack of time to focus on this goal
• Inadequate training
• Fear of antagonizing people
• A belief that focusing on risk reduction or on reduction of substance abuse is incompatible with most occupational therapy intervention goals
• A belief that people who abuse substances do not respond to intervention and that prevention efforts reap little benefit (Babor & Higgins-Biddle, 2001)

Each of these objections can be refuted and a case can be made for the likelihood of positive results occurring if evidence-based strategies are used to facilitate change. In terms of lack of time and being incompatible with other occupational therapy intervention goals, community-based occupational therapy programs should incorporate screening and brief interventions, because alcohol and drug use is a leading contributor to many other health and social problems and may be the underlying cause of the health, family, or employment problems requiring attention. Brief interventions do not have to be time-consuming and may range from not taking any of the therapist's time (e.g., providing relevant literature and screening tests in the form of pamphlets in waiting rooms and offering workbooks to clients willing to work on reducing alcohol and drug use) to spending 5 to 20 minutes talking to the client. Occupational therapy practitioners, especially those in practice areas other than mental health, often believe they lack the expertise to provide screening and intervention for risk of alcohol and drug abuse (Thompson, 2007). Moyers and Stoffel (1999) illustrated that an occupational therapist who worked in the office of a hand surgeon could be trained to incorporate screening and brief intervention strategies as a component of an effort to judge a client's health prior to hand surgery. In addition, occupational therapists are often in a position to identify misuse and abuse of prescription and nonprescription painkillers post-trauma or surgery by reviewing pain status and pain history with clients.

Antagonizing the client who comes to the therapist for other health-related reasons is of low risk during brief intervention when following principles of motivational interviewing, which incorporates a therapeutic style that avoids evoking denial and instead "rolls with resistance" (Miller & Rollnick, 2002) and promotes the person's responsibility for making change. Brief interventions have been found effective as noted in evidence-based literature reviews (Stoffel & Moyers, 2004), in treatment improvement protocols (Barry, 1999), and in occupational therapy practice guidelines (Stoffel & Moyers, 1997). The evidence-based section of this chapter analyzing prevention programs generally indicates the efficacy, and in some cases the cost-benefit, of such brief intervention programs.

Screening

Screening is the first step to bring about awareness of a possible alcohol or drug problem or as a way to facilitate movement into the preparation stage. Occupational therapists may find that doing a screening as part of an occupational profile to ascertain daily routines that contribute to health is a good fit regardless of the intervention setting. Such a screening process provides the basis for designing interventions with targeted outcomes.

When suspecting an alcohol problem, the CAGE (*C*ut down on drinking, being *A*nnoyed by someone criticizing the drinking, feeling *G*uilty about drinking, and having an *E*ye-opener in the morning; Ewing, 1984) and quantity and frequency (Q/F) questions may be used (Cooney, Zweben, & Fleming, 1995). One or more positive responses to the CAGE referring to the past year indicate a positive test. The sensitivity (true positives) and specificity (true negatives) of the CAGE range from 60% to 95% and from 40% to 95%, respectively (National Institute on Alcohol Abuse and Alcoholism [NIAAA], 1993). A corollary to the CAGE is the RAFFT for persons who use alcohol and/or drugs (Bastiaens, Riccardi, & Sakhrani, 2002). The five questions in the mnemonic are

- Do you drink/take drugs to *R*elax, feel better about yourself, or fit in?
- Do you ever drink/take drugs while you are by yourself, *A*lone?
- Do any of your close *F*riends drink/take drugs?
- Does a close *F*amily member have a problem with alcohol/drugs? and
- Have you ever gotten into *T*rouble from drinking/taking drugs?

The RAFFT has a sensitivity and specificity of 89% and 69%, respectively, with two positive answers.

Quantity and frequency (Q/F) questions are concerned with the number of days per week one has had a drink in the past month, number of drinks per drinking occasion, and the number of times in which one drank more than five drinks during the past month. Before obtaining answers to these Q/F questions, the person must be instructed in how much alcohol constitutes a "drink": one ordinary can of beer, a single shot of spirits (whiskey, gin, vodka, etc.), a glass of wine (140 mL), or a small glass of liqueur or aperitif (70 mL; Babor & Higgins-Biddle, 2001). On the Q/F screen, 14 or more drinks per week or 5 or more drinks per any given day equals a positive test for men under the age of 65. For women and men over age 65, seven or more drinks per week or four or more drinks per any given day equals a positive test. These quantity and frequency screening tests together have 90% accuracy in determining the existence of an alcohol problem (Cooney et al., 1995).

The Alcohol Use Disorders Identification Test (AUDIT; may be downloaded for free at http://whqlibdoc .who.int/hq/2001/WHO_MSD_MSB_01.6a.pdf; Sauders, Aasland, Babor, de la Fuente, & Grant, 1993) was developed for use by a range of health-care personnel and can be administered separately or combined with other questions, such as those from the occupational therapist's occupational profile (American Occupational Therapy Association [AOTA], 2008). This screening instrument has an interview format or a self-report version, consisting of 10 questions about recent alcohol use, alcohol dependence symptoms, and alcohol-related problems. Each question has a response ranging from 0 to 4, which are then added together for a total score.

Along with the AUDIT screen, the occupational therapist should implement an occupational profile (AOTA, 2002) to determine how the alcohol or drug use risk or problem currently affects occupational performance. Determining how the use has affected performance over time would necessitate conducting an occupational history (Moyers & Stoffel, 1999), such as the Occupational Performance History Interview (second version; Kielhofner et al., 1997). In order to determine how using the alcohol or drugs impacts occupational adaptation, the occupational therapy interview of choice might be the Occupational Circumstances Assessment—Interview Rating Scale (Haglund, Henriksson, Crisp, Friedheim, & Kielhofner, 2001).

Regardless of which instrument is used to discern the impact of alcohol and drug use on occupational performance and roles, the results should help the occupational therapist determine whether occupational performance is intact, whether there is risk for occupational alienation, whether occupational alienation is present, or whether occupational deprivation is occurring. If experiencing occupational alienation, the person would describe a loss of meaning on the occupational profile that was once associated with performance (Wilcock, 1998). The individual would still be engaging in those occupations but would report losing interest or would describe spending less time in healthy occupations. There would be a beginning pattern of spending more time in substance-using activities to maintain the addiction (e.g., raising money for drugs, protecting the supply from others, seeking persons with whom to use, and creating situations for using; Moyers & Stoffel, 2001).

As the occupational alienation process continues, substance-using activities may eventually take on greater meaning, such as fulfilling the need to "escape, have fun, relax and sleep, avoid physical and emotional pain, gain confidence, increase sexuality, feel less inhibited and more creative, or increase energy and activity levels" (Moyers & Stoffel, 2001, p. 325). The substance use may eventually impede engagement such that occupations are no longer meaningful and are no longer important to identity formation. These previously enjoyed occupations become a set of activities that one merely performs throughout the day, making the occupational alienation process complete. Over time, as performance continues to deteriorate, one is deprived of those once-important occupations necessary for a satisfying and meaningful life.

Occupational deprivation (Wilcock, 1998) occurs when individuals structure their substance-using activities into daily performance patterns that preserve the using routine and decrease participation in other occupations. The person habitually responds to alcohol or drug cues in the environment (e.g., driving past a bar, seeing beer in the refrigerator, or smelling marijuana) with craving or an increased desire to use alcohol or drugs. This desire to use activates physiological and psychological expectations regarding the potentially positive experience associated with using (Moyers & Stoffel, 2001). Long-term consequences of using the alcohol or the drug are ignored. Activities and occupations previously valued may in fact become barriers to using and are avoided so that the substance-using routines occur without disruption. Occupational participation, performance, performance patterns, and performance skills are all affected.

Intervention

If the screening is negative, the occupational therapist should still provide alcohol education about long-term health effects of using alcohol beyond moderation or about the potential safety, legal, and social problems occurring when alcohol and drug use begins to interfere with occupational performance and with engagement in valued occupations. The client is congratulated for currently using alcohol in moderation and is encouraged to remain within the guidelines for safe use. If clients do not use alcohol, they are told that they are among 40% of the U.S. population who abstain from alcohol (Babor & Higgins-Biddle, 2001). See Figure 15-2 for more information.

If the screens are positive, the intervention the occupational therapist provides can be associated with scores on the screening and with the results of the occupational profile. An AUDIT score up to seven suggests a need for alcohol education similar to that provided to those who received a negative screen, except the client is told that 40% of the U.S. population abstains and that 35% of the population are considered low-risk drinkers of which he or she would be a part (Babor & Higgins-Biddle, 2001). Typically, the occupational performance is intact, and there is engagement in desired and meaningful occupations. Discussion of the importance of continuing to engage in these occupations should also ensue along with emphasis that the client should remain in the abstainer or low-risk category.

An AUDIT score between 8 and 15 indicates that simple advice about the need for reduction of hazardous drinking should be given. There are signs the person is at risk for occupational alienation as time spent in drinking has the potential of eclipsing ability to spend time in desired and meaningful occupations. Although occupational performance is generally intact, performance patterns and skills may be affected. Simple advice involves giving feedback about the current level of risk. Clients are told that they are part of 20% of the U.S. population who are considered to be high-risk drinkers (Babor & Higgins-Biddle, 2001). The therapist should also provide information to the client in terms of the risks associated with drinking or using drugs. These risks include liver damage, reduced resistance to infection, increased risk of pneumonia, throat or mouth cancer, depression and nervousness, irrational and aggressive behavior, peripheral neuropathy, impaired sexual performance, heart muscle weakness, vitamin deficiency, inflammation of the pancreas, premature aging, breast cancer, and memory loss (Babor & Higgins-Biddle, 2001).

Next, the therapist encourages the client to set a goal to change drinking or using behavior as a targeted outcome. Goals range from abstinence to low-risk drinking. The low-risk drinking goal, however, may not be appropriate for persons with a prior history of alcohol or drug dependence, liver damage, or prior or current mental illness; women who are pregnant; and those who are taking medications that require total abstinence. When possible, most clients will pick a low-risk drinking goal. According to Babor and Higgins-Biddle (2001), no more than two standard drinks should be consumed per day over a 5-day period. The clients should understand that drinking should not occur in some situations, such as when needing to drive. The client receives information about what constitutes a standard drink.

The behavior of the therapist is important during the intervention. The therapist should be empathic and nonjudgmental while at the same time being authoritative. Having authority relates to knowledge of the problem and its impact on occupational performance and does not involve being confrontational. The therapist refrains from calling the person an alcoholic or a drug addict but engages the client in a joint decision-making process about how to reduce the risk that will occur if he or she continues to use in the manner described during the screening process. The client is also encouraged to reengage in the healthy occupations the individual used to engage in regularly, as this will involve the individual in something other than the growing engagement in alcohol or drug-using activities. Periodic follow-up of the client on the drinking or

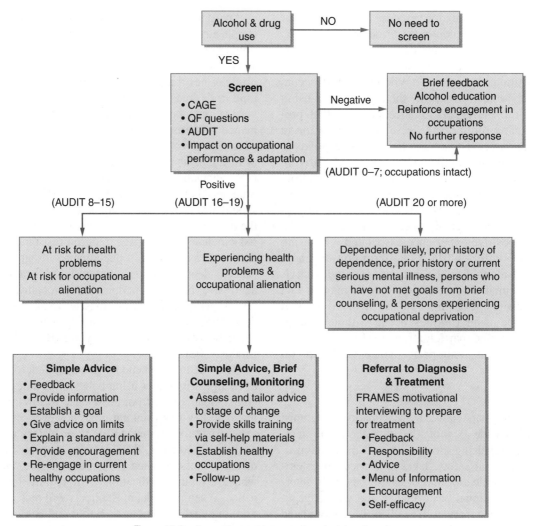

Figure 15-2   Screening and intervention decision flowchart.

drug-using problem is important to check on progress toward the goal. If the client is making progress, then encouragement to continue progress is given. Lack of progress indicates the need for a referral for further evaluation and in-depth intervention.

Brief intervention and continued monitoring is recommended for AUDIT scores between 16 and 19. The client is told that he or she is a part of 20% of the population who are high-risk drinkers (Babor & Higgins-Biddle, 2001). The risks for this level of use are reviewed as they were during the simple advice process. Current harm the client is experiencing should be discussed, as should the way in which engagement in occupations has changed. The occupational therapist should also consider administering the Readiness to Change Questionnaire (treatment version [RCQ-TV]; Heather, Luce, Peck, Dunbar, & James, 1999). Based on the results of

the Readiness to Change Questionnaire, the occupational therapist begins the intervention that matches the current stage. For instance, if the client is in the precontemplation stage, the emphasis of the intervention should be on feedback and providing information; if in the contemplation stage, the emphasis is on giving information and setting a goal; if in the preparation stage, the emphasis is on developing the goal, giving advice, and providing encouragement in implementing the steps to quit using; if in the action stage, the emphasis is on reviewing advice and giving encouragement to continue to implement the change process; and if in the maintenance stage, the emphasis is on giving encouragement to maintain the goal achieved.

After assessing the client's readiness to change, the occupational therapist can give the individual the self-help booklet found online that goes through the process of feedback, information, goal selection, advice, and encouragement (Babor & Higgins-Biddle, 2001). The occupational therapist can judge whether the client can work through the booklet independently or whether he or she would benefit from working on it with the therapist. Additionally, plans are developed and encouragement given to explore occupational interests and to engage in these important nonusing activities. Follow-up sessions are scheduled to determine progress toward the drinking goal and if not progressing, to initiate a referral to in-depth evaluation and intervention.

Clients with AUDIT scores of 20 or above are in need of further diagnostic evaluation and referral. The client should know that he or she is in the 5% of the U.S. population who are probably experiencing alcohol or drug dependence (Babor & Higgins-Biddle, 2001). In terms of the stages of change, the goal is to gradually move the client through preparation into action involving the individual seeking in-depth evaluation and treatment. The FRAMES (feedback, responsibility, advice, menu, empathy, self-efficacy; Miller & Sanchez, 1994) approach to motivational interviewing is used to help the client realize the need for the referral. The six parts of the FRAMES interview are

- feedback of personal risk or impairment (information indicating the client is in the 5% dependence category and information about the health, social, and legal complications that usually occur with dependence);
- emphasis on personal responsibility (the therapist acknowledges the client's right to decide what, if anything, will be done);
- clear advice to change (only abstinence will stop the problems associated with dependence and that withdrawing from the drug or alcohol requires medical intervention);
- a menu of alternative change options (where the client may go for an evaluation and for treatment recommendations);
- therapist empathy (the therapist recognizes the difficulty in making a change); and
- facilitation of client self-efficacy or optimism (the therapist expresses confidence in the client's success in taking action but schedules a follow-up to monitor what happens as the result of the evaluation and then to monitor the result of the intervention).

Conclusion

Occupational therapists and occupational therapy assistants have a responsibility to consider how drinking or using drugs affects their client's general health, wellbeing, quality of life, and occupational performance and role competence. In addition, it is important to consider strategies to facilitate community support for reducing risks for alcohol and drug use. The occupational perspective has much to offer to current health promotion programs that focus on improving the social competence of the individual at risk for abusing alcohol and drugs. Engagement in healthy occupations may have a positive influence on decreasing risk for substance use. Promoting engagement in desired occupations can occur as a part of downstream, midstream, and upstream programs.

Most of the discussion in this chapter about health promotion focused on midstream and upstream levels of program design. Midstream programming involves identifying at-risk individuals and using brief interventions and social competency training to reduce risk. The types of occupational interventions most often used in midstream programs include therapeutic use of self, occupations, education, and consultation. Upstream efforts focus more on the community level to improve the availability of healthy occupations and to decrease unhealthy occupations. This change in design of occupations occurring in a community is part of an extensive community mobilization effort. The idea is for the community to develop norms against risky alcohol- or drug-using behaviors and to provide support for alternative occupations that elicit healthy behaviors. This effort also includes the development of local government and organizational policies on alcohol and drug use, alcohol sales and service policies, and local regulation of alcohol. Community mobilization also involves the cooperation of the local media in creating community awareness about enforcement of laws related to drinking and driving, drug trafficking and purchasing of illegal substances, public intoxication, and disorderly conduct.

The chapter included a thorough discussion of how the occupational therapist designs a midstream program. The process of identifying risk includes using screening assessments that can be incorporated into the overall evaluation. Results of screening indicate the appropriate intervention that may involve substance education, simple advice, brief intervention, or referral for evaluation and in-depth intervention. A variety of screening instruments were described and resources indicated for obtaining these instruments. A screening and intervention flowchart illustrated the decision-making process for determining what to do if the screening is positive or negative. A focus on everyday occupations and their impact on health and wellbeing is the unique contribution occupational therapy practitioners can make to alcohol and drug abuse prevention efforts.

Case Study 15-1

An occupational therapist wants to begin working with a local industry's employee assistance program (EAP), which already offers a range of services for employees who have drug and alcohol problems and for their families. The industry contracts with a community mental health center to provide these services consisting of evaluation, substance withdrawal, inpatient and outpatient intervention, and follow-up. The center offers the services of a psychiatrist, other physicians, two nurse practitioners, nursing staff, psychologists, clinical counselors, lay counselors, and several social workers. The community mental health center is not sure what services the occupational therapist could add that are not already being provided; however, it is willing to entertain a proposal given that the industry is not satisfied with the record of return to work and is wanting the EAP to implement prevention strategies designed to reduce incidence of employee alcohol and drug abuse, which has resulted in excessive absenteeism, decreased productivity, an increase in on-the-job accidents and injuries, and incidents of workplace violence.

Questions

1. The current work of the community mental health center would be considered downstream interventions. What would occupational therapy add to the existing program to enhance return to work and prevention of relapse while working?
2. What midstream intervention could the occupational therapist suggest to address the need for prevention strategies that include an occupation-based perspective and incorporate evidence from the prevention literature?
3. What upstream interventions could the occupational therapist use to create supportive environments for sobriety within the community that would augment implementation of appropriate work behaviors at the local industry?

▶ For Discussion and Review

1. Think about how occupational deprivation might possibly lead to unhealthy habits in your own life. How might understanding this concept lead to more well-developed prevention strategies?
2. What are the differences between downstream, midstream, and upstream interventions (include the terms *primary, secondary,* and *tertiary prevention*)? Where do you feel occupational therapy practitioners might make their greatest impact? Support your position with opportunities you have observed in your own community.
3. How does the Transtheoretical Model of Behavior Change (TMBC) apply to prevention strategies? How might a practitioner's approach differ when interacting with an individual in the precontemplation stage versus the action stage?
4. Given the suggestions provided in this chapter, what do you see as facilitators and barriers for occupational therapy practitioners assuming an active role in their communities and workplaces related to the prevention of substance abuse?
5. What would be the initial steps an occupational therapy practitioner might take to aid in the prevention or reduction of substance abuse? What resources would you find most helpful in this effort?

▶ Research Questions

1. "Does a healthy pattern of performance in activities and occupations prevent substance abuse?" (Stoffel & Moyers, 2004, p. 582)
2. "In the situation where clients seek occupational therapy services for problems secondary to their substance-use problem (e.g., physical rehabilitation), does use of brief interventions (feedback, information about risk, and brief advice) lead to an improved readiness for changing their substance using behavior? Will these clients who address their underlying substance use be more likely to achieve their occupational therapy goals?" (Stoffel & Moyers, 2004, p. 581)
3. If screening, brief intervention, and referral for substance-related problems impacting occupational performance and quality of life were a part of every occupational therapy practitioner's standard procedure, would overall occupational therapy outcomes be significantly improved over those obtained through usual practice?

References

American Occupational Therapy Association. (2008). Occupational therapy practice framework: Domain and process. *American Journal of Occupational Therapy, 62*(6), 625–88.

Babor, T. F., Aguirre-Molina, M., Marlatt, G. A., & Clayton, R. (1999). Managing alcohol problems and risky drinking. *American Journal of Health Promotion, 14,* 98–103.

Babor, T. F., & Higgins-Biddle, J. C. (2001). *Brief intervention for hazardous and harmful drinking: A manual for use in primary care.* Geneva, Switzerland: World Health Organization. Retrieved July 30, 2008, from http://www.whqlibdoc.who.int/hq/2001/WHO_MSD_MSB_01.6b.pdf.

Bagnall, G. (1990). Alcohol education for 13 year olds, does it work? Results from a controlled evaluation. *British Journal of Addiction, 85,* 89–96.

Barry, K. L. (1999). *Brief interventions and brief therapies for substance abuse.* Rockville, MD: Center for Substance Abuse Treatment, Substance Abuse and Mental Health Services Administration.

Bastiaens, L., Riccardi, K., & Sakhrani, D. (2002). The RAFFT as a screening tool for adult substance use disorders. *American Journal of Drug and Alcohol Abuse, 28,* 681–91.

Botvin, G. J., Baker, E., Dusenbury, L., Botvin, E. M., & Diaz, T. (1995). Long-term follow-up results of a randomized drug abuse prevention trial in a white middle-class population. *Journal of the American Medical Association, 273,* 1106–12.

Botvin, G. J., Baker, E., Dusenbury, L., Tortu, S., & Botvin, E. M. (1990). Preventing adolescent drug abuse through a multimodal cognitive—behavioral approach: Results of a 3-year study. *Journal of Consulting and Clinical Psychology, 58,* 437–46.

Botvin, G. J., Eng, A., & Williams, C. L. (1980). Preventing the onset of cigarette smoking through life skills training. *Preventive Medicine, 9,* 135–43.

Botvin, G. J., Schinke, S. P., Epstein, J. A., Diaz, T., & Botvin, E. M. (1995). Effectiveness of culturally focused and generic skills training approaches to alcohol and drug abuse prevention among minority adolescents: Two-year follow-up results. *Psychology of Addictive Behaviors, 9,* 183–94.

Caplan, M., Weissberg, R. P., Grober, J. S., Sivo, P. J., Grady, K., & Jacoby, C. (1992). Social competence promotion with inner-city and suburban young adolescents: Effects on social adjustment and alcohol use. *Journal of Consulting and Clinical Psychology, 60,* 56–63.

Clark, F., Wood, W., & Larson, E. (1998). Occupational science: Occupational therapy's legacy for the 21st century. In M. E. Neistadt & E. B. Crepeau (Eds.), *Willard and Spackman's occupational therapy* (9th ed., pp. 13–21). Philadelphia: Lippincott-Raven.

Clayton, R. R., Cattarello, A. M., & Johnstone, B. M. (1996). The effectiveness of Drug Abuse Resistance Education (Project DARE): 5-year follow-up results. *Preventive Medicine, 25,* 307–25.

Collins, S. E., Carey, K. B., & Sliwinski, M. J. (2002). Mailed personalized normative feedback as a brief intervention for at-risk college drinkers. *Journal of Studies on Alcohol, 63,* 559–67.

Cooney, N. L., Zweben, A., & Fleming, M. F. (1995). Screening for alcohol problems and at-risk drinking in health-care settings. In R. K. Hester & W. R. Miller (Eds.), *Handbook of alcoholism treatment approaches effective alternatives* (2d ed., pp. 45–60). Boston: Allyn & Bacon.

Corral, M., Holguin, S. R., & Cadaveira, F. (2003). Neuropsychological characteristics of young children from high-density alcoholism families: A three-year follow-up. *Journal of Studies on Alcohol, 64,* 195–99.

DiClemente, C. C., & Prochaska, J. O. (1998). Toward a comprehensive, transtheoretical model of change: Stages of change and addictive behaviors. In W. R. Miller & N. Heather (Eds.), *Treating addictive behaviors* (2d ed., pp. 3–24). New York: Plenum Press.

Eisen, M., Zellman, G. L., Massett, H. A., & Murray, D. M. (2002). Evaluating the Lions-Quest "Skills for Adolescence" drug education program: First-year behavior outcomes. *Addictive Behaviors, 27,* 619–32.

Eisen, M., Zellman, G. L., & Murray, D. M. (2003). Evaluating the Lions—Quest "Skills for Adolescence" drug education program: Second-year behavior outcomes. *Addictive Behaviors, 28,* 883–97.

Epstein, J. A., Griffin, K. W., & Botvin, G. J. (2000). Role of general and specific competence skills in protecting inner-city adolescents from alcohol use. *Journal of Studies on Alcohol, 61,* 379–86.

Ewing, J. (1984). Detecting alcoholism: The CAGE questionnaire. *Journal of the American Medical Association, 252,* 1905–07.

Gutman, M., & Clayton, R. (1999). Treatment and prevention of use and abuse of illegal drugs: Progress on interventions and future directions. *American Journal of Health Promotion, 14,* 92–97.

Haglund, L., Henriksson, C., Crisp, M., Friedheim, L., & Kielhofner, G. (2001). *The Occupational Circumstances Assessment Interview and Rating Scale (OCAIRS)* (version 2.0). Chicago: Model of Human Occupation Clearinghouse, Department of Occupational Therapy, University of Illinois.

Heather, N., Luce, A., Peck, D., Dunbar, B., & James, I. (1999). The development of a treatment version of the Readiness to Change Questionnaire. *Addiction Research, 7*(1), 63–68.

Hingson, R. W., Heeren, T., Jamanka, A., & Howland, J. (2000). Age of drinking onset and unintentional injury involvement after drinking. *Journal of the American Medical Association, 284,* 1527–33.

Holder, H. D., Saltz, R. F., Grube, J. W., Voas, R. B., Gruenewald, P. J., & Treno, A. J. (1997). Section I. Overview. A community prevention trial to reduce alcohol-involved accidental injury and death. *Addiction, 92* (Supplement 2), S155–S171.

Kielhofner, G., Mallinson, T., Crawford, C., Nowak, M., Rigby, M., Henry, A., & Walens, D. (1997). *A user's guide to the Occupational Performance History Interview-II (OPHI-II)* (version 2.0). Chicago: Model of Human Occupation Clearinghouse, Department of Occupational Therapy, University of Illinois.

Lester, B. M., LaGasse, L. L., & Seifer, R. (1998). Cocaine exposure and children: The meaning of subtle effects. *Science, 282,* 633–37.

Miller, W. R., & Rollnick, S. (2002). *Motivational interviewing: Preparing people for change* (2d ed.). New York: Guilford Press.

Miller, W. R., & Sanchez, V. C. (1994). Motivating young adults for treatment and lifestyle change. In G. Howard (Ed.), *Issues in alcohol use and misuse by young adults* (pp. 55–82). South Bend, IN: University of Notre Dame Press.

Monti, P. M., Colby, S. M., Barnett, N. P., Spirito, A., Rohsenow, D. J., Myers, M., Woolard, R., & Lewander, W. (1999). Brief intervention for harm reduction with alcohol-positive older adolescents in a hospital emergency department. *Journal of Consulting and Clinical Psychology, 67,* 989–94.

Moyers, P. A., & Stoffel, V. C. (1999). Alcohol dependence in a client with a work related injury. *American Journal of Occupational Therapy, 53,* 640–44.

Moyers, P. A., & Stoffel, V. C. (2001). Community-based approaches for substance use disorders. In M. Scaffa (Ed.), *Occupational therapy in community-based practice settings* (pp. 318–42). Philadelphia: F. A. Davis.

National Institute on Alcohol Abuse and Alcoholism. (1993). *Eighth special report to the U.S. Congress on alcohol and health.* (NIH Pub. No. 94-3699). Bethesda, MD: National Institutes of Health.

National Institute on Drug Abuse. (2007). *Anabolic steroids.* Retrieved October 30, 2007, from http://teens.drugabuse .gov/facts/facts_ster1.asp.

O'Connor, M. J., Shah, B., Whaley, S., Cronin, P., Gunderson, B., & Graham, J. (2002). Psychiatric illness in a clinical sample of children with prenatal alcohol exposure. *American Journal of Drug and Alcohol Abuse, 28,* 743–54.

Oggins, J. (2003). Changes in health insurance and payment for substance use treatment. *American Journal of Drug and Alcohol Abuse, 29,* 55–74.

Palinkas, L. A., Atkins, C. J., Miller, C., & Ferreira, D. (1996). Social skills training for drug prevention in high-risk female adolescents. *Preventive Medicine, 25,* 692–701.

Pentz, M. A., Dwyer, J. H., MacKinnon, D. P., Flay, B. R., Hansen, W. B., Wang, E. Y., & Johnson, A. (1989). A multicommunity trial for primary prevention of adolescent drug abuse: Effects on drug use prevalence. *Journal of the American Medical Association, 261,* 3259–66.

Pierre, T. L., Kaltreider, D. L., Mark, M. M., & Aikin, K. J. (1992). Drug prevention in a community setting: A longitudinal study of the relative effectiveness of a three-year primary prevention program in Boys & Girls Clubs across the nation. *American Journal of Community Psychology, 20,* 673–706.

Reiss, A. J., Jr., & Roth, J. A. (1993–94). *Understanding and preventing violence.* Washington, DC: National Academy Press.

Saunders, J. B., Aasland, O. G., Babor, T. F., de la Fuente, J. R., & Grant, M. (1993). Development of the Alcohol Use Disorders Identification Test (AUDIT): WHO collaborative project on early detection of persons with harmful alcohol consumption. II. *Addiction, 88,* 791–804.

Smith, G. S., Branas, C. C., & Miller, T. R. (1999). Fatal non-traffic injuries involving alcohol: A meta-analysis. *Annals of Emergency Medicine, 33,* 659–68.

Spoth, R. L., Guyll, M., & Day, S. X. (2002). Universal family-focused interventions in alcohol-use disorder prevention: Cost-effectiveness and cost-benefit analyses of two interventions. *Journal of Studies on Alcohol, 63,* 219–28.

Spoth, R., Redmond, C., & Lepper, H. (1999). Alcohol initiation outcomes of universal family-focused preventive interventions: One- and two-year follow-ups of a controlled study. *Journal of Studies on Alcohol,* (Suppl 13), 103–11.

Spoth, R. L., Redmond, C., & Shin, C. (2001). Randomized trial of brief family interventions for general populations: Adolescent substance use outcomes 4 years following baseline. *Journal of Consulting and Clinical Psychology, 69,* 627–42.

Spoth, R., Reyes, M. L., Redmond, C., & Shin, C. (1999). Assessing a public health approach to delay onset and progression of adolescent substance use: Latent transition and loglinear analyses of longitudinal family preventive intervention outcomes. *Journal of Consulting and Clinical Psychology, 67,* 619–30.

Stoffel, V. C., & Moyers, P. A. (1997). *Occupational therapy practice guidelines for substance abuse disorders.* Bethesda, MD: American Occupational Therapy Association.

Stoffel, V. C., & Moyers, P. A. (2004). An evidence-based and occupational perspective of intervention for persons with substance-use disorders. *American Journal of Occupational Therapy, 58,* 570–86.

Substance Abuse and Mental Health Services Administration. (2002). *Results from the 2001 National Household Survey on Drug Abuse: Volume I. Summary of national findings.* Office of Applied Studies, NHSDA Series H-17, DHHS Publication No. SMA 02-3758. Rockville, MD.

Thompson, K. (2007). Occupational therapy and substance use disorders: Are practitioners addressing these disorders in practice? *Occupational Therapy in Health Care, 21*(3), 61–77.

U.S. Department of Health and Human Services. (2000). *Healthy People 2010: Understanding and improving health* (2d ed.). Washington, DC: Government Printing Office.

Velasquez, M. M., Maurer, G. G., Crouch, C., & DiClemente, C. C. (2001). *Group treatment for substance abuse: A stages-of-change therapy manual.* New York: Guilford Press.

Voas, R. B., Holder, H. D., & Gruenewald, P. J. (1997). Section II. Prevention components and results. The effect of drinking and driving interventions on alcohol-involved traffic crashes within a comprehensive community trial. *Addiction, 92*(Supplement 2), S221–S236.

Wagenaar, A. C., Murray, D. M., Gehan, J. P., Wolfson, M., Forster, J. L., Toomey, T. L., Perry, C. L., & Jones-Webb, R. (2000). Communities mobilizing for change on alcohol: Outcomes from a randomized community trial. *Journal of Studies on Alcohol, 61,* 85–94.

Weiss, R. D., Jaffee, W. B., de Menil, V. P., & Cogley, C. B. (2004). Group therapy for substance use disorders: What do we know? *Harvard Review of Psychiatry, 12*(6), 339–49.

Wilcock, A. A. (1993). A theory of human need for occupation. *Occupational Science: Australia, 1,* 17–24.

Wilcock, A. A. (1998). *An occupational perspective of health.* Thorofare, NJ: SLACK.

Wilcock, A. A. (2003). Population interventions focused on health for all. In E. B. Crepeau, E. S. Cohn, & B. A. B. Schell (Eds.), *Willard & Spackman's occupational therapy* (10th ed., pp. 30–45). Philadelphia: Lippincott, Williams & Wilkins.

Zador, P. L., Krawchuk, S. A., & Voas, R. B. (2000). Alcohol-related relative risk of driver fatalities and driver involvement in fatal crashes in relation to driver age and gender: An update using 1996 data. *Journal of Studies on Alcohol, 61,* 387–95.

Chapter 16

Promoting Sexual Health:
An Occupational Perspective

Michael A. Pizzi and S. Maggie Reitz

Healthy sexuality is a positive and life affirming part of being human. It includes knowledge of self, opportunities for healthy sexual development and sexual experience, the capacity for intimacy, an ability to share relationships, and comfort with different expressions of sexuality including love, joy, caring, sensuality, or celibacy. Our attitudes about sexuality, our ability to understand and accept our own sexuality, to make healthy choices and respect the choices of others, are essential aspects of who we are and how we interact with our world.

—Health Canada, 1999, p. 5

Learning Objectives

This chapter is designed to enable the reader to:

- Define and describe the complexity of sexual health, including cultural factors and influences such as gender and sexual identity.
- Discuss the developmental aspects of sexuality and the influence of sexual health on quality of life and engagement in occupation through the life span.

- Recognize the importance of sexual health for people with disabilities.
- Discuss the importance of prevention and health promotion for optimal sexual health through the life span.
- Identify potential contributions of occupational therapy to sexual health through the life span.

Key Terms

Gender identity

Heterosexism

Sexual activity

Sexual expression

Sexual health

Sexual identity

Sexuality

Sexually transmitted diseases

Sexually transmitted infections

Sexual orientation

Sexual rights

Sexual self-concept

Introduction

The occupational therapy profession's definition of **sexual expression** has been described in several ways. It was included in the second edition of the American Occupational Therapy Association's (AOTA) *Uniform Terminology for Occupational Therapy* as an area of occupational performance and was defined as the ability to "recognize, communicate, and perform desired sexual activities" (AOTA, 1989, p. 812). Five years later, in the third edition, it was defined primarily from a performance perspective as "engaging in desired sexual and intimate activities" (AOTA, 1994, p. 1052). The *Occupational Therapy Practice Framework* (referred

to as the *Framework*; AOTA, 2008) has replaced *Uniform Terminology* and focuses on occupational participation as it affects one's health, wellbeing, and quality of life. Within the occupational therapy profession, the term *sexual expression* has been replaced with the term *sexual activity*. **Sexual activity** is defined in the *Framework* as "engaging in activities that result in sexual satisfaction" (AOTA, 2008, p. 631). This chapter will address sexual health and sexual activity from the perspective of individuals, families, and populations with and without occupational performance limitations.

The World Health Organization (WHO) is dedicated to promoting health and examining the many cultural, social, and economic factors that can be barriers to health and healthy lifestyles. The WHO acknowledges that sexual health encompasses all aspects of sexuality, from infectious diseases and infertility to how disability or illness (e.g., cancer) affects sexual function.

> Sexual health can also be influenced by mental health, acute and chronic illnesses, and violence. Addressing sexual health at the individual, family, community or health system level requires integrated interventions by trained health providers and a functioning referral system. It also requires a legal, policy and regulatory environment where the sexual rights of all people are upheld. (WHO, n.d., ¶ 1)

Sexual health includes engaging in responsible sexual behaviors and being able to differentiate between responsible and irresponsible sexual behaviors. Access to information in order to make healthy sexual choices is a prerequisite of sexual health. *Healthy People 2010: Understanding and Improving Health* (U.S. Department of Health and Human Services [USDHHS], 2000) presented data regarding sexual health habits and sexually transmitted diseases, and summarized past research on the impact of interventions. According to this report, "the most effective school-based programs are comprehensive ones that include a focus on abstinence *and* condom use" (USDHHS, 2000, p. 35). Condom use among sexually active adults was maintained at a rate of 25% from 1995 to 2001. The total annual cost of unwanted adolescent pregnancies and sexually transmitted infections was estimated to range from $24 billion to $32 billion (USDHHS, 2000). Promoting healthy sexual behaviors across the life span is an important role for occupational therapists and occupational therapy assistants. Occupational therapy interventions and programming can promote sexual health and diminish the costs of sexual choices that have negative personal and societal consequences.

This chapter focuses on describing sexuality from a developmental perspective. Sexual activity will be viewed as much more than physically engaging in a sexual act. Prevention of disease and the promotion of sexual health are emphasized. Sexual health will be explored as an integral part of promoting a healthy lifestyle and wellbeing through old age. An effort has been made to offer an unbiased and nonjudgmental view of sex and sexuality, including the avoidance of **heterosexism,** which is the "belief that heterosexuality is the only 'natural' sexuality and that it is inherently healthier or superior to other types of sexuality" (Gay and Lesbian Medical Association [GLMA] and LGBT Experts, 2001, p. 446). As *health* is individually defined, each person uniquely defines his or her sexual health.

While this chapter defines *sexual health* and explores strategies for occupation-based interventions, it does not specifically address all issues related to sexuality that impact sexual health and quality of life, such as infertility, childhood sexual abuse, sexual harassment, sexual violence and rape, and sexual anomalies. Although these issues have a profound impact on sexual health, identity, and choices, they are beyond the scope of this chapter. Prevention of sexual violence is addressed in Chapter 18. This chapter focuses on sexual health as an important part of a person's overall wellbeing and quality of life.

Definitions of Sexuality Terminology

Several key terms that will be used throughout this chapter are defined in Content Box 16-1. Other key terms will be embedded throughout the chapter. The definitions of three of these terms—**sexuality, sexual health,** and **sexual rights**—are being developed and revised by experts identified by the WHO. However, these definitions should not be construed as official WHO definitions or as indicating a WHO position (WHO, n.d.).

A very important consideration when designing interventions or when working with individuals or groups on matters related to sexual activity is the preservation of dignity, respect, and human rights (WHO, n.d.). This is particularly relevant when a client's lifestyle or life choices with respect to sexual activity and intimacy, are different from that of the practitioner. This approach to care is well supported by AOTA's *Ethics Standards* (2004), which includes the *Occupational Therapy Code of Ethics* (AOTA, 2005b), the *Guidelines to the Occupational Therapy Code of Ethics* (AOTA, 2005a), and the *Core Values and Attitudes of Occupational Therapy Practice* (AOTA, 1993). In addition, it is supported by AOTA's statement of *Occupational Therapy's Commitment to Nondiscrimination and Inclusion* (Hansen & Hinojosa, 2004).

Sexual Health

There are many determinants of sexual health. These include the social and economic environment, one's innate capacities, strategies for coping, personal health practices, gender, and culture (Health Canada, 1999). Another determinant, which is closely aligned with the *Framework* (AOTA, 2008), is health services, "including services to promote, protect, maintain, and restore health" (Health Canada, 1999, p. 10). Figure 16-1 visually demonstrates the relationship between these

Content Box 16-1

Working Definitions of Sexuality, Sexual Health, and Sexual Rights

- *Sexuality* "is a central aspect of being human throughout life and encompasses sex, gender identities and roles, sexual orientation, eroticism, pleasure, intimacy and reproduction. Sexuality is experienced and expressed in thoughts, fantasies, desires, beliefs, attitudes, values, behaviors, practices, roles and relationships. While sexuality can include all of these dimensions, not all of them are always experienced or expressed. Sexuality is influenced by the interaction of biological, psychological, social, economic, political, cultural, ethical, legal, historical and religious and spiritual factors" (WHO Draft Working definition, 2002, ¶ 5).
- *Sexual health* "is a state of physical, emotional, mental and social wellbeing related to sexuality; it is not merely the absence of disease, dysfunction or infirmity. Sexual health requires a positive and respectful approach to sexuality and sexual relationships, as well as the possibility of having pleasurable and safe sexual experiences, free of coercion, discrimination and violence. For sexual health to be attained and maintained, the sexual rights of all persons must be respected, protected and fulfilled" (WHO Draft Working definition, 2002, ¶ 6).
- *Sexual rights* "embrace human rights that are already recognized in national laws, international human rights documents and other consensus documents. These include the right of all persons, free of coercion, discrimination and violence, to:
  - the highest attainable standard of health in relation to sexuality, including access to sexual and reproductive health care services;
  - seek, receive and impart information in relation to sexuality;
  - sexuality education;
  - respect for bodily integrity;
  - choice of partner;
  - decide to be sexually active or not;
  - consensual sexual relations;
  - consensual marriage;
  - decide whether or not, and when to have children; and
  - pursue a satisfying, safe and pleasurable sexual life" (WHO Draft Working definition, 2002, ¶ 7)

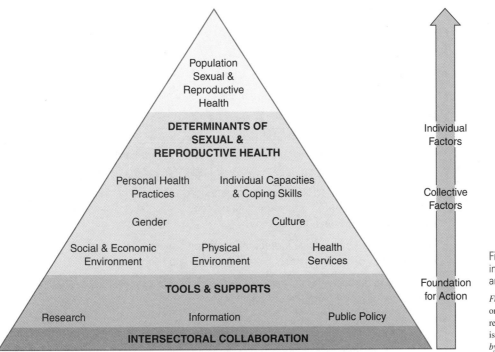

Those who have less power, who experience economic hardship, who have less access to information and services, and who live in marginalized circumstances tend to be most affected.

Figure 16-1 Factors that impact population sexual and reproductive health.

From: Report from consultations on a framework for sexual and reproductive health: What are the issues and challenges? *(p. 6), by Health Canada, 1999 ©, Ottawa, Ontario.* Reproduced with the permission of the Minister of Public Works and Government Services Canada, 2007.

determinants, policy, research findings, and health information and their joint impact on sexual and reproductive health. Health Canada (1999) discusses several factors related to sexual health:

- Youth from lower socioeconomic groups begin sexual activity at earlier ages and tend to engage in riskier sexual habits.
- Sexuality and sexual behavior, including opinions and choices about reproduction, are influenced by attitudes, values, and role expectations.
- High-risk behaviors are linked to educational levels, with less educated individuals seeing fewer benefits of postponing sex or engaging in safer sex practices.
- Healthy decisions about sexual health and reproduction are related to attitudes, competence, knowledge, and intentions.
- In nations where there is wide access to sex education, teen pregnancy and abortion rates are lower.

A Developmental Perspective on Sexual Health: Children and Adolescents

The capacity to learn, think critically, cope with stress, have good self-esteem, and make good decisions starts developing in early childhood. Healthy sexual development, including development of intimacy and trust, gender identification, and positive experience of sensual and sexual feelings, also begins in early childhood. These factors have a profound effect on healthy sexuality and sexual and reproductive decision making throughout life. (Health Canada, 1999, p. 16)

Sexuality and sexual health is important for sustaining quality of life throughout the life span. Table 16-1 details developmental milestones in sexual health, social influences, and key risks and issues for youth. The need for a society's youth to be educated regarding risk prevention and the importance of developing a

Table 16–1 Aspects of Sexual and Reproductive Health for Youth

Aspects	Descriptions
Developmental Milestones	• Capacity to use abstract reasoning and communicate with persons in close relationships
	• Development of meaningful relationships with peers
	• Puberty
	• Growing sense of self and establishment of values
	• Development of a sense of one's own body
	• Awareness of sexual feelings and responses
	• The ability to make decisions about sexual activity
Social Influences	• Young women often find it difficult to be assertive, but at the same time are given most of the responsibility for preventing pregnancy and sexually transmitted diseases.
	• Mass media images create and reinforce attitudes and values about gender roles and power; have powerful influences on attitudes about sexual attractiveness and body ideals; and create social expectations about acceptable choices regarding sex, sexuality, and reproduction.
	• Peer relationships also have a great influence on development of values and attitudes, and on decisions about sex, sexuality, and reproduction.
Key Risks and Issues	• Risky sexual practices by sexually active youth resulting in high rates of sexually transmitted diseases and teen pregnancies
	• High rates of violence in young people's intimate relationships
	• Negative and unrealistic images of sex and sexuality in the mass media
	• Negative social attitudes toward homosexuality that contribute to identity confusion, isolation, and rejection of gay, lesbian, and bisexual youth

From: *Report from consultations on a framework for sexual and reproductive health* (pp. 16–17), 1999 ©, by Health Canada, Ottawa, Ontario. Reproduced with the permission of the Minister of Public Works and Government Services Canada, 2007.

healthy appreciation for and understanding of their sexuality is clearly demonstrated by this table. This same type of information for adults and older adults will be summarized in other tables later in this chapter.

The Sexuality Information and Education Council of the United States (SIECUS) defined **sexual self-concept** as "an individual's evaluation of his or her sexual feelings and actions" (2001, ¶ 2) and described it as a key developmental task of adolescence. "During adolescence, young people tend to experience their first adult erotic feelings, experiment with sexual behaviors, and develop a strong sense of their own gender identity and sexual orientation" (SIECUS, 2001, ¶ 2). Sexual health interventions and education and the reduction of risky sexual practices need to be implemented early in development. Sexual practices, including unprotected sex, can begin in the preteen years (Content Box 16-2). "Teenagers whose parents have lower educational levels are more likely to be sexually active, and those who live with a single parent are more likely to have had multiple sex partners" (Health Canada, 1999, p. 10).

The National Association of School Nurses (2003) developed a position statement to support the provision of equitable services and equal opportunities to all students despite sexual orientation, gender expression, and gender identity. **Gender identity** is

an individual's basic self-conviction of being male or female. This conviction is not contingent upon the individual's biological gender. The exact process by which boys and girls come to see themselves as males or females is not known, but research indicates that gender identity develops some time between birth and age 3. (Child Welfare League of America, 2005, ¶ 13)

Sexual identity is a distinct concept that "evolves through a multistage developmental process, which varies in intensity and duration depending on the individual" (GLMA and LGBT Experts, 2001, p. 448). It includes how people think or label themselves (e.g., asexual, bisexual, gay, heterosexual, lesbian, queer, questioning, straight, undecided, undetermined) in terms of their sexuality (GLMA and LGBT Experts, 2001).

It is important to note that harassment, threats of physical violence, and actual physical assaults are frequently reported to have occurred at school by youth who are perceived to be gay or lesbian. Youth also report being subjected to homophobic comments while school employees and teachers ignore policies regarding antigay comments. In an effort to avoid this type of abuse, youth may engage in heterosexual sex behaviors that place them at risk for disease and pregnancy (Robins, 2006). If youth are engaging in these risky behaviors, they may also be compromising or denying their inherent sexual identities, which also can lead to future mental health issues.

Content Box 16-2

Youth Risk Behavior Surveillance— United States, 1999: Preteen and Teenage Sexual Health Facts

- Half (49.9%) of all students had had sexual intercourse during their lifetime. Hispanic male students (62.9%) were significantly more likely than Hispanic female students (45.5%) to have had sexual intercourse. Overall, black students (71.2%) were significantly more likely than Hispanic and white students (54.1% and 45.1%, respectively) to have had sexual intercourse.
- Nationwide, 8.3% of students had initiated sexual intercourse before age 13. Overall, male students (12.2%) were significantly more likely than female students (4.4%) to have initiated sexual intercourse before age 13. This significant sex difference was identified for all the racial/ethnic subpopulations and for students in grades 9, 10, and 12. Overall, black students (20.5%) were significantly more likely than Hispanic and white students (9.2% and 5.5%, respectively) to have initiated sexual intercourse before age 13, and Hispanic students (9.2%) were significantly more likely than white students (5.5%) to report this behavior.
- Nationwide, 16.2% of all students had had sexual intercourse during their lifetime with at least four sex partners. Overall, male students (19.3%) were significantly more likely than female students (13.1%) to have had at least four sex partners. This significant sex difference was identified for black and Hispanic students and students in grades 9 and 10. Overall, black students (34.4%) were significantly more likely than Hispanic and white students (16.6% and 12.4%, respectively) to have had at least four sex partners. Black male students (48.1%) were significantly more likely than Hispanic or white male students (23% and 12.1%, respectively) to have had at least four sex partners, and Hispanic male students (23.0%) were significantly more likely than white male students (12.1%) to report this behavior.

From "Youth risk behavior surveillance—United States, 1999," by L. Kann et al., 2000, *Morbidity and Mortality Weekly Report, 49*, p. 19. Atlanta, GA: Centers for Disease Control and Prevention.

Sexual Health Promotion and Youth

Development of occupation-based healt promotion interventions for children and adolescents can be challenging for practitioners, given the sensitivity of the topic, particularly when considering the age group. Some principles for programming can include the following:

- Recognize and incorporate the developmental level of the population during activity analysis and activity syntheses

- Select culturally sensitive occupation-based interventions and materials
- Incorporate the possibility that children and youth may have differing sexual orientations and require positive role models via the educational materials
- Understand the concepts of gender identity formation and sexual self-concept during sexual health interventions
- Recognize that adolescents with disabilities or chronic diseases are sexual beings and should have access to sexual health education and may need extra support to build a healthy sexual self-concept (Drench, Noonan, Sharby, & Ventura, 2006)
- Accept that a proportion of adolescents with disabilities will have sexual identities other than heterosexual and be able to address their concerns regarding sexual health (Drench et al., 2006)

The SIECUS (2004) has established a comprehensive manual of principles and guidelines for teaching, developing programs, and evaluating programs to promote healthy sexual behaviors for grades K–12. These guidelines were created to inform, educate, and provide insight in order to facilitate the development of responsible sexual behaviors.

A growing body of research is available to facilitate the development of efficacious sexual health promotion interventions. One area investigates the impact of parental involvement with sharing and encouraging safer sex behaviors. This is an important area of research, as public service announcements (PSAs) often encourage parents' involvement and imply it is their role and responsibility. Unfortunately, these often vague PSAs encourage parents to talk about "sex" and AIDS but do not provide the parents with the tools, skills, or knowledge to be effective health promotion agents with their children (Lefkowitz, Boone, Au, & Sigman, 2003). While most research to date investigating parent-child communication regarding sexual activity has been survey based, Lefkowitz and colleagues (2003) conducted a qualitative study of mother/adolescent dyads. Based on the results of this study and a review of other quantitative research, the researchers provided the following suggestions for developers of parent-based sexual health promotion for youth:

- Provide parents with specific prevention topics to discuss with their children (e.g., abstinence, prevention of HIV/AIDS, safer sex, pregnancy prevention)
- Provide information about these topics to the parents so they can be informed and feel competent to engage in the conversations
- Consider the religiosity of the parents to determine if both abstinence and safer sex should be components in the program

A careful balance needs to be made between parents' religiosity and adolescents' risk for pregnancy and sexually transmitted diseases. Encouraging parents to engage in conversations regarding dating relationships, dating safety, and disease prevention is important, but for some parents the addition of discussions of safer sex may cause them to withdraw from a program or these important conversations. However, if condoms are not discussed, adolescents may engage in unsafe sexual practices, even given their or their parents' religious values (Lefkowitz et al., 2003).

Research from the United Kingdom, which has some of the highest rates of sexually transmitted diseases and teen pregnancy in western Europe, indicates that the rates are cyclical and not constant. The rates spike after December and summer school holidays. Although these cyclical patterns are well established, rates have been dramatically increasing. Recent research (Bellis, Hughes, Thomson, & Bennet, 2004) indicates that the rising rates may be partially the result of cheaper airfare to international vacation destinations focusing on nightlife. The nightlife lifestyle promotes engagement in alcohol consumption and participation in unsafe sex. The availability of protective measures (e.g., condoms) may also be limited, and language may be a barrier to the use of safer sex techniques. These research results indicate the need to examine the preparation of students from other countries, including the United States, as they participate in study-abroad programs where a similar escalation of unsafe sexual behavior may also be present.

Additional research will help occupational therapists, public health workers, and other health professionals develop culturally sensitive prevention programs that will protect youth's overall health and wellbeing, including their sexual and future reproductive health. One such area of research that may assist in the development of health promotion programming for this age group is the identification of potential occupation-based protective factors, such as participation in school sports (Page, Hammermeister, Scanlan, & Gilbert, 1998) and other extracurricular school activities, religious groups, or community activism.

A Developmental Perspective on Sexual Health: Adults

As people sexually mature, they discover what is sexually pleasurable and gratifying, and usually become more comfortable with their sexual selves. People develop sexual relationships based on preferences and choices. Adult sexual expression and behaviors in which people engage are personally chosen. The social influences and key determinants guiding those sexual choices and other developmental aspects of adult sexuality are detailed in Table 16-2.

Knowledge about adult sexuality assists occupational therapy practitioners in discussing client concerns about sexual expression. In women, menopause can significantly change one's sexual desires or views on sexuality. Physical and emotional side effects occur, and estrogen replacement therapy may be needed. To make intercourse easier, vaginal lubricants can be used or other forms of sexual expression beside intercourse that are satisfying to the woman and her partner can be employed (Drench et al., 2006). Health professionals providing sexual health education need to continually review the research literature in order to communicate accurate, timely information, so individuals can make fully informed health decisions.

Adult men also experience changes in sexual function as they age. Some sexual health facts for men include the following:

- Testicles slow testosterone production after approximately age 25.
- Erections may occur more slowly once testosterone production slows.
- Men become less able to have another erection after an orgasm and may take up to 24 hours to achieve and sustain another erection.
- The amount of semen released during ejaculation also decreases, but men are capable of fathering a baby even when they are in their 80s and 90s. (Advocates for Youth, section on adult sexuality, 2005 ¶ 2)

Table 16–2 Aspects of Sexual and Reproductive Health for Adults

Aspects	Description

Developmental Milestones	- Sexuality is a continuing part of life for all adult men and women, whether or not they are sexually active
	- Sexuality may include sexual feelings and expression, sexual decision making
	- Sexual decision making may include:
	  - whether to make a longer-term commitment to a partner
	  - when to have children
	  - decisions involving pregnancy and childbirth
	  - decisions regarding contraceptive use and protection from sexually transmitted diseases and HIV/AIDS
	- Menopause
	- Coping with conditions and diseases that negatively affect sexual and reproductive health

Social Influences	- Gender roles and power continue to influence sexual and reproductive choices and health - Widespread homophobia - Media images often portray sex role stereotypes and violence, creating discord and dysfunction in sexual relationships - High rates of unintended or unwanted pregnancies
Key Risks and Issues	- High rates of sexually transmitted diseases - Infertility - Growing use of reproductive technologies to respond to infertility or manipulate the conception process - Risks during pregnancy linked to poor prenatal care, substance use and abuse, poverty and lack of social supports - Menopause and hormonal changes - Sexual violence - Reproductive cancers, including breast, cervical, and prostate cancer and other sexual and reproductive conditions and disorders

From: *Report from consultations on a framework for sexual and reproductive health* (p. 17), 1999 ©, by Health Canada, Ottawa, Ontario. Reproduced with the permission of the Minister of Public Works and Government Services Canada, 2007.

In adults, sexual orientation becomes clearer. **Sexual orientation** is defined as "the orientation within human beings that leads them to be emotionally and physically attracted to persons of one gender or both. One's sexual orientation may be heterosexual, homosexual, bisexual, or asexual" (Child Welfare League of America, 2005, ¶ 30). It is unclear how or when one's sexual orientation develops.

Sexual Health Promotion and Adults

During the adult years, humans become more sexually active, they develop sexual relationships, and intimacy with others becomes more predominant. Principles that should be considered when developing occupation-based interventions regarding sexual health include the following:

- The choice to be sexually active resides with each individual, with some people choosing a celibate or asexual lifestyle.
- Personal decisions about sexual health are an individual choice but can be guided by access to accurate and appropriate information.
- Information on sexual health should be imparted in a culturally sensitive format that is also targeted at the educational level(s) of the population being served.
- Health professionals should be knowledgeable in current evidence and literature on sexual health promotion and should be able to impart this knowledge in a positive and practical way.

If an occupational therapist or occupational therapy assistant is uncomfortable following the principles outlined above or imparting information on sexual health, or if he or she has a biased view on the subject, the practitioner should refer clients to others more comfortable and competent in meeting the clients' sexual health needs.

Culturally appropriate current educational materials on sexual health are important tools when implementing occupational therapy interventions with individuals, groups, families, or communities. However, these items are not always available. For example, while resources are available to help communicate specific information to individuals and heterosexual couples learning to manage the impact of new disabilities on sexual intimacy (Hebert, 1997; Kroll & Klein, 1992), similar resources, including visual educational materials that are inclusive of the gay, lesbian, bisexual, and transgender community have not been located. The *Healthy People 2010 Companion Document for Lesbian, Gay, Bisexual, and Transgender (LGBT) Health* (GLMA and LGBT Experts, 2001), available at http://www.nalgap.org/PDF/Resources/HP2010CDLGBTHealth.pdf, provides information to support health promotion program and policy development for LGBT individuals and groups. Knowledge of the client's sexual orientation and being nondiscriminatory in intervention can help promote more client-centered and compassionate care in occupational therapy.

An example from practice centers on a 38-year-old woman with cancer. The woman had a 20-year-old daughter living with her and was very active in her neighborhood, participating in daily life as much as her energy level allowed. The Pizzi Holistic Wellness Assessment (PHWA) was administered, along with a comprehensive occupational therapy evaluation. The PWHA (Pizzi, 2001) addresses a person's sexual health as one of eight areas of health, and she rated herself a two out of a possible ten. When discussing this issue with her, she related that she was a lesbian but was very private about her sexual orientation. She stated that she was very unhappy with her social worker, because there was an implicit assumption by the social worker that she was heterosexual. In her words, "because I have a daughter and was a former beauty queen, discussions of dating men were initiated by this other professional which told me the [other professional] didn't really know who I was as a person. I had a hard time really relating to that person after that and was concerned about discussing my orientation because I thought I might be judged by this person." The client stated she felt more comfortable relating her concerns and lack of participation in dating occupations with the occupational therapist than with anyone else because of the practitioner's openness and nonjudgmental attitude. This eventually led to the client developing a sustainable relationship over time with a woman who became her partner.

A Developmental Perspective on Sexual Health: Older Adults

Sexual activity, expression, and desire continue through the life span. Although men and women change as they age, they do not lose their desire for sexual expression. Even among the very old, the need for touch and intimacy remains, although the desire and ability to have sexual intercourse may lessen. Table 16-3 summarizes the developmental and social issues and the key determinants for this stage of sexual life. It is important to remember that individuals and couples will have differences in the need and desire for sexual expression.

As people age, acute illnesses, chronic conditions, medications, and a variety of other factors can become barriers to sexual expression and sexual intercourse. Past

Table 16-3   Aspects of Sexual and Reproductive Health for Older Adults

Aspects	Description
Developmental Milestones	• Men and women in their later years remain sexual beings and many people continue to be sexually active in later life • When sexual expression changes, sexual feelings and responses continue • Experience of sex and sexuality is influenced by the physical and emotional responses associated with hormonal changes and the process of aging • A sense of loss and grief related to changes in sexual functioning and expression, and to loss of partners and peers can be experienced
Social Influences	• Growing sense of freedom with the lessening of child rearing and job responsibilities • A more balanced appreciation of sexual and other personal relationships • Societal attitudes tend to deny the sexuality of older men and women, and do not value older adults as much as youth • Social views of femininity (e.g., youth, beauty) and masculinity (e.g., potency, control) that often decline with age can negatively impact self-esteem and health of older women and men
Key Risks and Issues	• Increasing rates of cancers of the reproductive system, especially for breast and prostate cancer • Violence directed toward older adults living in institutions • Other conditions and disorders such as arthritis, chronic back pain, diabetes, hypertension, incontinence, osteoporosis, and heart disease that may affect sexual functioning

From: *Report from consultations on a framework for sexual and reproductive health* (pp. 17–18), 1999 ©, by Health Canada, Ottawa, Ontario. Reproduced with the permission of the Minister of Public Works and Government Services Canada, 2007.

sexual enjoyment, loneliness, boredom, health status of partner, losses, fear of failure, lack of privacy, potency, use of drugs or alcohol, cognitive function, and depression (Heckheimer, 1989) can also impact the desire and potential to engage in sexual intimacy. Other factors that can influence sexual activity in the elderly include changes in hormonal levels and psychosocial conditions such as social isolation and poverty (Drench et al., 2006).

Besides physical changes and attitudes about sexuality, there may also be evidence of fear and anxiety about changes in bodily structures and sexual expression (Brewer, 2004; Spence, 1992). Some of these fears may be based on commonly held misconceptions that can be removed by education. Examples of these misconceptions include avoiding sex after a heart attack and the significance of penis size. It is important for clients with cardiac dysfunction and their partners to know that less than 1% of individuals experience sudden death during intercourse and that 80% of these deaths occur when the sex is with someone other than a spouse (Laflin, 2002). It is also important for men to understand that a common age-related change is a slight shrinkage in penis size. Heterosexual men of any age can benefit from knowing that penis size is less

important to women than they may think and has little or no impact on their ability to facilitate an orgasm in their female partners (Brewer, 2004).

Sexual Health Promotion and Older Adults

During discussions of sexuality and sexual health, occupational therapy practitioners need to consider that older adults, especially those growing up in the United States, lived in an era first of sexual repression, when homosexuality was considered a crime or a mental illness (Robins, 2006), then through a time of sexual liberation in the 1960s and 1970s. These temporal features will impact the views, biases, and sexual self-concept of this age group and need to be considered during interventions.

Kessel (2001) identified three current societal attitudes regarding sexuality and older adults:

1. Sexual expression is nonexistent among this population.
2. Sexuality is a source of ridicule through social media such as birthday cards.

3. Sexual expression in later life is viewed with disgust.

These negative attitudes regarding sex and older adults could impact this population's readiness to initiate or discuss questions regarding sexuality due to fear of a negative response from health-care professionals. The attitudes and values of the elderly must be acknowledged and become part of client-centered care.

Laflin (2002) encouraged the inclusion of a sexual history during ADL evaluation. This can be done simply by asking elder clients, "How do you view sex and sexuality as part of your overall health?" The answer and nonverbal cues in response to this question will help the interviewer determine the extent to which he or she can delve into sexual health in the discussion. Because this is often a topic health practitioners do not discuss readily with elderly clients, sensitivity to clients' reactions must be employed. Interview questions also can be introduced in terms of how one health area relates to another (e.g., alternate positions for a variety of activities, including sexual ones, can ease joint pain of arthritis), thereby diminishing the possibility of alienating the client.

As people age, their core sexual being does not necessarily change. While physical capabilities may diminish, sexual expression is retained. Some principles for sexual health and older adults that should be incorporated into occupation-based health promotion interventions include

- providing information on strategies to maintain sexual expression;
- suggesting alternatives to sexual expression, including safer sex for the newly widowed;
- sharing strategies to cope with new disabilities; and
- providing sexual health information in a sensitive way that is tailored to the cultural and educational levels of the older adult population, while also recognizing common physical and biological changes that occur with age (e.g., diminished hearing, vision, sensation).

Age Concerns (Brewer, 2004), an older adult advocacy and education group based in the United Kingdom, produced an excellent resource for older heterosexual couples regarding sexual health. There are also resources for occupational therapists and occupational therapy assistants. One such resource is a chapter in *Aging: The Health-Care Challenge* that provides diagrams of adapted sexual positions for heterosexual couples (Laflin, 2002).

There are many factors related to the development of sexual health throughout the life span, many of which were discussed above. Sexual health behaviors are learned behaviors, and caring for one's health includes caring for one's sexual being. The next section describes the importance of having knowledge about sexually transmitted infections and their impact on health.

Sexually Transmitted Infections (STIs) and Sexually Transmitted Diseases (STDs)

The terms **sexually transmitted infection (STI)** and **sexually transmitted disease (STD)** will be used throughout the rest of this chapter. While *STD* is the more familiar term, *STI* is a newer term and is beginning to replace *STD* in the public health literature (Content Box 16-3 defines these two terms). Public health experts support this change in language, since symptoms are not readily apparent in most infected persons for many STDs, and if there are symptoms, they are mild and often overlooked. In addition, in the case of some common STDs, such as herpes and chlamydia, "the sexually transmitted virus or bacteria can be described as creating 'infection,' which may or may not result in 'disease'" (American Social Health Association, 2006a, ¶ 2).

The Institute of Medicine (IOM) developed a report that declared STDs a major hidden epidemic that was having huge health and economic consequences for the United States (Eng & Butler, 1996). This report concluded that STDs could be managed but that some changes in the system of care were needed. These changes included

- development of "a much more effective national system for STD prevention, which takes into account the complex interaction between biological and social factors that sustain STD transmission in populations";
- a focus on preventing the disproportionate impact that STDs have on youth and underserved populations;

Content Box 16-3

Definitions of STDs and STIs

- *Sexually transmitted diseases* (*STDs*) are "the more than 25 infectious organisms transmitted primarily through sexual activity" and are "behavior linked diseases that result from unprotected sex" (USDHHS, 2000, p. 25-3).
- *Sexually transmitted infections* (*STIs*) are "acquired through sexual contact in a substantial number of cases" (American Social Health Association, 2006a, ¶ 34).

- application of "proven, cost-effective behavioral and biomedical interventions"; and
- recognition "that education, mass communication media financing and health care infrastructure policies must foster change in personal behaviors and in health care services" (USDHHS, 2000, pp. 25–33).

While this chapter does not focus on the medical management of STIs, readers are encouraged to seek medical information from their personal health professionals or university health center. Web resources such as Go Ask Alice! (http://www.goaskalice.columbia.edu) can be helpful to learn more about personal health, including sexual health and to enhance competence as a health care provider. If the interactions between biological and social factors relative to STIs are understood by occupational

therapists and occupational therapy assistants, more directed occupation and client-centered health promotion interventions may result. These factors are listed in Table 16-4. One of these factors is the shyness that many people in the United States exhibit when discussing sex, sexuality, and STIs with their partners or health professionals. Culturally sensitive health education materials must be developed and distributed. These materials should address this shyness in an open but sensitive manner, while again being culturally sensitive and culturally relevant. In addition, sexual health educational materials for youth must also address communication, especially negotiation, and relationship building and maintenance. This is important because many young people fail to use protection as they are too trustful of their partners and do not want to jeopardize relationships (AIDS Alert, 2002).

Table 16–4 Biological and Social Factors Related to STDs/STIs

Factors	Description
Biological Factors	
Asymptomatic nature of STDs/STIs	Since symptoms frequently are not detected or are very mild and thus ignored, STDs/STIs are often transmitted unknowingly to others.
Lag time between infection and complications	Serious health problems may not appear for years (e.g., "cervical cancer caused by human papillomavirus (HPV); infertility and ectopic pregnancy resulting from unrecognized or undiagnosed chlamydia or gonorrhea") (p. 25-4)
Gender and age	"Women are at higher risk than men for most STDs, and young women are more susceptible to certain STDs than older women" due to the presence of more susceptible cells on a younger cervix (p. 25-4).
Social and Behavioral Factors	
Poverty and marginalization	"STDs disproportionately affect disenfranchised persons and persons who are in social networks in which high-risk sexual behavior is common and either access to health care or health-seeking behavior is compromised" (p. 25-4).
Access to health care	Groups with the highest rates of STDs/STIs are often the same groups that have the least access to health services.
Substance abuse	Research has linked substance abuse with STDs. The "introduction of new illicit substances into communities often can drastically alter sexual behavior in high-risk sexual networks, leading to the epidemic spread of STDs" (p. 25-4).
Sex work	Sex work, substance abuse, and STDs often coexist.
Sexual coercion	Research indicates that women with a history of involuntary sexual intercourse are more likely to have voluntary intercourse at earlier ages, which is a known risk factor for STDs.
Sexuality and secrecy	In the United States, while sexuality is considered a normal part of human life, people are uncomfortable with open, frank discussions of sexual behavior and sexual health. This secrecy can lead to lack of communication about healthy sexuality and hamper sexual health education at the individual, couple, family, and population level.

Adapted from *Healthy People 2010: Understanding and improving health* (pp. 25-3–25-6), by U.S. Department of Health and Human Services, 2000, Washington, DC: U.S. Government Printing Office.

Accessibility to reproductive and STD clinics may be unavailable due to transportation issues or geography (e.g., rural living). When certain communities or populations lack power or equality, it is more difficult for their members to choose healthy sexual relationships and make healthy sexual choices. Women, in general, often have the least amount of power in primarily heterosexual relationships, and thus are at risk for impaired sexual health. "Members of certain groups often have less status and may be marginalized in terms of full participation in the social and economic benefits of society" (Health Canada, 1999, p. 11).

The USDHHS factors listed in Table 16-4 can be used as a first step in program development to ensure access to information and service, as in the fictitious example that follows. An occupational therapy student group makes diminishing the STD rate on their campus a priority for improving the health and wellbeing of students, faculty, and staff. Together with health education and nursing students, they research the prevalence rates of STDs on their campus, gather facts about STDs and STD prevention (including information in Table 16-4), conduct focus groups, and search for and critique brochures on sexual health for both men and women. They then develop culturally sensitive workshops on sexual expression and the prevention of STDs tailored to students, faculty, and staff, including lesbian, gay, bisexual, and transgendered (LGBT) individuals.

Human Immunodeficiency Virus (HIV)

HIV affects all of humanity. It affects not only persons infected with the virus but also their parents, siblings, friends, lovers, children, and coworkers. After being diagnosed as HIV positive, an individual can be immobilized and drastically alter his or her occupational performance and participation in society or the individual can treat the diagnosis as an impetus to act in positive, life-transforming ways. (Pizzi, 2004, p. 1194)

The prevalence of HIV has increased over the last 25 years into a global pandemic (Joint United Nations Programme on HIV/AIDS, 2004). While HIV is considered an STD, it warrants its own discussion in this chapter given its magnitude as a population-based problem. HIV is also the only STD typically addressed in the occupational therapy literature. Initially, the literature reflected the need for infection control, signs and symptoms, and basic biopsychosocial interventions (Denton, 1987; Giles & Allen, 1987; Gordon, 1987). From the early 1990s to the present, HIV has become an important public health issue to be addressed from a holistic occupational perspective (Bedell, 2000; Braveman, 2001; Gutterman, 1990; Johnson & Pizzi, 1990; Molineux, 1997; Pizzi, 1990a, 1990b, 2004).

Pizzi (1992) emphasized the role of health promotion programming for women with HIV and AIDS. Using an occupational science perspective, women living with HIV and AIDS were examined from a sociocultural perspective. Learning about sexual health, caring for oneself, and developing action plans toward optimal sexual health and self-empowerment were discussed as a means of preventing social and emotional deprivation. Wood and Aull (1990) also discussed empowering women with HIV and AIDS to participate in daily life occupations optimally throughout their lives. Barrett (1997) explored the socioeconomic disadvantage of rural African women and the impact on living and coping with HIV. The effects of the disease on their children and on their participation in meaningful occupations and occupational roles given their illness and poverty were discussed.

The National Center for HIV, STD and TB Prevention, a part of the Divisions of HIV/AIDS Prevention in the Centers for Disease Control and Prevention (CDC), is responsible for "helping control the HIV epidemic by working with community, state and international partners in surveillance, research, prevention and evaluation activities" (CDC, 2006, ¶ 1). Within the epidemic, sexually healthy individuals are those who recognize preventive strategies and practice these on a routine basis (which include all people who can be sexually active). However, it must also be recognized that sexually healthy choices can only be made when the opportunity for education about and access to preventive strategies exists. Health behavior interventions are often utilized to promote healthy sexual expression and sexual health. Behavioral recommendations from the CDC (2003) that promote sexual health for people with HIV are noted in Content Box 16-4. An additional source of HIV information from the CDC to share with clients and their families is a question-and-answer page located at http://www.cdc.gov/hiv/pubs/faqs.htm#prevention.

Occupational therapy has always been a leader among the health professions in recognizing the physical, social, emotional, and spiritual health concerns and needs of people with HIV and AIDS. Emphasis has been on helping clients to recognize ways to maintain quality of life through participation in meaningful and life-sustaining roles and occupations. Sexual health is a part of human occupational performance that can often be overlooked but is integral to fostering quality of life. The maintenance of sexual health is an area where occupational therapists and occupational therapy assistants can be of great service to those with HIV and to communities and populations that look for positive

Content Box 16-4

Recommendations for Behavioral Interventions to Reduce Human Immunodeficiency Virus (HIV) Transmission Risk

- Clinics or office environments where patients with HIV infection receive care should be structured to support and enhance HIV prevention.
- Within the context of HIV care, brief general HIV prevention messages should be regularly provided to HIV-infected patients at each visit or periodically, as determined by the clinician, and at a minimum of twice yearly.
- These messages should emphasize the need for safer behaviors to protect their own health and the health of their sex or needle-sharing partners, regardless of perceived risk.
- Messages should be tailored to the patient's needs and circumstances.
- Patients should have adequate, accurate information regarding factors that influence HIV transmission and methods for reducing the risk for transmission to others, emphasizing that the most effective methods for preventing transmission are those that protect noninfected persons against exposure to HIV (e.g., sexual abstinence; consistent and correct use of condoms made of latex, polyurethane, or other synthetic materials; and sex only with a partner of the same HIV status).
- HIV-infected patients who engage in high-risk sexual practices (i.e., capable of resulting in HIV transmission) with persons of unknown or negative HIV status should be counseled to use condoms consistently and correctly.
- Patients' misconceptions regarding HIV transmission and methods for reducing risk for transmission should be identified and corrected. For example, ensure that patients know that (1) per-act estimates of HIV transmission risk for an individual patient vary according to behavioral, biological, and viral factors; (2) highly active antiretroviral therapy (HAART) cannot be relied on to eliminate the risk of transmitting HIV to others; and (3) nonoccupational postexposure prophylaxis is of uncertain effectiveness for preventing infection in HIV-exposed partners.
- Tailored HIV prevention interventions, using a risk-reduction approach, should be delivered to patients at highest risk for transmitting HIV.
- After initial prevention messages are delivered, subsequent longer or more intensive interventions in the clinic or office should be delivered, if feasible.
- HIV-infected patients should be referred to appropriate services for issues related to HIV transmission that cannot be adequately addressed during the clinic visit.
- Persons who inject illicit drugs should be strongly encouraged to cease injecting and enter into substance abuse treatment programs (e.g., methadone maintenance) and should be provided referrals to such programs.
- Persons who continue to inject drugs should be advised to always use sterile injection equipment and to never reuse or share needles, syringes, or other injection equipment and should be provided information regarding how to obtain new, sterile syringes and needles (e.g., syringe exchange program).

From Table 4 in "Incorporating HIV prevention into the medical care of persons living with HIV," by Centers for Disease Control and Prevention, 2003, *Morbidity and Mortality Weekly Report, 52*(RR 12), p. 39.

health messages to prevent the spread of infection. For example, Phillips (2002) used a community wellness project to discuss strategies used by occupational therapy students in the area of HIV prevention. This project encourages HIV education and prevention among college students and demonstrates ways occupational therapy can make a difference in the community.

The possibilities for creative, culturally sensitive, occupation-based therapy health promotion interventions are numerous. In an urban population of young gay men, the intervention could include lectures, seminars, and workshops on healthy dating and connecting with others from an emotional, physical, and spiritual perspective at a popular entertainment venue. Role playing and open discussions of healthy sexuality, combined with health information about HIV and STDs, can be utilized as effective means of promoting safer sexual practices and preventing the spread of

infection. This intervention could be tailored to reach rural gay men via the Internet.

Occupational Therapy and Sexual Health

It is important for occupational therapists and occupational therapy assistants to understand sexual health as a part of client-centered care. Holism is inherent in occupational therapy practice, yet intervening in the area of sexual health remains uncomfortable for many practitioners. "Historically, sexuality has been, for the most part, left out of the occupational therapy profession" (Jackson, 1995, p. 675).

With their focus on holistic care, occupational performance, role maintenance, and adaptation of activity, it would seem that occupational therapists may have a positive role in sexual habilitation or rehabilitation. However, it is not clear if the profession regards sexual activity as much at the heart of its purpose as personal care, work, and leisure. (Couldrick, 1999, p. 496)

There are a variety of possible reasons for this apparent lack of attention to clients' sexual health and sexual activity by occupational therapists and occupational therapy assistants, including shyness, lack of knowledge, and belief in myths, among other factors. People with disabilities are not asexual, but many practitioners may have this misconception, which can reinforce a societal myth (Gender, 1992). Practitioners may also eliminate sexual health issues completely from their evaluation because of this misconception or because they feel uncomfortable, even if clients wish to discuss these issues as they relate to their emotional, social, and physical wellbeing. Client-centered care includes respect for individuals and their occupational needs. Sexual health is an important aspect of people's lives and requires the same attention as work and leisure issues, particularly if initiated by the client.

> Practitioners must examine both societal attitudes toward people with disabilities and their own beliefs, values and attitudes about sexuality. Cultural and religious biases must be put aside, and there must be an acknowledgement that there is no universal agreement about acceptable or unacceptable, right or wrong sexual behavior. (McKenna, 2003, p. 542, based on Couldrick, 1999)

In a review of the international occupational therapy literature using keywords *sexuality, sex behavior,* and *sex counseling,* the following general topics were found relative to sexual health (values in parentheses indicate the number of articles related to each topic):

- Physical disabilities (8)
- Sexual orientation (5)
- General uncategorized (3)
- Knowledge and attitudes (2)
- Childhood sexual abuse (1)
- Sexuality as ADL (1)
- Developmental disabilities (1)
- Mental health (1)
- Older adults (1)
- Sexual harassment (1)

None of the articles directly addressed health promotion issues; however, several articles discussed issues (e.g., self-esteem, life satisfaction, heterosexism) that could directly impact wellbeing and health in the area of sexuality, particularly for people with disabilities.

In a qualitative research study, Yallop and Fitzgerald (1997) analyzed data from five senior occupational

therapy students and five practicing therapists regarding comfort levels when addressing sexuality. From an analysis of these narratives, they concluded that there was a lack of knowledge, experience, and positive attitudes to effectively intervene with sexuality issues in a variety of settings. They also discovered a theme of power and control. If respondents felt a higher sense of power and control in a given situation (regarding sexual issues), then they experienced higher levels of comfort in addressing issues of sexuality.

Kingsley and Molineux (2000) investigated perspectives of occupational therapists regarding work with gay, lesbian, or bisexual clients. Four themes emanated from their research:

1. Being prepared and comfortable (related to feeling prepared and comfortable with gay, lesbian, and bisexual clients)
2. The missing link (related to being unprepared academically)
3. No different than anyone else (related to neglecting the impact of sexual orientation on one's occupational life)
4. A narrow view of occupation (related to having a diminished awareness of the complexity and holism of occupation)

This study, like that of Yallop and Fitzgerald (1997), highlights the importance of incorporating sexuality and sexual health into occupational therapy curricula so that students and future practitioners develop a beginning level of comfort. One of the earliest advocates for increased education about sexuality for occupational therapy students and practitioners was Miller (1984), who worked as an occupational therapist and sexual health clinician. Both Jackson (1995) and Kingsley and Molineux (2000) suggest that sexuality in its broadest sense be approached in the academic arena in order to help students see a link between sexuality and occupation, and thereby assist in examining occupation more holistically.

> For occupational therapists who aim to create accepting environments that encourage persons with disabilities to recreate their lives after a life disruption, knowledge about weaving one's lesbian, gay, or bisexual identity into daily occupations may be crucial to the rehabilitative process. (Jackson, 1995, p. 678)

There are multiple health disparities that exist due to one's sexual orientation, which is unto itself a major sexual health issue that is often not wholly recognized in practice. Some of these disparities and sexual health issues include lack of access to care, discrimination based on one's sexual orientation, fear of clients declaring their sexual orientation to health providers, and lack of cultural competence among health professionals (GLMA, 2000, 2004). Health promotion messages about sexual health need to be provided to all individuals at all developmental stages regardless of sexual orientation.

Occupational therapists and occupational therapy practitioners are keenly aware of the need for cultural sensitivity and client-centered care in practice. They are well positioned to be health advocates and leaders for individuals, communities, and populations requiring sexual health promotion interventions. There are several simple steps that occupational therapists and occupational therapy assistants can take wherever they may practice. One step is using their knowledge and appreciation of the importance of context in the delivery of occupational therapy services and health education—for example, displaying health promotion posters, pamphlets, and other health education materials that depict people from a variety of ethnic, religious, and minority backgrounds, including same-sex couples (Robins, 2006). Other important steps include consistently avoiding assumptions, stereotypes, and voyeurism; using gender-neutral language; requesting permission before identifying a client's sexual orientation in their medical or health record; referring clients and, where applicable, parents to appropriate support services (e.g., counselors, support groups); and educating both one's self and coworkers regarding the health and health promotion needs of sexual minorities (Robins, 2006).

Wherever occupational therapy services are offered, sexual expression and healthy sexual choices need to be discussed to holistically promote optimal quality of life. For example, in school systems, practitioners must have an awareness of sexual development, which can give them different insight into self-chosen play occupations and the need of children to express themselves in intimate ways. Healthy intimate expression can be fostered and developed safely and can include discussions with parents about burgeoning sexual expression and ways to allow children to express themselves in a safe environment that can also assist in developing boundaries.

Correctional facilities are another potential site for occupational therapy health promotion interventions that address sexual health. Male prisoners often engage in high-risk sexual behavior prior to and during their incarceration, putting themselves and their future partners at risk for STIs, including HIV (Toepell, 2003). In prisons, life skills in the area of sexuality can be taught, including the need to protect their "steady" partners to whom they will return. The life skills program should include joint sessions with the steady partner when they visit their significant others.

Prior to these joint sessions, the needs of women who are the incarcerated males' steady partners need to be addressed. First, they may need assistance in overcoming shyness and cultural norms regarding discussions about sex. Through participation in open, frank, health education sessions with peers, health educators, mental health counselors, and occupational therapy practitioners, they will gain a level of comfort to continue with the program. This infusion of confidence and knowledge can be built upon through occupation-based sessions to develop skills in condom access and use, self-advocacy, safer sex techniques, and other relationship issues. Research has indicated that in order to succeed, programs need to incorporate cultural realities and must maintain contact with the women (Toepell, 2003).

Working with couples who hold strong traditional gender beliefs, or where one partner has diminished power, can be difficult for occupational therapy practitioners who hold different beliefs. Still more difficult may be the realization that women can be trapped in abusive relationships by poverty and isolation. Providing short-term interventions or interventions without simultaneous interventions for the male partners or the expertise of other professionals may cause more harm than benefit. However, if these realities are addressed, the potential to impact longevity and quality of life for the women and their potential children will be tremendous.

In rehabilitation centers and supportive housing, the knowledge that clients may have differing viewpoints and lifestyles regarding sexuality (e.g., one may be heterosexual or not) can empower practitioners to be more client-centered and can help them develop occupational interventions that promote overall quality of life. With the elderly and others residing in assisted-living facilities and nursing home environments, sexual expression can be facilitated through provision of occupational opportunities that view the person as a sexual being. When practitioners become more comfortable with incorporating sexual health issues into evaluation and interventions, then clients in any setting will be more open to discussing this part of their lives.

Sexual Health Interventions

A review of government documents can provide guidance as to principles and goals of national sexual health agendas. Health Canada (1999) identifies eight basic principles that "should guide the actions to maintain, protect, and promote the sexual and reproductive health of all people" (p. 13). These principles are listed in Content Box 16-5. Based on these principles, occupational therapists and occupational therapy assistants have opportunities to enable optimal sexual health for individuals, communities, and populations, thereby enhancing their wellbeing and quality of life. While not all of these principles may apply to the practice of occupational therapy specifically, all are, at the very least, indirectly related to practice. A variety of U.S. national objectives related to sexual health appear throughout *Healthy People 2010* (USDHHS, 2000); a selection of which appears in Table 16-5.

The Permission, Limited Information, Specific Suggestions and Intensive Therapy (PLISSIT) Model (Annon, 1976) is often cited for use in sexuality counseling (McKenna, 2003). In the Permission step, an occupational therapist or occupational therapy assistant can begin to introduce sexuality as an important part of one's occupational being. The practitioner can guide this introduction, but careful active listening to the client can also provide an opening for discussion. In the

---

Content Box 16-5

Principles of Sexual Health

Principle 1	All individuals are sexual beings throughout their lives.
Principle 2	Individual autonomy and responsibility should guide all aspects of decision-making.
Principle 3	The promotion of sexual and reproductive health and prevention of problems will reap the greatest benefits.
Principle 4	Health interventions should be safe, effective, and evidence-based, and individuals should be fully informed before making decisions.
Principle 5	The simplest and least invasive intervention that is appropriate and effective should be used in delivering health care.
Principle 6	Access to sexual and reproductive health programs and services should be equitable, responsive to diversity, and not limited because of discrimination based on gender, age, race, ethnicity, marital status, sexual orientation, religion, culture, language, socioeconomic status, disability, or geographic location.
Principle 7	Individuals should be protected from diseases and hazardous environments that can adversely affect their sexual and reproductive health.
Principle 8	Families and communities share responsibility in providing a physical and psychosocial environment that enables all its members to maintain their sexual and reproductive health.

From *Report from consultations on a framework for sexual and reproductive health* (pp. 13–15), 1999 ©, by Health Canada, Ottawa, Ontario. Reproduced with the permission of the Minister of Public Works and Government Services Canada, 2007.

Limited Information step, the practitioner provides general factual information that can range from disease transmission to physiology of sexual issues (e.g., return to sexual activity postsurgery) to occupational performance (e.g., dating etiquette and safety). The Specific Suggestions step is focused on client issues and problems specific to the client's occupational lifestyle and body structures and functions. Finally, the Intensive Therapy step involves a referral to a sexual health specialist.

This model can support and guide occupational therapy sexual health promotion and prevention interventions. For example, during an occupational therapy evaluation, a client stated that she was concerned about the spread and prevention of STIs relative to her teenagers' health. It is evident the client has given permission to discuss the topic openly with the practitioner. Occupation-centered intervention would focus on the client's mental health related to the concerns she has as a parent and the impact on her own occupational lifestyle, including the impact on her family. Health information could be provided that focuses on STI prevention and teen sexual health issues to help ameliorate concerns. If the client is familiar with computers, legitimate websites (e.g., CDC, WebMD, Go Ask Alice!) can be provided for independent exploration. After increased familiarity and rapport have been established with the practitioner, the client may feel safer, and meaningful dialogue can be evoked to guide future intervention strategies. The client may, for example, be concerned about the sexual identity of one of her children, or may have provided clear abstinence education to them, yet believes they are sexually active, which is emotionally difficult for her.

The focus of occupational therapy sexual health promotion is to help clients prevent occupational impairment relative to sexuality issues. In this case, actively listening to the client's concerns, providing accurate sexual health education and resources, role-playing scenarios, and having the client practice problem-solving can be a major step toward empowering her to have important dialogues with her children. In this way, the health promotion program continues to be occupation and client-centered. This could lead to improved mental health of the client and the family system and could help promote healthy sexual behaviors for her teenagers.

Using the Transtheoretical Stages of Change Model (DiClemente et al., 1991; McKenzie & Smeltzer, 2001), which is described in detail in Chapter 3 of this text, practitioners can impact safer sex practices among adolescents. First, a determination needs to be made as to the stage of the population or designated target group in terms of seeking and using sexual health education. Then, specific actions can be designed to facilitate movement from stage to stage. For example, strategically placed health information can assist with the movement

Table 16-5 *Healthy People 2010* Objectives Related to Sexual Health

Objective Number	Objective
7-2	Increase the proportion of middle, junior high, and senior high schools that provide school health education to prevent health problems in the following areas: unintentional injury; violence; suicide; tobacco use and addiction; alcohol and other drug use; unintended pregnancy, HIV/AIDS, and sexually transmitted disease (STD) infection; unhealthy dietary patterns; inadequate physical activity; and environmental health
13-5	(Developmental) Reduce the number of cases of HIV infection among adolescents and adults
13-6	Increase the proportion of sexually active persons who use condoms
13-7	(Developmental) Increase the number of HIV-positive persons who know their serostatus
13-8	Increase the proportion of substance abuse treatment facilities that offer HIV/AIDS education, counseling, and support
13-9	(Developmental) Increase the number of state prison systems that provide comprehensive HIV/AIDS, STDs, and tuberculosis (TB) education
13-10	(Developmental) Increase the proportion of inmates in state prison systems who receive voluntary HIV counseling and testing during incarceration
13-12	(Developmental) Increase the proportion of adults in publicly funded HIV counseling and testing sites who are screened for common bacterial STDs (chlamydia, gonorrhea, and syphilis) and are immunized against hepatitis B virus
13-13	Increase the proportion of HIV-infected adolescents and adults who receive testing, treatment, and prophylaxis consistent with current Public Health Service treatment guidelines
13-17	(Development) Reduce new cases of perinatally acquired HIV infection
25-1	Reduce the proportion of adolescents and young adults with *Chlamydia trachomatis* infections
25-12	(Developmental) Increase the number of positive messages related to responsible sexual behavior during weekday and nightly prime-time television programming
25-13	Increase the proportion of tribal, state, and local sexually transmitted disease programs that routinely offer hepatitis B vaccines to all STD clients
25-14	(Developmental) Increase the proportion of youth detention facilities and adult city or county jails that screen for common bacterial STDs within 24 hours of admission and treat STDs (when necessary) before persons are released
24-15	(Developmental) Increase the proportion of all local health departments that have contracts with managed care providers for the treatment of nonplan partners of patients with bacterial STDs (gonorrhea, syphilis, and chlamydia)
25-19	(Developmental) Increase the proportion of all STD clinical patients who are being treated for bacterial STDs (chlamydia, gonorrhea, and syphilis) and who are offered provider referral services for their sex partners

From *Healthy People 2010: Understanding and improving health,* by U.S. Department of Health and Human Services, 2000, Washington, DC: Government Printing Office.

from the precontemplation stage to contemplation such as in bus and train stations, bathrooms in coffee shops and bars, and other areas where adolescents gather (Fig. 16-2). A focus group may assist in determining what is and is not understood about safer sex practices by the targeted adolescents. (No actions may have been taken, as the population of adolescents may have had little knowledge.) In the contemplation and preparation stages, the broader group can be engaged in an educational series using a variety of teaching methods

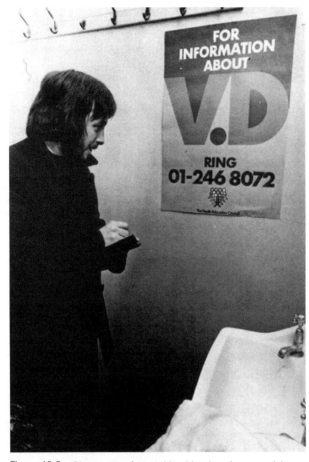

Figure 16-2   Placement of sexual health education materials promotes contemplation.

Reprinted with permission from the World Health Organization. Available from the National Library of Medicine.

(e.g., audiovisuals, lecture, peer educators, peers with STIs). The action stage focuses on goal planning regarding how and when to engage in safer sex and STI prevention, while the maintenance stage focuses on continuing to be vigilant about safer sex practices. Involving the population of adolescents in this type of occupational therapy program creates a client-centered focus.

Newly divorced or single adults may also benefit from occupational interventions to promote healthy dating and relationship building. Reentering the dating scene may be complicated and potentially overwhelming. Readiness to do so may depend upon the length of time away from dating, the individual's personality, current societal dating practices, and other factors. Prevention of STDs/STIs and HIV and a review of dating safety and etiquette can be helpful for this population as they navigate the possibilities for developing new partners.

Conclusion

This chapter included definitions of key terms related to sexual health and described implications for occupational therapy. The importance of being knowledgeable about STIs, including HIV and AIDS, was emphasized in order for occupational therapists and occupational therapy assistants to develop and implement effective educational occupation-based programs for individuals, communities, and populations. Disease prevention was discussed as a primary means for optimizing sexual health. A few key concepts are summarized here:

- Sexual expression begins in childhood and is a developmental process throughout one's lifetime.
- Personal responsibility for one's sexual health lies with each individual.
- There are many forms of sexual expression.
- Sexuality and sexual health are important for sustaining quality of life throughout the life span.
- In order to be optimally effective, sexual health information must be relevant to the culture, orientation, and level of understanding of targeted individuals, communities, and populations.
- Occupational therapy can develop a prominent role in the promotion of sexual health locally, nationally, and globally through occupation and client-centered programming.

Under the section "Areas of Occupation" in the *Framework, sexual activity* is defined as "engaging in activities that result in sexual satisfaction" (AOTA, 2008, p. 631). This definition can encompass activities of sexual expression, communication, and intimacy. However, a health-focused definition is needed if occupational therapists and occupational therapy assistants are to view sexual health in a holistic way and as an important contributor to a person's quality of life.

A definition of *sexual health* within the practice of occupational therapy is offered: Sexual health is that area of human function reflected in a person's ability to relate, communicate, express, be intimate, and engage in sexually satisfying ways consistent with the developmental level of the individual and the cultural norms of the society. These activities of sexuality affirm an individual's right to be a sexual being throughout the life span and are not limited to the sexual act. Sexually healthy individuals choose sexual activities that are meaningful to their lives, that are health promoting for oneself, and that are not harmful to others. A healthy society that promotes sexual health provides its members with the right, if they choose, to engage in healthy sexual relationships without being coerced, discriminated against, or have acts of violence thrust upon them because of their choices. This type of society promotes

Betty is a 52-year-old newly divorced executive with osteoarthritis, who has been referred to occupational therapy. During the evaluation, Betty states that during sexual intercourse, she has increased joint pain and asks for some suggestions. While the occupational therapist discusses adaptive positioning to ease her pain and increase sexual satisfaction, she also sees an opportunity to discuss how Betty is coping with daily life since her divorce as well as with her renewed occupation of dating. Betty explains that she feels more attractive when men wish to "sleep with me" and states that she only has sexual intercourse with men over 50 because "they are less prone to have a disease." She also states that she does not always have them use a condom, especially when the men ask nicely and tell her they are disease free.

From actively listening to Betty and asking questions that address all areas of occupational performance, the occupational therapist recognizes that Betty requires education on STIs, how to communicate with partners, and how to protect herself (and her partner). She also has a need for psychosocial interventions around issues of self-esteem and self-image, which can be hidden barriers to protecting herself

(e.g., if she feels "needed" and attractive, she may be less prone to using protection).

This example is used to demonstrate the necessity for occupational therapists to be holistic in their practice, to understand the need for broad interventions, and to understand how both sexual health promotion and positioning are important for Betty. There are multiple interventions possible in the area of sexual health. Improving the education of occupational therapy students regarding sexual health issues increases the likelihood that future practitioners will feel comfortable and capable of addressing the sexual health needs of clients.

Questions

1. What theoretical frameworks would support your evaluation and subsequent interventions?
2. What types of psychosocial interventions would you implement to help Betty?
3. Research women's health issues online and develop a prevention program for Betty.
4. What educational materials might you present to Betty to help her best understand the possible consequences of her actions? How might you make them occupation centered?

---

self-empowerment through chosen sexual activities and optimal sexual health.

> Because of the critical and life affirming significance of sexual and reproductive health for individuals, families, and society as a whole, it is important to ensure the conditions required to promote, protect, and maintain it are in place. Healthy societal values and attitudes about sexuality and reproduction, family, and community networks and supports, educational and economic opportunities, a healthy physical environment, and access to effective services all enable sexual and reproductive health. Investing in policies, programs, and initiatives to positively influence these conditions will offer excellent returns, now and far into the future. (Health Canada, 1999, p. 5)

▶ For Discussion and Review

1. Do you think people remain sexual throughout the life span? What is the evidence?
2. Why do you think the content on sexual behavior and health in *Healthy People 2010* is focused on

the adolescent/young adult population? Is there research to support your ideas?
3. What might be some occupational therapy interventions/health messages for an individual, community, and population regarding HIV and STI prevention? How might these health messages/interventions differ from other disciplines?
4. How is a person's health—sexually, emotionally, mentally, spiritually, and physically—affected when one experiences barriers that prevent communicating, performing, or engaging in sexual activities? Describe occupational therapy interventions that may be helpful in this situation.

▶ Research Questions

1. How does the sexual health of people with disabilities compare with nondisabled peers of similar backgrounds (e.g., age, ethnicity, educational backgrounds, income levels)?
2. According to the WHO (2002, ¶ 2),

> sexuality research must go beyond concerns related to behavior, numbers of partners and practices, to the

underlying social, cultural and economic factors that make individuals vulnerable to risks and affect the ways in which sex is sought, desired and/or refused by women, men and young people. Investigating sexuality in this way entails going beyond reproductive health by looking at sexual health holistically and comprehensively.

Reflecting on this recommendation, design an occupation-based sexual health research question that would address this concern.

References

Advocates for Youth. (2005). *Sexual development through the life cycle.* Retrieved April 7, 2005, from http://www.advocatesforyouth.org/lessonplans/sexdevelop.htm.

AIDS Alert. (2002, September). Unwitting trust of partners result in infection: Study shows how youth perceive trust. *Supplement to AIDS Alert, 17*(9), 113–14.

American Occupational Therapy Association. (1989). Uniform terminology for occupational therapy (2d ed.). *American Journal of Occupational Therapy, 43*(12), 808–15.

American Occupational Therapy Association. (1993). Core values and attitudes of occupational therapy practice. *American Journal of Occupational Therapy, 47,* 1085–86.

American Occupational Therapy Association. (1994). Uniform terminology for occupational therapy (3d ed.) *American Journal of Occupational Therapy, 48*(11), 1047–54.

American Occupational Therapy Association. (2004). *Commission on standards and ethics, standard operating procedures.* [Revised and adopted by Representative Assembly May, 2004]. Bethesda, MD: Author.

American Occupational Therapy Association. (2005a). *Guidelines to the occupational therapy code of ethics.* Retrieved January 23, 2006, from http://www.aota.org/members/area2/index.asp#7.

American Occupational Therapy Association. (2005b). Occupational therapy code of ethics (2005). *American Journal of Occupational Therapy, 59*(6), 639–42.

American Occupational Therapy Association. (2008). Occupational therapy practice framework: Domain and processes (2d ed.). *American Journal of Occupational Therapy, 66,* 625–83.

American Social Health Association. (2006a). *Sexual health glossary, R–Z.* Retrieved January 25, 2006, from http://www.ashastd.org/learn/learn_glossary_R_Z.cfm.

American Social Health Association. (2006b). *STD/STI Statistics: STD vs. STI.* Retrieved January 25, 2006, from http://www.ashastd.org/learn/learn_statistics_vs.cfm.

Annon, J. S. (1976). The P-LI-SS-IT model: A proposed conceptual scheme for the behavioral treatment of sexual problems. *Journal of Sexuality Education Therapy, 2,* 1–15.

Barrett, H. R. (1997). Women, occupation and health in rural Africa: Adaptation to a changing socioeconomic climate. *Journal of Occupational Science: Australia, 4,* 93–105.

Bedell, G. (2000). Daily life for eight urban gay men with HIV/AIDS. *American Journal of Occupational Therapy, 54,* 197–206.

Bellis, M. A., Hughes, K., Thomson, R., & Bennett, A. (2004). Sexual behavior of young people in international tourist resorts. *Sexually Transmitted Infections, 80,* 43–47.

Braveman, B. H. (2001). Development of a community-based return to work program for people with AIDS. *Occupational Therapy in Health Care, 13*(3/4). 113–31.

Brewer, S. (2004). *Intimate relations: Living and loving in later life.* London: Age Concern.

Centers for Disease Control and Prevention. (2003). Incorporating HIV prevention into the medical care of persons living with HIV. *Morbidity and Mortality Weekly Report, 52*(RR 12). Retrieved March 8, 2005, from http://www.cdc.gov/mmwr/preview/mmwrhtml/rr5212a1.htm.

Centers for Disease Control and Prevention. (2006). *Division of HIV/AIDS Prevention.* Retrieved January 17, 2006, from http://www.cdc.gov/hiv/dhap.htm.

Child Welfare League of America. (2005). *GLBTQ terminology.* Retrieved April 2, 2005, from http://www.cwla.org/programs/culture/glbtqterminology.htm.

Couldrick, L. (1999). Sexual issues within occupational therapy, part 2: Implications for education and practice. *British Journal of Occupational Therapy, 62,* 26–30.

Denton, R. (1987). AIDS guidelines for occupational therapy intervention. *American Journal of Occupational Therapy, 41,* 427–32.

DiClemente, C. C., Prochaska, J. O., Fairhurst, S. K., Velcier, W. F., Velasquez, M. M., & Rossi, J. S. (1991). The process of smoking cessation: An analysis of precontemplation, contemplation, and preparation stages of change. *Journal of Consulting and Clinical Psychology, 59,* 295–304.

Drench, M. E., Noonan, A. C., Sharby, N., & Ventura, S. H. (2006). Sexuality. In *Psychosocial aspects of health care* (2d ed., pp. 213–28). Upper Saddle River, NJ: Prentice Hall.

Eng, T. R., & Butler, W. T. (Eds.). (1996). *The hidden epidemic: Confronting sexually transmitted diseases.* Washington, DC: Institute of Medicine. Retrieved January 25, 2005, from http://books.nap.edu/html/epidemic/.

Gay and Lesbian Medical Association. (2000). *Elimination of health disparities based upon sexual orientation: Inclusion of sexual orientation as a demographic variable in Healthy People 2010 objectives.* Retrieved October 30, 2005, from http://www.glma.org/policy/hp2010/hp2010final.shtml.

Gay and Lesbian Medical Association. (2004). *Strategic Plan 2004–2007.* Retrieved October 30, 2005, from http://www.glma.org/images/GLMA_Strat_Plan_04.pdf.

Gay and Lesbian Medical Association and LGBT Experts. (2001). *Healthy People 2010 companion document for lesbian, gay, bisexual, and transgender (LGBT) health.* San Francisco: Gay and Lesbian Medical Association. Retrieved January 27, 2008, from http://www.nalgap.org/PDF/Resources/HP2010CDLGBTHealth.pdf.

Gender, A. R. (1992). An overview of the nurse's role in dealing with sexuality. *Sexuality and Disability, 10,* 71–79.

Giles, G. M., & Allen, M. E. (1987). AIDS, ARC and the occupational therapist. *British Journal of Occupational Therapy, 50,* 120–23.

Gordon, L. (1987). An occupational therapy protocol for the AIDS patient. *Physical Disabilities Special Interest Section Newsletter, 10*(3), 4–5.

Gutterman, L. (1990). A day treatment program for persons with AIDS. *American Journal of Occupational Therapy, 44,* 234–37.

Hansen, R. H., & Hinojosa, J. (2004). Occupational therapy's commitment to nondiscrimination and inclusion (edited 2004). *American Journal of Occupational Therapy, 58*(6), 668.

Health Canada. (1999). *Report from consultations on a framework for sexual and reproductive health.* Retrieved January 22, 2006, from http://www.hc-sc.gc.ca/hppb/srh/pubs/report/index.html.

Hebert, L. A. (1997). *Sex & back pain: Advice on restoring comfortable sex lost to back pain* (3d ed.). Bangor, ME: IMPACC.

Heckheimer, E. F. (1989). *Health promotion of the elderly in the community.* Philadelphia: Saunders.

Jackson, J. (1995). Sexual orientation: Relevance to occupational science and the practice of occupational therapy. *American Journal of Occupational Therapy, 49*(7), 669–79.

Johnson, J. A., & Pizzi, M. (Eds.). (1990). *Productive living strategies for people living with AIDS.* Binghamton, NY: Haworth Press.

Joint United Nations Programme on HIV/AIDS. (2004). *UNAIDS 2004 Report on the global AIDS epidemic.* Retrieved February 20, 2009, from http://www.unaids .org/bangkok2004/report_pdf.html.

Kann, L., Kinchen, S. A., Williams, B. I., Ross, J. G., Lowry, R., Grunbaum, J. A., Kolbe, L. J., & State and Local YRBSS Coordinators. (2000). Youth Risk Behavior Surveillance— United States, 1999. *Morbidity and Mortality Weekly Report, 49*(SS05), 1–96.

Kessel, B. (2001). Sexuality in the older person. *Age & Aging, 30*(2), 121–24.

Kingsley, P., & Molineux, M. (2000). True to our philosophy? Sexual orientation and occupation. *British Journal of Occupational Therapy, 63*(5), 205–10.

Kroll, K., & Klein, E. L. (1992). *Enabling romance: A guide to love, sex, and relationships for the disabled (and for the people who care about them).* New York: Woodbine House.

Laflin, M. (2002). Sexuality and the elderly. In C. B. Lewis (Ed.), *Aging: The health-care challenge* (4th ed., pp. 278–300). Philadelphia: F. A. Davis.

Lefkowitz, E. S., Boone, T. L., Au, T. K., & Sigma, M. (2003). No sex or safe sex? Mothers' and adolescents' discussions about sexuality and AIDS/HIV, *Health Education Research, 18*(3), 341–51.

McKenna, K. (2003). Sexuality and disability. In E. B. Crepeau, E. S. Cohn, & B. A. B., Schell (Eds.), *Willard and Spackman's occupational therapy* (10th ed., pp. 541–46). Philadelphia: Lippincott.

McKenzie, J. F., & Smeltzer, J. L. (2001). Theories and models commonly used for health promotion interventions. In J. F. McKenzie & J. L. Smeltzer (Eds.), *Planning, implementing, and evaluating health promotion programs: A primer* (pp. 137–69). Needham Heights, MA: Allyn & Bacon.

Miller, W. T. (1984). An occupational therapist as a sexual health clinician in the management of spinal cord injuries [Abstract]. *Canadian Journal of Occupational Therapy, 51*(4), 172–75. Retrieved March 10, 2005, from http://www.ncbi.nlm.nih.gov/entrez/query.fcgi?cmd= Retrieve&db=PubMed&list_uids=10268922&dopt=Abstract.

Molineux, M. (1997). HIV/AIDS: A new service continuum for occupational therapy. *British Journal of Occupational Therapy, 60*(5), 194–98.

National Association of School Nurses. (2003). *Position statement: Sexual orientation and gender identity/ expression.* Retrieved January 23, 2006, from http://www .nasn.org/Portals/0/positions/2003pssexual.pdf.

National Library of Medicine. (n.d.). *Whispers and shyness will not control AIDS; Education will!!* Retrieved February 2, 2006, from http://wwwihm.nlm.nih.gov/cgi-bin/gw_44_3/ chameleon.

Page, R. M., Hammermeister, J., Scanlan, A., & Gilbert, L. (1998). Is school sports participation a protective factor against adolescent health risks? *Journal of Health Education, 29*(3), 186–92.

Phillips, I. (2002). Occupational therapy students explore an area for future practice in HIV/AIDS community wellness [Abstract]. *AIDS Patient Care and STDS, 16,* 147–49.

Pizzi, M. (1990a). Nationally speaking: The transformation of HIV infection and AIDS in occupational therapy: Beginning the conversation. *American Journal of Occupational Therapy, 44*(3), 1–5.

Pizzi, M. (Ed.) (1990b). *Special issue of the American Journal of Occupational Therapy on HIV and AIDS.* Bethesda, MD: American Occupational Therapy Association.

Pizzi, M. (1992). Women, HIV infection and AIDS: Tapestries of life, death and empowerment. *American Journal of Occupational Therapy, 46,* 1021–27.

Pizzi, M. (2001). The Pizzi Holistic Wellness Assessment. *Community Occupational Therapy Education and Practice, 13*(3/4), 51–66.

Pizzi, M. (2004). HIV infection and AIDS. In H. Pendleton & W. Schultz-Krohn (Eds.), *Pedretti's occupational therapy: Practice skills for physical dysfunction* (6th ed., pp. 1193–1203). St. Louis, MO: Elsevier,

Robins, S. (2006). Understanding sexual minorities. In M. Royeen & J. L. Crabtree (Eds.), *Culture in rehabilitation: From competency to proficiency* (pp. 357–76). Upper Saddle River, NJ: Prentice Hall.

Sexuality Information and Education Council of the United States. (2001). *Lesbian, gay, bisexual and transgender youth issues.* Retrieved March 30, 2005, from http://63.73.227.69/pubs/fact/fact0013.html.

Sexuality Information and Education Council of the United States. (2004). *Guidelines for comprehensive sexuality education: Grades K through 12* (3d ed.). New York: Author. Available at http://www.siecus.org/pubs/fact/fact0003.html.

Spence, S. H. (1992). Psychosexual dysfunction in the elderly. *Behaviour Change, 9,* 55–64.

Toepell, A. R. (2003). The health belief model and safer sex: Implications for women's health. *Women's Health and*

Urban Life: An International and Interdisciplinary Journal, 2(1), 22–41.

U.S. Department of Health and Human Services. (2000). *Healthy People 2010: Understanding and improving health.* Washington, DC: U.S. Government Printing Office.

Wood, W., & Aull, M. R. (1990). Women and AIDS: Implications for occupational therapists. *Occupational Therapy in Health Care, 7*(2/3/4), 151–60.

World Health Organization. (n.d.). *Gender and reproductive rights: Sexual health.* Retrieved January 16, 2006, from http://www.who.int/reproductive-health/gender/sexual _health.html.

World Health Organization. (2002). *Working definition.* Retrieved January 16, 2006, from http://www.who.int/ reproductive-health/gender/sexual_health.html.

Yallop, S., & Fitzgerald, M. H. (1997). Exploration of occupational therapists' comfort with client sexuality issues. *Australian Occupational Therapy Journal, 44,* 53–60.

Chapter 17

Promoting Mental Health and Emotional Wellbeing

Marjorie E. Scaffa, Michael A. Pizzi, and S. Blaise Chromiak

The voices of the resilient send a powerful message: Personal perceptions and responses to stressful life events are crucial elements of survival, recovery, and rehabilitation, often transcending the reality of the situation or the interventions of others. The inner life . . . holds the potential for transforming traumas into varying degrees of triumph. Ironically, these same phenomena are often ignored in the clinical reasoning and practice of many health professions, including our own.

—Fine, 1991, p. 493

Learning Objectives

This chapter is designed to enable the reader to:

- Define mental health and identify its characteristics.
- Describe the emerging science of positive psychology.
- Discuss the implications of the Ryff and Keyes's (1995) Model of Complete Mental Health.
- Identify a variety of mental health promotion approaches.
- Discuss the role of occupational therapy in mental health promotion.
- Utilize the concept of resilience in clinical reasoning and practice to promote mental health.

Key Terms

Agency thinking	Emotional understanding	Mental health	Resilience
Allostatic load	Emotional wellbeing	Mental health promotion	Resiliency
Attachment	Goals thinking	Optimism	Self-efficacy
Emotional intelligence	Learned optimism	Pathways thinking	Social support
Emotional management		Positive psychology	Spirituality

Introduction

Historically, mental health promotion in occupational therapy can be traced to the roots of the profession and the advent of moral treatment. Moral treatment was a humanistic view of the human being as a person who had reason and ability and who could survive in the world given the right opportunities. Both Pinel and Tuke, moral treatment advocates, recognized the power of occupation to help restore health and wellbeing to people with mental illness. The basic principles of occupational therapy at the time included

- a belief in the uniqueness of each human being;

- a clear focus on the power of meaningful occupational participation to improve health; and
- a holistic perspective of the person in context in order to enable participation (Bing, 1981).

Although the moral treatment philosophy was applied to interventions for persons with mental illness, the principles are also relevant for promoting mental health for all persons.

In any given year, approximately 20% of the U.S. population are affected by mental illness. Mental disorders affect all ethnic and racial groups and persons of every socioeconomic level across the life span. Depression, the most common mental health disorder, is a leading cause of disability and premature death in the United States, ranked second only to heart disease (U.S. Department of Health and Human Services [USDHHS]), 2000). The impact of mental illness on physical health and productivity is often severely underestimated. Based on measures of disability-adjusted life years, mental illness is responsible for at least 10% of the global burden of disease, and this is predicted to increase to 15% by the year 2020. Clearly, mental illness is a significant threat to individual and community quality of life and public health throughout the world (Herrman, 2001; World Health Organization [WHO], 2004).

Although treatments, medications, and psychological therapy for mental disorders like depression are highly effective, questions remain: Can mental disorders, particularly depression, be prevented? Can overall mental health and resilience be enhanced in order to prevent the development of certain mental illnesses? Research is beginning to demonstrate that mental health promotion can be effective in enhancing resilience, coping, and adaptation to adversity. According to *Healthy People 2010,* "Promising universal and targeted preventive interventions, implemented according to scientific recommendations, have great potential to reduce the risk for mental disorders and the burden of suffering in vulnerable populations" (USDHHS, 2000, p. 18-9).

The U.S. Surgeon General's report regarding mental health emphasizes the interdependent nature of physical and mental health and wellbeing and focuses attention on the mental health needs of persons across the life span. The report is based on the best available scientific evidence and addresses the unique mental health needs of children, adolescents, adults, and the elderly. Each stage of life is associated with specific vulnerabilities for mental illness and distinct capacities for mental health. Children and adolescents with positive mental health "have a sense of identity and self-worth, sound family and peer relationships, an ability to be productive and to learn, and a capacity to tackle developmental challenges and use cultural resources to maximize growth" (WHO, 2005, p. 2, ¶ 1). Also in the U.S. Surgeon General's report, mental health is viewed as a dynamic phenomenon that reflects an individual's genetic predispositions, life experiences, and social environment (USDHHS, 1999).

This chapter focuses on the definitions and characteristics of mental health, the emerging science of positive psychology, research on mental health promotion, and strategies for promoting mental health. This chapter will not consider treatment of mental illness. There are many other occupational therapy texts that provide this information. However, the principles of positive psychology and the development of resilience discussed here are very applicable to persons with disabilities and those with mental disorders. The main purpose of this chapter is to describe concepts of mental health promotion and their efficacy to enhance psychological and emotional wellbeing for all persons.

Definitions of Mental Health

There are many definitions of mental health, but they all have one thing in common: They recognize that mental health is not simply the absence of mental illness. This idea parallels the World Health Organization's position that health is not simply the absence of illness and disease (WHO, 1946). Rather, mental health is a state where a set of wellbeing characteristics is present, at a specific level and for a specified duration. These characteristics coincide with distinctive emotional, psychological, and social functioning (Keyes & Lopez, 2005).

In *Healthy People 2010,* **mental health** is defined as "a state of successful performance of mental functioning resulting in productive activities, fulfilling relationships with other people, and the ability to adapt to change and cope with adversity" (USDHHS, 2000, p. 18-3). With a similar emphasis, the WHO (2001) defines mental health as "a state of wellbeing in which the individual realizes his or her own abilities, can cope with the normal stresses of life, can work productively and fruitfully, and is able to make a contribution to his or her community" (¶ 2).

The term *positive mental health,* often used synonymously with *subjective wellbeing,* has been studied as a cluster of specific dimensions of wellbeing rather than as a complete entity. These dimensions include the perceptions and evaluations of individuals regarding their own lives in three areas: emotional wellbeing, positive psychological functioning, and positive social functioning (Keyes & Lopez, 2005). **Emotional wellbeing** is comprised of positive affect and overall life satisfaction. The Successful Midlife in the U.S. (MIDUS) study (MacArthur Foundation, 1995) supported the above dimensions and the finding that satisfaction and happiness are related but distinct constructs.

Positive psychological functioning is generally viewed as having six dimensions: self-acceptance, personal growth, purpose in life, environmental mastery, autonomy, and positive relations with others (see Content Box 17-1). These dimensions of psychological wellbeing are accepted as reliable and well validated, and the MIDUS study confirmed the usefulness of the six-factor structure in a large representative and random sample of adults in the United States (Keyes & Lopez, 2005).

Positive social functioning includes five dimensions indicating social wellbeing: social coherence, social actualization, social integration, social acceptance, and social contribution (see Content Box 17-2). These dimensions derive from individuals' evaluations and

Content Box 17-1

Dimensions of Psychological Wellbeing

- *Self-acceptance:* One has a positive appraisal of self, past life, and the multiple aspects of oneself.
- *Personal growth:* One has a sense of personal effectiveness and an openness to continued development, fulfillment of potential, and new experiences.
- *Purpose in life:* One has goals and beliefs that give a sense of direction and purpose to life.
- *Environmental:* One has an ability to respond to environmental demands and mastery to choose personally meaningful contexts.
- *Autonomy:* One has an ability to make decisions independently and adheres to standards over social pressure.
- *Positive:* One has an ability to develop and maintain caring relationships and is able to exhibit affection, empathy, and intimacy with others.

Adapted from "Toward a science of mental health: Positive directions in diagnosis and interventions" by C. L. Keyes & S. J. Lopez, 2005, in C. R. Snyder & S. J. Lopez (Eds.), *Handbook of positive psychology* (pp. 45–59). By permission of Oxford University Press, Inc.

Content Box 17-2

Dimensions of Social Wellbeing

- *Social coherence*   One generally envisions a logical and predictable social world and cares about society.
- *Social actualization*   One has a generally positive world view where society is believed to be growing in a positive direction.
- *Social integration*   One generally has a sense of belonging to, and receives support from the community.
- *Social acceptance*   One is generally accepting of and positive toward others.
- *Social contributions*   One generally believes in the value of one's contributions to society.

Adapted from "Toward a science of mental health: Positive directions in diagnosis and interventions" by C. L. Keyes & S. J. Lopez, 2005, in C. R. Snyder & S. J. Lopez (Eds.), *Handbook of positive psychology* (pp. 45–59). By permission of Oxford University Press, Inc.

have been confirmed as reliable and valid constructs (Keyes & Lopez, 2005). Mental health, subjective wellbeing, and positive psychological and social functioning have been topics of study in the field of positive psychology.

Positive Psychology

Martin Seligman is frequently considered to be one of the founders of positive psychology. His work shifted the focus of psychology from a pathology-based perspective to a strength-enhancing practice. This movement has been embraced by the American Psychological Association and is certainly a paradigm shift in psychology that should resonate with occupational therapy practitioners. **Positive psychology** focuses on positive subjective experiences, including quality of life, happiness, satisfaction, wellbeing, optimism, hope, and joy. The practice of positive psychology is about identifying and nurturing positive qualities and helping people find the best possible environments in which to live, happily and productively, using their strengths. The scientific discipline of positive psychology is concerned with individual human traits and social or civic values that enhance wellbeing. According to Seligman (2005),

> Psychology is not just the study of disease, weakness and damage; it is also the study of strength and virtue. Treatment is not just fixing what is wrong; it is also building what is right. Psychology is not just about illness or health; it is also about work, education, insight, love, growth and play. (p. 4)

Positive human traits can act as buffers to prevent the development of mental illness. Therefore, cultivating personal and social strengths may be an effective prevention approach.

Mental health treatments have traditionally been aimed at symptom reduction. This was believed to be the best primary goal, especially when the community mental health system was not nearly as available as it is today. The positive psychology movement endeavors to open the mental health field toward finding ways to measure client wellbeing and to diagnose states of mental health. This paradigm shift envisions the pursuit of loftier goals for individuals, such as the promotion of quality of life and even the attainment of flourishing in life (Keyes & Lopez, 2005).

The interchange that has been stimulated reflects a move to connect diagnosis and treatment. This trend shifts diagnostic systems and introduces alternative treatment options to the field. This shift is envisioned as an additive change process rather than as keeping the status quo of problem management and symptom relief. A new outlook is emerging, and it may force fresh ideas on issues such as how to choose persons as candidates for psychotherapeutic interventions; what constitutes a successful treatment outcome for an individual; and what promotes growth, change, and wellbeing (Keyes & Lopez, 2005).

The system changes in mental health have been helped along by several trends in the real world, including the notion that clients are active seekers of health, are agents in their own change, and even are self-healers capable of reaching their optimum health status (Keyes & Lopez, 2005). The notion of clients as self-healers, seekers of health, and personal change agents, combined with the push to destigmatize mental illness, has also caused a paradigm shift in the approach to treating mental illness.

Clients now are not viewed as passive receivers of the "healing magic" of psychology professionals but actually assume the bulk of "change responsibility" (Keyes & Lopez, 2005). In the working relationship of the client and the socially sanctioned healer, positive change is not just hoped for but expected. This "new direction" of care focuses on the strengths and resources of clients rather than on their weaknesses and limitations. The emphasis has shifted from where people have been to where they want to go (Keyes & Lopez, 2005).

The self-help movement also fosters the view of the Keyes model, which holds that people move through stages of being and healing. Clinicians are more aware that the individual focus of treatment must shift to a prevention approach, where effecting change in the environment, as well as individuals, is needed (Keyes & Lopez, 2005). One of the ways prevention may work to decrease the prevalence (number of cases) and the incidence (number of new cases) is to bring a broader view of what is considered effective life functioning. In the *DSM-IV-TR* (American Psychiatric Association, 2000), the Global Assessment of Functioning (GAF) scale measures change in symptoms and vitality. A score of 100 means "superior functioning in a wide range of activities, life's problems never seem to get out of hand, is sought out by others because of his or her many positive qualities" (p. 34).

It is clear that there is more to moving toward healthy functioning than just alleviating symptoms. A model of mental health, as opposed to one focused on mental illness, is explained in more depth below. This model details how prevention can block declines in health, how intervention can eliminate barriers to growth and wellbeing, and how health promotion can help people go beyond their baseline functioning to a more optimal life state even after a mental health decompensation (Keyes & Lopez, 2005).

A Model of Complete Mental Health

A model for mental health and mental illness that uses two separate but interacting continua is Ryff and Keyes's (1995) Model of Complete Mental Health. Here, the mental health and mental illness dimensions are combined, and two states of mental health and two states of mental illness are postulated. There is a complete state and an incomplete state of both mental health and mental illness (see Fig. 17-1).

These authors posit that mental health is not simply the absence of mental illness and not simply the presence of subjective wellbeing. This model accounts for more variation in the level of mental health and mental illness of individuals, and it is therefore more reflective of real life. It allows for individuals to move among the four states and reflects that sometimes coping is good,

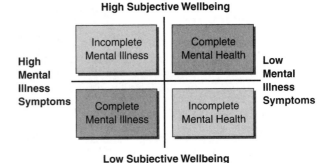

Figure 17-1 Model of Complete Mental Health.

Adapted from "Toward a science of mental health: Positive directions in diagnosis and interventions" by C. L. Keyes & S. J. Lopez, 2005, in C. R. Snyder & S. J. Lopez (Eds.), Handbook of positive psychology *(pp. 45–59). By permission of Oxford University Press, Inc.*

and sometimes there is decompensation from complete mental health or incomplete compensation from complete mental illness, where coping levels are poor (Keyes & Lopez, 2005).

The states of complete mental health and complete mental illness are easier to identify. Complete mental health combines the absence of recent mental illness and high levels of emotional, psychological, and social wellbeing. Thus, mentally healthy adults will exhibit high psychological and social functioning and emotional vitality, with high levels of life satisfaction and happiness (Ryff & Keyes, 1995).

Complete mental illness states combine high levels of mental illness symptoms, a recent diagnosis of a mental condition, and low levels of emotional, psychological, and social wellbeing. For example, with depression, mentally unhealthy adults will exhibit the signs of depression, will usually be unhappy and feel poorly about their lives, and will be functioning poorly in the psychological and social areas (Ryff & Keyes, 1995).

In the other two areas—incomplete mental health and incomplete mental illness—the state of incomplete mental health includes persons, with the absence of recent mental illness, who combine low levels of wellbeing in the psychological, social, and emotional areas. This group may include chronic malcontents and complainers, the "worried well," or those "in a rut" (Keyes & Lopez, 2005).

The state of incomplete mental illness is where mental illness symptoms, or a recent mental illness episode, join with the individual's perception of relative happiness and satisfaction with their lives, and they appear to be functioning at an adequate to fairly high level in the psychological and social areas. This group includes apparently high-functioning persons who may have serious substance-use issues and yet may be able to perform well enough at work to retain their jobs (Keyes & Lopez, 2005).

Keyes (2002, 2005) defines these groups more thoroughly: The completely mentally healthy are described as *flourishing* and the completely mentally ill as *floundering*. A person who is flourishing experiences high levels of emotional wellbeing and attains high levels of positive psychological and social functioning. Keyes (2002) describes persons with incomplete mental health as *languishing*. These individuals experience low levels of emotional wellbeing and attain low levels of positive functioning. Languishing is associated with significant levels of impairment in daily living and work productivity. In a study of over 3000 adults, 12% met the criteria for languishing. These are individuals who are not diagnosed with mental illness yet experience emotional distress that limits their effective participation in occupations. Another 14% met the *DSM-IV TR* (American Psychiatric Association, 2000) criteria for major depressive episode (Keyes, 2002). Keyes and Haidt (2003) describe individuals categorized with incomplete mental illness as *struggling* with life.

This conceptualization of mental health and mental illness has several implications. First, it is possible to be diagnosed with a mental illness and still have a reasonably good level of mental health and wellbeing; second, although a mental illness may not be curable, it is possible and desirable to promote the mental health and wellbeing of persons with mental disorders; and third, many people without diagnosed mental disorders are not, by virtue of this lack of pathology, mentally healthy and are in need of mental health promotion services to enhance their subjective wellbeing and optimal development (Tudor, 1996).

Characteristics of Mentally Healthy People

Mentally healthy individuals demonstrate a variety of common characteristics. Typically they perceive and exercise some control over their lives; they demonstrate the ability to learn, grow, and develop; and they feel loved, understood, and valued. In general, mentally healthy people have a zest for life, are self-accepting, and have a healthy level of self-esteem; they are resilient, optimistic, and hopeful. However, no two people are identical, and each of us will manifest characteristics of mental health in different ways at different times. No one can be expected to demonstrate all the characteristics all the time. Mental health is a fluid condition, not constant, static, or rigid. However, the number of characteristics displayed and their frequency

and duration may be a good measure of a person's mental health at any given moment in time (Donnelly, Eburne, & Kittleson, 2001).

According to the National Mental Health Association (1996), mental health encompasses feelings people have about themselves and about others and the ability to meet and handle the demands of life. Regarding feelings about the self, mentally healthy people

- have a realistic view of themselves, including their talents and abilities;
- effectively cope with success and disappointment;
- accept their limitations;
- experience reasonable pride in their accomplishments;
- have a high level of self-awareness; and
- appreciate their emotions rather than being troubled by them.

With respect to other people, mentally healthy people

- are able to establish and maintain meaningful relationships;
- give and receive love;
- respect others' differences;
- have the capacity to focus on the needs and interests of others; and
- demonstrate a healthy sense of caring toward others.

In meeting and handling the demands of life, mentally healthy people

- accept responsibilities and plan effective strategies to meet these obligations;
- do not fear the future;
- make the best use of their talents and abilities;
- plan for the future and set realistic goals; and
- are able to manage the unexpected.

The typologies of mental health characteristics are nearly limitless. For example, Carl Rogers (1961), an early proponent of the human potential movement, advocated for a positive perspective on mental health and described the characteristics of the *fully functioning human being*. According to Rogers (1961), the fully functioning person seeks and welcomes new experiences, is spontaneous and adaptable, has the capacity to make choices free from past constraints, trusts their feelings and impressions, and is creative in meetings life's challenges. More recently, Tudor (1996) identified eight elements of mental health and viewed these as potential targets for health promotion: coping, stress management, self-concept, self-esteem, self-development, autonomy, change, and social support. Donnelly and colleagues (2001) identify 10 characteristics:

- A generally positive outlook on life
- Realistic expectations

- Effective management of emotions
- Ability to have satisfying relationships with others
- Healthy and reasonable appetites for enjoyment
- Effective coping skills
- Spirituality or sense of purpose in life
- Honest self-appraisal and self-esteem
- Accurate and realistic perception of the world, past, present, and future
- Ability to gain support from others without becoming overly dependent

Assessing Mental Health

A holistic evaluation of mental health requires a multi-faceted approach that assesses the person's strengths, limitations, and interaction with the environment. In traditional psychiatry and psychology, the practitioner attempts to identify pathology and categorize a person's dysfunction in order to develop a treatment plan to remediate these deficits. However, from a positive psychology perspective, assessment is designed not only to identify the limiting characteristics or deficiencies of the individual (client weaknesses) but also

- the person's strengths and assets—for example, motivation, coping, and cognitive resources (client assets);
- the resources and opportunities in the environment—for example, family networks, social support, community and church groups (environmental assets); and
- the deficiencies, barriers, and destructive factors in the environment (environmental limitations).

This is referred to as the Four-Front, or Four-Level Matrix, approach to assessment (Snyder, Ritschel, Rand, & Berg, 2006; Wright & Lopez, 2005). The Four-Level Matrix has two dimensions: valence (assets and weaknesses) and source (the individual and the environment). The result is a four-cell matrix (Fig. 17-2). Snyder, Ritschel, and colleagues (2006) advocate the systematic application of this matrix during assessment, asking questions and making observations about all four cells and organizing and recording the results directly on the matrix.

The environment is a key component (50%) of the matrix assessment. Human beings live, work, and play in a variety of contexts. On a daily basis, individuals use a combination of strengths and weaknesses to function in a variety of environments. Therefore, in order to adequately understand a person's behaviors, one must explore the environments in which these behaviors occur. Attributing all of a person's problems to the individual without consideration of the contexts in which they must function leads to victim

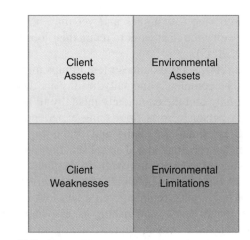

Figure 17-2 Four-cell matrix.

From "Twenty-first century graduate education in clinical psychology: A four level matrix approach" by C. R. Snyder & T. R. Elliott, ©2005, Journal of Clinical Psychology, 61*(9), 1033–54. Reproduced with permission of John Wiley & Sons, Inc.*

blaming. Unhealthy environments may be a source of the person's problems, so the environment may be a target for intervention in order to improve quality of life and emotional wellbeing. In addition, evaluating the environment "helps delineate how pervasive or circumscribed any particular problem might be" by determining the degree to which a person alters or fails to alter their behavior across situations (Snyder, Ritschel, et al., 2006, p. 35).

Some challenges involved in using the matrix include distinguishing between characteristics of the individual and aspects of the environment, and determining the extent to which certain characteristics are strengths or weaknesses. Due to the interaction between individuals and their environment, it may be difficult to determine the source of the strength or weakness. For example, a person who reports marital discord may have personality characteristics that interfere with optimal dyadic functioning (an aspect of the individual), or a family-in-law that is intrusive and causes conflict in the marital relationship (an aspect of the environment), or a combination of the two. In addition, some characteristics may be adaptive in some settings and maladaptive in others. Strengths may become weaknesses if they are overused, used inappropriately, or used in the wrong context. For example, the attribute of empathy is a valued strength but when misdirected may produce inappropriate boundary-crossing behavior in professional relationships.

One goal of assessment is to facilitate the development and implementation of an optimal intervention. This includes identifying "assets (psychological or environmental) that can help the person to be more resilient when encountering future challenges" (Snyder, Lopez, Edwards, et al., 2003, p. 33). It is important to recognize that strengths and limiting factors, both internal and external to the individual, are not all-or-nothing phenomena; rather, these characteristics occur on a continuum from very high levels to very low levels.

Assessing only a client's problems and deficits can have multiple negative consequences. It may lead to blaming the victim, having a negative bias toward the client, and introducing a destructive self-fulfilling prophecy in which the client acts and the practitioner responds in accordance with the negative label. On the other hand, inquiring about a client's strengths can have multiple beneficial effects. It indicates to the client that the practitioner is concerned about the whole person and not solely their diagnosis. This can facilitate rapport and trust in the therapeutic relationship. In addition, it encourages the client to examine their assets and determine how best to utilize them to enhance their mental health. This enables the client to reclaim some self-worth and empowers them to act on their own behalf (Snyder, Ritschel, et al., 2006).

Evaluation data can be gathered through a variety of assessment techniques, including interviews, checklists, observation, questionnaires, and psychological tests. Integrating all these data can be challenging, as the internal and external assets and liabilities are interdependent and in constant interaction. There are many assessments designed to identify psychological deficits and mental disorders but few that measure psychological strengths and global mental health. One instrument that shows promise is the Values in Action Inventory of Strengths (VIA-IS) developed by Peterson and Seligman (2004). The VIA-IS was designed to assess individual character strengths on continua from high levels to low levels of each trait. The latest version of the tool consists of 240 items assessing 24 strengths using a five-point Likert scale. It is available in paper-and-pencil and online versions and takes approximately 30 minutes to complete. A report is generated that identifies the person's top five strengths, which are referred to as *signature strengths* (Snyder & Lopez, 2007).

In addition to the VIA-IS, a variety of assessment tools exist to measure individuals' specific character strengths, such as optimism, self-efficacy, creativity, resilience, emotional intelligence, hope, and other positive psychological attributes. A sampling of these assessments can be found in Table 17-1. At present, assessments that measure environmental assets and limitations are few. However, instruments exist that measure family environment, organizational climate in work settings, and instructional environments in schools. It is important to not only assess the properties of home, work, and school environments, but also the client's perceptions of these contexts (Lopez & Snyder, 2003).

Mental Health Promotion

Everyone has mental health needs, regardless of whether or not they have a diagnosis of a mental disorder; therefore, mental health promotion applies to the whole population in the context of everyday life. Mental health needs are met, or not met, within families, through friendships, at school and work, and in communities. Although the need for mental health promotion is universally relevant, little attention has been devoted to enhancing mental health in any systematic way. **Mental health promotion** consists of any actions, activities, and strategies designed to foster, protect, and enhance the mental wellbeing of individuals, families, groups, or communities and to build individual and community capacity for positive mental health. The potential benefits of mental health promotion include

- enhanced physical and mental health and wellbeing;
- increased emotional resilience;
- reduced incidence of mental disorders;
- improved quality of life;
- higher productivity;
- greater social inclusion and participation; and
- increased mental health literacy and decreased stigma.

Principles of Mental Health Promotion

The promotion of mental health and the prevention and treatment of mental illness are complementary goals, but the methods used to achieve these ends are different. Prevention activities are often categorized by stage of intervention. For example, primary prevention focuses on preventing the onset of disease or illness, secondary prevention focuses on minimizing the duration and disability associated with disease, and tertiary prevention focuses on reducing negative sequelae. Health promotion activities are often categorized based on risk level; approaches directed at an entire population to enhance wellbeing are described as *universal,* while health promotion strategies that are directed at higher risk population subgroups are called *selective.* Health promotion efforts are considered *indicated* if they are targeted at high-risk individuals who are in the early stages of symptom development (Herrman, 2001).

Evidence regarding risk and protective factors is particularly strong with respect to the impact of early childhood experiences. It is believed that

good mental health in childhood is a prerequisite for optimal psychological development, productive social relationships, effective learning, an ability to care for self, good physical health and effective economic participation as adults. This can be done by reducing the impact of risk factors on the one hand,

Table 17–1 **Positive Psychological Assessments**

Name of Instrument	Description
Attributional Style Questionnaire (ASQ)	Measures how people explain negative events or to what they attribute these events. Presents 12 hypothetical events (6 positive and 6 negative) that are rated on a seven-point scale that measures the degree to which the attributed cause is internal/external, stable/unstable, and specific/global.
Children's Attributional Style Questionnaire (CASQ)	Measures how children (aged 8 to 14) explain negative events or to what they attribute these events. Presents 48 hypothetical events (24 positive and 24 negative) in a forced choice format.
Life Orientation Test (LOT)	Measures levels of optimism and pessimism. Consists of eight coded items plus fillers; half are framed in an optimistic manner, the others in a pessimistic manner. The respondent indicates their level of agreement/disagreement with each item.
Adult State Hope Scale	A six-item self-report scale that measures goal-directed thinking at any given point in time. Includes agency and pathways thinking subscores.
Children's Hope Scale	Consists of six items, designed for children aged 7 to 16. Ratings are on a six-point scale.
Problem Solving Inventory	This is a self-appraisal or personal perception of problem-solving ability and behaviors and attitudes associated with problem-solving. Assesses problem-solving confidence, approach-avoidance style, and personal control.
Torrance Tests of Creative Thinking (TTCT)	Available in two forms, nonverbal and verbal. Assesses four creative abilities: fluency, flexibility, originality, and elaboration. The nonverbal form requires respondents to draw additional lines to elaborate on a shape and to draw as many different pictures as possible using the same shape. The verbal version requires respondents to generate questions, alternative uses, and guesses in response to six activities.
Rosenberg Self-Esteem Scale	Measures global self-esteem using a 10-item scale that the respondent rates on a strongly agree to strongly disagree scale.
Mayer-Salovey-Caruso Emotional Intelligence Test	Assesses four aspects of emotional intelligence: perceiving emotion, using emotion to facilitate thought, understanding emotion, and managing emotion. Uses photographs and scenarios to measure emotional intelligence skills.

From *Positive psychological assessment: A handbook of models and measures* by S. J. Lopez & C. R. Snyder, 2003, Washington, DC: American Psychological Association.

and by enhancing the effects of protective factors on the other. (WHO, 2005, p. 7, ¶ 4)

Risk and protective factors fall into several categories: individual factors, family factors, school context, life events and situations, and community and cultural factors (United Kingdom, Department of Health, 2001). Examples of risk and protective factors well supported in the literature can be found in Table 17-2. The evidence on risk and protective factors can provide a foundation

for designing mental health promotion interventions for schools, workplaces, and communities.

Research demonstrates that stressful life events are risk factors that influence the onset and outcome of a variety of disorders, both physical and mental. These events, in the presence of certain predisposing vulnerabilities, can lead to significant impairment. A goal of mental health promotion is to decrease the number and severity of life stressors and increase the capabilities of individuals and communities to respond effectively

Table 17–2 Evidence-Based Risk and Protective Factors for Mental Health

Category	Risk Factors	Protective Factors
Individual	Prematurity, low birth weight, or other birth complications	Adequate nutrition
	Poor health in infancy	Attachment to family
	Insecure attachment to parents	School achievement
	Difficult temperament	Internal locus of control
	Poor social skills	Social competence
	Low self-esteem	Optimism
	Impulsivity	Problem-solving skills
	Alienation	Adaptive coping style
	Hopelessness	Positive self-related cognitions
		Feeling respected, valued, and supported
Family	Having a teenage mother	Supportive, caring parent
	Absence of father in childhood	Secure, stable family
	Family violence and disharmony	More than 2 years between siblings
	Marital discord in parents	Strong family norms and morality
	Poor supervision and monitoring of child	Family harmony
	Long-term parental unemployment	
	Parental substance abuse	
	Harsh or inconsistent discipline style	
	Social isolation	
	Lack of warmth and affection	
School Context	Bullying	Sense of belonging
	Peer rejection	Positive peer group
	School failure	Opportunities for success
	Deviant peer group	Recognition of achievement
	Poor attachment to school	Positive school climate
Life Events and Situations	Physical, psychological, and sexual abuse	Economic security
	Divorce	Good physical health
	Death of a family member	Involvement with significant others
	Homelessness	
	Poverty	
	War or natural disasters	
	Frequent moves and school transitions	
Community and Cultural Factors	Discrimination	Sense of belonging
	Isolation, alienation	Participation in community organizations
	Neighborhood violence and crime	Access to support services
	Poor housing conditions	Attachment to community
	Lack of support services in community	Strong community networks
	Rapid social change	

Adapted from *Making it happen: A guide to delivering mental health promotion*, United Kingdom, Department of Health, 2001, London: Crown Copyright.

to these inevitable events. Mental health promotion also strives to enhance resiliency or protective factors and reduce risk factors at individual community and policy levels.

The underlying principles of mental health promotion are the same as those of health promotion in general and include the following:

- A holistic, biopsychosocial orientation to health
- Promoting health and quality of life, as well as preventing illness
- Intervening at a variety of levels, including community and policy levels, and not exclusively focused at the individual level
- Establishing collaborative partnerships and alliances, bringing together diverse constituencies for a common goal
- Client and community participation in program design, implementation, and evaluation (Secker, 1998)

Comprehensive mental health promotion approaches include a balance of interventions designed to strengthen individuals and families, strengthen communities, and reduce societal and structural barriers to mental health. All these interventions can apply to the general population, vulnerable groups, high-risk individuals, and persons with mental disorders. Examples of each of these areas of intervention are provided in Content Box 17-3.

Content Box 17-3

Examples of Mental Health Promotion Interventions

Strengthen Individuals and Families
- Life skills and coping training
- Self-esteem development
- Relationship and parenting skills
- Adaptive coping
- Domestic violence prevention
- Physical activity and recreation programs

Strengthen Communities
- Increasing social inclusion and participation
- Enhancing neighborhood environments
- Appropriate childcare
- Self-help programs
- School violence prevention
- Community safety
- Social support

Reduce Societal and Structural Barriers
- Meaningful employment
- Housing
- Access to high-quality education

Strategies for Promoting Mental Health

Although the research on the efficacy of mental health promotion is limited, there is scientific evidence that mental health can be enhanced through public health and social interventions (WHO, 2004). Programs and strategies that show promise include

- early childhood and preschool psychosocial interventions;
- school and community violence-prevention programs;
- school-based mental health promotion activities;
- mental health interventions in the workplace (e.g., stress management);
- intergenerational, bereavement, and social support programs for the elderly;
- economic and social empowerment programs for women;
- postdisaster psychological and social preventive interventions; and
- community development initiatives (WHO, 2004).

Snyder and Lopez (2005) created a typology for positive psychological approaches and mental health promotion. They categorized strategies into emotion-focused, cognitive-focused, self-based, interpersonal, and biological approaches. Examples of targets of intervention in each of these approaches are provided in Content Box 17-4. It is beyond the scope of this chapter to describe all the intervention strategies; however, a few will be described here for potential use in occupation-based mental health promotion. These include the concepts of resilience, emotional intelligence, self-efficacy, learned optimism, hope, social support, and spirituality as they relate to mental health.

Resilience

Resilience is "characterized by patterns of positive adaptation in the context of significant adversity or risk" (Masten & Reed, 2005, p. 75). Positive adaptation consists of two components: internal adaptation (a positive psychological adjustment as opposed to emotional distress and dysfunction) and external adaptation (positive and effective behavioral responses to extenuating circumstances). Adversity can manifest as a single event that overwhelms a person's ability to cope, such as a disaster, or as an accumulation of stressors and risk factors over time.

Resilience can also be described as "a force within everyone that drives them to seek self actualization, altruism, wisdom, and be in harmony with a spiritual

Content Box 17-4

Examples of Mental Health Promotion Concepts by Category

Emotion-Focused Approaches
- Subjective wellbeing
- Resilience
- Self-esteem
- Positive affectivity
- Emotional intelligence
- Flow

Cognitive-Focused Approaches
- Creativity
- Self-efficacy
- Learned optimism
- Problem-solving
- Hope theory
- Personal causation

Self-Based Approaches
- Reality negotiation
- Authenticity
- Humility
- Uniqueness seeking

Interpersonal Approaches
- Compassion
- Forgiveness
- Gratitude
- Social support
- Empathy and altruism
- Moral motivation

Biological Approach
- Hardiness

Specific Coping Approaches
- Personal narrative
- Overcoming loss
- Pursuit of meaningfulness
- Humor
- Meditation
- Spirituality

Data from *Handbook of positive psychology* by C. R. Snyder & S. J. Lopez. (Eds.), 2005, New York: Oxford University Press.

factors, or resources, included competence (positive social, academic, and physical skills and self-worth), positive coping styles, sense of humor, connectedness (with parents or adults who demonstrate caring), and knowledge of health behaviors and health risks. The YRF describes these protective factors as they relate to adolescent development and how best to fortify them with strategies for developing resilience. According to Rew and Horner (2003), "early interventions that enhance protective resources, in spite of multiple individual and sociocultural risk factors, must be developed and tested to promote the health and well-being of adolescents" (p. 386). Much research has examined the individual and environmental factors that have a protective effect during times of adversity and that enhance resilience. A sampling of factors that enhance resilience in children is listed in Content Box 17-5.

Waite and Richardson define **resiliency** as "the process and experience of being disrupted by change, opportunities, stressors and adversity and, after some introspection, ultimately accessing gifts and strengths (resilience) to grow stronger through the disruption" (2004, p. 178). They identify three waves of inquiry regarding human resiliency. The first wave defines characteristics of people (e.g., internal locus of control, self-efficacy, self-esteem)

Content Box 17-5

Factors for Resilience in Childhood

Characteristics of the Child
- Effective problem-solving skills
- Adaptable personality
- Positive self-concept and self-efficacy
- Effective emotional self-regulation
- Perceives meaning in life
- Sense of humor

Characteristics of the Family
- Positive relationships with caregivers
- Low parental discord
- Organized home environment
- Parenting style high on warmth, expectations, and monitoring
- Positive socioeconomic indicators

Characteristics of the Community
- Presence of competent, caring, and supportive adults
- Prosocial peer groups
- Organizations that provide activities for children
- High level of public safety
- High-quality, accessible health services
- Effective schools

Adapted from "Resilience in development" by A. S. Masten & M. G. Reed, 2005, in C. R. Snyder & S. J. Lopez (Eds.), *Handbook of positive psychology.* By permission of Oxford University Press, Inc.

source of strength" (Richardson, as cited in Waite & Richardson, 2004, p. 179). From a developmental perspective, resilience is the ability to achieve age-related developmental milestones and tasks under harsh stressful conditions. In order to identify sociocultural risk factors and protective resources that influence health outcomes in adolescence, Rew and Horner (2003) developed the Youth Resilience Framework (YRF). The primary risk factors identified in their research included gender, childhood distress, trauma (which includes divorce or death of a loved one), difficult temperament, and poor school performance. The protective who cope and work through daily life disruptions. The second wave is more process oriented, determining how people acquire these characteristics. The third wave explores innate resilience, or the mechanisms within certain people that motivate them to cope and overcome adversity.

Approaches for fostering resilience can be conceptualized in three categories: risk-focused strategies, asset-focused strategies, and process-focused strategies. Risk-focused strategies are designed to reduce exposure to negative experiences by preventing or lowering risks and stressors. Examples of this approach include parenting skills training to decrease child abuse, community policing to reduce crime and violence, and community recreation programs to prevent adolescent alcohol and drug abuse. Asset-focused strategies are designed to increase the development of, and access to, the resources needed to respond effectively to challenging situations. It attempts to improve social capital. Providing tutors, recreational programs, and enrichment opportunities are examples of this approach. Process-focused strategies attempt to influence processes that impact people's lives and mobilize adaptational systems—for example, building self-efficacy through a series of graded experiences of success, fostering mentoring relationships, and supporting cultural traditions that provide social support. Effective interventions to increase resiliency use a combination of these three types of strategies (Masten & Reed, 2005).

Susan Fine first introduced resilience to the occupational therapy profession in her 1990 Slagle lecture, in which she asks the profession to consider "Who rises above adversity?" She noted that resilience is a concept aligned more closely with a health and wellness perspective than with the medical model. The definition of *mental health* above incorporates the term *resilience* as a characteristic of mental health. The focus of resilience research and subsequent interventions is on exploring "good psychosocial capacities such as competence, coping, creativity, and confidence" (Anthony & Cohler, as cited in Fine, 1991, p. 496). Fine (1991) states that "resilience is made operational by cognitive and coping skills and the recruitment of social support" (p. 496) and that "resilience is often measured behaviorally on the basis of the person's competence and success in meeting society's expectations despite great obstacles" (p. 497).

In their study of 232 allied health workers in a large government organization, Waite and Richardson (2004) examined the impact of resilience training. Random assignment was made to a control group and the experimental group (training group). Results of the repeated measures analysis of variance (ANOVA) tests and paired samples t-test showed positive and significant changes in the experimental group after the training. Waite and Richardson state that, in light of the ongoing changes in health care, "allied health professionals in hospitals and other settings may need to become more resilient themselves" (2004, p. 182).

Emotional Intelligence

Emotional intelligence (EI) refers to the ability to effectively process information that is emotion-laden. This skill allows an individual to use emotional intelligence as a guide for problem-solving and other cognitive activities and as a means of focusing energy on required behaviors. Specifically, emotional intelligence is the ability to

- "perceive, appraise, and express emotion accurately and adaptively;
- understand emotion and emotional knowledge;
- access and/or generate feelings when they facilitate cognitive activities and adaptive action; and
- regulate emotions in oneself and others" (Salovey, Mayer, & Caruso, 2005, p. 159).

The concept of emotional intelligence has a long history. The ancient Greek school of thought (Stoic) believed that emotions, being individualistic and self-absorbed, were unreliable as a guide to insight and wisdom. This contrasted with the later view of the European Romantic movement in the late 18th and early 19th centuries that empathy and intuition rooted in emotion could provide insights not possible through logic alone. The Romantic movement stimulated more modern conceptualizations of EI as an ability to understand feelings in oneself and others and using these feelings as information that shapes one's thinking and actions.

Emotional intelligence has four branches (Salovey et al., 2005). The first is emotional perception and expression, which involves the recognition and intake of verbal and nonverbal information into the emotion system. This ability comprises attending to, registering, and deciphering emotional messages, such as in body language, tone of voice, and facial expressions, as well as those implied by cultural differences. Missing these signals may determine the difference between success and failure in life tasks.

The second branch of EI is the emotional facilitation of thought, or using emotions as a part of cognitive processes like creativity and problem-solving. This emotional facilitation of cognitive processes has implications for more effective problem-solving, reasoning, decision-making, and creative activity. The emotions may either disrupt cognition or focus attention on what is important and on what tasks one performs best in a given mood. Emotions like anxiety, sadness, or fear may interfere with factors like motivation, self-esteem, confidence, or drive related to the expression or performance of these activities. Shifting an individual's view from more skeptical (negative) to more accepting (positive) may produce multiple vantage points for thinking and creativity (Salovey et al., 2005).

The third branch of EI involves the cognitive processing of emotion, where insight and knowledge impact the feelings of individuals. This is called **emotional understanding** and is the ability to label emotions with words and to recognize levels of emotion. This is how a particular spectrum of emotion may evolve under certain circumstances—for example, when feelings of annoyance or irritation evolve into rage if the offending stimulus is not removed, or when the feeling of envy evolves into the more destructive emotion of jealousy. The ability to understand the meaning, the blending in context, and the time progression of emotions appears to have a significant impact on interpersonal relationships (Salovey et al., 2005).

The fourth and final branch in this model is **emotional management**. This is the ability to regulate emotions and, by itself, is what most people would identify as emotional intelligence. Emotional management may lead individuals to attempt to control others' moods as well as their own. Excessive control of one's emotions may actually stifle EI, and having a positive effect on others' emotions is more likely achieved by harnessing, not suppressing, their emotions. Positive mood-control techniques include exercise, positive affirmations, self "pep talks," and participation in hobbies (socializing, reading, writing, art and music, and sports events). These involve active energy expenditure that combines varied degrees of relaxation, stress management and reduction, cognitive effort, social support, and self-soothing behaviors. Counterproductive emotional management strategies include social withdrawal and isolation, and escape into potentially addictive substances (alcohol, drugs, caffeine) and behaviors (excessive television watching or computer use, overeating, oversleeping, or sexual fantasy and acting-out behavior).

Healthy emotional self-management relies on the ability to reflect on and manage emotions. Emotional disclosure, the act of disclosing one's emotional experiences, has a positive effect on an individual's physical and mental health. For the purpose of healing, it may not matter what the method is in which this disclosure occurs, whether in writing or through psychotherapy, a religious experience, or a spiritual program (Salovey et al., 2005).

A more daunting task is measuring EI and designing reliable and valid instruments. Research, in early and preliminary stages, may have some practical relevance. For example, increased emotional intelligence is believed to be associated in children with increased prosocial behaviors as noted by teacher reports, and similar results are found in college students who exhibit fewer antisocial behaviors when observed by their peers (Salovey et al., 2005).

In other studies in school systems, emotional intelligence was also associated with decreased smoking of tobacco, decreased use of alcohol, and increased belief in the importance of doing well in school (Salovey et al., 2005). Emerging studies support positive results associated with EI training in schools. The development and utilization of EI training curricula in schools is usually incorporated into broader programs that are called Social and Emotional Learning (SEL). Various amounts of instruction time and levels of depth are associated with topics like problem-solving skills in specific social situations, conflict-resolution strategies, and character development. The New Haven, Connecticut, school system has a program from grades K to 12 that integrates the development of social and emotional skills in the context of various prevention programs. Topics include the prevention of HIV, drug use, and teen pregnancy. Concepts like self-monitoring, feelings of awareness, empathy (perspective taking), anger management, and understanding nonverbal communication are covered in 25 to 50 hours of highly structured classroom instruction. Preliminary results of testing every 2 years show positive trends in the reduction of school violence and feelings of hopelessness (Salovey et al., 2005).

Another EI curriculum is Self Science, utilized in Hillsborough, California, in grades one through eight. This flexible course includes 54 lessons organized around 10 goals. There are three main assumptions: (1) there is no thinking without feeling and no feeling without thinking; (2) the more conscious one is of what one is experiencing, the more learning is possible; and (3) self-knowledge is an integral component of the learning process. Some of the topics include

- talking about feelings and needs;
- listening to and sharing with others;
- including and comforting others;
- learning to grow from conflict and adversity;
- setting goals and prioritizing activities;
- making conscious decisions; and
- giving time and resources to the larger community (Salovey et al., 2005).

The workplace is another area where progress is being noted from EI training. This training was associated with the increased effectiveness of managers and team leaders in guiding their team to improved performance in customer service. However, EI did not lead to greater speed in handling customer complaints (Salovey et al., 2005). Workplace interventions spurred by EI training include the Weatherhead MBA program at Case

Western Reserve University in Cleveland and the Emotional Competency Training Program for American Express Financial Advisors. These programs are unique and are not reworked versions of formerly used training sessions on human relations, achievement motivation, stress management, and conflict resolution.

The Weatherhead MBA program incorporates into the curriculum training in social and emotional competency for future business leaders. The experiences are related to emotions and are designed to promote flexibility, empathy, persuasiveness, self-confidence, self-control, achievement drive, networking, and group-management skills (Salovey et al., 2005).

The American Express program trains managers to be "emotional coaches" for their employees. The goal is to gain awareness of how one's own emotional reactions and the emotions of others affect management practices. The company believes its internal data shows a higher business growth rate for financial advisors whose managers had participated in the training than for those whose managers had not taken the training (Salovey et al., 2005).

These authors have observed a limited number of similar approaches to emotional coaching in the business world, in companies that span the gamut from network marketing, to insurance and financial services, to the airline industry, to grocery stores and other service-related fields. Note has been made that even in the training and continuing education of physicians, there are an increasing number of courses on communication, empathy, and emotion-related skills development (Salovey et al., 2005).

Self-Efficacy

Self-efficacy is one of the constructs of social cognitive theory and is the belief in one's capabilities to produce desired effects through one's own actions (Bandura, 1997). Self-efficacy impacts psychological adjustment, mental and physical wellbeing, and health behavior change. It is not a genetically controlled trait; rather, it is a belief that develops over time through interaction with the world. The predisposing conditions for the development of self-efficacy are the ability to enact symbolic thought, particularly cause-and-effect thinking, and the capacity for self-reflection. In addition, the social environment influences the development of self-efficacy. Environments that are responsive to a person's attempts at mastery enhance the development of self-efficacy, while unresponsive environments inhibit its development (Maddux, 2005).

Persons with high levels of self-efficacy are more resilient, have healthier relationships, and express more life satisfaction. They are more likely to adopt healthy behaviors and maintain them in spite of adversity. In addition, they tend to more effectively manage stress. Persons with low levels of self-efficacy are more vulnerable to depression. They often feel impotent to change or control things in their environment and lack the psychic energy to manage difficult life situations. Depressed persons often approach situations with apprehension, which in turn disrupts performance and decreases the likelihood of a positive outcome. The negative outcome then diminishes their sense of self-efficacy, and a dysfunctional cycle has been initiated. Self-efficacy also influences goal setting and goal attainment. The higher the level of self-efficacy, the loftier the goals set and the more persistent the pursuit. Self-efficacious persons are typically better problem-solvers and decision-makers than their low-self-efficacy counterparts. Better problem-solving and decision-making frequently results in better outcomes, which in turn increases self-efficacy, and a positive cycle is initiated (Maddux, 2005).

Strategies to enhance self-efficacy include

- providing tangible evidence of success;
- experiencing a sense of mastery;
- challenging dysfunctional beliefs and attitudes;
- encouraging the adoption of adaptive beliefs and realistic expectations;
- modeling and social support for behavior change;
- practicing cognitive rehearsal and imagery; and
- employing techniques to reduce emotional arousal and decrease performance anxiety—for example, meditation, biofeedback, and relaxation training (Maddux, 2005).

Self-efficacy research is about human potential and possibilities and has demonstrated that self-confidence, effort, and perseverance are more important than innate ability in achieving success, happiness, and wellbeing.

Learned Optimism

Optimism can be defined as "the tendency to look on the more favorable side of events or conditions, the belief that good will ultimately triumph over evil" (Random House Webster's Dictionary, 1998, p. 505). How people respond to adversity and cope with stress is somewhat determined by their outlook on life. Optimists tend to approach challenges with self-confidence and persistence, whereas pessimists are doubtful and hesitant. Optimism and pessimism are basic personality characteristics that "influence how people orient to events in their lives" (Carver & Scheier, 2005, p. 233). Research indicates that optimism is associated with lower levels of psychological stress, an enhanced ability to cope with adversity, greater life satisfaction, and fewer symptoms of depression. Optimists use more problem-focused coping strategies and positive reframing and less denial and attempts to distance oneself from a problem than do pessimists. In addition, optimists are more likely to engage in proactive, positive health behaviors. Pessimists, on the other hand, are less likely to take action to ensure their wellbeing and are more likely to engage in maladaptive behaviors (Carver & Scheier, 2005). As a result, these individuals have an increased likelihood of premature deaths, particularly from accidents (Peterson & Steen, 2005).

According to Seligman, Reivich, Jaycox, and Gillham (1995), optimism arises from four potential sources: genetics, environment (particularly parental influence), feedback received during childhood, and life experiences that promote either helplessness or mastery. Secure attachments and the development of a sense of trust in childhood appear to be particularly important to the development of optimism. **Learned optimism** refers to transforming negative thought processes into positive ones that enhance flexible thinking and resilience (Keyes & Lopez, 2005). Learned optimism training can transform negative thinking into positive cognitive processes. There are three components of explanatory style in learned optimism interventions: permanence, pervasiveness, and personalization. These components are modified with cognitive techniques to help people respond in a healthier manner to daily events, regardless of their positive or negative outcome.

The prevention benefits of learned optimism training were demonstrated in a study of 70 fifth graders at risk for depression. The children learned ways to change their style of explaining situations and experienced significantly fewer depressive symptoms following the study as compared with a control group. In addition, for 2 years afterward (with 6-month follow-ups), the children who completed the training were half as likely to develop depression than the control group (Keyes & Lopez, 2005).

Hope

Although many authors characterize hope as an emotion (Farina, Hearth, & Popovich, 1995), Snyder, Rand, and Sigmon (2005) emphasize the thought processes involved. Hope is goal-directed thinking and "the belief that one can find pathways to desired goals and become motivated to use those pathways" (Snyder et al., 2005, p. 257). Hope involves three types of thinking:

1. Goals thinking
2. Pathways thinking
3. Agency thinking

An assumption underlying hope theory is that most of human behavior is focused on goal pursuits. Goals are what a person desires to experience, create, do, or become. "Stretch goals" are those that are slightly more challenging than previously achieved goals and therefore require individuals to stretch beyond their comfort zone (Snyder, Lopez, Shorey, Rand, & Feldman 2003). **Goals thinking** refers to the ability to clearly conceptualize and delineate goals toward which to target their purposeful efforts. **Pathways thinking** refers to the ability to generate reasonable strategies or pathways to achieve these goals, which requires a perception of causality. High-hope persons are able to generate multiple pathways toward their goals. **Agency thinking** refers to the person's motivation or capacity to implement the identified pathways or strategies for goal attainment under normal and impeded conditions, which requires the ability to see oneself as a causal agent. Agency thinking provides the energy that initiates and sustains action toward one's goals. It is the perception of successful goal pursuit that causes the emotional reaction associated with hope. The process is iterative with past goal attainment experiences influencing present pathways and agency thinking. Hope is learned through interactions with peers, caregivers, and teachers throughout one's lifetime (Snyder et al., 2005).

Hope is significantly correlated with other positive psychology constructs, although their factor structures differ. For example, measures of hope are correlated with optimism (0.50) and with self-esteem (0.45). In addition, hope correlates highly with meaning in life (0.70 to 0.76) and self-actualization (0.79). Self-efficacy is also related to hope and is a measure of a person's perception of their ability to perform in a specific context, whereas hope is a measure of the person's perception that they will perform. *Ability* refers to the capacity to act, while the will to act reflects intentionality. Hope impacts many areas of life, including academics, athletics, physical health, and emotional wellbeing. Hope is correlated with higher test scores and better academic achievement and is not significantly related to intelligence (Snyder, McDermott, Cook, & Rapoff, 2002). High-hope athletes perform better than low-hope athletes even when the variance in natural ability is accounted for. High-hope individuals engage in more preventive health behaviors and adjust better to chronic health conditions than persons with low hope. For example, Everson and colleagues (1996) found that hopelessness predicted later cardiovascular disease and cancer among middle-aged men even when risk factors were controlled for statistically. High hope is also related to positive affect, effective coping skills, and healthy interpersonal relationships.

Hope can be conceptualized as a relatively stable personality trait or as a transient state of mind. It can be related to goals in general, to domain-specific goals (e.g., school achievement), or to one goal in particular. Assessments are available for children, adolescents, and adults that measure various aspects of hope (trait, state, and domain). These assessment tools can identify which of the three components of hope (goals thinking, pathways thinking, and agency thinking) is most affected. Interventions can then be tailored to meet individual needs. A basic outline for developing hope interventions can be found in Content Box 17-6.

Social Support

Humans are by nature social creatures. Living in small groups, families, large groups, and communities has offered physical protection and social support. Social contact has been shown to enhance health and wellbeing and to provide a buffer during times of stress. In addition, social support (perceived or actual) facilitates routine activities and reduces activity restrictions in elders (Williamson, 2005). Social isolation is a significant risk factor for morbidity and mortality. Attachment to others is a key component of wellbeing. **Social support** can be defined as the provision of information, practical assistance, companionship, emotional concern, and affirmation. It fulfills our basic need to belong (Turner, Barling, & Zacharatos, 2005).

Attachment refers to "the tendency to seek closeness with particular others and to feel more secure in their

presence" (Taylor, Dickerson, & Klein, 2005, p. 557). Long separations from primary caregivers both in baby monkeys (Harlow & Harlow, 1962) and in human infants (Bowlby, 1973) can produce fearful and aggressive behaviors; emotional disturbance, particularly depression; and failure to thrive. In childhood, the quality of the caregiver-infant relationship is critical for normal development and for physical and mental health. In addition to the psychological benefits of social support, it appears that social relationships also exert physiological and neuroendocrine effects that moderate stress responses and enhance immune function (Taylor et al., 2005).

The research is consistent in its findings that females are more likely to develop social networks and seek social support in times of stress than are males. This appears to be a cross-cultural phenomenon. Positive social contact has been shown to increase the secretion of endogenous opioid peptides, which provide a sense of wellbeing through their effects on the brain. In addition, prolonged social isolation can reduce brain serotonin activity and thereby produce symptoms of depression. The gender differences may be due in part to the hormone oxytocin. Mothers of many species secrete oxytocin immediately after giving birth. This hormone is believed to facilitate attachment behaviors and increase prosocial behaviors in response to stress (Taylor et al., 2005).

The benefits of social support are not tied to the number of social relationships one has but rather to the quality of those relationships (Holahan, Moos, Holahan, & Brennan, 1996). A sense of belonging and security with others is a key dimension of mental health. Social support groups offer the opportunity to share concerns, offer suggestions, and provide role models for health behavior change. Alcoholics Anonymous and other 12-step programs have a strong social support component.

Ryff and Singer (2005) describe the cumulative effect of social relationships on wellbeing. They differentiate between positive and negative relationship pathways. A positive relationship pathway indicates that an adult has had at least one parent who was caring, supportive, and affectionate and has experienced at least one of two forms (emotional/sexual and intellectual/recreational) of adult spousal intimacy. A negative relationship pathway indicates that a person had negative bonds with both parents or had negative experiences with both forms of spousal intimacy. These researchers found that adults with positive relationship pathways had lower allostatic loads, as measured by physiological stress markers, than those with negative relationship pathways. **Allostatic load** is "a measure of cumulative wear and tear on numerous physiological systems" (Ryff & Singer, 2005, p. 548). This suggests that having positive and supportive social relationships may actually protect the individual's health

---

Content Box 17-6

Basic Components of Hope Interventions

Administer Appropriate Hope Assessments
- Review results with client
- Educate client about basic concepts in hope theory

Facilitate Client's Goal Selection and Definition
- Identify highly valued goals
- Establish an ideal challenge level
- Specify measurable subgoals

Facilitate Client's Pathways Thinking
- Visualize paths to the goals
- Generate several strategies or pathways to achieve the goal
- Identify alternative routes if the original pathways are blocked or not effective

Facilitate Client's Agency Thinking
- Increase positive self-talk
- Evaluate progress made toward goals
- Celebrate accomplishments
- Practice basic health habits, good nutrition, physical activity, and adequate sleep

Adapted from "Hope for rehabilitation and vice versa" by C. R. Snyder, K. A. Lehman, B. Kluck, B., & Y. Monsson, 2006, *Rehabilitation Psychology, 51*(2), 89–112.

through physiological mechanisms. Interestingly, this effect was stronger for males than it was for females (Ryff & Singer, 2005).

Spirituality

The power, functional importance, and impact of spirituality on mental health is often underestimated. There is growing evidence that spirituality and religious participation have beneficial effects on mental health. For example, persons with a spiritual or religious affiliation are significantly less likely (approximately 40%) to develop major depressive disorder during their lifetimes and may recover faster when they do experience depression than those without such an affiliation. In addition, religious and spiritual commitment correlates with lower levels of substance abuse. One of the mediating variables appears to be the acceptance and support people experience from their faith communities during times of stress (Hartz, 2005).

Spirituality is often confused with religiosity. Although overlapping, they are distinct concepts. Both constructs can be expressed individually and socially, and both have the capacity to improve or impair wellbeing. Although there are probably an infinite number of meanings for the term **spirituality,** for the purposes of this chapter, it will be defined as a "search for meaning and purpose in ways related to the sacred or to ultimate reality" (Hartz, 2005, p. 4). Spirituality may include experiences of transcendence, connectedness to the sacred, awe, reverence, a sense of wholeness, and profound love. Spirituality can be experienced through religious activities; however, religion has some attributes that spirituality does not—for example, theology, moral codes, rituals, and institutions. One can practice spirituality without belonging to any particular religion (Hartz, 2005).

The search for spirituality is a process that involves effort to discover sacred truths and apply them to one's life. Spiritual pathways may include traditional religious institutions; newer spirituality movements (e.g., feminist, goddess, spiritual ecologists); and nontraditional spiritual groups, associations, and programs (e.g., 12-step programs, meditation centers). Spiritual practices may include the traditional (prayer, rites of passage, reading and studying of holy books), as well as other forms of human activity whose goal is finding and experiencing the sacred, such as meditation, music, art, yoga, social action, and sensing the divine in nature and everyday experiences. Prayer may have several goals, but meditative prayer—in which the person spends time just "being in" the presence of God—is more strongly related to measures of wellbeing and a sense of closeness to God than other types of prayer (Pargament & Mahoney, 2005).

Spirituality has been connected in many studies to individuals' social, psychological, and physical health. College students who reported spiritual striving in their list of personal goals were correlated more highly with measures of wellbeing than those striving for any other type of goals. Other studies show that persons who perceive God to be a loving, compassionate, and responsive figure express higher levels of wellbeing than those who describe God in terms of a more distant, fearful, harsh, or punitive being. The latter view is correlated with higher levels of psychic distress. In studying religious coping, it was found that people who see God as a partner in the problem-solving process of life report better mental health, while those who tend to defer controllable problems to God show lower levels of mental health. These studies give support to the idea that the helpfulness or harmfulness of people's perception of the divine being and the kind of relationship formed with their God significantly impacts their mental health (Pargament & Mahoney, 2005).

Crisis situations that are reframed in spiritually meaningful terms offer an opportunity for growth. Studies show that the individual who sees or believes there is a spiritual design in tragedy is helped to preserve their beliefs in a benevolent divine being despite adversity, and this view leads to better overall life adjustment. These findings were echoed in studies of hospice cancer patients. Those who reframed their experience in spiritual terms had greater coping efficacy, greater purpose in life, and more positive outcomes. This effect was also seen in medical rehabilitation patients who improved over a 4-month period when they could reframe their situation as a positive. Those who were angry with God experienced a significant decline in function after a 4-month period. Negative forms of religious reframing are correlated with increases in depression, distress, physical symptoms, and maladjustment to life stressors (Pargament & Mahoney, 2005).

Individuals seem to choose spiritual stability rather than change when confronted with major life stresses or traumatic events. Studies show that levels of faith and religious beliefs and practices are largely unchanged or strengthened during war, accidental injuries, or death of loved ones (Pargament & Mahoney, 2005). In addition, life cycle issues (discovering, conserving, redefining, rediscovering) and traumatic life events and experiences (trauma, illness, death) impact the perception and expression of spirituality and can promote or trigger what is variously called a religious conversion, a cosmic healing, an oceanic experience (Pargament & Mahoney, 2005), or a spiritual awakening (Alcoholics Anonymous, 2001, p. 60).

Conclusion

There are many ways to enhance mental health, and no one intervention is appropriate for everyone. Positive psychology research provides some insight regarding the characteristics of mental health and how these characteristics can be developed. Occupational therapy practitioners, like other health-care professionals, sometimes fall into the trap of focusing exclusively on a person's deficits and dysfunction. Positive psychology reminds us

to consider the whole person and utilize a person's strengths to maximize their function. Focusing on the development of hope, resilience, emotional intelligence, and optimism can do more to enhance quality of life than simply reducing symptoms and remediating deficits. These principles can be applied to individuals with and without disabilities and to families, social groups, communities, and populations. Mental health promotion programs based on these concepts have been demonstrated to be efficacious, but more research is needed.

Case Study 17-1

Sheila is a very successful and prominent professor at a private college in a large metropolitan area. She is in her midforties, married with two children (Matt who is 17 and Sydney who is 12), and has many friends. She is closely connected with family, and a year ago she lost her mother, with whom she had a very tight bond. Sheila has always struggled with weight issues and has tried "every diet on the planet." She complains of sometimes-strained relationships with her husband and has lost interest in sex. Sheila states their arguments are often about her being a workaholic, her lack of focus on home life, and her inability to balance the many projects for which she often complains she has little time.

Sheila is a community volunteer with the homeless, works with her local political party, often writes for professional publications, and is president of the board for her local community theater. She used to be a weekly participant in her knitting group, played canasta on Mondays, and used to bowl weekly, but she has given up all fun activities for the past 2 years.

Sheila recently has been experiencing migraines, which she never had before. She feels overwhelmed, and her

normal routines are often lately in disarray (her routines and habits used to help organize her day). She has been overeating and becomes more easily frustrated with issues and events with which she previously easily coped. Sheila spends little time with her children and sees her husband in passing. She does not identify any health concerns but is aware that she has changed her behaviors recently, as her best friend pointedly discussed these with her. Sheila has not spoken to her friend for 3 months due to the anger she felt when confronted (her perception).

Questions

1. Identify at least seven potential mental health issues experienced by Sheila using the *ICF*, the Practice Framework, and the model described in this chapter.

2. Name two assessments you would use. What is your rationale for their use?

3. How would you describe Sheila in the context of positive psychology?

4. How would you use the model described in the chapter to create a health and wellness intervention plan for Sheila?

Case Study 17-2

Mark is a 17-year-old high school student with a history of an auditory processing disability. He has received therapy services his entire school life up until ninth grade, and he had a difficult time transitioning to high school. He is well liked by his fellow students and teachers but is often bullied. Mark's grades recently began to plummet much to the dismay of his single mom, who often berates him for being "not like a boy should be."

Mark is active at school, is involved in the Key Club, and spends much time volunteering in the community. He is also a cheerleader and is loved by his squad and by some

of the football players, some of whom try to protect him. Mark is involved with the theater group and recently landed his first role in the community play. Despite his being loved by many, he is having a difficult time paying attention in class, is constantly anxious, and recently began experimenting with marijuana, which he says takes the edge off and helps him enjoy life. Mark has begun dating but does not really enjoy the company of girls. He had his first gay experience with a college sophomore who convinced Mark that protection was not needed because he had no sexually transmitted diseases.

Questions

1. Use your knowledge of adolescence and mental health. What are some identifiable issues Mark is facing and some potential issues he may face in young adulthood?

2. Name two assessments you might use to help Mark identify his issues if he came for occupational therapy. Why would you use them?

3. In what areas would occupational therapy help Mark (a) remediate current mental health issues and (b) prevent future mental health issues?

4. Develop a health, wellness, and prevention intervention plan for Mark. Are there certain areas that would be more important than others? What factors would you consider in developing this plan?

5. How might you work with Mark's mother? His teachers? Should they even be part of the intervention plan? Why or why not?

▶ For Discussion and Review

1. Do you think mental health is an inborn trait, or is it the product of one's life experiences? Justify your answer.

2. What are some strategies that could be used in occupational therapy to enhance mental health?

3. Which of the positive psychology concepts is most relevant in your life and why?

4. What are the benefits and limitations of using positive psychology principles in occupational therapy practice?

5. What is the role of spirituality in mental health? Is spirituality an aspect of health that occupational therapists ought to address? Why or why not?

▶ Research Questions

1. How can occupational therapists enhance resilience in their clients?

2. What is the relationship between hope and resilience?

References

Alcoholics Anonymous. (2001). *The big book of AA* (4th ed.). New York: A.A. World Services.

American Psychiatric Association. (2000). *Diagnostic and statistical manual of mental disorders* (4th ed., text revision). Washington, DC: Author.

Bandura, A. (1997). *Self-efficacy: The exercise of control.* New York: Freeman.

Bing, R. K. (1981). Eleanor Clarke Slagle Lectureship—1981—Occupational therapy revisited: A paraphrastic journey. *American Journal of Occupational Therapy, 35*(8), 499–518.

Bowlby, J. (1973). *Attachment and loss.* New York: Basic Books.

Carver, C. S., & Scheier, M. F. (2005). Optimism. In C. R. Snyder & S. J. Lopez (Eds.), *Handbook of positive psychology* (pp. 231–43). New York: Oxford University Press.

Donnelly, J. W., Eburne, N., & Kittleson, M. (2001). *Mental health: Dimensions of self-esteem and emotional wellbeing.* Boston: Allyn & Bacon.

Everson, S. A., Goldberg, D. E., Kaplan, G. A., Cohen, R. D., Pukkala, E., Tuomilehto, J., & Salonen, J. T. (1996). Hopelessness and risk of mortality and incidence of myocardial infarction and cancer. *Psychosomatic Medicine, 58,* 113–21.

Farina, C. J., Hearth, A. K., & Popovich, J. M. (1995). *Hope and hopelessness: Critical clinical constructs.* Thousand Oaks, CA: Sage.

Fine, S. (1991). Resilience and human adaptability: Who rises above adversity? *American Journal of Occupational Therapy, 45,* 493–503.

Harlow, H. F., & Harlow, M. K. (1962). Social deprivation in monkeys. *Scientific American, 207*(5), 136–46.

Hartz, G. W. (2005). *Spirituality and mental health: Clinical applications.* New York: Haworth Press.

Herrman, H. (2001). The need for mental health promotion. *Australian and New Zealand Journal of Psychiatry, 35,* 709–15.

Holahan, C. J., Moos, R. H., Holahan, C. K., & Brennan, P. L. (1996). Social support, coping strategies, and psychosocial adjustment to cardiac illness: Implications for assessment and prevention. *Journal of Prevention and Intervention in the Community, 13,* 33–52.

Keyes, C. L. (2002). The mental health continuum: From languishing to flourishing in life. *Journal of Health and Social Research, 43,* 207–22.

Keyes, C. L. (2005). Mental illness and/or mental health? Investigating axioms of the complete state model of health. *Journal of Consulting and Clinical Psychology, 73*(3), 539–48.

Keyes, C. L., & Haidt, J. (2003). *Flourishing: Positive psychology and the life well-lived.* Washington, DC: American Psychological Association.

Keyes, C. L., & Lopez, S. J. (2005). Toward a science of mental health: Positive directions in diagnosis and interventions. In C. R. Snyder & S. J. Lopez (Eds.), *Handbook of positive psychology* (pp. 45–59). New York: Oxford University Press.

Lopez, S. J., & Snyder, C. R. (2003). *Positive psychological assessment: A handbook of models and measures.* Washington, DC: American Psychological Association.

MacArthur Foundation. (1995). *Midlife in the United States: A study of health and well-being.* Retrieved March 1, 2008, from http://www.midus.wisc.edu/midus1/.

Maddux, J. E. (2005). Self-efficacy: The power of believing you can. In C. R. Snyder & S. J. Lopez (Eds.), *Handbook of positive psychology* (pp. 277–87). New York: Oxford University Press.

Masten, A. S., & Reed, M. G. (2005). Resilience in development. In C. R. Snyder & S. J. Lopez (Eds.), *Handbook of positive psychology* (pp. 74–88). New York: Oxford University Press.

National Mental Health Association. (1996). *Characteristics of mentally healthy people.* Alexandria, VA: Author.

Pargament, K. I., & Mahoney, A. (2005). Spirituality: Discovering and conserving the sacred. In C. R. Snyder & S. J. Lopez (Eds.), *Handbook of positive psychology* (pp. 646–59). New York: Oxford University Press.

Peterson, C., & Seligman, M. E. P. (2004). *Character strengths and virtues: A handbook and classification.* Washington, DC: American Psychological Association.

Peterson, C., & Steen, T. A. (2005). Optimistic explanatory style. In C. R. Snyder & S. J. Lopez (Eds.), *Handbook of positive psychology* (pp. 244–56). New York: Oxford University Press.

Random House Webster's Dictionary. (1998, 3d ed.). New York: Ballantine Books.

Rew, L., & Horner, S. D. (2003). Youth resilience framework for reducing health-risk behaviors in adolescents. *Journal of Pediatric Nursing, 18*(6), 379–88.

Rogers, C. (1961). *On becoming a person.* Boston: Houghton Mifflin.

Ryff, C. D., & Keyes, C. L. (1995). The structure of psychological wellbeing revisited. *Journal of Personality and Social Psychology, 69,* 719–27.

Ryff, C. D., & Singer, B. (2005). From social structure to biology: Integrative science in pursuit of human health and wellbeing. In C. R. Snyder & S. J. Lopez (Eds.), *Handbook of positive psychology* (pp. 541–55). New York: Oxford University Press.

Salovey, P., Mayer, J. D., & Caruso, D. (2005). The positive psychology of emotional intelligence. In C. R. Snyder & S. J. Lopez (Eds.), *Handbook of positive psychology* (pp. 159–71). New York: Oxford University Press.

Secker, J. (1998). Current conceptualizations of mental health and mental health promotion. *Health Education Research, 13*(1), 57–66.

Seligman, M. (2005). Positive psychology, positive prevention and positive therapy. In C. R. Snyder & S. J. Lopez (Eds.), *Handbook of positive psychology.* New York: Oxford University Press.

Seligman, M., Reivich, K., Jaycox, L., & Gillham, J. (1995). *The optimistic child.* Boston: Houghton Mifflin.

Snyder, C. R., & Elliott, T. R. (2005). Twenty-first century graduate education in clinical psychology: A four level matrix approach. *Journal of Clinical Psychology, 61*(9), 1033–54.

Snyder, C. R., Lehman, K. A., Kluck, B., & Monsson, Y. (2006). Hope for rehabilitation and vice versa. *Rehabilitation Psychology, 51*(2), 89–112.

Snyder, C. R., & Lopez, S. J. (Eds.) (2005). *Handbook of positive psychology.* New York: Oxford University Press.

Snyder, C. R., & Lopez, S. J. (2007). *Positive psychology: The scientific and practical explorations of human strengths.* Thousand Oaks, CA: Sage.

Snyder, C. R., Lopez, S. J., Edwards, L. M., Pedrotti, J. T., Prosser, E. C., Walton, S. L., Spalitto, S. V., & Ulven, J. C. (2003). Measuring and labeling the positive and the negative. In S. J. Lopez & C. R. Snyder (Eds.), *Positive psychological assessment: A handbook of models and measures.* Washington, DC: American Psychological Association.

Snyder, C. R., Lopez, S. J., Shorey, H. L., Rand, K. L., & Feldman, D. B. (2003). Hope theory, measurements, and application to school psychology. *School Psychology Quarterly, 18,* 122–39.

Snyder, C. R., McDermott, D., Cook, W., & Rapoff, M. (2002). *Hope for the journey* (revised ed.). Clinton Corners, NY: Percheron Press.

Snyder, C. R., Rand, K. L., & Sigmon, D. R. (2005). Hope theory: A member of the positive psychology family. In C. R. Snyder & S. J. Lopez (Eds.), *Handbook of positive psychology.* New York: Oxford University Press.

Snyder, C. R., Ritschel, L. A., Rand, K. L., & Berg, C. J. (2006). Balancing psychological assessments: Including strengths and hope in client reports. *Journal of Clinical Psychology, 62*(1), 33–46.

Taylor, S. E., Dickerson, S. S., & Klein, L. C. (2005). Toward a biology of social support. In C. R. Snyder & S. J. Lopez (Eds.), *Handbook of positive psychology.* New York: Oxford University Press.

Tudor, K. (1996). *Mental health promotion: Paradigms and practice.* London: Routledge.

Turner, N., Barling, J., & Zacharatos, A. (2005). Positive psychology at work. In C. R. Snyder & S. J. Lopez (Eds.), *Handbook of positive psychology* (pp. 715–30). New York: Oxford University Press.

United Kingdom, Department of Health. (2001). *Making it happen: A guide to delivering mental health promotion.* London: Crown Copyright.

U.S. Department of Health and Human Services. (1999). *Mental health: A report of the surgeon general.* Rockville, MD: U.S. Department of Health and Human Services, Substance Abuse and Mental Health Services Administration, Center for Mental Health Services, National Institutes of Health, National Institute of Mental Health.

U.S. Department of Health and Human Services. (2000). *Healthy People 2010: Understanding and improving health* (2d ed.). Washington, DC: Government Printing Office.

Waite, P. J., & Richardson, G. E. (2004). Determining the efficacy of resiliency training in the work site. *Journal of Allied Health, 33*(3), 178–83.

Williamson, G. M. (2005) Aging well: Outlook for the 21st century. In C. R. Snyder & S. J. Lopez (Eds.), *Handbook of positive psychology* (pp. 676–86). New York: Oxford University Press.

World Health Organization. (1946). *Constitution of the World Health Organization.* New York: Author.

World Health Organization. (2001). *Mental health: strengthening mental health promotion.* Retrieved August 10, 2006, from http://www.who.int/mediacentre/factsheets/fs220/en/print.html.

World Health Organization. (2004). *Promoting mental health: Concepts, emerging evidence, practice. Summary report.* Geneva, Switzerland: Author.

World Health Organization. (2005). *Child and adolescent mental health policies and plans.* Retrieved June 10, 2005, from http://www.who.int/mental_health/policy/Child%20%20 Ado%20Mental%20Health_final.pdf.

Wright, B. A., & Lopez, S. J. (2005). Widening the diagnostic focus: A case for including human strengths and environmental resources. In C. R. Snyder & S. J. Lopez (Eds.), *Handbook of positive psychology.* New York: Oxford University Press.

Chapter 18

Unintentional Injury and Violence Prevention

Marjorie E. Scaffa, S. Blaise Chromiak, S. Maggie Reitz, Angela Blair-Newton, Lynne Murphy, and C. Barrett Wallis

The risk of injury is so great that most persons sustain a significant injury at some time during their lives. Nevertheless, this widespread human damage too often is taken for granted, in the erroneous belief that injuries happen by chance and are the result of unpreventable 'accidents.' In fact, many injuries are not 'accidents,' or random, uncontrollable acts of fate; rather, most injuries are predictable and preventable.

—U.S. Department of Health & Human Services [USDHHS], 2000, p. 15-3.

Learning Objectives

This chapter is designed to enable the reader to:

- Discuss the range and magnitude of unintentional injuries.
- Discuss the range and magnitude of injuries due to violence.
- Describe the three Es of injury prevention.
- Identify federal agencies with responsibilities for injury and violence prevention.
- Apply Haddon's matrix to injury prevention planning.
- Identify the characteristics of effective injury and violence prevention strategies.
- Describe the mental health consequences of unintentional injury and violence.

Key Terms

Bullying	Ergonomics	Poison	Violence
Cyberbullying	Family violence	Secondary trauma	Years of potential life lost (YPLL)
Elder abuse	Hazard	Sexual violence	
Enforcement	Homicide	Suicide	
Engineering/ environmental modification	Injury	Three Es	
	Intimate partner violence	Unintentional injury	

Introduction

In the United States, unintentional and intentional injuries are leading causes of death and disability, especially in children, young adults, and older adults. Over 5 million people in this country are coping with chronic disability as a result of an injury (USDHHS, 2006). **Injury** is defined as "unintentional or intentional damage to the body resulting from acute exposure to thermal, mechanical, electrical, or chemical energy or from the absence of such essentials as heat or oxygen" (USDHHS, 2000, p. 15–55).

According to the National Center for Health Statistics (2007), the four leading mechanisms-of-injury death in 2005 accounted for 73.4% of all injury deaths and were (in rank order)

- motor vehicle crashes (25.1%);
- poisoning (18.8%);
- firearms (17.7%); and
- falls (11.8%)

Approximately two-thirds of overall injury-related deaths are classified as unintentional, and one-third are due to an act of violence. Of intentional injury deaths due to violence, approximately 60% are attributed to suicide and 40% are classified as homicide (Centers for Disease Control and Prevention [CDC], 2005; USDHHS, 2000).

Injuries are a central factor in the health profile of the United States and a major threat to wellbeing and quality of life. They are clearly a public health concern and a highly preventable source of morbidity and mortality. Millions of people are temporarily incapacitated or permanently disabled due to unintentional injury and violence. Particularly vulnerable are the young and elderly. Human behavior is often a contributing factor in injuries and is therefore an essential target for intervention. For example, the use of alcohol, tobacco, and other drugs by adolescents, or substance use by their parents, have been associated with the increased risk of youths committing violent acts (National Center for Injury Prevention and Control [NCIPC], 2007a).

Certain groups experience a disproportionate share of particular types of injury over the life span. For example, African Americans have higher death rates from unintentional injuries than all other groups, and homicide rates are higher among African American and Hispanic youth than among whites (USDHHS, 2000). Figure 18-1 displays the 10 leading causes of injury (unintentional and violence-related) death by age group in 2005. Occupational therapists and occupational therapy assistants need to be aware of these data and similar state and local data in order to direct interventions toward the populations in greatest need and structure those interventions appropriately to reflect the needs and culture of the target group.

This chapter addresses both unintentional and intentional injuries, and describes injury-prevention principles and strategies as well as the role of occupational therapy in injury and violence prevention and intervention. The general public commonly refers to intentional injuries as *violence;* both terms will be used within this chapter. The first section of the chapter will address

10 Leading Causes of Injury Deaths, United States 2005, All Races, Both Sexes

Rank	<1	1–4	5–9	10–14	15–24	25–34	35–44	45–54	55–64	65+	All Ages
					Age Groups						
1	Unintentional Suffocation 748	Unintentional Drowning 493	Unintentional MV Traffic 560	Unintentional MV Traffic 763	Unintentional MV Traffic 10,657	Unintentional MV Traffic 7,047	Unintentional Poisoning 6,729	Unintentional Poisoning 6,983	Unintentional MV Traffic 4,287	Unintentional Fall 15,802	Unintentional MV Traffic 43,667
2	Unintentional MV Traffic 140	Unintentional MV Traffic 489	Unintentional Fire/burn 138	Suicide Suffocation 172	Homicide Firearm 4,499	Unintentional Poisoning 4,386	Unintentional MV Traffic 6,491	Unintentional MV Traffic 6,179	Suicide Firearm 2,470	Unintentional MV Traffic 7,048	Unintentional Poisoning 23,618
3	Homicide Unspecified 129	Unintentional Fire/burn 208	Unintentional Drowning 121	Homicide Firearm 143	Unintentional Poisoning 2,484	Homicide Firearm 3,780	Suicide Firearm 2,855	Suicide Firearm 3,472	Unintentional Poisoning 2,007	Unintentional Unspecified 5,069	Unintentional Fall 19,656
4	Homicide Other Spec., classifiable 99	Homicide Unspecified 153	Unintentional Other Land Transport 47	Unintentional Drowning 132	Suicide Firearm 1,962	Suicide Firearm 2,269	Homicide Firearm 2,010	Suicide Poisoning 1,707	Unintentional Fall 1,451	Suicide Firearm 3,889	Suicide Firearm 17,002
5	Unintentional Drowning 64	Unintentional Pedestrian, Other 129	Homicide Firearm 44	Unintentional Fire/burn 85	Suicide Suffocation 1,570	Suicide Suffocation 1,524	Suicide Suffocation 1,670	Suicide Suffocation 1,197	Suicide Poisoning 852	Unintentional Suffocation 3,271	Homicide Firearm 12,352
6	Undetermined Suffocation 50	Unintentional Suffocation 126	Unintentional Suffocation 44	Suicide Firearm 84	Unintentional Drowning 649	Suicide Poisoning 757	Suicide Poisoning 1,456	Unintentional Fall 1,181	Suicide Suffocation 575	Adverse Effects 1,708	Suicide Suffocation 7,248
7	Unintentional Fire/burn 36	Homicide Other Spec., classifiable 74	Unintentional Pedestrian, Other 25	Unintentional Other Land Transport 63	Homicide Cut/pierce 528	Undetermined Poisoning 564	Undetermined Poisoning 944	Homicide Firearm 1,097	Unintentional Suffocation 509	Unintentional Fire/burn 1,178	Unintentional Unspecified 6,551
8	Undetermined Unspecified 30	Unintentional Natural/Environment 38	Unintentional Natural/Environment 17	Unintentional Suffocation 59	Suicide Poisoning 361	Homicide Cut/pierce 474	Unintentional Fall 607	Undetermined Poisoning 1,026	Homicide Firearm 405	Unintentional Natural/Environment 1,069	Unintentional Suffocation 5,900
9	Homicide Suffocation 27	Homicide Firearm 37	Unintentional Poisoning 17	Unintentional Firearm 37	Unintentional Other Land Transport 298	Unintentional Drowning 385	Unintentional Drowning 497	Unintentional Fire/burn 506	Unintentional Fire/burn 405	Unintentional Poisoning 931	Suicide Poisoning 5,744
10	Unintentional Unspecified 22	Unintentional Fall 34	Three Tied 15	Unintentional Poisoning 34	Undetermined Poisoning 292	Unintentional Fall 295	Homicide Cut/pierce 426	Unintentional Drowning 492	Unintentional Natural/Environment 376	Suicide Poisoning 603	Unintentional Drowning 3,582

WISQARS™ Produced By: Office of Statistics and Programming, National Center for Injury Prevention and Control, Centers for Disease Control and Prevention

Data Source: National Center for Health Statistics (NCHS), National Vital Statistics System

Figure 18-1   Ten leading causes of injury deaths by age group—United States, 2005.

From 10 leading causes of death by age group, United States—2004, *National Center for Injury Prevention and Control, 2007. Retrieved December 16, 2007, from http://www.cdc.gov/ncipc/osp/charts.htm.*

unintentional injury prevention, and the second section will focus on violence prevention. Data on the occurrences and cost of injury will be provided in each respective section. This data helps provide context for the discussion of specific prevention strategies and the role of occupational therapy that follows. The goal of this chapter is to serve as an overview; it is not an authoritative source of the latest injury statistics. For the most current data, please consult the websites of the National Center for Health Statistics (NCHS) at http://www.cdc.gov/nchs/ and the National Center for Injury Prevention and Control (NCIPC) at http://www.cdc.gov/injury/. Prior to addressing specific unintentional injuries, explore the need for investing in prevention strategies as the primary public health approach is explored.

A Public Health Perspective

Traditionally, injuries have been viewed as accidental and thus not preventable. This perspective allowed injuries to be seen as isolated problems of individual victims instead of as a public health concern. However, prevention is now viewed as the best strategy to address this problem. This shift in thinking is reflected in changing terminology; for example, what were previously described as auto accidents are increasingly being referred to as auto crashes. Stewart and Lord (2002) asserted that the term

> motor vehicle crash should replace motor vehicle accident in the clinical and research lexicon of traumatologists. Crash encompasses a wider range of potential causes for vehicular crashes than does the term accident. A majority of fatal crashes are caused by intoxicated, speeding, distracted, or careless drivers and, therefore, are not accidents. (p. 333)

In the case of motor vehicle crashes, improvements in roadways and vehicle design have lowered fatality rates. Public outcry, especially from the group Mothers Against Drunk Driving (MADD), has led to increased emphasis on designated drivers, imprisoning and restricting impaired drivers, and avoiding impaired driving (Christoffel & Gallagher, 2006). The U.S. government is developing policies to lessen injuries and to assure the public that programs are in place to decrease the incidence and cost of injuries to society. These initiatives consist of a variety of strategies, including education of the general public and target groups; encouragement of community organizations to implement prevention plans; modifications that improve the safety of consumer products and the environment; and laws that, when heeded and enforced, limit the number of injuries.

Public health models have been helpful in this effort, although much more remains to be done. Evidence of the potential contributions of health professionals, such as occupational therapists and occupational therapy assistants, needs to be gathered and communicated. Successful strategies developed by the World Health Organization (WHO) or other countries need to be identified and studied to determine if they can be utilized or adapted for implementation. In addition, prevention programs will be more effective as they receive more money and attention commensurate with the magnitude and scope of the injury problem. The goal is for injury to be viewed as a phenomenon that is highly preventable, in ways that are understood and achievable.

According to the *Occupational Therapy Practice Framework,* injury and disability prevention is both an intervention approach and an outcome that can be derived from occupational therapy intervention and is therefore of great interest to the practitioners. Prevention may take the form of training in proper lifting techniques to reduce the incidence of back injuries, providing wrist supports to prevent repetitive stress injury, and providing a parenting class to decrease the rates of child abuse. Prevention activities enhance the health and wellbeing of individuals, families, organizations, and the community as a whole (American Occupational Therapy Association [AOTA], 2008).

The next section of this chapter will focus on unintentional injuries. However, the distinction between unintentional and intentional injury is sometimes artificial. Intent is only one relevant factor for injuries. Other factors include access to the means of injury, injury countermeasures, and medical response. In most cases, deaths from drowning, poisoning, or fire are classified as either unintentional or intentional based on the circumstances. The overwhelming majority of falls (95%), fire (90%), and drowning (84%) fatalities are unintentional deaths. The data for poisonings show a somewhat different pattern, with 63% of these deaths categorized as unintentional and the remaining 37% classified as intentional (Christoffel & Gallagher, 2006). It is important to note that "although the events leading to an intentional and an unintentional injury differ, the outcomes and extent of the injury are similar" (USDHHS, 2000, p. 15-4).

Unintentional Injury

Unintentional injuries occur without purposeful intent; however, this does not imply that they are not preventable. Unintentional injury is the fifth leading cause of death overall and is the leading cause of death for those aged 1 to 44 (NCIPC, 2007b). These injuries are likely to result from one of the physical forms of energy in the environment (i.e., kinetic, chemical, thermal, electrical, radiation) or are due to the lack of a needed energy element, such as oxygen during drowning or heat during hypothermia (Christoffel & Gallagher, 2006).

Injuries affect younger age groups disproportionately, causing premature death and the loss of years and quality of life even for survivors. **Years of potential life lost (YPLL)** is a statistic to measure premature death that is calculated by subtracting the age of an individual at death from their life expectancy. For the purpose of calculating YPLL, the CDC uses 75 years of age as the average life expectancy (USDHHS, 2000). Prior to age 65, unintentional injuries result in the loss of more years of productive life than any other cause, with nearly 2.3 million potential years of life lost per year, accounting for 19.4% of the total YPLL in 2005 (CDC, 2005). Of YPLL due to unintentional injuries, motor vehicle crashes account for approximately 50% and poisoning accounts for just under 25% (CDC, 2005). Besides lost years of life and productivity for fatalities, costs for disabled survivors include medical treatment and medications, rehabilitative care, and lost income (NCIPC, 2001).

Intentional and unintentional death rates vary by age, gender, income, geographic location, and race. Unintentional injury death rates are highest for those aged 85 and older and are second highest for those aged 15 to 24. Other groups with high rates are those aged 1 to 9 and aged 75 to 84 (NCHS, 2007). Death rates for unintentional injury are higher in infancy than for young children, then increase again for teens to young adults in their midtwenties. The rates then decline through middle age and rise again for the elderly (Content Box 18-1).

Motor Vehicle Injuries

Motor vehicle crashes account for 25% of all injury deaths. This category comprises the number one cause of total injury deaths and unintentional injury deaths for those aged 5 to 34 (CDC, 2005). Statistics indicate that more than 80% of those injured in motor vehicle crashes are vehicle occupants, with the other 20% comprised of pedestrians, motorcyclists, and bicyclists. Death rates are the highest for the very young and the second highest for the very old (Christoffel & Gallagher, 2006). Approximately 25% of the deaths occur for those aged 15 to 24, and men are three times as likely to die from motor vehicle injuries as women. Fatal injuries are much more likely in rural than in urban areas, whereas nonfatal injuries are the reverse (Christoffel & Gallagher, 2006).

Motor vehicle crashes result in more than 500,000 hospital admissions and over 5 million persons with injuries not requiring hospital admission each year. Motor vehicle crashes are the number one cause of serious and permanent brain and spinal cord injuries. The elderly have the highest ratio of death rate to injury rate; however, school-age children account for the largest number of overall deaths and injuries (Christoffel & Gallagher, 2006).

Motor vehicle crash injuries are also the number one cause of fatalities on the job (Christoffel & Gallagher, 2006). Recent debate on increasing the limits on hours per day and per week for commercial truck and vehicle drivers has been newsworthy. This change could result in more crashes and higher rates of vehicular death and injury due to increased exposure time on the road and by increasing the likelihood of drowsiness in commercial drivers. Some solutions include team driving, requiring more frequent breaks during driving shifts, and legislating longer rest periods between long driving shifts.

Prevention strategies have focused on postcrash, crash survivability, and precrash factors. Postcrash prevention involves better vehicle engineering that distributes the mechanical energy of the crash over space and time. Improved crash survivability is particularly evident in the improvements in response times and the skills of emergency medical and hospital trauma teams.

The most difficult factor is changing the behavior of drivers before crashes occur. Precrash strategies include decreasing speed limits with increased enforcement, lessening of auto and truck traffic, safer roadway and walkway designs, and the research and development of more crashworthy vehicles. Driver-calming techniques have been useful, including the timing of stoplights and placement of speed bumps and rest areas. Seat restraints and airbags, child seats, placing children in the rear seat, helmet laws for bicyclists and motorcyclists, and better driver testing have improved safety and decreased injury rates and severity.

Other precrash factors have also lowered crash rates, such as stricter requirements for new drivers and a decrease in the teenage population. Other factors include raising the minimum age for driving and limiting teen driving to daylight hours unless a special work or travel permit is issued. These are examples of Graduated Driver Licensing (GDL) laws, which, as of January 2006, had been adopted by 44 states and the District of Columbia.

Content Box 18-1

Top 10 Causes of Unintentional Injury Deaths for 2005

1. Motor vehicle traffic
2. Poisoning
3. Falls
4. Unintentional unspecified
5. Suffocation
6. Drowning
7. Fire/burns
8. Natural/environment
9. Other land transport
10. Other

Data from *Web-based injury statistics query and reporting system (WISQARS)*, Centers for Disease Control and Prevention, 2005. Retrieved January 28, 2008, from www.cdc.gov.ncipc/wisqars.

Included is the incentive of increased federal funding for enactment (National Highway Transportation Safety Administration [NHTSA], 2006).

Another area of precrash prevention involves the restriction and revocation of driving privileges for disabled and elderly persons who have become unsafe on the road. Causes of impairment that lead to the inability to drive safely can be categorized in four areas:

- Chronic physical and systemic medical disorders
- Sensory impairment, including decreased vision and hearing
- Impairment of coordination and reaction times, especially with neurological disorders that affect motor function and sensation
- Decline in judgment and decision-making ability, especially from traumatic brain injury (TBI), dementia, and mental illness

Sleep and alertness factors also influence highway safety. Prescription and over-the-counter medications that induce drowsiness now have warning labels to inform users of their effects on the person's ability to safely operate a motor vehicle.

Older Drivers

Motor vehicle crashes are the leading cause of accidental death for those aged 65 to 74. The percentage of drivers over age 65 is increasing dramatically due to the aging of the baby boomers. In 2004, there were approximately 28 million licensed older drivers. This represents a 17% increase since 1994 (NCIPC, 2007c). Nationally, older drivers (over 65 years of age) are expected to number 70 million and comprise at least 26% of the driving population by 2030. This means that one in every four drivers on the road will be over age 65. The motor vehicle death rate for persons over age 70 is approximately 23 per 100,000. In 2005, 79% of auto fatalities among older adults over age 65 occurred in the daytime and 73% on the weekends, and 73% of the crashes involved another vehicle (NHTSA, 2006).

Chronic disease and disabling conditions can affect an older person's ability to drive, thus jeopardizing their own safety and that of others. It has been estimated that one-third of persons over age 65 have functional limitations, particularly cognition, psychomotor, and sensory-perceptual deficits, that impair their ability to perform numerous activities of daily living (ADLs). In a telephone survey of adults with elderly parents, 25% of the respondents believed their parents should voluntarily impose driving restrictions on themselves and 10% said that their parents should have some mandatory restrictions or not be driving at all (Knowledge Networks, 2009).

Driving is an important instrumental ADL that contributes to an older person's autonomy, quality of life, and social participation. Occupational therapists can promote older driver safety and contribute to prevention efforts through CarFit assessments and older driver screenings and comprehensive evaluations. CarFit is an educational program developed by the American Society on Aging in collaboration with the American Automobile Association (AAA), the American Association of Retired Persons (AARP), and AOTA. The goals of CarFit are to assess older drivers' fit with their personal vehicles, and recommend actions that can be taken to improve the driver-vehicle fit and to initiate information exchange regarding driver safety and community mobility (CarFit, 2007).

Older driver screenings can be done using the Assessment of Driving-Related Skills (ADReS) developed by the American Medical Association. This brief assessment targets essential abilities that are needed for safe driving (e.g., motor, sensory, and cognitive functions). Occupational therapists can help older adults develop personal driving plans that voluntarily restrict driving under certain conditions based on their functional limitations (e.g., nighttime, inclement weather, and major highways). If it is deemed necessary for a person to cease driving due to conditions that impair safe vehicle operation, then the occupational therapist can assist the individual to develop a personalized community mobility plan using alternative transportation options to meet his or her needs.

Poisoning

Poisoning is the second most frequent cause of unintentional deaths overall. It is responsible for over 250,000 hospital admissions a year. A **poison** is "any substance that is harmful to your body when ingested (eaten), inhaled (breathed), injected, or absorbed through the skin" (NCIPC, 2008, ¶ 1). The number one cause of unintentional poisoning deaths is drugs, both legal and illegal. It is impossible to determine how many of these deaths are suicides. Carbon monoxide poisoning is the number one cause of intentional poisoning deaths (Christoffel & Gallagher, 2006).

Over 90% of poisonings occur in the home, and one-fourth of home injury deaths involve poisoning. The highest fatality rates are in adults aged 20 to 49 (McDonald & Gielen, 2006). For children, over 50% of poisonings occur in those under age 6 and are usually caused by cleaners, cosmetics, personal care products, and medications. Prevention measures include child-proof packaging, lockboxes, and locking cabinets. Reports have indicated that "Mr. Yuk" labels have had no effect on prevention of poisoning in children under age 2, and these colorful labels may actually attract young children. Syrup of ipecac is now contraindicated for use in children because of lack of efficacy and the risk of further harm by use after the ingestion of caustic chemicals (McDonald & Gielen, 2006).

For the elderly, prevention of poisoning includes decreasing the number and frequency of both prescription and over-the-counter (OTC) medications and removing outdated or unused medications from the home. Close monitoring of medications that have severe adverse effects—such as anticoagulants (i.e., blood thinners), which increase the risk of hemorrhage, and a large group of centrally acting drugs that cause sedation and increase the risk of falls—has lowered the risk of poisoning in the elderly.

Carbon Monoxide

Poisoning with carbon monoxide (an odorless, colorless gas) is responsible for 15,000 emergency department visits and about 440 deaths per year (NCIPC, 2007d). These deaths are classified as unintentional and nonfire related, and they are more likely to result at home than anywhere else. The average number of deaths per month is typically greatest in January, which is consistent with the high use of fossil fuels and natural gas for heating. High rates of carbon monoxide (CO) poisoning are more likely in workplaces that utilize carbon-based fuels; internal combustion engines; and forges, blast furnaces, and coke ovens (Occupational Safety and Health Administration [OSHA], 2002).

Carbon monoxide poisoning mimics flu and other viral illnesses and may result in initial misdiagnosis. Acute carbon monoxide poisoning may result in cardiac, pulmonary, neurological, and other complications, including myocardial infarction, retinal hemorrhages, memory loss, and rhabdomyolysis-induced renal damage (Tomaszewski, 1999). Severe neurological sequelae are possible, including permanent memory loss, chronic behavioral and learning disabilities in children, and incapacitating motor disorders.

Prevention of carbon monoxide poisoning includes education of the public to the hazards at home, regular inspection of gas heaters and appliances, adequate ventilation of indoor gases and fireplaces, keeping outdoor smoke outdoors, and use of CO alarms that are in good working order. Workplace safety starts with the preventive measures used in homes and adds employer and employee education, compliance with OSHA standards, and use of personal CO alarms and appropriate respirator masks and oxygen supply systems (OSHA, 2002).

Lead Poisoning

Although a single high toxic dose of lead can manifest in severe emergency symptoms and rarely in death, lead poisoning is usually the result of prolonged or repeated exposure to smaller amounts of lead dust that accumulates in the body. Children, and their developing nervous systems, are particularly susceptible to the effects of lead exposure, leading to symptoms and toxicity (Mayo Clinic, 2007). Symptoms of lead poisoning in children include irritability, decreased appetite and energy, weight loss, developmental delay or regression, anemia with pallor, constipation, and vomiting. Lower intelligence scores, learning difficulties, and poor school performance are often observed with abnormal serum lead levels.

Symptoms of lead poisoning in adults include headache, pain/numbness/tingling of the extremities, muscle weakness, memory loss, mood disorders, and abnormal fertility. The first sign of a high toxic dose of lead may be abdominal pain, followed later by vomiting, ataxic gait, increased muscle weakness, seizure, and coma (Mayo Clinic, 2007).

Sources of contamination include dust from soil near highways and construction sites that has been polluted by leaded gasolines and paints; water from lead pipes and solder for plumbing uses; old buildings with lead paint where children eat the lead chips; children's toys and ceramics; imported canned foods, and cosmetics. Children are most at risk, because they tend to put objects into their mouths. Adults at highest risk are those who breathe lead dust in their job or hobby (usually construction or making stained glass or refinishing furniture).

Although there is treatment, prevention by removing sources of exposure and cleaning up the environment is preferred. Preventive measures include lead inspection and risk assessment, hand washing before meals and after play, removing unused lead-based substances from the home, running tap water at least 1 minute before using in buildings with old pipes and fixtures, and using caution when working with or in areas that have old lead paint.

Falls

Falls are the third leading cause of unintentional injury deaths but are the most frequent cause of nonfatal injuries. Five percent of all persons residing in the United States receive emergency department treatment for fall injuries in their lifetime. One-third of falls occur in those over age 85 and are responsible for 87% of fractures in the elderly. One-third of falls are from heights, and these occur in the extremely young or old; in those impaired by alcohol, drugs, and mental and medical conditions; and at work (Christoffel & Gallagher, 2006). The risk of fatality from falls increases with height of fall, with age over 60, with unforgiving surface, and with a direct fall on the head (McDonald & Gielen, 2006).

Falls in those aged 65 and older account for 60% of deaths, which are declining overall. Factors that increase fall risk in the elderly are a prior fall; cognitive impairment; chronic illness; balance or gait impairment; decreased body-mass index (BMI); osteoporosis; increased frailty; female gender; certain home hazards; and use of certain medications, such as diuretics, vasodilators, anticholinergic drugs and sedatives, as these drugs may cause dehydration, orthostatic hypotension, drowsiness, and loss of balance (Christoffel & Gallagher, 2006).

Prevention measures for the elderly include weight-bearing exercise, activity, environmental modification, avoiding offending medications, and treatment with bone-strengthening agents such as calcium. In long-term care centers and nursing homes, fall prevention measures may also include use of bed alarms, nonslip bathtub surfaces, scheduled voiding, and frequent nursing rounds. In addition, good lighting, stair railings, colored nonslip step strips, and bath and bed grab bars may be useful. For further information on preventing falls in the elderly, see Chapter 24.

For children, ways to prevent falls or lessen their impact include window guards in high-rise buildings, gates on stairways, and energy-absorbing surface materials in playgrounds and play areas. Avoiding the use of baby walkers has also been very effective. Educating and counseling parents and caretakers on safety issues and remaining vigilant result in better fall prevention for children.

Suffocation

Suffocation is the fifth leading cause of unintentional deaths, and the term implies unintentional asphyxiation or choking (CDC, 2005). Unintentional deaths due to suffocation can occur due to

- obstruction in the respiratory tract by nonfood objects (e.g., toy parts, balloons, coins);
- inhaled, ingested, or regurgitated food in the respiratory tract; and
- mechanical obstruction from items like plastic bags and balloons (Christoffel & Gallagher, 2006).

For children under 1 year of age, suffocation accounts for 69% of unintentional injury deaths (USCDC, 2005). To prevent these unfortunate deaths, consumer product safety improvements have been made. Toys are larger and more difficult to swallow, and they have better warning labels. Fewer balloons are in use, and those that are in use are now more difficult to burst. There has also been a decline in children accidentally strangled by window cords, as more blinds utilize twist-turn handles. Negative media attention, lawsuits, and stricter laws that make it easier to remove unsafe products from the market, or prevent manufacturers from making them at all, have also proved useful. The training of adults in first aid, with recognition of choking and the use of the

Heimlich maneuver, has saved many lives (Heimlich & Patrick, 1990). For those with difficulty swallowing, cutting food into smaller pieces, pureeing food, alternating sips and bites, and using thickening agents for liquids has helped to decrease choking and aspiration (Paik, 2006).

Drowning

Drowning is the sixth leading cause of unintentional death overall but is the second leading cause for infants and children up to 14 years old. Drowning rates vary by gender, race, and ethnicity. Males are three and a half times more likely than females to die by drowning. Asian Americans and Native Americans have the highest rates, and African Americans are one and a half times as likely as whites to die by drowning (Christoffel & Gallagher, 2006).

Children under age 1 are most likely to drown in bathtubs, buckets, or toilets. Most drowning cases in children aged 0 to 4 years occur in residential swimming pools (NCIPC, 2007e). For those over 15 years of age, recreation in natural water settings, such as lakes, rivers, or the ocean, represents the majority of drownings. Most boating fatalities are the result of drowning, and 87% of those victims were not wearing life jackets. Alcohol use is implicated in up to 50% of water recreation deaths (NCIPC, 2007e).

Use of preventive education, training, and environmental modifications are recommended. Prevention measures include fencing off swimming pools on all four sides, using personal flotation devices, and swimming training. These precautions also apply to adults, and the latter two may prove especially useful offshore. For diving, the implementation of safety measures, avoidance of impaired diving, and common sense cannot be emphasized enough. For boating, knowledge from safety courses and the avoidance of impaired boating decreases the risk of drowning (NCIPC, 2007e).

Fires and Burns

Although fires and burns are the seventh leading cause of unintentional deaths (Christoffel & Gallagher, 2006), many are preventable. Higher-risk groups include the extremely young; the elderly; the disabled and those with medical impairments; the poor; smokers; and intoxicated persons, especially those using alcohol (McDonald & Gielen, 2006).

House fires are responsible for 80% of unintentional fire deaths and are the location for 76% of structural fires. Deaths are more likely (69%) from smoke (fumes, smoke inhalation, and carbon monoxide) than from burns (15%; McDonald & Gielen, 2006). "Alcohol impairment contributed to 40% of residential fire deaths," and cigarettes contributed to 25% of all fire deaths (Christoffel

& Gallagher, 2006, p. 85). Low-income areas, including substandard housing and mobile homes, were five times more likely than high-income areas to have fire death. Fires occur more often in the winter due to the use of home heating and cooking equipment (Christoffel & Gallagher, 2006).

Other causes of injury and death include flame; scalding; electrical, chemical, and ultraviolet radiation; and smoke inhalation (toxic gases). Burns can be thermal (heat), electrical, or chemical. Thermal burns include flame, scalding with hot liquid or steam, and ultraviolet radiation. Burns are classified in two ways: by the percentage of body surface involved (Rule of 9s) or by the depth of skin involvement (first- to fourth-degree burns). The Rule of 9s refers to dividing the body into approximately 11 regions each representing 9% of the body's surface in order to make it easier to estimate the percentage of the body that is burned (Livingston & Lee, 2000). Depth factors include temperature, characteristics of skin and coverings, and duration of exposure to heat source (McDonald & Gielen, 2006).

In 2005, burns caused 3299 deaths, with the highest fatality rates in adults over age 65 and children under 5 years. The highest injury rate for burns is in children aged 0 to 4 years, followed by persons 15 to 19 years, and then 20 to 24 years (McDonald & Gielen, 2006). The age group with the lowest injury rate from burns is 80 to 84 years. Cooking is the leading cause of injuries from home fires (McDonald & Gielen, 2006).

Prevention measures include use of smoke detectors, which must have working batteries or a power system. When tested, only 50% of home smoke alarms were in working order (McDonald & Gielen, 2006). Presetting water heaters to 125°F and below; having laws requiring both smoke detectors and preset water heaters; paying attention to burning stoves, ovens, and outdoor and grill fires; and avoiding smoking indoors help prevent fires. Programs that distribute smoke alarms are helpful but are too few. Lives have been saved when families prepare and practice a fire escape plan. For businesses, the use of sprinkler systems and rapid response of fire departments are helpful in decreasing fire damage and spread.

Sports Injuries

The overall number one cause of nonfatal injuries is sports activities, both organized and spontaneous. There were over 4 million nonfatal sports injuries in 2003, and over 1 million were listed as serious (Christoffel & Gallagher, 1999). Fortunately, there are relatively few deaths, but they are often dramatic in nature. The majority of high school sport injuries occur in football. Other sports with high injury rates include basketball, gymnastics, ice hockey, and wrestling. The

most common causes of injury are due to "falls, from being struck by an object, or from overexertion" (Christoffel & Gallagher, 2006, p. 87).

The scope of this concern is magnified because 30 million children play sports. Injury rates are highest overall for boys age 10 to 14 years, and injury is the number one cause for discontinuing participation in sports. Children under age 15 account for 40% of all sports- and recreation-related emergency department visits, and those aged 15 to 24 account for another one-third of these visits (McDonald & Gielen, 2006). By type of sport, playground and bicycle injuries are the majority for those aged 0 to 9 years. For boys aged 10 to 19, football, baseball, and bicycling injuries are predominant, and for girls aged 10 to 19, basketball is the leading sport for injuries (McDonald & Gielen, 2006).

Prevention includes better equipment; game rules and training, especially for cycling, football, and hockey; and the use of proper techniques, especially for tackling in football. Other measures are grouping players in contact sports by ability and improving the medical response to injury, including medical personnel overseeing practices and participating in emergency readiness and procedure training (Christoffel & Gallagher, 2006).

Work Injuries

Work injuries are a significant cause of lost productivity, increased costs, disability, and death in the workplace. Despite advances in ergonomics, workplace management and engineering safety measures, industrial hygiene, and equipment to lessen work hazard exposure, the number and extent of work injuries and their consequences still exacts an enormous social and economic burden on workers and their families, businesses, and insurance companies. Yearly total deaths have dropped from 20,000 per year in the early 1900s to less than 5113 per year in 2005 (NCHS, 2007), but this total is still believed to be too high. The decline is steeper for deaths from motor vehicles, machines, and electrocutions and is less steep for falls.

A study of records from 2005 for U.S. hospital emergency departments showed that approximately 11,000 workers per day were treated and 200 were hospitalized, while 36,000 were injured and 16 were killed each day (McDonald & Gielen, 2006). In 2006, 2.1 million workplace injuries resulted in days lost from work, job transfer, or work restrictions, which represented a rate of 2.3 cases per 100 workers. Figure 18-2 illustrates the industries with the highest rates of workplace injuries (Bureau of Labor Statistics, 2007).

In 2004, workers under age 25 had higher rates than those over age 25 of work-related injury. Overall, males have higher rates (3 per 100 full-time equivalent workers) of nonfatal occupational injuries than females

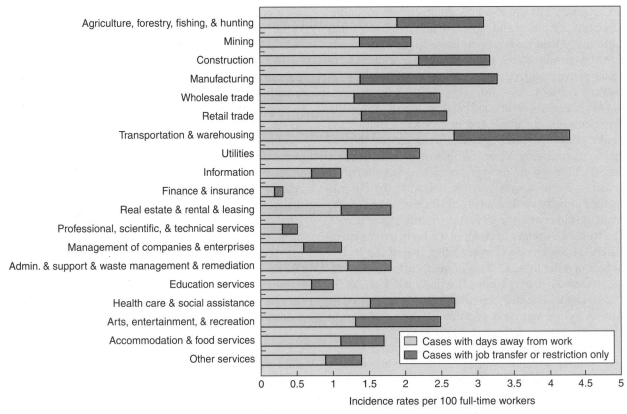

Figure 18-2 Workplace injuries by type of industry.

From Workplace injuries and illnesses in 2006 *(p. 4), Bureau of Labor Statistics, 2007, Washington, DC: U.S. Department of Labor.*

(1.9 per 100). Males between the ages of 18 and 19 had the highest rates (7 per 100). More than 75% of all workplace injuries were the result of contact with objects or equipment; bodily exertion, such as a sprain or strain; and falls (CDC, 2007a).

Ergonomics is the field devoted to the study of preventing and reducing work injury by improving body mechanics, machine design, and work techniques. Attention to body mechanics has helped reduce repetitive use injuries, such as carpal tunnel syndrome. Machine designs, including computer keyboards, have been changed to facilitate job performance with fewer injuries. Education in body mechanics, including lifting techniques that reduce stress on the back, neck, and joints of the extremities, has been helpful. Equipment such as lifting belts, joint braces, and eye and hearing protection has prevented significant injury and disability in the workplace. Job hazard analysis is a useful tool in worksite injury prevention and "focuses on the relationship between the worker, the task, the tools, and the work environment" (OSHA, 2002). Identifying job hazards is the first step to eliminating or reducing them in order to prevent injury.

An Example of Injury Prevention in the Workplace

Ergonomics, as it applies to the practice of occupational therapy, has been defined as "the science of fitting the task to the worker and not the worker to the task" (Fenton & Gagnon, 2003, p. 343). Jacobs (1999) describes ergonomics as "the study of work performance with an emphasis on worker safety and productivity" (p. 9). It is the task of the occupational therapist to accurately evaluate a person's ability to function in his or her work environment and to develop any necessary recommendations to modify the individual's work practices, the work environment, or the work task itself to facilitate safety, to prevent injury, and to improve productivity on the job.

Ergonomic consulting is often a routine expectation of the occupational therapist in many industrial rehabilitation settings. The work settings are anything but typical and may include a variety of jobs in a variety of industries and businesses. Many laborers learn how to reduce their risk of back or other musculoskeletal injuries through the interventions of occupational therapists. Office workers can benefit from an occupational therapist's ergonomic consultation by learning to reduce their risk of cumulative trauma disorders, especially those associated with the rapid and repetitive pace of data entry on computer systems and keyboarding functions.

At Towson University, occupational therapy faculty members provide ergonomic consulting services throughout the university community. Currently, on-site computer workstation evaluations are offered to faculty and staff across the campus. See Appendix D for recommended computer workstation guidelines. A partnership has been developed between the university's Department of Environmental Health and Safety (EHS) and the Department of Occupational Therapy and Occupational Science (DOTOS). This partnership has resulted in additional opportunities for faculty and staff members to participate in work-site evaluations that identify situations and equipment that put them at risk for discomfort or injury and to improve their workstations to promote safety and productivity. Whenever possible, a safety manager from EHS collaborates with the occupational therapist during the consultation.

The ergonomic consultation consists of a work-site visit, observation, and measurement of the employee's computer workstation and related equipment, and recommendations are made for any changes that could improve work performance safety. General education is also provided related to recommended safe working positions and general resources, including the federal ergonomic guidelines available from OSHA's website (OSHA, n.d.a, n.d.b). Follow-up with a brief written report and e-mails to check on implementation of recommendations is also routinely conducted.

In addition to individual workstation evaluations, faculty in the DOTOS have presented recommended computer workstation arrangements to the larger campus community through a variety of staff training opportunities. The topic of promoting an ergonomically safe workstation has been presented at staff conferences and during faculty retreats. By providing the general education regarding a safe workstation, workers are empowered to make the changes on their own and accept responsibility for their safety and productivity. Presentations have been made to the campus ACCESS committee (ACCessibility and Education for Students and Staff/faculty), *Healthy Campus Task Force,* and Staff Council Workshops. Individuals in the University Office for Disability Support Services and the University Fair Practices Officer have made direct referrals for services.

Injuries Due to Violence

We can have justice whenever those who have not been injured by injustice are as outraged by it as those who have been. (Solon, Greek philosopher, ca. 640–559 BC)

Violence has become pervasive in U.S. society and comes in a variety of forms, including homicide, suicide, domestic and family violence, sexual violence, and youth and school violence. On an average day in the United States, 70 persons die of homicide, 84 persons die of suicide, and a minimum of 18,000 persons survive interpersonal assaults (USDHHS, 2000). Elders, women, and children are most frequently the targets of violence, and the perpetrators are often people they know. In addition, people with disabilities are more often the targets of violence than their nondisabled counterparts. The social context of disability, including factors such as poverty, isolation, and dependence on support services, significantly increases a person's risk for abuse.

Violence can be defined as "the intentional use of physical force or power, threatened or actual, against another person or against oneself or against a group of people, that results in or has a high likelihood of resulting in injury, death, psychological harm, maldevelopment, or deprivation" (USDHHS, 2000, p. 15-56). Although the media often portrays violence perpetrated by strangers, in reality the majority of violence occurs within families and among acquaintances (Christoffel & Gallagher, 2006). See Content Box 18-2.

A public health approach to violence is to identify risk and protective factors, to design programs based on epidemiological data, to evaluate program effectiveness, and to modify prevention strategies based on evidence. Risk factors associated with violence include personal factors such as male gender, alcohol abuse, and childhood trauma, and environmental and social factors such as access to guns and poverty (Gellert, 2002).

Homicide

Homicide is "death resulting from injuries inflicted by another person with the intent to injure or kill" (Christoffel & Gallagher, 2006, p. 106). It occurs when

---

Content Box 18-2

Top 10 Causes of Violence-Related Injury Deaths (2005)

1. Suicide with a firearm
2. Homicide with a firearm
3. Suicide by suffocation
4. Suicide by poisoning
5. Homicide—cut/pierce
6. Homicide unspecified
7. Suicide by fall
8. Homicide by suffocation
9. Suicide—cut/pierce
10. Homicide—other

Data from *Web-based injury statistics query and reporting system (WISQARS)*, Centers for Disease Control and Prevention, 2005. Retrieved January 28, 2008, from www.cdc.gov.ncipc/wisqars.

"a person knowingly, purposefully, recklessly or negligently causes the death of another human being" (Gellert, 2002, p. 240). In 2002, 17,638 deaths, or an average of 48 per day, were attributable to homicide. Firearms are used in approximately 70% of murders. Although homicide rates overall are dropping, homicide is the second leading cause of death for Hispanic Americans aged 15 to 34 and the leading cause of death for African Americans aged 15 to 24. Males are most often the perpetrators and victims. When the effects of socioeconomic status are controlled for, the rates of homicide among whites, Hispanics, and African Americans are nearly identical—the risk factor appears to be poverty, not race (Christoffel & Gallagher, 2006). Other risk factors include discrimination, lack of education, and lack of employment opportunities (USDHHS, 2000).

Most homicides are not the result of organized criminal activity but rather are the result of family dysfunction, alcohol and drug use, and poverty. It is estimated that 40% of homicides are perpetrated by friends or acquaintances, 15% by family members, and the remaining 45% by strangers. Homicides occur 2.5 times more frequently in low-income neighborhoods than in high-income areas. Social disorganization in neighborhoods is a risk factor for violence, while social cohesion is a protective factor. Alcohol and drugs are frequently associated with homicide deaths. Approximately 10% of homicides are related to illicit drug use. In addition, alcohol is often present in both the perpetrator and the victim (Christoffel & Gallagher, 2006). The rate of homicide for young males in the United States is 10 times higher than in Canada and 15 times higher than in Australia (USDHHS, 2000).

Suicide

Suicide is "death from intentional self-inflicted injury" (Christoffel & Gallagher, 2006, p. 103) and is the cause of over 30,000 deaths annually. Every 17 minutes in the United States, a person commits suicide. Suicide occurs twice as often as homicide (Bergen, Chen, Warner & Fingerhut, 2008). The vast majority of suicides are committed with firearms. The next two most frequent means of suicide are suffocation and poisoning, respectively. Persons living in households that contain guns have five times greater suicide risk than those living in households without firearms. Other risk factors include previous suicide attempts; psychiatric disorders, especially depression; alcohol and substance abuse; family history of suicide or abuse; physical illness; feelings of hopelessness or isolation; and emotional or financial loss, among others. Males are four times more likely than females to die from suicide, yet females make suicide attempts more often. Whites account for 90% of all suicides (Christoffel & Gallagher, 2006).

Among teenagers, suicide is the third leading cause of death; only homicides and injuries kill adolescents more frequently. In 2005, fifty-five thousand adolescents in 42 states were screened for mental illness. Of these, about one-third rated positive on the questionnaire, and half of those were clinically significant enough to be referred for further evaluation (Friedman, 2006). Among youth, the most common correlates of suicide are depression, behavioral problems, impulsivity, neurocognitive difficulties, family adversity, substance abuse, and the availability of guns. Firearms are involved in 60% of adolescent male and 47% of adolescent female suicides (Brent & Mann, 2006). The elderly are also at high risk for suicide, particularly males over the age of 50 who have been recently widowed. Male U.S. veterans "are twice as likely to die by suicide as males without military service" (Suicide Prevention Advocacy Network USA [SPAN USA], 2007, ¶ 3).

Suicide is a public health problem that requires community-based prevention strategies. The warning signs of suicide are thoughts or threats of harming oneself, substance abuse, anxiety, withdrawing from family and friends, anger, reckless behavior, dramatic mood changes, feeling trapped, no sense of purpose in life, and hopelessness (American Association of Suicidology, 2006). Effective suicide prevention programs share certain characteristics:

- Designed to enhance protective factors, reduce risk factors, and increase help-seeking behavior
- Long-term with repeated interventions
- Family focused
- Adapted to address the specific problems in a community or population
- Age-specific, developmentally appropriate
- Culturally relevant (SPAN USA, 2001)

Funding is needed to support the development of suicide prevention programming. Advocacy groups have been successful in seeking and obtaining federal legislation to gain financial resources for suicide intervention and prevention. In 2004, the Garret Lee Smith Memorial Act was passed, releasing $82 million to communities and states for a 3-year period to fund programs related to youth suicide (Christoffel & Gallagher, 2006). More recently, in 2007, President Bush signed into law the Joshua Omvig Veterans Suicide Prevention Act, Public Law 110-110 (SPAN USA, 2007).

Domestic and Family Violence

Statistics indicate that 30% of women will experience violence from an intimate partner at some point in their lives (McAllister, 2000). However, women are not the only ones at risk for experiencing abusive situations. In some U.S. communities, child mortality is more common from violence than disease, with most of these occurring in domestic cases (Veenema, 2001). For the households in which domestic violence occurs between husband and wife, children are 15 times more likely to suffer physical abuse than those in nonviolent families (McAllister, 2000). These numbers may only approximate the true occurrence within the United States, because domestic violence often remains hidden within the community.

Several factors are believed to put persons at increased risk of falling victim to domestic violence. Because abuse has been shown to occur in cycles, those who have suffered abuse as children are at increased risk of fostering violent households of their own. Also, women who have been abused are likely to return to yet another violent relationship after a previous violent relationship ends. It is believed that those experiencing these or similar scenarios may be limited by psychosocial, environmental, socioeconomic, and/or developmental problems (McAllister, 2000). Regardless of the causes of domestic violence, the results of abuse may be devastating in many ways. **Family violence** includes child abuse and neglect, intimate partner violence, and elder abuse. Each of these will be discussed briefly.

Child Abuse and Neglect

In 2005, out of 1000 children under age 18, 12.1 were reported victims of child maltreatment. This same year, 1.96 children per 100,000 died of abuse. For these children, maltreatment was evident in several forms, including physical abuse (17%), sexual abuse (9%), emotional abuse (7%), and neglect (63%). Overall, girls are at slightly higher risk for child maltreatment than boys. The highest rate of child maltreatment is for children from birth to 3 years of age, and the rates decline as children get older (CDC, 2007b). In most cases, the perpetrator of child abuse is a family member. In 75% of the cases, the parents were the abusers and 10% were other relatives (USDHHS, 2000). Child abuse can be found in all socioeconomic groups, and family stress, particularly economic stress, is a major determinant in abuse. Children who are abused often become abusive parents themselves and also have a higher likelihood of committing other violent acts (Christoffel & Gallagher, 2006).

A variety of factors increase a child's risk for abuse or neglect. Children from unplanned pregnancies, children of single parents, children who are adopted, and children who have disabilities are all at higher risk. Family factors that predispose children to abuse include social isolation, family disruption, and poverty. According to Gellert (2002), "In homes where child abuse occurs, violence among siblings is not uncommon" (p. 27). Children who are being abused can be identified by a wide range of signs and symptoms. Physical signs

of broken bones, lacerations, and bruises may be infrequent. More subtle signs may include malnutrition, failure of the child to develop properly, bed-wetting, thumb-sucking, poor school performance, and difficulty forming meaningful relationships (Gellert, 2002).

Through studies of children's play habits, it has been found that an abused child's play tends to be impulsive, disorganized, and lacking a play theme (Cooper, 2000), in comparison to the play of a nonabused child. This is of great concern, because for young children, play is the most important means of adapting and developing skills needed to prepare for more advanced tasks. School-age children often continue to have problems and exhibit difficulty concentrating in the classroom, which leads to poor academic performance (Davis, 1999).

Abused children are also at an increased risk for behavioral problems. The child's behavioral repertoire may be limited, and this can often be seen at a young age by a skilled observer. The child may engage in stereotypic repetitive play, and such repetitious behavior can continue in other areas as the child gets older (Caughey, 1991; Mann & McDermott, 1983). When a child is unable to escape this situation, exploration, which is normally a vehicle for learning, may remain at a minimal level. When children find themselves in unfamiliar environments, they may not exhibit appropriate behavior and in turn may experience stress.

Abused children often present with an assortment of psychosocial problems. They may have difficulty expressing themselves appropriately, and, consequently, they may show aggressive play themes (Cooper, 2000). These children often have a low self-concept and experience feelings of self-blame for situations in which they find themselves. As a result, abused children have much higher rates of depression that, left untreated, could persist later in life (Veenema, 2001).

Occupational therapists and occupational therapy assistants are mandated as health-care providers to report suspected child abuse and neglect. This is a serious legal and ethical responsibility. Procedures for reporting may vary across health-care facilities and from state to state, so the practitioner must familiarize themselves with state law and regulatory acts. Reports of child abuse and neglect should always be documented.

Intimate Partner Violence (IPV)

Intimate partner violence (IPV) refers to "actual or threatened physical or sexual violence or psychological and emotional abuse by an intimate partner" (USDHHS, 2000, p. 15-56). Intimate partners include, but are not limited to, spouses, former spouses, opposite sex and same-sex partners, or former partners. Partners need not be cohabitating or engaging in sexual activities to be considered intimate partners (USDHHS, 2000). Intimate partner violence may be physical, psychological, or sexual. IPV includes physical assault; verbal abuse; sexual coercion; intimidation; destruction of personal property; restriction of freedom to participate in everyday activities; isolation; stalking; and withholding of resources, especially financial (National Coalition Against Domestic Violence, n.d.). Domestic violence affects not only the direct victim of the violence, but also "the children witnessing it, the family and friends of the survivor and the communities in which it occurs" (AOTA, 2007, p. 704).

Women are the victims of reported abusive behavior 85% of the time, which means that in 15% of cases, men are the victims. One in every four women has experienced IPV in her lifetime, and one in seven men have been victims. In 2003, IPV against women resulted in approximately 2 million injuries and 1300 deaths (Breiding, Black, & Ryan, 2008; NCIPC, 2003). Intimate partner homicides accounted for one-third of the murders of women in 2000. Women aged 16 to 24 are most at risk, and disabled, pregnant, and postpartum women are particularly vulnerable. Approximately 70% of men who abuse their female partners also abuse their children. IPV occurs in all social, economic, racial, ethnic, and religious groups and occurs in heterosexual and homosexual relationships at nearly the same rate (AOTA, 2007; Bryant, 2005; McDonnell, Burke, Gielen, & O'Campo, 2006).

The aftermath of domestic violence involves several negative consequences for those who have been victimized. The survivors typically exhibit limitations in daily life skills, particularly in leisure participation, home management, parenting, work performance, financial management, and educational participation. These limitations are often due to difficulty with decision-making, problem-solving, following directions, task initiation, and judgment. Problems with self-confidence, interpersonal relationships, stress management, and coping skills are also prevalent (AOTA, 2007; Gorde, Helfrich, & Finlayson, 2004). Limitations may also exist in important prevocational skills, such as acquiring and maintaining a job to provide for the family. Children exposed to IPV frequently have sleep and eating disturbances and have difficulty self-calming. In addition, they may exhibit developmental delay, maladaptive behaviors, limited social skills, and poor academic performance (AOTA, 2007).

Elder Abuse

The burgeoning elderly population includes 45 million people over age 60 and three million over age 85. By the year 2030, the elderly will comprise 20% of the population. With the increasing recognition of neglect and abuse of the elderly, and the lack of adequate funding of services for this population, this problem will likely remain significant for years to come (Gorbien & Eisenstein, 2005).

Elder abuse takes several forms, including physical abuse, emotional or psychological abuse, sexual abuse, financial or material exploitation, abandonment, neglect, and self-neglect (Content Box 18-3). Since elder abuse and neglect is underreported, particularly for emotional and financial abuse, numbers vary among studies. An estimate is that over 2 million elderly adults are mistreated each year, with a prevalence rate of 32 per 1000 adults (Gorbien & Eisenstein, 2005). The majority of abused elders are physically maltreated by their children and are often living with their abusers. Those 75 years and older are most at risk to be victimized (Conoley & Goldstein, 2004).

Risk factors for mistreatment include the following: increasing age, lack of access to resources, low income and education levels, minority status, social isolation, functional or cognitive impairment, substance abuse by elder or caregiver, previous history of family violence, history of psychological problems, and caregiver stress. Women are victimized more often than men, often suffer physical abuse, and are almost always the victims in sexual abuse (Gorbien & Eisenstein, 2005).

Recent research has shed light on both understanding and recognizing abusers. Adult children are more likely to abuse their elder parent than spouses are to abuse their mate (50% vs. 20% to 40%). Males are

---

Content Box 18-3

Types of Elder Abuse—Definitions

- *Physical abuse:* The use of physical force that might result in bodily injury, physical pain, or impairment. Physical punishments of any kind are examples of physical abuse.
- *Emotional or psychological abuse:* The infliction of anguish, pain, or distress.
- *Sexual abuse:* Nonconsensual sexual contact of any kind with an elderly person.
- *Financial or material exploitation:* The illegal or improper use of an elder's funds, property, or assets.
- *Abandonment:* The desertion of an elderly person by an individual who had physical custody or otherwise had assumed responsibility for providing care for an elder, or by a person with physical custody of an elder.
- *Neglect:* The refusal or failure to fulfill any obligations or duties to an elder.
- *Self-neglect:* The behaviors of an elderly person that threaten his or her health or safety. The definition of *self-neglect* excludes a situation in which a mentally competent older person who understands the consequences of his or her decisions makes a conscious and voluntary decision to engage in acts that threaten his or her own health or safety.

Adapted from "Elder abuse and neglect: An overview" by M. J. Gorbien & A. R. Eisenstein, 2005, *Clinics in Geriatric Medicine, 21*, 279–92.

abusers more frequently than females, and the abuser often depends financially on the victim. Previous abuse and a poor long-standing relationship between caregiver and victim are also significant risk factors. Alcohol abuse is the most common risk factor for physical violence (Gorbien & Eisenstein, 2005).

Ramsey-Klawsnik (2000) divided abusers into five types (Content Box 18-4): the overwhelmed, the impaired, the narcissistic, the domineering or bullying, and the sadistic or sociopathic. The overwhelmed group is generally well intentioned and qualified to provide care but may be verbally or physically abusive if care needs exceed their ability. The impaired group is well intentioned but has physical or mental problems that become barriers to providing adequate care, so neglect is more common in this group. The other three types of abuser are more predatory and try to use victims to meet their needs and to feel powerful. Domineering types are

prone to neglect and financially abuse others. They are also the most likely to engage in sexual abuse.

Improving the identification and reporting of elder abuse is essential to lessen the impact of this problem. Identification includes having consistent definitions, standard laws, and improved training of social service and health professionals and health workers. Improvements in screening instruments, long-term and nursing home care, and awareness of physical indicators of elder abuse are needed. Lafata and Helfrich (2001) created an Occupational Therapy Elder Abuse Checklist specifically for use by occupational therapy practitioners. The checklist is available in two forms, one for elders who live alone and one for elders who live with others. It is administered to both the elder and his or her caregiver in order to compare their perceptions of the home environment. The instrument addresses health issues, caregiver attitudes, financial issues, support systems for the client and caregiver, and safety issues.

Although there are mandatory reporting laws for child abuse, and Child Protective Services can take children away from their abusive caregivers, few such protections exist for victims of elder abuse. One innovative program, the Coalition for the Rights of the Infirm Elderly, develops training methods to prevent abusive behavior by nursing home personnel (Gorbien & Eisenstein, 2005).

Sexual Violence and Assault

Sexual violence is defined in the WHO's *World Report on Violence and Health* as

> any sexual act, attempt to obtain a sexual act, unwanted sexual comments or advances, or acts to traffic a person's sexuality, using coercion, threats of harm or physical force, by any person regardless of relationship to the victim, in any setting, including, but not limited to home and work. (WHO, 2004, p. 1)

Both males and females can be the victims or perpetrators of sexual violence. Perpetrators may be a family member, spouse/significant other, acquaintance, or stranger to the victim. However, in the case of rape, 8 out of 10 victims know the perpetrator (Tjaden & Thoennes, 2000).

Women are more likely to become victims of sexual violence than men. Statistics indicate that 87% of the sexual assaults reported in the National Crime Victimization Survey were women, and 13% were men (U.S. Department of Justice [USDOJ], 2005). According to the National Violence Against Women survey, 1 in 6 women and 1 in 33 men in the United States have been victims of attempted or completed rape (Tjaden & Thoennes, 2000). Although sexual violence occurs across the life span, the majority of rapes involve minors as victims, with 54% of rapes occurring in women

---

Content Box 18-4

Types of Abusers of the Elderly

The first two categories are nonpredatory; the last three categories exhibit predatory behavior.

1. *The overwhelmed:* This well-intentioned group is generally qualified to provide care. When care needs exceed what they can provide, they may abuse verbally or physically, but they do not look for victims.
2. *The impaired:* This is a well-intentioned group who have mental or physical problems that prevent them from delivering care. They may be unaware of the deficits in their care delivery. They may tend to control the victim through abuse; neglect is more common in this group.
3. *The narcissistic:* These caregivers enter into caregiving relationships in order to meet their needs. They are more likely to steal from elders and neglect them. They view the relationship as a means to an end and may be attracted to nursing homes or care centers where they can enter into relationships with vulnerable adults.
4. *The domineering or bullying:* This group feels entitled to exert power and authority. They may have narcissistic tendencies and often feel that the victim deserved the mistreatment. This type of offender may honor limits in other settings and has insight into the nature of their maladaptive behavior. This offender is prone to neglect and financial abuse and may engage in sexual abuse.
5. *The sadistic or psychopathic:* This type of offender takes pleasure in mistreating their victim. They have feelings of power and importance when they abuse others.

Adapted from "Elder-abuse offenders: A typology" by H. Ramsey-Klawsnik, 2000, *Generations, 2,* 46–51. In "Elder abuse and neglect: An overview" by M. J. Gorbien & A. R. Eisenstein, 2005, *Clinics in Geriatric Medicine, 21,* 279–92.

before the age of 18 and 22% before the age of 12 (Tjaden & Thoennes, 2000). Risk factors that may increase the chance of victimization include young age, use of drugs and alcohol, previous history of sexual violence, having multiple sex partners, and poverty (NCIPC, 2004). Violence during dating has been reported by 22% of high school students and by 32% of college students (Christoffel & Gallagher, 1999).

Symptoms and behavioral indicators that may be exhibited in victims of sexual violence include deficits in interpersonal and intrapersonal skills, such as an inability to engage in appropriate social activities, difficulty recognizing unsafe situations, confusing sexual acts with affection, and engaging in unsafe sex. In addition, victims of sexual violence often lack a supportive network and have a decreased sense of personal boundaries that allows others to violate their personal rights, thereby increasing their likelihood of revictimization (Gutman & Swarbrick, 1998).

According to NCIPC (2004) statistics, consequences of sexual violence/abuse may be physical, psychological, social, and emotional. Victims of sexual violence often experience long-term effects such as anxiety, sleep disturbances, depression, and sexual dysfunction. Physical symptoms resulting from sexual violence may be acute or chronic and may include increased risk of urogenital infections, chronic pelvic pain, gastrointestinal disorders, pelvic inflammatory disease, and migraine and other headaches (Coker, Smith, Bethea, King & McKeow, 2000). Contracting sexually transmitted diseases and becoming pregnant are also physical consequences associated with sexual violence. Statistics indicate that between 4% and 30% of rape victims will contract a sexually transmitted disease (NCIPC, 2004).

The immediate psychological symptoms resulting from sexual violence may include shock, disbelief, denial, fear, confusion, anxiety, and withdrawal (Herman, 1992a). In addition to these symptoms, victims of sexual violence often experience symptoms of acute stress disorder, such as emotional detachment, sleep disturbances, and flashbacks. Statistics (NCIPC, 2004) show that in approximately one-third of victims experiencing sexual violence, psychological symptoms will continue for 3 months or become chronic, leading to the long-term psychological and emotional effects of post-traumatic stress disorder (PTSD). Other consequences of sexual violence include an increased likelihood of drug and alcohol abuse and concomitant psychological and emotional disorders. Often, victims of sexual violence turn to drug and alcohol abuse as a means of avoiding the pain and coping with the abuse (Gutman & Swarbrick, 1998).

Occupational therapy practitioners play an important role in their clients' lives and often assist with private and personal areas of their occupational functioning.

Because of this, many clients may feel more comfortable opening up to their occupational therapist concerning their experience with sexual abuse/violence. Reports of sexual violence should always be documented.

Youth and School Violence

Youth are frequently both the perpetrators and victims of violence (USDHHS, 2000). The U.S. Department of Justice (USDOJ) receives reports of nearly 3 million crimes annually at or near schools. This is approximately 16,000 per school day nationwide, or one every 6 seconds that school is in session (Conoley & Goldstein, 2004). There are many correlates to school violence. One is the size of the school, with larger schools experiencing higher ratios of incidents of violence per student. Crowding is another such correlate, as acts of school violence occur more frequently in crowded hallways, cafeterias, and stairways than in less crowded classroom environments. For unknown reasons, more episodes of school violence seem to occur during the spring rather than fall term. According to Stephens (1997), school violence is not "confined to any socioeconomic group, cultural group, or ethnic community" (p. 72).

Approximately one-third of children who are physically abused at home become perpetrators of violence themselves. Conoley and Goldstein (2004) believe that acts of school violence are but one manifestation of the violence that characterizes much of present-day life and that "aggression is primarily learned behavior" (p. 11). Although teachers are occasionally the victims of school violence, most student aggression is directed at their peers. The greatest increases in violence are occurring among elementary school-age children. However, older adolescents are more frequently both the aggressor and the victim. Often, it is the case of extreme violence that is brought to the attention of the public, but lower levels of aggressive behavior are far more prevalent. If lower levels of aggressive behavior are tolerated, it invites students to further challenge the limits of acceptable behavior. See Content Box 18-5 for a list of categories of aggressive behaviors displayed in schools.

Children and adolescents who commit violent acts share several common risk factors: poor supervision or monitoring, parental alcohol or drug abuse, social cognitive deficits, academic failure, association with delinquent peers, and exposure to violence. Violence prevention strategies advocated by the USDOJ that may be of interest to occupational therapy practitioners include youth and parent life skills training, job training and placement, street outreach services, gang intervention strategies, youth conflict resolution training, and mentoring programs for at-risk youth (Gellert, 2002).

From *School violence intervention: A practical handbook* (2d ed., pp. 10–11) by J. C. Conoley & A. P. Goldstein, 2004, New York: Guilford Press.

Content Box 18-5

Categories of School Violence

The following is ordered from least aggressive to most aggressive:

- Horseplay
- Rule violation
- Disruptiveness
- Cursing
- Bullying
- Sexual harassment
- Refusal/defiance
- Threats
- Vandalism
- Out-of-control behavior
- Student-student fights
- Attacks on teachers
- Use of weapons
- Collective violence

Bullying

Bullying is fairly prevalent among students of all ages, with nearly half of all children and adolescents reporting being the victim of bullying at least once during their school years (American Academy of Child & Adolescent Psychiatry [AACAP], 2008). In one study of playground behavior, Craig and Pepler (2000) observed one incident of bullying every 7 minutes, with adult intervention occurring in only 4% of these incidents. **Bullying** "occurs when a student or group of students targets an individual repeatedly over time, using physical or psychological aggression to dominate the victim" (Brewster & Railsback, 2001, p. 12). It can take the form of name-calling, racial slurs, spreading rumors, insults, threats, physical attacks, and theft. Children who are victims of bullying experience significant fear and anxiety that can interfere with academic achievement and social-emotional development (AACAP, 2008).

Bullying is an attempt to gain power and influence over others. Bullies view aggressive behavior as an acceptable means of resolving disputes and handling problems. The vast majority of bullying incidents occur in school corridors and on the playground. Some researchers believe that bullying is an early precursor of adult criminal behavior (Gellert, 2002); therefore, it should receive greater attention than is typically given by parents and school officials (Conoley & Goldstein, 2004). Nansel and colleagues (2003) warn that "bullying should not be considered a normative aspect of youth development, but rather a marker for more serious violent behaviors, including weapon carrying, frequent fighting, and fighting-related injury."

A fairly recent phenomena is **cyberbullying,** or electronic bullying, which refers to using e-mail, chat rooms, websites, instant messaging, text messaging, and other electronic methods of communication to repeatedly intimidate and cause emotional distress. It is estimated that over 90% of adolescents aged 12 to 18 years, use the Internet. This is the most "wired" generation to date, and therefore the most vulnerable to cyberbullying (Kowalski & Limber, 2007).

Risk and Protective Factors for Youth Violence

"The concepts of risk and protection are integral to public health. A risk factor is anything that increases the probability that a person will suffer harm. A protective factor is something that decreases the potential harmful effect of a risk factor" (USDHHS, 2001, p. 57). Risk and protective factors that have been identified in *Youth Violence* (USDHHS, 2001) are displayed in Table 18-1. These data clearly demonstrate the need for parent education and support.

Strategies for Preventing School Violence and Enhancing Safety

Safe schools are secure; well supervised; and free of sexual harassment, drugs, weapons, gangs, crime, and violence (Stephens, 1997). The three approaches to preventing school violence are based on the three levels of prevention. Providing school safety programming for an entire population of students is an example of primary prevention, or a compensatory approach. Targeting students who are at high risk for aggression or victimization is considered a protective approach, or secondary prevention (Morrison, Furlong, D'Incau, & Morrison, 2004). Addressing issues related to school violence after an incident has occurred is tertiary prevention and is obviously the least desirable approach.

Effective strategies for increasing school safety include controlling campus access, developing a comprehensive school safety plan, requiring picture identification for all students and staff members, modifying school environments to prevent crime, creating a climate of ownership and school pride, developing and enforcing a school dress code, providing adequate adult supervision, and encouraging multicultural understanding. Other strategies offered by Stephens (1997) that are particularly relevant for occupational therapy are

- establishing interesting and challenging extracurricular activity programs;
- incorporating life skills training focused on decision-making, conflict resolution, anger management, social interaction, and responsibility;

Table 18–1 **Early and Late Risk Factors for Violence at Age 15–18 and Proposed Protective Factors, by Domain**

Domain	RISK FACTOR Early Onset (Age 6–11)	Late Onset (Age 12–14)	Protective Factor*
Individual	General offenses	General offenses	Intolerant attitude toward deviance
	Substance use	Psychological condition	High IQ
	Being male	Restlessness	Being female
	Aggression**	Difficulty concentrating**	Positive social orientation
	Psychological condition	Risk-taking	Perceived sanctions for transgressions
	Hyperactivity	Aggression**	
	Problem (antisocial) behavior	Being male	
	Exposure to television violence	Physical violence	
	Medical, physical	Antisocial attitudes, beliefs	
	Low IQ	Crimes against persons	
	Antisocial attitudes, beliefs	Problem (antisocial) behavior	
	Dishonesty**	Low IQ	
		Substance use	
Family	Low socioeconomic status/poverty	Poor parent-child relations (e.g., harsh, lax discipline; poor monitoring, supervision)	Warm, supportive relationships with parents or other adults
	Antisocial parents	Low parental involvement	Parents' positive evaluation of peers
	Poor parent-child relations (e.g., harsh, lax, or inconsistent discipline)	Antisocial parents	Parental monitoring
	Broken home	Broken home	
	Separation from parents	Low socioeconomic status/poverty	
	Other conditions	Abusive parents	
	Abusive parents	Other conditions	
	Neglect	Family conflict**	
School	Poor attitude, performance	Poor attitude, performance	Commitment to school
		Academic failure	Recognition for involvement in conventional activities
Peer Group	Weak social ties	Weak social ties	Friends who engage in conventional behavior
	Antisocial peers	Antisocial, delinquent peers	
		Gang membership	
Community		Neighborhood crime, drugs	
		Neighborhood disorganization	

*Age of onset not known.
**Males only.
From Box 4-1 from *Youth Violence: A report of the surgeon general* (p. 58). U.S. Department of Health and Human Services, 2001, Washington, DC: U.S. Government Printing Office.

- encouraging active student participation in promoting school safety; and
- developing peer counseling and peer mediation programs, and training students to fulfill these roles.

Prevention strategies for school violence that have little or no research-evidence support include suspension from school, "boot camp" programs, and corporal punishment (penalizing someone for an offense by inflicting pain or imposing confinement). A listing of model and promising youth violence programs is provided in Table 18-2.

Violence Prevention on a College Campus

University and college administrators are increasingly monitoring and addressing campus violence, which includes violence perpetrated by outsiders as well as members of the academic community. The publication of *Healthy Campuses: Making It Happen* (American College Health Association [ACHA], 2002) provided a framework and set of priorities to assist postsecondary educational institutions in such efforts. The ACHA's National College Health Assessment (NCHA) collects data on the violence rate among young adults on university and college campuses. Figures 18-3 and 18-4 display data from the Spring 2003 survey (*n* = 19,497).

An initiative that has been successful in facilitating preventive health education and policy implementation for academic communities can serve as a model for future efforts. Fostering collaborative ventures among parents, students, administrators, and faculty makes campuses not only safe places for students, but also places to learn to become engaged in promoting health among individuals and society. In 1986, the nonprofit organization Security On Campus, Inc., was founded by parents of a first-year university student who was the victim of brutal violence that led to her death. Her assailant was another student attending the same educational institution (Security On Campus, 2004, ¶ 1). The mission of Security On Campus is to make campuses safer for students. The specific goals that support this mission appear in Content Box 18-6.

This organization was responsible for the passage of the Campus Security Act, a landmark federal law now known as the Jeanne Clery Disclosure of Campus Security Policy and Campus Crime Statistics Act. The passage of this act and five additional related federal laws has impacted crime investigation and reporting, as well as how survivors of campus sexual assault are treated at most college and university campuses nationwide. Since passage of this legislation, administrators at colleges and universities have been increasingly more proactive in the area of violent crime prevention.

Table 18–2 Rating Prevention Programs

Model
Level 1 (Violence Prevention)
- Seattle Social Development Project
- Prenatal and Infancy Home Visitation By Nurses
- Multidimensional Treatment Foster Care

Level 2 (Risk Prevention)
- Life Skills Training
- The Midwestern Prevention Project

Promising
Level 1 (Violence Prevention)
- School Transitional Environmental Program
- Syracuse Family Development Research Program
- Perry Preschool Program
- Striving Together to Achieve Rewarding Tomorrows
- Intensive Protective Supervision Project

Level 2 (Risk Prevention)
- Promoting alternative thinking strategies
- I Can Problem Solve
- Iowa Strengthening Families Program
- Preparing for the Drug-Free Years
- Linking the Interests of Families and Teachers
- Bullying Prevention Program
- Good Behavior Game
- Parent-Child Development Center Programs
- Parent-Child Interaction Training
- Yale Child Welfare Project
- Families and Schools Together
- The Incredible Years Series
- The Quantum Opportunities Program

Does Not Work
- Drug Abuse Resistance Education
- Scared Straight

From *Youth violence: A report of the surgeon general*, 2001, U.S. Department and Health and Human Services, Washington, DC: U.S. Government Printing Office.

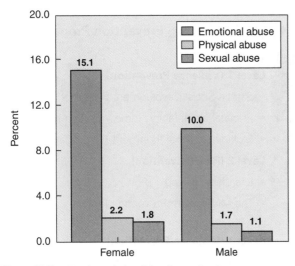

Figure 18-3   Abusive relationships: Last school year.

From Figure 7 National College Health Assessment Web Summary, *by American College Health Association. National College Health Assessment Web Summary, 2004, Baltimore, MD. The figure reflects students' self-reported data from the spring 2003 NCHA survey (n = 19,497).*

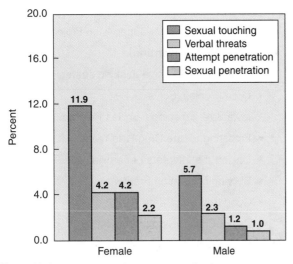

Figure 18-4   Sexual abuse/assault: Last school year.

From Figure 6 National College Health Assessment Web Summary, *by American College Health Association. National College Health Assessment Web Summary, 2004, Baltimore, MD. The figure reflects students' self-reported data from the spring 2003 NCHA survey (n = 19,497).*

Mental Health Aspects of Unintentional Injury and Violence

Psychological and emotional effects of unintentional injury or violence may be short- or long-term. Due to the differing circumstances, the severity of symptoms may differ for unintentional injury and violence; however, the basic mental health responses are similar.

Content Box 18-6

Mission of Security On Campus, Inc.

- To educate prospective students, parents and the campus community about the prevalence of crime on our nation's college and university campuses.
- To compassionately assist victims and their families with guidance pertaining to laws, victims' organizations, legal counsel and access to Security On Campus, Inc., files.
- To foster security improvements through campus community initiatives.
- To provide effective procedures and programs to reduce alcohol and drug abuse.

From *About Security On Campus, Inc., our mission* (¶ 1), by Security On Campus, Inc., 2004, King of Prussia, PA.

Individuals—children and adults—who have experienced severe injury, who have witnessed a traumatic event such as a fatal motor vehicle crash, or who are victims of violence may develop symptoms consistent with acute stress disorder (ASD) and PTSD. The likelihood of developing either or both of these anxiety disorders depends on the intensity, severity, and duration of the traumatic event and the physical proximity of exposure to it. Lifetime prevalence of PTSD is approximately 12% among women and 6% among men. Persons with ASD or PTSD typically react to the traumatic event with intense fear, helplessness, or horror. Nearly two-thirds of persons with PTSD also present with comorbid conditions, most frequently substance abuse, depression, bipolar disorder, or anxiety disorders (Sadock & Sadock, 2003).

In acute stress disorder, the person develops anxiety and dissociative symptoms within 1 month after experiencing a traumatic event. The symptoms may include difficulty concentrating, feeling guilty about engaging in normal everyday activities, decreased emotional responsiveness, difficulty recalling important aspects of the traumatic event, inability to enjoy pleasurable activities, and a sense of detachment or numbing (American Psychiatric Association [APA], 2000). Other symptoms indicative of anxiety include difficulty sleeping, irritability, hypervigilance, psychomotor agitation, and an exaggerated startle response. In addition, the individual frequently re-experiences the event through flashbacks, images, and dreams, and avoids any stimuli associated with the trauma. ASD causes significant emotional distress and impairment in social and occupational function. The symptoms may last for a minimum of 2 days up to a maximum of 4 weeks. After 4 weeks, the person may meet the diagnostic criteria for PTSD (APA, 2000).

Of those with ASD, approximately 80% will eventually meet the diagnostic criteria for PTSD. The symptoms of PTSD are virtually identical to those of ASD; however, they persist for more than 1 month. Other symptoms that can occur include paranoia, self-destructive and impulsive behavior, somatic complaints, outbursts of anger, social withdrawal, and changes in personality. Symptoms usually become apparent within 3 months of the traumatic event, but there may be a delayed onset of months or years. Symptoms can last for years, but approximately half of those affected recover within 3 months of symptom emergence. Persons who have experienced PTSD are at high risk of recurrence, as new traumatic events or life stressors can reactivate PTSD symptoms (APA, 2000). Risk factors for PTSD include childhood trauma, personality disorders, inadequate family or peer support, recent stressful life changes, family history of psychiatric disorders, and an external locus of control (Sadock & Sadock, 2003).

Herman (1992b) describes three posttraumatic stages of recovery typically experienced by victims of severe injury or violence. Directly following the injury/assault, many victims experience an acute crisis phase, which may involve experiencing feelings of terror, helplessness, rage, humiliation, shame, and guilt. During this first stage, the injury/violence is often relived through flashbacks and nightmares. The first stage of recovery can last days to years, depending on the severity of the trauma. The primary task of this stage is to establish physical and emotional safety. Victims often experience a loss of control and may feel unsafe in their own bodies. At this time, it is critically important to prevent secondary trauma and retraumatization. **Secondary trauma** refers to trauma that occurs after the event and that is associated with responses toward the victim—for example, law enforcement questioning the victim's behaviors as a cause of the trauma or well-meaning family members and friends telling the victim that they were fortunate because the trauma could have been worse. Relaxation strategies, exercise, medications, unconditional positive regard, consistency, and boundary setting can relieve symptoms and increase the victim's sense of safety.

The second stage is characterized by grieving. The primary task of this stage is telling one's story. There is a need to acknowledge the traumatic event, revisit it, and assign meaning to the experience. The victim often feels powerless at this stage, and it is important to reframe the mourning process as evidence of the person's strength and courage. Focusing on the person's assets, abilities, and strengths re-empowers them and enables them to assimilate the traumatic experience. A nonjudgmental attitude and compassion toward the person is most helpful at this stage.

In the third stage of recovery, reconnecting with ordinary life is the primary task. The victim builds a new identity and a new life that incorporates the positive and negative elements of the trauma. Re-education about what is normal and ordinary may be useful, as the trauma has taken them out of the usual, everyday experience. During this stage, the person regains their sense of power and self-efficacy. Some victims transcend the trauma and develop survivor missions—for example, developing support services or prevention programs for others in similar circumstances (Herman, 1992b).

Principles of Unintentional Injury and Violence Prevention

The public health approach to unintentional injury and violence prevention is typically interdisciplinary. Prevention approaches can take the form of education, engineering/environmental modification, and enforcement. These are often referred to as the **three Es** of injury prevention. Public health education is designed to increase knowledge and skills, change attitudes, encourage safe behaviors, remind people of recognized risks, and reduce risky behaviors. Educational strategies can be targeted not only at individuals, but also at high-risk groups, health professionals, schools, the media, businesses, policymakers, and the general public.

Engineering/environmental modification refers to producing products and environments that are safer with fewer hazards and that make behavior change easier or unnecessary. The environment has both physical and sociocultural elements. The physical environment includes natural and human-made objects and settings. The sociocultural environment relates to public perceptions, beliefs and attitudes, and social norms. In addition to producing safer products and environments, operating practices and protocols (e.g., at worksites) can also be modified to minimize injuries, and safety equipment can be provided. Any or all of these aspects of environment can be targeted for modification.

Enforcement refers to modifying behavior through compulsory public health measures, statutes, and regulations. These legal approaches "can be directed at individual behavior (people), at products (things), or at environmental conditions (places)" (Christoffel & Gallagher, 2006, p. 217). For example, seat belt and helmet use, compulsory immunization, and child restraint laws are targeted at the behavior of individuals. Motor vehicle safety standards, laws requiring child-proof caps on medications, and regulations regarding storage of flammable materials are directed at products, and building codes and airport safety regulations are directed at places.

Many federal agencies have responsibilities in this area, including the National Highway and Traffic Safety Administration (NHTSA); the Occupational Safety and Health Administration (OSHA); the Food and Drug

Administration (FDA); the Consumer Product Safety Commission (CPSC); the Federal Aviation Administration (FAA); the Bureau of Alcohol, Tobacco and Firearms (ATF); and the Centers for Disease Control and Prevention (CDC). In addition, state governments can enact and enforce injury prevention laws, statutes, and regulations. For example, Massachusetts has over 100 state and local laws addressing unintentional injury to children (Christoffel & Gallagher, 2006).

Haddon's Matrix

Developed by William Haddon, Jr., physician and engineer, this matrix conceptualizes injury as occurring in three phases: preinjury event, injury event, and postinjury event, in interaction with human factors, an agent or vehicle, and physical and sociocultural environments. Levels of prevention correspond to the phases of the matrix. In the preinjury event phase, primary prevention efforts are appropriate; for example, speed limit enforcement to reduce motor vehicle crashes. During the injury event phase, secondary prevention is the focus; for instance, air-bag deployment to reduce injury. In the postinjury event phase, tertiary prevention approaches are most relevant; for example, shortening emergency response times and improving the efficacy of rehabilitation (Christoffel & Gallagher, 2006).

Haddon identified 10 categories of injury prevention strategies focused on addressing hazards. A **hazard** is defined as the potential to cause harm, or a condition or activity, which if left uncontrolled, could result in illness or injury (OSHA, 2002). Hazards typically fall into four broad categories: physical, chemical, biological, and psychological. Physical hazards include such things as radiation, noise, and poor working conditions. Chemical hazards may be naturally occurring or human-made, such as vapors and gases from industry and tobacco smoke. Biological hazards take the form of allergens, bacteria, viruses, and other microbiological organisms. Psychological hazards are typically occurrences that induce unreasonably high levels of stress, such as exposure to violence (Agius, 2001).

Haddon's categories of injury prevention strategies, known as the Haddon Ten, include

1. preventing the initial creation of a hazard;
2. reducing the amount of energy a hazard contains;
3. preventing the release of existing hazards;
4. modifying the rate or distribution of a hazard;
5. separating the hazard, by time or space, from the person;
6. using material barriers to prevent exposure to a hazard;
7. modifying qualities of a hazard to reduce its impact;
8. increasing the person's resistance to damage from a hazard;
9. countering the damage already done as quickly as possible; and
10. stabilizing, repairing, and rehabilitating the damage produced by a hazard (Christoffel & Gallagher, 2006, p. 158).

The most effective unintentional injury and violence prevention programs address all three phases (i.e., preevent, event, and postevent) and components that could be changed (i.e., human factors, agent or vehicle, physical environment, and sociocultural environment) of the Haddon matrix, and use a combination of education, engineering/environmental modification, and enforcement strategies (Christoffel & Gallagher, 2006). Some of the most successful interventions to prevent unintentional injury include bicycle helmet education and laws, child safety restraints, traffic calming measures (e.g., speed bumps), free provision of smoke detectors, child-resistant containers to prevent poisoning, window bars and stair gates to prevent falls, and enforcing rules protecting player safety in sports (Christoffel & Gallagher, 2006; Harvard Injury Control Research Center, 2003–2007).

Role of Occupational Therapy in Unintentional Injury and Violence Prevention

As in most areas of prevention, identification of risk and protective factors is critical. In injury prevention, occupational therapists are uniquely equipped to analyze daily activities in work, leisure, and self-care; to identify potential risk and protective factors; and to then design strategies to reduce risk of injury. These strategies may include modifying environmental, equipment, and activity variables to increase safety in occupational performance, decreasing individual risk factors for injury, and increasing protective factors. For example, in falls prevention, environmental and activity modifications and improving an individual's protective factors (motor strength and balance) decreases the risk of falls. Occupational therapists can also provide risk reduction education and train persons to engage in activities in the safest manner possible. These strategies can be used as primary prevention (prior to the occurrence of any injury) and as secondary prevention to reduce the likelihood of reinjury.

For primary prevention of violence, a focus on decreasing risk factors and increasing protective factors is also appropriate. Improving assertiveness and interpersonal skills, increasing safety awareness, and building self-defense skills are protective factors that offer appropriate prevention opportunities for occupational therapy. These decrease personal vulnerability and the likelihood of becoming a victim of violence. Life skills training, anger management, conflict resolution, and coping and relaxation skill development may decrease the probability of some forms of violence by providing the potential perpetrator with alternative strategies for dealing with stress. These approaches can also be used for victims and perpetrators of violence as secondary prevention to reduce the likelihood of reoccurrence.

As was mentioned earlier, serious injury and violence often have significant psychological and emotional health consequences. If left unaddressed, these emotional symptoms and responses can result in long-term psychological sequelae that negatively impact a person's occupational and social functioning. It is therefore important to address these issues and mediate these emotional responses in order to prevent occupational dysfunction and to rebuild a sense of empowerment and self-worth. Expressive therapy techniques such as music, dance, drawing, painting, journaling, and so on, are particularly beneficial for this purpose.

Conclusion

Occupational therapists and occupational therapy assistants have the opportunity to utilize their skills in activity analysis, environmental modification, and life skills training to decrease the risk of unintentional injury and violence. The provision of psychosocial occupational therapy interventions to victims of injury and violence can lessen the negative impact of these incidents on social, emotional, and occupational functioning. In order to be maximally effective, occupational therapy injury and violence prevention efforts should not focus solely on individuals. Due to the inextricable links between persons and their environments, prevention strategies should also address families, groups, organizations, communities, and policymakers. Occupational therapists can be advocates for, and designers of, safer work and play environments and better-designed toys, leisure, and work equipment.

Research on the relationship between occupation and injury and occupation and violence, articulation of the role of occupational therapy, and demonstrations of effective preventive interventions are essential if the profession is to become a key contributor in these areas of public health. In addition, occupational therapists and occupational therapy assistants need to use appropriate public health and injury and violence prevention terminology, be cognizant of the literature of these fields, and apply known public health principles in occupational therapy prevention interventions.

Case Study 18-1

Injury Prevention

Nationally, the proportion of older drivers (over 65 years of age) continues to increase dramatically. Elderly drivers are expected to number 70 million and comprise at least 26% of the driving population by 2030. A community located in the southern United States near the Gulf of Mexico is experiencing a significant growth in the older adult population, as it is a haven for retirees. With this change in demographics, the community has also experienced an increase in motor vehicle crashes involving older adults. According to the U.S. Census Bureau, in 2006, this community had 63,721 older adults, which represented 13.4% of the population, exceeding the national average of older adults, which is 12.4% of the population. Of the 60 and older population, 28% are minorities, 17% live in rural areas, 25% live alone, and 14% live below the poverty level.

You have been asked to serve on the Mayor's task force on older drivers to assist in the development of a prevention and intervention program to reduce motor vehicle crashes and the morbidity and mortality associated with them. The task force consists of health-care professionals, area agency on aging personnel, representatives from the transportation industry, local members of AARP, and the state licensing board.

Questions

1. What additional information do you need about this community and population to design an appropriate prevention and intervention program? How will you collect this information?
2. List three potential long-term goals for this older driver program.
3. Describe the basic components of a comprehensive older driver crash prevention and intervention program.
4. What is the role of the occupational therapist in older driver crash prevention programs? What services might occupational therapists provide?
5. How would you evaluate the effectiveness of the program?

Case Study 18-2

Violence Prevention

The school board of an affluent county, located close to a large prosperous urban area, was shocked by video footage of a group of varsity high school girl field hockey players planning and participating in a hazing incident at a county park. As a result of this incident, three junior varsity players were hospitalized for head injuries and other physical trauma. Five additional junior varsity players, who sustained multiple fractures to the elbows, wrists, and hands, were treated in the emergency room and released.

The school board was pressured by the media and victims' parents to establish a commission to investigate the incident and review county policy with the goal of preventing future occurrences. The school board worked in collaboration with the victims' parents to determine the appointments to the commission. Cindy, one of the parents whose daughter was receiving occupational therapy for head and hand injuries, was appointed to the commission. She was very impressed with the occupational therapist, Juanita, who was addressing not only the physical issues but also resultant psychosocial issues due to the victimization experience. Cindy was so impressed with Juanita's holistic, occupation-centered intervention that she sought to have her appointed to the commission. At first, the school board was hesitant, not believing an occupational therapist could make contributions to the group. However, after hearing of Juanita's graduate occupational therapy project at a domestic violence shelter, she was appointed to the commission.

The commission was slated to start meeting the following autumn. In order to prepare for her role on the commission, Juanita knew she had to update her knowledge on population-based models and become acquainted with literature regarding bullying and hazing. Juanita contacted the local university and chose a graduate student interested in youth violence prevention. The student worked with Juanita to review the literature as a directed readings elective course over the summer. Based on the results of the directed reading course, Juanita was well prepared for her role from an evidence and theoreti-

cal perspective. The student was excited to see her work being used to impact a social issue in her community.

At the first commission meeting in the fall, Juanita was pleased at being able to effectively participate in discussions regarding which approach to use in examining the issue. The selected approach was the PRECEDE-PROCEED Model. The parents on the committee encouraged Juanita to conduct individual and focus group meetings with the perpetrators, hazing targets, and parents of both groups to explore the factors contributing to the hazing event.

Questions

1. Was hazing or bullying an issue in your school or in the community where you grew up? Did it ever result in prolonged intimidation or physical violence? Were adult leaders in the community aware of the existence of the problem?
2. If you had been invited to join a commission or advocacy group to decrease this type of behavior, what might you have suggested? Which of the solutions could be generalized to other communities and which might not work elsewhere? Why?
3. Which occupational therapy model do you think would be helpful in the development of a hazing/bullying prevention program for a local middle school? Sketch the main theory-based components of the program. Would this program need to be modified for a high school population? Why or why not?
4. Does your institution have a program and policies in place to report and decrease violence on campus? If so, are they easily accessible to prospective students, current students, staff, and faculty? What, if any, information is missing or unclear?
5. Compare your institution's Web-based communications in this area with two other institutions. Describe how these efforts were similar and how they were different. What steps can you take as an occupational therapy student to improve communication about violence prevention and safety on your campus?

▶ For Discussion and Review

1. How might occupational therapists apply their skills of occupational analysis to the reduction of sports injuries among school-age children?
2. What are reliable sources of information on unintentional injury and violence prevention?

3. What are the characteristics of effective injury and violence prevention programs?
4. How could Haddon's Matrix be applied to the problem of falls in the elderly?
5. What are some risk factors and protective factors for motor vehicle injuries? What purpose might

occupational therapy serve in motor vehicle injury prevention?

▶ Research Questions

1. Do occupational therapy driving evaluations and interventions decrease the incidence of motor vehicle crashes involving elderly drivers?
2. Are persons who have received ergonomic consultations implementing the resulting recommendations after 1 month, 6 months, 1 year?
3. Does universal design decrease the risk of injury for persons with disabilities? For persons without disabilities?
4. What is the relationship between occupational deprivation and violence?
5. What factors contribute to a person's ability to overcome the emotional and psychological consequences of severe injury and violence?

References

Agius, R. (2001). *Hazard and risk.* Retrieved January 3, 2007, from www.agius.com/hew/resource/introeh.htm.

American Academy of Child & Adolescent Psychiatry. (2008). *Facts for families: Bullying.* Retrieved March 31, 2008, from http://www.aacap.org/cs/root/facts_for_families/bullying.

American Association of Suicidology. (2006). *How do you remember the warning signs of suicide?* Retrieved November 28, 2006, from www.suicidology.org.

American College Health Association. (2002). *Healthy Campus 2010: Making it happen.* Baltimore: Author.

American College Health Association. (2004, June). *National College Health Assessment Web summary.* Retrieved November 28, 2004, from http://www.acha.org/projects _programs/ncha_sampledata_public.cfm.2004.

American Occupational Therapy Association. (2007). Occupational therapy services for individuals who have experienced domestic violence. *American Journal of Occupational Therapy, 61*(6), 704–09.

American Occupational Therapy Association. (2008). Occupational therapy practice framework: Domain & process. *American Journal of Occupational Therapy, 62*(6), 625–88.

American Psychiatric Association. (2000). *Diagnostic and statistical manual of mental disorders* (4th ed., text revision). Washington, DC: Author.

Bergen, G., Chen, L. H., Warner, M., & Fingerhut, L. A. (2008). *Injury in the United States: 2007 chartbook.* Hyattsville, MD: National Center for Health Statistics.

Breiding, M. J., Black, M. C., & Ryan, G. W. (2008). Prevalence and risk factors of intimate partner violence in eighteen U.S. states/territories, 2005. *American Journal of Preventive Medicine, 34*(2), 112–18.

Brent, D. A., & Mann, J. J. (2006). Familial pathways to suicidal behavior: Understanding and preventing suicide among adolescents. *New England Journal of Medicine, 355*(26), 2719–21.

Brewster, C., & Railsback, J. (2001). *Schoolwide prevention of bullying. By Request Series.* Portland, OR: Northwest Regional Educational Laboratory. Available through ERIC at http://eric.ed.gov.

Bryant, G. A. (2005). *Spousal and partner abuse—Intimate partner violence (IPV): Detection, assessment and intervention strategies.* GSC Home Study Courses.

Bureau of Labor Statistics. (2007). *Workplace injuries and illnesses in 2006.* Washington, DC: U.S. Department of Labor.

CarFit. (2007). *Program goals and outcomes.* Retrieved April 10, 2009, from http://www.car-fit.org.

Caughey, C. (1991). Becoming the child's ally: Observations in a classroom for children who have been abused. *Young Children, 46*(4), 22–28.

Centers for Disease Control and Prevention. (2005). *Web-based injury statistics query and reporting system (WISQARS).* Retrieved January 28, 2008, from www.cdc.gov.ncipc/wisqars.

Centers for Disease Control and Prevention. (2007a). Nonfatal occupational injuries and illnesses—United States, 2004. *Morbidity and Mortality Weekly Report, 56*(16), 393–97.

Centers for Disease Control and Prevention. (2007b). *Child maltreatment: Facts at a glance.* Retrieved March 31, 2008, from http://www.cdc.gov/ncipc/dvp/CMP/default.htm

Christoffel, T., & Gallagher, S. S. (1999). *Injury prevention and public health: Practical knowledge, skills and strategies.* Gaithersburg, MD: Aspen.

Christoffel, T., & Gallagher, S. S. (2006). *Injury prevention and public health: Practical knowledge, skills and strategies* (2d ed.). Gaithersburg, MD: Jones and Bartlett.

Coker, A. L., Smith, P. H., Bethea, L., King, M. R., & McKeown, R. E. (2000). Physical health consequences of physical and psychological intimate partner violence. *Archives of Family Medicine, 9,* 451–57.

Conoley, J. C., & Goldstein, A. P. (2004). *School violence intervention: A practical handbook* (2d ed.). New York: Guilford Press.

Cooper, R. J. (2000). The impact of child abuse on children's play: A conceptual model. *Occupational Therapy International, 7*(4), 259–76.

Craig, W., & Pepler, D. (2000). Observations of bullying in the playground and in the classroom. *School Psychology International, 21*(1), 22–37.

Davis, J. (1999). Effects of trauma on children: Occupational therapy to support recovery. *Occupational Therapy International, 6,* 126–41.

Fenton, S., & Gagnon, P. (2003). Section III—Work activities. In E. B. Crepeau, E. S. Cohn, & B. A. Schell, *Willard & Spackman's occupational therapy* (10th ed., pp. 342–46). Philadelphia: Lippincott, Williams & Wilkins.

Friedman, R. A. (2006). Uncovering an epidemic: Screening for mental illness in teens. *New England Journal of Medicine, 355*(26), 2717–19.

Gellert, G. A. (2002). *Confronting violence* (2d ed.). Washington, DC: American Public Health Association.

Gorbien, M. J., & Eisenstein, A. R. (2005). Elder abuse and neglect: An overview. *Clinics in Geriatric Medicine, 21,* 279–92.

Gorde, M. W., Helfrich, C. A., & Finlayson, M. L. (2004). Trauma symptoms and life skills needs of domestic violence victims. *Journal of Interpersonal Violence, 19,* 691–708.

Gutman, S. A., & Swarbrick, P. (1998). The multiple linkages between childhood sexual abuse, adult alcoholism, and traumatic brain injury in women: A set of guidelines for occupational therapy practice. *Occupational Therapy in Mental Health, 14*(3), 33–64.

Harvard Injury Control Research Center. (2003–2007). *Success stories.* Retrieved December 9, 2007, from http://www.hsph .harvard.edu/research/hicrc/success-stories/index.html.

Heimlich, H. J., & Patrick, E. A. (1990). Heimlich maneuver: Best technique for saving any choking victim's life. *Postgraduate Medicine, 87*(6), 38–53.

Herman, J. (1992a). Complex PTSD: A syndrome in survivors of prolonged and repeated trauma. *Journal of Traumatic Stress, 5*(3), 377–91.

Herman, J. (1992b). *Trauma and recovery.* New York: Basic Books.

Jacobs, K. (1999). *Ergonomics for therapists* (2d ed.). Boston: Butterworth-Heinemann.

Knowledge Networks. (2008). *Mature drivers survey: Final report. Retrieved* April 10, 2009, from http://downloads.nsc .org/pdf/MatureDriversSurveyReport.pdf.

Kowalski, R., & Limber, S. (2007). Electronic bullying among middle school students. *Journal of Adolescent Health, 41*(6), S22–S30.

Lafata, M. J., & Helfrich, C. A. (2001). The occupational therapy elder abuse checklist. *Occupational Therapy in Mental Health, 16*(3/4), 141–61.

Livingston, E. H., & Lee, S. (2000). Percentage of burned body surface area determination in obese and nonobese patients. *Journal of Surgical Research, 91*(2), 106–10.

Mann, E., & McDermott, J. (1983). Play therapy for victims of child abuse and neglect. In C. E. Schaefer & K. J. O'Connor (Eds.), *Handbook of play therapy* (pp. 283–307). New York: John Wiley & Sons.

Mayo Clinic. (2007). *Lead poisoning.* Retrieved January 1, 2008, from www.mayoclinic.com/health/lead-poisoning/ FL00068.

McAllister, M. (2000). Domestic violence: A life span approach to assessment and intervention. *Lippincott's Primary Care Practice, 4*(2), 174–89.

McDonald, E. M., & Gielen, A. C. (2006). House fires and other unintentional home injuries. In A. C. Gielen, D. A. Sleet, & R. J. DiClemente (Eds.), *Injury and violence prevention: Behavioral science theories, methods and applications* (pp. 274–96). San Francisco: Jossey-Bass.

McDonnell, K. A., Burke, J. G., Gielen, A. C., & O'Campo, P. J. (2006). Intimate partner violence. In A. C. Gielen, D. A. Sleet, & R. J. DiClemente (Eds.), *Injury and violence prevention: Behavioral science theories, methods and applications* (pp. 323–45). San Francisco: Jossey-Bass.

Morrison, G. M., Furlong, M. J., D'Incau, B., & Morrison, R. L. (2004). The safe school: Integrating the school reform agenda to prevent disruption and violence at school. In J. C. Conoley & A. P. Goldstein (Eds.), *School violence intervention: A practical handbook* (2d ed., pp. 256–96). New York: Guilford Press.

Nansel, T. R., Overpeck, M. D., Hyanie, D. L., Ruan, W. J., & Scheidt, P. C. (2003). Relationships between bullying and violence among U.S. youth. *Archives of Pediatric and Adolescent Medicine, 157,* 348–53.

National Center for Health Statistics. (2007). *Deaths: Preliminary data 2005.* Retrieved January 28, 2008, from http://www.cdc .gov/nchs/products/pubs/pubd/hestats/prelimdeaths05/ prelimdeaths05.htm.

National Center for Injury Prevention and Control. (2001). *Injury factbook 2001–2002.* Atlanta, GA: Centers for Disease Control and Prevention.

National Center for Injury Prevention and Control. (2003). *Costs of intimate partner violence against women in the United States.* Atlanta, GA: Centers for Disease Control and Prevention.

National Center for Injury Prevention and Control. (2004). *Sexual violence: Fact sheet.* Retrieved November 22, 2004, from http://www.cdc.gov/ncipc/factsheets/svfacts.htm.

National Center for Injury Prevention and Control. (2007a). *Youth violence prevention scientific information: Risk and protective factors.* Retrieved December 16, 2007, from http://www.cdc.gov/ncipc/dvp/YVP/YVP-risk-p-factors.htm.

National Center for Injury Prevention and Control. (2007b). *10 leading causes of death by age group, United States— 2004.* Retrieved December 16, 2007, from http://www.cdc.gov/ncipc/osp/charts.htm.

National Center for Injury Prevention and Control. (2007c). *Older adult drivers: Fact sheet.* Retrieved February 9, 2008, from http://www.cdc.gov/ncipc/factsheets/older.htm.

National Center for Injury Prevention and Control. (2007d). *10 leading causes of injury death by age group; highlighting unintentional injury deaths, United States—2003.* Retrieved December 16, 2007, from http://www.cdc.gov/ncipc/osp/charts.htm.

National Center for Injury Prevention and Control. (2007e). *Water-related injuries: Fact sheet.* Retrieved January 28, 2008, from http://www.cdc.gov/ncipc/factsheets/ drown.htm.

National Center for Injury Prevention and Control. (2008). *Poisoning in the United States: Fact sheet.* Retrieved February 8, 2008, from www.cdc.gov/ncipc/factsheets/poisoning.htm.

National Coalition Against Domestic Violence. (n.d.). *What is battering?* Retrieved November 15, 2006, from http://www.ncadv.org.

National Highway Transportation Safety Administration. (2006). *Traffic safety facts: Laws—Graduated driver licensing system.* Retrieved November 3, 2006, from http://www .nhtsa.dot/gov/staticfiles/DOT/NHTSA/rulemaking/ articles.htm.

Occupational Safety and Health Administration. (2002). *Job hazard analysis.* Retrieved January 3, 2007, from www.osha.gov/Publications/osha3071.html.

Occupational Safety and Health Administration. (n.d.a). *E-tools: Computer workstations.* Retrieved February 22, 2005, from http://www.osha.gov/SLTC/etools/computerworkstations/ index.html.

Occupational Safety and Health Administration. (n.d.b). *Effective ergonomics: Strategies for success.* Retrieved February 22, 2005, from http://www.osha.gov/SLTC/ergonomics/index.html.

Paik, N. J. (2006). *Dysphagia.* Retrieved February 8, 2008, from http://www.emedicine.com/pmr/topic194.htm.

Ramsey-Klawsnik, H. (2000). Elder-abuse offenders: A typology. *Generations, 2,* 17–22. [See also Gorbein, M. J. & Eisenstein, A. R. (Eds.). (2005).]

Sadock, B. J., & Sadock, V. A. (2003). *Synopsis of psychiatry* (9th ed.) Philadelphia: Lippincott, Williams & Wilkins.

Security On Campus, Inc. (2004). *About Security On Campus, Inc., our mission.* Retrieved November 28, 2004, from http://www.securityoncampus.org/aboutsoc/index.html.

Solon (594 BC). When asked how social justice could be achieved in Athens. Retrieved February 24, 2009, from http://quotes.liberty-tree.ca/quotes_by/solon.

Stephens, R. D. (1997). National trends in school violence: Statistics and prevention strategies. In A. P. Goldstein & J. C. Conoley (Eds.), *School violence intervention: A practical handbook* (pp. 72–92). New York: Guilford Press.

Stewart, A. E., & Lord, J. H. (2002). Motor vehicle *crash* versus *accident*: A change in terminology is necessary. *Journal of Traumatic Stress, 15,* 333–35.

Suicide Prevention Advocacy Network USA. (2001). *Suicide prevention: Prevention effectiveness and evaluation.* Atlanta, GA: SPAN USA.

Suicide Prevention Advocacy Network USA. (2007). *President signs Omvig Suicide Prevention Bill into law.* Retrieved December 9, 2007, from http://www.spanusa.org/.

Tjaden, P., & Thoennes, N. (2000). Prevalence and consequences of male-to-female and female-to-male intimate partner violence as measured by the National Violence Against Women Survey. *Violence Against Women, 6*(2), 142–61.

Tomaszewski, C. (1999). Carbon monoxide poisoning. *Postgraduate Medicine, 105*(1), 39–52.

U.S. Department of Health and Human Services. (2000). *Healthy People 2010: Understanding and improving health* (2d ed.). Washington, DC: U.S. Government Printing Office.

U.S. Department of Health and Human Services. (2001). *Youth violence: A report of the surgeon general.* Washington, DC: U.S. Government Printing Office.

U.S. Department of Health and Human Services. (2006). *Healthy People 2010 midcourse review.* Retrieved December 16, 2007, from http://www.healthypeople.gov/data/midcourse/html/focusareas/FA15Introduction.htm.

U.S. Department of Justice. (2005). *Crime Victimization Survey.* Retrieved January 8, 2007, from www.ojp.gov/bjs/abstract/cvus/gender780.htm.

Veenema, T. G. (2001). Children's exposure to community violence. *Journal of Nursing Scholarship, 33*(2), 167–74.

World Health Organization. (2004). *World report on violence and health, Chapter 6: Sexual violence.* Retrieved November 22, 2004, from http://www.who.int/violence_injury_prevention/violence/interpersonal/ip3/en/print.html.

Health Promotion and Prevention From an Occupational Therapy Perspective

Health Promotion for People With Disabilities

Michael A. Pizzi

> Health is created and lived by people within the settings of their everyday life; where they learn, work, play, and love. Health is created by caring for oneself and others, by being able to make decisions and have control over one's life circumstances. Caring, holism, and ecology are essential issues in developing strategies for health promotion and wellness.
> —Ottawa Charter for Health Promotion, World Health Organization [WHO], 1986, p. 1

Learning Objectives

This chapter is designed to enable the reader to:

- Discuss how health promotion and wellbeing can be addressed with and for people with disabilities and are supported by the American Occupational Therapy Association's (AOTA) *Occupational Therapy Practice Framework: Domain and Processes (2008)* (referred to as the *Framework*).
- Examine the evaluation process and occupational assessments in view of health promotion and prevention to meet the occupational and health needs of those with disabilities.

- Develop interventions that promote healthier lifestyles and aim to prevent secondary conditions related to a primary disability.
- Discuss occupational therapy and interdisciplinary research that supports health promotion for children and adults with disabilities.

Key Terms

Health	High-level wellness	Secondary conditions
Health determinants	Learned helplessness	Wellness

Introduction

The purpose of this chapter is to inform and educate the reader about health promotion and wellbeing for people with disabilities in order to create a paradigm shift within the profession of occupational therapy. After a brief review of the prevalence of disabilities within the United States and world populations, several key terms are defined. The chapter presents a review of several crit-

ical concerns that impact the participation and quality of life for individuals with disabilities. These include describing the disparities in the health status of individuals with disabilities and the limited attention given to the importance of preventing secondary conditions in these individuals. Next, models for interventions from related disciplines are presented and research in this area is summarized. This is followed by a review of assessments and a description of potential occupation-based and client-centered occupational therapy health promotion interventions for individuals with disabilities.

There are large numbers of individuals living with disabilities both within the United States and around the world. According to 2006 U.S. Census Bureau data, the percentage of children aged 5 to 20 living with a disability ranged from a low of 4% in Nevada to highs of approximately 10% in both Maine and Puerto Rico. Unsurprisingly, the percentages increase with age. The rates ranged from a low of 34.8% of people over age 65 living with a disability in Wisconsin to highs of 52% in Mississippi and 62.7% in Puerto Rico (U.S. Census Bureau, 2006). The World Health Organization (WHO) estimates that 650 million people worldwide are living with disabilities (WHO, 2008). This indicates that much must be done at both the individual and population levels in terms of advocacy.

Occupational therapists and occupational therapy assistants need to be knowledgeable of and use the language of the WHO's *International Classification of Functioning, Disability and Health (ICF)* (WHO, 2001). It is important to use internationally recognized language and classification systems to advocate for the availability of services that facilitate independence in activities of daily living (ADLs) and when advocating for policies and programs that promote participation in society for individuals with disabilities. An example of the need for this type of advocacy is clearly articulated by Rimmer (2005). According to Rimmer, in order for individuals with disabilities to have equal opportunities to engage in physical activity, changes must be made to the built environments (e.g., fitness facilities, pools) and the manufacturing of exercise equipment.

Definitions of *wellness* and *high-level wellness* are inclusive of individuals with disabilities. In 1985, Johnson defined **wellness** as "a context for living . . . a state of being, a place from which to come as we commit ourselves to improving life for all humanity . . . It is available to all" (cited by Johnson, 1986a, p. 14). **High-level wellness** is "an integrated method of functioning that is oriented toward maximizing the potential of which the individual is capable" and "requires that the individual maintain a continuum of balance of purposeful direction with the environment where he or she is functioning" (Dunn, 1961, pp. 4–5). It is achieved by being actively engaged in occupations to foster changes in the society one lives in to create conditions that allow the attainment of health by all its members. Health professionals are becoming more aware of the need to address high-level wellness, health promotion, and wellbeing with people with disabilities:

> Although health promotion activities have been investigated in a number of groups, including working adults, recovering cancer patients and the elderly, the health promotion of the disabled has not been a focus of research or practice for health care professionals. (Stuifbergen, Becker, & Sands, 1990, pp. 11–12)

Interventions should address the management of the disease or disability and should facilitate clients reaching their fullest potential. Thus, interventions need to integrate the mind, body, and spirit in order to optimize health and prevent further disabling secondary conditions. Tingus (2003) believes that wellness is an appropriate aspiration for individuals with disabilities, as "they may meet all the criteria for physical, emotional, social, and spiritual health in the context of their condition" (p. 98).

Health-promoting behaviors and developing healthy, lifestyle-based routines can best be realized when a person, group, or community develops an overall attitude of wellness. *Wellness* is often defined by the person, group, or community as they actively pursue occupational balance (Neufeld & Kniepmann, 2001). Scaffa, Van Slyke, and Brownson (2008) state that optimal balance, use, choice, and opportunity in occupations are crucial for optimal health and wellbeing. Wilcock (1998) discusses potential occupation-based risk factors for health problems, such as occupational imbalance, deprivation, and alienation.

Until recently, health promotion for people with disabilities has been neglected in the general health community (U.S. Department of Health and Human Services [USDHHS], 2000). Researchers, funding agencies, healthcare providers, and consumers are leading an effort to establish higher-quality health care for the estimated 54 million people with disabilities living in the United States (USDHHS, 2000). This includes not only tertiary prevention, or rehabilitation, but also the integration of health promotion interventions. These interventions complement therapy interventions and assist people in their awareness of the need for prevention and maintaining healthy lifestyles within the context of living with a disability. Occupational therapists and occupational therapy assistants play a prominent role in prevention with a variety of secondary problems (Finn, 1972; Johnson, 1993; Johnson & Jaffe, 1989; Kniepmann, 1997; Missiuna & Pollock, 1991; Neufeld & Kniepmann, 2001; Pizzi, 2001; Reitz, 1992, 1999; Renwick, Brown, & Nagler, 1996; Scaffa, 2001; West, 1969; Wiemer, 1972). However, occupational therapy practitioners often neglect the promotion of health and wellbeing for clients with disabilities. A first step to rectify this is changing the approach to intervention, which may increase the number of occupational therapists and occupational therapy assistants who further empower people with disabilities toward managing their own health.

Fearing, Law, and Clark (1997) state, "The art of occupational therapy includes the ability to create healthy environments where clients can grow and change while remaining firmly grounded within the context of their own lives" (p. 12). West (1968) and Finn (1972) were among the first to examine the role of occupational therapists as health agents.

> In order for a profession to maintain its relevancy it must be responsive to the trends of the times. The trend today in health services is the prevention of disability. Occupational therapists are being asked to move beyond the role of the therapist to that of health agent. This expansion in role identity will require a reinterpretation of current knowledge, the addition of new knowledge and skills, and the revision of the educational process. (Finn, 1972, p. 59)

Justice for Individuals With Disabilities

Occupational therapists and occupational therapy assistants need to be aware of injustices commonly faced by individuals with disabilities. These injustices are many and include limited access to health care, housing, employment, and social participation (USDHHS, 2000, pp. 6–8). The focus of this next section will be limited to health issues. However, the reader is encouraged to remember the broader array of inequities that impact occupational engagement.

Health Disparities for Individuals With Disabilities

There are notable health status disparities between people with and without disabilities delete reference. Numerous reports demonstrate that people with disabilities as a group experience worse health than the rest of the population. According to *Healthy People 2010: Understanding and Improving Health* (USDHHS, 2000), people with disabilities are more likely to have early deaths, chronic conditions, and preventable secondary conditions, and make more emergency room visits. They also have less health insurance coverage and less overall use of the health-care system (as indicated by numbers of Pap tests, mammography, and oral health exams). One indicator of the health disparities experienced by people with disabilities is that the rate of diabetes among this group is 300% higher than among the general population (Krahn, 2003, p. 14). In 2001, the U.S. Census Bureau indicated that people with a disability reported worse health status than people without disabilities, and those with more severe disabilities were likely to report more health problems. Individuals aged 25 through 65 who had a severe disability were five times less likely to report their health as "very good" or "excellent" compared with respondents with no disability (15% vs. 75%) (Krahn, 2003).

Health professional involvement with people with disabilities needs to be broadened to routinely include an emphasis on developing healthy behaviors and routines. This can help people maintain wellbeing both during and after a traditional rehabilitation program, decrease obesity, diminish sedentary lifestyle choices, decrease alcohol and tobacco use, and prevent secondary disabilities (Krahn, 2003).

Occupational therapy health promotion interventions can assist with decreasing the disparities faced by individuals with disabilities. The role of occupational therapy is to create opportunities for occupational engagement and to help people with disabilities improve their own awareness of their individual and collective health and occupational needs. AOTA's *Framework* (2008) supports this role, which can empower individuals with disabilities to become advocates and health agents for themselves and thereby take responsibility for their own health care.

For example, in an occupational therapy evaluation, it is discovered that Mabel does not take her insulin on a regular basis. Upon further examination, the occupational therapist recognizes that health literacy and economics play an important role in Mabel's irregular health patterns, which prevent her from optimally participating as her own health agent. The occupational therapist, in collaboration with the nurse and social worker, help Mabel better understand her diabetes and ways to manage her health to prevent secondary conditions.

Prevention of Secondary Conditions

In 1948, the WHO defined **health** as "a state of complete physical, mental, and social wellbeing and not merely the absence of disease or infirmity" (p. 1). Krahn (2003) states that actualization of these health beliefs requires health practitioners' understanding that health and wellness are related to one's lived experiences and that people with disabilities can be healthy and well. Rimmer (1999) believes that health promotion programs aim to reduce secondary conditions and maintain functional independence. He also states that an improved quality of life and opportunities for improved life satisfaction and leisure pursuits are more readily available when involved with health promotion.

Secondary conditions can be defined as "those physical, medical, cognitive, emotional, or psychosocial consequences to which persons with disabilities are more susceptible by virtue of an underlying impairment, including adverse outcomes in health, wellness, participation and quality of life" (Hough, 1999, p. 162). Community-based health promotion initiatives must be emphasized for people with disabilities in order to achieve the objective of optimizing health and preventing secondary conditions (Rimmer, 1999). Health and wellbeing are a part of the life story of a person living with a disability.

Wiemer (1972) identified five stages on the preventative health-care continuum: promotion, protection, identification, correction, and accommodation, with the latter three stages relating to managing and minimizing secondary conditions. Weimer also provided helpful suggestions that encouraged occupational therapists to consider new or additional interventions in order to minimize the impact of secondary conditions. (For a more thorough description of these stages and other related information, refer to Chapter 1 of this text.) Occupational therapy philosophical beliefs and principles support the hypothesis that teaching a wellness ideology (i.e., the value and knowledge of health habits and strategies) can enhance adaptation to future illness or disability. Furthermore, it can be hypothesized that those individuals who embrace this ideology will be able to adapt and will do so at a higher level than those without such an ideology. In addition, this ideology may create less stress and improve mental health during an illness or disability.

Unfortunately, this ideology is often not supported by the U.S. health-care system, particularly since the advent of managed care programs, which changed the landscape of the health-care system. Rehabilitation services for adults and children are often limited (i.e., capped) by funding availability. As a result, pressure is placed on practitioners to accelerate clients' rates of progress. This faster pace fosters a reductionistic view of care, with little or no time for discussion of health promotion strategies, including prevention of secondary conditions. In addition, clients are sometimes discharged prematurely with many unmet functional and health needs. Federal efforts in health promotion and disease prevention have focused on primary prevention for the general, nondisabled population and on strategies that promote and maintain healthy living (USDHHS, 2000). Unfortunately, specific attention to prevention strategies for people with disabilities has not received sufficient attention, which compromises health outcomes.

Patrick, Richardson, Starks, and Ros (1994) make a clear distinction regarding prevention for people with and without disabilities. For people without disabilities, prevention starts with the individual being absent of disease and includes efforts to eliminate or reduce the risk of disease or disability. For people with disabilities, primary and secondary prevention addresses efforts to diminish the possibilities of secondary conditions associated with the lifestyle of the disabled (e.g., inactivity secondary to a disability).

The prevention of secondary conditions through health promotion interventions applies to all people with disabilities, yet "health promotion programs have largely neglected people with intellectual and developmental disabilities (I/DD); and the widening inequities in health care services for people with I/DD compared to their non-disabled peers is resulting in poorer health outcomes" (Marks & Heller, 2002, p. 2). Frey, Szalda-Petree, Traci, and Seekins (2000) also make a strong argument for developing a paradigm shift to incorporating health promotion as central to maintaining independence and inclusion for people with developmental disabilities, particularly from the public health perspective. The authors cite several secondary conditions that may be preventable, such as pressure sores, urinary tract infections, and psychosocial adjustment.

> Therefore, having a disability is viewed as increasing one's risk for a variety of preventable problems that can limit health, functional capacity, participation in life activities and independence. A prevention framework that incorporates rehabilitation interventions and themes of consumer empowerment can be offered using a public health orientation. (Frey et al., 2000, p. 362)

Frey and colleagues (2000) noted that the few studies examined that met the study criteria (i.e., articles pertaining to the prevention of secondary health conditions in the population of adults with developmental disabilities) focused on decreasing duration of secondary conditions. The majority of these conditions were self-abuse or self-injurious behaviors (SIB). It is evident from this research that occupational therapists and occupational therapy assistants can work from a health promotion framework with a behavioral focus. Health behaviors would include not only healthy occupational patterns of living (e.g., physical activity, proper nutrition, self-esteem, and confidence-building occupations) but also behavioral interventions that can diminish SIB.

Bird, Sperry, and Carreiro (1998) support this type of intervention. They developed a comprehensive assessment and living support system. People who demonstrated SIB were evaluated with this assessment and provided support, goals, and skill training (not limited to decreasing SIB). A client-centered approach was used, and they asked for goal input from consumers. The outcomes included decreased hospitalization, significant reduction in maladaptive behaviors, and increased time spent in the community. Participants reported increased degree of satisfaction, perceived productivity, independence, and community integration. These health outcomes demonstrate the importance of shifting how occupational therapists think about health versus improving function and offer insight into developing a more comprehensive view of practice that impacts individuals at the participation level as described by the *ICF* (WHO, 2001).

There are many benefits noted for people with I/DD who participate in health promotion (e.g., decreased inequities in health, empowerment toward self-responsibility to the extent possible), but health determinants must be considered. **Health determinants** are conditions that influence positive or negative health behaviors and outcomes and include

1. biology/physiology;
2. health and medical care and public health services;
3. health behaviors such as eating habits; tobacco, alcohol, and drug use; physical fitness;
4. the interrelationship of individuals within their environments; and
5. social/societal influences (Tarlov, 1999, cited in Marks & Heller, 2002, p. 4).

The social and societal factors are major overarching concerns that influence the other four areas and must be attended to if attempts are made to effect change in those other areas.

Hough (1999) views the change in thinking from disability prevention to prevention of secondary conditions as a massive paradigm shift. In his paradigm shift, he envisions that the environment needs to play an important role in ameliorating or preventing secondary conditions. He states that "secondary prevention of the secondary conditions of disabilities must be elevated to high priority . . . to prepare for the needs of larger number of persons who will experience a disability within their lifetime, regardless of the etiology of such disabilities" (pp. 187–88).

His concerns seem to be addressed by the description of health promotion for people with disabilities as articulated in *Healthy People 2010:*

1. The promotion of healthy lifestyles and a healthy environment
2. The prevention of health complications and further disabling conditions
3. The preparation of the person with a disability to understand and monitor his or her own health and health-care needs
4. The promotion of opportunities for participation in commonly held life activities (USDHHS, 2000).

There are several objectives identified in *Healthy People 2010* that relate to the promotion of health, well-being, and quality of life (QOL) of people with disabilities and that address the overarching goal to "promote the health of people with disabilities, prevent secondary conditions, and eliminate disparities between people with and without disabilities in the U.S. population"

(USDHHS, 2000, p. 6-3). Several are directly related to the domain of occupational therapy and concern mental health issues of adults and children, social participation, self-reported life satisfaction, employment, education, accessibility, assistive devices and technology, and caregiver health. These objectives support the need for occupational therapy involvement in health promotion and prevention of secondary conditions for people with disabilities throughout the life span.

Impact of Secondary Conditions

People with disabilities often experience limitations in social roles and participation. The ability to engage in occupations and roles within the community can be limited by psycho-emotional and physical barriers. These barriers limit socialization, and occupational therapists empower clients to develop and redevelop social roles and community participation. An example of social role and community participation impairment is the case of Phil, a 20-year veteran of the police department who was shot and subsequently wheelchair bound. After completing a rehabilitation program, Phil refused to leave his apartment despite encouragement from family and friends. Occupational therapy home care evaluation revealed that he was embarrassed that "a man like me" would get shot, let alone be in a wheelchair. He also felt like he was a burden on his family and became depressed. Psychosocial and community-based occupational interventions that included his family and friends, police department colleagues, and members of his local church eventually empowered Phil to venture out and rediscover ways to become a community activist and participant. With the help of the occupational therapist, Phil developed a community safety program and bilingual educational manuals around issues of violence, safety, and security and developed a role as a community leader and speaker.

Models for Health Promotion

Four models are introduced here to provide a variety of frameworks for readers to consider when reflecting upon their practice. These models are not exhaustive but have been selected as examples that further illuminate the content of this chapter.

Socioecological Perspective

Kickbusch (1997) views health and health promotion from a socioecological perspective. In this view, health promotion is seen as a theory-based process of social change contributing to the goal of human development, building on many disciplines and applying interdisciplinary knowledge in a professional, methodical, and creative way. Kickbusch (1997) also views health promotion as "determinants based," rather than evidence-based. Health promotion "bases its strategies on best knowledge of how health is created and how social and behavioral change is best effected" (Kickbusch, 1997, p. 267). Health is seen as needing to be maintained as a resource. Kickbusch asks health professionals to reflect on the following questions:

1. What creates health?
2. Which investment creates the largest health gain?
3. How does this investment help reduce health inequities and ensure human rights?
4. How does this investment contribute to overall human development? (p. 267)

Responses to these questions may infuse a socioecological perspective into the clinical reasoning of occupational therapists and occupational therapy assistants in their work with people with disabilities. It may also help the occupational therapy profession to keep asking the question whether occupational therapy should view health promotion as determinants-based or evidence-based practice.

While there are individuals and organizations that view health as determinants-based, it will be the evidence in occupational therapy, the outcome of research, which will justify the need for occupational therapy in health promotion for people with disabilities. Current practice needs to be strengthened, both academically and clinically, by engaging in such research.

Conceptual Model of Health Promotion and Quality of Life for People With Chronic and Disabling Conditions

Stuifbergen and Rogers (1997) propose a conceptual model of health promotion and QOL for people with chronic and disabling conditions. The model is comprised of three stages: antecedents, selection and use of health promoting behaviors, and outcomes. This model incorporates health-promotion concepts and theories and can be adapted for use in occupational therapy programming for people with disabilities. The first stage, *antecedents,* includes the concepts of barriers, resources, and perceptual factors that serve as precursors to the second stage.

Barriers include those factors that limit health promotion, such as unavailability of a program or an inconvenience (e.g., inability to access transportation). Resources are factors such as income and social support, which can assist in selecting and maintaining health-promoting behaviors. Perceptual factors are those issues perceived by an individual, group, or community that may limit engagement in health promotion. These include self-efficacy for health practices (Stuifbergen & Rogers, 1997).

In addition, emotional support has been linked to healthy family function and utilization of health-promoting behaviors (Stuifbergen, 1995). People with disabilities may develop **learned helplessness,** the state in which one adapts to being passive and disengaged (Seligman, 1972). This can be a direct result of cultural influences; societal perceptions; family influences; health-care sick-role expectations, despite positive experiences in the rehabilitation environment; and even a secondary learned behavior toward health professionals, including therapists, from a lack of client-centered care to authoritarian attitudes.

The second stage relates to the selection and use of health-promoting behaviors. In this stage, occupational therapists examine the individual's behavioral, cognitive, and emotional activities in order to promote health and wellbeing. Research documents the desire of people with disabilities for health promotion services. Persons with spinal cord injury request health-promotion services, such as exercise, nutrition, and stress management, more often than they request medical services (Stuifbergen & Rogers, 1997). Individuals with multiple sclerosis who conducted self-assessments and health monitoring had fewer hospitalizations and office visits for health care than research participants who did not perform similar assessments. The frequency of engaging in health-promoting behaviors has been correlated with perceived QOL (Gulick, 1991; Stuifbergen, 1995).

The third stage is *outcomes.* In the proposed model, QOL is the outcome of integrating health promotion with rehabilitation. While creating a quality of life for themselves, "people living with a chronic disabling condition thus must manage a wide variety of disease-related, intrapersonal, and environmental demands. Engaging in health promoting behaviors is one strategy recommended to manage disease symptoms and enhance QOL" (Stuifbergen & Rogers, 1997, p. 5).

Preliminary studies provide information about how health-promoting behaviors impact perceived QOL. However, it remains unclear how symptoms of illness and the experience of chronicity (e.g., fatigue, time constraints, uncertainty of long-term prognosis) influence health-promoting behaviors and how participation in these behaviors may be influenced by contextual factors unique to this population (Stuifbergen & Rogers, 1997). Perceived outcomes of health-promoting behaviors often include improved QOL and health. Related to this is that improved psychosocial adaptation can be realized when people with disabilities, such as multiple sclerosis populations, are in contact with "healthy" people and have perceived support of others (Stuifbergen & Roberts, 1997). In a study by Wineman (1990), purpose in life, related to perceived supportiveness of interactions and functional disability, affected psychosocial adaptation.

Holistic Vision of Disability

Another model that can be used in occupational therapy is one proposed by Patrick, Richardson, Starks, & Rose (1994). This model presents a holistic vision of disability and includes the prevention of disabling conditions and prevention of progression toward further disability. The model is built on five areas that, together, describe the person's life. The five areas include environment, human development, the disabling process, opportunity, and quality of life (QOL). The first area is *environment,* which encompasses biological, physical, social, economic, and cultural spheres of living. The risk factors for further disablement can be reduced to the degree that prevention is realized and the promotion of opportunity for participation exists.

The second area is *human development.* Disability can occur at any stage of life, which then affects occupational performance at current and future levels of development. Occupational therapy practitioners are encouraged to address not only current but also future occupational functioning so that health can be realized at all stages of life as people age.

The *disabling process* is the third area of the life of a person with disability. The transition from disease or injury to becoming a person with a disability has a profound effect on a person's mental, physical, emotional, and spiritual health. In occupational therapy, it is vital to bear in mind that prevention in any area of a disability (e.g., body functions and structures, mental functions, or social role impairment) can promote health, occupational engagement, and participation.

Opportunity is the fourth area. This recognizes that, despite a disability, people need to be provided opportunities for participation. The Americans with Disabilities Act of 1990 and the Independent Living Movement both assist individuals with disabilities in creating opportunities (Schlaff, 1993). Occupational therapists and occupational therapy assistants are skilled practitioners in developing and adapting contexts, performance skills, habits, routines, and roles in order for people with disabilities to have greater opportunity to engage in meaningful living experiences. This promotes a higher level of health and wellbeing on physical, psychosocial, emotional, and spiritual levels.

The final area in this holistic model of disability examines the *QOL* from the perspective of the person with disability. This refers to perception of one's position in life relative to culture and their value system. This is also related to personal goals, expectations, standards, and concerns. Perceptions of various factors in one's life are developed over time and through experiences. Thus, for a person with a disability, these can include experiences of the disability, contacts with the health-care system, and environmental contexts (Patrick et al., 1994). This client-centeredness is well established in occupational therapy (AOTA, 2008; Law, 1998; Peloquin, 1990, 1993).

Transtheoretical Model

The Stages of Change, or Transtheoretical, (TTM) Model developed by Prochaska and DiClemente (1992) is cited as a primary model that guides assessment and intervention to assist individuals in changing habits and maladaptive patterns, and encourages and reinforces newly learned health-promoting behaviors (this model is explained and depicted in Chapter 3). When a person is in the earlier stages of the model (e.g., contemplation), self-efficacy is often low.

Occupational therapists and occupational therapy assistants can assist in empowering individuals through reframing perceived barriers and problems and setting a direction for goal achievement (Cardinal & Cardinal, 1997; Lee, 1993). This approach requires a focus on mental and physical health and calls for occupational therapy practitioners to be holistic and systems oriented.

Cardinal (2003) studied which constructs from the TTM (e.g., behavioral and cognitive processes of change, decisional balance, and self-efficacy), along with exercise barriers, affect the exercise behaviors of individuals with disabilities. This survey of 322 adults was the first study to examine stages of change for exercise behavior among adults with physical disabilities using all constructs of the TTM as well as exercise barriers.

> Overall, the results are in general agreement with existing evidence among non-disabled populations. Behavioral strategies derived from TTM, such as being moved emotionally, being rewarded, being a role model, developing a healthy self-image, gathering information, getting social support, making a commitment, making substitutions, taking advantage of social mores, and using cues may all facilitate exercise behaviors of adults with physical disabilities. (Cardinal, 2003, p. 46)

The TTM is a viable model for people with physical, psychosocial, and cognitive disabilities. Interventions that begin with assisting individuals in becoming aware of their own health needs (i.e., precontemplation and contemplation stages) and then help them maintain healthy lifestyles (maintenance stage) is consistent with the occupational therapy intervention process. Clients can become more independent health agents when they have an awareness of their own health needs.

When people have increased awareness of goals to improve QOL, healthier lifestyles are the outcome. Tailoring health promotion programs to client or community needs and interests can promote greater follow-through toward healthy living (Bulger & Smith, 1999). When developing programs of health and behavior change, occupational therapists need to be client-centered and aware of the level of understanding and stage of change of those being served.

Sneed and Paul (2003) conducted a survey of 250 people with congestive heart failure (CHF) to identify the stage of readiness for change in six lifestyle behaviors important in the management of CHF. The study was based on the TTM and revealed that this theoretical framework may not work as well as hoped, perhaps due to the complexity and number of changes needed to promote health, wellbeing, and optimize QOL in individuals with CHF. Interestingly, there was a significant difference ($p = 0.001$) between what respondents thought they were consistently doing to optimize health and the actual reporting of these behaviors (e.g., thinking that they were reducing sodium in the diet while reporting that they ate things within the last 24 hours that contained sodium and were not recommended for people with CHF). The model may assist people with CHF if the numbers of recommended changes are kept to a minimum. Once each change is habituated, subsequent changes could be made. This would decrease the feelings of being overwhelmed, as reported by many of the participants.

The views of how health professionals think about living well with disabilities are evolving with the development of new models of health and wellness. There is increasing awareness that, despite disability of any kind, people have aspirations, goals, and needs to live a life with integrity, dignity, and quality. If open to rethinking terms such as *physically or emotionally challenged* and *disability,* health professionals can avoid stereotyping and learn strategies for wellbeing and health through actively listening to people with disabilities.

Research in Health Promotion and People With Disabilities

There is little research, let alone discussion, in the occupational therapy literature that relates to the direct use and utilization of health promotion theory and interventions for people with disabilities, with a few exceptions, such as Johnson (1986b), White (1986), Kniepmann (1997), Reitz (1999), and Scaffa (2001). The profession is currently incorporating health promotion and wellness into practice and researching its effectiveness. The following are some instances of research in health promotion for people with disabili-

ties from which the occupational therapy profession can begin to develop an evidence base.

Stuifbergen and Rogers (1997) interviewed 20 individuals with multiple sclerosis (MS) who shared their stories about health promotion, QOL, and factors that affected these areas of health. They identified six life domains related to QOL: family (most frequently identified domain), functioning to maintain independence, spirituality, work, socioeconomic security, and self-actualization. Six broad themes also emerged related to health-promoting behaviors: exercise or physical activity, nutritional strategies, lifestyle adjustment, maintaining a positive attitude, health responsibility behaviors, and seeking and receiving interpersonal support.

Harrison and Stuifbergen (2002) noted that parents, particularly mothers with disabilities, need special attention to prevent depression related to concern for their children. Their exploratory analysis of mothers with MS noted that disability and concern for their children are independent predictors of depressive symptoms, and social support can help to mediate the effect of concern for children on depressive symptoms.

Neufeld and Kniepmann (2001) describe a community-based program that was developed in collaboration with the National Multiple Sclerosis Society (NMSS). They discuss issues of language and power, paths and directions, the model design, and evaluation and negotiating expansion as the journey of establishing collaboration. Language and power relate to understanding each other's shared meanings and ideologies. "Collaboration . . . becomes a process of aligning and realigning power through ways of talking and ways of knowing" (p. 71). In order to choose paths and partners, Neufeld and Kniepman (2001) conducted a needs assessment to explore possibilities for development of a wellness program to promote healthier daily living for people with MS. For example, they examined environments that promoted wellbeing to set up programming (e.g., hospital context connotes illness).

A needs assessment and the literature on wellness and health promotion were used to create the Gateway to Wellness program. This program had the following four objectives for participants:

1. Demonstrate skills to manage the consequences of MS
2. Demonstrate confidence in skills to manage the consequences of MS
3. Identify options and adopt a healthy lifestyle
4. Build networks with individuals and community agencies for continued support and education (Neufeld & Kniepmann, 2001, p. 75)

Neufeld and Kniepmann provided strategies for occupational therapists to become involved and to develop collaborative partnerships with organizations. They also articulated how health promotion can be integrated into programming for those with chronic illness using an occupation-centered and population-based approach.

Ho (2003) examined the factors associated with health behaviors of adults with diabetes-related functional limitations. The target population was individuals who were aged 18 and older and who resided in the community. The sample included 2285 cases of an estimated 13 million individuals with diabetes. Three specific aims were to examine

1. the characteristics of adults with diabetes and diabetes-related functional limitations;
2. the differences in personal characteristics and health behaviors between adults with and without functional limitations; and
3. factors that are associated with health behaviors in adults who have diabetes and functional limitations.

Compared to people with diabetes without functional limitations, people with diabetes with functional limitations were more likely to be older, female, poorer, less educated, and not married. They were also more likely to perceive their health as poor or fair, to have higher rates of chronic medical conditions, to be more frequently engaged in risky health behaviors, and to require adaptive equipment more often. Individuals with diabetes and functional limitations participated less frequently in leisure-time physical activities than their counterparts without functional limitations. Most had weight concerns, with at least half of them obese or overweight. They also had higher rates of tobacco and alcohol use compared to diabetics without functional limitations (Ho, 2003). People with diabetes with functional limitations tended to use more health services than did those without functional limitations. Although they have higher health-care utilization rates, they also identify barriers to accessing timely medical care. For instance, there was a large percentage of people needing medications, eyeglasses, and transportation to access health care (Ho, 2003).

Tudor-Locke, Myers, and Rodger (2001) described an approach to developing a physical activity intervention for sedentary individuals with type 2 diabetes. The researchers used a theory-driven approach to organize and explain the program and its outcomes, as well as the circumstances that were identified to contribute to lack of exercise. Sedentary lifestyle and attrition from a structured exercise program were factors ranked highest in those identified as lacking exercise. It was also discovered that instructions and guidelines for implementation of programs are often vague and confusing. Tudor-Locke and colleagues (2001) offer six

critical elements to consider for programming that can better ensure successful outcomes:

1. Problem identification (e.g., sedentary lifestyles)
2. Critical inputs (e.g., walking, self-monitoring)
3. Mediating processes (e.g., health theories that underlie implementation, such as social cognitive theory or the TTM)
4. Expected outcomes (e.g., increased walking behaviors, decreased cardiovascular risk factors)
5. Extraneous factors (e.g., social support)
6. Implementation issues (e.g., recruitment, documentation, and follow-up contacts)

Carleton and Henrich (1998) used the Stevens Point Multidimensional Model for Wellness to support their wellness program. They studied the usefulness of this program to determine exercise adherence. This model includes the physical, spiritual, occupational, social, emotional, and intellectual dimensions of wellness. Courses were developed around each area relative to exercise and exercise adherence. Results showed the students had a significant increase to exercise adherence and reported improved sense of wellbeing after participation. The holism inherent in the program was cited as an important component to exercise adherence.

A landmark study that supports occupational therapy health promotion interventions for people with disabilities (although not conducted by occupational therapists) explored the life stories and narrative of people with disabilities and their perceptions of health and wellbeing (Putnam et al., 2003). Nineteen focus groups comprised of people with long-term disabilities were asked to define health and wellness and the barriers and facilitators of health and wellness. The themes generated suggested that health and wellness, for this group of participants, demanded an interplay between person, community, and the health-care system. Focus group participants described health and wellness as

• being able to function and having the chance to do what you want to do;
• being independent and having self-determination regarding choices, opportunities, activities;
• having physical and emotional states of wellbeing; and
• not being held back by pain (Putnam et al., 2003).

For many participants, having the capacity to perform necessary or desired ADLs and instrumental activities of daily living (IADLs), being independent and self-determined, and feeling in control of their life were important measures of health and wellness. According to participants, health and wellness necessitated physical and emotional wellbeing. Other participants expanded this definition to include spirituality and contextual factors, such as community, family, friends, and work (Putnam et al., 2003). One participant described this succinctly:

> Well, for me, it [health and wellness] encompasses several things: physical health, emotional health, spiritual health . . . when I feel that I have a good balance in these three areas, I feel that I've achieved a good level of health and wellness. (Putnam et al., 2003, p. 39)

Participants also shared their opinions about differences between themselves and nondisabled peers regarding health and wellbeing. They believed that being adaptable to social and physical barriers was vital. They also felt that people needed to understand that *health and wellness exist within the experience of disability* and that people with disabilities need to promote and maintain their health and wellness on a daily basis. They also felt more susceptible to increased health challenges, including the development of secondary conditions. A majority of participants believed that their disability was distinctly separate from health and wellbeing (Putnam et al., 2003).

Other ways they promoted and maximized personal health and wellbeing included

- developing coping strategies;
- having contact with peers;
- staying as active as possible, through participation in sports and exercise;
- contributing to society through work or volunteerism; and
- setting personal goals and embracing challenges (Putnam et al., 2003).

Emphasis was also placed on the importance of feeling valued and supported by family and friends and being treated as a whole person by health-care professionals. Putnam and colleagues (2003) concluded that

> definitions of health and wellness that people living with disability have may be much broader and more complex than those held by persons who are not disabled. In their conceptualizations, health and wellness is not just a personal issue, but one that is dependent on interactions with other people and health, financial and regulatory systems. (p. 44)

There are many ways to influence health and wellbeing for people with disabilities; five recommendations derived from this study are summarized in Content Box 19-1.

The participants were aware of their needs and desires as well as the barriers they face in achieving their health and wellness goals. Findings documented their ability to appreciate, understand, and clearly articulate their lived experiences. Maintaining high levels of

---

Content Box 19-1

Recommendations to Influence Health and Wellness for People With Disabilities

1. Expand definitions of *wellness* and *health promotion* for persons with disabilities to include preservation of function and prevention of secondary conditions.
2. Explore, through research, the individual, family, community, and systems level barriers and facilitating factors to health and wellness for persons with disabilities, particularly the efficacy of occupational engagement as a health promotion intervention.
3. Create client-centered and occupation-based materials that educate persons with disabilities on health promotion strategies, community health and wellness resources, and access to health promotion opportunities.
4. Increase health-care providers' knowledge of best practices in health promotion, and improve their ability to effectively respond to the health and wellness needs of persons with disabilities.
5. Identify and reduce systems barriers that limit health and wellness opportunities for people with disabilities, particularly poor environmental accessibility, social stigma and discrimination, and financial unaffordability.

Adapted from "Health and wellness: People with disabilities discuss barriers and facilitators to well being," by M. Putnam, S. Geenen, L. Powers, M. Saxton, S. Finney, & P. Dautel, 2003, *Journal of Rehabilitation, 69*(1), 37–45.

---

health and wellness were clearly important to them. Occupational therapy practitioners can facilitate health and wellbeing by increasing clients' self-advocacy and assertiveness and by improving their awareness of healthier living strategies.

Padilla (2003) utilized a phenomenological approach with a 21-year-old woman disabled from a head injury. Throughout the interview and transcription process, Padilla noted several emerging themes from the data that included nostalgia, abandonment, and hope. He described each theme using quotes from the subject, "Clara," to elucidate her identity as a disabled person. Hope, the final theme that emerged, helped to renew meaning in life and overcome her disability. "Clara" offers an insight into her own discovery of wellness:

> I tried, I really tried hard all those years [to let go of the sense of abandonment]—I tried to do everything people told me would be good for me, but didn't realize that it wasn't important what I did or even how I did it. What was important wasn't "doing" at all. It was that through doing I could realize I could be myself,

and be someone who, like others, continues to live and change and grow. (Padilla, 2003, p. 419)

According to Oleson (1990), commonly used measures of QOL are often objective in nature, thus they fail to demonstrate how individuals actually perceive their lives. Subjective evaluations of QOL represent individuals' perceptions of life domains important to them, and satisfaction with those domains are subjectively judged as critical to their personal QOL (Oleson, 1990). Bostick (1977) found that groups of people with and without disabilities had similar responses when asked to describe the domains of QOL. In a study of 227 adults with chronic illness, independence (i.e., being able to do for oneself) was the one theme generated in verbal responses that could not be placed within the domains of the Flanagan Quality of Life Scale (Burckhardt, Woods, Schultz & Ziebarth, 1989).

The implications of narrative and other research with people with disabilities relative to health promotion and wellbeing are vast. The narratives clearly speak about the correlation between being active and engaging in social and physical activity, and the positive mental health outlook engendered by occupational engagement relative to clients' subjective definitions of health promotion and wellbeing. It behooves occupational therapy practitioners to begin making that paradigm shift and transition from defining oneself as a rehabilitation specialist to a specialist in occupation, health promotion, and wellbeing, using occupation to facilitate healthy living. Through listening to the narratives of people with disabilities and chronic illnesses and engaging in client-centered evaluation and interventions, occupational therapists and occupational therapy assistants can assist them in maximizing QOL and participation in society.

Occupational Perspective on Health Promotion and Disability

The official AOTA *Occupational Therapy in the Promotion of Health and the Prevention of Disease and Disability Statement* (Scaffa, Van Slyke, Brownson, & American Occupational Therapy Association Commission on Practice, 2008, p. 694) states the following:

> The American Occupational Therapy Association . . . supports and promotes involvement of occupational therapists and occupational therapy assistants in the development and provision of health promotion and disease or disability prevention programs and services.

Health promotion programs and services may target individuals, organizations, communities and populations, and policymakers. The focus of these programs is to

- prevent or reduce the incidence of illness or disease, accidents, injuries, and disabilities in the population;
- reduce health disparities among racial and ethnic minorities and other underserved populations;
- enhance mental health, resiliency, and quality of life;
- prevent secondary conditions and improve the overall health and well-being of people with chronic conditions or disabilities and their caregivers; and
- promote healthy living practices, social participation, *occupational justice,* and healthy communities, with respect for cross-cultural issues and concerns. (Scaffa et al., 2008, p. 695)

Wilcock (1998) defines *health* from an occupational perspective, which supports the promotion of health and wellbeing lifestyles for all clients, including those with disabilities (Content Box 19-2). Johnson (1993) discusses health as composed of balance and participation, which she believes are key ingredients for healthy living. Transforming one's life through these two principles of occupational therapy help one to engage more fully in life. People of any age with disabilities are often limited in achieving balance in their lives by the very nature of their disability. Likewise, a disability impedes occupational performance and can thereby impede health management and maintenance as well as normal development.

Yerxa (1998) states that health can be viewed as an encompassing, dynamic state of "wellbeingness," reflecting adaptability, a good quality of life, and satisfaction in one's own activities. She says, "This perspective of health does not exclude persons with disabilities" (p. 412) and cites Pörn (1993), who believes that people with disabilities have the potential to be healthy by developing and using skills to achieve goals. Pörn examines relationships between happiness; goal achievement; balance between

---

Content Box 19-2

Wilcock's Characteristics of Health From an "Occupational Perspective"

- The absence of illness but not necessarily disability
- A balance of physical, mental, and social wellbeing attained through socially valued and individually meaningful occupation
- Enhancement of capacities and opportunity to strive for individual potential
- Community cohesion and opportunity
- Social integration, support, and justice, all within and as part of a sustainable ecology (Wilcock, 1998, p. 110)

environment, abilities, and goal realization; and their total relationship to living a healthy lifestyle. He believes that one can be disabled yet achieve a level of health through adaptation in life. Health, thereby, can be perceived as having a set of skills that enable people to achieve their goals in their own environment (Pörn, as cited in Yerxa, 1998).

In 1921, Meyer (1977) presented a paper articulating the developing beliefs of a new association being developed called the National Society for the Promotion of Occupational Therapy. Reitz (1992), in an historical perspective on preventive health and wellness in occupational therapy, cites four examples of these beliefs:

1. An active interaction with reality (i.e., the environment) maintains and balances the individual.
2. The mind and body work in unison, and this link must be studied and appreciated.
3. Natural rhythms have a positive effect on wellbeing and human performance.
4. There is a need for balance in all spheres of occupation. (p. 50)

The attainment of balance in the lives of people with disabilities appears to be a major construct in the literature that relates directly to the promotion of health and wellbeing. Lanig, Chase, Butt, and Hulse (1966) and Kailes (2000) state that, despite a disability, health can be viewed as being evident through

• maximizing one's potential along various dimensions;
• balancing physical, social, emotional, spiritual, and intellectual factors;
• functioning effectively in given environments; and
• fulfilling needs and helping one to adapt to major stresses.

When viewed from this perspective, people with disabilities can also be considered healthy.

Client-Centered Health Promotion for People With Disabilities

Renwick and colleagues (1996) stated that "rehabilitation has strong potential as a collaborator in the process of making health promotion people-centered in that it has collective expertise in client-centeredness at the individual level of analysis and application" (p. 366). Law (1998) summarized constructs of a client-centered approach after analyzing six frameworks or models (Content Box 19-3). It is the client-centeredness of occupational interventions that can have the most impact on health behavior change for people with disabilities. Client-centered approaches are foundational to occupational therapy practice.

Content Box 19-3

Concepts of Client-Centered Practice Common to All Models

• Respect for clients and their families, and the choices they make
• Clients and families have the ultimate responsibility for decisions about daily occupations and occupational therapy services.
• Provision of information, physical comfort, and emotional support
• Emphasis on person-centered communication
• Facilitation of client participation in all aspects of occupational therapy service
• Flexible, individualized occupational therapy service delivery
• Enabling clients to solve occupational performance issues
• Focus on the person-environment-occupation relationship

From *Client-centered occupational therapy* (p. 9) by M. Law (Ed.), 1998, Thorofare, NJ: SLACK. Copyright © 1998 by SLACK Incorporated. With permission.

Occupational therapy practitioners develop a collaborative relationship with clients in order to understand their experiences and desires for intervention (AOTA, 2008, p. 647).

According to AOTA's (2008) *Framework*, the client is not always an individual but can also be an organization, community, family member, or others who receive occupational therapy services.

Schlaff (1993) makes assumptions about people with disabilities that reflect independent living and that people with disabilities can be empowered through a change in societal attitudes:

It is preferable for persons with disabilities to view themselves as being consumers (not patients), adults (not perpetual children), capable of independent living with supports (not in need of institutionalization), contributors to society (not burdens), self-directed (not controlled by others), in need of personal assistance services (not caregiving), and in need of rights (not cures). (p. 943)

She asserts that occupational therapists can make a difference in promoting healthier states of wellbeing by being advocates for people with disabilities and helping them develop a sense of self that overcomes any disability. Community-based services help to empower people with disabilities and redefine disability. Advocacy is an important service for occupational therapy practitioners to deliver (Schlaff, 1993).

Padilla (2003) challenges occupational therapists to work with clients as "co-investigators of the meaning of their life experience rather than recipients of the expert knowledge of the able-bodied" (p. 422). Another role for occupational therapists and occupational therapy assistants is to challenge expert thinking by inquiring into the experiences and lives of the disabled and discover their perceived sense of wellness and how they promote health in their daily habits and routines. The practitioner can then allow client responses to guide or, at the very least, inform interventions. Client-centered practice can empower people with disabilities; motivate individuals to follow through with health promotion interventions; and positively influence client wellbeing, including self-esteem, self-worth, and self-concept.

The next section of this chapter focuses on the occupational therapy health promotion needs of children and youth with disabilities. This is followed by a broader discussion of assessment issues and interventions strategies that address all ages.

Health Promotion for Children and Youth With Disabilities

Given that 12% of all children under 18 years of age have a disability (USDHHS, 2000), there is tremendous need to advocate for their health promotion. Table 19-1 displays *Healthy People 2010* objectives designed specifically for children and youth. Occupational therapy practice for children and youth with disabilities has long emphasized improving occupational performance to enable fuller participation in life as well as promote primary skill building that is developmentally appropriate. There is little in the interdisciplinary literature that speaks to the issue of promoting health and wellness from this occupational performance and developmental perspective. Due to high rates of disability among youth, occupational therapy services that address all aspects of health and wellbeing, including promoting health, preventing secondary conditions, and removing environmental barriers, are essential.

Schaaf and Davis (1992) encourage collaboration with those intimately involved with a disabled child's care or with children who are at risk for disability. Schaaf and Davis developed goals for occupational therapy "to promote health and wellness for children and families in any setting" (Kniepmann, 1997, p. 548). Play deprivation could result in secondary disability on physical, social, and emotional levels. Missiuna and Pollock (1991) identified barriers to free play, which can be perceived as risk factors that occupational therapists could address via consultation with parents, teachers, and caregivers. Community outreach activity groups for at-risk mothers and children and community-based, play-focused intervention for mothers of

Table 19–1 **Examples of *Healthy People 2010* Objectives for Children and Youth**

Objective Number	Objective
6-2	Reduce the proportion of children and adolescents with disabilities who are reported to be sad, unhappy, or depressed.
6-7	Reduce the number of people with disabilities in congregate care facilities, consistent with permanency planning principles.
6-7b	Persons aged 21 years and under in congregate care facilities.
6-9	Increase the proportion of children and youth with disabilities who spend at least 80 percent of their time in regular education programs.

Data from *Healthy People 2010: Understanding and improving health,* by U.S. Department of Health and Human Services, 2000, Washington, DC: Government Printing Office.

preschoolers also reflect the opportunities occupational therapists and occupational therapy assistants have to promote health and wellness for children and youth (Esdaile, 1996).

> In a child with a chronic disability, individual abilities and disabilities may be confined to one domain (physical, cognitive, psychosocial) but more likely will touch several or all domains of performance. . . . Does the play of children with chronic disabilities include the qualities of play and playfulness, or does the nature of the specific disabling problem and the daily occupations that are in place to address them in some way prevent sufficient involvement in the world of play? (Burke, 1996, p. 416)

Occupational therapists and occupational therapy assistants possess valuable knowledge and skill in human development and play development. Use of these skills and knowledge enable children and youth with disabilities to more actively participate in the world and will help children transcend disability and foster significant health and wellbeing. To become more active in the world instills confidence, self-esteem, and a sense of competence that should not be relegated only to nondisabled children and youth.

Although there have been studies examining the role of health-care professionals, especially physicians, and the dissemination of health promotion information to the general population, there is little research regarding such dissemination for people with disabilities (Krahn, 2003; Wechsler, Levine, Idelson, Rohman, & Taylor, 1983; Wechsler, Levine, Idelson, Schor, & Coakley, 1996). Krahn (2003) examined the health promotion practices of primary care physicians as they relate to adults and children with physical disabilities. The survey results indicated that pediatricians across the United States gather more information on behavior problems, accidental injuries, sleep, parenting, abuse/neglect, social support, depression, and stress for children with disabilities than for those without, and they refer disabled children less for preventive and early detection tests. They also gather less information on adolescents with disabilities on smoking, alcohol/drug use, and sexual activity.

In terms of actual practices, pediatricians again report gathering information about health promotion behaviors more often than adult care providers, but these differences are only significant for their care of typical patients and not for children/adolescents and adults with disabilities. The findings of this survey of adult care physicians corroborates what surveys of people with disabilities have reported regarding referrals for preventive and early detection tests—that they are referred at lower rates than their nondisabled counterparts. The study represents one of the first of physician practices on health promotion for children with disabilities (Krahn, 2003).

The implications for occupational therapists during evaluation and intervention with children and youth are manifold. Practitioners can incorporate the questions asked in the above study and can then begin to develop occupation-based assessments of children and youth with disabilities using a health promotion approach. These assessments can help pediatricians, teachers, and parents or primary caregivers better understand the importance of an occupational therapy program as it relates to *health* outcomes and not just activities of daily living, fine motor skills, or socialization. This approach to occupational history will also help occupational therapists and occupational therapy assistants develop a paradigm shift for themselves and their colleagues and help to alter occupational therapy practice to be health outcomes oriented.

Evaluation and Assessment

Occupational therapists can participate in the development of programs like those mentioned earlier in this chapter using occupation-based holistic assessments such as the Pizzi Holistic Wellness Assessment (Pizzi, 2001) and the Lifestyle Performance Interview (Velde &

Fidler, 2002). These assessments can be used to gather data and design client-centered health promotion interventions related to improving occupational performance and participation in society. These tools provide a multidimensional evaluation of wellbeing and utilize an occupation and client-centered approach. The development of specific, client-chosen occupational habits and routines, combined with occupational coaching from a skilled professional, seems to be the key to successful outcomes in the promotion of healthier lifestyles.

The Pizzi Holistic Wellness Assessment (Pizzi, 2001; see Chapter 10 and go to http://www.michaelpizzi.com) can be a useful assessment of primary caregivers of people with disabilities when exploring caregiver health issues and programming that is more systems and social sciences oriented. From a systems perspective, if the health of primary caregivers is compromised in any way, then the health and wellbeing of the person with disabilities will also be affected. McGuire, Crowe, Law, and VanLeit (2004) engaged in a phenomenological study of mothers with children with disabilities. Their needs, time use, and occupational wellbeing were clearly seen as impacting the therapy process. This study supports the need to include parents and primary caregivers in the evaluation and intervention process.

During the occupational evaluation process, the following questions need to be addressed: "With the disability that my client has, what are some questions and interventions that can promote healthier living and engage the person in developing a healthy lifestyle that can be self-maintained?" and "What are some secondary conditions that may be prevented through occupational therapy?" Preventive or *futuristic* (*conditional*) clinical reasoning is essential for completing the occupational therapy evaluation and future interventions where the focus is on occupational adaptation to facilitate QOL and wellbeing (Benamy, 1999).

Health promotion concepts can be integrated into rehabilitation, as in the following brief example. In home care, a 17-year-old with paraplegia was living with her single mom on the second floor of an apartment building in New York City. She was able to propel her own chair. The referral for occupational therapy was to evaluate and treat ADL deficits. The ADL assessment included the following questions: "Do you smoke and, if so, how much? Do you drink alcohol and if so, how much? What is your typical diet like? What are your thoughts on your daily habits? Are there any things you might want to change? Do you feel you can make those changes on your own or might you need support?"

This addition to the occupational history revealed an intelligent young woman who smoked a pack of cigarettes per day, smoked marijuana 1 to 2 times per week, drank with friends in the park after school on occasion, and who was beginning to gain weight. The client implemented the interventions in mobility, home management, and ADLs. She also discussed her daily habits and additionally described the changes she would like to make because she was interested in dating. This provided an opportunity to discuss safer sex and dating as a person with disabilities. The effects of some of her health behaviors on her physical condition and cardiovascular system (e.g., the hidden damaging effects) were also discussed.

Once she recognized the ill effects of these health behaviors, she began to make subtle and slow changes. Occupational changes and changes in health status that affected her lifestyle were clearly documented. Social work and nursing were informed routinely about the occupational therapy program and progress. After 8 weeks of occupational therapy, she had reduced alcohol consumption, began to read about Alcoholics Anonymous (her absent father and her mother were alcoholics), and cut her smoking of both cigarettes and marijuana by 75%. These were considered significant improvements given her life story and living situation. At discharge, while having improved in health management and maintenance and home management, she was also provided other resources and collaborated with the author on self-improvement goals that she could work toward on her own over the next 6 months.

During the occupational therapy process, the client's mother was also evaluated for occupational risks, occupational dysfunction, and areas of wellbeing. Caregivers also need occupational interventions in order to assist them in developing performance skills, habits, routines, roles, and healthy lifestyles to promote their own wellbeing. These health promotion and prevention strategies help caregivers to organize time and activity for both themselves and the person they are caring for. Maintaining people with disabilities in the community requires wellness and health promotion interventions and programs for caregivers. The interdependence between caregiver and the person with disability requires that caregivers also embrace and engage in a wellness lifestyle. Chapter 20 of this text provides more information on health promotion and caregivers.

Education of both client and caregivers is needed around the issue of preventive occupation, which is defined as "the application of occupational science to prevent disease/disability and promote the health and wellbeing of persons and communities through meaningful engagement in occupations" (Scaffa, Desmond, & Brownson, 2001, p. 44). Preventive occupations are those that clients with disabilities engage in to prevent the development of secondary conditions. It will take a prevention focus of occupational therapists and occu-

pational therapy assistants to develop and maintain this shift in clinical reasoning.

Health Promotion and Occupational Interventions

Drum (2003) views intervention from a systems perspective. He believes that health promotion is supported by personal, communal, and systemic factors. Stuifbergen, Gordon, and Clark (1998) emphasize the need for health practitioners to integrate health promotion strategies in neurorehabilitation for people with stroke. They view health promotion as emphasizing self-care, self-monitoring, developing a healthy lifestyle, moving toward health and wellbeing (as opposed to avoiding illness), and promoting individual control over health behaviors.

Interventions can include enhancing awareness of opportunities for health, facilitating behavior change, and establishing the value of a supportive environment. While nurses often explore some of these issues with clients, the occupational therapist can create opportunities for occupational engagement. In so doing, they challenge themselves and their clients to examine occupational patterns, contexts, and activities that both support health and may be barriers to health. For example, if people with stroke were overeating or smoking cigarettes, an exploration of their patterns of eating and smoking, the cues to action for these behaviors, and the barriers to diminishing these behaviors could be incorporated into home management or goal planning for future sessions. These can contribute to a more holistic program that is client-centered and focused on health during traditional rehabilitation programming. However, it needs to be emphasized that it will take the individual therapist or assistant to integrate health promotion into the delivery of rehabilitation services. Once the reframing from a health promotion and wellness perspective has taken place, the interventions toward healthy living and not simply improved function will flow.

Nutrition is also a misunderstood and often needed intervention for people with disabilities. Occupational therapists and occupational therapy assistants are often involved with meal preparations and home and food management interventions that can be adapted to the occupational demands of the activity and can involve a nutritional component that helps to promote healthier eating and prevent secondary conditions. For example, in people with Down's syndrome, cerebral palsy, and spinal cord injury, a premature onset of osteoporosis is common (Angelopoulou et al., 2000; Kocina, 1997; Turk, Geremski, Rosenbaum, & Weber, 1997). Knowledge of nutritional needs can enable occupational therapy practitioners to develop occupation-based interventions that incorporate nutritional strategies to aid in the prevention of the secondary condition osteoporosis.

Physical activity and exercise are often cited as primary strategies that facilitate wellness and promote health. Walking is often recommended as the best exercise for people to prevent health problems; however, this may be a very inappropriate recommendation for persons with disabilities. When mobility patterns are impaired, physical activity and exercise involving intact body parts can be health-promoting interventions.

Functional skills training, while seen as rehabilitation in tertiary prevention, can be viewed from a social systems perspective to help children and adolescents with disabilities develop necessary skills to manage daily living in self-care, work, and leisure (Brollier, Shepherd, & Markley, 1994). These "necessary skills" include the psychosocial and emotional coping skills needed simultaneously with the physical motor skills for occupational performance. When health promotion is the overarching framework for skill development and training, disabled children can also learn lifelong habits and routines that can optimize health throughout the life span.

Exercise as a health-promoting behavior can be key to symptom management for people with chronic disability. However, occupational patterns and routines often require adaptation. Reynolds (2001) provides an overview of facilitating physical activity to enhance wellbeing. She notes that the literature consistently lists the following as effective in assisting individuals to adopt a healthier lifestyle: exploring barriers to physical activity, promoting self-efficacy for exercise, providing educational interventions, maximizing rewards, encouraging goal setting, enhancing resistance to relapse, building social support, and providing reminders or cues to action. However, despite the *Surgeon General Report on Physical Activity and Health* (USDHHS, 1994), which strongly suggests regular physical activity for all people as a preventive measure, people with disabilities often lead more sedentary lifestyles and cannot or do not pursue the recommended amount of physical activity necessary to prevent the occurrence of secondary conditions.

In *Healthy People 2010: Understanding and Improving Health* (USDHHS, 2000), it is stated that significantly more people with disabilities reported having no leisure time physical activity (56%) than those who had no disability (36%). The lower rate of participation may be due to several factors including environmental and architectural barriers, organizational policies and practices, discrimination, and social attitudes. Individuals with activity limitations "report having had more days

of pain, depression, anxiety, and sleeplessness and fewer days of vitality during the previous month than people not reporting activity limitations" (USDHHS, 2000, p. 6-4). Occupational therapists are skilled at engaging people with disabilities in meaningful pursuits that promote ongoing participation in life and utilizing skills in adapting environments according to need. Heightened awareness by health professionals is the key to change.

Marks and Heller (2002) propose that the Ottawa Charter guidelines for health promotion (WHO, 1986) be used to develop and implement health promotion strategies for people with I/DD and others. These five action areas consist of

1. establishing community-based health promotion policies;
2. creating supportive environments for health;
3. strengthening communities;
4. developing personal skills; and
5. recruiting health services.

Within each of these areas, occupational therapists and occupational therapy assistants have ample opportunity to work from an occupation- and client-centered perspective to promote health behaviors that optimize daily occupational living. While traditional occupational therapy may be to develop life skills and optimize occupational performance within one's cognitive limitations, a health promoting framework can be utilized to assist in training people with I/DD in the creation of healthy living. Marks and Heller (2002) propose four key principles to ensure that programs are successful:

1. Build from a base of community ownership and partnership
2. Target specific behaviors
3. Incorporate sound theoretical frameworks as a basis for program plans
4. Consider the types of interventions that work best given the specific populations and circumstances (Marks & Heller, 2002, pp. 15–16)

It is recommended that occupational therapy interventions be community-based whenever possible, reflect the needs of the individual for community integration, be specific and understandable to the clients, and be theory-based and client- and occupation-centered. In 2004, the World Federation of Occupational Therapists (WFOT) released a position paper on community-based rehabilitation (CBR). This paper supports and encourages the participation of occupational therapists to collaborate with people who experience disabilities and their families and communities. This would help to demonstrate the global power of occupational therapy through the support of "people with disabilities' needs and rights of dignity and inclusion, in both developing and developed societies" (WFOT, 2004, p. 1).

Conclusion

According to the WHO (1986), health promotion is

> the process of enabling people to increase control over, and to improve, their health. To reach a state of optimal physical, mental and social wellbeing, an individual or group must be able to identify and to realize aspirations, to satisfy needs, and to change or cope with the environment. Health is, therefore, seen as a resource for everyday life, not the objective of living. (p. iii)

This conceptualization of health and health promotion is as appropriate for people with disabilities as it is for persons without disabilities.

People with disabilities, like their nondisabled counterparts, have aspirations for living a quality life and must cope and adapt to changes in their environments and lifestyles. This chapter was designed to heighten awareness of the need to integrate health promotion strategies into the practice of occupational therapy for people with disabilities. Newer frameworks, models, assessments, and intervention strategies have been discussed that relate to a paradigm shift. This shift involves changes in clinical reasoning and approaches to clients, consumers, and families, and it incorporates occupation- and client-centered care to achieve positive health outcomes.

A major focus of occupational therapy for people with disabilities is utilizing health promotion interventions to prevent secondary conditions. These conditions can be physical (e.g., decubiti), psychosocial (e.g., developing depression), spiritual (e.g., loss of meaning in daily activity), or social (e.g., disengaging from previous activity with friends and family). Occupational therapy health promotion interventions for people with disabilities should be holistic in nature and occupation- and client-centered. Traditional occupational therapy assessments and interventions may need to be modified to incorporate

lifestyle factors that may impede or support health and wellbeing for people with disabilities. Social support, health beliefs, and health-focused occupational habits and routines of people with disabilities are essential elements to address, as they can act as facilitating factors or barriers to health and wellbeing. Occupational strategies to empower people with disabilities to become their own health agents are crucial interventions to prevent disabling secondary conditions and promote health and healing. In addition, enhancing quality of life for people with disabilities is a legitimate outcome of occupational therapy health promotion interventions (AOTA, 2008).

Occupational therapy can be a leader in the provision of services that promote healthy lifestyles for people with disabilities throughout the life span. The profession has always advocated for and engaged in promoting public health policy and community health initiatives that advance health. Training and education in human development, psychosocial aspects of disability, social systems approaches to health and wellbeing, and the development of adaptive capacities for all people positions occupational therapy practitioners to become leaders in health promotion.

Occupational therapists must begin to examine how health promotion, which starts with the evaluation process followed by recommendations of preventive occupations, can enhance the care provided to people with disabilities. As children and youth age and mature, positive occupational patterns learned and habituated early in childhood will significantly impact their future occupational participation as active adults in the community and may diminish secondary conditions as they age.

Health status is critically important to experiencing QOL, maintaining independence, and participating fully in society. For the more than 54 million people in the United States with disabilities (USDHHS, 2000), maintaining health and wellness is essential to reduce the impact of impairment on functioning and to foster positive development. Additionally, as persons with disabilities live longer, long-term health promotion and QOL issues will need to receive greater attention.

Case Study 19-1

Joe is a 50-year-old man with multiple sclerosis (MS). He is married, with a 14-year-old son. Both Joe and his wife, Ann, are blue-collar workers with high school educations. Joe lives with his family in a rented, ranch-style home with 10 stairs to the basement, where Joe likes to play his electric guitar on Saturday nights. They cannot afford to move. Joe works for an auto parts store full-time, making less than $25,000 per year, and he stands most of the time to assist customers. He sits occasionally for some computer work. Joe's hobbies include anything to do with rock and

roll, eating out, and watching television. On the weekdays, he usually gets up at 5:30 a.m. and returns home at 7:00 p.m. (he drives 1 hour to work each way) and is exhausted when he arrives home. Joe participates in no structured exercise or activity during the week and occasionally will do some light yard work or household chores.

Ann works two jobs in order to pay the bills. She is overweight and is often under tremendous pressure to "keep things going" in the home. She has a tendency to take over many tasks in and around the house, because she is "afraid

Joe might fall." Over the past 5 years, Joe has developed lower extremity weakness and requires a cane much of the time to walk. He has difficulty ascending and descending stairs while carrying anything over 10 pounds. About twice a year, Joe experiences an exacerbation of symptoms and is bedbound for a week at a time. He states that he often gets depressed about his situation, not feeling like a "man" and unable to do many things with his son.

Questions

1. What may be some signs and symptoms of MS about which Joe may not be aware? Develop three educational sessions for Joe and his wife with goals

and interventions to promote healthy living both during and after an exacerbation in order to maximize occupational participation.

2. Are there some health promotion strategies that can help Joe prevent mental health problems related to his situation? What might a mental health prevention intervention consist of? Would it include physical interventions? Why or why not?

3. Can Joe's wife do anything to help promote a healthier lifestyle for both of them? What might an occupational therapy health promotion intervention with Joe and his wife consist of?

▶ For Discussion and Review

1. How might an occupational therapist gather and analyze narrative information about people with disabilities and their perceptions about health and wellness?
2. What areas of health and wellness for people with disabilities could occupational therapists explore more in depth? How would they go about it?
3. How does a physical disability impair occupational roles, routines, and performance of meaningful occupations? How do these disruptions impact the person's overall health?
4. Is wellness a concept that "fits" within the context of living with a disability? How does it fit or not fit?
5. Choose three different disabilities. How would each be viewed under the functional and social conceptualization of disability as defined in this chapter? What health promotion interventions for each conceptualization could you develop?

▶ Research Questions

1. How is meaningfulness of life activity perceived by people with disabilities?
2. Is a person more adaptive throughout their lifetime if they develop a disability in childhood? If so, what might create that adaptability?
3. What are society's expectations of people with disabilities, and how is that similar or different from the perspectives of people with disabilities?

References

American Occupational Therapy Association. (2008). Occupational therapy practice framework: Domain and process (2d ed.). *American Journal of Occupational Therapy, 62,* 625–83.

Americans with Disabilities Act, 1990. (Public Law 101-336), 42 U.S.C.A. §12101.

Angelopoulou, N., Matziari, C., Tsimaris, V., Sakadamis, A., Souftas, V., & Mandroukas, K. (2000). Bone mineral density and muscle strength in young men with mental retardation (with and without Down syndrome). *Calcified Tissue International, 66,* 176–80.

Benamy., B. C. (1999). *Developing clinical reasoning skills: Strategies for the occupational therapist.* San Antonio, TX: PsycCorp.

Bird, F. L., Sperry, J. M., & Carreiro, H. L. (1998). Community habilitation and integration of adults with psychiatric disorders and mental retardation: Development of a clinically responsive environment. *Journal of Developmental and Physical Disabilities, 10,* 331–48.

Bostick, R. M. (1977). Quality of life survey among a severely handicapped population. *Dissertation Abstracts International, 38,* 1946-B (University Microfilms No. 77-20).

Brollier, C., Shepherd, J., & Markley, K. F. (1994). Transition from school to community living. *American Journal of Occupational Therapy, 48,* 346–53.

Bulger, D. W., & Smith, A. B. (1999). Message tailoring: An essential component for disease management. *Disease Management Health Outcomes, 5,* 127–34.

Burckhardt, C., Woods, S., Schultz, A., & Ziebarth, D. (1989). Quality of life of adults with chronic illness: A psychometric study. *Research in Nursing and Health, 12,* 347–54.

Burke, J. (1996). Variations in childhood occupations: Play in the presence of chronic disability. In R. Zemke & F. Clark (Eds.), *Occupational Science: The evolving discipline* (pp. 413–18). Philadelphia: F. A. Davis.

Cardinal, B. (2003). *Transtheoretical strategies for physical activity.* Paper presented at the Changing Concepts of Health & Disability: State of the Science Conference & Policy Forum, Bethesda, MD. Retrieved April 8, 2006, from http://www.healthwellness.org/archive/training/sciconf/sciconf.htm.

Cardinal, B. C., & Cardinal, M. (1997). Changes in exercise behavior and exercise identity associated with a 14-week aerobic exercise class. *Journal of Sport Behavior, 20*(4), 377–86.

Carleton, B. H., & Henrich, T. W. (1998). A qualitative and quantitative analysis of the impact of a multidimensional wellness program. *Hong Kong Journal of Sports Medicine and Sports Science, 7,* 50–55.

Drum, C. (2003). *Behavioral risk factor surveillance system project-health status & disability.* Paper presented at the Changing Concepts of Health & Disability: State of the Science Conference & Policy Forum, Bethesda, MD. Retrieved April 8, 2006, from http://www.healthwellness .org/archive/training/sciconf/sciconf.htm.

Dunn, H. L. (1961). *High level wellness.* Arlington, VA: R.W. Beatty.

Esdaile, S. A. (1996). A play focused intervention involving mothers of preschoolers. *American Journal of Occupational Therapy, 50,* 113–23.

Fearing, V. G., Law, M., & Clark, J. (1997). An occupational performance process model: Fostering client and therapist alliances. *Canadian Journal of Occupational Therapy, 64,* 7–15.

Finn, G. (1972). The occupational therapist in prevention programs. *American Journal of Occupational Therapy, 26,* 59–66.

Frey, L., Szalda-Petree, A., Traci, M. A., & Seekins, T. (2000). Prevention of secondary health conditions in adults with developmental disabilities: A review of the literature. *Disability and Rehabilitation, 23*(9), 361–69.

Gulick, E. E. (1991). Self-assessed health and use of health services. *Western Journal of Nursing Research, 13,* 195–219.

Harrison, T., & Stuifbergen, A. (2002). Disability, social support and concern for children: Depression in mothers with multiple sclerosis. *Journal of Obstetric, Gynecologic and Neonatal Nursing, 31*(4), 444–53.

Ho, P. (2003). *Determinants of health behaviors in adults with diabetes.* Paper presented at the Changing Concepts of Health & Disability State of the Science Conference & Policy Forum, Bethesda, MD. Retrieved April 8, 2006, from http://www.healthwellness.org/archive/training/ sciconf/sciconf.htm.

Hough, J. (1999). Disability and health: A national public health agenda. In R. J. Simeonsson & D. B. Bailey (Eds.), *Issues in disability and health: The role of secondary conditions and quality of life* (pp. 161–203). Chapel Hill, NC: North Carolina Office on Disability and Health.

Johnson, J. A. (1986a). *Wellness: A context for living.* Thorofare, NJ: SLACK.

Johnson, J. (1986b). Wellness and occupational therapy. *American Journal of Occupational Therapy, 40*(11), 753–58.

Johnson, J. (1993). Wellness programs. In H. S. Hopkins & H. D. Smith (Eds.), *Willard and Spackman's occupational therapy* (8th ed., pp. 843–52). Philadelphia: Lippincott.

Johnson, J., & Jaffe, E. (Eds.). (1989). *Health promotion and preventive programs: Models of occupational therapy practice.* Binghamton, NY: Haworth Press.

Kailes, J. I. (2000). *Can disability, chronic conditions health and wellness coexist?* Retrieved October 20, 2003, from http://www.ncpad.org.

Kickbusch, I. (1997). Think health: What makes the difference. *Health Promotion International, 12*(4), 265–72.

Kniepmann, K. (1997). Prevention of disability and maintenance of health. In C. Baum & C. Christiansen (Eds.), *Occupational therapy: Enabling function and wellbeing* (2d ed., pp. 531–55). Thorofare, NJ: SLACK.

Kocina, P. (1997). Body composition of spinal cord injured adults. *Sports Medicine, 23,* 48–60.

Krahn, G. (2003). *Keynote: Changing concepts in health, wellness, and disability.* Paper presented at the Changing Concepts of Health & Disability: State of the Science Conference & Policy Forum, Bethesda, MD. Retrieved April 8, 2006, from http://www.healthwellness.org/archive/ training/sciconf/sciconf.htm.

Lanig, I. S., Chase, T. M., Butt, L. M., & Hulse, K. L. (1966). *A practical guide to health promotion after spinal cord injury.* Gaithersburg, MD: Aspen.

Law, M. (Ed.). (1998). *Client-centered occupational therapy.* Thorofare, NJ: SLACK.

Lee, C. (1993). Attitudes, knowledge and stages of change: A survey of exercise patterns in older Australian women. *Health Psychology, 12*(6), 476–80.

Marks, B. A., & Heller, T. (2002). Bridging the equity gap: Health promotion for adults with intellectual and developmental disabilities. *Nursing Clinics of North America, 38*(2), 205–28.

McGuire, B. K., Crowe, T. K., Law, M., & VanLeit, B. (2004). Mothers of children with disabilities: Occupational concerns and solutions. *OTJR: Occupation, Participation and Health, 24*(2), 54–63.

Meyer, A. (1977). The philosophy of occupation therapy. *American Journal of Occupational Therapy, 31*(10), 639–42. (Original work published in 1922.)

Missiuna, C., & Pollock, N. (1991). Play deprivation in children with physical disabilities: The role of the occupational therapist in preventing secondary disability. *American Journal of Occupational Therapy, 45,* 882–88.

Neufeld, P., & Kniepmann, K. (2001). Gateway to wellness: An occupational therapy collaboration with the National Multiple Sclerosis Society. *Occupational Therapy in Health Care, 13*(3/4), 67–84.

Oleson, M. (1990). Subjectively perceived quality of life. *Image: Journal of Nursing Scholarship, 22,* 187–90.

Padilla, R. (2003). Clara: A phenomenology of disability. *American Journal of Occupational Therapy, 57*(4), 413–23.

Patrick, D. L., Richardson, M., Starks, H. E., & Rose, M. A. (1994). A framework for promoting health of people with disabilities. In D. J. Lollar (Ed.), *Preventing secondary conditions associated with spina bifida and cerebral palsy: Proceedings and recommendations of a symposium* (pp. 3–16). Washington, DC: Spina Bifida Association of America.

Peloquin, S. (1990). The patient-therapist relationship in occupational therapy: Understanding visions and images. *American Journal of Occupational Therapy, 44*(1), 13–21.

Peloquin, S. (1993). The depersonalization of patients: A profile gleaned from narratives. *American Journal of Occupational Therapy, 47*(9), 830–37.

Pizzi, M. (2001). The Pizzi Holistic Wellness Assessment. *Occupational Therapy in Health Care, 13*(3/4), 51–66.[For more information, go to http://www.michaelpizzi.com.]

Pörn, I. (1993). Health and adaptedness. *Theoretical Medicine, 14,* 295–303.

Prochaska, J. O., & DiClemente, C. C. (1992). Stages of change in the modification of behavior problems. In M. Hersen, R. M. Eisler, & P. M. Miller (Eds.), *Progress in behavior modification* (pp. 184–214). Sycamore, IL: Sycamore Press.

Putnam, M., Geenen, S., Powers, L., Saxton, M., Finney, S., & Dautel, P. (2003). Health and wellness: People with disabilities discuss barriers and facilitators to well being. *Journal of Rehabilitation, 69*(1), 37–45.

Reitz, S. (1992). A historical review of occupational therapy's role in preventive health and wellness. *American Journal of Occupational Therapy, 46*(1), 50–55.

Reitz, S. M. (1999). Cardiac rehabilitation: An opportunity for promoting wellness. *Physical Disabilities Special Interest Section Quarterly, 22*(2), 1–4.

Renwick, R., Brown, I., & Nagler, M. (Eds.). (1996). *Quality of life in health promotion and rehabilitation: Conceptual approaches, issues and application.* Newbury Park, CA: Sage.

Renwick, R., Brown, I., Rootman, I., & Nagler, M. (1996). Conceptualization, research and application: Future directions. In R. Renwick, I. Brown, & M. Nagler (Eds.) *Quality of life in health promotion and rehabilitation: Conceptual approaches, issues and application* (pp. 357–67). Newbury Park, CA: Sage.

Reynolds, F. (2001). Strategies for facilitating physical activity and wellbeing: A health promotion perspective. *British Journal of Occupational Therapy, 64*(7), 330–36.

Rimmer, J. H. (1999). Health promotion for people with disabilities: The emerging paradigm shift from disability prevention to prevention of secondary conditions. *Physical Therapy, 79,* 495–502.

Rimmer, J. H. (2005). The conspicuous absence of people with disabilities in public fitness and recreations facilities: Lack of interest or lack of access? *American Journal of Health Promotion, 19*(5), 327–29.

Scaffa, M. (2001). *Occupational therapy in community-based practice settings.* Philadelphia: F. A. Davis.

Scaffa, M., Desmond, S., & Brownson, C. A. (2001). Public health, community health, and occupational therapy. In M. Scaffa (Ed.), *Occupational therapy in community-based practice settings* (pp. 35–50). Philadelphia: F. A. Davis.

Scaffa, M. E., Van Slyke, N., Brownson, C. A., & American Occupational Therapy Association Commission on Practice. (2008). Occupational therapy in the promotion of health and the prevention of disease and disability statement. *American Journal of Occupational Therapy, 62*(6), 694–703.

Schaaf, R. C., & Davis, W. S. (1992). Promoting health and wellness in the pediatric disabled and "at risk" population. In J. Rothman & R. Levine (Eds.), *Prevention practice: Strategies for physical and occupational therapy.* Philadelphia: W. B. Saunders.

Schlaff, C. (1993). From dependency to self-advocacy: Redefining disability. *American Journal of Occupational Therapy, 47*(10), 943–48.

Seligman, M. E. P. (1972). Learned helplessness. *Annual Review of Medicine, 23,* 407–12.

Sneed, N. V., & Paul, S. C. (2003). Readiness for behavioral changes in patients with congestive heart failure. *American Journal of Critical Care, 12*(5), 444–53.

Stuifbergen, A. (1995). Health promoting behaviors and quality of life among individuals with multiple sclerosis. *Scholarly Inquiry for Nursing Practice, 9*(1), 31–50.

Stuifbergen, A. K., Becker, H., & Sands, D. (1990). Barriers to health promotion for people with disabilities. *Family and Community Health, 13*(1), 11–22.

Stuifbergen, A., Gordon, D., & Clark, A. P. (1998). Health promotion: A complementary strategy for stroke rehabilitation. *Topics in Stroke Rehabilitation, 5*(2), 11–18.

Stuifbergen, A. K., & Roberts, G. J. (1997). Health promotion practices of women with multiple sclerosis. *Archives of Physical Medicine and Rehabilitation, 78* (Supplement 5), S3–S9.

Stuifbergen, A., & Rogers, S. (1997). Health promotion: An essential component of rehabilitation for persons with chronic disabling conditions. *Advances in Nursing Science, 19*(4), 1–20.

Tarlov, A. R. (1999). Public policy frameworks for improving population health. *Annals of the New York Academy of Sciences, 896,* 281–93.

Tingus, S. (2003). *Keynote: NIDRR's future directions in health and wellness.* Paper presented at the Changing Concepts of Health & Disability: State of the Science Conference & Policy Forum, Bethesda, MD. Retrieved April 8, 2006, from http://www.healthwellness.org/archive/training/sciconf/sciconf.htm.

Tudor-Locke, C., Myers, A., & Rodger, N. (2001). Development of a theory-based daily activity intervention for individuals with type-2 diabetes. *Diabetes Educator, 27*(1), 85–93.

Turk, M. A., Geremski, C. A., Rosenbaum, P. F., & Weber, R. J. (1997). The health status of women with cerebral palsy. *Archives of Physical Medicine, 78,* S10–S17.

U.S. Census Bureau. (2006). *Disability: 2006 American Community Survey.* Retrieved April 27, 2008, from http://www.census.gov/hhes/www/disability/2006acs.html.

U.S. Department of Health and Human Services. (1994). *Physical activity and health: A report of the surgeon general executive summary.* Washington, DC: U.S. Government Printing Office.

U.S. Department of Health and Human Services. (2000). *Healthy People 2010: Understanding and improving health* (2d ed.). Washington, DC: U.S. Government Printing Office.

Velde, B., & Fidler, G. (2002). *Lifestyle performance: A model for engaging the power of occupation.* Thorofare, NJ: SLACK.

Wechsler, H., Levine, S., Idelson, R. K., Rohman, M., & Taylor, J. O. (1983). The physician's role in health promotion—A survey of primary-care practitioners. *New England Journal of Medicine, 308,* 97–100.

Wechsler, H., Levine, S., Idelson, R. K., Schor, E. L., & Coakley, E. (1996). The physician's role in health promotion revisited—A survey of primary care practitioners. *New England Journal of Medicine, 334,* 996–98.

West, W. (1968). Professional responsibility in times of change. *American Journal of Occupational Therapy, 22,* 231–49.

West, W. (1969). The growing importance of prevention. *American Journal of Occupational Therapy, 23,* 226, 231.

White, V. (1986). Promoting health and wellness: A theme for the eighties. *American Journal of Occupational Therapy, 40*(11), 743–48.

Wiemer, R. B. (1972). Some concepts of prevention as an aspect of community health. *American Journal of Occupational Therapy, 26*(1), 1–9.

Wilcock, A. A. (1998). *An occupational perspective of health.* Thorofare, NJ: SLACK.

Wineman, N. (1990). Adaptation to multiple sclerosis: The role of social support, functional disability and perceived uncertainty. *Nursing Research, 39,* 294–99.

World Federation of Occupational Therapists. (2004). *WFOT position paper on community based rehabilitation.* Retrieved October 1, 2006, from www.wfot.org/documents .asp?state=&name=&id=&pagenum=4.

World Health Organization. (1948). *Preamble to the Constitution* as adopted by the International Health Conference. (Official Record of the World Health Organization, no. 2, p.100.)

World Health Organization. (1986). *Ottawa charter for health promotion: The first international conference on health promotion meeting in Ottawa.* Retrieved January 4, 2004, http://www.who.int/hpr/NPH/docs/ottawa_charter_hp.pdf.

World Health Organization. (2001) *International classification of functioning, disability and health.* Retrieved October 1, 2006, from http://www3.who.int/icf/icftemplate.cfm.

World Health Organization. (2008). *Disability and rehabilitation.* Retrieved April 27, 2008, from http://www.who.int/ disabilities/en/index.html.

Yerxa, E. J. (1998). Health and the human spirit for occupation. *American Journal of Occupational Therapy, 52*(6), 412–18.

Chapter 20

Promoting Health and Occupational Participation With Caregivers

Michael A. Pizzi

> Family caregivers are less likely than peers of the same age to engage in health-promoting behaviors that are important for chronic disease prevention and control. Given that the demands of caring for a loved one may compromise caregiver health and functioning and increase caregivers' risk of developing physical health problems, there is a pressing need to encourage family caregivers to engage in activities that will benefit their own health, wellbeing, and longevity.
>
> —U.S. Department of Health and Human Services (USDHHS), 2003, ¶ 4

Learning Objectives

This chapter is designed to enable the reader to:

- Describe the caregiving role and challenges of caregivers.
- Discuss characteristics of family systems and caregiver dynamics.
- Identify caregiver needs, including respite.
- Integrate current occupational therapy knowledge of health promotion to more holistically evaluate and intervene with caregivers.

Key Terms

Caregiver	Family processes
Caregiving	Family structure
Care of others	Health-promoting self-care

Respite	Self-efficacy
Self-care self-efficacy	Support group

Introduction

Caregiver health is often compromised when caring for an ill loved one and often goes unnoticed by health professionals as well as the caregivers themselves (Acton, 2002). While caregivers are in need of health-promoting self-care interventions, it is the loved one with a health impairment who receives services, often with little inclusion or recognition of health issues of caregivers. Occupational therapy interventions focus on facilitating health and wellbeing, with a resultant outcome of improved quality of life (QOL) for caregivers and clients. The health and wellbeing of the family system is dependent on the level of understanding by health professionals of the many challenges each family and its members encounter, and the interventions implemented that facilitate wellbeing.

According to the American Occupational Therapy Association's (AOTA) *Occupational Therapy Practice* *Framework: Domain and Process* (referred to as the *Framework*), the term client is used to name "the entity that receives occupational therapy services" (AOTA, 2008, p. 669). In the *Framework,* caregivers are included in the description of *client:* "Clients may include (1) individuals and other persons relevant to the individual's life, including family, caregivers, teachers, employers, and others who may help or be served indirectly . . ." (AOTA, 2008, p. 669). For the purposes of this chapter, a **caregiver** is defined as an individual, usually a family member, who has the principal responsibility of caring for a child or dependent adult in the home. In the *Framework,* **caregiving** as an occupation is subsumed under areas of occupation/instrumental activities of daily living (IADLs). It is identified as "**care of others** (including selecting and supervising caregivers)" and is defined as "arranging, supervising, or providing care for others" (AOTA, 2008, p. 631). Outcomes of care include engagement in occupation that supports participation, thus outcomes for caregiver interventions can include, for example, enhancing health and wellbeing, improving QOL, or preventing psychosocial disruption. When these outcomes are achieved, then caregiving occupations can be better supported.

Caregiving and the caregiver experience will be described in this chapter. Conceptual frameworks for caregiving and the family life cycle are discussed relative to occupational participation. Challenges of caregiving, health promotion, evaluation of caregivers, and interventions from an occupational perspective are presented in order to provide readers with strategies for empowering caregivers to have healthy lifestyles.

Conceptual Frameworks for Caregiving

Family systems theories help organize and shape occupational therapy assessment and intervention with caregivers and families. While these theories differ in approach, all are valuable when families and caregivers are helped to view life in a healthier and more positive way despite impairments in wellbeing or QOL. Some of these theories and models are briefly described below.

Behavioral family therapy has a reward and punishment focus and is guided by the principle that "behavior is determined more by its consequences than by its antecedents" (Becvar & Becvar, 1993, p. 257). The goal is increasing the frequency of positive behaviors.

Another model is the communications approach to family therapy, which focuses on the "redundant patterns of communication and interaction between and within systems" (Becvar & Becvar, 1993, p. 211). The underlying belief of this approach is that clear and congruent messages are essential for healthy relationships in the family. Incongruent styles include: placating; blaming; or being super-reasonable, irrelevant, or distracting.

A third approach is contextual family therapy, which focuses on fairness in family relationships, equitability, trustworthiness, and loyalty. It seeks to uncover "obligations" and "debts" accrued over time and discusses loyalty and legacy, with the thrust being to establish trustworthiness in family relationships. The therapist is not in a prescriptive, reframing, or restructuring role; instead, therapy elicits family members' thinking about the other person's perspectives as well as their own (Becvar & Becvar, 1993).

Perhaps the two most influential theorists in family therapy are Minuchin and Bowen. Minuchin developed structural family therapy, whereby the therapist plays a directive and manipulative role. Therapists identify and name human behaviors in reference to alignment, power, and boundaries within the family structure and use three challenging strategies to address the family's symptoms, structure, and reality as grounded in structural work. A spin-off of Minuchin's work is that of Haley, who developed strategic, or problem-solving, family therapy. The guiding principle of this therapy is that change occurs not through insight or understanding, but through the process of the family carrying out directives issued by the therapist (Becvar & Becvar, 1993). This style is mostly concerned with symptoms, metaphors, hierarchy, and power.

Finally, the approach developed by Bowen is based on nine concepts, which include differentiation of self, triangles, multigenerational transmission process, sibling position, emotional cutoff, nuclear family, emotional system, family projection process, and societal regression. "All of these concepts in Bowen's model are linked by the presence of and the family's reaction to heightened, uncontrolled anxiety" (Glasscock & Hales, 1998, p. 38). Bowen's therapy is an outgrowth of psychoanalytic theory and offers the most comprehensive view of human behavior and problems of any approach to family therapy. The core goal underlying the Bowenian model is differentiation of self, namely the ability to remain oneself in the face of group influences, especially the intense influence of family life. This model also considers the thoughts and feelings of each family member as well as the larger contextual network of family relationships that shapes the family's life. The family is viewed as the client, and the family is the center of care.

The concept of client-centered care used in occupational therapy can be applied to family caregivers as clients. Assessing caregiver wellbeing and providing interventions aimed at caregiver health improves QOL and wellbeing for both the client and the caregiver. Improving the health of caregivers supports and promotes ongoing, effective, and healthful caregiving.

Bowen developed his model and approach using general systems theory as a foundation. This theory recognizes that each system and subsystem is part of a whole, broader system. All these systems are dynamic in nature, with the foundational concept being that a change in one part of the system affects the whole. In terms of family systems, one person with an illness, impairment, or disability will affect the entire family unit, depending on the relationships with that person. Caregiving and the caregiver will be affected by the dynamic that occurs within that family system.

Hall and Kirschling (1990) proposed a framework based on systems theory and family development for end-of-life care (ELC) and the hospice caregiver. These authors believe that when the family is viewed as a system in need of care, hospice professionals are better equipped to help both the care recipient and the family cope with the many issues the dying process evokes. Through interacting with the family, the professional caregiver and other involved health professionals will be able to gain an understanding and appreciation of the family and its unique habits, division of roles, and perspective on the illness and its expected trajectory. With this knowledge, the professional caregiver and health professional can better serve both the patient and the family.

Within the conceptual framework thus far articulated, Hall and Kirschling described both the structure and process of families, which "serve as the locus of family strengths and/or limitations or dysfunctions" (1990, p. 4). **Family structure** refers to a static arrangement of the family's parts at a given moment in time (Bertrand, as cited in Hall & Kirschling, 1990). Illness, disability, and death are viewed as a disruption in the structure, and families both anticipate and experience structural changes.

Family processes are a "series of changes which are arranged in a special order that occur continuously through time, both within the family and between the family and its environment" (Hall & Kirschling, 1990, p. 10). These changes include adaptation, integration, and decision-making. In order for the family to continuously function and survive a crisis of health, adaptation is necessary. Hall and Kirschling (1990) illustrate caregiving and family dynamics/family challenges related to the dying process. However, the basic concepts are applicable to any caregiver situation. Knowledge of family dynamics and how families meet challenges can inform occupational therapy evaluation and intervention.

The Family Life Cycle

Carter and McGoldrick (1988) conceptualized six developmental stages in the family life cycle. When there is a disruption in the natural timing of a family life cycle, then stress will be more profound during that transition between one stage and another. These six stages are family systems–oriented and not chronological age–determined:

1. Between families—single young adult
2. Joining of families though marriage
3. Families with young children
4. Families with adolescents
5. Families launching children
6. Families in later life

The following is an example of how a life event affects the family at specific stages of the family life cycle:

Hospice caregivers may be called upon to assist families at all stages of the family life cycle. The stage in which the death occurs determines the family and individual developmental tasks, which are most likely to be interrupted. The death of a parent may stall the launching of the young adult, making it difficult for him or her to establish a separate existence. The death of a spouse in young families has a profound effect not only on the marriage partner but also on the quality of the parenting available for young children. Death of a child is especially hard for families to accept, for parents do not expect to bury their young as was common in past generations. Although the unexpected, off-schedule death is often the most stressful, even the expected death of a grandparent can be difficult for the family. Regardless of the stage of the family life cycle or whether the death was expected or unexpected, a death reverberates through the entire system. (Hall & Kirschling, 1990, p. 21)

Any disability or impairment of participation, not just death and the dying process, can disrupt the family life cycle. This creates a need for occupational adaptation. Identifying a family's stage in the life cycle enhances the development of effective interventions.

Caregiver Health

Women are usually the primary caregivers in the United States (Aneshensel, Pearlin, Mullan, Zarit, & Whitlatch, 1995). Disabled spouses, especially men, are typically cared for by their wives in heterosexual relationships. In gay and lesbian relationships, partners also are usually the caregivers. However, with a diagnosis of AIDS, for example, people with no partner or social network may return to their place of origin, often to their parents, for support and caregiving (Shernoff, 1997). Alternatively, as children become older, with increasing obligations and needs to balance occupations and roles, the role of caregiver for elderly parents or others may be added. The extent of caregiving and the ability to provide care may also depend on the relationships and rituals among family members (e.g., children who are emotionally distant from a parent, a father who disowns his gay son, a close-knit Italian family that had Sunday dinner together throughout their lives). These distinct relationships and rituals within families need to be acknowledged and included in the occupational therapy intervention plan.

Caretaking takes a toll on the provider of care. In their study of rural, female, informal caregivers, Blakley and Jaffe (2000) found that 30% believed there was nothing that could make caregiving tasks less difficult. The women reported that the demands of caregiving in a rural community limited their social lives, interfered with their work lives, and reduced their own health. Emanuel and colleagues (2000) examined the economic and other burdens of the terminally ill and their caregivers. They generated a model that applies to all terminal illnesses. This model shows that increased economic burden and decreased physical functioning of people with terminal illness impose great psychosocial stress on caregivers. Other research supports this model and discusses other challenges of caregiving. When people at the end of life experience poor physical function, are of an advanced age, incontinent, or have decreased socioeconomic status, then there are greater care needs, which also increase psychosocial burdens on caregivers, including depression (Covinsky, Padgett, Schlesinger, Cohen, & Burns, 1994; Siegel, Raveis, Houts, & Mor, 1991).

In a 1997 study on preventive health behaviors, Burton, Newson, Schulz, Hirsch, and German (as cited in Acton, 2002) compared spousal caregivers with a spouse experiencing at least one activity of daily living (ADL) impairment to a matched demographic group. Results showed that such care "significantly increased the risk for not getting enough rest, not having enough time to exercise, not being able to take enough time to recuperate from illness, and forgetting to take prescription medications" (Burton et al., 1997, as cited in Acton, 2002, p. 74). Follow-up studies by occupational therapists using both a functional restorative program of self-care combined with health promotion intervention for caregivers could prove beneficial in producing evidence for occupational therapy health promotion interventions.

Challenges of Caregiving

One of the most comprehensive and overreaching studies on caregiving was conducted under the auspices of the National Alliance for Caregiving and American Association of Retired Persons (NAC & AARP, 2004). The purpose of this study was to update and expand knowledge about the activities caregivers perform, the perceived impact of caregiving on their daily lives, and the unmet needs of caregivers. People were randomly telephoned, and of those contacted, 1247 caregivers were identified. For this study, caregivers were defined as being at least 18 years old, living in the United States, and performing one or more ADLs or IADLs for someone 18 years of age or older (NAC & AARP, 2004). Some of the findings from this study included the following:

• The average length of caregiving is 4.3 years.
• Caregivers tend to live near the people they care for.
• Nearly 4 in 10 caregivers are men.
• Overall, female caregivers are providing more hours of care, and they are providing a higher level of care than male caregivers.

• Women are more likely to report experiencing emotional stress as a result of caregiving than men.
• Women and men report equal proportions of physical strain (NAC & AARP, 2004, pp. 6–9).

The report also describes the caregiver level of burden on a scale of five levels. The Level of Burden Scale incorporates ADLs, IADLs, and amount of time devoted to caregiving (NAC & AARP, 2004). Occupational therapists and occupational therapy assistants can help reduce the burden of caregiving (AOTA, 2007). When practitioners have knowledge of how caregiving impacts occupational participation, intervention can become more client-centered to help remediate problems and enhance the health and wellness of caregivers. For example, having a simple but indirect conversation with a caregiver about the many roles one must balance or the amount of care being provided can help caregivers reveal how time is used and their frustrations about not engaging in their own occupations. A compassionate, empathic response with some practical suggestions to participate in meaningful occupations other than caregiving can be as important as working directly with the client.

Caregiver burden or impairment in occupational participation and role strain, real or perceived, are often universally experienced to some degree no matter the context of caregiving. Specific issues related to caregiving for persons with varying needs include caregiving for children with disabilities, persons with serious and persistent mental illness, persons with other chronic conditions, persons with dementia, and persons at end of life.

Caregiving for Children With Disabilities

A child with a disability can be an emotional and physical challenge for parents or the child's primary caregivers. While caregivers may feel a host of emotions, from anger and resentment to despair and depression, there can also be a transformation within a family system to hope and joy. "Mothers of children with disabilities report more stress than fathers, whereas fathers report more trouble forming bonds with their children" (Beckman et al. as cited in Cohn, Henry, & Marks, 2003, p. 547). Occupational therapists and occupational therapy assistants can help facilitate an adaptive process for providing care for children with disabilities.

Scorgie and Sobsey (2000) reported parents feeling enlivened and enriched through attending and lecturing at health conferences for parents of children with disabilities or writing about their experiences. The emotional and intellectual connection with others in similar situations provided strength and support in times of crisis, and adaptation to a different view on life occurred as a result.

The importance of occupational therapy for parents with more severely impaired children is essential for improved family health and improved care of and interactions with the child. Psychosocial and social rehabilitation interventions would be very appropriate for these caregivers, such as providing outlets for emotional needs or helping caregivers create different daily routines to improve occupational balance.

Carey (2004) reported on a study conducted by Epel and Blackburn of the University of California at San Francisco. Blood samples from 58 young and middle-aged mothers, with 39 as primary caregivers of a child with a chronic disability, had white blood cell DNA analyzed. The longer the women had cared for their disabled children, the greater the negative impact was found relative to increased stress and premature aging. Epel also stated that "some of the women who had a lot of objective, real stress also had a low perceived amount of stress, and the next step is trying to understand what it is that promotes this kind of resilience" (Carey, p. 2). The implications for occupational therapy are to produce both quantitative and qualitative evidence that supports occupational therapy interventions to reduce caregiver stress and optimize participation to promote health and wellbeing.

Navaie-Waliser, Spriggs, and Feldman (2002) studied gender differences in informal caregiving. In a randomly selected nationwide telephone interview, they found that women were primarily the caregivers, they provide intensive and complex care, they have difficulty with role balance, and they contend with poorer emotional health secondary to caregiving. While women are often the primary caregivers in Western society, a cultural and societal shift has taken place since the 1990s, with fathers being more intimately involved in caregiving occupations (Lamb, as cited in Cohn et al., 2003). Occupational therapy practitioners must identify who is designated as the primary caregiver, have an understanding of some of the characteristics listed here, and develop services to meet specific needs of that caregiver while acknowledging the social and cultural differences inherent in each family.

Caregiving for Persons With Serious and Persistent Mental Illness

Care for severely mentally ill individuals living in the community may carry a heavy caregiver burden, which is particularly true for close family members such as parents, many of whom take care of their mentally ill children for long periods of time (Lefley, 1996). Well-being can become impaired for both caregivers and the persons for whom care is provided (Rudnick, 2004).

A study was implemented to measure the burden of caregivers for people with mental illness within a participatory action research framework (Rudnick, 2004). Fifty-three family members participated, all of whom reported moderate burden overall. A sense of being in danger was the mildest sense of burden, while worry about the person with mental illness was deemed severe. Female caregivers, regardless of age, perceived the most burden.

According to the Mental Illness Fellowship of Australia, Inc. (2005), there are various stages of coping for caregivers of people with mental illness. Initially, there is *crisis and stabilization,* where the client may enter into an acute phase of mental illness. The goal is to respond proactively, with reassurance and practical information (for both the client and caregiver), while the caregiver experiences emotional reactions such as fear, anxiety, disbelief, and shock. The next phase is categorized as *growing awareness,* whereby caregivers begin to recover and restructure their lives, learning how to incorporate mental illness into their occupational living, while also experiencing and fluctuating between grief and hope, despair and anxiety, frustration, and guilt. Support groups that can validate one's experiences, provide practical help, and instill hope for a positive future are crucial. The final phase of the emotional journey of caregivers is *recovery and hope.* It is in this phase that caregivers can look to a brighter future, having more fully integrated a loved one's mental illness into their daily routines. While the caregiver may experience some relief in developing this new routine and role, the relief is often accompanied by grief due to the losses, suffering, and human costs of mental illness.

Caregiving for Persons With Chronic Illnesses

A study of caregivers of people with cancer in Hong Kong discussed the risk these caregivers face for both physical and, increasingly, psychological problems (Chan & Chang, 1999). These risks are directly correlated with caregiver tasks and the stressors related to the caregiver role. When caregivers reported feeling tired most of the time, the researchers propose it may be more from devoting care to the relative than from being busy. There was little worry about a caregiver's personal health; however, within the cultural context of the Chinese family, there is great joy in being occupied with caregiving and little time and energy left for self.

Similar findings were discovered in the stroke literature and have implications for occupational therapy interventions. Stroke is the third leading cause of adult disability, with 23% of stroke survivors having multi-infarct dementia. After hospitalization and rehabilitation,

80% of stroke survivors become community dwellers once again and rely on family members for emotional, informational, and instrumental support for daily living (Anderson, Linto, & Stewart-Wynne, 1995). Evidence exists that depression in stroke caregivers worsens depression in clients and thus predicts poor responses of patients to rehabilitation (Glass, Matchar, Belyea, & Feussner, 1993). It has been noted that there is a higher rate of depression among stroke caregivers than non-stroke caregivers. With fewer social contacts, caregivers were more likely to be depressed, and caregivers with more stress-related physical symptoms were also more likely to be depressed (Han & Haley, 1999). In a study by Dennis, O'Rourke, Lewis, Sharpe, and Warlow (1998), 55% of the caregivers studied ($n = 246$) indicated emotional distress as a caregiver. Caregivers were more likely to be depressed if the patients were severely dependent or emotionally distressed themselves. Female caregivers reported more anxiety than male caregivers.

Although people with stroke in these studies survived, there is still profound loss, grief, and bereavement that families must go through to reach a place of equanimity, much like that of caregivers coping with family members approaching the end of life. Loss of function, meaning, purpose, and daily occupational performance—and the daily reminder of these losses—may exacerbate or be the direct cause of caregiver anxiety, depression, and emotional distress. Holistic assessment and interventions that are family/caregiver-centered and occupation-focused can assist in alleviating some of these challenges. The many mental health challenges faced by caregivers need to be considered by therapists working in stroke rehabilitation and in all arenas of occupational therapy, from the first encounter through the last.

Caregiving for Persons With Dementia

Corcoran (2001) described family caregivers of people with dementia as experiencing poor health, depression, burden, and stress. These caregiver characteristics match those of caregivers in end-of-life care. She also recommended that health professionals assess a family's patterns of care and beliefs about caregiving in order to stay family-centered. Corcoran stated that "how care is provided and who provides care are based on the family's definition of disability, health and responsibility" (p. 295). She described holistic assessment for caregivers of people with dementia and suggested several areas for intervention, including understanding the physical, emotional, and social health of caregivers; their patterns of care and caregiving; and the culture of the caregiver and care recipient. Corcoran emphasized two methods to assess care: (1) having caregivers describe their day from beginning to end, and (2) direct observation of care being provided. These two methods can help occupational therapists provide best practice in the area of dementia and assist caregivers in improving their own QOL.

Schulz and colleagues (2003) examined the effects of bereavement on family caregivers of persons with dementia who are also at the end of life. They found that caregivers exhibited high levels of depressive symptoms while providing care but became quickly resilient after the death. They concluded that caregivers of people with dementia require interventions before the person's death to decrease the burden of caregiving and to enable health and wellbeing. The caregivers reported considerable relief at the death itself, due to the ongoing loss and grief experienced daily during the dying process. Occupational therapists have opportunities in dementia care to help decrease caregiver burden through, for example, reconnecting caregivers to meaningful occupations they relinquished in order to provide care.

Dooley and Hinojosa (2004) explored caregiver burden and QOL of people with Alzheimer's disease living in the community relative to the adherence to occupational therapy recommendations. A pretest-posttest control group design was used, and the Assessment of Instrumental Function (AIF) was administered to two groups of people with Alzheimer's disease in their own homes. Caregivers were given measures of feelings of burden and QOL. They concluded that individualized occupational therapy intervention, which was theory-based (person-environment fit), appeared effective for caregivers and clients.

Butin, Miller, Maultsby, and Winter (1996) described a pilot program called Caregiver Options for Practical Experiences (COPE). A sample size of six caregivers and their relatives with dementia took part in a 10-week activity group. The first part of a two-part program was to empower caregivers in managing daily care issues and enhance coping. The program was designed using a participative model of problem-solving. The second part was an occupation-based group involving caregivers and care recipients. This was "specifically tailored to the needs of each pair in order to improve communication and reestablish involvement in daily activities" (p. 598). The outcomes included less disruptive behaviors of care recipients as reported by caregivers, as well as an increase in activity levels of both caregivers and care recipients.

Caregiving and End-of-Life Care (ELC)

As hospice and palliative care ideology, including the hospice philosophy of the family as the unit of care, becomes increasingly acknowledged to be the foundation for best practice in ELC (Doyle, Hanks, & Mac-Donald, 1998; Jones, Moga, & Davie, 1999; Koff,

1980), the need for continued research and practical application for practice is growing relative to caregivers' needs and challenges. It has been noted that most studies on caregiver needs and challenges seldom focus solely on the caregiver. Common caregiver needs identified in studies included physical care of the client, family counseling, and community resources (Harrington, Lackey, & Gates, 1996).

McGrath's (2001) research focused on caregivers' insights on the dying trajectory in hematology-oncology, a very high-tech practice. The participants were 10 caregivers, 9 of whom were women, caring for someone at the end of life and identified as the primary caregiver. The dominant themes that emerged from the caregiver interviews were caregiver demands, advocacy, the patient-caregiver dyad, informational issues, nurse communications, and doctor communication. Similarly, Harrington and colleagues (1996) emphasized the importance of good communication between health professionals and caregivers. Health messages about prevention and empowering the client or caregiver to participate can promote positive emotional, social, spiritual, and mental health in times of family crisis, such as chronic or life-threatening illness.

The caregivers in the McGrath (2001) study also reported high demands of self-care activities, transportation, and coping with emotional distress of the client, and they noted that they were developing stress-related illnesses secondary to caregiving. These and many other stressors caused many of the caregivers to experience posttraumatic stress (McGrath, 2001). Prevention of posttraumatic stress can be an important intervention for caregivers. Occupational therapy interventions focused on these stressors can assist caregivers in developing a balance in their lives that is needed in this time of crisis.

Stetz and Hanson (1992) examined perceptions of the demands of caregiving and found that caregivers of people at the end of life experience emotional distress, depression, anxiety, and a multitude of other psychoemotional issues. One daily occupation noted for caregivers became "constant vigilance" and "standing by" waiting for death to approach. This is a very unique occupation for this group of caregivers and one that practitioners should consider when developing intervention plans.

In this study, 50% of caregivers expressed regrets over not seeking out and utilizing more resources to aid in caregiving. The implications for occupational therapy practice include helping caregivers work through anticipatory grief, identifying and coping with lesser demands that may become important later (e.g., positioning), and addressing the issue of regrets. Providing permission to caregivers to "not be strong" may enable them to seek out and accept more help when the help is accessible and

available. These psychosocial rehabilitation interventions can help caregivers facilitate a "good death" (see Chapter 25 of this text for a description of this term) of their loved one and can help the caregiver cope with the loss.

Social support has been determined to be health promoting and helps restore a sense of wellbeing (Broadhead et al., 1983). Kirschling, Tilden, and Butterfield (1990) explored dimensions of social support in the experience of hospice family caregivers using the Cost and Reciprocity Index (CRI). This self-report assessment examined both the positive and negative aspects of social networks and yields scores for social support, reciprocity, cost, and conflict (Tilden, 1986). Three major implications for practice evolved from this work. First, hospice team members should explore the positive and negative aspects of social support available to the caregiver, relative to cost, reciprocity, and conflict. For example, before suggesting the caregiver's daughter come in to help, health professionals need to explore the emotional and financial cost and the potential aid or conflict that may result from the daughter being present. Second, the size of the social network does not necessarily equate with the quality of the social support provided. Third, hospice team members need to work within the social context of the support network and remember that it is this network that will be present for the caregiver long after the health professional has left.

While emotional support was characterized as a time-consuming and difficult occupational task for caregivers, the literature also revealed other life stressors and challenges. In a qualitative study of hospice caregiving families, Hull (1990) identified three general sources of stress: patient symptoms, interactions with others, and concerns for self. As patients began to demonstrate decreasing cognitive skills over time, the rudimentary communications with someone "they once knew" were difficult to sustain over time and became very stressful. Increased dependence for basic ADLs was also noted to be stressful as symptoms increased. In interactions with others, although people were "well-meaning," the need to interact became stressful. This was often complicated by having to maintain traditional family roles and having to engage in the new caregiver role, which became increasingly difficult as the care recipient deteriorated. The caregivers in this study identified five areas of concern:

- Putting one's life on hold
- Personal health
- Feelings of guilt
- Isolation from family and friends
- Lack of time for themselves

The theme of time was dominant in a study by Rose (1998), which identified the practical, emotional, and outside demanding tasks that can become burdens to caregivers of people at the end of life. She recognized the need for health professionals to help caregivers manage and plan time around daily activities that need attention and to help caregivers achieve some balance in their daily lives. Occupational therapists are skilled in helping people organize time and space to promote health. Balancing occupational obligations, needs, and wants—not just for loved ones but also for oneself as a caregiver—is crucial to healthy living. While time and place are important to understand relative to ELC, these are critical concepts for all occupational therapy practitioners to integrate when working with caregivers, no matter the diagnosis.

Bakas, Lewis, and Parsons (2001) described family caregiver perceptions of time spent and difficulty in certain caregiving tasks for people with lung cancer. Emotional support, finding transportation, and monitoring symptoms were the most time-consuming tasks reported for adult children and spouses, while the most difficult tasks were providing emotional support, behavioral management, monitoring symptoms, and household tasks. In a study by Carey, Oberst, McCubbin, and Hughes (1991), providing emotional support was also identified as one of the most draining stressors for caregivers. Yang and Kirschling (1992) reported that having to provide what was termed the "little extra tasks" (e.g., housekeeping and financial, legal, and health tasks) occurred more frequently than providing personal care to hospice patients. Thus, providing emotional support is one of the most draining stressors for caregivers, which is only compounded by the multiple other stressors experienced by caregivers of persons with terminal illnesses. Psychosocial and physical interventions, including conserving energy, managing time, adapting performance patterns (i.e., habits, roles, and routines), and using proper body mechanics, for example, can help decrease the stress of caregiving and promote a healthier context for care.

Occupational therapists and occupational therapy assistants can promote health and wellbeing for caregivers and improve occupational participation by recognizing caregivers' concerns. The next section of this chapter will discuss health promotion and wellbeing issues for caregivers, followed by assessment and interventions from an occupational therapy perspective.

Health Promotion and Wellbeing Issues for the Caregiver

If strategically implemented, the paradigm shift from the client being a person to the client being the entire family or caregiver can enhance the overall health and wellbeing and participation of the entire family system

and can support holistic interventions. Acton (2002) compared health-promoting self-care behaviors in family caregivers with caregivers matched demographically to investigate if these behaviors mediated the relationship between stress and wellbeing. **Health-promoting self-care** is defined as "those actions persons take to improve their health, maintain optimal functioning, and increase general wellbeing" (Acton, 2002, p. 73).

Acton's study was based on the variables of health developed by Pender (1996), which include perceived importance of health promotion, barriers to health promotion, self-efficacy for health promotion, health responsibility, physical activity, nutrition, spiritual growth, interpersonal relations, stress management, hours of sleep, and number of prescription medications taken. Pender's model is important for occupational therapists invested in evidence-based practice. The outcomes are focused on the likelihood of engaging in health-promoting, self-care behaviors rather than the experience of general health or wellbeing.

Family caregivers scored significantly lower on all variables mentioned above except in the areas of nutrition and number of medications. Engaging in health-promoting self-care activities significantly reduced the stress of caregiving and improved overall wellbeing (Acton, 2002). A study by Yates, Tennstedt, and Chang (1999) was comparable in that results "showed that the quality of caregiver-care received relationship mediated the relationship between caregiving stress and caregiver depression" (as cited in Acton, 2002, p. 83).

Hasselkuss, an occupational therapist, discussed themes of meaning crucial to understanding the caregiver experience (Hasselkuss, 1988, as cited by Rogers, 1996). These included "(1) sense of self . . . (2) sense of managing . . . (3) sense of future . . . (4) sense of fear or risk and (5) sense of changes in role and responsibilities" (p. 251). "The goals of caregiving were conceptualized as getting things done, and achieving a sense of health and wellbeing for the caregiver and the care recipient" (Hasselkuss, 1989, as cited in Rogers, 1996, p. 251).

Meyers and Gray (2001) drew many conclusions regarding hospice family caregivers and the relationship between care, QOL, and burden. Their findings indicated the following:

- A loved one's functional status is not correlated with caregiver QOL.
- "At-risk" caregivers are those who are still working, have been providing care for a long time and live in a rural locale.
- The longer the dying process is, the harder the experience is on caregivers. (Meyers & Gray, 2001, p. 79)

These findings indicate that caregiver burdens must be carefully assessed, and these factors need consideration. It should not be assumed that the caregiving role or associated activities are necessarily a burden or strain. Although this study is specific to hospice family caregivers, it is worthy of replication for nonhospice-related family caregiving relative to chronic illness.

Some studies have shown that caregivers may be at risk for poorer health outcomes than noncaregiving peers (Schulz, O'Brien, Bookwala, & Fleissner, 1995; Wright, Clipp, & George, 1993). Researchers have reported that the caregiving experience is affected by not only the patient's physical health but also the anxiety and mood of the patient and partner (Moen, Robinson, & Dempster-McCain, 1995), as well as the coping responses of the caregiver.

There has been some research on **self-efficacy** (defined as people's confidence in their capability to accomplish specific behaviors) related to caregiving. Several researchers have suggested that patients' self-efficacy mediates the relationship between family caregivers' stressors and outcomes (Solomon & Draine, 1995). More assistance needed by care recipients who have diminished self-efficacy increases caregiver burden. As patients' self-efficacy decreases, most family caregivers perceived burden increases due to the patient's perception that he or she is unable to perform self-care or other activities.

Lev (1997) cited the work of Bandura, who reported that perceptions of self-efficacy impact general performance of daily living tasks. Positive perceived self-efficacy can be thought to have beneficial health effects and mediate stress. According to self-efficacy theory, knowledge itself may not be associated with changing behavior, but a person's perception of his or her capabilities is an important characteristic to consider in predicting behavioral responses (Mowat & Laschinger, 1994). Bandura suggested that a sense of perceived control over life can buffer negative health effects of stress. Like perceived control, self-efficacy mediates the relationship between health-related stressors and outcomes (Mowat & Laschinger, 1994). Although a threat to health may be present, the threat is transformed to something more tangible with which one can more easily cope when a perception of being in control occurs. People with self-efficacy, confident in their ability to perform a specific behavior, are likely to perform the behavior; people without self-efficacy related to a specific behavior are not likely to perform the behavior.

In a study of family caregivers of cancer patients, Lev and Owen (2003) noted that caregivers who adapt poorly may be more vulnerable to psychological and physical distress and may be less capable of providing high-quality patient care. Therefore, "maximizing long-term mental and physical health outcomes for caregivers may prevent the negative health effects associated with caregiver experiences" (Lev & Owen, 2003, p. 10).

Their study integrated self-efficacy theory, QOL issues, and holistic health concerns of family caregivers. The results suggested that aspects of a patient's **self-care self-efficacy,** defined as an individual's confidence in using strategies to promote health, may mediate caregiver stress.

Scott (2000) noted a similar self-efficacy correlation in her study on caregiving among the technologically dependent, heart-failure population. She noted that caregiver mental health and self-esteem were identified as significant predictors of health-related quality of life (HRQOL). "This implies that caregivers' psychological wellbeing and confidence in their performance (self-efficacy) enhance perceptions of HRQOL and may even ameliorate the negative consequences associated with technological caregiving" (p. 92). Scott also identified both positive and negative reactions to caregiving. She revealed the positive as being the desire to provide care and fulfill the caregiver role, and the negative aspects included effects on daily schedules, health, and finances. It appears that health professionals need to constantly consider all aspects of social support and the caregiver role to assist caregivers in maintaining healthy lifestyles while defining oneself as a caregiver.

Tang and Chen (2002) implemented a home interview with 134 primary caregivers of people with stroke. The study was to "explore the relationship between and among the caregiver's personal factors, the care recipient's functional status, the caregiver's perceived self-efficacy, social support, reactions to caregiving, and health promotion behaviors" (Tang & Chen, 2002, p. 329). Findings showed that the healthier the caregiver, the stronger his or her self-efficacy for caregiving occupations. A higher level of caregiver strain existed when self-perceived caregiver health was compromised. A "caregiver's social support and the care recipient's functional status made significant contributions in explaining the caregiver's health promotion behaviors" (Tang & Chen, 2002, p. 329).

The results of these studies clearly illustrate the need for health professionals, particularly occupational therapists, to be as involved with caregiver health as client health. As a health team member, in conjunction with nursing and social work service providers, occupational therapists help promote caregiver health through some of the following (which is not an all-inclusive list):

- Improved self-efficacy through validating caregivers' abilities in the caregiving process
- Health education strategies to increase caregiver awareness of the need to care for their own physical, emotional, social, and spiritual health

- Development of a caregiver "schedule" that includes times for caregiver leisure and balance of work and play
- Finding out the meaningful and important caregiver occupations and helping caregivers to rediscover the joy of participating in them

A focus on families as a unit, no matter how those families are comprised, can help both the caregiver and the client understand health in the context of their intermeshed lives. Occupation and balance in life can be the best mediators of illness and promote healthier lifestyles for all concerned.

Evaluation and Assessment of Caregivers

Holistic, health, and occupation-based assessment of the caregiver will help determine caregiver burden. Some of the research cited above has indicated that there are both perceived burdens on caregivers and real threats to their health and wellbeing, especially during a long illness (Meyers & Gray, 2001). There are many caregiver burden assessments available that are both generic and specific to various diseases or illnesses. A list of nine such assessments has been identified by the Center to Improve Care of the Dying (2004) (available at http://www.gwu.edu/~cicd/toolkit/caregive.htm). Occupational therapists need to begin evaluating the health and wellbeing of the caregiver as well as the client.

Pizzi (1994) developed the Pizzi Social Environment Interview (PSEI) to assess caregiver levels of wellbeing and health as related to occupational participation. The assessment was based on the principle of treating the family as the unit of care. "It is an often stated health care assumption that when one cares for him/herself, one can better care for others" (Pizzi, 1994, p. 87). Original development of this interview is traced back to 1984; when working as a practitioner in a nursing and rehabilitation center, Pizzi became acutely aware of the caregiver burden placed on the daughter of a woman dying of cancer. The dying woman spoke about her concern for her daughter's health, as her daughter was neglecting her own family, work, and leisure. Pizzi developed an interview (Content Box 20-1) to assess the real and perceived caregiver issues related to occupational participation that supported or hindered the caregiver's health and wellbeing. The outcomes of that assessment resulted in both the client being relieved about her daughter's wellbeing (while she was dying, she was still engaged in her occupational role of mother) and the caregiver's improved occupational health, particularly in the areas

---

Content Box 20-1

Pizzi Social Environment Interview (PSEI)

Interview Questions

1. What was your daily routine like before the diagnosis of your family member? After the diagnosis, and currently?
2. How do you currently manage your own time? Do you feel productive?
3. Are you involved with any leisure activities, hobbies, or do things for fun?
4. Have you altered your activity level since diagnosis of your family member? How do you feel about this alteration? What would you change, if anything, regarding your own activity participation?
5. How has this current situation affected your work? Productivity level? Your relationships? Your daily responsibilities and their performance? Your communication with others in your life?
6. Do you feel competent in your caring for your loved one? In what areas, if any, do you feel you need assistance and/or support?

From *HIV infection and AIDS: A professional's guide to wellness, health and productive living* by M. Pizzi, 1994, Positive Images and Wellness, Inc.: Silver Spring, MD. (Copies of the manual can be obtained from the author.)
Author note: The PSEI was originally developed in 1984 with caregivers of people with life-threatening illness but not published until 1994, as noted by the reference.

---

of her self-management of time spent in occupations (apart from caregiving) that had personal meaning.

This assessment provides a quick overview of occupational areas that the caregiver may or may not perceive as challenges. The goal of the assessment is to increase awareness of potential or real changes in one's occupational participation and its relationship to time spent with caregiving. Following the assessment interventions are designed to help caregivers begin to establish balance in their lives. The PSEI has been subsequently used in a variety of settings, including with caregivers who were parents of children with disabilities, friends of people living with mental illness, spouses of people with dementia, and partners of men and women with AIDS.

The Caregiver Burden Scale (CBS) has two subscales—relationship and personal consequences (Montgomery, Gonyea, & Hooyman, 1985). It is scored on a five-point Likert scale and asks questions addressing social, recreational, occupational, and emotional factors. It is a phenomenological measure of how much time people perceive they have to engage in certain occupations and how burdened they may feel in their caregiving occupations. This sample was tested on informal caregivers of psychogeriatric clients. (The CBS can be downloaded at http://www.nysaaaa.org/Caregiver_Forum/Caregiver ForumErieHandout09.pdf; no permission is required to use the tool.)

Robinson (1983) reported on another tool that can be used by occupational therapists—the Caregiver Strain Index (CSI). A sample of 132 caregivers of recently hospitalized older adults receiving help was used as the basis of the CSI's development. It is a 13-item tool that identifies families who are stressed by and have problems coping with caregiving. Domains that items examine include employment, financial, physical, social, and time. The greatest level of strain is indicated by positive responses to seven or more items on the index. This instrument can be used to assess individuals of any age who have assumed the role of caregiver for an older adult. The CSI is a brief, easily administered tool that can identify families who may benefit from further assessment and intervention.

Caregivers require self-care and self-management of their lives but often are not aware of the need due to their involvement in caregiving. Occupational therapists and occupational therapy assistants may provide tips for self-assessment. This can lead to caregivers initiating discussion around the burden of caregiving, which can then lead to the initiation of more formal caregiver assessment. (Tips for caregivers can be downloaded at http://www.partnersincare.msu.edu/selfassessmentscontent.asp?ID=4.)

Interventions for Caregivers

Thus far, this chapter has addressed several challenges and difficulties caregivers face. Promoting health for caregivers and family systems has been explored. Interventions for caregivers are as crucial for their health and wellbeing as are interventions for the client. The following are intervention guidelines and strategies that can assist occupational therapists and occupational therapy assistants in helping caregivers achieve optimal wellbeing during the caregiving experience. Health-promotion activities can enhance health and wellbeing (Pender, 1996). Sufficient rest, proper nutrition, and appropriate exercise can better help remediate the stress caused by memory and behavior problems of care recipients.

Corcoran and Gitlin (2001) studied caregiver acceptance of recommended physical and social environmental adaptations to ease the burden of caregiving for people with dementia. They concluded that a high percentage of caregivers actually implement recommended interventions, and occupational therapists need to include caregivers and their occupational challenges in the occupational therapy plan.

Andershed and Ternestedt (1998) examined the concept of coherence developed by Antonovsky (1996) relative to the impact of meaningful relationships between caregivers and health professionals. One's sense of coherence "can be profoundly shaken by traumatic events and unresolved chronic problems. Such events and problems may assault the very foundation of one's entire action agenda and raise broad questions about one's life that threaten behavior controls" (Van Egeren, 2000, p. 457).

Antonovsky's concept of coherence helps explain how the client or caregivers will deal with difficulties confronting them. The three key components of this model include comprehensibility, manageability, and meaningfulness. Andershed and Ternestedt's participants were relatives of clients with serious, incurable cancer with an expected short period of survival. The authors suggested that the Antonovsky model is helpful in being a foundation to guide interventions. The more the caregivers comprehended, recognized, and used the resources available (manageability) and the more they developed a strong sense of coping with the situation, the stronger the sense of coherence overall. The Antonovsky model can also be applied by occupational therapists for all caregivers in order to optimize meaningful participation with the client while simultaneously caring for one's own health.

Pearlin, Mullan, Semple, and Skaff (1990) suggested that stressors caregivers perceive as problematic (e.g., indicators of patients' physical and psychological status) explain variation in caregiver stress. They report that patients' coping and social support were mediators of caregiver stress. These are two vital areas for assessment and intervention for the occupational therapist to consider in program planning, whether on an individual level or for community outreach groups whose members are caregivers, both past and present.

The literature on self-efficacy and caregiving supports occupational therapy interventions aimed at caregiver-centered care. Scott (2000) proposed two major interventions. First, fulfilling family obligations, especially when caregivers derive esteem from such, may serve to enhance wellbeing and self-esteem. The caregiver may feel there is a purpose to his or her existence in the time of a health crisis and experience a sense of productivity. Second, when purpose is discovered from the caregiving role, unknown strengths and abilities can emerge that promote deeper satisfaction with the role of caregiver and improve HRQOL. The end result is that caregivers can find the experience of caregiving more meaningful than burdensome.

Cohn and colleagues (2003) suggested that caregiving be assessed using a family-centered approach by being partners with the caregivers. They stated that the goal of assessment is "identifying family strengths, priorities and values as well as daily challenges associated with caregiving" (p. 549). They listed several areas of skills training (intervention) for parents of children with disabilities (Content Box 20-2).

Chen (1999) described the effectiveness of health promotion counseling for family caregivers provided by homecare nurses. Eighty-four family members of people with disabilities living in Taipei, China, were randomly assigned to two groups: the health promotion counseling group or the control group, who received no counseling but who were in traditional homecare. Findings of a preassessment and postassessment showed that persons in the health promotion group were more empowered to lead healthier lifestyles. Implications of this research for occupational therapy practitioners are to begin integrating more health promotion interventions in direct care services to both clients and their caregivers to promote healthy living, which can support occupational participation. Care must be taken to acknowledge the cultural differences in both the dissemination and receipt of information by caregivers in the United States.

Rando (1984) proposed that health professionals develop plans for intervention during the dying process, at the time of death, and after the death. This enables

family systems to adapt more easily during this crisis in their lives and promotes healthier relationships, communication, and connectedness. More than physical distress, caregivers often feel the emotional and psychological stress of caregiving. Rando (1984) provided suggestions for easing the suffering of caregivers and enhancing their sense of empowerment. Health-care professionals can

- legitimize caregivers' feelings of anger, sadness, and fear and acknowledge the intensity of these feelings;
- assist caregivers and family members to process their uncomfortable feelings in a positive way;
- enhance caregivers' ability to engage the person who is dying in meaningful activity;
- convey a calm, reassuring, empathic manner;
- facilitate improved coping capacity; and
- enable caregivers and family members to experience the joys and pleasures that are still available to them (Rando, 1984).

Rando's suggested interventions can also be adapted for any age or health issue that impairs caregiving occupations and the caregiver role. Although people at the end of life require some unique interventions, Rando's observations and suggestions apply to all caregivers.

Caregiver Respite

An often underutilized but important intervention is educating caregivers about the need for respite. **Respite** "refers to an opportunity for rest, cessation or reprieve from the ordinary duties of life" (Reinhard, Bemis, & Huhtala, 2005, p. 2). Often, caregivers sense an obligation to care for a loved one or experience a host of emotions connected to the need to enact the role of caregiver. Boundaries are often not set. "Not knowing or acknowledging these limits results in otherwise responsible people making poor choices or engaging in self-defeating behaviors" (Smalley, 1990, p. 7).

Respite can be experienced in a variety of ways for caregivers. Formal paid assistance for a few hours a week can help re-energize caregivers. Having a loved one cared for outside the home (e.g., day program, halfway house, nursing home, hospice) for a few days a week or a few hours per day can assist with diminishing caregiver burden and role strain. Depending on the needs and perceptions of caregivers, a schedule of daily occupations for the caregiver, developed by the occupational therapist or occupational therapy assistant, can be sufficient respite.

Inpatient, short-term hospital stays for people with Alzheimer's can be beneficial for caregivers; however,

---

Content Box 20-2

Interventions for Parents of Children With Disabilities

- Teaching parenting skills (e.g., home maintenance, time and money management, child behavior management, and advocacy for services).
- Teaching parents to support their child's development and to nurture their relationship with the child.
- Helping parents communicate with children about disability.
- Environmental adaptations may include the following:
  - Creating play spaces in the home that are accessible for family members with disabilities.
  - Helping parents access human and nonhuman resources.
  - Designing adapted baby-care equipment.
  - Designing environments to minimize fatigue.
- Support services may include the following:
  - Providing support groups for family caregivers or parents with disabilities.
  - Accessing naturally occurring resources (e.g., friends, neighbors, and community services).

From "Childrearing and care giving" by E. S. Cohn, A. D. Henry, & K. Marks, 2003, in E. B. Crepeau, E. S. Cohn, & B. A. B. Schell (Eds.), *Willard & Spackman's occupational therapy*, 10th ed. (pp. 549–50). Philadelphia: Lippincott, Williams & Wilkins. Copyright © 2003, by Lippincott, Williams & Wilkins. Reprinted with permission.

the risk of diminished capacity and occupational performance for the client secondary to a changed environment exists (Larkin & Hopcroft, 1993). Hospice laypersons (volunteers or paid help) can stay with the client, allowing caregivers to obtain sleep, which decreases the exhaustion factor and allows caregivers to maintain a level of healthfulness during the caregiving process (Bramwell, MacKenzie, Laschinger, & Cameron, 1995).

The role of caregiver and their respite needs are unique to each individual and family. Practitioners need to honor caregivers' choices. If the choice continues to be potentially unhealthy (e.g., caregiver loses too much weight or begins to smoke because of the stress of caregiving), innovative and adaptive strategies for them to discover the need for respite can be developed and suggested over time.

Support Groups for Caregivers

A **support group** is a group of people with a problem or concern in common who meet regularly to discuss their challenges and to support one another. There are support groups for nearly every medical diagnosis, and their importance should not be underappreciated. Hospice care always has formal and informal support groups for caregivers of people with terminal illness. For caregivers of people with dementia, Alzheimer's, and related illnesses, there are various person-to-person and online support groups available. The National Alliance for Mental Illness (NAMI) provides support for caregivers coping with mental illness in their lives.

The common thread that weaves support groups together is they all provide caregivers a sense of not being alone. This web of humanity is often a much-needed factor in the lives of caregivers. Occupational therapy practitioners can provide caregivers with resources to help them learn that life can be less difficult when challenges are shared, even with people one does not know.

Conclusion

Assisting caregivers who are coping with caregiving challenges, whether chronic or acute, can be of enormous benefit to enhancing the life and QOL of both the caregiver and the client. Promoting health in caregivers can be the single most important intervention to assist in promoting health within the care system, namely the family. Holistic evaluation and assessments that explore participation (or barriers to participation) in meaningful occupations important to the caregivers, and subsequent interventions that caregivers deem as important to their life situation, are essential in the

practice of occupational therapy. There is increasing evidence that caregiver burden affects both caregivers and the care recipient. Future occupational therapy research on caregiver health and wellbeing will provide payers, like insurance companies, the evidence that care for the caregiver is essential and that occupational therapists and occupational therapy assistants possess the skills and knowledge to promote caregiver health. Gitlin eloquently states, "Informal caregiving has serious consequences on the health and wellbeing of families. . . . This is a serious societal and public health concern for which occupational therapists can have an important impact" (Glomstad, 2004, p. 14).

The research and case studies presented in this chapter demonstrate that caregivers have many needs that often remain unmet for a variety of reasons, including lack of communication about those needs, lack of time provided by professionals, or lack of resources. Many times caregivers feel they "must be strong" or "no one can do as good a job as me." Thus, they do not communicate issues openly and directly to health professionals. Occupational therapists and occupational therapy assistants can assist families and paid and unpaid caregivers through understanding caregiver burden, recognizing the health needs of caregivers throughout the caregiving process, and helping caregivers prioritize needs of caregiving, which include the need to care for themselves.

No matter the diagnosis or the context of caring for another, occupational therapy has an important role in helping caregivers cope with the multitude of caregiving challenges. Caregiver health is as vital to the care recipient as any intervention provided by health professionals. It is the caregiver who is with the client most of the time, thus it is important that the caregiver's health status is acknowledged and integrated into the occupational therapy plan.

Case Studies

From pediatrics to end-of-life care, there are numerous issues with which caregivers must cope. Importantly, it is vital that each caregiver situation be seen as individually as one sees a client. Each caregiver brings different issues to the occupational therapy process, all of which impact intervention. Two case studies are presented to further illustrate the needs of caregivers and the potential contributions of occupational therapy interventions. The first case study concerns a caregiver and her husband as he faces the end of life; the second involves a young child following a motor vehicle crash.

Hospice and Terminal Illness

Bill is a 45-year-old man with terminal prostate cancer. His 40-year-old wife is named Mary. Assisting in Bill's care was a 4-hour-per-day home health aide and a private-duty 6-hour-per-day aide. During the occupational therapy evaluation, the therapist discovered that Mary was so involved in his care that the two aides felt as though they could do nothing right and were both ready to quit the case.

Bill expressed his concern for his wife's mental health, which depressed him further, as he recognized that his life-threatening illness was causing her great concern. In several occupational therapy sessions, the therapist, attempted to empower Mary to recognize the contributions of the two aides and their excellent care of Bill. The therapist shared the perspective of how the aides provided caregiver respite, which allowed her to engage in meaningful occupations of her own. Mary was given the PSEI to complete, which she refused to do, stating that she was managing just fine. One day, the occupational therapist had a "checking in" session with Mary alone, over coffee, in her backyard. This relaxed atmosphere (environmental influence) enabled Mary to discuss more openly what was most meaningful to her and how Bill's dying influenced her daily occupations and occupational engagement. It was discovered that she refused to leave his side for fear that he will die when she is out shopping, and she "supervised" every detail of his care because she needed to do everything "perfectly" in her own life or else she felt like a failure (the other outcome of this was her not-so-perfect treatment of the home health aides). This information was shared with the hospice team, who

became much more understanding of a woman about to lose the most important person in her life.

Mary and the occupational therapist, in conjunction with Bill, developed a plan that included her going out for short periods of time but with her cell phone always available so she could call occasionally (a limit was set on the number of calls per hour). A session was held with the aides to discuss how best to communicate the needs of everyone involved and to organize a routine for Bill so that his needs and those of all the caregivers were met. These interventions, while seeming to focus on the caregivers, directly impacted Bill and his mental, physical, spiritual, and social health. The outcomes of this case included a much more relaxed environment for all concerned, a more actively engaged Mary, and a less stressed Bill, who loved his wife and was happy to see her participating in important and meaningful occupations. As the end of his life neared, Bill whispered in my ear that he was most grateful for the care and concern expressed for his wife. It gave him great comfort to see that she could and would live on without him, which helped him ease more comfortably into a meaningful death.

Questions

1. What occupational interventions can help Mary stay in control of the situation? Why would an occupational therapy practitioner want to address that?
2. What are some psychosocial issues Mary is dealing with, and how would you evaluate and intervene other than ways already mentioned in the case?
3. What are some potential physical and spiritual interventions that could benefit both Mary and Bill?

Young Child With a Traumatic Injury

This case involves a 2-year-old named Maya and her mother and grandmother. Maya and her mom were driving one day, and their car was hit head-on. Mom was buckled up, but Maya was in an unbuckled car seat and went through the windshield at 60 miles per hour. They were going a half mile for some milk. While Mom was unharmed, Maya became a quadriplegic and was seen by me in homecare for many months after several months in a rehabilitation facility.

The family was very poor, uneducated, and had no health insurance, and Maya, Mom, and Grandmother lived

together in a one-bedroom apartment. Mom worked at night as a prostitute (her primary work role) to make ends meet and had a problem with substances prior to the crash. After the crash, she was admitted to drug rehab and was thus able to take Maya home as long as the grandmother lived with them as well.

Initially, visits with Maya included only her and the occupational therapist together, engaging in her favorite play occupations adapted to her physical needs. She was a joyful child whose smile would light up the sky and whose laughter was infectious. While her physical health was obviously compromised, the environment in which she lived and the people with whom she interacted were beginning to compromise her social and emotional health. Mom was rarely seen, and Grandmother spoke little English and mainly watched television. When Mom did appear, she was often tired, seemingly depressed, and rarely interactive. One day, when working with Maya, she was engaging with typical 2-year-old flair, not attending much to me or the activity we designed together. Mom came over to Maya, slapped her hand, and told her to "listen" Maya responded with a downtrodden look that led to a torrent of tears. The occupational therapist recognized that, in order to positively impact Maya, Mom's behavior needed to change.

In a discussion with Mom away from Maya, the therapist and Mom discussed how she thought she was doing with Maya's care and her love for her daughter. Mom burst into tears and said the occupational therapist was the only person who even cared to ask her. She felt the other health professionals judged her for who she was and didn't see her as a person who felt anything for her daughter. She discussed her guilt over the crash and how Maya was an unplanned birth but that she felt proud that she went through with the pregnancy. She felt Maya was something good that she did in the world, and after the crash, she felt like God punished her. She recognized that her life and lifestyle were unhealthy and very risky for herself and her family. She had little sleep and was trying to make ends meet. She did not see any other means to making life work for herself and her daughter, and she felt like a victim.

The therapist shared with Mom the positive interactions with Maya in order to prevent potential abuse and to help Mom recognize signs and symptoms of caregiver burden and distress that may lead to abuse. Mom did state there were times after the crash that she didn't think she could "take it" anymore and "came close . . . ." This health promotion intervention in and of itself was very important to help Mom begin to recognize characteristics within herself and their impact on her interactions. It provided a strategy that helped increase her awareness of healthier forms of communicating and being in the world and provided something over which she could take control to help prevent unhealthy behaviors. This educational strategy also strengthened the "victor" in her

and diminished a sense of victimization she had felt for most of her life.

The importance of her interacting regularly with Maya was stressed as the reciprocal relationship would be beneficial to both Mom and Maya, as Mom could learn healthy parenting skills while Maya benefited from positive interactions with her mother. The grandmother also started to participate in Maya's care and learned several therapeutic activities. Over time, Mom began to smile more appreciably and she began to understand human development better as Maya's "terrible twos" stage was discussed despite dealing with quadriplegia. The more knowledgeable she became, the more interactive and less fearful she became of hurting her daughter.

Over the several months of working together, both with and without Maya, Mom revealed that she quit smoking, began to take better care of her physical health, and began to consider getting her GED. Mom started to benefit from health promotion strategies designed collaboratively with the occupational therapist and began her development of redesigning her life on several levels. Some of this redesign she initiated, demonstrating an ongoing sense of developing resilience.

Tragically, Maya spiked a fever one night and died 3 days later. Mom was with her every last moment of Maya's life. At the funeral, Mom and Grandmother both hugged the occupational therapist, and Mom shared her memories of therapy time. As she squeezed one of Maya's favorite toys into the occupational therapist's hands for him to keep, she stated she was continuing to change her life and recognized that she needed more help and was seeking that help. The case of Maya highlights the impact occupational therapy can have on changing the life of the caregiver.

Questions

1. List at least three other health promotion and wellness interventions for Mom. How would you introduce them with? What is the rationale for each intervention?
2. Would Grandmother be considered another caregiver in this case? How might the occupational therapist intervene with her? What might the occupational therapist ask Grandmother?
3. How might the Stages of Change Model apply in this case?

▶ For Discussion and Review

1. What may be some challenges of caregiving for people with disabilities, an aging relative, a friend with HIV, and a spouse of a person with a mental illness? How could occupational therapy be helpful?

2. In end-of-life care, are there particular challenges for caregivers? What might those be, and how would occupational therapy benefit the family system?
3. What are some family-centered theories that can prove helpful when evaluating and intervening with family systems?

▶ Research Questions

1. What are the long-term impacts on health and occupational engagement for caregivers of children who lost a parent during the terrorist attacks on 9/11? What are the benefits of an occupation-based intervention for the caregiver and the children?

2. What occupation-based interventions are most effective in decreasing the burden and improving the quality of life of family members providing care for a loved one with dementia?

References

Acton, G. J. (2002). Health promoting self care in family caregivers. *Western Journal of Nursing Research, 24*(1), 73–86.

American Occupational Therapy Association. (2008). Occupational therapy practice framework: Domain and process (2d ed.). *American Journal of Occupational Therapy, 62,* 625–83.

American Occupational Therapy Association. (2007). *AOTA's societal statement on family caregivers. American Journal of Occupational Therapy, 61* (6), 710.

Andershed, B., &. Ternestedt, B. (1998). Involvement of relatives in the care of the dying in different care cultures: Involvement in the dark or in the light? *Cancer Nursing, 21*(2), 106–11.

Anderson, C., Linto, J., & Stewart-Wynne, E. G. (1995). A population-based assessment of the impact and burden of caregiving for long term stroke survivors. *Stroke, 26,* 843–49.

Aneshensel, C. S., Pearlin, L. I., Mullan, J. T., Zarit, S. H., & Whitlatch, C. J. (1995). *Profiles in caregiving: The unexpected career.* San Diego: Academic Press.

Antonovsky, A. (1996). The salutogenic model as a theory to guide health promotion. *Health Promotion International, 11,* 11–18.

Bakas, T., Lewis, R. R., & Parsons, J. E. (2001). Caregiver tasks among family caregivers of patients with lung cancer. *Oncology Nursing Forum, 28*(5), 847–54.

Becvar, D., & Becvar, R. (1993). *Family therapy: A system integration* (2d ed.). Boston: Allyn & Bacon.

Blakley, B., & Jaffe, J. (2000). Coping as a rural caregiver: The impact of health care reforms on rural women informal caregivers. *Centres of Excellence Research Bulletin, 1*(1), 1–4.

Bramwell, L., MacKenzie, J., Laschinger, H., & Cameron, N. (1995). Need for overnight respite for primary caregivers of hospice clients. *Cancer Nursing, 18*(5), 337–43.

Broadhead, W. E., Kaplan B. H., James, S. A., Wagner, E. H., Schoenback, V. L., Grimson, R., Heyden, S., Tibblin, G., & Gehlbach, S. H. (1983). The epidemiologic evidence for a relationship between social support and health. *American Journal of Epidemiology, 11*(7), 521–37.

Butin, D. N., Miller, P. A., Maultsby, P., & Winter, N. (1996). COPE (Caregiver Options for Practical Experiences): An activity group for caregivers with relatives with dementia. In K.O. Larson, R. G. Stevens-Ratchford, L. Pedretti, & J. L. Crabtree (Eds.), *ROTE: The role of occupational therapy with the elderly* (pp. 597–609). Bethesda, MD: American Occupational Therapy Association.

Carey, B. (2004, November 30). Too much stress may give genes gray hair. *New York Times.* Retrieved November 30, 2004, from http://www.nytimes.com/2004/11/30/health/30age.html.

Carey, P. J., Oberst, M. T., McCubbin, M. A., & Hughes, S. H. (1991). Appraisal and caregiving burden in family members caring for patients receiving chemotherapy. *Oncology Nursing Forum, 18,* 1341–48.

Carter, B., & McGoldrick, M. (1988). Overview: The changing family life-cycle. In B. Carter & M. McGoldrick (Eds.), *The changing family life cycle: A framework for family therapy.* New York: Gardner Press.

Center to Improve Care of the Dying. (2004). *Toolkit of instruments to measure end-of-life.* Retrieved December 3, 2004, from http://www.gwu.edu/~cicd/toolkit/caregive.htm.

Chan, C. W. H., & Chang, A. M. (1999). Stress associated with tasks for family caregivers of patients with cancer in Hong Kong. *Cancer Nursing, 22*(4), 260–65.

Chen, M. (1999). The effectiveness of health promotion counseling to family caregivers. *Public Health Nursing, 16*(2), 125–32.

Cohn, E. S., Henry, A. D., & Marks, K. (2003). Section IV: Childrearing and care giving. In E. B. Crepeau, E. S. Cohn, & B. A. B. Schell (Eds.), *Willard & Spackman's occupational therapy* (10th ed, pp. 546–54). Philadelphia: Lippincott, Williams & Wilkins.

Corcoran, M. (2001). Dementia. In B. Bonder (Ed.), *Functional performance in older adults* (2d ed., pp. 287–304). Philadelphia: F. A. Davis.

Corcoran, M., & Gitlin, L. (2001). Family caregiver acceptance and use of environmental strategies provided in an occupational therapy intervention. *Physical & Occupational Therapy in Geriatrics, 19*(1), 1–20.

Covinsky, K. E., Padgett, D. K., Schlesinger, H. J., Cohen, J., & Burns, B. J. (1994). The impact of serious illness on patients' families. SUPPORT Investigators. Study to Understand Prognoses and Preferences for Outcomes and Risks of Treatment. *JAMA, 272,* 1839–44.

Dennis, M., O'Rourke, S., Lewis, S., Sharpe, M., & Warlow, C. (1998). A quantitative study of the emotional outcome of people caring for stroke survivors. *Stroke, 29,* 1867–72.

Dooley, N. R., & Hinojosa, J. (2004). Improving quality of life for persons with Alzheimer's disease and their family caregivers: Brief occupational therapy intervention. *American Journal of Occupational Therapy, 58,* 561–69.

Doyle, D., Hanks, G., & MacDonald, N. (1998). *Oxford textbook for palliative medicine.* Oxford, UK: Oxford Medical.

Emanuel, E. J., Fairclough, D. L., Slutsman, J., Alpert, H., Baldwin, D., & Emanuel, L. L. (2000). Understanding economic and other burdens of terminal illness: The experience of patients and their caregivers. *Annals of Internal Medicine, 132*(6), 451–59.

Glass, T. A., Matchar, D. B., Belyea, M., & Feussner, J. (1993). Impact of social support on outcome in first stroke. *Stroke, 24,* 64–70.

Glasscock, F., & Hales, A. (1998). Bowen's family systems theory: A useful approach for a nurse administrator's practice. *Journal of Nursing Administration, 28*(6), 37–42.

Glomstad, J. (2004). A perfect fit. *Advance for Occupational Therapy Practitioners, 20*(24), 12–14.

Hall, J. E., & Kirschling, J. M. (1990). A conceptual framework for caring for families of hospice patients. *Hospice Journal: Family Based Palliative Care, 6*(2), 1–28.

Han, B., & Haley, W. E. (1999). Family caregiving for patients with stroke: Review and analysis. *Stroke, 30*(7), 1478–85.

Harrington, V., Lackey, N. R., & Gates, M. F. (1996). Needs of caregivers of clinic and hospice cancer patients. *Cancer Nursing, 19*(2), 118–25.

Hull, M. M. (1990). Sources of stress for hospice caregiving families. *Hospice Journal, 6*(2), 29–54.

Jones, A., Moga, D., & Davie, K. (1999). Transforming end-of-life care for the 21st century: The hospice vision. *Journal of Palliative Medicine, 2*(1), 9–14.

Kirschling, J. M., Tilden, V. P., & Butterfield, P. G. (1990). Social support: The experiences of hospice family caregivers. *Hospice Journal, 6*(2), 75–93.

Koff, T. H. (1980). *Hospice: A caring community.* Cambridge, MA: Winthrop.

Larkin, J. P., & Hopcroft, B. M. (1993). In-hospital respite as a moderator of caregiver stress. *Health and Social Work, 18*(2), 132–38.

Lefley, H. P. (1996). *Family caregiving in mental illness.* Thousand Oaks, CA: SAGE.

Lev, E. L. (1997). Bandura's theory of self-efficacy: Applications in oncology. *Scholarly Inquiry for Nursing Practice: An International Journal, 11,* 21–36.

Lev, E. L., & Owen, S. V. (2003). Association of cancer patients' quality of life, symptoms, moods and self-care self-efficacy with family caregivers' depression, reaction and health. *International Orem Society Newsletter, 10*(2), 3–12.

McGrath, P. (2001). Caregivers' insights on the dying trajectory in hematology oncology. *Cancer Nursing, 24*(5), 413–21.

Mental Illness Fellowship of Australia. (2005). *Feeling the impact of mental illness: The emotional journey.* Retrieved March 23, 2006, from http://www.schizophrenia.org.au/pdfs/Feeling the Imapact of MI.pdf.

Meyers, J. L., & Gray, L. N (2001). The relationships between family primary caregiver characteristics and satisfaction with hospice care, quality of life and burden. *Oncology Nursing Forum, 28*(1), 73–82.

Moen, P., Robinson, J., & Dempster-McCain, D. (1995). Caregiving and women's wellbeing: A life course approach. *Journal of Health and Social Behavior, 36,* 259–73.

Montgomery, R. J. V., Gonyea, J. G., & Hooyman, N. R. (1985). Caregiving and the experience of subjective and objective burden. *Family Relations, 34,* 19–26.

Mowat, J., & Laschinger, H. K. (1994). Self-efficacy in caregivers of cognitively impaired elderly people: A concept analysis. *Journal of Advanced Nursing, 19,* 1105–13.

National Alliance for Caregiving & American Association for Retired Persons. (2004). *Caregiving in the U.S.* Retrieved January 30, 2005, from http://www.caregiving.org/04finalreport.pdf.

Navaie-Waliser, M., Spriggs, A., & Feldman, P. H. (2002). Informal caregiving: Differential experiences by gender. *Medical Care, 40*(12), 1249–59.

Pearlin, L. I., Mullan, J. T., Semple, S. J., & Skaff, M. M. (1990). Caregiving and the stress process: An overview of concepts and their measures. *Gerontologist, 30,* 583–91.

Pender, N. J. (1996). *Health promotion in nursing practice.* Stamford, CT: Appleton & Lange.

Pizzi, M. (1994). *HIV infection and AIDS: A professional's guide to wellness health and productive living.* Silver Spring, MD: Positive Images and Wellness. (Copies of the manual can be obtained from the author.)

Rando, T. A. (1984). *Grief, dying and death: Clinical interventions for caregivers.* Champaign, IL: Research Press.

Reinhard, S. C., Bemis, A., & Huhtala, N. (2005). *Defining respite care.* Retrieved October 30, 2005, from http://www.cshp.rutgers.edu/TACCMSconfPapers/ReinhardRespite.pdf.

Robinson, B. C. (1983). Validation of a caregiver strain index. *Journal of Gerontology, 38,* 344–48.

Rogers, J. C. (1996). Section 5: Ability and disability: The performance areas. In K. O. Larson, R. G. Stevens-Ratchford, L. Pedretti, & J. L. Crabtree (Eds.), *ROTE: The role of occupational therapy with the elderly* (pp. 230–62). Bethesda, MD: American Occupational Therapy Association.

Rose, K. E. (1998). Perceptions related to time in a qualitative study of informal caregivers of terminally ill cancer patients. *Journal of Clinical Nursing, 7*(4), 343–51.

Rudnick, A. (2004). Burden of caregivers of mentally ill individuals in Israel: A family participatory study. *International Journal of Psychosocial Rehabilitation, 9*(1), 147–52.

Schulz, R., Mendelsohn, A., Haley, W. E., Mahoney, D., Allen, R. S., Zhang, S., et al. (2003). End-of-life care and the effects of bereavement on family caregivers of persons with dementia. *New England Journal of Medicine, 349*(20), 1936–42.

Schulz, R., O'Brien, A. T., Bookwala, J., & Fleissner, K. (1995). Psychiatric and physical morbidity effects of Alzheimer's disease caregiving: Prevalence, correlates and causes. *Gerontologist, 35,* 771–91.

Scorgie, K., & Sobsey, D. (2000). Transformational outcomes associated with parenting children who have disabilities. *Mental Retardation, 38,* 195–206.

Scott, L. D. (2000). Caregiving and care receiving among a technologically dependent heart failure population. *Advances in Nursing Science, 23*(2), 82–97.

Shernoff, M. (1997). Gay men with AIDS in rural America. *Journal of Gay and Lesbian Social Services, 7*(1), 73–86.

Siegel, K., Raveis, V. H., Houts, P., & Mor, V. (1991). Caregiver burden and unmet patient needs. *Cancer, 68,* 1131–40.

Smalley, S. (1990). Chronic illness and codependence: The caring role. *Occupational Therapy Practice, 2*(1), 1–8.

Solomon, P., & Draine, J. (1995). Subjective burden among family members of mentally ill adults: Relations to stress, coping and adaptation. *American Journal of Orthopsychiatry, 65,* 419–27.

Stetz, K. M., & Hanson, W. (1992). Alterations in perceptions of caregiving demands in advanced cancer during and after the experience. *Hospice Journal, 8*(3), 21–34.

Tang, Y., & Chen, S. (2002). Health promotion behaviors in Chinese family caregivers of patients with stroke. *Health Promotion International, 17*(4), 329–39.

Tilden, V. P. (1986). *CRI.* Portland, OR: Oregon Health Sciences Center.

U.S. Department of Health and Human Services. (2003). *Ensuring the health and wellness of our nation's family caregivers.* Retrieved December 5, 2005, from http://aspe.hhs.gov/daltcp/CaregiverEvent/overview.htm.

Van Egeren, L. (2000). Stress and coping and behavioral organization. *Psychosomatic Medicine, 62,* 451–60.

Wright, L. K., Clipp, E. C., & George, L. K. (1993). Health consequences of caregiver stress. *Medicine, Exercise, Nutrition and Health, 2,* 181–95.

Yang, C. T., & Kirschling, J. M. (1992). Exploration of factors related to direct care and outcomes of caregiving. *Cancer Nursing, 15,* 173–84.

Yates, M. E., Tennstedt, S., & Chang, B. (1999). Contributors to and mediators of psychological wellbeing for informal caregivers. *Journal of Gerontology: Psychological Sciences, 54B,* 12–22.

Chapter 21

Health Promotion for Families

Karen Goldrich Eskow and M. Beth Merryman

> After a few minutes, a woman from the hospital tells Liz and me it is time to say good night. I don't see how I can leave. That's my son, and he doesn't know anyone here. Standing in the empty hallway, I hear the cold, metallic clang of a bolt as the door is locked . . . it is the most forlorn sound I have ever heard. Liz and I walk separately, back toward the hospital entrance, not speaking. I'm crying, and I'm embarrassed. I don't look at her. Alex is alone on the other side of that locked door, without me, and I do not have the key.
>
> —Raeburn, 2004, p. 5

Learning Objectives

This chapter is designed to enable the reader to:

- Discuss issues and challenges that arise during each stage of the family life cycle.
- Describe how family functioning impacts family health.
- Apply family theories and models to specific family situations.

- Discuss the impact of disability on family life.
- Describe how mental illness and substance abuse impact family functioning.
- Discuss the roles of occupational therapists and occupational therapy assistants working with families across the life span.

Key Terms

Adaptability	Family cohesion	Family quality of life	Internal boundaries
Collaboration	Family dynamics	Family resilience	Morphogenesis
External boundaries	Family household	Family system	Morphostasis
Family	Family life cycle	Horizontal stressor	Vertical stressors

Introduction

The shift to a client-centered model of care has challenged health-care providers to examine the wants and needs of the recipient of services in the context of their recovery (Law & Mills, 1998). A family-centered approach has been adopted for populations such as children with developmental disabilities, where the primary recipient of care either lives with or is dependent on the family for care (Lawlor & Mattingly, 1998). Public policy supports individual rights of self-determination and community-based services over institutional care in the United States. This policy is made explicit in several of the *Healthy People 2010: Understanding and Improving Health* objectives (U.S. Department of Health and Human Services [USDHHS], 2000), particularly in Section 6, "Disability and Secondary Conditions," Objectives 6-4, 6-7, and 6-12. These objectives address increasing social participation among adults with disabilities, reducing the number of children and adults with disabilities living in congregate care homes or institutions, and reducing environmental barriers to activity participation in the community (USDHHS, 2000). The health-care community has recognized this change through the development of several policies that are shifting care to supporting individuals and families in environments of their choice.

This philosophical shift to family-centered care is supported by language in both international and professional documents. The World Health Organization's (WHO) *International Classification of Functioning, Disability and Health (ICF)* includes language related to identifying and removing environmental barriers to social participation rather than terminology that solely focuses on skill deficits (WHO, 2001). The American Occupational Therapy Association (AOTA) broadly defines environment and context within the *Occupational Therapy Practice*

Framework: Domain and Process (referred to as the *Framework*) (AOTA, 2008). The environment includes both "the external physical and social environments that surround the client and in which the client's daily life occupations occur" (AOTA, 2008, p. 645). Four interrelated elements comprise context: cultural, personal, temporal, and virtual (AOTA, 2008). These comprehensive definitions help alert occupational therapists and occupational therapy assistants to the variety of contextual factors that may either facilitate occupational performance of a family or that may act as barriers to full social participation

Family-Centered Care in Occupational Therapy

The AOTA *Framework* embraces a client-centered model of practice throughout the evaluation and intervention process and in the identification of desired outcomes. The evaluation consists of an occupational profile that first asks, "Who is the client (person, including family, caregivers, and significant others; populations; or organization)?" and leads to the question "Why is the client seeking services, and what are the client's current concerns relative to engaging in occupations and daily activities?" (AOTA, 2008, p. 650). With these questions, the occupational therapist is challenged to see the impact of intervention from the client's view and that of the broader family unit. The *Framework* language specifically identifies instrumental activities of daily living (IADLs) as possibly including the care of others. This category also includes many other activities for which satisfactory completion could depend on the interdependence of a family, further highlighting the importance of viewing the family as a cultural construct embedded in context. Therefore, occupational therapists and occupational therapy assistants must have a broader and deeper understanding of family structure and function, both in times of health and illness, in order to provide more effective interventions.

Several articles serve to highlight the demand for increased knowledge of family dynamics when working with families. These include articles about occupational therapists working with families in homeless shelters (Schultz-Krohn, 2004), families of children with autism (Werner DeGrace, 2004), and families of adults with mental illness (Abelenda & Helfrich, 2003). Hinojosa, Sproat, Mankhetwit, and Anderson (2002) examined parent-therapist partnerships in work with preschool children with developmental disabilities and found that working with parents in partnership contributed the greatest impact on a child's progress. The evidence demonstrates that engaging

families is critical to the health and wellbeing of all family members.

The family is a critical social network, yet many health-care professionals have ignored or blamed families for contributing to a member's illness (Johnson, 1987). The literature on families and members with health-care issues includes family burden, family dynamics, and family resilience. This chapter addresses general family knowledge, the dynamics of family life when a health issue arises, and collaboration between families and the health-care professional. In order to provide health promotion services for families, it is necessary to understand how families are defined and to understand the typical and stress-related dynamics of families.

Defining the Family

The definition of *family* has objective and subjective components. There is an observable structure to families as well as a process that is less obvious. It is a common misconception that individuals understand families simply because they have had experience in one. Understanding the family as a unit and families as a community in U.S. society involves a very complex process that addresses multiple contextual factors. Knowledge about family process is a basic prerequisite in promoting health for families.

The definition of *family* also varies by the context and circumstances in which it is defined; it is impacted by societal and political trends that are translated into laws and policies. An example is the debate about same-sex marriages. In 2004, the U.S. Supreme Court decided not to review the decision of the Massachusetts Supreme Judicial Court's ruling that gays and lesbians have the legal right to marry thereby constituting a family (Associated Press, 2004a, 2004b).

The definition of *family* is also unique to an individual and evolves and changes over time. For instance, admission to a hospital identifies the next of kin, the family member to notify in case of an emergency, and the person responsible for paying the bill. Any definition of *family* must incorporate relationship dimensions in addition to biological ties. The core values of the profession (AOTA, 1993) and the changing nature of families requires that the occupational therapist and occupational therapy assistant maintain an open mind regarding the various definitions of family in order to provide unbiased health promotion interventions.

Again, it is important to view the term **family** from multiple perspectives. In 1990, the U.S. Census Bureau (USCB) defined it as follows:

A family consists of a householder and one or more other persons living in the same household who are related to the householder by birth, marriage, or adoption. All persons in a household who are related to the householder are regarded as members of his or her family. A household can contain only one family for purposes of census tabulations. Not all households contain families since a household may comprise a group of unrelated persons or one person living alone. (USCB, 1990, Glossary)

In the 2000 Census, the term **family household** was used and defined as follows:

A "family household" consists of a householder and one or more people living together in the same household who are related to the householder by birth, marriage, or adoption—it may also include people unrelated to the householder. If the householder is married and living with his/her spouse, then the household is designated a "married-couple household." The remaining types of family households not maintained by a married couple are designated by the sex of the householder. (USCB, 2001, p. 2)

The evolution of the term *family* since the 1990 U.S. Census Bureau definition includes a shift in the definition of *family household*. This shift moves from a household unit that must be related by blood or legal ties to a definition of family household that includes people unrelated to the householder. This change is consistent with how individuals define their own families in today's society. Groups of people who consider themselves a family may have other characteristics than a blood or legal relationship. The definition of family is personal, and the recent U.S. Census Bureau definition allows for varied group compositions.

This general definition gives a basic understanding of what constitutes a family. However, obtaining a definition that reflects a perspective that is most relevant for client-centered care involves asking individuals to describe their family. How the individual family member defines his or her family is influenced by individual characteristics, perspectives of other family members, perspective of the family unit (i.e., nuclear and extended family), and other community and cultural considerations. It is important to remember that not all members will define the family in the same way. This adds to the complexity of understanding the family unit.

A family can be conceptualized as a system. A **family system** is a collection of family members with particular relationships who share a common history of successes, failures, and aspirations. In family systems theory, family processes are explained using three core constructs: organization, morphostasis, and morphogenesis. Family systems exhibit organization in the "consistent, repetitive and predictable patterns of inter-

action that underlie the rules and relationships within the family" (McKenry & Price, 2005, p. 407). Three constructs underlie family organization: wholeness, boundaries, and hierarchy. *Wholeness* refers to the fact that each family is unique, and the whole of the family is greater than and cannot be explained by the sum of the individual family members. The behavior of one family member affects all members because of their interdependence. *Boundaries* delineate who is in the family and who is not, and *hierarchy* describes the power differentials among family members and family subsystems (McKenry & Price, 2005).

Morphostasis is how the family system maintains itself in the face of change. A family monitors signs of change in the environment and modifies its behavior in order to maintain as much stability and constancy as possible in family structure, patterns, and roles. **Morphogenesis** provides the mechanism for family systems to change, grow, and adapt. There are two types of morphogenesis: first-order change and second-order change. First-order change is a temporary reaction to stress, while second-order change involves reorganization of family life and redefinition of family rules, roles, and boundaries (McKenry & Price, 2005).

Family Life Cycle

To understand the physical, developmental, psychological, and emotional health of the family unit, the health factors for the various individuals and those of the group must be examined. Family health cannot be viewed as a single moment in time. The "slice of life" approach offers too simplistic a view of a family's health (Carter & McGoldrick, 1999). Families, like individuals, develop in stages; therefore, the family life cycle must be considered to more fully understand family health. The **family life cycle** framework includes those "processes in the multigenerational system as it moves forward over time" (Carter & McGoldrick, 1999; Walsh, 2003, p. 8). This framework takes into account the complexity through which families evolve. The development of the individual units within a family (Table 21-1) is considered within the culture in which they exist and with sensitivity toward the many types of families in today's world. For example, 50% of married partners do not grow old together, so one must consider divorce, remarriage, and stepfamilies in the life cycle.

Dynamics of Family Life

Family process is complex and requires consideration of the needs of each individual, as well as the needs of the group as a whole. Family groups differ from other

Table 21–1 **Understanding Families at Different Stages of the Life Cycle**

Individual Life Stage	Family Factors to Consider
Infants	• Need to attach to a significant other • High dependency needs • Need for stable, safe, and nurturing environment • Parental role adjustment as infant's needs predominate
Children	• Beginning to be aware of self as separate from significant others • Beginning to develop relationships outside family • Parents begin the process of letting go and respecting the individuality of the child • Parents encourage self-initiative, independence but are available for children to come back to
Adolescence	• Develop interpersonal competency outside the family • Importance of peers, managing peer pressure • Begin transition from reliance on family for attachment to a combination of family and friends who meet emotional needs • Activities reflect physical, social, and emotional independence • Parents learn balance between letting go and providing structure and support
Young adulthood	• Individuates self from family of origin—identity • Family of origin in supportive versus prominent role
Later young adulthood	• Self-focus bridges into relationship with significant other • Builds nuclear family and integrates with family of origin
Early middle adulthood	• Depended upon by others • Contributes to family and community • Focus is on others rather than self • Blends intergenerational families • Time of productivity
Later middle adulthood	• Independent again! • Shift in family focus—children leave and focus is on couple-hood • Adult relationships with adult children • Family expansion to include in-laws and grandchildren • May care for parents and deal with their mortality
Early older adulthood	• Opportunity to review the past • Relationships with grandchildren and great-grandchildren • Potential to connect with children • Friendships emerge as important social connections

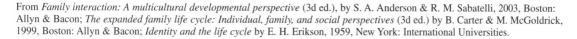

Table 21–1 Understanding Families at Different Stages of the Life Cycle—cont'd

Individual Life Stage	Family Factors to Consider
Later older adulthood	• Death of loved ones
	• Potential dependence
	• Family history dominates, rather than potential for family
	• Potential for unique view of life as a reflective process over the life span
	• Opportunity for younger generations to gain practical and familiar wisdom

From *Family interaction: A multicultural developmental perspective* (3d ed.), by S. A. Anderson & R. M. Sabatelli, 2003, Boston: Allyn & Bacon; *The expanded family life cycle: Individual, family, and social perspectives* (3d ed.) by B. Carter & M. McGoldrick, 1999, Boston: Allyn & Bacon; *Identity and the life cycle* by E. H. Erikson, 1959, New York: International Universities.

groups. In addition to the fact that a family group exists over time, it is important to realize that members may not be part of a family by choice. According to the biological definition of the family, relationships begin with birth and end with death. It is easier to terminate a legal family relationship, but it still involves far more than walking away from a social group to which one no longer wants to belong.

When attempting to understand how the family form influences its function, it is helpful to identify the roles of the various family members, how decisions are made, the rules of the family, the power balance, and how problems are solved. These dynamics are outlined in Content Box 21-1.

Family history, communication, stress, and other issues that are process-based, and thus not evident to most observers, further influence family dynamics. **Family dynamics** refers to the interactions and relationships among the people who are part of the family unit. Several models have been developed to explain family dynamics. This chapter addresses a few, including the Circumplex Model, the ABCX Crisis Model, a Competency-Based Family Resilience Model, and the Family FIRO Model.

Circumplex Model

Process in family relationships can be understood by exploring closeness and distance, flexible and rigid boundaries, and response to change. Balance across each of these areas is critical. For example, one needs enough of a boundary to provide structure but still allow for natural or crisis-determined growth. The combination and interaction among the dimensions of communication, family cohesion, and adaptability is shown as the Circumplex Model (Anderson & Sabatelli, 2003; Olson & Gorall, 2003). *Communication* serves as the conductor for flexibility and cohesion. As discussed by Anderson and Sabatelli (2003), families that can communicate

effectively are more likely to have appropriate balance along the other two dimensions. **Family cohesion** is defined as "the emotional bonding members have with one another and the degree of individual autonomy a person experiences in the family system" (Olson, Sprenkle, & Russell, 1979, p. 5). **Adaptability** is defined as "the ability of a marital/family system to change its power structure, role relationships and relationship rules in response to situational and developmental stress" (Olson & McCubbin, 1983, p. 62).

Understanding Families Under Stress

Stress is a significant factor that impacts family health. There are several models that discuss stress and the family. Carter and McGoldrick (1999) identify vertical and horizontal stresses inherent in all families across time (Fig. 21-1). The **vertical stressors** include family patterns, secrets, and legacies. The **horizontal stressors** include life cycle transitions that are normative and occur throughout the life cycle, as well as unexpected stressors. The unexpected stressors may include traumatic life experiences, such as untimely death, chronic illness, and accidents. These stressors impact all levels of the family system. The family deals with these stressors through involvement in multiple systems, which include individuals, nuclear and extended families, communities, work environments, friends, and broader societal systems (cultural, political, and economic).

ABCX Crisis Model

McCubbin and Patterson (1983) describe how families cope with stress. This model presents a useful template when trying to understand how different families cope with stress. It can be used to understand factors that may determine why coping with a particular stressor is more difficult for some families than others. McCubbin and Patterson (1983) describe the ABCX Crisis Model: "A (the stressor event)—interacting with B (the family's

Content Box 21-1

Dynamics of Family Life

Roles
- Understanding roles
  - Societal norms
  - Cultural norms
- Multiple family roles
  - Roles of significant others (i.e., spouse, parent)
  - Permanent or situation specific
  - Interaction (complementary = team, conflict = stress)
- Function of the role
  - Supportive
  - Productivity (manage activities—i.e. childcare, basic resources, etc.)
  - Support/productivity

Decision-Making
- Identify and articulate the decision to be made
  - Do both parties understand the decision to be made and want the same thing?
- Consider:
  - Communication styles and interaction patterns of decision-makers
  - The beliefs, values, and family-of-origin components an individual brings to a decision
  - The process used to make decisions
- Desired involvement of various parties
- Resources
  - Time
  - Information
- Various external factors that influence decisions
- History of decisions and the decision-making process

Rules
- Explicit rules
- Implicit rules
- Are rules the same for all family members?
- Cultural rules

- Religious-based rules
- Function of rules: provide structure and regulation for the family system

Power
- Status—control, influence
- Interaction based
- Situation based
- Cultural base
- Static and/or changing over time
- Internal sense of power
- External perception of power
- Authoritative vs. complementary

Problem-Solving
- Identify and articulate the problem to be solved.
  - Is there agreement that a problem exists, and is the problem defined the same by family members?
- Is there a desire to resolve the problem among family members?
- Brainstorm possible strategies to address the problem.
  - Identify the strengths and weaknesses of different strategies.
  - Identify a preferred strategy.
- Create an action plan based on the preferred strategy selected.
  - Break down the plan to include tasks, person (people) responsible for task completion, time frame anticipated for each task, and any anticipated challenges.
- Evaluate whether the strategy was effective in solving the problem. If problem persists, one must consider two things:
  - Accurate definition of the problem
  - Review of other problem-solving strategies

From *Family communication: Cohesion and change* (6th ed.), by K. M. Galvin, C. L. Bylund, & B. J. Brommel, 2004, Boston: Allyn & Bacon.

crisis meeting resources)—interacting with C (the definition the family makes of the event)—produce X (the crisis)" (p. 12).

The schematic that appears in Figure 21-2 illustrates the Double ABCX Crisis Model (McCubbin & Patterson, 1983). The precrisis aspect of the diagram reflects the ABCX model, and the postcrisis part of the diagram represents the double ABCX model discussed below.

Stressors can include a normative life event or an unexpected event. Family resources include factors related to internal family dynamics; external family supports and relationships; and material resources such as those related to money, food, transportation, and shelter. Each family defines a life situation differently. The combination of the stress, the family resources, and the way the family defines the situation determine if the event is a

crisis. A crisis exists when the family cannot resolve the issue and regain a sense of balance; the family system may then change (McCubbin & Patterson, 1983).

Double ABCX Model: Family Adaptation

To further understand the potential for health in a family unit, one may consider what McCubbin and Patterson identify as the Double ABCX Model: Family Adaptation (refer to Fig. 21-2). This model goes beyond the event-specific crisis to the ability of a family to integrate stressful events over time. The "Double A" aspect of this model refers to the pile of multiple stresses over time. McCubbin and Patterson (1983) identify five types of stressors that contribute to a "pileup": the initial stressor, normative transitions, prior strains, the consequences of family efforts to

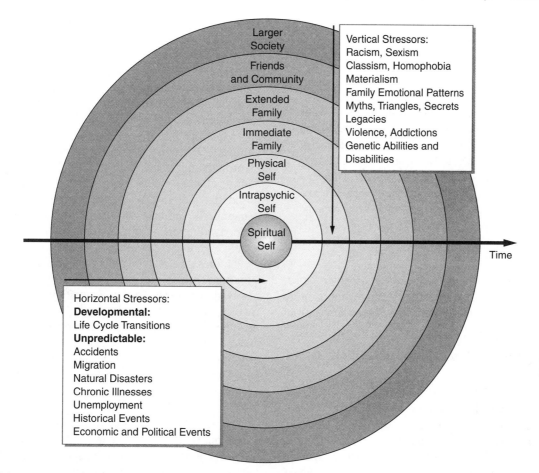

Figure 21-1 The context for assessing problems.

From "The family life cycle" by M. McGoldrick & B. Carter, 2003, in F. Walsh (Ed.), Normal family processes: Growing diversity and complexity *(3d ed., pp. 375–98). New York: Guilford Press.*

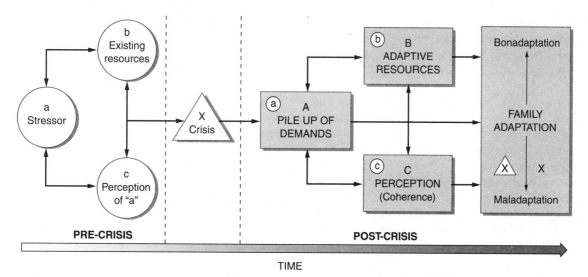

Figure 21-2 The Double ABCX Model.

From "The Double ABCX Model of Family Stress and Adaptation: An empirical test by analysis of structural equations with latent variables" by Y. Lavee, H. I. McCubbin, & J. M. Patterson, 1985, Journal of Marriage and Family 47(4), p. 812. Copyright © 1985 by National Council on Family Relations. Reproduced with permission from Blackwell Publishing Ltd.

cope, and ambiguity. The adaptive resources, or the "Double B" component of this model, involve the individual members, the family's internal supports, and social supports. Critical resources include flexibility, adaptability, and appropriate boundaries.

> Two types of family boundaries exist: external boundaries and internal boundaries. **External boundaries** delineate the family from other systems. They determine family membership by delineating who is in, and out, of the family. External boundaries also regulate the flow of information between the family and other social systems. **Internal boundaries** regulate the flow of information between and within family subsystems. In addition, they influence the degree of autonomy and individuality permitted within the family. (Anderson & Sabatelli, 2003, p. 13)

Boundaries that promote health are open to closeness but are not so close that they exclude others or are stifling. External support can be a huge asset and an important resource.

A Competency-Based Family Resilience Model

Abelenda and Helfrich (2003) describe a model of family resilience developed by Marsh and colleagues (1996) in which a competence paradigm is adopted. Competency-based models highlight the positive qualities of each family member and identify specific strengths that indicate capacity to make needed changes to support family adaptation. These models embrace the notion that families need information, coping skills to enable their support of the primary recipient of service, and support for themselves (Marsh, 1998). **Family resilience** is a multidimensional construct that examines several dimensions of family coping and adaptation (Marsh et al., 1996), including family burden, coping skills, adaptive capacity, among others. Five characteristics are suggested to enhance family resilience: highlighting positive qualities rather than fostering helplessness; engaging in collaborative decision-making; meeting the information, coping, and support needs of the family; acknowledging and addressing the needs of each family member; and encouraging and reinforcing the potential for family resilience. Resilience is a dynamic and contextual process, dependent in part on the fit between family strengths and resources with a particular challenge at a particular time (Abelenda & Helfrich, 2003). It is important to acknowledge that some situations may enable family resilience and others may not.

Family Fundamental Interpersonal Relations Orientation (FIRO) Model

Schaber (2002) describes the Family FIRO Model (Doherty, Colangelo, & Hovander, 1991) as a means to understand what drives an individual's behavior in family situations. A major premise is that people have three interpersonal needs (stages)—to belong (inclusion), to feel some degree of power (control), and to feel emotional closeness (intimacy). The model is sequential, in that inclusion precedes control, which precedes intimacy. In addition, the model is cyclical: Interactions occur where the unit has the most concern at the time. The value is in knowing both the sequential and cyclical features so that the current stage can be identified and issues relevant to that stage can be addressed and actively facilitated. Schaber (2002) proposed that applying this model to a family dealing with a member's serious, long-term illness would enable understanding of anxieties among family members and enable effective collaboration.

Families give meaning to single or ongoing stressful situations. Stresses may turn into crises or they may be resolved. The meaning that a situation has to the family ultimately influences the family's adjustment. Some people view difficult situations as challenges, and others define the smallest inconvenience as a crisis. A challenge represents an obstacle to overcome and can be interpreted as a call to action. On the other hand, a crisis can refer to something that exists and should be responded to rather than overcome.

The models described above are complex in presentation, understanding, and application. In addition, they are influenced by other factors, such as multiple stressors occurring simultaneously or in rapid succession (Burr, Klein, & Associates et al., 1994, as cited in Galvin, Bylund, & Brommel, 2004). In addition, the stages of family crisis can influence the stress response and adaptation. The stages of family crisis include "shock, recoil, anger, confusion, blaming, guilt and bargaining, depression and reorganization resulting in acceptance and recovery" (Galvin et al., 2004, p. 320). These stages can be used to understand another aspect that influences family health as individuals within the family and the family as a unit navigate typical and unexpected stresses. Health does not require one to be free of stressors but rather to be able to cope with stressors in a flexible manner. This involves being open to adaptation and being able to benefit from the emotional closeness and support of others.

Families and Community Life

The models discussed in the preceding sections recognize the family as a system related to the larger community. Family groups are further complicated by interaction with and being part of a community. For example, the community of a family with an infant is different than the community of two aging individuals residing in assisted living. See Content Box 21-2 for examples of five different family structures.

Content Box 21-2

Variety of Family Structures

Consider these questions as you read the descriptions of family structures below.

1. Who are the people who would be considered the nuclear family for this group?
2. Who are the people who would be considered part of the extended family of this group?
3. What types of relationships are possible between the nuclear and extended group?
4. How would one define the community that the family interacts with? Is it a school community? One based on social service? A neighborhood? One based on religious practices?
5. How do the layers of the family group interact with the social system? Are there financial needs? Are there educational needs? Are there health-care needs? Do these needs require that the family interact with the social system?
6. Brainstorm a list of potential stressors that may impact the family, resources that a family may utilize, and different ways the family could define their life situation.

Family Structure 1

Alison is a single mother. She has a 13-year-old daughter and a 2-year-old son. She has never been married but has had two long-term relationships with the father of each of her children. The fathers see the children two or three times a year. They provide financial support when they have the money. Alison lives in government-subsidized housing. She has very close relationships with several of the families in her building. Due to urban renewal, Alison's building is being torn down, and she has to find a new housing situation.

Family Structure 2

Leslie and Lee are recently married. They have both been previously married. Leslie's ex-husband lives 500 miles away. Their three children reside with Leslie and Lee for the academic year and spend summers with their father, his wife, and her two children from her first marriage. The children range in age from 3 to 17 years. Lee's former wife lives in the same neighborhood, and they have joint custody of the children. His children live with their mother for half the week and then with Lee and Leslie for the rest of the week. Leslie and Lee both work full-time and are saving money to add an addition onto their current home. The 17-year-old is investigating college possibilities. A good athlete with a history of learning disabilities and attention deficit disorder, he wants to attend a university across the country. Leslie and Lee are opposed to this idea.

Family Structure 3

Hal is 80 years old and lives in an assisted-living facility. His wife died 3 years ago. Hal is on a fixed income. His three daughters and their families (which include 11 grandchildren) live within 4 hours of his home. Hal's neighbor is worried about him, because he seems to be more easily fatigued and forgetful lately.

Family Structure 4

Stacy is 19 years old. She works full-time and goes to school part-time. She shares an apartment with her two best friends from high school. Her hometown is 100 miles away, where her parents, grandparents, and two younger brothers live. Her roommate has been binge eating and purging throughout the semester and has not attended classes for the past 2 weeks. Stacy observes her in bed when she leaves for work in the morning and when she returns from classes at 7:00 p.m.

Family Structure 5

Kate and Bill, both 29, married 2 years ago and are the parents of a newborn diagnosed with spina bifida. Both have graduate degrees in a health-care field. They just bought Kate's childhood home that is near the church she attended as a child. Kate's sister lives three blocks away, and her parents live within walking distance. The neighborhood is child-centered and retains many traditions from Kate's childhood.

Fully understanding a family and factors that influence health requires not only consideration of the immediate community, but also the society in which they live. For example, unemployment impacts family access to resources such as health insurance, and living in a geographic region that has few health-care providers may further negatively impact family health. Social systems permeate and influence all aspects of the family. The ultimate goal for a family is to live a productive life in a civil society and provide a structure for functional and civil societal relationships. Families are considered the building blocks of communities, and communities are the building blocks of society.

Society can and often does seem overwhelming and beyond the control of most individual and family units. In response to this feeling of being overwhelmed, people form subgroups of connectedness and intimacy that, ultimately, define the larger society. Subgroups can be based on a variety of social and political factors. The most personal subgroups involve those identified as family. The role of the family in promoting health ranges from instrumental support, such as transportation, to social and emotional support, such as listening as an aid to decision-making around a needed medical intervention or participation in preventive behaviors.

Impact of Physical Disability on the Health of a Family

Families impact the health of individuals, and the health of family members impacts the family as a whole. Defining *disability* varies with each family member. The child with cerebral palsy has a different impact on her brother than she does on her mother or father or grandparents. The person with a disability impacts the individuals in the family; the family unit; and subgroups within the family, such as parents or siblings. There are many factors that combine with a disability that may enhance or create barriers in an individual's or family's quality of life (QOL). The impact of disability on a family's health has been studied from various perspectives. The quality-of-life concept is widely used to evaluate the long-term impact of interventions or perception of daily life with a chronic illness (Liddle & McKenna, 2000; Mayers, 1995; Pain, Dunn, Anderson, Darrah, & Kratochvil, 1998; Park, Turnbull, & Turnbull, 2000; Parkin et al., 1997; University of Toronto, n.d.). Definitions that pertain to QOL have components such as emotional health, social relationships, physical health, and productivity. Additional characteristics may include spirituality, independence, privacy, and financial wellbeing. The WHO defines *quality of life* as

> an individual's perception of their position in life in the context of the culture and value systems in which they live and in relation to their goals, expectations, standards and concerns. It is a broad ranging concept affected in a complex way by the person's health, psychological state, personal beliefs, social relationships and their relationship to salient features of their environment. (WHO, 1997, p. 1)

The Beach Center on Disability (2004) discusses the concept of **family quality of life** (FQOL). The Beach Center website statement on FQOL indicates that families experience a high quality of life when

- family members' needs are met;
- family members enjoy their time together; and
- family members are able to do things that are important to them.

According to this definition, family quality of life involves issues of concern for the family as a unit and for the individual family members.

Understanding both the health of a family and the impact of disability on a family requires input from various family members. The information shared must then be understood from perspectives held by two or more of the individuals identified as family members. This is a complex process that if done comprehensively would take much time. To understand family health, it is critical to be aware of the number and complexity of these factors. Family health issues may change frequently. As individuals enter new stages of development, new issues may emerge. For example, families with children diagnosed with spina bifida were interviewed using the Beach Center's FQOL definition (Poston et al., 2003). Selected for the interview were three families belonging to three different age groups of children: early childhood, early adolescence, and late adolescence. The age ranges were chosen to capture various developmental stages of the families and the key issues that described their family's quality of life. Results of multiple case studies indicated that while some FQOL domains were similar for all families, others were identified for families with teenagers. Table 21-2 presents evidence of factors or domains that describe the perspectives of QOL for a small group of families in three different age groups.

Areas related to family interaction and to emotional and social wellbeing were identified by all families. As the children grew older, issues related to community-based interaction emerged. The oldest group discussed issues pertaining to the status of the adolescent who is preparing to leave the family unit and the protection of public education laws. These families talked about productivity, health, and relationships with professionals and the schools. This time of transition creates another lens through which to view health for a family with a child with a disability. The reality of a child creating an independent and meaningful life becomes more significant after puberty. For instance, consider the daily life of a family with a young boy who has physically matured. His mother, who has always assisted with his catheterization, is faced with a new dilemma. Issues of privacy and boundaries between a mother and a young man are different than between a mother and a boy (Moran, 2001).

Impact of Mental and Substance Abuse Disorders on the Health of a Family

Family occupations have been identified as being together, sharing, and affording learning opportunities (Segal, 1999). Each of these is affected when mental health or substance abuse issues are present. Mondimore (2002) discusses typical parent roles to include nurturing, protecting, and supervising children. He also identifies typical family roles such as supporting, understanding, and encouraging members. These roles

Table 21–2 **Identified Components That Contribute to Family Quality of Life for Families With Children With Spina Bifida**

Description of Families	Family Identified Quality of Life Domains Shared by All Three Families
Children Ages: 5–7 • Family members: Two parents and siblings in each household • Home: single family or town house • Schooling: public or home school	• Family interaction • Social wellbeing • Emotional wellbeing
Children Ages: 11–13 • Family members: biological parents, biological mother and stepfather, biological grandparents • Home: single family or town house • Schooling: public or private middle school	• Family interaction • Emotional wellbeing • Social wellbeing • Barriers • Community supports • Advocacy • Transitions
Adolescents Ages: 16–18 • Family members: single parents—mothers and siblings in each household • Home: apartment, duplex, town house • Schooling: public high school or entering college	• Family interaction • Parenting • Emotional wellbeing • Productivity • Health • Social wellbeing • Family/professional partnerships • School

From *Family quality for children with spina bifida: A family perspective* by L. Gore, L. Graves, T. Henry, & K. Goldrich Eskow, May 2002. Poster session presented at the American Occupational Therapy Association Annual Meeting, Miami, FL; *Family quality for children with spina bifida: A family perspective* by C. Englar, K. Graham, K. Krupinski, & K. Goldrich Eskow, May 2002. Poster session presented at the American Occupational Therapy Annual Meeting, Miami, FL; *Family quality for children with spina bifida: A family perspective* by S. Gore, J. Moran, T. O'Brien, & K. Goldrich Eskow, May 2002. Poster session presented at the American Occupational Therapy Annual Meeting, Miami, FL.

are magnified and challenged in families where a child has a mental disorder or substance abuse problem. Among the additional challenges to parents in this situation are observing subtle behavioral changes, analyzing information to decide actions, managing treatment schedules, administering medications, and negotiating the education and health-care systems (Schumacher, Stewart, Archbold, Dodd, & Dibble, 2000). In the case of a child or adolescent with a mental health or substance abuse problem, the parent experiences great stress supporting healthy development (educational, physical, social) while simultaneously advocating for the child's mental health needs. Parents often experience isolation and loss of social support

due to lack of understanding and social stigma related to childhood mental disorders. Mondimore (2002) clarifies the effects of childhood mental illness on parents by identifying ways that parents support the child's recovery. These include recognizing when actions are symptoms of the illness rather than assuming that the child has control of his or her behavior; getting involved in treatment while navigating how much involvement is appropriate; and monitoring the child's safety in terms of mood, use of substances, and risk of violence. Because parenting in this situation adds stress, it is also recommended that the parents and family members get the support they need to cope with the child's condition. This may include attending support groups, engaging in valued routine activities, and becoming educated with resources related to the illness.

Larson (2006) examined the extra challenges that mothers of children with autism experienced relative to developing and monitoring family routines. Of particular note were the child's preferences for routine but unpredictability in carrying them out and the mother's management of irregular household routines. Orsmond, Lin, and Seltzer (2007) examined maternal and family wellbeing in families in which more than one sibling had a disability. The most common disabilities were attention deficit disorder with hyperactivity and autism spectrum disorders. These families had higher levels of depressive and anxious symptoms and lower family cohesion. These studies have implications for occupational therapists providing family-centered care.

Olson (2006) developed a parent-adolescent activity group to provide a vehicle to address the challenging interactions between children with mental illness and their parents. Results of her qualitative study of the group effects revealed that the greatest benefit was that the group "opened a door to positive interaction" not present before. A study of mothers of sons with schizophrenia emphasized the value of addressing the ongoing emotional aspects of caregiving for a child with a chronic, unpredictable, and stigmatizing condition as well as the mothers' occupational needs. The use of occupational history interviewing with the mothers provided a means to understand and support them in the care of their sons (Chaffey & Fossey, 2004). A community capacity-building project was developed to assist the transition to adulthood of a population of youth with developmental disabilities. The involvement of the youth and parents using a participatory approach empowered both groups (Wynn, Sewart, Law, Burke-Gaffney, & Moning, 2006). These approaches have promise for occupational therapists interested in supporting community integration and family quality of life.

Influence of Health-Care Practitioners on the Family's Adaptation

A paradigm shift in health-care recognizes the family as the critical unit to focus on when providing care. This shift has required changes in the perspectives of various professionals toward their work with families. Perhaps most notable is the continued focus on family professional relationships as identified in the document *Achieving and Measuring Success: A National Agenda for Children with Special Health Care Needs* (Maternal and Child Health Bureau, 2005)—a 10-year action plan

to accompany *Healthy People 2010* (USDHHS, 2000). Legislation related to the passage of Public Law 99-457, which mandated that families become actively involved in developing education plans for their children with special needs, is also relevant. Under this law, schools have been required to work with families in developing plans for their children. The initial law has been updated several times, and implementation remains an area of concern. Recent literature in the professional journals of educators and related professions in the school system indicates that the goal of the law has not been fully realized (Brown, Humphrey, & Taylor 1997; DeChillo, 1993; Doherty, 1995; Dunst, Trivette, Starnes, Hamby, & Gordon, 1994; Gill, 1993; Lawlor & Mattingly, 1998; McWilliams, Snyder, Harbin, Porter, & Munn, 2000).

The growing population of individuals with chronic, progressive diseases such as Alzheimer's disease and the impact of care relative to family burden and social and financial costs has led to studies that address issues of quality of life (Baum, 1995; Corcoran & Gitlin, 2001; Dooley & Hinojosa, 2004; Rogers et al., 1999). It has been found that the QOL of caregivers of individuals with Alzheimer's disease is reflective of the QOL of those for whom they are providing care (Dunkin & Anderson-Hanley, 1998). A recent study found that maintaining everyday occupations was beneficial for both caregivers and care receivers with Alzheimer's disease (Hasselkus & Murray, 2007). A qualitative study of individuals with Parkinson's disease and their family members found that both experienced anxiety and stress related to alterations in daily routines and increased social isolation. Providing psychological support and generating strategies for daily life routines were viewed as beneficial (Wressle, Engstrand, & Granérus, 2007). Salmon (2006) used autoethnography to describe her caregiving process as she supported her mother who was awaiting nursing home placement. The coping and grieving processes of the caregiver are particularly emphasized. Typical caregiver involvement by occupational therapists includes family education and environmental modification to enable the highest level of independent function and quality of life. These studies have implications for occupational therapists working with families relative to collaboration and support of the family unit.

Ideally, family members and professionals work together as a team. The roles the various team members play and how they interact is further complicated by the fact that the team often includes multiple professionals who work separately with the family. Doherty (1995) introduced levels of training required for various types of family partnerships. This demarcation was reviewed and elaborated upon by Brown and colleagues (1997).

At the core of both articles is the discussion of the practitioner's role as she or he engages the family. Family and therapist roles are complex and can be understood along a developmental continuum. Content Box 21-3 presents two perspectives: one that focuses on professional training and the other that focuses on role of the family. The left-hand column outlines professional competencies and specialized training needed to work with families. The skills range from the ability to impart information and advice to the ability to use effective communication skills such as reflective listening and sincere empathy, both of which are needed to demonstrate competence in "Level III: Feelings and Support." The highest levels in this column require advanced professional training, as they include intervention skills to enhance family functioning. The right-hand column identifies how a therapist can choose to involve the family in service provision. This column focuses on the type of relationship a professional can develop with family members. Skills in family-professional collaboration are needed for effective family involvement (Blue-Banning, Summers, Frankland, Nelson, & Beegle, 2004). Each perspective must be adapted to the specific family and situation. Both perspectives are grounded in innate skills and common sense, and they require active engagement and specific skill sets. Taken together, the information supplies the reader with perspectives for therapist competencies and levels of family participation. Both are necessary as professionals explore the types of relationships they would like to have with the families with whom they work.

Family-professional relationships are important to clients and can impact health care. Often neither the occupational therapist nor the various family members come to treatment with preparation on how to utilize the professional relationship in the intervention process. In order for the therapist to engage a family as a co-client and understand the family in context, they must know the range of questions to ask. Occupational therapy practitioners must have training in the types of interventions that would be effective in a family system once they know a family's dynamics. Content Box 21-4 describes several situations to consider. Each situation reflects a health challenge and is followed with questions that professionals should consider in determining their role when developing a relationship with the family.

All participants in a relationship are responsible for their individual area of expertise. Therapists must be competent in their professional area of expertise. The family member is an expert in his or her role within the family unit. The family member knows strengths and weaknesses, daily family routines, family relationships, areas of support, and areas of need for each family member.

Content Box 21-3

Perspectives of Family-Professional Relationships

Focus on Professional Training	Focus on Role of the Family
Level I: Minimal Emphasis on Family	Level I: No Family Involvement
Level II: Information and Advice	Level II: Family as Informant
Level III: Feelings and Support	Level III: Family as Therapist's Assistant
Level IV: Brief Focused Intervention	Level IV: Family as Co-Client
Level V: Family Therapy	Level V: Family as Consultant
	Level VI: Family as Team Collaborator
	Level VII: Family as Director of Service

From "A model of the nature of family-therapist relationships: Implications for education" by S. Brown, R. Humphrey, & E. Taylor, 1997, *American Journal of Occupational Therapy, 51*(7), 597–603; "Boundaries between parent and family education and family therapy: The levels of family involvement model" by W. J. Doherty, 1995, *Family Relations, 44*, 353–58.

Content Box 21-4

Situations for Reflection

Situation 1

A parent is having a difficult time getting her child to use his adaptive device. Consider these questions: How much training does the therapist have in helping the parent adjust a parenting style? How much does the therapist know about how the family system functions? Does the therapist have the knowledge base to assess the family problems in such a way that he or she can introduce effective intervention? What training is required before a therapist can engage the parent as a consultant?

Situation 2

The adult daughter of an elderly client who is post-stroke continues to perform ADLs that the client is able to manage. The therapist would like the client to increase functional independence. Consider these questions: What knowledge base and practical skills does the therapist have to understand why the adult daughter continues to perform for her parent the activities he can do alone? What knowledge does the therapist have to help her understand the motivation or habits behind this family's behaviors?

The answer to many of these questions is that the therapist requires focused training to work with families at Level IV (see Content Box 21-3) for either situation.

Each participant is responsible for communication, which involves sharing thoughts and feelings (as appropriate) in a way that the receiver can understand. Listening is also a critical component of the communication process. An ongoing dialogue should involve speaking, listening, responding, and confirming perceptions with intentions. It is imperative that the listener hears the speaker's intended message. A knowledge base and evidence of good communication skills are essential for competence in Levels I and II (see Content Box 21-3). Often therapists and families/clients assume that they are better communicators than they really are. The process of listening, clearly and without bias, is critical to supporting the feelings of another person and when attempting to solve problems. One must be able to fully understand the complexity of a presented problem before any shared intervention can be discussed. Basic responsibilities include having a sound and grounded knowledge base and knowing and using effective communication skills.

In addition, a professional must be able to engage in introspective thinking. Self-awareness must precede effective use of self. An honest assessment of one's personal and professional values will help the practitioner develop effective partnerships with families. Eskow (2001) developed a vehicle for self-assessment that involved analyzing one's own family and the dynamics of those relationships. While it is true that developing relationships requires responsive interactions, the therapist is in the position to begin this process. The relationship between professional and client/family is not an equal one. The individual with a health-care need is seeking a service and is usually paying a fee for it, while the role of the health-care professional is to engage in and develop a relationship with a client that involves the client's family.

There are many levels of collaboration that can define a relationship. Mattingly and Lawlor (2003) define **collaboration** as a "series of complex interpretive acts in which the practitioner must understand the meanings of interventions, the meanings of illness or disability in a person and family's life, and the feelings that accompany these experiences" (p. 70). An important aspect of this relationship is to spend time understanding the type of relationship that the client wants and then identify the type of relationship you as a professional want to engage in. The relationship should unfold in a way that meets the goals of the individual, the family, and the professional.

To build a team, one must consider the participants who are actively involved in intervention sessions and those who are actively involved in the client's life but not present in the intervention session with the specific therapist. The other team members may include other professionals, a biological parent or stepparent, siblings, grandparents, neighbors, clergy, and friends. The grocery store clerk who wraps bundles in a specific way to ease an elderly customer's burden may be a critical member of the nonvisible team. There are many people who influence day-to-day functioning and help enhance or detract from the health of a family. An example of this is the contrast between the situations of Lisa and Mary, which follow.

Lisa, a 40-year-old woman whose mother and sister have been successfully treated for breast cancer, was tested and found to have a genetic malformation that puts her at high risk for breast cancer. She has friends who are very active in breast cancer research who helped her get involved in an MRI study to enhance early detection of breast cancer. She also decided to have her ovaries removed as further protection from breast cancer. Through her job at a major hospital and with the help of her friends, she built connections with physicians and related personnel. She was carefully monitored and developed a collaborative relationship with the radiologist who, when a biopsy came back "not quite right," advocated for additional testing. As a result, an aggressive form of breast cancer was detected earlier, and this action could very well have saved Lisa's life or eased the type of treatment required.

Mary is a 44-year-old woman who has been complaining of severe abdominal pain for over a year. She has limited financial resources. Mary saw a nurse practitioner for her gynecological care, but she needed further testing. After searching for a while, she found a sliding scale clinic at a local hospital. Several tests were performed that indicated the presence of abdominal growths. While the test results were available on January 6, she was told she had to wait until January 29 for the next appointment. Mary was in tremendous pain with few resources and felt she had no option but to wait.

In these examples, Lisa was able to build a health-care team through her supportive friends and better insurance coverage. Her relationships enhanced her health emotionally and physically. In addition to poor financial resources, Mary had few emotionally supportive relationships. Accessing care can be enhanced through family and friends who are often important resources to effect positive outcomes.

Conclusion

This chapter introduced the construct of the family as it relates to health promotion. In particular, the complexity of understanding family functioning under various conditions was described. Occupational therapists are interested in facilitating engagement in valued occupations and social participation in environments of choice (AOTA, 2008). Embracing a social model of understanding health promotion, illness, and disability requires knowledge beyond just engaging the individual but also supporting families and communities. In this chapter the authors described several parameters to understand families in context. These included a discussion of what constitutes a family from various perspectives, such as the U.S. Census Bureau and other sociopolitical views. In addition, the family life cycle was discussed from the perspective of several models, including the Circumplex Model (Anderson & Sabatelli, 2003), which addresses family function relative to three dimensions. Other models described families under stress and include the ABCX Crisis Model (Olson & McCubbin, 1983), the Competency-Based Family Resilience Model (Abelenda & Helfrich, 2003), and the Family FIRO Model (Doherty et al., 1991). Although each model is well developed, all share the notion that family education and support are key to successful adaptation to life crises.

The role of families in the larger community and factors that enable families to contribute to the livelihood of their communities were also discussed. The impact of broad social forces, such as the closing of a factory in a small community, was addressed as was the value of developing social subgroups within the community to promote health. The role of health-care providers in the adaptation process of a family dealing with a health crisis was reviewed. The life stages of each family member were also discussed in terms of impact. Using literature on family quality of life (FQOL) to frame the discussion, several case scenarios were used to examine the impact of disability on a family's health (Park et al., 2000; WHO, 1993).

A discussion of knowledge and skills necessary for occupational therapy practitioners to work effectively with families across the life span is provided through focused reflection questions, case studies, and self-awareness activities for the learner.

Case Studies

The situations presented below involve families configured at different points across the life span. To fully understand each situation requires awareness of factors associated with human development and family life across the life span. Reflective questions were generated to help the reader explore and appreciate the complexity of family health. Critical components include defining the family unit, describing the impact of the event on each family member and the unit as a whole, and examining the community context and the broader social forces that represent barriers and possible supports.

Reflective Questions for All Cases

1. What are the stressors that the family member or family unit is dealing with now?
2. What stressors have they dealt with in the past? How are stressors dealt with?
3. What are the important issues to an individual member and to the family group?
4. What are the habits of the family—what is a typical day like?
5. What are some of the challenges for the individual? For the family?
6. What are the communication patterns of the family group?

Case Study 21-1

Life Stage: Young Adulthood

In her late 20s, Stephanie was diagnosed with a malignant brain tumor. At the time of diagnosis, she was the mother of a 2-year-old and was 6 months pregnant with her second child. Surgery was performed successfully, and Stephanie completed her pregnancy and delivered a healthy baby. Five months later, the tumor returned. Stephanie needed surgery and now needs 8 weeks of daily radiation treatment. The radiation treatment occurs at a hospital 1 hour from her home. In this situation, health must be viewed from multiple perspectives.

Questions

1. Stephanie had assistance from her husband when she first came home, but he now must return to work to maintain financial stability in the home and thus cannot drive her to her radiation appointments. How much help can he realistically provide to Stephanie and the children?
2. Stephanie is on medical leave from her full-time job. How long will the company hold her job open?

Case Study 21-2

Life Stage: Late Middle Adulthood

Pam and Mark, a couple in their late 50s, moved to an upper-middle-class suburb. Pam recently was diagnosed and treated for encephalitis. She had been an active and well-known anesthesiologist prior to her illness. While Mark recognizes that his wife has limitations, he continues his practice as a physician and assumes that Pam can manage on her own during the daytime hours. As they are new to the community, there are few people who they know on a personal level.

The following events unfold over a 3-month time frame. The dog that Mark got to keep Pam company is often seen roaming the neighborhood on its own. The dog has chased and nipped the neighbor's young children. Often mail and service delivery personnel ring a neighbor's door, because Pam seems fearful of strangers and answering her door. One early morning, a neighbor hears faint cries for help. He goes into Pam's backyard to see if someone is in need of assistance and is greeted by an aggressively barking dog. Pam is in the deep end of the swimming pool unable to swim or get herself out. Fortunately, the neighbor is able to pull her out of the pool.

Questions

1. What factors must be considered to promote Pam's health within her current situation?
2. What options do she and Mark have to resolve these issues?

Case Study 21-3

Life Stage: Adulthood in a Single-Parent Household

Ben is a single father of two sons. One child is in elementary school, and the other is in middle school. The middle-school child is a talented musician but struggles with ADHD. He has a history of disorganization, disruptive behavior, and poor follow-through with homework.

Ben's wife, Donna, recently died from lung cancer at the age of 40 after a 2-year battle. Donna had never been a smoker, so the diagnosis was completely unexpected.

Questions

1. How can the family and school work together to help the middle-school child achieve a productive level of functioning?
2. How does the death of the mother change your perspective of this situation or the questions you would ask?

Case Study 21-4

Life Stage: Older Adulthood

Marlene and Tom are a retired couple in their late 70s. They live in an apartment in a town just outside a major city. Marlene has been diagnosed with arthritis in her spine. She also has a long list of other medical problems, including tuberculosis, high blood pressure, blood clots in the lungs, and depression. She takes 15 pills a day, and neither she nor Tom is certain what each pill is for. Tom suffered a heart attack 15 years ago and had quadruple bypass surgery 10 years ago. Tom continued to work through last year, when the company he worked for closed. His work role was a major source of motivation and gratification for him.

Marlene received two steroid injections to relieve arthritic back pain. She refused physical therapy, because she feared it would make her worse. Marlene and Tom have two grown children who live over 6 hours away and who have jobs and families of their own. The goal is to keep the couple as independent in their apartment as long as possible.

Questions

1. What criteria would you use to understand the meaning of health for this couple?
2. What additional information would be needed to more fully understand the situation?
3. What potential barriers to intervention might be encountered?

▶ For Discussion and Review

1. Identify someone you know at a particular stage of the family life cycle, and discuss issues and challenges that may arise.
2. Describe and discuss the impact of a serious health condition on family quality of life and occupational engagement:
   a. Physical health condition
   b. Mental health condition
   c. Developmental disability
3. Use the Family Resilience Model and FIRO to discuss the role of the occupational therapy provider in the following:
   a. Early childhood education of a boy with autism
   b. Transitioning-age (21) female with cerebral palsy leaving the education system
   c. Thirty-year-old returning war veteran with a traumatic brain injury
   d. Elderly couple both of whom are Holocaust survivors, where husband is the care provider and the wife requires standby to moderate assistance to complete activities of daily living

▶ Research Questions

1. How do perceptions of family quality of life change over time?
2. What perspectives of quality of life does each family member identify, and how does the perspective of one family member compare to the perspectives of other family members?
3. What is the relationship between perceived family quality of life and perceived health?
4. What components of family quality of life impact health of the individual with a medical condition or disability?
5. What aspects of family professional relationships are perceived as enhancing family quality of life?

References

Abelenda, J., & Helfrich, C. A. (2003). Family resilience and mental illness: The role of occupational therapy. *Occupational Therapy in Mental Health, 19*(1), 25–39.

American Occupational Therapy Association. (1993). Core values and attitudes of occupational therapy practice. *American Journal of Occupational Therapy, 47,* 1085–86.

American Occupational Therapy Association. (2008). Occupational therapy practice framework: Domain and process (2d ed.). *American Journal of Occupational Therapy, 62*(6), 625–83.

Anderson, S. A., & Sabatelli, R. M. (2003). *Family interaction: A multicultural developmental perspective* (3d ed.). Boston: Allyn & Bacon.

Associated Press. (2004a, November 30). Court rejects challenge to gay marriage. *Washington Post,* A03. Retrieved December 6, 2004, from http://www.washingtonpost.com/wp-dyn/articles/A19677-2004Nov29.html.

Associated Press. (2004b, November 29). High court won't review Mass. gay marriage law. *MSNBC News: U.S. News.* Retrieved December 6, 2004, from http://www.msnbc.msn.com/id/6607648/.

Baum, C. M. (1995). The contribution of occupation to function in persons with Alzheimer's disease. *Journal of Occupational Science: Australia, 2*(2), 59–67.

Beach Center on Disability. (2004). *Research: Family quality of life.* Retrieved March 2, 2004, from http://www.beachcenter.org.

Blue-Banning, M., Summers, J. A., Frankland, H. C., Nelson, L. L., & Beegle, G. (2004). Dimensions of family and professional partnerships: Constructive guidelines for collaboration. *Exceptional Children, 70*(2), 167–84.

Brown, S., Humphrey, R., & Taylor, E. (1997). A model of the nature of family-therapist relationships: Implications for education. *American Journal of Occupational Therapy, 51*(7), 597–603.

Burr, W. R., Klein, S., et al. (1994). Reexamining family stress. In K. M. Galvin & B. J. Brommel (Eds.), *Family communication: Cohesion and change* (4th ed., 1996). New York: HarperCollins College.

Carter, B., & McGoldrick, M. (1999). *The expanded family life cycle: Individual, family, and social perspectives* (3d ed.). Boston: Allyn & Bacon.

Chaffey, L., & Fossey, E. (2004). Caring and daily life: Occupational experiences of women living with sons diagnosed with schizophrenia. *Australian Occupational Therapy Journal, 51,* 199–207.

Corcoran, M. A., & Gitlin, L. N. (2001). Family caregiver acceptance and use of environmental strategies provided in an occupational therapy intervention. *Physical and Occupational Therapy in Geriatrics, 19*(1), 1–20.

DeChillo, N. (1993). Collaboration between social workers and families of patients with mental illness. *Families in Society: The Journal of Contemporary Human Services, 2,* 104–15.

Dixon, L., Adams, C., & Lucksted, A. (2000). Update on family psychoeducation for schizophrenia. *Schizophrenia Bulletin, 26,* 5–20.

Doherty, W. J. (1995). Boundaries between parent and family education and family therapy: The levels of family involvement model. *Family Relations, 44,* 353–58.

Doherty, W. J., Colangelo, N., & Hovander, D. (1991). Priority setting in family change and clinical practice: The family FIRO model. *Family Process, 30,* 227–40.

Dooley, N. R., & Hinojosa, J. (2004). Improving quality of life for persons with Alzheimer's disease and their family caregivers: Brief occupational therapy intervention. *American Journal of Occupational Therapy, 58,* 561–69.

Dunkin, J. J., & Anderson-Hanley, C. (1998). Dementia caregiver burden: A review of the literature and guidelines for assessment and intervention. *Neurology, 51*(Suppl 1), S53–S60.

Dunst, C. J., Trivette, C. M., Starnes, A. L., Hamby, D. W., & Gordon, N. J. (1994). *Building and evaluating family support initiatives: A national study of programs for persons with development disabilities.* Baltimore: Paul H. Brooks.

Englar, C., Graham K., Krupirski, K., & Goldrich Eskrow, K. (May 2002). *Family quality for children with spina bifida: A family perspective.* Poster session presented at the American Occupational Therapy Association Annual Meeting, Miami, FL.

Erikson, E. H. (1959). *Identity and the life cycle.* New York: International Universities.

Eskow, K. G. (2001). *Family self analysis.* Unpublished manuscript, Family Studies Department, Towson University, Towson, MD.

Galvin, K. M., Bylund, C. L., & Brommel, B. J. (2004). *Family communication: Cohesion and change* (6th ed.). Boston: Allyn & Bacon.

Gill, K. M. (1993). Health professionals' attitudes toward parent participation in hospitalized children's care. *Children's Health Care, 22,* 257–71.

Gore, L., Graves, L., Henry, T., & Goldrich Eskow, K. (May 2002) *Family quality for children with spina bifida: A family perspective.* Poster session presented at the American Occupational Therapy Association Annual Meeting, Miami, FL.

Gore, S., Moran, J., O'Brien, T., & Goldrich Eskow, K. (May 2002). *Family quality for Children with spian bifida: A family perspective.* Poster session presented at the American Occupational Therapy Association Annual Meeting, Miami, FL.

Hasselkus, B. R., & Murray, B. J. (2007). Everyday occupation, well-being, and identity: The experience of caregivers in families with dementia. *American Journal of Occupational Therapy, 61,* 9–20.

Hinojosa, J., Sproat, C. T., Mankhetwit, S., & Anderson, J. (2002). Shifts in parent-therapist partnerships: Twelve years of change. *American Journal of Occupational Therapy, 56*(5), 556–63.

Johnson, D. (1987). Professional-family collaboration. In A. Hatfield (Ed.), *Families of the mentally ill: Meeting the challenges* (pp. 73–80). San Francisco: Jossey-Bass.

Larson, E. (2006). Caregiving and autism: How does children's propensity for routinization influence participation in family activities? *OTJR: Occupation, Participation and Health, 26,* 69–79.

Lavee, Y., McCubbin, H. I., & Patterson, J. M. (2003). The Double ABCX Model of Family Stress and Adaptation. In P. Boxx (Ed.), *Family stress: Classic and contemporary readings* (pp. 123–41). Thousand Oaks, CA: Guilford. (Reprinted from *Journal of Marriage and the Family.* November 1985, pp. 811–25.)

Law, M., & Mills, L. (1998). Client-centered occupational therapy. In M. Law (Ed.), *Client-centered occupational therapy.* Thorofare, NJ: SLACK.

Lawlor, M. C., & Mattingly, C. F. (1998). The complexities embedded in family-centered care. *American Journal of Occupational Therapy, 52,* 259–67.

Liddle, J., & McKenna, K. (2000). Quality of life: An overview of issues for use in occupational therapy outcome measurement. *Australian Occupational Therapy Journal, 47,* 77–85.

Marsh, D. T. (1998). *Serious mental illness and the family.* New York: Wiley.

Marsh, D., Lefley, H., Evans-Rhodes, D., Ansell, V., Doerzenbacher, B., LaBarbera, L., & Paluzzi, J. (1996).

The family experience of mental illness: Evidence for resilience. *Psychiatric Rehabilitation Journal, 20,* 3–12.

Maternal and Child Health Bureau. (2005). *Achieving and measuring success: A national agenda for children with special health care needs.* Retrieved March 14, 2005, from http://www.mchb.hrsa.gov/programs/specialneeds/ measuresuccess.htm.

Mattingly, C. F., & Lawlor, M. C. (2003). Disability experience from a family perspective. In E. B. Crepeau, E. S. Cohn, & B. A. Boyt-Schell (Eds.), *Willard and Spackman's occupational therapy* (10th ed., pp. 69–79). Philadelphia: Lippincott, Williams & Wilkins.

Mayers, C. A. (1995). Defining and assessing quality of life. *British Journal of Occupational Therapy, 58*(4), 146–50.

McCubbin, H. I., & Patterson, J. M. (1983). Family transition: Adaptation to stress. In H. I. McCubbin & C. R. Figley (Eds.), *Coping with normative transitions* (vol. I, pp. 5–25). New York: Brunner/Mazel.

McGoldrick, M., & Carter, B. (2002). The family life cycle. In F. Walsh, *Normal family processes: Growing diversity and complexity* (3d ed., pp. 375–98). New York: Guilford Press.

McKenry, P. C., & Price, S. J. (2005). *Families and change* (3d ed.). Thousand Oaks, CA: Sage.

McWilliams, R. A., Snyder, P., Harbin, G. L., Porter, P., & Munn, D. (2000). Professionals' and families' perceptions of family-centered practice in infant-toddler services. *Early Education and Development, 11,* 519–38.

Mondimore, F. M. (2002). The role of the family. *Adolescent depression: A guide for parents* (pp. 238–48). Baltimore: Johns Hopkins University Press.

Moran, J. (2001). *Family quality of life: Perspectives from families of early adolescents with spina bifida.* Unpublished master's project, Towson University, Towson, MD.

Olson, D. H., & Gorall, D. M. (2003). Circumplex Model of marital and family systems. In F. Walsh (Ed.), *Normal family processes* (pp. 514–48). New York: Guildford Press.

Olson, D. H., & McCubbin, H. I. (1983). The Circumplex Model of marital and family systems VI: Application to family stress and crisis intervention. In H. I. McCubbin, A. E. Cauble, & J. M. Patterson (Eds.), *Family stress, coping, and social support* (p. 62). Springfield, IL: Charles C. Thomas.

Olson, D. H., Sprenkle, D. H., & Russell, C. S. (1979). Circumplex Model of marital and family systems I: Cohesion and adaptability dimensions, family types and clinical applications. *Family Process, 18,* 3–28.

Olson, L. (2006). What do we know about the daily interaction between children with mental illness and their parents? *Occupational Therapy in Mental Health, 22,* 11–22.

Orsmond, G. I., Lin, L., & Seltzer, M. M. (2007). Mothers of adolescents and adults with autism: Parenting multiple children with disabilities. *Intellectual Developing Disabilities, 45,* 257–70.

Pain, K., Dunn, M., Anderson, G., Darrah, J., & Kratochvil, M. (1998). Quality of life: What does it mean in rehabilitation? *Journal of Rehabilitation, 64,* 5–11.

Park, J., Turnbull, A. P., & Turnbull, H. R. (2000). Impacts of poverty on quality of life in families of children with disabilities. *Exceptional Children, 68*(2), 151–70.

Parkin, P. C., Kripalani, H. M., Rosenbaum, P. L., Fehlings, D. L., Van Nie, A., Willan, A. R., & King, D. (1997). Development of a health-related quality of life instrument for use in children with spina bifida. *Quality of Life Research, 6,* 123–32.

Poston, D., Turnbull, A., Park, J., Mannan, H., Marquis, J., & Wang, M. (2003). Family quality of life: A qualitative inquiry. *Mental Retardation, 41*(3), 313–28.

Raeburn, P. (2004). *Acquainted with the night: A parents' quest to understand depression and bipolar disorder in children.* New York: Broadway Books.

Rogers, J. C., Holm, M. B., Burgio, L. D., Ganieri, E., Hsu, C., Hardin, M. J., et al. (1999). Improving morning care routine of nursing home residents with dementia. *Journal of Advanced Nursing, 36,* 573–82.

Salmon, N. (2006). The waiting place: A caregiver's narrative. *Australian Occupational Therapy Journal, 53,* 181–87.

Schaber, P. L. (2002). FIRO Model: A framework for family-centered care. *Physical & Occupational Therapy in Geriatrics, 20*(3/4), 1–18.

Schultz-Krohn, W. (2004). The meaning of family routines in a homeless shelter. *American Journal of Occupational Therapy, 58*(5), 531–42.

Schumacher, K. L., Stewart, B. J., Archbold, P. G., Dodd, M. J., & Dibble, S. L. (2000). Family caregiving skill: Development of the concept. *Research in Nursing and Health, 23,* 191–203.

Segal, R. (1999). Doing for others: Occupations within families with children who have special needs. *Journal of Occupational Science, 6,* 53–60.

University of Toronto. (n.d.). *Quality of life.* Retrieved on March 2, 2004, from http://www.utoronto.ca/qol/concepts.htm.

U.S. Census Bureau. (1990). *Census of population: Summary tabulation file.* Retrieved March 2, 2004, from http://factfinder.census.gov.

U.S. Census Bureau. (2001, September). *Census 2000 brief—Households and families.* Retrieved February 2, 2004, from http://www.census.gov/prod/2001pubs/c2kbr01-8.pdf.

U.S. Department of Health and Human Services. (2000). *Healthy People 2010: Understanding and improving health* (2d ed.). Washington, DC: U.S. Government Printing Office.

Walsh, F. (Ed.). (2003). *Normal family processes: Growing diversity and complexity* (3d ed.). New York: Guilford Press.

Werner DeGrace, B. (2004). The everyday occupation of families with children with autism. *American Journal of Occupational Therapy, 58*(5), 543–50.

World Health Organization. (1993). Study protocol for the World Health Organization project to develop a quality of life assessment instrument (WHOQOL). *Quality of Life Research, 2,* 153–59.

World Health Organization. (1997). *Programme on Mental Health: WHOQOL Measuring Quality of Life* (WHO/MSA/MNH/PSF/97.4). Geneva, Switzerland: World Health Organization, Division of Mental Health and Prevention of Substance Abuse.

World Health Organization. (2001). *International classification of functioning, disability, and health.* Geneva, Switzerland: Author.

Wressle, E., Engstrand, C., & Granérus, A. (2007). Living with Parkinson's disease: Elderly patients' and relatives' perspectives on daily living. *Australian Occupational Therapy Journal, 54,* 131–39.

Wynn, K., Stewart, D., Law, M., Burke-Gaffney, J., & Moning, T. (2006). Creating connections: A community capacity-building project with parents and youth with disabilities in transition to adulthood. *Physical & Occupational Therapy in Pediatrics, 26,* 28–103.

Chapter 22

Health Promotion for Individuals and Families Who Are Homeless

Georgiana Herzberg and Theresa M. Petrenchik

> Give me your tired, your poor,
> Your huddled masses yearning to breathe free,
> The wretched refuse of your teeming shore.
> Send these, the homeless, tempest-tost to me,
> I lift my lamp beside the golden door!
>
> —Emma Lazarus (November 2, 1883; on the Statue of Liberty, New York City Harbor)

Learning Objectives

This chapter is designed to enable the reader to:

- Discuss the impact of poverty on health and occupation.
- Define and contextualize the problem of homelessness.
- Analyze environmental and personal factors that predispose persons to homelessness.
- Describe the roles of occupational therapists with the homeless population.
- Discuss the importance of building partnerships when providing services to homeless populations.
- Describe needs assessment strategies that can be used to measure the perceived needs of service recipients and service providers.
- Develop client-centered, occupation-based interventions for persons and families who are homeless.

Key Terms

Client-centered practice	Empowerment	Mainstream intervention resources	Proprietary consultant role
Community-based practice	Environmental press		Pro bono
	Homeless	Occupation-based practice	Service learning
Community-built practice			

Introduction

Homelessness is a nationwide problem. It is estimated that at least 2.3 million individuals experience homelessness at some time during an average year, and 6% to 8% of U.S. adults are likely to experience homelessness at some point in their lives (Burt, Aron, Lee, and Valente, 2001; Toro & Warren, 1999). On any given night in the United States, an estimated 842,000 people sleep homeless (or approximately 1% of the U.S. population over a 1-year period); of these, 39% are children (National Coalition for the Homeless, 2006a, 2006b; Urban Institute, 2000). Currently, between 900,000 and 1.4 million children are homeless each year, with more than half of these children being under 6 years of age (Burt, 2001b). Putting these figures into larger perspective, the estimated number of U.S. residents who experience homelessness in any given year currently exceeds the combined annual incidence of new and recurrent cases of coronary attack and stroke (U.S. Centers for Disease Control and Prevention [CDC], 2005a, 2005b).

The need for occupational therapy interventions with the homeless population and the agencies that provide services to them is great. Within the trap of poverty and homelessness, one finds virtually every imaginable human difficulty. Rates of disability, disease, substance abuse, mental illness, trauma and abuse, and serious head injury are disproportionately high in the homeless population when compared with the general population (Broward Coalition to End

Homelessness, Inc., 2002; Health Care for the Homeless (HCH), 2003; Petrenchik & Herzberg, 2002). In addition, the personal histories of women and children who are homeless overflow with accounts of abuse, trauma, housing insecurity, and social isolation.

Because occupational therapy practitioners grasp the health-related significance of participation and occupation, they can make a valuable contribution to the health and wellbeing of men, women, and children who are homeless. Occupational therapists and occupational therapy assistants understand the meaning and consequences of being without the security of a home. They are aware of the damage that stigma, discrimination, and stereotyping can do to a person's quality of life and general wellbeing. As health promoters and advocates, occupational therapists recognize the fundamental importance of social and community participation to a person's overall health and development.

In this chapter, the importance of client-centered, occupation-based interventions that help to provide persons who are homeless with greater resources and opportunities for social and community participation is discussed. The problem of homelessness is defined and contextualized, and environmental factors and personal vulnerabilities known to influence the occurrence of homelessness are reviewed. The remainder of the chapter elaborates on several of the many roles, program development processes, and intervention strategies used by occupational therapists working with this population. In the intervention section, programs to empower and build the personal skills and capacities of individuals and families in homeless shelters are described, and strategies for building the skills and capacities of agencies serving this population are discussed. Recent research and the community-based experiences of the authors are presented in order to provide insights that guide interventions that are occupation-based and client-centered.

Homelessness: Definition, Context, and Characteristics

The enactment of the Stewart B. McKinney Homeless Assistance Act in 1987, a predecessor of the current McKinney-Vento Act (P.L. 100-77), gave the nation the first federal definition of *homelessness*. In addition, the McKinney Act mandated 15 programs to provide a range of services to people who are homeless, including the Continuum of Care Programs: the Supportive Housing Program, the Shelter Plus Care Program, the Single Room Occupancy Program, and the Emergency Shelter Grant Program.

According to federal legislation, a person or family is **homeless** if they

- lack a fixed, regular, and adequate nighttime residence;
- share the housing of other persons due to loss of housing, economic hardship, or a similar reason;
- live in emergency or transitional shelters; or
- have a primary nighttime residence that is a public or private place not ordinarily used as a regular sleeping accommodation for human beings.

Families and individuals who meet the federal definition of homelessness qualify for services legislated under the McKinney-Vento Act (P.L. 100-77). A complete definition and related laws are available at http://www.hud.gov/offices/cpd/homeless/rulesandregs/laws/index.cfm.

In 1988, the Health Care for the Homeless (HCH) program was created under Title IV of the Stewart B. McKinney Homeless Assistance Act. HCH is a federally administered, competitive grant program for the provision of health care to homeless individuals. The goal of HCH is to improve the health status of individuals and families by improving access to primary health care, mental health services, and substance abuse treatment. These programs increase health-care access and decrease service fragmentation through a combination of outreach, case management, and linkages to services such as housing, benefits, and other critical supports. In 2004, HCH grantees served more than 600,000 men, women, and children who were homeless. In 2005, federal appropriations for HCH were $145 million, an all-time high (Bureau of Primary Health Care, 2006).

The McKinney-Vento Homeless Education Assistance Act defines children and youth who are homeless and ensures that they can attend school and preschool. This act gives them rights to enroll in school, stay in school, and get transportation to school, and it encourages success in school. In accordance with this legislation, local school districts are responsible for organizing services for homeless children and youth. Occupational therapy practitioners working within school systems may provide services to these children.

Poverty: The Defining Context of Homelessness

Although income poverty and homelessness are not synonymous, the two problems are interrelated. For most, the experience of becoming homeless is rooted in economic disadvantage. Poverty status dramatically increases the likelihood of experiencing at least one episode of homelessness (Burt, 2001a). Once a person becomes homeless, income poverty and the social problems that coalesce in an environment of poverty increase the probability of experiencing repeat episodes of homelessness, particularly among female-headed single-parent families (Burt, 2001a).

In a large national study of homelessness, income levels for surveyed single adults and families were well below the federal poverty line (Burt et al., 2001). The federal poverty measure was developed in the 1960s as a method for tracking poverty in America. It is a threshold used to distinguish those who are poor from those who are able to meet the basic necessities of life (Institute for Research on Poverty [IRP], 1998). Each year, the poverty line is adjusted for inflation. The 2006 poverty guidelines appear in Table 22-1.

Demographic Characteristics

Because the majority of people who are homeless are also poor, their demographic characteristics are most similar to those living in poverty and differ significantly from the overall population (Burt et al., 2001). Data from the 1996 National Survey of Homeless Assistance Providers and Clients (Burt, 2001a) show that homeless people are more likely to be African American than white or Hispanic. Historically, minorities are overrepresented in the homeless population (Burt, 1999). When compared with housed peers, people who are homeless are more likely to live in an urban central city and be middle aged and single. Educational attainment among the two groups is similar, with the majority of both groups having at least a high school degree or an equivalent.

Although regional differences in the composition of the homeless population are commonplace, single men comprise the largest proportion of the homeless population nationwide (Burt, 2001a). However, during the past 10 years, family homelessness has become increasingly more common, and nearly 43% of the homeless population is now comprised of families with children. While the numbers and characteristics of homeless persons vary by community and change over time (Fosburg & Dennis, 1999), the defining characteristics of people who are homeless are that they are poor, lack adequate housing, and lack sufficient income to meet their needs (NCH, 2006b).

Health Disparities and Barriers to Care

Homelessness is strongly associated with poor physical, mental, and behavioral health. People who are homeless experience health problems at more than twice the rate of persons in stable housing (Gelberg & Arangua, 2001). Forty-two percent report activity limitations, and 46% have chronic health conditions such as arthritis, diabetes, high blood pressure, or cancer (National Rehabilitation Hospital Center for Health & Disability Research, 2002; Urban Institute, 2000). The prevalence of communicable diseases, such as tuberculosis (32% to 43%) and HIV infection (6% to 9%), among those who are homeless is higher than in the housed population.

In terms of mental and behavioral health, one person in four or five who is homeless will have a diagnosable mental illness (Federal Task Force on Homelessness and Mental Illness, 1992). One person in every two (50%) will have a history of alcohol abuse or dependence, and one person in three (33%) will have a history of drug abuse or dependence (Rosencheck, Bassuk, & Salomo, 1999). As many as 7 out of 10 people in this population struggle with substance abuse or

Table 22–1   2006 Poverty Guidelines (by Income)

Persons in Family or Household	48 Contiguous States and D.C.	Alaska	Hawaii
1	$ 9,800	$12,250	$11,270
2	13,200	16,500	15,180
3	16,600	20,750	19,090
4	20,000	25,000	23,000
5	23,400	29,250	26,910
6	26,800	33,500	30,820
7	30,200	37,750	34,730
8	33,600	42,000	38,640
For each additional person, add	3,400	4,250	3,910

From *Federal Register Part V: Department of Health and Human Services: Annual update of the HHS poverty guidelines*, U.S. Department of Health and Human Services, 2006, Washington, DC: National Archives and Records Administration.

dependence (Toro et al., 1997), and one in five will struggle with both mental illness and substance abuse (Toro & Warren, 1999).

Although exposure to violence often precipitates and accompanies homelessness, the systematic study of head injury among the homeless population has received little attention in the literature. Two recent cross-sectional survey studies of homelessness found an unusually high incidence of head injury among adults surveyed. Self-reports of serious head injury were 24% in a large regional sample of adults in a southeastern metropolitan area (Broward Coalition to End Homelessness, 2002) and ranged between 33% and 45% in two probability samples of adults in two northern metropolitan areas (HCH, 2003). Comparatively, head injury occurs in approximately 1% of the general population (National Center for Injury Prevention and Control, 2007). When compared with their homeless peers, adults in the southeast who reported a head injury showed significantly higher rates of self-reported disability, drug and mental health problems, prolonged unemployment, and chronic and repeat episodes of homelessness (Petrenchik & Herzberg, 2002).

Women who are homeless experience poorer physical health than women in the general population, and more than 87% have a history of severe physical violence or sexual assault (Bassuk et al., 1996). Given this level of violence, the high rates of depression and posttraumatic stress disorder reported by homeless women are not surprising. Women who are homeless report poorer overall health and greater lung and stomach problems, anemia, arthritis, and physical limitations than their housed peers (Bassuk et al., 1996; Rog, McCombs-Thornton, Gilbert-Mongelli, Brito, & Holupka, 1995).

Children who are homeless share many of the same risks as children growing up in poverty, including increased risk for adverse health and developmental outcomes. Although controlled studies of the social, emotional, and cognitive development of children in homeless shelters are relatively few in number, studies indicate these children have disproportionately higher rates of developmental delay, learning disabilities, social and emotional problems, cognitive impairments, and behavioral problems than children in the general population (Fosburg & Dennis, 1999; United States Department of Health and Human Services [USDHHS], 1998). Infants in families who are homeless have higher rates of low birth weight and need special care more often than other children (Better Homes Fund, 1999; Shinn & Weitzman, 1996). Nearly one-third of these children lack essential immunizations (Better Homes Fund, 1999). As a result of poor living conditions, these children are at greater risk for chronic respiratory problems and lead poisoning. Children who are homeless often lack proper nutrition and go hungry twice as often as low-income housed children (National Center on Family Homelessness [NCFH], n.d.).

Studies of preschoolers, school-age children, and adolescents who are homeless indicate these children have delays in cognitive, social, and language development, with language delays most prominent (Rosencheck et al., 1999; USDHHS, 1998). These children are more often diagnosed with learning delays, need more special education services, and have repeated a grade more often than other children (Better Homes Fund, 1999; Masten, 1992; Rosencheck et al., 1999; USDHHS, 1998). Likewise, homeless children have more stress exposure and significantly more behavioral and emotional problems than children in the general population (Masten, 1992; Rosencheck et al., 1999; Weinreb, Goldberg, Bassuk, & Perloff, 1998).

Unfortunately, existing services do not match the needs reported by homeless individuals and families (Herman, Struening, & Barrow, 1994). People who are homeless experience barriers to mainstream services, including insensitive service providers (e.g., lack of respect, workers' negative attitudes); negative policies and procedures (e.g., age discrimination, dehumanizing rules and regulations); and problems with inaccessibility, inadequate services, and a generally discouraging social services system (Applewaite, 1997). This indicates the need to be client-centered when considering developing new programs and services for this population (Finlayson, Baker, Rodman, & Herzberg, 2002). People who are homeless need health promotion services and preventative health care, and their physical and mental disabilities may benefit from the skills and knowledge of occupational therapists (Heubner & Tryssenaar, 1996; Tryssenaar & Clarke, 1996; Tryssenaar, Jones, & Lee, 1999).

Person-Environment Factors Affecting the Occurrence of Homelessness

Over the past two decades, researchers have come to recognize that the risk factors for becoming homeless are a complex interaction of structural factors and personal vulnerabilities (Petrenchik, 2006). Structural factors are the social/environmental infrastructure in which people conduct their lives. As shown in Content Box 22-1, factors that comprise this infrastructure are the quantity, quality, and price of housing; prevalence of jobs across a range of education and training levels; health and diversity of the local economy; stability of that economy; and average pay compared with federal minimum wage. Few people would be homeless without the structural systems factors that set the stage for becoming homeless. Within the context of these social-environmental conditions, the vulnerabilities and characteristics of individuals affect

Content Box 22-1

Personal and Structural Factors Associated With the Occurrence of Homelessness

Personal Factors
Poverty in combination with

- limited education
- poor skills
- mental illness
- physical disability
- lack of social support
- alcohol or drug abuse
- domestic violence

Structural Factors
- Lack of affordable housing
- Fewer employment opportunities for people with a high school education or less
- Unlivable minimum wage
- Removal of institutional supports for people with severe mental illness
- Decline in public assistance

Adapted from "Homelessness in America: Perspectives, characterizations, and considerations for occupational therapy" by T. Petrenchik, 2006, *Occupational Therapy in Health Care, 20*(3/4), 9–30.

their ability to effectively manage their environment. When social conditions worsen, even those who are most able or least vulnerable become susceptible to crises that may precipitate a homeless episode (Burt et al., 2001).

Occupational Therapy Roles

Like U.S. society, the population of citizens who are homeless is composed of culturally and ethnically diverse groups of men, women, and children. Each of these groups—including veterans, the elderly, single adults (male and female), families, and youth—has unique needs and faces distinct challenges (Rosencheck et al., 1999). Recognizing this diversity, a report of the 1998 National Symposium on Homelessness Research (Fosburg & Dennis, 1999) recommends that each community collect its own data on the needs of its homeless population and use this information to develop interventions uniquely appropriate to their situation. Occupational therapists in these communities must tailor their roles and interventions accordingly.

The occupational therapist's roles in serving people who are homeless are also based upon how the client is defined. In working with the homeless population, clients are typically identified as

- individual direct service recipients,
- intervention groups, and
- service provider agencies and public/private organizations.

Individual direct service recipients and intervention groups may include families with and without children, single adults, veterans, runaway and homeless youth, persons with mental health or substance abuse problems, people whose resources have been depleted by medical costs, and persons who have lost their employment—and ultimately their homes—due to economic downturns or natural disasters. Systems-level clients may include private and public service agencies, their staff, their governing boards, multiagency service centers, or their boards of directors. An ecological, empowerment approach to practice informs and guides both levels of practice, direct service, and systems change. The core dimensions of this empowerment approach to person-environment practice appear in Table 22-2.

In the next section, occupational therapy roles are discussed from the perspectives of persons or families who are homeless and from that of a systems or secondary services provider.

Direct Services Roles

Characteristics of the identified population or population subgroup and the environment in which services are provided influence the occupational therapist's choice of direct service role(s). In addition, the organizational culture and mission of the service provider agency in which the occupational therapist works will influence role identification and implementation. The physical setting of the agency, staffing patterns, and available resources will also influence occupational therapist roles. As shown in Content Box 22-2, individualized direct services may be delivered in a variety of programs.

Within program settings, the special strengths and complex characteristics and needs of the direct services recipient must be identified, respected, and addressed. Some people who are homeless will require limited assistance, while others will require extensive, and possibly long-term, support. Each person's needs, skills, and abilities will change over time in response to the interventions provided and the occupational performance demands of the environments in which they must function.

Direct services roles of the occupational therapist are

- intervention specialist with a focus on occupational analysis, skill building, and environmental adaptation;
- life skills program group leader or coordinator;
- vocational evaluator;
- job developer or vocational coach;

Table 22–2 **Core Dimensions of an Ecological Empowerment Approach to Practice With Persons Who Are Homeless and the Agencies That Serve Them**

Core Dimensions	Characteristics
Participation	• *Client-therapist partnerships:* Collaborative, nonhierarchical roles; active client participation in goal identification, program planning, and service delivery
	• *Client-client partnerships:* Development of mutual and reciprocal alliances between and among clients and consumers
Education	• Education is a central feature of empowerment practice
	• An emphasis on client and family education, participatory action research, and capacity building
Critical Reflection	• Provide clients with opportunities for "reflection on action" in the context of occupational performance and participation
	• Occurs most powerfully through action in combination with dialogue with others
Transformation of Perspectives	• To act differently in the environment requires the belief that this is possible
	• *Key elements:* Self-efficacy, assertiveness, realistic appraisal of self and environment
	• Anchoring interventions in meaningful tasks and occupations gives clients ownership of the process
Competence-Building in Clients and Communities	• *Ecological competence:* Skills required for effective action in one's environment or life space
	• *Participatory competence:* Three interconnected dimensions of personal competence, critical understanding of the sociopolitical environment, and development of personal and collective resources for action
Social/Environmental Action	• Efforts at the local level must be linked with larger efforts to increase social equity and access

Adapted from *Person-environment practice: The social ecology of interpersonal helping* by S. P. Kemp, J. K. Whittaker, & E. M. Tracy, 1997, New York: Aldine de Gruyter.

Content Box 22-2

Program Settings for Direct Service Roles

• Emergency shelters
• Transitional housing
• Permanent housing
• Single residency occupancy units
• Food pantries
• Mobile food programs
• Soup kitchens/meal-distribution programs
• Physical health-care programs and clinics
• Mental health programs
• Alcohol and drug programs
• HIV/AIDS programs
• Outreach programs
• Drop-in centers
• Jails and detention centers

Adapted from *Helping America's homeless: Emergency shelter or affordable housing?* by M. Burt, L. Aron, E. Lee, & J. Valente, 2001, Washington, DC: Urban Institute Press. With permission.

• advocate; and
• case manager.

The emphasis of these roles is to foster occupational performance that enables meaningful participation in everyday occupations and in occupations that assist the client in community reintegration. Occupational therapists are skilled in providing direct services designed to capitalize on client strengths and minimize deficits.

Systems Roles

Occupational therapists may also choose roles that indirectly impact the person or family who is homeless. Roles that provide a secondary service impact and focus on systems change are advocate, program consultant, community educator, staff training facilitator, researcher, and community board member. These roles address the recommendations of the 1998 National Symposium on Homelessness Research (Fosburg & Dennis, 1999) for the collection of local data on needs and the development of interventions that are uniquely appropriate to the local situation.

Occupational therapists select and implement these roles to empower clients by acting on the local system(s) that administrate, guide, or fund direct services. In the public health literature, **empowerment** is defined as "a social action process by which individuals, communities, and organizations gain mastery over their lives in the context of changing their social and political environment to improve equity and quality of life" (Minkler, 1997, p. 7). It is important to recognize and implement roles that define the client at a macro level of intervention as does the public health sector. As McColl (1998) notes, "it seems essential that we prepare occupational therapy students to work with communities and with organizations of persons with disabilities and not simply with individuals" (p. 17). Baum and Law (1998) support her sentiments, stating, "Occupational therapy practitioners can contribute to those challenges [of the Healthy Communities Movement, sponsored by the World Health Organization (1990)] and help to change the environment and social policy in communities rather than changing the individual" (p. 8).

Occupational therapists are encouraged to seek out private and public service agencies serving people who are homeless. Clients in these system settings include administrators, staff, governing boards, oversight centers or groups, and educational institutions that collaborate in providing direct services. In these venues, assessing organizational culture, resource availability, and the agency's mission and philosophy helps the occupational therapist to understand what programming is likely to be implemented and sustained. Systems level assessment of the characteristics, service usage, and service needs of the local homeless population helps to ensure that proposed interventions have meaning and impact.

At the direct service level, assessment of environmental stresses experienced by people who are homeless, as well as their individual strengths and challenges, helps the occupational therapy professional to develop client-centered interventions. In contrast, needs assessments that include the perspectives of multiple stakeholders are the key to developing systems-valued interventions. Occupational therapy interventions that facilitate or implement such systems changes are discussed in the following section.

Partnership Building

Partnership building is a first step in establishing collaborations to promote the health and wellbeing of individuals and families who are homeless. Establishing open communication and a shared culture of client-centeredness among partners is essential for the survival and growth of such partnerships. Within this process, the occupational therapist considers client-identified service needs and preferences, the philosophical compatibility between the occupational therapist and the environmental press of the agency/organization, and the culture and context where services will be provided. **Environmental press** can be defined as the impact and demands of the combined social, emotional, cultural, and physical factors in the individual's perceived immediate environment. Each environment provides certain expectations for behavior and occupational performance, and this is referred to as *press* (Kielhofner, 1985). An understanding of an agency's mission, philosophy, and culture is essential to developing occupational therapy programs that meet the needs of both service recipients and agencies.

The choice of a community partner is an important one because an agency's culture and service delivery model establishes which types of occupational therapy interventions are most likely to be congruent with the agency's standard operating procedures. For example, it may be challenging for occupational therapists to develop a client-centered health education and advocacy program in an agency that typically delivers intensive behavior modification and rehabilitation services.

In working with underserved populations in community settings, occupational therapists use client-centered, process-oriented models of intervention. Current thinking and best practice approaches for community interventions recommend the use of this type of approach over that of an expert or a community-based model (Minkler, 1997). However, in practice, community interventions include a continuum of **community-based** to **community-built** models (see definitions in Content Box 22-3).

Community-built programs and community-based programs meet different community needs, serve different functions, and use different formats for interventions. Some community agencies demonstrate a clear preference for community-based programs, while others use a community-built approach. Both types of programs are needed to address the diverse needs of people who are homeless. Both types of programs appropriately offer occupational therapy interventions. However, in a community-practice paradigm, the client is the expert on his or her situation and makes the final decisions on services (Scaffa, 2001).

The client, or recipient of services, may be an individual, family, group, or agency/organization that is the primary stakeholder in the identified occupational therapy intervention. **Client-centered practice** refers to interventions negotiated between the occupational therapist

Definitions of Community-Based and Community-Built Practice

Community-Based Practice

Skilled services delivered by a health practitioner(s) using an interactive model with clients. This model emphasizes the strengths of a specific profession in eliminating or remediating the problems of the client. Typically this type of practice is medical system initiated, relies on referrals from other professionals, and is ongoing over time.

Community-Built Practice

Skilled services delivered by a health practitioner(s) using a collaborative and interactive model with clients. This model emphasizes the strengths of the client and is wellbeing oriented. Typically such a practice eliminates or resolves client issues by providing expert knowledge that is not otherwise available to the client, is issue based, and ends when the client-defined community has effectively built the capacity for empowerment.

From *Stedman's Medical Dictionary* (27th ed.). Philadelphia: Lippincott, Williams & Wilkins.

and the client that maximize the potential of the client for occupational performance now and in the future. Partnership agencies may or may not share the occupational therapist's beliefs about the value and necessity of client-centered practice. Therefore, establishing and maintaining open communication and a shared culture of client-centeredness among partners is essential to the long-term success of occupational therapy collaborations to promote the health and wellbeing of persons who are homeless.

Once partnerships are formed, working relationships with agency administrators and staff must be developed and maintained. In the initial phases of program development, when an occupational therapist is working to establish their intra-agency roles and services, communication and collaboration with agency staff is essential to promoting a client-centered context for service provision. For example, an agency partner required that all residents of the shelter obtain some form of paid employment within 8 days of acceptance into the shelter, regardless of skills or local economy considerations. This condition of work in exchange for housing at the shelter reflected staff beliefs that residents must demonstrate their commitment to helping themselves in breaking the cycle of homelessness. Those who did not earn wages within an 8-day period were evicted.

Another agency mandated that its residents work only in shelter-related jobs/tasks for a 3-month period while living at the shelter. One can argue that all work

provides useful learning experiences, both positive and negative, that can be used in building future job success. It can also be argued that people become unable to envision themselves moving beyond these experiences when they become dependent on minimum wage or sheltered job situations. The disadvantage to both of these well-intentioned but paternalistic and coercive approaches is that the strengths and job skills of the individual client are not necessarily maximized.

At one agency, occupational therapists facilitated the institution of team meetings; the development of policies regarding the participation of clients in team meetings; the education of staff about the value of client-centered service delivery; and the fashioning of graded programs of interventions to build on individual client strengths, skills, and needs. For example, one client who had extensive waitstaff experience but a poor record of work stability for more than 6 months indicated to a staff member other than his case manager that his dream job was to become a chef. An analysis of the job activity, client strengths, and occupational performance issues was conducted and the shelter's chef was convinced to collaborate on a graded internship plan to build the mandatory skills and work history for this client to become employed as a line chef.

The success of this collaboration served as an example of the value of client-centered, occupation-based interventions that could lead to career choices rather than meaningless, dead-end jobs. Staff and clients profited from this demonstration of the effectiveness of client-staff collaboration in setting and achieving goals that served both the purposes of the individual who was homeless and the agency attempting to break the cycle of homelessness.

Other examples of the importance of communication and compatible philosophy of intervention are the importance of spirituality or religious traditions in times of stress and the use of psychotropic medications among shelter residents. In times of personal challenge, clients often put additional emphasis on spirituality or religious traditions to help overcome adversity. Spirituality is an appropriate area of assessment and intervention for the occupational therapist (McColl, 2003). However, the occupational therapist must be aware of the mandated and cultural expectations within the service agency regarding spirituality and religion. In some faith-based agencies, client access to housing, clothing, food, and employment skills training requires participation in religious services. In one setting, agency staff assumed/expected that the occupational therapist would help to maintain this policy. Governmental agencies, on the other hand, may expressly forbid religion or spiritually oriented groups, even when shelter residents request and act to organize them.

In these instances, active negotiation for mutually acceptable compromises that respect the values of all stakeholders is warranted. Some programs are directed toward the development of routines and rituals that support people in their faith. However, discussions of spirituality and spiritual practices are always client-directed and nonsectarian. The occupational therapist's role as mediator between a shelter resident's personal beliefs on the one hand and agency expectations on the other can be rewarding and helpful.

Programs that provide services to homeless persons with substance abuse problems or mental illness are not uncommon. Twelve-step programs such as Alcoholics Anonymous or Narcotics Anonymous can be an effective but highly structured intervention for people with substance abuse problems. Twelve-step programming may be specifically offered as an intervention or may underlie interventions in some shelters. Some shelter programs interpret the 12-step prohibition on mind-altering drugs to also include prescribed psychotropic medications. People with mental illnesses utilize psychotropic drugs for symptom control and management. When not taking medications, they may have symptoms or cognitive deficits that interfere with their ability to accurately assess reality.

Research with people with mental disorders indicates that they are more apt to benefit from programs that support medication compliance and offer flexible and supportive approaches that shape behavior more gradually than classic behavior-modification approaches. Although well intentioned, the program policies that prohibit the on-site use of prescription medications for symptom control and management may be counterproductive and potentially harmful. In such instances, occupational therapists assume the role of educator, consultant, advocate, and possibly mediator, facilitating the use of evidence-based and best-practice approaches in community settings. These roles are especially important in community agencies, particularly those that are poorly funded, understaffed, and heavily reliant upon the services of volunteers.

Establishing and maintaining a client-centered intervention philosophy in community agencies can be challenging. While all communal living facilities have rules and policies, homeless shelters tend to be fairly restrictive environments. The rules governing shelter life serve two primary functions: (1) maintaining order and control within the shelter and (2) superimposing structure and organization onto the lives of residents (DeOllos, 1997). While rules and procedures are necessary for maintaining order and safety in shelters, gross power imbalances can aggravate the tension between staff and residents. Purposeful resistance to staff demands or inadvertent violations of facility rules can lead to the sanctioning of privileges and restricting a resident's social and community participation.

Staff responses to rule infractions may include spontaneous reactions to a perceived offense and can result in the immediate removal of privileges. Sometimes these decisions do not include an appeal process. To address this problem, one intervention was to establish an orientation group for residents to provide discussion of agency expectations and policies. Orientation handouts included simple strategies and suggestions to help new residents adjust to life in this specific shelter. The handouts were a useful educational tool because they could be reviewed when new residents were less stressed and better able to concentrate. Handouts helped to increase communication and cooperation among residents and to decrease the novelty of the shelter environment.

Establishing a resident advisory board achieved the same goals of enhanced communication and consistency by focusing on current client needs and identifying resources to meet these needs. For example, in one shelter, staff traditionally offered residents the option of requesting a shelter-prepared lunch to take when they are out on a job. Through participation in the advisory board, residents were able to share that they routinely missed breakfast at the shelter, because local transportation issues forced them to leave for work before breakfast was served. As a result, residents were eating their lunches for breakfast. With this knowledge, takeaway breakfasts and lunches were provided. Another effective intervention was the development of a client-run peer center where residents share their knowledge of computer skills, job search techniques, safe housing areas, and public transportation routes, in addition to encouraging others through stories of personal achievements while living at the shelter.

In summary, collaborations to promote the health and wellbeing of individuals and families who are homeless begin with partnership building. Open communication among partners influences the development and success of interventions. Occupational therapists can bring people together and facilitate an open dialogue among all partners to ensure that everyone's concerns are addressed even if they cannot be immediately met. Successful community collaboration programs benefit all participants—people who are homeless, the agencies that provide services, the agency staff, and the occupational therapist. By promoting a shared culture of client-centeredness and open communication, occupational therapists can establish effective interventions that meet the needs of multiple stakeholders. Careful analysis of the culture and environmental press within an agency helps an occupational therapist to identify valued and effective roles within the partnership and to implement programs responsive to client-identified needs and preferences. The next section discusses the process of analyzing cultural/environmental press and determining occupational therapy roles.

Needs Assessment

An initial step in formulating community intervention programs is information gathering and analysis of context (Fazio, 2001). One place to begin is to determine the community needs where services are being considered. Identifying the specific needs of the target population includes the perceived needs of service recipients and service providers and the objective needs of clients. Determining discrepancies between objective and felt concerns helps the occupational therapist to identify unmet needs. Existing community resources and programs must be identified to determine services currently available and whether these services are accessible and effective. Conceptualizing occupational therapy interventions within a continuum of care or network of services is essential to identifying and implementing useful and effective occupational therapy roles.

Identifying Direct Service Needs

In the spring of 1999, the authors conducted a needs assessment to facilitate development of an occupation-based program at a homeless shelter in Florida (Finlayson, Baker, Rodman, & Herzberg, 2002). **Occupation-based practice** provides goal-directed interventions focused on the meaningful and purposeful everyday activities of a client. Research supported the notion that interventions are most effective when both direct services and systems needs are considered. This qualitative study used participant observation, focus groups, and reflective journals from direct services recipients, agency staff, and occupational therapy students. Three primary themes emerged from the data: the "hunt for meaning and focus," "get a job," and "uncommon ground." The "hunt for meaning and focus" theme predominated for the shelter residents, while "get a job" predominated for the staff. Herzberg and Finlayson (2001) provide a detailed history of the process and outcomes of this study. Finding meaning and focus in their lives was the main concern of the shelter residents. These people expressed the desire to get more out of life while recognizing that identified basic needs must be met in order for this to happen. A significant part of this theme was the clients' readiness to change their own situation, to seek assistance, and to accept assistance to get where they wanted to be. While the "hunt for meaning and focus" was strong in helping clients set direction for their lives, it was

apparent that this drive was also very fragile. Clients talked about how difficult it was to maintain hope and courage when they were not seeing rapid progress toward their goals.

The ups and downs inherent in breaking any cycle led to a narrow focus of intervention by both clients and staff—that of getting a job. The overriding theme emerging from the staff focus group was the message that the primary focus for people living at the shelter should be to get a job. Embedded within this message was a secondary theme that having a job, regardless of type, was going to end a person's experience with homelessness.

The occupational therapy students' journals, on the other hand, reflected concerns that getting a job is a complex process that involves many aspects of the person—their skills and abilities, their hopes and dreams, and the realities of the environment. Journal entries reflected the students' discomfort and confusion with the focus on getting a job rather than on building skills that would serve the client in the longer term (Finlayson et al., 2002). The students recognized that people under stress have increased difficulty in prioritizing tasks and following through. In addition, verbal and behavioral skill sets that facilitate survival on the streets by keeping others away (to ensure personal safety) are not necessarily compatible with the skill sets needed for success on a job.

It is not uncommon for clients and staff to assume that if clients had a job and were earning money, they would not be homeless. Individualized services are needed because physical or mental disability may limit the ability to engage in the quantity or quality of work necessary to secure or maintain gainful employment. That said, systems factors completely out of the control of the homeless person may make quick reentry into the job market impossible even if the person were to surmount personal barriers. One consideration is that the available jobs may not provide a living wage in that locale. Jobs that are available may not offer health benefits adequate for the current and future needs of people who are homeless and more likely to be living with chronic disability or disease. For these reasons, occupational therapists must recognize the need for client advocacy and staff education roles that support direct services interventions. Anecdotal practice experience and health promotion research (Smedley & Syme, 2000) indicate that direct service interventions alone are insufficient.

Like the findings of previous studies (Toro et al., 1997; Toro & Warren, 1999), the needs assessment found that both residents and staff were aware of the added challenges presented by substance abuse and dependence within the cycle of homelessness. Occupational therapists have a history of providing direct services interventions to people with substance abuse and substance dependence problems, although typically these services are provided at inpatient units that control patient interactions with the outside world. Working with people who are homeless and have addictions requires assessment of systems demands and of the individual's personal strengths and vulnerabilities.

In many shelters, residents must be out of the shelter during the day but remain substance free. This creates added stress for those residents who must deal with the physical and psychological assaults of substance withdrawal. These residents must implement new, substance-free ways of coping with the frustrations that are a part of normal daily life, adjust to the dependence and rules of living in a shelter, and find a job. Interactions between people who are homeless and agency staff are further complicated by the fact that shelter staff members must enforce abstinence rules for the safety and wellbeing of others living in the shelter environment. In most shelter settings, clients under the influence of a substance are automatically denied entry. An individual who is free of overt symptoms of drug use when they enter the shelter environment may still be excluded from staying at the shelter on the basis of results of random drug tests. There are few, if any, concessions made that allow shaping of behavior. Occupational therapists can adopt advocacy and education roles to mediate this discordance and to support direct services interventions.

Building the personal and employment-related skills of persons who are homeless is not the only means to promoting health and wellbeing in this population. While the needs and challenges of these persons are great, much work is needed in addressing the societal factors that create the conditions for homelessness to occur. Without such efforts, homelessness and its concomitant health problems are likely to persist. An Institute of Medicine review of social and behavioral health promotion research (Smedley & Syme, 2000) concluded that

> while some behavioral interventions have succeeded in improving health behaviors, many narrow, individually focused models of behavior change have proven insufficient in helping people to change high-risk behavior. . . . It is unreasonable to expect that people will change their behavior easily when so many forces in the social, cultural, and physical environment conspire against such change. If successful programs are to be developed to prevent disease and improve health, attention must be given not only to the behavior of individuals, but also to the environmental context within which people live. (p. 4)

As professionals concerned with optimizing health and wellbeing through occupation and participation, it is vital to understand that addressing the needs of people who are homeless is far more complex than simply evaluating education and technical skill levels or having the ability to communicate appropriately with supervisors and peers, to sustain work quantity or quality, or to comprehend and solve problems. Direct services interventions must help the individual to find meaning and focus and to satisfactorily meet current and anticipated environmental demands for occupational performance, and the interventions must support and nurture fragile hopes, dreams, and successes. However, the components of occupational performance must be examined against a contextual backdrop of service agency culture and the local economy. Occupational therapists must be aware of the need for advocacy and education to mediate and improve direct services environments and to impact policy.

Systems Level Analysis

Occupational therapists can collaborate with municipal agencies, community organizations, service providers, and consumers in planning and evaluating the delivery of health and human services for individuals and families experiencing homelessness. Collecting and analyzing local data for the purpose of service planning and delivery for persons who are homeless is considered a best-practice approach in communities nationwide (Fosburg & Dennis, 1999). Technical and research assistance in conducting and analyzing biennial countywide census survey and needs assessment for the Broward Coalition to End Homelessness, Inc., is a systems level occupational therapy approach. In this intervention, the client is defined as a 50-member, countywide, umbrella coalition of private- and public-sector agencies serving people who are homeless. Occupational therapists facilitated the occupational performance of this coalition in a systems level intervention. Some of the data resulting from this intervention are presented here to lay the groundwork for the direct service interventions discussed next.

Every other year, using current U.S. Housing and Urban Development (HUD) guidelines for determining homelessness, the Broward Coalition to End Homelessness, Inc., collects survey data to identify characteristics, service usage, and service needs of their local homeless population. In 2002 and 2004, the survey data were analyzed to identify the unique needs of our local population. In 2004, they found that 54% of the population had been homeless for less than 6 months. Twenty-two percent reported being homeless for less than 30 days with an additional 32% reporting homelessness of 1 to 6 months' duration. Eleven percent of our population reported homelessness of 5 or more years' duration (Broward Coalition to End Homelessness, Inc.,

2002). The stresses for each of these groups, and their intervention needs, are different. Table 22-3 shows responses of individuals and Table 22-4 shows the responses of families regarding services used and needed but not currently perceived to be accessible. This information is of particular interest to occupational therapists.

A subanalysis of the data found that services used and needed by survey respondents differed by sheltered versus unsheltered status, as well as by individuals and families with minor children. A finding of importance to occupational therapists was that approximately 24% of all respondents reported they had sustained a severe head injury in the past. This finding is clearly different from the incidence of acquired brain injury in the general population of approximately 1%. Further analyses

of this finding are currently being conducted to learn how respondents defined a severe head injury and how they acquired it. Possible causes that have ramifications for the direction of occupational therapy direct services interventions are domestic violence, substance abuse, aggressive interpersonal behaviors, susceptibility to street violence, and inadequate problem-solving skills that create a hazard to personal safety. Service providers need to know if there is a need for adapted case management and educational or skills programming for some or all of these individuals who may have cognitive deficits.

The report was distributed to all member agencies to assist in the coordination and planning of intervention services. Even though occupational therapists are not involved in direct services with the majority of these

Table 22–3 2002 Broward Coalition to End Homelessness Census Survey: Selected Services Used and Needed but Not Currently Perceived Accessible by Sheltered and Unsheltered Individuals

Services	SHELTERED (N = 540)		UNSHELTERED (N = 1001)	
	% Used	% Needed	% Used	% Needed
Meals	59	6	53	20
Mental health outpatient	27	4	11	9
Substance abuse outpatient	26	1	9	7
Life skills training	29	6	5	10
Job training	11	14	6	22
General medical care	35	9	11	18

Table 22–4 2002 Broward Coalition to End Homelessness Census Survey: Selected Services Used and Needed but Not Currently Perceived Accessible by Sheltered and Unsheltered Families

Services	SHELTERED (N = 81)		UNSHELTERED (N = 207)	
	% Used	% Needed	% Used	% Needed
Meals	23	0	22	17
Mental health outpatient	10	4	7	8
Substance abuse outpatient	10	4	6	9
Life skills training	15	2	4	11
Job training	9	9	7	18
General medical care	15	9	8	17

agencies, this systems level needs analysis allows occupational therapy input. These analyses are valuable to the coalition-member client in planning meaningful and purposeful direct service interventions.

In summary, occupational therapists facilitate occupational performance and participation based on needs assessment at the systems level and at that of the individual recipient of services. Assessing environmental context, resources, and intervention philosophy helps to understand what programming is likely to be implemented and sustained. Systems level assessment of the characteristics, service usage, and service needs of the local homeless population helps to ensure proposed interventions have meaning and impact. At the direct service level, assessment of environmental stresses experienced by people who are homeless, in addition to assessment of individual strengths and challenges, helps to develop client-centered interventions. Needs assessments that include the perspectives of multiple stakeholders are the key to developing systems-valued interventions. The next section provides specific examples of interventions that are based on needs assessments and are guided by an empowerment approach and the Canadian Model of Occupational Performance (Townsend, 1997).

Sample Occupational Therapy Interventions

Since 1998, Nova Southeastern University Department of Occupational Therapy faculty, students, and graduates have filled various volunteer and paid roles at a local emergency homeless shelter. Direct service roles include intervention specialist focusing on occupational analysis, skill building, or environmental adaptation; life skills program group leader or coordinator; vocational evaluator; job developer or vocational coach; advocate; and case manager. Systems change roles are those of advocate, program consultant, community educator, staff training facilitator, researcher, and coalition board member.

Occupational therapists are known for client-centered interventions that help people to move from "where they are" to where they would like to be in terms of meaningful engagement and participation in all aspects of life. Occupational therapy theories and frameworks help to guide goal-directed interventions, and theory facilitates the ability to articulate the benefits and the uniqueness of occupational therapy interventions to both service recipients and agency staff. Adherence to the Canadian Model of Occupational Performance (CMOP) as a theoretical perspective ensures greater coherence in interventions and

helps maintain the focus of full participation by clients (Herzberg & Finlayson, 2001).

The CMOP was chosen for use at the shelter because of its emphasis on the dynamic interaction between person/environment/occupation and client-centered occupational performance. The CMOP emphasis on spirituality at the core of the physical, cognitive, and affective performance components was culturally relevant for both the direct services clientele and the service agency. The emphases of the CMOP facilitate communication that allows people to make a cost-benefit analysis regarding their participation in interventions. In this section, information is provided on the kinds of direct service group programming and developmental screenings that were conducted. In addition the substance and importance of systems level interventions are discussed.

Interventions With Adults

Maslow's hierarchy states that basic needs for food, shelter, and safety must be resolved successfully before attention can be directed to other tasks (Maslow, 1971). Uncertainty regarding one's ability to meet basic needs, the physical dislocation from where one was living, and the psychological effects of loss of home and personal expectations of one's success and competency can result in nonclinical and clinical depressive states. Consequently, direct service occupational therapy interventions must carefully consider the individual's stabilization, the client's expressed needs and goals, and the individual's current ability to engage in tasks or learning that go beyond the demands of basic survival.

The first step is to identify purposeful and meaningful occupations in which the client chooses or is expected to engage. One of the key areas of discordance between shelter residents and staff was perceptions of the residents' productivity needs and how these needs were best addressed (Finlayson et al., 2002). Residents identified that they needed better skills to find a job and needed confidence for job interviews. They talked about not knowing how to deal with a criminal background when filling out job applications. Residents also expressed a desire to learn more about computers and to gain computer skills that would help them find a job. Staff members also raised the same issues of knowledge and confidence. Throughout the data, it was apparent that both clients and staff recognized the small steps that needed to be addressed before clients could get and keep a job. Nevertheless, the here-and-now focus of the shelter's clients and staff was on "get a job."

Many group interventions are themed around "get a job" but also address the underlying prevocational skills of effective communication; the ability to work with consistency, care, and attention to quality of effort; coping skills; and the appropriate exercise of judgment and problem-solving skills. Discussions and activity groups themed around issues of self-disclosure of problems with substance abuse or dependence, mental illness, current living situation (i.e., the shelter), self-concept, legal issues, or dysfunctional relationships or activities are conducted after assessment of resident interest and abilities.

Some groups are gender specific and address sexuality, relationships, parenting issues, self-esteem, and assertiveness. Other groups build specific skills, such as filling out job applications, interviewing, dressing for job success, clarifying supervisor communication, dealing with conflict, managing anger, and improving coping skills. Some groups address time management, use of energy and resource management, money management and budgeting, productive and satisfying use of leisure time, goal setting, building friendships and effective personal support systems, and giving back/making a meaningful contribution to the lives of others. See Content Box 22-4 for an overview of themes of groups conducted by the occupational therapists.

For persons with disabilities who live at the shelter, occupational therapists provide screening, individualized consultation for activity, and environmental adaptation with agency staff regarding disability limitations

and needed accommodations. They also provide educational information on disease processes and management for staff and residents when appropriate.

All groups include an activity component in which the participants are called upon to demonstrate the principles or themes of the session. Because of the identified incidence of head injury, student group leaders prepare modifications to planned activities to ensure successful inclusion of people with varying levels of ability. Typically, a theme is emphasized during a 1- to 2-hour session with a series of activities. These activities move from simple to complex, from low interpersonal demand to higher interpersonal demand, and from concrete to abstract thinking. To reinforce the session theme, each session ends with verbal reflection from participants. The group members reflect on

- what each participant liked or disliked and why,
- what each participant learned from the session, and
- what he or she will take from the session to help him or her in the future.

While topics differ from session to session, the format remains consistent. The session topics and format support an empowerment approach and are consistent with the theoretical base of the Canadian Model of Occupational Performance.

Session participants report high levels of satisfaction with these client-centered, occupation-based interventions. They report feeling that their input and participation are respected and valued. This in turn facilitates the educational aspects of the session. Residents value the opportunity to practice skills, work collaboratively with health-care professionals, and share communication and successes in a supportive environment.

Interventions to Empower Parents

A direct service that is provided for families living at the shelter is developmental screening of their children. Poverty and homelessness increase risk factors for developmental delays. In addition, the physical and psychological stressors associated with experiencing homelessness may negatively impact a parent's ability to meet the parenting and developmental needs of their children. The purpose of these screenings is to provide parents with a baseline measure of their child's development that educates and empowers. Through these developmental screenings, the occupational therapy faculty and students disseminate knowledge about normal developmental milestones, teach skills, support parental efforts to facilitate normal development, alert parents to developmental delays, and generate documentation that allows parents to access mainstream intervention resources. **Mainstream intervention resources** are

---

Content Box 22-4

Themes of Group Interventions With Adults

- Stress management (leisure skills, time management, coping skills)
- Self-care training (nutrition/cooking, health and safety, medication management, hygiene, grooming, dressing)
- Community living skills training (clothing care, money management, shopping, public transportation, landlord and roommate issues, room maintenance, community resources)
- Prevocational services (task skills, aptitude testing, job structuring, interviewing and application activities, job coaching)
- Social and interpersonal skills (assertiveness, self-expression, conflict resolution, basic conversational skills, friendships)
- Home and neighborhood familiarization for those individuals transitioning into permanent housing to increase knowledge of local resources and transportation
- Individualized assistance to secure needed home items (furniture, bedding, kitchen items, etc.) and create a pleasant, livable, and personalized environment

those that accommodate or mediate identified categories of disabilities or disabling circumstances and are widely known to the general population (i.e., specialized school programs or intervention services).

Another purpose of the screenings is to provide a faculty-supervised service learning experience for first-year, graduate-level occupational therapy students who are studying assessment and evaluation. **Service learning** refers to educational experiences meeting the learning requirements of the student while providing needed services to another individual or agency. Second-year students also volunteer to participate to gain more experience with testing, interviewing, and interacting with parents and to demonstrate leadership and role modeling for first-year students. The students practice the professional skills that will help them to empower their future clients and these families.

Parents request evaluation via a consent form that identifies basic demographic information on the child and allows identification of any specific parent concerns. The supervising therapist returns a copy of this form to the parent with type of screening conducted, screening results, recommendations for follow-up if needed, and directions on how to arrange follow-up.

The Denver II (Frankenburg, Dodds, Archer, Shapiro, & Bresnick, 1992) screening tool has been used for children from birth to 6 years of age, and the FirstStep Screening Test for Evaluating Preschoolers (Miller, 1999) has been used to screen children from 2.9 to 6.2 years of age. Both tests were selected for their ease of administration and their visual representation of results. The selection of an assessment is based on the child's age and the occupational therapy supervisor's clinical judgment. In part, this choice is influenced by the therapist's judgment of its usefulness as a teaching tool for the parent. Some parents are better able to understand normal development using the age and behavior cues on the Denver II, with its contextual reference of the expected behaviors of children within the age range it covers.

Children 6.2 years and older are screened with an observational tool that the authors developed, which allows assessment of gross and fine motor skills, visual-perceptual skills, ability to conceptualize and execute an idea, and psychosocial issues. The children respond positively to it, often asking when they can return to "play some more games" with the occupational therapy students. It allows the observation and discussion of child behavior with the parent as it occurs, in addition to educating the parent on normal developmental behavior.

Screenings are conducted at the shelter between 6:30 and 8:30 p.m. twice per month. Since residents are expected to leave the shelter by 7:00 a.m. and may not return to the shelter until after 5:00 p.m., families may have already had a very long day prior to the scheduled screening. Children who are obviously tired are rescheduled for another time.

After completion of the appropriate screen, the supervising therapist signs the dual purpose consent/recommendations form and provides the parent with a copy. Handouts to educate and enrich parent-child interactions and directions for individualized follow-up, if needed, concludes the screening session.

Systems Level Interventions

Public funding for services for people who are homeless is usually very limited, and programs rely heavily on faith-based interventions and volunteer staff. Agencies often utilize less well-trained staff to provide direct services. Community-university partnerships are one solution to improving the quality of services to homeless people by improving the knowledge level of agency staff. Contractually or as a part of the university service mission, Nova Southeastern University faculty consult on specific clients or topics and provide evaluation services or educational experiences tailored to the needs of agency staff. In the local area, on both a pro bono and a consultant basis, occupational therapists associated with the university provide staff education on

- how to respond therapeutically to anxious individuals and those experiencing posttraumatic stress disorders, cognitive deficits, major mental illnesses, or substance abuse problems;
- techniques for helping clients engage in goal-directed activities;
- how to maintain therapeutic roles and personal equilibrium;
- principles of needs assessment; and
- documentation skills.

The community-university partnership began with proprietary and pro bono occupational therapy consultant roles. In the **proprietary consultant role,** services are provided on a fee-for-service basis with the intent of producing a profit. **Pro bono** refers to services provided without cost to the client.

The community-university partnership evolved to include master's level occupational therapy students as part of a 4-year training grant (1-D37-HP-00755-01) funded by the U.S. Department of Health and Human Services, Health Resources and Services Administration (HRSA). The grant provided interdisciplinary training experiences for students to build team- and discipline-specific technical skills; to develop applied research skills via data gathering, analysis, and dissemination; and to make an important contribution to the health and wellbeing of this population. It provided required and volunteer experiences for students from occupational therapy, communications disorders (speech-language pathology and audiology), optometry, and conflict analysis and resolution. Faculty-supervised professional services are provided via this "wraparound partnership" that applies state-of-the-art theory and techniques to services for people who would otherwise have had little or no access to them.

Outcomes research on student perceptions of this program's impact is very positive. Students reported that while they may not seek initial employment with agencies specifically serving underserved or minority populations, the learning experiences at the homeless shelter were valuable to them. Students report that this experience helped them to become more knowledgeable, empathetic, and client-centered. They report it changed how they perceived their professional role and how interventions should be selected and implemented.

Because homelessness is a growing social concern, states have developed oversight or coordinating boards from city, county, and state-level coalitions of public and private services agencies. These boards benefit from interactions with occupational therapists who choose to implement advocacy, educational, or consultant roles at this level. In the community consultant role, the occupational therapists note effectiveness in serving the information and research needs of the local coalition of homeless service provider agencies. Identification of the patterns of needs and services provided and desired now influences service planning and funding in the county.

This evidence helps coalitions and individual agencies to negotiate outside services and funding. It also helps local agencies to evaluate changing use and need patterns. The analyses of client-reported challenges to successful occupational performance are also used to define local need for state and federal funding opportunities. As a result of these efforts, an occupational therapy faculty member was invited to join the board of directors of the local county coalition of providers. This is a direct result of the value accorded the community-university partnership and, specifically, the occupational therapy component of this partnership.

Conclusion

In this chapter, the federal definition of *homelessness* and the characteristics and context of homelessness were discussed. Person-environment factors that influence the occurrence of homelessness in the United States were introduced, and the direct services and systems roles that occupational therapists fill in working with this population were outlined.

In the needs analysis and interventions sections, environmental factors were described that influenced program design and implementation. Client-centered and occupation-based programs to empower and build the skills and capacities of clients were discussed. Those clients may be individuals; families; organizations; or local, regional, state, or national groups or boards.

People who are homeless benefit from direct service interventions and systems change interventions designed by occupational therapists. Research in the field was presented along with experiences and interventions for underserved shelter residents who previously had little, if any, contact with an occupational therapist. The authors hope other therapists will benefit from the knowledge gained and will be encouraged to develop additional programs to optimize health and wellbeing through occupation and participation for persons who are homeless.

Case Study 22-1

John, a 24-year-old male, received an honorable discharge from the U.S. Army 1 year ago following 4 active years of service. While in the military, John spent a 15-month tour in Fallujah and Baghdad, Iraq. While there he lost three platoon members and was forced to shoot and kill several suspected terrorists. He has been transferred to the Individual Ready Reserve (IRR) for the remainder of his military service obligation. This means he can be recalled to active duty during a time of war or natural emergency until the 8 years have expired.

Over the past year, John has been staying on his single mother's couch of her cramped one-bedroom apartment. Beth, John's mother, has noticed him displaying some odd behaviors ever since he returned home from active duty. She often cries herself to sleep because she misses the sweet boy who left her straight out of high school 5 years ago to pursue his dreams of becoming an infantry soldier and one day attending college. John has not been able to hold a steady job over the past year; he has a hard time concentrating and sleeping and often wakes up in the middle of the night making noise around the apartment. He has not displayed any positive or loving feelings toward his mom since his return. John's mother, thinking some tough love will bring him to reality, forces John to find his own place to live and to get a steady job.

Continued

John started off doing well on his own and was able to keep a job for 2 months. One day, while John was walking into work, a car on the nearby street loudly backfired, and John dropped down on his hands and knees in the middle of the busy sidewalk seeking refuge. This was not the first time something like this has happened, so John decided to seek help for his problem. John does not have medical coverage through his current job and sought treatment at a local Veterans Administration (VA) clinic. There he was misdiagnosed with adjustment disorder and a preexisting mental condition, neither of which allows him to collect disability. He did not receive appropriate psychiatric treatment, and his mental condition worsened. He simply cannot hold down a job any longer, he cannot collect disability, and he has been unable to find a place where he can afford to live. Having already overstayed his welcome at his mother's apartment, he has no place to go. John shows up at a local VA homeless shelter looking for help.

Questions

1. As an occupational therapist at a Health Care for Homeless Veterans (HCHV) program that offers case management services; mental health services such as the integrated mental illness, addictions, posttraumatic stress disorder program; and vocational rehabilitation, what type of intervention would you provide for John?
2. List which of the areas of occupation you would address in John's intervention plan and briefly describe to what extent you would address each occupation.
3. What types of community resources could you suggest to John?

Case Study 22-2

Margaret is a 38-year-old female who has been homeless for the past 2 years. Her husband passed away 5 years ago due to a motor vehicle crash. Margaret is the mother of two children: Joshua, age 11, and Madison, age 9. Both children are enrolled in a local elementary school and participate in after-school activities. Before her husband's death, Margaret was enrolled in college part-time to become an interior decorator. She spent the remainder of her time taking care of household duties and caring for her children.

After her husband's death, she had difficulty coping with the loss and depended on alcohol to cope with her feelings of abandonment and grief. She reported that she has been dependent on alcohol for a couple of years, and "she can't live without it." Her dependency on alcohol has caused her to sever relationships with close family members, including two brothers and a sister who live 2 hours away. She is currently employed as a cashier at a local grocery store but is on the verge of being fired. Customers and coworkers have reported that Margaret frequently shows up to work with a disheveled appearance and impoverished hygiene. Her employer has warned her on several occasions about her appearance and the effect it has on customer service.

Previously, she and her children stayed with friends until they outstayed their welcome, which resulted in her finding a new residence. They currently reside in Life Hope homeless shelter located in an urban area within her community. The program director reports that Margaret is a caring person and does whatever she can to provide for her children. The homeless shelter has just contracted an occupational therapist to assist residents with regaining independence and increasing quality of life.

Questions

1. What areas should the occupational therapist address to assist Margaret in regaining independence and establishing positive health behaviors? Briefly describe interventions to address deficits in each area.
2. What are some recommended services or strategies, if any, the occupational therapist might suggest for Margaret?
3. Identify protective and risk factors for Margaret's children and interventions the occupational therapist can implement.

Acknowledgment

Case studies were submitted by Julie Tatonetti and Marvin Williams, while occupational therapy students at the University of South Alabama.

▶ For Discussion and Review

1. Visit a homeless shelter or soup kitchen in your area. Conduct a stakeholder needs assessment by respectfully asking the people using those services about their plans for the future and the services or interventions that they feel are needed to help them achieve these plans.
2. Calculate the cost and availability of fair market rent housing in your area. Use this information to plan a budget based on the monies earned from a job that pays minimum wage.
3. Find out what services are provided in your community for people who are homeless, the amount of professional services provided in addition to those that meet basic needs for food and shelter, and what local initiatives exist to end homelessness.
4. Discuss the needs of children who are homeless and how occupational therapists working in the school system might address these needs.
5. Describe the application of the Canadian Occupational Performance Measure for persons who are homeless.
6. What other theoretical models might be useful for planning interventions for the homeless population, and how could they be applied?

▶ Research Questions

1. What roles do occupational therapists perceive for themselves in interventions that benefit people who are homeless, and to what extent do they implement them?
2. What adaptations improve the occupational performance of people who are homeless and report having had a severe head injury?
3. What occupational therapy interventions are most effective in reducing psychological stress of people who are homeless after first episodes of 1-month, 6-month, and 1-year duration?
4. How do in vivo experiences with people who are homeless affect later practice patterns of occupational therapy students?

References

Applewaite, S. (1997). Homeless veterans: Perspectives on social services use. *Social Work, 42*(1), 19–30.

Bassuk, E. L., Weinreb, L. F., Buckner, J. C., Browne, A., Salomon, A., & Bassuk, S. S. (1996). The characteristics and needs of sheltered homeless and low-income housed mothers. *Journal of the American Medical Association, 276,* 640–46.

Baum, C., & Law, M. (1998). Nationally speaking: Community health: a responsibility, an opportunity, and a fit for occupational therapy. *American Journal of Occupational Therapy, 52,* 7–10.

Better Homes Fund. (1999). *America's homeless children: New outcasts.* Newton, MA: Author.

Broward Coalition to End Homelessness. (2002). *Census survey.* Ft. Lauderdale, FL: Author.

Bureau of Primary Health Care. (2006). *Health care for the homeless information resource center.* Retrieved June 10, 2006, from http://www.bphc.hrsa.gov/hchirc/.

Burt, M. (2001a). Homeless families, singles, and others: Findings from the 1996 national survey of homeless assistance providers and clients. *Housing Policy Debate (Fannie Mae Foundation), 12,* 737–80.

Burt, M. (2001b). *What will it take to end homelessness?* Retrieved June 29, 2006, from the Urban Institute website: http://www.urban.org/publications/310305.html.

Burt, M., Aron, L., Lee, E., & Valente, J. (2001). *Helping America's homeless: Emergency shelter or affordable housing?* Washington, DC: Urban Institute Press.

Burt, M. R. (1999). Demographics and geography: Estimating needs. In L. B. Fosburg & D. L. Dennis (Eds.), *Practical lessons: The 1998 National Symposium on Homelessness Research.* Washington, DC: U.S. Department of Housing and Urban Development and the U.S. Department of Health and Human Services.

DeOllos, I. Y. (1997). *On becoming homeless: The shelterization process for homeless families.* Lanham, MD: University Press of America.

Fazio, L. (2001). *Developing occupation-centered programs for the community: A workbook for students and professionals.* Upper Saddle River, NJ: Prentice Hall.

Federal Task Force on Homelessness and Mental Illness. (1992). *Outcasts on Main Street: Report of the Federal Task Force on Homelessness and Severe Mental Illness.* Washington, DC: Interagency Council on the Homeless.

Finlayson, M., Baker, L., Rodman, L., & Herzberg, G. (2002). Process and outcomes of a multi-method needs assessment at a homeless shelter. *American Journal of Occupational Therapy, 56,* 313–21.

Fosburg, L. B., & Dennis, D. L. (Eds.) (1999). *Practical lessons: The 1998 National Symposium on Homelessness Research.* Retrieved June 29, 2006, from U.S. Department of Housing and Urban Development and the U.S. Department of Health and Human Services website: http://aspe.hhs.gov/progsys/homeless/symposium/toc.htm.

Frankenburg, W. K., Dodds, J., Archer, P., Shapiro, H., & Bresnick, B. (1992). The Denver II: A major revision and restandardization of the Denver developmental screening test. *Pediatrics, 89,* 91–97. Test available from Denver Developmental Materials for online purchase at http://www.denverii.com.

Gelberg, L., & Arangua, L. (2001). Homeless persons. In R. Andersen, T. H. Rice, & G. F. Kominski (Eds.), *Changing the U.S. health care system* (2d ed., pp. 332–86). San Francisco: Jossey-Bass.

Health Care for the Homeless (HCH) Clinicians Network. (2003). Dealing with disability: Cognitive impairments and homelessness. *Healing Hands, 7*(1), 1–6. Available at http://www.nhchc.org/Network/HealingHands/2003/hh-0303.pdf.

Herman, D. B., Struening, E. L., & Barrow, S. M. (1994). Self-reported needs for help among homeless men and women. *Evaluation and Program Planning, 17,* 249–56.

Herzberg, G., & Finlayson, M. (2001). Development of occupational therapy in a homeless shelter. *OT in Health Care 13*(3/4), 133–47.

Heubner, J. E., & Tryssenaar, J. (1996). Development of an occupational therapy practice perspective in a homeless shelter: A fieldwork experience. *Canadian Journal of Occupational Therapy, 63,* 24–32.

Institute for Research on Poverty. (1998). Revising the poverty measure. *Focus, 19*(2).

Kemp, S. P., Whittaker, J. K., & Tracy, E. M. (1997). *Person-environment practice: The social ecology of interpersonal helping.* New York: Aldine de Gruyter.

Kielhofner, G. (1985). *A model of human occupation: Theory and application.* Baltimore: Williams & Wilkins.

Maslow, A. (1971). *The farther reaches of human nature.* New York: Viking.

Masten, A. S. (1992). Homeless children in the United States: Mark of a nation at risk. *Current Directions in Psychological Science, 1*(2), 41–44.

McColl, M. A. (1998). What do we need to know to practice occupational therapy in the community? *American Journal of Occupational Therapy, 52,* 11–18.

McColl, M. A. (2003). *Spirituality and occupational therapy.* Ottawa: Canadian Association of Occupational Therapists.

Miller, L. J. (1999). *FirstStep screening test for evaluating preschoolers* (manual edition). San Antonio, TX: Psychological Corporation, Harcourt Assessment. Test available for online purchase from Harcourt Assessment at http://harcourtassessment.com.

Minkler, M. (Ed.) (1997). *Community organizing and community building for health.* New Brunswick, NJ: Rutgers University Press.

National Center on Family Homelessness. (n.d.). *America's homeless children: Fact sheet.* Retrieved May 18, 2006, from http://familyhomelessness.org/ fact_children.pdf.

National Center for Injury Prevention and Control. (2007). *Traumatic brain injury.* Retrieved December 26, 2007, from http://www.cdc.gov/ncipc/factsheets/tbi.htm.

National Coalition for the Homeless. (2006a). *How many are homeless?* (NCH Fact Sheet #2). Retrieved June 29, 2006, from http://www.nationalhomeless.org/publications/facts/How_Many.pdf.

National Coalition for the Homeless. (2006b). *Who is homeless?* (NCH Fact Sheet #3). Retrieved June 29, 2006, from http://www.nationalhomeless.org/publications/facts/Whois.pdf.

National Rehabilitation Hospital Center for Health & Disability Research. (2002, November). *Homeless and disabled: Focusing on the health and healthcare needs of an underserved population.* Retrieved June 29, 2006, from the National Rehabilitation Hospital Center for Health & Disability Research website: http://www.nrhrehab.org/documents/Research/brief_housing.pdf.

Petrenchik, T. (2006). Homelessness in America: Perspectives, characterizations, and considerations for occupational therapy. *Occupational Therapy in Health Care, 20*(3/4), 9–30.

Petrenchik, T., & Herzberg, G. (2002). *Incidence of self-reported head injury and associated health disparities for persons who are homeless in Broward County, FL. A summary report for the Broward County Homeless Initiative Partnership Administration.* College of Allied Health and Nursing, Nova Southeastern University, Ft. Lauderdale, FL.

Rog, D. J., McCombs-Thornton, K. L., Gilbert-Mongelli, A. M., Brito, M. C., & Holupka, C. S. (1995). Implementation of the homeless families program: 2. Characteristics, strengths, and needs of participant families. *American Journal of Orthopsychiatry, 65*(4), 514–23.

Rosencheck, R., Bassuk, E., & Salomon, A. (1999). Special populations of homeless Americans. In L. B. Fosburg & D. L. Dennis (Eds.), *Practical lessons: The 1998 national symposium on homelessness research* (pp. 2:1–2:31). Washington, DC: U.S. Department of Housing and Urban Development.

Scaffa, M. (2001). *Occupational therapy in community-based practice settings.* Philadelphia: F. A. Davis.

Shinn, M. L., & Weitzman, B. C. (1996). Homeless families are different. In J. Baumohl (Ed.), *Homelessness in America* (pp. 109–22). Phoenix, AZ: Orynx.

Smedley, B. D., & Syme, S. L. (Eds.). (2000). *Promoting health: Intervention strategies from social and behavioral research.* Washington, DC: National Academy Press.

Stedman's Medical Dictionary (27th ed.). Philadelphia: Lippincott, Williams & Wilkins.

Toro, P., Rabideau, J., Bellavia, C., Daeschler, C., Wall, D., Thomas, D., & Smith, S. (1997). Evaluating an intervention for homeless persons: Results of a field experiment. *Journal of Consulting and Clinical Psychology, 65*(3), 476–84.

Toro, P., & Warren, M. (1999). Homelessness in the United States: Policy considerations. *Journal of Community Psychology, 27,* 119–36.

Townsend, E. (Ed.) (1997). *Enabling occupation: An occupational therapy perspective.* Ottawa, ON: CAOT Publications ACE.

Tryssenaar, J., & Clarke, F. (1996). Occupational performance needs of a shelter population. *Canadian Journal of Occupational Therapy, 66,* 188–95.

Tryssenaar, J., Jones, E. J., & Lee, D. (1999). Occupational performance needs of a shelter population. *Canadian Journal of Occupational Therapy, 66,* 188–95.

Urban Institute. (2000). *A new look at homelessness in America, February 01, 2000.* Retrieved June 29, 2006, from http://www.urban.org/publications/900302.html.

U.S. Centers for Disease Control and Prevention. (2005a). *Preventing heart disease and stroke.* Retrieved October 1, 2005, from http://www.cdc.gov/nccdphp/bb_heartdisease/index.htm.

U.S. Centers for Disease Control and Prevention. (2005b). *Stroke fact sheet.* Retrieved October 1, 2005, from http://www.cdc.gov/cvh/library/pdfs/fs_stroke.pdf.

U.S. Department of Health and Human Services. (1998). *Advisory committee on homeless families: Meeting summary February 27, 1998.* Rockville, MD: Author.

U.S. Department of Health and Human Services. (2006). *Federal Register Part V: Department of Health and Human Services: Annual update of the HHS poverty guidelines.* Washington, DC: National Archives and Records Administration.

Weinreb, L., Goldberg, R., Bassuk, E., & Perloff, J. (1998). Determinants of health and service use patterns in homeless and low-income housed children. *Pediatrics, 102,* 554–62.

Chapter 23

Promoting Successful Aging Through Occupation

Michael A. Pizzi and Theresa M. Smith

There is a fountain of youth: It is your mind, your talents, the creativity you bring to your life and the lives of the people you love. When you learn to tap into this source, you will truly have defeated age.

—Sophia Loren

Learning Objectives

This chapter is designed to enable the reader to:

- Describe the aging process and the development of healthy and successful aging.
- Analyze theories of aging and their relevance to successful aging.
- Discuss current models of successful aging.
- Identify the health risks and health behaviors of older adults.
- Determine opportunities and barriers to occupational participation that support successful aging.
- Appraise methods used by occupational therapists in promoting health and wellness with the elderly.

- Apply the Transtheoretical Model (TTM) to healthful behavior changes for the elderly.
- Discuss the role of occupational therapy in current health promotion programs that maintain healthy and successful aging as supported by the *Occupational Therapy Practice Framework: Domain and Processes* (referred to as the *Framework*) developed by the American Occupational Therapy Association (AOTA).
- Explain the importance of health literacy as a determinant of implementing successful aging interventions.

Key Terms

Aging in place

Functional health
    literacy

Health literacy

Health mentor

Life review
    reminiscence

Lifestyle Redesign

Optimal aging

Positive spirituality

Successful aging

Universal design

Introduction

The normal aging process, age-related factors, and pathology may adversely affect older adults' occupational performance. Occupational therapists and occupational therapy assistants are adept at promoting engagement in occupation through remediation, modification, or adaptation of mitigating factors. In this chapter health promotion interventions that support engagement in occupation and social participation to achieve successful aging are examined.

Individuals in the United States are living longer than ever before due to an improved standard of living, better nutrition, prevention and treatment of disease, and medical and technological advances. In the year 2000, persons over the age of 65 made up greater than 12% of the U.S. population, and by 2015 that number is expected to grow to well over 14% (Kinsella & Velkoff, 2001). Although this group comprises just over 12% of the population, it accounts for one-third of health-care dollars spent (U.S. Centers for Disease Control and Prevention [CDC], 2003). Chronic disease is common among this population and includes by rank of prevalence the following conditions: arthritis, heart disease, hearing impairment, high blood pressure, orthopedic impairment, and cataracts (Fulmer, Wallace, & Edelman, 2002).

These physical problems may inhibit a person's ability to participate in everyday activities, as may psychological disorders for which older adults are at risk such as depression, schizophrenia, anxiety states, or substance abuse. In addition, social stressors such as changes in roles, difficulty negotiating the environment, and difficulties in performing daily activities may lead to decreased life satisfaction for older adults (Clark et al., 1997). Age-related changes vary from individual to individual and may be influenced by genetic factors and exposure to injury, illness, genetics, stress, or other factors (Fulmer et al., 2002). However, when older people are asked to self-rate levels of physical, emotional, and social aspects of health, a positive correlation exists between self-ratings of good to excellent health and decreased mortality (Idler & Benyamini, 1997). This means that people who rate themselves positively in these areas tend to live more successfully as they age.

Content Box 23-1 presents population-based statistics to assist occupational therapy practitioners in the promotion of successful aging and wellbeing. The profession of occupational therapy must create strategies and help support policies that enable older people to age successfully in order to promote their participation in daily life and society. It is incumbent upon the profession of occupational therapy to continue to become more sensitive to diversity and diverse needs of a growing older population in order to best serve them. It is also crucial that occupational therapists and occupational therapy assistants work diligently to provide up-to-date health education and develop community-based health promotion programs that help the elderly maintain and optimize health, wellness, and quality of life (QOL).

Content Box 23-1

Statistics on Aging

- "The older population in 2030 is projected to be twice as large as their counterparts in 2000 . . . representing nearly 20 percent of the U.S. Population" (p. 2).
- "The population age 85 and older could grow from 4.2 million in 2000 to nearly 21 million by 2050" (p. 2).
- "Older women were more than twice as likely as older men to live alone (40% and 19%, respectively)" (p. 8).
- "As the older population grows larger, it will also grow more diverse. The older Hispanic population is projected to grow the fastest (from 2 million to 15 million)" (p. 4).
- "The gender gap in completion of a college education will narrow in the future because men and women in younger cohorts are earning college degrees at roughly the same rate" (p. 6).

From *Older Americans 2004: Key indicators of well-being* by Federal Interagency Forum on Aging Related Statistics, 2004, Washington, DC: Author.

The profession of occupational therapy is committed to occupation and client-centered approaches to help people achieve, restore, and maintain participation in everyday activities. Occupation has been defined as the "ordinary and familiar things that people do every day" (Christiansen, Clark, Kielhofner, & Rogers, 1995, p. 1015). Since its inception, occupational therapy has relied on the principles of occupation and participation to promote health and wellbeing (Baum, 2003), with health being defined as a "complete state of physical, mental, and social well-being, not just an absence of disease or infirmity" (World Health Organization [WHO], 1947, p. 29). It is the unique perspective of occupational therapy that "engaging in occupations structures everyday life and contributes to health and well-being" (AOTA, 2008, p. 628).

Successful Aging

The CDC (2004) has proposed health promotion, prevention, maintenance of ability, and enhancement of QOL as the primary methods to support successful aging. A CDC advisory committee identified five roles for the CDC to promote health and prevent disease in older adults:

1. To provide high-quality health information and resources to public health professionals, consumers, health-care providers, and aging experts
2. To support health-care providers and health-care organizations in prevention efforts
3. To integrate public health-prevention expertise with the aging services network
4. To identify and implement effective prevention efforts
5. To monitor changes in the health of older adults.

These roles will require new efforts to address the special needs of older adults and to deliver programs in communities in which older adults work, reside, and congregate. Existing public health programs will be required to examine whether they meet the needs of an aging population. (CDC, 2003, pp. 104–05)

Vaillant (2002), director of the Harvard Study of Adult Development, the longest longitudinal study of aging, synthesized data from the study for his ground-breaking book *Aging Well*. The study examined three distinctly different groups: The Harvard Cohort (i.e., male Harvard graduates studied from 1939 to present or until death), the Inner City Cohort (i.e., 456 men from inner-city Boston), and the Terman Women Sample (i.e., a female cohort from Stanford University that acted as a comparison group to the Harvard men). Content Box 23-2 displays the major findings of this study. Through these findings, the reader can determine qualities a person may possess for successful aging.

Successful aging from an occupational therapy perspective, is having the physical, emotional, social, and spiritual resources, combined with an ability to adapt to life changes, in order to engage in meaningful and important self-selected occupations of life as one ages. The following section describes a number of theories of successful aging.

Aging and Successful Aging Theories

Older adults have reached the human development stage of maturation. Theorists generally group aging issues into categories such as physical, mental, or social changes associated with aging. Despite the existence of over 300 theories of aging (Ashok & Ali, 1999), no single theory explains all aging phenomena. Content Box 23-3 identifies notable theories of biological aging and socioemotional aging, and theories from health psychology that can be applied to older adults. Biological aging theories conceptualize aging as "a progressive physiological deterioration that results in

---

Content Box 23-3

Select Theories on Aging

Biological Aging Theories
- Rate of living theory (Pearl, 1928)
- Caloric restriction (Carlson & Riley, 1998)
- Free-radical theory (Harman, 1956)
- Cross-linkage theory (Bjorksten, 1976)
- Somatic mutation theory (Curtis, 1961)
- Error catastrophe theory (Orgel, 1963)
- Hormonal theory (Walford, 1974)

Socioemotional Aging Theories
- Erikson's theory of eight stages of the human life span (Erikson, 1982)
- Peck's reworking of Erikson's final stage (Peck, 1968)
- Disengagement theory (Cummings & Henry, 1961)
- Activity theory (Neugarten, Havighurst, & Tobin, 1968)
- Socioemotional selectivity theory (Carstensen, 1991)

Health Psychology Theories
- Transtheoretical Model (Prochaska, 1979)
- Transformational Learning (Mezirow, 1991)
- Social Cognitive Theory (Bandura, 1997)
- Ecologic Well-Being Model (Ruffing-Rahal, 1991)

---

increased vulnerability to stress and an increased probability of death" (Cristofalo, Tresini, Francis, & Volker, 1999, p. 98). Socioemotional developmental theorists hypothesize that humans have predetermined tasks at different points of life.

For occupational therapists to engage in theory and evidence-based health promotion practice, they must appreciate the necessity of being knowledgeable of and skilled at facilitating change in health behaviors. Health promotion interventions not only encourage continuing and improving healthy behaviors, but also entail changing unhealthy dominating habits and instituting new healthy habits. For example, this can include cessation of some behaviors (e.g., smoking) or commencing others (e.g., increasing physical activity). According to Belmont and Harris, "The leading causes of premature death and premature disability in industrialized countries are heart disease, cerebrovascular disease, cancer, and trauma—conditions largely influenced by lifestyle factors such as stress, diet, exercise, and smoking" (2002, p. 195).

One of the most current theories of successful aging was developed by Rowe and Kahn (1997). In their theory of successful aging, maintaining interpersonal relations and skills and actively engaging in productive activities that are meaningful (paid or unpaid), in

---

Content Box 23-2

Major Findings of the Harvard Study of Adult Development

- It is bad not the things that happen to us that doom us; it is the good people who happen to us at any age that facilitate enjoyable old age.
- Healing relationships are facilitated by a capacity for gratitude, for forgiveness, and for taking people inside (becoming eternally enriched by loving a particular person).
- A good marriage at age 50 predicted positive aging at 80. Surprisingly, low cholesterol levels at age 50 did not.
- Alcohol abuse—unrelated to unhappy childhood—consistently predicted unsuccessful aging, in part because alcoholism damaged future social supports.
- Learning to play and create after retirement and learning to gain younger friends as we lose older ones add more to life's enjoyment than retirement income.
- Objective good physical health was less important to successful aging than subjective good health.

From *Aging well* (p.13), by G. E. Vaillant, 2002, New York: Little Brown and Company. Copyright © 2002 by George E. Vaillant, MD. By permission of Little Brown & Company.

combination with lack of disease and good function (cognitive and physical), are integral to successful aging. The model is hierarchical, with Rowe and Kahn stating that

> the absence of disease and disability makes it easier to maintain mental and physical function. And maintenance of mental and physical function in turn enables (but does not guarantee) active engagement with life. It is the combination of all three—avoidance of disease and disability, maintenance of cognitive and physical function, and sustained engagement with life—that represents the concept of successful aging most fully. (1997, p. 39)

Their theory demonstrates successful aging as an outcome if the conditions set forth are met. Rowe and Kahn acknowledge that disease and disability are not wholly under one's control but emphasize that individual choice and effort throughout a life can determine successful aging (Rowe & Kahn, 1997).

Crowther, Parker, Achenbaum, Larimore, and Koeni (2002) assert that Rowe and Kahn's successful aging model is useful in helping to develop interventions to support successful aging. However, they add a positive spirituality dimension to expand the model. **Positive spirituality** is defined as involving "a developing and internalized personal relation with the sacred or transcendent that is not bound by race, ethnicity, economics, or class and promotes wellness and welfare of self and others" (Crowther et al., p. 614).

There are also those who view successful aging as including (and adapting to) disease and disability. Chapter 19 emphasizes that health and wellbeing can be achieved despite living with a disability. For the older adult, many of whom cope with some type of disease and disability, successful aging can still be achieved.

Other models and definitions of successful aging need further exploration. Inui (2003) indicates successful aging as "not adequately understood as mere longevity, but implies sufficient well-being in a number of spheres (mental, physical, social, spiritual, economic) to sustain a capacity to function successfully in the changing circumstances of one's life" (p. 391).

> The determinants of such well-being and functional status are manifold and include the genetic endowment, physical environment, social environment, population and individual responses to challenges, the occurrence of disease, availability and effectiveness of health care, and personal prosperity. (Inui, 2003, p. 391)

He further elaborates that successful aging can include disease and disability, and emphasis should be placed on preserving capacity to perform meaningful activity.

Kane (2003) stated that the potential to successfully age with a disability is more likely if health care shifts focus from an emphasis on cure to an emphasis on care, which "implies placing greater emphasis on preventing the transition from disease to dysfunction" (p. 461). Minkler and Fadem (2002) examined the Rowe and Kahn (1997) model with a disability perspective. They concluded that the model can lead to stigmatization and marginalization of the underserved, the disabled, and those who live in impoverished environments. They argued for broadening the model to include an "ecological approach, one that stresses environmental accommodations and policy change and acknowledges that gains as well as losses are a critical part of the aging process" (Minkler & Fadem, 2002, p. 229).

Baltes (1997), a life-span theorist, developed a model of successful aging called the *selection-optimization-compensation (SOC) theory*. Selection is related to the types of activities people choose, or select, while optimization makes the most of one's resources in creating opportunities for oneself. Compensation is related to adaptation and focuses on how one may choose a new strategy for goal attainment if a formerly successful strategy fails to work. Baltes and Baltes (1990) used the term **optimal aging** instead of *successful aging* and defined it as "a kind of utopia, namely aging under development-enhancing and age-friendly environmental conditions" (Baltes & Baltes, 1990, p. 8). This environmental perspective closely aligns with the thinking in occupational therapy relative to active and ongoing participation in society. When social and physical environments can be adapted to accommodate disability, then active engagement with life, also emphasized by Rowe and Kahn, can be maintained. Unlike the Rowe and Kahn (1997) model, however, Baltes theorized that one can still successfully age with a disability. More research is needed with both models in order to build an inclusive model that fosters and promotes active and ongoing participation in society and engagement with life. Occupational therapists should be major contributors to theory in successful aging, given their expansive knowledge base in health, wellness, QOL, and participation.

Menec (2003) viewed activity as integral to successful aging and studied successful aging indicators such as wellbeing, function, and mortality and their relationship to everyday activities. The study concluded that

- overall activity was positively related to happiness;
- activity level corresponded to improved function and reduced mortality;
- prevention of functional decline was positively correlated to engagement in social and productive activity; and
- although activity levels declined with age, older age was not related to a diminution in happiness levels.

Menec also studied the importance of solitary versus social activities and their impact on wellbeing, function, and mortality. She concluded that solitary activity is important to successful aging in the psychosocial domain of happiness. "It makes intuitive sense that reading the newspaper, writing letters, or listening to music would be related to a more specific measure that captures, in part, interest in life" (Menec, 2003, p. S79).

The gerontology theory base in occupational therapy is growing rapidly, integrating theories from health education, health psychology, and other disciplines. Emerging theories of successful aging contribute enormously to existing theory and practice in occupational therapy. The understanding and integration of such is crucial to better understanding the aging process and occupational participation.

Health promotion appears to be the key to unlocking the mystery of how people age successfully. Occupational therapists and occupational therapy assistants work with the elderly in a variety of settings, including nursing and rehabilitation centers, acute care hospitals, assisted-living facilities, day-care centers, in-home care, and community-based programs. In all of these contexts, the need to understand and appreciate the current and potential health risks and behaviors of the elderly can support occupational therapy evaluation and interventions. It can also assist in helping other disciplines and society understand the impact of occupation in promoting health and preventing disability. In addition, it can assist the profession to be contributors to interdisciplinary efforts to promote continued participation in society.

Health Risks and Behaviors in Aging

In order to promote successful aging, occupational therapists and occupational therapy assistants need to be aware of the health risks that can impede successful aging and the health behaviors that can be fostered through occupation-centered interventions. The following section discusses some of these health risks and behaviors and how they impact occupational and social participation.

Social interactions enable older people to maintain physical and mental health and help prevent the need for health services (Federal Interagency Forum on Aging Related Statistics [FIFARS], 2004). Social activity includes activity that encompasses interactions with significant others, including family and friends.

Physical activity has also been noted to help people successfully age (Menec, 2003; Tabbarah, Crimmins, & Seeman, 2002; Vaillant, 2002). However, there are certain populations that experience numerous barriers of time, money, accessibility, or interest that limit engaging in physical activity of any kind. Content Box 23-4 identifies populations in the United States with low rates of physical activity. Occupational therapists can do much to increase the physical health of the elderly within the context of their living situation. Research has shown that physical activity improves mobility and overall functioning in even the frailest of individuals (Albert, 2004; Fiatarone et al., 1990, 1994; U.S. Department of Health and Human Services [USDHHS], 1996, 2000). It can prevent depression, reduce risk of some chronic conditions, and improve independent living and overall QOL (Butler, Davis, Lewis, Nelson, & Strauss, 1998). Introducing the elderly to the concept of engaging in physical meaningful occupations as health maintenance and prevention strategies can be the beginning of an occupational therapy prevention program regardless of the context in which therapy occurs.

Mental health of the elderly population is severely compromised by several losses experienced throughout the aging process. These can include loss of

---

Content Box 23-4

Populations in the United States With Low Rates of Physical Activity

- Women generally are less active than men at all ages.
- People with lower incomes and less education are typically not as physically active as those with higher incomes and higher education.
- African Americans and Hispanics are generally less physically active than whites.
- Adults in northeastern and southern states tend to be less active than adults in north central and western states.
- People with disabilities are less physically active than people without disabilities.

From *Healthy People 2010: Understanding and improving health* (2d ed., Populations with low rates of physical activity, ¶ 1), USDHHS, 2000, Washington, DC: U.S. Government Printing Office.

social support, occupational roles, meaningful occupational performance, and familiar environments. Depression can be a major psychosocial issue and is the most frequently occurring mental illness for the older adult. Depression in this population "may be due to changes such as: the loss of a spouse, the loss of peers, social isolation, stress of concurrent illnesses, retirement, the loss of one's home, and drug interactions" (Lewis, 2003, p. 75). The presence of depressive disorders and syndromes is as high as 20% to 25% for community-dwelling older adults and at least 25% for nursing home residents older than 65 (Riley, 2001). Depression is one of the most common negative outcomes of the caregiving process (Pruchno & Resch, 1989). Other factors can also lead to compromised mental health, especially depression, in older adults:

> Adults and older adults have the highest rates of depression. Major depression affects approximately twice as many women as men. Women who are poor, on welfare, less educated, unemployed, and from certain racial or ethnic populations are more likely to experience depression. In addition, depression rates are higher among older adults with coexisting medical conditions. For example, 12 percent of older persons hospitalized for problems such as hip fracture or heart disease are diagnosed with depression. Rates of depression for older persons in nursing homes range from 15 to 25 percent. (USDHHS, 2000, Populations with high rates of depression, ¶ 2)

Older adults are also at higher risk for viral infections. "In 1998, influenza immunization rates were 64 percent in adults 65 and older—almost double the 1989 immunization rate of 33 percent. In 1998, 46 percent of persons aged 65 years and older had never received a pneumococcal vaccine" (USDHHS, 2000, ¶ 3).

People with lower SES tend to have poorer eating habits, with some not being able to afford nutritious foods (Federal Interagency Forum on Aging Related Statistics, 2000).

> Nutrition is a key factor in growth, development, the maintenance of health, the recovery from acute illness, and the management of chronic disease. Throughout the life cycle, nutrition is essential to vitality and health. Building muscle strength, developing antibodies to potential invading microorganisms, maintaining immune function, preserving cellular integrity, healing wounds, and experiencing a general sense of well-being and an active lifestyle are all dependent on maintaining nutritional health. (Chernoff, 2001, p. 43)

The implications for occupational therapists and occupational therapy assistants include interventions that incorporate health information to help prevent health problems. In home management, interventions can be adapted based on knowledge of the client's SES, affordability of nutritious food items, and the impact of such on occupational habits, roles, and overall performance.

Factors Inhibiting Access to and Participation in Occupation

A selection of personal and environmental factors that are potential barriers to participation has been listed above. This is not an exhaustive list but illustrates factors that must be addressed in occupational therapy evaluation and interventions to promote health, wellbeing, and QOL for elderly individuals and the communities in which they reside. Other potential barriers that inhibit access to and participation in occupation are identified below.

Personal Factors

Personal factors can include but are not limited to client factors, roles, socioeconomic factors, disability, and psychosocial functioning. Client factors such as sensory functions of seeing and hearing, neuromusculoskeletal and movement-related functions, and cardiovascular function can affect functional performance (AOTA, 2008). Near vision declines starting around age 40, and the prevalence of eye diseases (e.g., diabetic retinopathy, age-related macular degeneration, glaucoma, cataracts) increases with age. In the United States, over 1 million persons aged 40 and over are currently blind, and approximately 2.4 million are visually impaired (National Eye Institute, 2002). In addition, the prevalence of general hearing loss increases from 25% for those aged 65 to 74 years to 40% for those older than 75 years (Hooper, 1994). Neuromusculoskeletal and movement-related functions affected by aging include functions of joints and bones, muscles, and movement. There is a slow progressive decline in muscle mass and strength with age. By age 75, muscle mass has decreased by half with associated declines in muscle strength (Evans, 1995). Muscle weakness can lead to impaired mobility and balance, thereby increasing the chance of falls.

Cardiovascular changes include the age-related anatomical and physiological changes of the heart and blood vessels. These changes result in reduced capacity for oxygen transport at rest, and during the movement needed to perform activities of daily living (ADLs), there is a greater need for oxygen (Dean, 1994).

Roles

Roles change throughout the life span and may be significantly different for the older adult. At 50 to 64 years of age, 80% of persons are in the workforce in the United States. This number drops to 56.4% for those aged 55 to 64 and then to 11.3% for those aged 65 to 74 (Sterns, Junkins, & Bayer, 2001). Losing the role of worker can contribute to financial decline and decreased feelings of productivity. Older adults may experience role reversal with children secondary to declining health or financial constraints. Major roles can be lost to the older adult due to death of loved ones. The major role of husband, wife, or partner is lost with the death of a significant other. Statistically, women outlive men by 7 years (Bonder, 2001) and widows are more likely to remain single for the rest of their lives. Contemporaries die, too, and friendships formed years ago are irreplaceable. In addition to role losses, role changes may occur. For example, a spouse may have assumed a caregiver role. Caregivers have been found to suffer burnout from stress, and stress, physical illness, and psychological distress have all been linked to the caregiver's role (Riley, 2001). This makes caregiver health and wellness an important concern for occupational therapists (see Chapter 20). Aged caregivers may be in fragile health themselves and may have limited resources to share their caregiving responsibilities. They may also have had to forgo paid employment to care for the spouse full-time, thereby adding to financial distress.

Current State of Practice in Occupational Therapy

As stated earlier, occupational therapists are well equipped to address adaptation, modification, and compensation for environmental and personal factors inhibiting the aging adult. The occupational therapy profession is familiar with concepts such as aging in place, universal design, Lifestyle Redesign, and life review reminiscence, which are briefly reviewed here.

Aging in Place

Aging in place allows the older adult to remain in his or her present residence as long as possible. In 1995, the American Association of Retired Persons (AARP) reported 28% of those over age 60 have lived in their current residence for more than 30 years. Usually older adults need to make modifications to their current residence to allow for age-related changes. Environmental factors can facilitate occupational participation (Law, 2002), and home modifications that promote livability or a good "person-environment" fit can help elders age in place (Liebig, 1999). These modifications can include handrails, grab bars, ramps, wide doorways, and seating in showers or tubs.

Universal Design

Unlike the aging-in-place concentration on the older adult, universal design focuses on the needs and abilities of all people throughout the life span (Rosto, 2003). The Institution of the Americans with Disabilities Act in 1990 established universal design standards. **Universal design** is a means of planning by "taking into consideration the needs and abilities of all people throughout the life span, regardless of age, stature, size or disability" (Rosto, 2003, p. 59). Universal design generally encompasses abilities in broad contexts such as housing, public buildings, and parks rather than on an individual level (Ringaert, 2002).

Lifestyle Redesign

Lifestyle Redesign is a preventive occupational therapy process in which clients are guided through an "occupational self-analysis" (Jackson, Carlson, Mandel, Zemke, & Clark, 1998, p. 330) in order to modify patterns of occupational engagement to maximize quality of life and health. Actual engagement in occupations is a critically important aspect of the process. The term *Lifestyle redesign* was developed during a significant occupational therapy research investigation known as the Well Elderly study, which will be discussed later in this chapter. This and subsequent efforts have shown the technique to be an efficacious and cost-effective preventive occupational therapy intervention with well, older adults (Clark et al., 2001; Clark, Carlson, Jackson, & Mandel, 2003). A practical manual is available that provides details about philosophical and theoretical foundations of the process, as well as tools for developing interventions to enhance independence and quality of life in older adults (Mandel, Jackson, Zemke, Nelson, & Clark, 1999).

Life Review Reminiscence

Life review reminiscence allows the older adult to reexamine important events, role transitions, and coping strategies used in adjusting to life's changes (Stevens-Ratchford, 1996). Stevens-Ratchford (1993) and Burnside (1994) indicate life review reminiscence to be a positive and worthwhile experience for older persons. Lewis (2003) suggests groups may be helpful in promoting the life review process. Groups recommended include

- collage group of an important positive experience;
- quilting group of life's experiences;

- development of life story photograph albums;
- "drawing or painting of an important moment in one's life" (Lewis, 2003, p. 178); and
- "writing or taping one's life story" (Lewis, 2003, p. 178).

Health Promotion and Participation

Bonder (2001) points out that the majority of factors that promote good health, such as good nutrition, exercise, and avoidance of harmful substances, are within the control of the individual. Other factors associated with good health are a good social support system, a sense of spiritual fulfillment, positive coping mechanisms, and a satisfying array of occupations (Bonder, 2001).

Older adults often develop acute, then chronic, conditions such as heart disease, arthritis, osteoporosis, and weight problems. Over the years, they become habituated to living with a "few aches and pains" and may have difficulty changing occupational routines, habits, and patterns to accommodate preventive occupations. Often, getting a person to recognize the health benefits of preventive occupations is one of the most difficult tasks of an occupational therapy practitioner.

Motivation for changing habits and unhealthy occupational patterns include

1. perceived threats to health (having diabetes with increasing complications may provoke a change in behavior);
2. perceived benefits (achieving the goal of not becoming diabetic through weight loss); or
3. beliefs about personal skills, the ability to change, and the ability to overcome barriers (Prochaska, 1979).

These motivators are reflected in the Stages of Change Theory, or Transtheoretical Model (TTM) developed by Prochaska (1979). (See Chapter 3 for more details on this model.) Tables 23-1 and 23-2 provide examples of the TTM as related to behavior change in the elderly.

Health Promotion Program Examples

There are numerous health promotion programs developed and implemented by occupational therapists, occupational therapy assistants, and nonoccupational therapists who are committed to promoting successful aging. Several of them are described here.

Most occupational therapists are now familiar with the Well Elderly study. It was based on the premise that the ability to experience meaning in the context of one's occupations is a key component of successful aging (Clark et al., 1991; Jackson, 1996). Results from the Well Elderly study suggested that preventative occupational therapy programs might moderate against the health risks of independent-living older adults (Clark et al., 1997). Elders in the study receiving lifestyle redesign, a preventative occupational therapy technique, demonstrated significant benefits in health, function, and QOL. Whereas, in areas of significant benefits, control subjects who participated in a social activity program or who received no treatment tended to decline over the 9-month study period (Clark et al., 1997).

The Senior Wellness Project (CDC, 2004) uses both a client- and occupation-centered approach to enrich the lives of the elderly. It is a low-cost behavioral change program that includes exercise programs and classes on self-management of chronic conditions. A study undertaken by the Northshore Senior Center initiated the Lifetime Fitness Program, developed from such positive results as decreased physical pain and depression among participants.

The Health Enhancement Program was developed from a University of Washington study. Participants were referred from various local sources and were seen by a registered nurse and social worker. Participants were provided with a health self-evaluation, and the nurse practitioner helped participants identify self-determined health goals. Every 6 months there is a health program update for the participant and the physician. Available to participants is the nurse, social worker, and a health mentor. The **health mentor** is "a trained community-based volunteer who may accompany the participant to exercise classes, provide weekly calls and support, or engage in other activities supporting the participant in reaching health goals" (CDC, 2004, Phase 2, Senior Wellness Project, p. 1). The fee is sliding scale donations, and the health department pays for a nurse at five sites and interpreters as needed. In addition, a "University of Washington geriatrician assists in evaluating the program. Program outcome data is analyzed separately at the University. The results of the study found a 72 percent decrease in length of hospital stay and a 38 percent reduction in cases of hospitalization" (CDC, 2004, Phase 2, Senior Wellness Project, p. 1).

A chronic disease self-management program is based on a research model of self-management for chronic conditions (CDC, 2004). It is a 6-week course taught by peers who are usually older adults with chronic conditions. "The course helps participants develop short-term goals; provides information on nutrition, exercise and relaxation techniques; and acts as an educational group. It is designed to enhance

Table 23–1 **Stages of Behavior Change According to the Transtheoretical Model (TTM)**

Description	Motivational Issues	Techniques for Moving to Next Stage	Descriptive Phrases	Time
Precontemplative Stage The individual is not thinking about change and may not even want to know about the health issue; defensive.	The individual may be unaware of the health issues, demoralized over past failures; negative aspects of the change are more evident than the benefits.	Especially defensive when presented with action statements such as "quit smoking." Family or friends expressing how this behavior affects them may effect change. Individuals may be emotionally moved by the death of a loved one from a similar illness. Success in changing one behavior may influence changing others.	I won't.	This stage may be extended over months and years. People may leave and return to this stage.
Contemplative Stage The individual is thinking about change but is still ambivalent. Problem behavior is under examination.	An individual may not know how to change the behavior or how to begin the change.	Reinforcement for change from all sectors.	I may.	This stage may also take a long time. People may cycle in and out many times.
Preparation Stage The individual begins weighing the pros and the cons. As the pros become more compelling, the person begins to think about the advantages of behavior change. Plan of action unites with intent.	There may be fear about ability to enter the action phase or there may be grieving.	Often coming to classes and seeking information supports the change.	I will.	Action comes within a month. Again, time varies depending on moving to another stage and returning.
Action Stage The individual begins to perform the behavior and feels in control. Individual frequently turns to others for assistance and support.	A need to specify the terms for success becomes important to see the advantages of the behavior. Develop specific goals such as 20 minutes of exercise 3 times per week.	At this point, making environment as encouraging as possible to reach success is most important.	I am now.	This stage lasts approximately 6 months. The individual may cycle in and out of it.

Table 23–1 Stages of Behavior Change According to theTranstheoretical Model (TTM)—cont'd

Precontemplative Stage

Description	Motivational Issues	Techniques for Moving to Next Stage	Descriptive Phrases	Time
Maintenance Stage Individual is preventing relapse to past habits.		Providing rewards and incentives and sharing successes help encourage continuation of the new healthy behavior. Incentives can include becoming a teacher for this particular behavior change or serving as a role model.	I have.	Doing the behavior for more than 6 months. Lapses may occur, but generally the individual maintains a health routine.

From "Chapter 1: Introduction, stages of behavior change" in *Blue print for health promotion* by the American Society on Aging, n.d., U.S. Centers for Disease Control and Prevention. Copyright © 2002–2006, by the American Society on Aging. Available at http://www.asaging.org/cdc/module1/home.cfm. Adapted with permission.

Table 23–2 Three Required Conditions Necessary for Change

	Key Questions	Sample Questions	Resolution
Importance of the Change	*Why?* Why should I do it? What are the benefits? What are the costs?	How severe is the problem? Will it hurt me? What is the risk for me? Is it likely that this will affect me? What are the advantages to changing my behavior?	If the following conditions are met, there is reason to change: 1. The disease seems harmful. 2. The person's susceptibility is high. 3. The benefits are worthwhile. 4. The pros outweigh the cons.
Confidence in the Ability to Change	*What? How?* Am I able to do this? How can I do this? What will change?	What are the barriers to changing? What will make it difficult? Am I able to make this change? Will I be able to follow through?	If a person believes that he or she is capable of (1) making the change and (2) coping with the difficult aspects, it is likely that person will change.
Readiness to Change	*When?* At what time? What are my present priorities?	When are the changes easiest and most difficult to make? What makes this change important now?	The older person must 1. Feel prepared to make the change. 2. Decide when to change. 3. Give the change a priority.

From "Chapter 1: Introduction, Ripening the conditions for change" in *Blue print for health promotion* by the American society on Aging, n.d., U.S. Centers for Disease Control and Prevention. Copyright © 2002–2006, by the American Society on Aging. Adapted with permission.

regular treatment and to educate older adults on techniques for managing chronic conditions" (CDC, 2004, Phase 2, Senior Wellness Project, p. 1).

OASIS HealthStages is the health promotion strategy for OASIS, a national program designed to enrich the lives of older adults. HealthStages includes three components:

1. A state-of-the-art curriculum
2. An implementation model that is tailored to meet the needs and interests of the program's 25 local sites
3. A comprehensive evaluation model. HealthStages includes health curricula in seven areas: physical activity, nutrition, mental wellness, memory, sensory health, disease management, and general health promotion

The program emphasizes healthy aging by helping participants set personal goals and develop self-management skills through a combination of local OASIS health classes and national HealthStages courses. HealthStages provides a variety of learning opportunities for people at different stages of readiness to make health behavior changes. Course offerings are categorized by goal: awareness, knowledge, skill building, or maintenance of behavior change (CDC, 2004). Table 23-3 highlights topics in classes offered and the stage of the TTM model to which it relates.

Social influences can impact transforming illness to wellness through engaging in health-promoting behaviors. Other influences include personal exploration (i.e., assessing one's health values and priorities) and the timing of interventions (e.g., low self-efficacy and lack of confidence that a certain behavior can be changed might indicate decreasing the time spent on that intervention until such time as the older person indicates some readiness).

A pilot occupational therapy wellness program called Designing a Life of Wellness was developed by Matuska, Giles-Heinz, Flinn, Neighbor, and Bass-Haugen (2003). The program had 65 older adults (aged 70 to 92), participants from three different senior apartment complexes, and individuals living in the community in the Midwest. The program lasted for 6 months and consisted of weekly 1-hour educational classes taught by occupational therapy faculty members with the

Table 23–3 OASIS HealthStages Course Topics Related to the TTM Model

	STAGE			
Class Level	**Awareness (Precontemplation/ Contemplation)**	**Knowledge (Contemplation/ Preparation)**	**Skill-Building/ Behavior Change (Action)**	**Maintenance (Maintenance)**
General Health Promotion		Taking Charge of Your Health	Healthy Body, Healthy Mind	
Physical Activity/Fitness		Staying on Your Feet	Building Bones Exerstart! Improving Your Balance	
Nutrition	Personal Eating Plan (PEP)		Food Fitness	
Mental Health/Wellness		It's the Thought That Counts	Positive Attitudes, Positive Aging	
Disease Management		Medication Matters	Exercising Control: Managing Your Diabetes	
Memory			Memory Dynamics	
Sensory Health			Staying Active	

From "Chapter 1: Introduction, Example 2-OASIS HealthStages" in *Blue print for health promotion* by the American Society on Aging, n.d., U.S. Centers for Disease Control and Prevention. Copyright © 2002–2006, by the American Society on Aging. Adapted with permission.

assistance of occupational therapy students on their Level II fieldwork experience. The focus of the program was on teaching the importance of engagement in meaningful occupations to improve QOL and the removal of personal and environmental barriers to participation. Results from this pilot study, using pretest and posttest scores of the SF-36 Health Survey, demonstrated significantly increased QOL in vitality, social functioning, and the mental health summary score. Overall, the mean standard scores in all eight subscales of the SF-36 increased. In addition, the number of participants who communicated with family, friends, or support persons at least three times a week increased from 47% to 56%; participation in social or community activities rose from 47% to 66%. Participants who were able to drive yet had low attendance in the wellness program increased activities with family. Overall satisfaction with the program was rated as good or excellent by 87% of respondents. This study provides additional evidence of the benefits of health-promotion programs provided by occupational therapy students and faculty teams with the elderly.

Occupational therapists can work from an environmental perspective and explore contextual factors that may impede participation and that impact health-promoting behaviors. An older person may limit going out to shop or when using public transportation because of the safety factors involved within a community. Social support and context (i.e., social, physical, cultural, personal, spiritual, temporal, virtual) can contribute to a positive self-image, a sense of purpose, and empowerment. This can support occupational engagement.

Health Literacy

Health literacy is important to consider in occupational therapy health promotion assessment and interventions, particularly when promoting successful aging.

> Appropriate health literacy is essential to health promotion, particularly as we address issues of primary prevention. A health literate individual is more apt to know how to answer the question "How do I keep myself well?" Adequate health literacy may be of even greater importance in secondary prevention, as ineffective communication between health providers and patients can result in medical errors due to misinformation about medications and self-care instructions. (Selden, Zorn, Ratzan, & Parker, 2000, Health Literacy, ¶ 4)

Healthy People 2010 defines **health literacy** as the degree to which individuals have the capacity to obtain, process, and understand basic health information and services needed to make appropriate health decisions (USDHHS, 2000, Chapter 11, Health Communication). Specifically, **functional health literacy** is defined as

"the ability to read and comprehend prescription bottles, appointment slips, and the other essential health related materials required to successfully function as a patient" (American Medical Association, 1999, p. 552).

> Health literacy is increasingly vital to help people navigate a complex health system and better manage their own health. Differences in the ability to read and understand materials related to personal health as well as navigate the health system appear to contribute to health disparities. People with low health literacy are more likely to report poor health, have an incomplete understanding of their health problems and treatment, and be at greater risk of hospitalization. (USDHHS, 2000, Chapter 11, Health Communication)

Occupational therapists are expert in developing and transmitting health-promoting information. Elderly people may benefit from both auditory and visual cues to reinforce learning. Some strategies can include the following:

- Supplement text with pictures
- Tailor medication schedules or health promotion activities to fit a person's daily routine, using daily events as reminders
- Use clear captions, ample white space, and pictures or diagrams to attract the reader's attention and reinforce the message
- Limit a publication to one or two educational objectives
  - What the reader will learn
  - What the reader will do after reading the publication (CDC, 2004)

Conclusion

The future of occupational therapy in supporting successful aging rests with educators to adequately train for future practice with practitioners to open their hearts, and minds to integrate health and wellness in practice with older adults, and with researchers to explore relationships between meaningful occupational engagement and successful aging. The time has come to shape the profession's future and powerfully support the development of a healthier society in which older people can thrive and flourish. Care needs to be taken to

> be more creative and effective in developing intervention programs to encourage successful aging . . . to develop effective programs, . . . to train a whole new generation of experts to be a different kind of expert—an expert who not only provides people with information but also, with humility, helps people achieve the goals they care about most in their lives. (Syme, 2003, p. 402)

The key points to remember about promoting healthy and successful aging are the following:

- Successful aging from an occupational therapy perspective is having the physical, emotional, social, and spiritual resources, combined with an ability to adapt to life changes, in order to engage in meaningful and important self-selected occupations of life as one ages.
- Maintaining interpersonal relations and skills and actively engaging in productive activities that are meaningful (paid or unpaid), in combination with lack of disease and good function (cognitive and physical), are integral to successful aging.
- Potential to successfully age with a disability is likely if health care shifts focus from cure to care, which implies placing greater emphasis on preventing further dysfunction.
- Occupational therapy practitioners need to be knowledgeable about health risks and behaviors in order to best intervene with the elderly and promote successful aging.
- Health literacy is increasingly vital to help people navigate a complex health system and better manage their own health.
- It is crucial that occupational therapists and occupational therapy assistants work diligently to provide up-to-date health education and develop community-based health promotion programs that help the elderly maintain and optimize health, wellness, and QOL.

Case Study 23-1

Part I

Helen is a 79-year-old woman living in her own home that she bought with her husband of 60 years. They live in an urban area where all the conveniences needed for daily living are within walking distance. There is a park three blocks from their home.

Helen is usually an optimistic person, one who has always believed that when "life hands you lemons, you make a lot of lemonade." Recently, Helen chooses to access a community-based occupational therapy office that specializes in health and wellness. Her primary reason for this is to "stay healthy as long as I can because I have to care for my husband, who is ill."

Questions

1. What questions would you ask Helen in the initial occupational history interview? Present a rationale for each one.
2. What theoretical approach would you use to frame your questions and potential interventions? Why?

Part II

You discover that Helen presents with a past history of osteoarthritis and cardiomegaly and smokes 10 cigarettes per day. She is short of breath climbing only 5 stairs (she has 12 to the second floor of her home). Helen's primary interests have included gardening, boating, writing nonfiction, and playing bridge. She used to go to Bingo three times a week but has given up much of her leisure activity because "I don't want to leave Henry alone for too long," even though he has a full-time aide.

Questions

1. From this new information, what can you glean of Helen's background? Do you think it is important to ask questions of her early history? Why or why not?
2. What health and wellness interventions would you discuss with Helen? Provide at least five with a rationale for each.
3. How would you communicate their importance to the client?
4. What are some psychosocial issues with which Helen is coping? How would you incorporate Helen's own beliefs into the psychosocial interventions?
5. What theoretical model(s) might you use to support your interventions?
6. From the chapter, what are at least four principles of successful aging from which Helen can benefit?

▶ For Discussion and Review

1. How is successful aging defined by various age groups and ethnic communities?
2. What habits and occupational patterns have you developed that can lead to your own successful aging?
3. What habits and occupational patterns might you wish to change and why? How do these affect your emotional, physical, social, spiritual, and other areas of health?
4. If you interviewed someone in your life that you consider has successfully aged, what advice do you believe they would provide?

▶ Research Questions

1. How effective is an occupation-based program as compared to a non-occupation-centered program in the promotion of successful aging?
2. Is successful aging determined by personal choice, beliefs, habits, context, or a combination of these factors? Which factors exert the greatest influence?
3. What evidence exists for aging in place, Lifestyle Redesign, and other occupation-based health promotion programs?

References

Albert, S. M. (2004). *Public health and aging: An introduction to maximizing function and well-being.* New York: Springer.

American Association of Retired Persons. (1995). *Understanding senior housing for the 1990's: Survey of consumer preferences, consensus, and needs.* Washington, DC, PF4522 (593)D 13899.

American Medical Association, Council on Scientific Affairs Ad Hoc Committee on Health Literacy. (1999). Health literacy: Report of the Council on Scientific Affairs. *Journal of the American Medical Association (JAMA), 281*(6), 552–57.

American Occupational Therapy Association. (2002). Occupational therapy practice framework: Domain and process. *American Journal of Occupational Therapy, 56,* 609–39.

American Society on Aging. (n.d.). *Blueprint for health promotion.* Retrieved April 26, 2008, from http://www.asaging.org/cdc/module1/phase1/index.cfm.

Ashok, B. T., & Ali, R. (1999). The aging paradox: Free radical theory of aging. *Experimental Gerontology, 34,* 293–303.

Baltes, P. B. (1997). On the incomplete architecture of human ontogeny: Selection, optimization, and compensation as foundation of developmental theory. *American Psychologist, 52,* 366–80.

Baltes, P. B., & Baltes, M. M. (1990). Psychological perspectives on successful aging: The model of selective optimization with compensation. In P. B. Baltes & M. M. Baltes (Eds.), *Successful aging: Perspectives from the behavioral sciences* (pp. 1–34). Cambridge, UK: Cambridge University Press.

Bandura, A. (1997). Self-efficacy: Toward a unifying theory of behavioral change. *Psychological Review, 84*(2), 191–215.

Baum, M. C. (2003). Editorial: Participation: Its relationship to occupation and health. *Occupational Therapy Journal of Research, 23*(2), 46–47.

Belmont, M. F., & Harris, A. (2002). Health promotion for elderly clients. In C. B. Lewis (Ed.), *Aging: The healthcare challenge* (4th ed., pp. 193–203). Philadelphia: F. A. Davis.

Bjorksten, J. (1976). The cross linkage theory of aging: Clinical implications. *Comprehensive Therapy II,* 65–74.

Bonder, B. R. (2001). Wellness. In B. R. Bonder & M. B. Wagner (Eds.), *Functional performance in older adults* (2d ed., pp. 321–38). Philadelphia: F. A. Davis.

Burnside, I. (1994). Reminiscence and life review: Therapeutic interventions for older people. *Nurse Practitioner,* 55–61.

Butler, R. N., Davis, R., Lewis, C. B., Nelson, M. E., & Stauss, E. (1998). Physical fitness: Benefits of exercise for the older patient. *Geriatrics, 53*(10), 46–62.

Carlson, J. C., & Riley, J. C. M. (1998). A consideration of some notable aging theories. *Experimental Gerontology 33,* 127.

Carstensen, L. L. (1991). Selectivity theory: Social activity in life-span context. *Annual Review of Gerontology and Geriatrics, 11,* 195–217.

Centers for Disease Control and Prevention. (2003, February 14). Public health and aging: Trends in aging—United States and worldwide. *Morbidity and Mortality Weekly Report, 52*(06), 101–06.

Centers for Disease Control and Prevention. (2004). *Live well, live long: Health promotion and disease prevention for older adults.* Retrieved August 16, 2004, from http://www.asaging.org/cdc/module1/phase1/phase1_2b.cfm.

Chernoff, R. (2001). Nutrition. In E. A. Swanson, T. Tripp-Reimer, & K. Buckwalter (Eds.), *Health promotion and disease prevention in the older adult.* New York: Springer.

Christiansen, C. H., Clark, F., Kielhofner, G., & Rogers, J. (1995). Position paper: Occupation. *American Journal of Occupational Therapy, 49*(10), 1015–18.

Clark, F., Azen, S. P., Carlson, M., Mandel, D., LaBree, L., Hay, J., et al. (2001). Embedding health promotion changes into the daily lives of independent-living older adults: Long-term follow-up of occupational therapy intervention. *Journal of Gerontology: Psychological Sciences, 56*(1) 60–63.

Clark, F., Azen, S. P., Zemke, R., Jackson, J., Carlson, M., Mandel, D., et al. (1997). Occupational therapy for independent-living older adults. *Journal of the American Medical Association (JAMA), 278*(16), 1321–26.

Clark, F. A., Carlson, M., Jackson J., & Mandel, D. (2003). Lifestyle redesign: Improves health and is cost effective. *OT Practice 8,* 9–13.

Clark, F. A., Parham, D., Carlson, M. E., Frank, F., Jackson, J., Pierce, D., et al. (1991). Occupational science: Academic innovation in the service of occupational therapy's future. *American Journal of Occupational Therapy, 45,* 300–10.

Cristofalo, V. J., Tresini, M., Francis, M. K., & Volker, C. (1999). Biological theories of senescence. In V. L. Bengtson & K. W. Schaie (Eds.), *Handbook of theories of aging* (pp. 98–112). New York: Springer Publishing.

Crowther, M. R., Parker, M. W., Achenbaum, W. A., Larimore, W. L., & Koenig, H. G. (2002). Rowe and Kahn's model of successful aging revisited: Positive spirituality—The forgotten factor. *Gerontologist, 42*(5), 613–20.

Cummings, E., & Henry, W. E. (1961). *Growing old and the process of disengagement.* New York: Basic Book.

Curtis, H. J. (1961). Biological mechanisms underlying the aging process. *Science, 141,* 686–94.

Dean, E. (1994). Cardiopulmonary development. In B. R. Bonder & M. B. Wagner (Eds.), *Functional performance in older adults* (2d ed., pp. 86–120). Philadelphia: F. A. Davis.

Erikson, E. H. (1982). *The life cycle-review.* New York: W. W. Norton.

Evans, W. J. (1995). Effects of exercise on body composition and functional capacity of the elderly. *Journal of Gerontology, 50*(A), 147–50.

Federal Interagency Forum on Aging Related Statistics. (2004). *Older Americans 2004: Key indicators of well-being.* Washington, DC: Author.

Fiatarone, M. A., Marks, E. C., Ryan, N. D., Meredith, C. N., Lipsitz, L. A., & Evans, W. J. (1990). High intensity strength training in nonagenarians: Effects on skeletal muscle. *Journal of the American Medical Association, 263,* 3029–34.

Fiatarone, M. A., O'Neil, E. F., Ryan, N. D., Clements, K. M., Solares, G. R., & Nelson, M. E. (1994). Exercise training and nutritional supplementation for physical frailty in very elderly people. *New England Journal of Medicine, 330,* 1769–75.

Fulmer, T., Wallace, M., & Edelman, C. L. (2002). Older adult. In C. L. Edelman & C. L. Mandle (Eds.), *Health promotion throughout the lifespan* (pp. 709–46). St Louis, MO: Mosby.

Harman, D. (1956). A theory based on free radical and radiation chemistry. *Journal of Gerontology, 11,* 298–300.

Hooper, C. R. (1994). Sensory and sensory integrative development. In B. R. Bonder & M. B. Wagner (Eds.), *Functional performance in older adults* (2d ed., pp. 121–37). Philadelphia: F. A. Davis.

Idler, E. L., & Benyamini, Y. (1997). Self-reported health and mortality: A review of twenty-seven community studies. *Journal of Health and Social Behavior, 38,* 21–37.

Inui, T. S. (2003). The need for an integrated biopsychosocial approach to research on successful aging. *Annals of Internal Medicine, 139,* 391–94.

Jackson, J. (1996). Living a meaningful existence in old age. In R. Zemke & F. Clark (Eds.), *Occupational science: The evolving discipline* (pp. 339–61). Philadelphia: F. A. Davis.

Jackson, J., Carlson, M., Mandel, D., Zemke, R., & Clark, F. (1998). Occupation in lifestyle redesign: The Well Elderly Study Occupational Therapy Program. *American Journal of Occupational Therapy, 52*(5), 326–36.

Kane, R. L. (2003). The contribution of geriatric health services research to successful aging. *Annals of Internal Medicine, 139,* 460–62.

Kinsella, K., & Velkoff, V. A. (2001). *U.S. Census Bureau, Series P95/01-1, An aging world: 2001.* U.S. Government Printing Office. Retrieved October 31, 2003, from http://quickfacts.census.gov/qfd/states/00000.html.

Law, M. (2002). Participation in the occupations of everyday life. *American Journal of Occupational Therapy, 56*(5), 640–48.

Lewis, S. C. (2003). *Elder care in occupational therapy.* Thorofare: NJ: SLACK.

Liebig, P. S. (1999). Using home modifications to promote self-maintenance and mutual care: The case of old-age homes in India. In E. D. Taira & J. L. Carlson (Eds.), *Aging in place: Designing, adaptation, and enhancing the home environment* (pp. 79–99). New York: Haworth Press.

Mandel, D., Jackson, J., Zemke, R., Nelson, L., & Clark, F. A. (1999). *Lifestyle redesign: Implementing the Well Elderly Program.* Bethesda, MD: American Occupational Therapy Association.

Matuska, K., Giles-Heinz, A., Flinn, N., Neighbor, M., & Bass-Haugen, J. (2003). Outcomes of a pilot occupational therapy wellness program for older adults. *American Journal of Occupational Therapy 57,* 220–24.

Menec, V. H. (2003). The relation between everyday activities and successful aging: A 6-year longitudinal study. *Journal of Gerontology: Social Sciences, 59B*(2), S74–S82.

Mezirow, J. (1991). *Transformative dimensions of adult learning.* San Francisco: Jossey-Bass.

Minkler, M., & Fadem, P. (2002). Successful aging: A disability perspective. *Journal of Disability Policy Studies, 12*(4), 229–35.

National Eye Institute. (2002). *More Americans facing blindness than ever before.* Retrieved July 28, 2002, from http://www.nih.gov/news/pr/mar2002/nei-20.htm.

Neugarten, B. L., Havighurst, R. J., & Tobin, S. S. (1968). Personality and patterns of aging. In B. L. Neugarten (Ed.), *Middle age and aging.* Chicago: University of Chicago Press.

Orgel, L. E. (1963). The maintenance of the accuracy of protein synthesis and its relevance to aging. *Proceedings of the National Academy of Science USA, 49,* 517–21.

Pearl, R. (1928). *The rate of living.* New York: Alfred Knoph.

Peck, R. C. (1968). Psychological developments in the second half of life. In B. L. Neugarten (Ed.), *Middle age and aging.* Chicago: University of Chicago Press.

Prochaska, J. O. (1979). *Systems of psychotherapy: A transtheoretical analysis.* Homewood, IL: Dorsey Press.

Pruchno, R., & Resch, N. L. (1989). Husbands and wives as caregivers: Antecedents of depression and burden. *Gerontologist 29,* 159–65.

Riley, K. P. (2001). Depression. In B. R. Bonder & M. B. Wagner (Eds.), *Functional performance in older adults* (2d ed., pp. 305–18). Philadelphia: F. A. Davis.

Ringaert, L. (2002). Universal design and occupational therapy. *OT NOW. Chronicle of the World Health Organization, 1*(1), 29–40.

Rosto, L. (2003). Designing for life. *Advance for directors in rehabilitation 1*(1), 59–60; 79.

Rowe, J. W., & Kahn, R. L. (1997). Successful aging. *Gerontologist, 37,* 433–40.

Ruffing-Rahal, M. A. (1991). Rationale and design for health promotion with older adults. *Public Health Nursing, 8,* 258–63.

Selden, C. R., Zorn, M., Ratzan, S. C., & Parker, R. M. (2000). Current bibliographies in medicine 2000–2001. Retrieved August 30, 2004, from http://www.nlm.nih.gov/pubs/cbm/hliteracy.html#04.

Sterns, H. L., Junkins, M. P., & Bayer, J. G. (2001). In B. R. Bonder & M. B. Wagner (Eds.), *Functional performance in older adults* (2d ed., pp. 179–95). Philadelphia: F. A. Davis.

Stevens-Ratchford, R. G. (1993). The effect of life review reminiscence activities on depression and self-esteem in older adults. *American Journal of Occupational Therapy, 47*(5), 413–20.

Stevens-Ratchford, R. G. (1996). Occupational therapy services within the rehabilitation health care system. In K. O. Larson, R. G. Stevens-Ratchford, L. Pedretti, & J. L. Crabtree (Eds.), *The role of OT with the elderly* (2d ed., pp. 307–28). Bethesda, MD: American Occupational Therapy Association.

Syme, S. L. (2003). Psychosocial interventions to improve successful aging. *Annals of Internal Medicine, 139,* 400–02.

Tabbarah, M., Crimmins, E. M., & Seeman, T. E. (2002). The relationship between cognitive and physical performance: MacArthur studies of successful aging. *Journal of Gerontology: Medical Sciences, 57A*(4), M228–M235.

U.S. Department of Health and Human Services. (1996). *Physical activity and health: A report of the Surgeon General.* Atlanta: Centers for Disease Control and Prevention, National Center for Chronic Disease Prevention and Health Promotion.

U.S. Department of Health and Human Services. (2000). *Healthy People 2010: Understanding and improving health* (2d ed.). Washington, DC: U.S. Government Printing Office.

Vaillant, G. E. (2002). *Aging well.* New York: Little, Brown & Company.

Walford, R. L. (1974). The immunologic theory of aging: Current status. *Federal Proceedings 33,* 2020.

World Health Organization. (1947). Constitution of the World Health Organization. *Chronicle of the World Health Organization, 1*(1), 29–40.

Chapter 24

Preventing Falls Among Community-Dwelling Older Adults

Kimberly Mansfield Caldeira and S. Maggie Reitz

> Globally, an estimated 391,000 people died due to falls in 2002, making it the 2nd leading cause of unintentional injury death globally after road traffic injuries.
>
> In all regions of the world, adults over the age of 70 years, particularly females, have significantly higher fall-related mortality rates than younger people.
>
> —World Health Organization (WHO), 2006, ¶ 2

Learning Objectives

This chapter is designed to enable the reader to:

- Describe the epidemiology of falls and fall-related injuries.
- Discuss the costs of falls and fall-related injuries among older adults at the individual, community, and society levels.
- Identify the risk factors associated with falls among community-dwelling older adults.
- Apply the evidence on fall risk factors to a comprehensive occupational therapy evaluation.

- Identify the elements of effective fall prevention interventions.
- Apply the evidence on fall prevention interventions to occupation-based interventions.
- Explain the role of occupational therapy in an interdisciplinary, health promotion approach to fall prevention.

Key Terms

Behavioral risk factors	Intrinsic risk factors	Near-fall	Slip
Environmental press	Multifactorial	Orthostatic hypotension	Targeted intervention
Extrinsic risk factors	Multifactorial intervention	Polypharmacy	Trip
Fall		Situational factors	Untargeted intervention

Introduction

In the United States, fall prevention has been identified as a national priority for health promotion and prevention. Recognizing that "falls are the most common cause of injuries and hospital admissions for trauma among elderly persons," the U.S. Department of Health and Human Services (USDHHS) calls for a reduction in the rate of hip fractures for men and women aged 65 years and older (USDHHS, 2000, p. 15–39). The target is a 61% reduction for women (from 1056 to 416 per 100,000) and an 88% reduction for men (from 593 to 74 per 100,000). The foundation necessary for the development of an occupation-based approach to fall prevention for older adults living in the community is provided in this chapter. The numerous and often interrelated factors contributing to falls are explained, followed by a review of evidence-based guidelines for effective interventions and a discussion of the role of occupational therapy in fall prevention.

Without disregarding the problem of falls among older adults in hospitals, nursing homes, and other institutional settings, this chapter focuses on risk factors and programmatic issues specific to community-dwelling older adults, who reside in houses, apartments, or other homes privately owned or rented by themselves, their family, or their friends. Health promotion programs that incorporate fall prevention in community-based settings are a vital part of national public health efforts to enable the growing population of older adults to maintain independent, active, healthy lifestyles while remaining in their own homes as they age. Furthermore, although the prevention of falls among other age groups is a worthwhile pursuit as a component of general injury-prevention programs, it is beyond the scope of this chapter.

Background of the Problem

Each year an estimated 30% to 60% of community-dwelling older adults experience a fall, and about half of these experience multiple falls (Rubenstein & Josephson, 2002). Although other populations such as children and athletes have a higher incidence of noninjurious falls, falls are a more serious concern among older adults because of the high prevalence of chronic illness and age-related changes that make even minor falls potentially disastrous (Rubenstein & Josephson, 2002). In fact, the rate of fall-related deaths in the United States is over three times higher for adults aged 65 to 84 and nearly 23 times greater for adults 85 years and older, as compared to the overall population rate (USDHHS, 2000).

Terminology

In general, a **fall** can be defined as a loss of balance resulting in a person suddenly and unintentionally coming to rest on the floor, ground, or other lower surface, with or without ensuing injury. Often this definition excludes falls that involve loss of consciousness, acute medical conditions such as cerebrovascular accidents (CVAs) or myocardial infarction, or traumatic environmental events such as motor vehicle crashes. Syncope, also known as *fainting, loss of consciousness,* or *blacking out,* occurs when there is decreased blood flow to the brain and can be caused by a number of conditions (Mathias, Deguchi, & Schatz, 2001). Falls resulting from syncope are more difficult to document due to memory lapses and poor recall. Some studies have suggested that syncopal falls are more likely to result in serious injuries than nonsyncopal falls (Rubenstein & Josephson, 2002). Prevention of syncope requires specific medical interventions and therefore is not emphasized in this discussion of fall prevention.

Many falls result from slips and trips. A **slip** occurs when the foot slides out from underneath the person, while a **trip** occurs when the person stumbles over an object obstructing their pathway (Steinberg, Cartwright, Peel, & Williams, 2000). Normally in a slip or trip, the person regains balance before falling, so the event is called a **near-fall.** A fall only results when balance cannot be regained. Note that falls and near-falls can also be caused by a loss of balance associated with other activities such as reaching, rushing, or other imprudent maneuvering.

Economic Cost

Falls are a costly problem among older adults, in terms of both personal costs to the individual and economic costs to society. On the personal level, falls result in injuries ranging from minor (e.g., bruises and lacerations) to severe (e.g., fractures and head injuries), many of which are costly in terms of losses in functional independence and quality of life (QOL). While the majority of falls do not result in injury requiring medical attention, approximately 20% to 30% of falls produce moderate to severe injuries (Englander, Hodson, & Terregrossa, 1996; Tinetti, Speechley, & Ginter, 1988), and 5% to 10% produce serious injuries (Rubenstein & Josephson, 2002). Falls are responsible for the majority of fractures and a large proportion of the spinal cord injuries and traumatic brain injuries that occur among older adults (Desai, Zhang, & Hennessy, 1999). Falls also frequently result in a loss of independence, with 50% of fall-related hospital admissions resulting in nursing home placement (Sattin et al., 1990). Hip fractures are one of the most frequent and devastating consequences of falls among older adults. About half of patients who sustain a hip fracture never regain their former level of function (Desai et al., 1999), and 20% to 30% of them do not survive past the first year following their hip fracture (Magaziner et al., 1990, cited in Rubenstein & Josephson, 2002). Even noninjurious falls can have serious consequences such as increased fear of falling, which subsequently contributes to decreased QOL and further illness and injury.

Substantial economic costs to society are another consequence of fall-related injuries and deaths among older adults. "In 2000, the total direct cost of all fall injuries for people 65 and older exceeded $19 billion" (Stevens, Corso, Finkelstein, & Miller cited by Centers for Disease Control and Prevention, 2008, ¶ 1). As the baby-boomer generation matures to retirement age, this figure is projected to increase by 60% by the year 2020, when it will exceed $32 billion (Englander et al., 1996).

Mortality Rates

The cost of falls to individuals and families is often measured in terms of the number of lives lost. Unintentional injuries are the fifth leading cause of death among older adults, and falls account for two-thirds of those unintentional injury deaths (Desai et al., 1999). In 2003, fall-related injuries accounted for 13,700 deaths among older adults and 1.8 million visits to emergency rooms (Stevens, Ryan, & Kresnow, 2006). The rate of deaths due to falls increases with advancing age and is higher for men than women, possibly because men are more likely than women to have other comorbid conditions, although women have more nonfatal falls than men. Fall-related deaths are also higher among whites than African Americans (Stevens et al., 2006), due in part to the lower bone densities that make whites more likely to sustain hip fractures. Moreover, the rate of deaths due to falls appears to be on the rise, in part because medical advances have caused a reduction in deaths due to chronic illnesses (Desai et al., 1999).

Risk Factors for Falls

The identification of risk factors is a critical first step in preventing falls. A great many risk factors have been associated with falls and are usually categorized as either intrinsic or extrinsic. **Intrinsic risk factors,** also known as *personal* or *host factors,* are the physical, psychological, neurological, and sensory qualities that make a person more likely to fall. In the language of the *Occupational Therapy Practice Framework* (referred to as *Framework;* American Occupational Therapy Association [AOTA], 2008) and the *International Classification of Function, Disability and Health* (*ICF*) developed by the WHO (2001), intrinsic factors are known as client factors and include both body functions and body structures. Intrinsic risk factors can be related to medical disorders, drugs (Beers et al., 2005), impaired mental status, incontinence, history of previous falls, seizure disorder (Texas Department of Aging and Disability Services, 2003), and mental health disorders such as depression, dysthymia, dementia, anxiety, and phobias (Kelley, 2003).

Intrinsic risk factors are complex. For example, impaired mental status could be the result of medication regimen changes; sleep disturbances; acute illness (Cole, Ryan, Adrean, & Silver, 2001), such as an ear infection, cold, or the flu; excessive alcohol use; or mixing alcohol with over-the-counter or prescription drugs. In addition, ear infection, cold, or the flu could also lead to vestibular problems that affect balance and equilibrium. There is some discrepancy as to whether certain factors are identified as intrinsic, extrinsic, or behavioral factors. For instance, use of an assistive device could be considered an intrinsic risk factor (device needed due to a disease process), extrinsic factor (device contributed to a trip), or a behavioral risk factor (if the activity is completed too quickly due to increased confidence as a result of having a mobility aide). Content Box 24-1 provides a classification of risk factors as either intrinsic, extrinsic or, both.

Extrinsic risk factors consist of the situations and conditions outside the individual that increase one's opportunity for falls (Carter, Kannus, & Khan, 2001) and correspond to contextual factors in the *ICF* and *Framework.* Table 24-1 lists extrinsic factors and

---

Content Box 24-1

Classification of Common Risk Factors for Falls in Community-Dwelling Elderly

Risk Factor	Intrinsic vs. Extrinsic
• Muscle weakness	• Intrinsic
• History of falls	• Intrinsic
• Gait deficit	• Intrinsic
• Use of assistive devices	• Intrinsic and extrinsic
• Visual deficit	• Intrinsic
• Arthritis	• Intrinsic
• Impaired ADL	• Intrinsic
• Depression	• Intrinsic
• Cognitive impairment	• Intrinsic
• Age >80 years	• Intrinsic
• Medication use	• Intrinsic and extrinsic
• Environmental hazards	• Extrinsic
• Fear of falling	• Extrinsic

Data from Table 1 in *The effect of reducing falls on long-term care expenses: Literature review* (p. 8) prepared for the Office of Disability, Aging, and Long-Term Care Policy, U.S. Department of Health and Human Services, 2004, Contract #HHS-100—3-0008.

---

actions to minimize risk from these factors. **Behavioral risk factors** are sometimes recognized as a third category of risk factors and represent specific interactions between the individual and his or her environment (Clemson, Cumming, & Heard, 2003; Connell, 1996). In a national survey of approximately 2000 injurious falls among older adults,

- 59% resulted from slipping, tripping, or stumbling;
- 22% resulted from loss of balance, dizziness, syncope, or seizure; and
- 19% resulted from some other cause (Kochera, 2002).

Behavioral risk factors are key to an occupation-centered understanding of falls. Some sources refer to these risk factors as *situational factors.* **Situational factors** have been defined as activities or decisions that

> may increase the risk of falls and fall-related injuries. Examples are walking in stocking feet or in footwear with high heels, rushing to the bathroom (especially at night when not fully awake or when lighting may be inadequate), and rushing to answer the telephone. (Beers et al., 2005, ¶ 10)

Risk Factor Interaction

Many risk factors are reversible, in that they can be modified through therapeutic interventions such as strength training or assistive devices, while other risk factors are irreversible and may require adaptive strategies (Carter et al., 2001). Although irreversible risk

Table 24–1 Extrinsic Risk Factors and Recommended Modifications

Location	Hazard	Correction	Rationale
General household			
Lighting	Too dim	Provide ample lighting in all areas	Improves visual acuity and contrast sensitivity
	Too direct, creating glare	Reduce glare with evenly distributed light, indirect lighting, or translucent shades	Improves visual acuity and contrast sensitivity
	Inaccessible light switches	Provide night-lights or touch-activated lights	Reduces risk of tripping over or bumping into unseen obstacles in a dark room
		Install switches that are immediately accessible when entering room or motion sensors that activate lights	
Carpets, rugs, linoleum	Torn	Repair or replace torn carpet	Reduces risk of tripping and slipping, especially for people who have difficulty stepping
	Slippery	Provide rugs with nonskid backs	Reduces risk of slipping
	Curled edges	Tack or tape down rugs or linoleum to prevent curling	Reduces risk of tripping
		Replace rugs or linoleum	
Chairs, tables, other furnishings	Unstable	Provide furniture stable enough to support the weight of a person leaning on table edges or chair arms and backs	Increases support for people with impaired balance and helps with transferring
		Do not use chairs that have wheels or that swivel	
		Repair legs that are loose	
	Chairs without armrests	Provide chairs with armrests that extend forward enough to provide leverage when getting up or sitting down	Helps people with proximal muscle weakness and helps with transferring
	Obstructed pathways	Arrange furnishings so that pathways are not obstructed	Reduces risk of tripping over or bumping into obstacles, making movement in the home easier and safer, especially for people with impaired peripheral vision
		Remove clutter from hallways	
Heating	Too cool	Maintain temperature at 22.2°C in winter	Reduces risk of falls secondary to hypothermia
Wires and cords	Exposed in pathways	Tack cords above the floor or run beneath floor coverings	Reduce risk of falls secondary to tripping
Kitchen			
Cabinets, shelves	Too high	Keep frequently used items at waist level	Reduces risk of falls due to frequent reaching or standing on unstable ladders or chairs
		Install shelves and cupboards at an accessible height	

Continued

Table 24–1 **Extrinsic Risk Factors and Recommended Modifications—cont'd**

Location	Hazard	Correction	Rationale
Floors	Wet or waxed	Place rubber mat on floor in sink area	Reduces risk of slipping, especially for people with a gait disorder
		Wear rubber-soled shoes in kitchen	
		Use nonslip wax or buff paste wax thoroughly	
Gas range	Dial difficult to see	Clearly mark "on" and "off" positions on dials	Reduces risk of gas asphyxiation, especially if sense of smell is impaired
Table	Wobbly, unstable	Provide table with sturdy legs of even length	Increases support, especially for people with a gait disorder
		Do not use tripod or pedestal tables	
Bathroom			
Bathtub	Slippery tub floor	Install skid-resistant strips or rubber mat	Reduces risk of sliding on wet tub floor and risk of falls (eg, a bath seat enables people with impaired balance to sit while showering)
	Need to use the side of the bathtub for support or transfer	Use shower shoes or bath seat	
		Use a portable grab bar on the side of the tub	
		Take grab bar on trips	Helps with transferring
Towel racks, sink tops	Unstable for use as support while transferring from the toilet	Fasten grab rails to wall studs next to the toilet	Helps with transferring to and from the toilet
Toilet seat	Too low	Use elevated toilet seat	Helps with transferring to and from the toilet
Medicine cabinet	Inadequate lighting	Install brighter lighting	Helps avoid incorrect use of drugs, especially for people with visual impairment
	Drugs inadequately labeled	Label all drugs according to need for internal or external use	Helps avoid incorrect use of drugs, especially for people with visual impairment
		Keep magnifying glass in or near cabinet	
Door	Locks	Remove locks from bathroom doors or use locks that can be opened from both sides of door	Enables other people to enter if a person falls
Stairways			
Height	Height of steps too high	Correct step height to <15 cm	Reduces risk of tripping, especially for people who have difficulty stepping
Handrails	Missing	Install and anchor rails well on both sides of stairway	Provides support and enables people to grasp rail with either hand
		Use cylindrical rails placed 2.5–5 cm from wall	

Table 24–1 **Extrinsic Risk Factors and Recommended Modifications—cont'd**

Location	Hazard	Correction	Rationale
	Too short and end of rail unclear	Extend beyond top and bottom step, and turn ends inward	Signals that top or bottom step has been reached
Configuration	Too steep or too long	Install landings on stairways	Provides rest stop, especially for patients with heart or pulmonary disorders
Condition	Slippery	Place nonskid treads securely on all steps	Prevents slipping
Lighting	Inadequate	Install adequate lighting at both top and bottom of stairway	Outlines location of steps, especially for people with impaired vision or perception
		Provide night-lights or bright-colored adhesive strips to clearly mark steps	

From "Falls" by M. H. Beers & R. Berkow (Eds.), 2005, in *Merck manual of geriatrics* (3d ed.). Whitehouse Station, NJ: Merck & Co. Retrieved March 25, 2006, from http://www.merck.com/mrkshared/mmg/sec2/ch20/ch20a.jsp. Copyright © 2000 by Merck & Co., Inc. Reprinted with permission.

factors may not be treatable per se (e.g., history of previous falls), they may be useful in identifying "at-risk" populations who are likely to have other risk factors that are reversible (Tinetti et al., 1988). Therefore, irreversible risk factors should not be overlooked in the screening process. The advantage of identifying multiple risk factors for falls is that it increases the number of opportunities for intervention. Intrinsic, extrinsic, and behavioral risk factors should all be evaluated and incorporated into a fall prevention program.

Most falls are **multifactorial,** originating from a combination of multiple factors rather than one single factor (Campbell, Borrie, & Spears, 1989; Tinetti et al., 1988). There is evidence to suggest that risk factors interact in a synergistic way, such that a person's risk of falling increases sharply with the accumulation of risk factors (Rubenstein & Josephson, 2002).

Frequently, when asked about the cause of a recent fall, an older adult will first implicate an obstacle or other environmental condition. It is therefore incumbent upon the occupational therapist to probe more deeply to identify the multifactorial nature of the fall. For example, a fall resulting from a trip over an uneven threshold may actually have been caused by a combination of several intrinsic and extrinsic factors, such as a visual impairment that interfered with seeing the threshold, behavioral issues such as being in a hurry, confusion brought on by a new medication, lower extremity weakness related to a sedentary lifestyle, and poor lighting over the threshold.

Perhaps the most important risk factor for falling is having a history of a previous fall. Older adults who

have fallen in the past are three times more likely than nonfallers to experience future falls (Rubenstein & Josephson, 2002), and half of those who fall in a given year are repeat fallers (Moreland et al., 2003). Clearly, an accurate falls history is critical in identifying high-risk populations, yet underreporting of falls is a persistent problem for several reasons. First, providers may not include a falls history as part of their routine evaluation, and many falls do not result in visible injuries, such as bruises or scars that would trigger further assessment. Also, noninjurious falls may not be perceived as a cause for concern by the faller, or they may be interpreted as an inevitable result of aging. On the other hand, people who are troubled about their fall may not disclose that information out of fear of losing their independence, being institutionalized, or having their activities restricted (Gallagher et al., 2001).

Risk Factor Research

Intrinsic Risk Factors

In a meta-analysis of 16 epidemiological case-control studies, Rubenstein and Josephson (2002) analyzed the importance of several of the most consistently reported intrinsic risk factors for falling. They found that, on average, falls are four times more likely among older adults with lower extremity weakness, and three times more likely among those with gait disorders, balance problems, or a history of prior falls. Visual impairment, arthritis, and use of an assistive device each carry a two-and-a-half-fold increase in fall risk. Finally, older adults were twice as likely to fall if they had depression, cognitive impairment, or difficulties with activities of daily living (ADLs). Other well-established risk factors include chronic illness, polypharmacy, urinary incontinence, sensory deficits, orthostatic hypotension, social isolation, and others described below. While some of these intrinsic risk factors may be irreversible, such as arthritis or a prior history of falling, early identification of any risk factors provides the best opportunity to design interventions to prevent falls.

Gait impairments and lower-extremity muscle weakness are among the most well-established causes of falls. Some gait changes and loss of strength are generally associated with normal aging, but for many older adults the changes are related to inactivity and disease processes such as CVAs, Parkinson's disease, and arthritis (Rubenstein & Josephson, 2002). An estimated 49% of community-dwelling older adults have grossly detectable weakness of the lower extremities (Campbell et al., 1989), and gait disorders affect between 20% and 50% of older adults (Rubenstein & Josephson, 2002).

The risk of falls is thought to increase along with various age-related changes in the sensory mechanisms that regulate postural control. The vestibular, visual, and somatosensory systems all deteriorate to some extent with age, causing decreases in peripheral vision, proprioception, and the ability to detect changes in head position and acceleration (Carter et al., 2001). These changes can make it more difficult to recover quickly from a trip, slip, or other loss of balance before a fall occurs.

Sensory changes in vision and hearing present additional problems. Age-related changes such as reduced contrast sensitivity and heightened glare sensitivity make it more difficult to perceive the edges of carpets, stairs, thresholds, curbs, and other potentially hazardous footing. Approximately 18% of older adults report having a visual impairment, 24% report having cataracts, and 33% report having a hearing impairment (Campbell, Crews, Moriarty, Zack, & Blackman, 1999). Older adults with visual or hearing impairments are more likely than others to report difficulties performing a number of ADLs and instrumental activities of daily living (IADLs), especially functional and community mobility (including getting in and out of a chair or bed, walking, and getting outside), medication management, and meal preparation (Campbell, Crews, et al., 1999). Therefore, visual and hearing impairments not only interfere with the ability to avoid trip and slip hazards in the environment, but can also increase the risks for physical inactivity, adverse medication effects, and inadequate nutrition, all of which contribute to falls. Social isolation, another risk factor for falls, is also slightly more likely among those with visual impairments (Campbell, Crews, et al., 1999).

Chronic illness is a significant contributor to falls, and the risk for falling increases with the number of illnesses a person has (Campbell et al., 1989; Tinetti et al., 1988). Conditions such as osteoarthritis, chronic obstructive pulmonary disease (COPD), congestive heart failure, and coronary artery disease are frequently implicated in falls (Fortin, Yeaw, Campbell, & Jameson, 1998). Many chronic illnesses can contribute to balance problems, reduce strength and endurance, and diminish general conditioning due to extended periods of inactivity. A history of CVAs is strongly associated with falling, especially if there are residual neurological deficits affecting motor control and visual and sensory awareness (Campbell et al., 1989).

Furthermore, the side effects associated with some medications prescribed to treat chronic illnesses can also contribute to falls. Unwanted or harmful side effects of medications are also known as *adverse drug reactions,* which may include fall risk factors such as dizziness, confusion, orthostatic hypotension, and urinary frequency. The ability to metabolize medications effectively declines with age, especially if pathological conditions such as cardiac, renal, and hepatic insufficiency are present; older adults, therefore, are more susceptible than others to adverse drug reactions (Rosedale, 2001; Schmucker, 2001). Furthermore, older adults have been severely underrepresented in the clinical trials of most pharmaceuticals, so the age-specific effects of most medications are poorly understood (Schmucker, 2001). Psychotropic medications are especially notorious in contributing to falls because of their detrimental effects on balance, reaction time, and postural hypotension (Shaw, 2002). One survey estimated that 59% of community-dwelling older women take medications likely to cause postural hypotension, and 32% take at least one psychotropic medication (Campbell et al., 1989).

Polypharmacy is the term for taking a regimen of multiple medications simultaneously. Polypharmacy entails an elevated risk for adverse effects from drug interactions, and it is fairly common, with an estimated 26% of older adults taking more than three medications (Campbell et al., 1989). Drug interactions can cause cognitive impairment, hypotension, and other conditions that may increase the risk of falling (Pollow, Stoller, et al., 1994 as cited in Enevold & Courts, 2000). Polypharmacy appears to be a factor for the vast majority of older adults who fall, with 48% taking three or more medications (Cumming et al., 1991) and 26% taking 8 to 14 medications (Fortin et al., 1998). Unfortunately, it can be difficult for a prescribing physician to be aware of all the medications a person is on, particularly if that patient is seeing several specialists or taking additional over-the-counter (OTC) medications, which patients may forget to mention. Therefore, "brown bag" medication checks, where older adults are invited to bring in all their prescription and nonprescription drugs to be checked for possible interactions by a physician or pharmacist, are a frequently recommended intervention (Pollow, Stoller et al., 1994 as cited in Enevold & Courts, 2000).

Urinary incontinence is an intrinsic condition with behavioral consequences that can contribute to falls—for example, it may cause urgent situations in which the individual has to rush to the bathroom (Mosley, Galindo-Ciocon, Peak, & West, 1998; Rosedale, 2001). Despite significant underreporting of this condition (only half of those affected consult their physician), up to one-third of community-dwelling older adults are believed to experience some level of urinary incontinence (Merkelj, 2001). Older adults can reduce the risks associated with incontinence by planning ahead for nighttime visits to the toilet. For example, proper footwear such as secure slippers with nonskid soles (instead of socks or bare feet) can be kept at the bedside, and a night-light can provide adequate lighting (Mosley et al., 1998). Other strategies include keeping the pathway to the bathroom unobstructed and using a bedside commode.

Orthostatic hypotension affects between 5% and 25% of healthy community-dwelling older adults (Alagiakrishnan, Masaki, Schatz, Curb, & Blanchette, 2001; Rubenstein & Josephson, 2002) and is implicated in many instances of unexplained falls or syncope. **Orthostatic hypotension,** also known as *postural hypotension,* is defined by a drop of at least 20 mm Hg in systolic blood pressure or 10 mm Hg in diastolic blood pressure persisting for 3 minutes after moving from supine to an upright posture (Alagiakrishnan et al., 2001), resulting in dizziness, collapse, or even loss of consciousness (syncope). The prevalence of this condition increases with age and is even more common among older adults with medical issues such as hypovolemia, parkinsonism, and cardiovascular problems. Orthostatic hypotension is a common side effect of many medications, especially antihypertensives, vasodilators, antidepressants, psychotropics, and sedatives (Rubenstein & Josephson, 2002). Behavioral strategies (e.g., learning to get up slowly in the morning) can be adopted by some individuals to minimize the effects of orthostatic hypotension, but medical management of the underlying cause(s) of the condition is recommended.

Psychosocial Factors

A variety of psychosocial and psychiatric issues constitute important intrinsic factors related to falls, with fear of falling among the most widespread. An estimated 40% to 73% of recent fallers and 20% to 46% of non-fallers acknowledged they had a fear of falling (King & Tinetti, 1995). Women are more likely than men to report fear of falling, but the prevalence and extent of fear of falling increases with age and level of frailty for both genders (Arfken, Lack, Birge, & Miller, 1994). Fear of falling often develops in response to a firsthand experience of a fall or near-fall, or even from knowing someone else who has fallen. While appropriate levels of caution can be helpful in avoiding a fall, fear of falling is actually an important contributor to falls, because it results in self-imposed restrictions on physical activity. In this way, people who are afraid of falling are at risk for loss of strength, flexibility, endurance, and other necessary components of functional mobility. In addition, reduced activity can result in social isolation, diminished engagement in occupation, reduced quality of life, anxiety, and depression, which then further exacerbate the fear (Arfken et al., 1994; Walker & Howland, 1991). Ultimately, this condition can escalate over time and set the stage for future falls and illness (Steinmetz & Hobson, 1994).

Mental health disorders such as depression, dysthymia, dementia, anxiety, phobias, and alcohol/sedative/hypnotic abuse are increasingly prevalent among older adults (Kelley, 2003) and can contribute to falls if left untreated. These conditions are often marked by lethargy, agitation, or reduced motivation, all of which can increase the risk of falling. Yet providers may avoid prescribing psychotropic medications to treat these conditions in older adults because of the potential for side effects, such as sedation, dizziness, and gait instability. While psychotropic medications are generally considered a fall risk factor, many newer medications have fewer side effects, so the association between falls and psychotropic medications remains controversial (Rosedale, 2001).

One of the more difficult risk factors to address in fall prevention is cognitive impairment, which may or may not constitute dementia. Persons with dementia exhibit a progressive decline in cognitive functions such as memory, problem-solving, language, math, and sequencing (Kelley, 2003). Dementia and other forms of cognitive impairment affect an estimated 25% of older adults (Graham & Rockwood, 1997), and falls may be as much as twice as frequent among this population compared with cognitively normal older adults (Shaw, 2002). Cognitive impairment is associated with recurrent falling but not with one-time falls. One-time falls may be the result of chance happenings, while repeated falls may be indicative of an inability to map a safe route through the environment (Fletcher & Hirdes, 2002). Cognitively impaired older adults who experience a fall are more likely than other fallers to sustain a serious injury and subsequently have poorer prognosis for making a functional recovery (Shaw, 2002). They also are less likely than cognitively normal older adults to benefit from fall prevention programs (Shaw et al., 2003).

Cognitive impairment appears to increase the risk of falls through both direct and indirect mechanisms. Intact cognitive function underlies the capacity to see one's physical capacities and limitations, and the ability to recognize environmental hazards and identify and adopt appropriate protective behaviors. Cognitive impairments can make it difficult for a person to follow safety precautions, while also interfering with the ability to process and integrate the perceptual information necessary for maintaining postural stability (Shaw, 2002) and orienting oneself geographically (Rubenstein & Josephson, 2002). As a result, cognitive impairment tends to increase susceptibility to environmental hazards that otherwise might not cause a fall (Clemson, Cumming, & Roland, 1996). More indirectly, cognitive impairment is associated with changes in gait and balance that exceed those expected in the normal aging process (Shaw, 2002), which further increases the risk of falling. In general, both cognitive impairments and mental health disorders can increase disability and the risk for falling by eroding a person's ability to self-manage physical limitations or disease processes as they arise over the life span (Kelley, 2003).

Behavioral Risk Factors

Intrinsic and extrinsic risk factors can be better appreciated by considering the behavioral factors associated with them. Hurrying; carelessness; ineffective mobility behaviors such as low stepping height, being distracted by other elements of the environment, lack of confidence, overexertion, and not scanning the path ahead are frequently cited behavioral risk factors, especially in falls that occur outside the home (Clemson, Manor, & Fitzgerald, 2003). In one study of healthy older adults living in the community (Reinsch, MacRae, Lachenbruch, & Tobis, 1992), approximately one-third of falls occurred during activities associated with inattention (e.g., tripping over a large object or looking somewhere else), while another third occurred during imprudent activities (e.g., slipping on a wet surface, rushing, or lifting heavy objects).

Other behavioral factors include the use of mobility devices and choice of footwear. Mobility devices such as canes and walkers seem to have mixed results in fall prevention. On the one hand, their proper use is meant to improve functional mobility among people with impairments in strength, balance, or other body structures and functions, most of which are also risk factors for falling. Many older adults are aware of the benefits of such devices in increasing stability and preventing falls, yet they refuse to adopt their use because of the symbolic and stigmatizing associations of those devices with old age and disability (Aminzadeh & Edwards, 1998). On the other hand, the use of a mobility device is associated with an increased risk of falling (Rubenstein & Josephson, 2002). It is unclear how often assistive devices actually contribute to falls. In some cases, improper use of devices poses a direct fall hazard (Fortin et al., 1998; Rosedale, 2001), but in other cases, the increased fall risk may only be associated with the underlying impairments. Assistive devices are known to cause a shift in one's center of gravity and bring about a change in posture. They also are often used incorrectly and are frequently not adjusted to the correct height. These factors require a person using a new assistive device to make adjustments in mobility and other habits and routines to accommodate the device.

The choice of footwear also can be seen as a behavioral risk factor. Footwear that is slippery (such as socks and stockings) or unstable (such as flip-flops or high-heeled shoes) can contribute to a fall. Ideal footwear should fit securely on the foot. This may require a podiatric consult for therapeutic footwear if bunions or other foot disorders interfere with a proper shoe fit (Tideiksaar, 2002). The insole should provide firm support without too much cushioning, which could interfere with proprioceptive feedback regarding changes in footing. It is important to promote proprioceptive cues; shoes should not decrease this process more than is necessary. A slip-resistant sole is important, but it should not be so grippy as to catch on carpets and floors. The appropriate degree of grippiness depends on the individual's gait pattern and step height as well as the type of floor surface; therefore, footwear assessment and recommendations should be based on individual observation (Tideiksaar, 2002). Clients may benefit from situation-specific footwear recommendations, such as using nonskid slippers at night when crossing a linoleum floor to reach the toilet, using smooth-soled loafers in the daytime around the house over carpeted surfaces, and using lightly cushioned sneakers for outdoor use on surfaces that might be uneven or slippery.

The development of assessments and continued research will help determine risk factors that should be addressed in prevention programs and fall prevention program evaluations. An assessment specifically focusing on behavioral risk factors has been jointly developed by Clemson, an occupational therapist and lecturer in occupation and leisure sciences; Cumming, a professor in public health; and Heard, a lecturer in behavioral sciences (Clemson, Cumming, et al., 2003). This instrument, the Falls Behavioral (FaB) Scale for Older People, shows promise. The results of the initial study suggest that the scale will be a time-efficient, reliable, and valid tool for behavioral fall interventions and for research on the effectiveness of such interventions.

Extrinsic Risk Factors

Between 25% and 45% of falls implicate environmental hazards as a contributing factor (Rubenstein & Josephson, 2002). Yet it is important to remember that most falls in this category actually result from the interaction of the individual with the environment, such that the intrinsic risk factors resulting from disease or normal aging limit the individual's capacity to adjust to and compensate for any unexpected elements in the environment.

Any environmental element that creates an opportunity for a fall is an extrinsic risk factor, such as electrical cords or furniture crowding a walkway. Other hazards are posed by the absence of a safety feature, such as adequate lighting or grab bars in the bathroom. Still other hazards are posed by faulty or inappropriate items, such as furniture that is too soft or too low, unstable footstools, stairs in disrepair, or loose rugs and carpet edges. Many hazards contribute to slips and trips, which are frequent precursors to falls in the home. Content Box 24-2 identifies common household hazards that may contribute to falls.

Content Box 24-2

Common Home Hazards

These environmental hazards are widely recognized in most home evaluations:

- Absence of grab bars next to toilet and in tub
- Absence of nonskid strips or mat in tub
- Absence of sturdy footstool in places where reaching is necessary
- Cabinet storage that requires frequent reaching to low or high places
- Cluttered stairs and pathways, especially between the bed and bathroom
- Inadequate lighting, especially over stairways and thresholds and in hallways
- Exposed extension, telephone, or computer cords in pathways
- Furniture for sitting too high, too low, too soft, or lacking armrests for steady transfers
- Glare from shiny floors and surfaces or direct light sources such as unshaded windows
- Stairs that are too steep, that lack sturdy railings, or are in need of repair
- Toilet seat too low
- Uneven or unstable floor coverings, such as
  - Slippery throw rugs
  - Loose floorboards or tiles
  - Torn, wrinkled, or puckered carpet
- Unstable furniture prone to tipping when used for support

Few studies have investigated the connection between environmental hazards and falls, and the findings are mixed (Connell, 1996). Some studies have found that the risk of falling is not increased by the presence of one or more home hazards (Gill, Williams, & Tinetti, 2000), while other studies have shown that environmental hazards in the home are a significant predictor of falls (Connell, 1996) and differentiate one-time fallers from repeat fallers (Fletcher & Hirdes, 2002). It is also important to consider environmental hazards outside the home and in transition areas around the home, such as patios, entrances, and garages, which are often characterized by glare and rapid changes in illumination (Reinsch et al., 1992).

It is clear that environmental factors cannot be completely separated from intrinsic and behavioral factors, which vary from person to person and over time for an individual. The level of perceived risk, which is influenced by the level of impairment, determines the level of caution an individual will exercise in any situation, which either reduces or increases the risk of falling. Extrinsic risk factors seem to play a more important role in falls among younger, healthier individuals, while intrinsic factors become more important as frailty and age increase (Reinsch et al., 1992; Steinmetz & Hobson, 1994). This association may be mediated by certain behavioral choices; for example, having more frail individuals (i.e., those with the greatest intrinsic risks) deliberately avoid obvious hazards such as stairs and activities that could cause a loss of balance. On the other hand, vigorous adults take greater risks in their activities and therefore encounter more environmental hazards that could cause falls. This pattern may partially explain Tinetti and colleagues' finding (1988) that falls among healthier, more vigorous individuals tended to occur on stairs, away from home, and in activities that challenge balance; whereas falls among frailer individuals tended to occur in the home during routine, less-demanding activities.

Furthermore, one must consider the familiarity of the environment. A person living in a cluttered home full of throw rugs, extension cords, and other trip and slip hazards might be very successful negotiating those hazards quite safely because they are so familiar. Yet those same hazards in less familiar locations such as a store, church, or friend's home might pose a much greater threat. While familiarity does not excuse the need to eliminate obvious hazards whenever they are found, it does reveal the importance of behavior as a mediating factor in the relative risk posed by environmental hazards. Evaluation of individuals by an occupational therapist within their unique home environments may be more likely to result in changes that actually prevent falls than a simple home safety checklist used in isolation (Cumming et al., 1999).

The concept of environmental press is useful in thinking about the role of home hazards in fall prevention. **Environmental press** refers to the interaction between a person's competence to perform a given task and the specific demands required by the environment to carry out that task (Connell, 1996; Lawton, 1980). For instance, a person may possess a certain level of competence in descending a flight of stairs. But if the stairs are in disrepair, unevenly spaced, or poorly lit, or if there are other distractions in the environment, then the environmental demands may be so high that they exceed the person's competence. The construct of environmental press offers an explanation for why so many falls occur at home, in an environment that is utterly familiar to the individual, in which their competence is usually adequate for successful occupational performance. A person who has lived in a home for many years without incident may not recognize age-related changes in competence and continue interacting with their home environment in the same accustomed ways. Yet as that person's competence begins to drop below the demands of the environment, he or she may continue functioning without a fall but with increasing dependence in one or more activities. At this marginal level of functioning, the slightest distraction, disruption in routine, or onset of a new impairment is likely to result in an adverse outcome such as a fall (Connell, 1996). In assessing the person-environment fit, the occupational therapist must recognize when environmental press exceeds competence and must intervene with strategies to reduce excessive environmental demands and increase competence by modifying intrinsic and behavioral risk factors.

Guidelines for Evidence-Based Evaluation

Moreland and colleagues (2003) present a set of evidence-based guidelines for management of community-dwelling older adults with a history of falling. Elements that should be included in an occupational therapy evaluation for fall prevention are mental status; depression; postural hypotension; vision; hearing; psychotropic medications; polypharmacy; balance; muscle strength; transfers; activities of daily living; environmental hazards, including medical equipment; gait; use of mobility devices; urinary incontinence; dizziness; lower extremity coordination; and social isolation. In addition, the level of physical activity should be evaluated to determine whether it is inadequate, excessive, or optimal. Moderate levels of physical activity have been shown to be protective against falling, while too much or too little physical activity is associated with increased fall risk (Moreland et al., 2003).

Guidelines for Evidence-Based Interventions

Evidence suggests that the most effective approach to fall prevention is a program of individualized, targeted, multifactorial interventions, which may include exercise, home modification, education, and other intervention strategies. These and other guidelines for evidence-based interventions are detailed below.

First, interventions must be tailored to meet the needs of each client (Moreland et al., 2003; Rosedale, 2001; Steinmetz & Hobson, 1994), according to the needs identified in the individualized evaluation. If universal components such as group education sessions or exercise programs are to be used, they will be most effective as part of an individually tailored intervention plan (Gardner, Robertson, & Campbell, 2000).

Second, for the greatest impact, interventions should target populations with one or more identified risk factors for falling. A **targeted intervention** is one that screens for certain risk factors as criteria for program enrollment and then addresses those specific impairments in the intervention. This method ensures that the program targets a high-risk population. **Untargeted interventions** deliver a more generic package of interventions to a population without regard to their specific risk factors for falling (Moreland et al., 2003). In comprehensive reviews, both Cumming (2002) and Moreland and colleagues (2003) found that most of the successful trials have targeted a population with at least one identified risk factor for falling, such as history of previous falls, advanced age, lower extremity weakness, or gait impairment. Untargeted interventions were almost uniformly unsuccessful in reducing the risk of falling. Therefore, programs that target high-risk populations are more likely to demonstrate measurable reductions in the risk of falling, whether the intervention is exercise, home modification, education, or a multifactorial combination.

Third, interventions should be multifactorial (Brouwer, Walker, Rydahl, & Culham, 2003; Cumming, 2002; Desai et al., 1999; Moreland et al., 2003; Steinmetz & Hobson, 1994). Although there are examples of single intervention programs that have produced statistically significant results, the preponderance of evidence suggests that multifactorial interventions have a greater impact because they can address more risk factors for each client. It is worth noting that successful single intervention programs have incorporated other key strategies for success, such as targeting high-risk populations (Cumming et al., 1999; Gardner, Robertson, McGee, & Campbell, 2002; Wolf et al., 1996), individualizing the intervention (Cumming et al., 1999), or targeting self-selected populations that have an interest in reducing their risk (Thompson, 1996).

Multifactorial Interventions

The multifactorial approach to fall prevention has long been regarded as the industry standard, although specific program components have varied considerably. Because the risk of falling increases linearly with the number of risk factors (Tinetti et al., 1988), multifactorial interventions appear to hold the greatest potential for reducing the risk of falling by modifying multiple risk factors. **Multifactoral interventions** combine a variety of strategies offered by an interdisciplinary team, often with a portion of the program including strategies directly targeted to individual needs. Care must be taken in directly comparing research results across studies, as operational definitions of *multifactoral intervention* can vary. For example, Davison, Bond, Dawson, Steen, and Kenny (2005) included three specific disciplines as the multifactorial intervention (i.e., medicine, occupational therapy, and physical therapy) in a randomized control study of frequent fallers. In a review of this study, Lever (2005) noted that Davison and colleagues did not include nursing, whereas other previous similar studies did include nursing as part of multifactoral interventions.

The first multifactorial intervention trial shown to actually reduce the risk of falling was conducted by Tinetti and others (1994). This trial targeted community-dwelling older adults who had at least one of several selected risk factors for falling (e.g., postural hypotension, polypharmacy, home hazards, gait impairments, lower extremity weakness, etc.). Participants received interventions such as home-based gait training, medication review, transfer training, and home modifications in an individualized plan designed to target their individual risk factors. This multifactorial intervention produced a 31% reduction in falls. Close and colleagues (1999) provided additional evidence in support of multifactorial interventions among high-risk older adults in a trial that involved a comprehensive geriatric evaluation and occupational therapy home visits.

Brouwer and others (2003) demonstrated the value of a multifactorial approach in addressing fear of falling from a variety of perspectives simultaneously. Overall, balance confidence was improved by both an educational and an exercise intervention. Psychosocial health was improved in the education group due to opportunities to talk about fear of falling and to learn strategies to reduce risk, and perceived health status was improved in the exercise group.

Exercise Interventions

Exercise is a common component of fall prevention programs and can address multiple goals. Exercise programs can be designed to modify many of the intrinsic risk factors associated with falls, such as strength and flexibility of the lower extremities, balance, coordination, gait, and reaction time, and these programs may also affect self-perceived health status, self-efficacy, and fear of falling. Moreover, physical activity benefits participants' overall health and wellbeing, both physically and mentally. However, despite numerous studies testing the outcomes of a variety of exercise programs, no single type of exercise or program format has clearly emerged as the optimal approach for preventing falls (Carter et al., 2001; Cumming, 2002). In fact, findings have been quite mixed regarding the effectiveness of exercise in preventing falls. Comprehensive literature reviews by Cumming (2002) and by Gardner and colleagues (2000) have summarized these findings, noting that while successful exercise programs have produced statistically significant reductions in the risk of falling by up to 49%, many programs have shown no effect at all. Since these reviews were conducted, new research indicates that exercises promoting ankle strength (Hong & Robinovitch, 2003) can improve older persons' ability to regain balance after being challenged. In addition, a 6-month randomized control trial found that both intense strength training and agility training were successful in reducing falls among older adults (Liu-Ambrose, Khan, Lord, & McKay, 2003).

In their guidelines for fall prevention, Moreland and colleagues (2003) recommend a program of balance exercises nearly universally, even when the only risk factor is a history of falling. The exercise program should include balance exercises involving tai chi movements or equilibrium-control exercises on firm and soft surfaces (Moreland et al., 2003). Additional exercises for gait and strength training and flexibility, provided as part of an individualized home-based intervention plan, are also recommended for women over 80 years of age (Campbell et al., 1997; Moreland et al., 2003). However, practitioners are cautioned against making untargeted recommendations for older adults to increase their level of physical activity, as unprepared elders can increase their risk, especially if they take that recommendation to the extreme (Moreland et al., 2003). Furthermore, not all forms of exercise are effective in reducing falls, and therefore fall prevention programs should not simply recommend that older adults increase their physical activity (Cumming, 2002). Overall, research suggests that exercise has the greatest impact on fall prevention among high-risk older adults whose functional mobility is below a certain threshold (Robertson, Campbell, Gardner, & Devlin, 2002) or on the verge of serious decline (Buchner et al., 1997) and that the effect is mediated primarily by improvements in balance (Cumming, 2002; Day et al., 2002; Moreland et al., 2003).

The Cawthorne and Cooksey exercises were developed in the 1940s by a physician and a physical therapist (Cawthorne, 1945; Cooksey, 1946; McGee, 2000). Recent research has demonstrated that the use of

Cawthorne and Cooksey exercises in 1-hour sessions, three times a week, for a 3-month period enhanced balance in a group of healthy older women as measured by the Berg Balance Scale (Ribeiro & Pereira, 2005). The same technique, applied in a group format, was also shown to be effective for elderly women with benign paraoxysmal positional vertigo, as measured by increased ADL performance and enhanced quality of life (Resende, Taguchi, de Almeida, & Fujita, 2003). Timely initiation of the exercises for unilateral peripheral vestibular disorders has been linked with higher compliance and lower self-reported disability scores, supporting the need for prompt vestibular rehabilitation referral (Bamiou, Davies, McKee, & Luxon, 2000). Corna and colleagues (2003) found both the Cawthorne and Cooksey exercises and a course of rehabilitation effective interventions for improving balance in individuals with unilateral vestibular deficit. However, the rehabilitation approach (i.e., supervised balance activities on a moveable platform) appeared to be more effective in improving balance control.

Additional exercises have been described in the literature. The efficacy of each varies with the type of vestibular dysfunction, whether they were supervised or unsupervised, and whether they had been customized. Readers are encouraged to carefully study the most recent evidence-based research literature, including review articles (Cohen, 2006; Herdman, Blatt, & Schubert, 2000), and to seek mentoring before engaging in vestibular rehabilitation. While improving balance is an important aspect of fall prevention, for individuals with or without a vestibular disorder, it is only one of many factors that must be addressed.

Gardner and colleagues (2000) outlined additional recommendations for exercise. First, exercises must be intense enough to produce measurable modifications to the factors associated with falls, such as strength, flexibility, and balance. Second, whenever possible, participants should be offered the choice of a group or home-based format, to increase the program's acceptability to people with different personal preferences and functional capacities. While the group format offers the added benefits of social interaction, the home-based format may be more appropriate for participants who are frailer or who have difficulty accessing transportation (Gardner et al., 2000).

Many lessons learned from unsuccessful exercise programs have provided other helpful recommendations. Some programs have been ineffective because other risk factors not affected by exercise were more significant in those populations (Gardner et al., 2000). For instance, balance deficits resulting from polypharmacy would not be reduced by physical activity. Therefore, exercise as part of a multifactorial intervention may have the best chance of success, because more risk factors can be modified concurrently.

Poor compliance with exercise programs has also frequently been implicated in unsuccessful exercise programs (Gardner et al., 2000). As with any other population, successful exercise programs for older adults must be appealing, motivating, enjoyable, and easy to follow. One strategy to enhance compliance is to incorporate accountability elements into the program, such as having participants log their exercise sessions on a calendar and providing regular "checkup" phone calls from program staff to monitor program compliance (Gardner et al., 2002). Also, recognizing that illness is a common reason for noncompliance, programs with built-in flexibility and choice can optimize compliance by allowing participants to easily stop and restart the program around periods of short-term illness (Gardner et al., 2002).

One form of exercise that is recommended for fall prevention is tai chi. This Chinese martial art involves a series of slow, fluid movements of every part of the body (Wu, 2002), continuous shifting of the body weight, and a coordination of breathing with movement (Kessenich, 1998). Tai chi is popular for fall prevention because it can improve balance, strength, posture, and concentration, and it can be practiced alone or in groups. In one large trial, participants in a tai chi program demonstrated a 48% reduction in their risk of falls and a significant reduction in the fear of falling (Wolf et al., 1996). Yet, as with other kinds of exercise programs, there are several important considerations in designing a tai chi program for the purpose of preventing falls. For instance, balance improvements resulting from this exercise may be more likely when it is practiced over a long period of time (i.e., at least 40 sessions) and among populations with mild balance problems (Wu, 2002). Furthermore, it is important to choose the most appropriate style of tai chi, as some styles are more challenging to strength and balance, while other styles may be easier to learn and therefore more attractive to beginners (Wu, 2002).

Home Modification Interventions

Environmental modifications often play a central role in fall prevention programs (Steinmetz & Hobson, 1994), and this type of intervention offers several advantages. First, most home modifications are relatively easy, cost-effective, and feasible (Connell, 1996; Plautz, Beck, Selmar, & Radetsky, 1996; Salkeld et al., 2000), especially compared to interventions aimed at modifying other risk factors. Second, home modifications may have a synergistic benefit when combined with other interventions to reduce intrinsic risk factors (Connell, 1996). Yet even as an isolated intervention, some home modifications serve as visual cues (e.g., grab bars) that reinforce safer behaviors and a heightened awareness of the risk of falling. Therefore, environmental modifications may provide both direct and indirect benefits by contributing to behavioral changes while reducing environmental hazards (Thompson, 1996). Third, environmental modifications outside the home can have a broader impact by reducing the risk of falling for all people who use the space (Connell, 1996).

The nature of home modifications can vary widely, depending on the needs of the individual and the financial resources available. The modifications mentioned most frequently in the literature include removing throw rugs, reducing clutter, adding slip-resistant bath mats or adhesive strips, securing loose rugs, and installing stair railings (Cumming et al., 1999; Plautz et al., 1996; Salkeld et al., 2000). Less common modifications include installing grab bars near the toilet and bath, moving electrical cords, adding night-lights, making exterior repairs to pathways and stairs, making interior repairs to flooring, and installing brighter lighting (Cumming et al., 1999; Salkeld et al., 2000). Adding touch lighting (Beers et al., 2005) by the bed for persons who awaken in the middle of the night to use the bathroom is another easy modification to prevent falls due to diminished visibility, although care must be taken to ensure the light is neither too bright nor too dim.

To date, only one randomized trial of home modifications for fall prevention has been published (Cumming et al., 1999). Home visits by an occupational therapist were associated with a 36% reduced risk of falling among those who had a previous fall (Cumming et al., 1999). The program was designed to identify home hazards and recommend modifications, yet unexpectedly, the program reduced falls both inside and outside the home, suggesting that the occupational therapist actually helped participants increase their personal awareness of fall risks and adopt behavioral changes to live more safely in all available contexts. This finding highlights the importance of therapeutic interaction with a skilled practitioner, relative to the value of a generic home-safety checklist administered by the client or an unskilled volunteer. Interestingly, the program had no effect among those who had no history of a prior fall, which supports the notion that environmental hazards pose the greatest danger when combined with intrinsic risk factors. As a result of this significant study, home evaluations by an occupational therapist have been recommended in the medical literature for all older adults with a history of previous falls (Moreland et al., 2003).

On the other hand, other, less rigorous research suggests that home modifications administered by unskilled paraprofessionals may also reduce falls, especially if the interventions are targeted to populations with a strong interest in making changes for risk-reduction (Thompson, 1996). Older adults who seek out a fall prevention program advertised in the community already have a heightened interest in fall prevention and thus a greater willingness to follow recommendations and make changes to their home and their behaviors. Therefore, a presentation on fall prevention delivered in community venues likely to attract interested older adults, such as places of worship and senior centers, may be an effective recruitment strategy for reaching elders with the highest interest, if not the highest risk (Thompson, 1996).

Nevertheless, the body of literature on home modifications is mixed (Connell, 1996) and has several implications for practice. Home-safety checklists should be used cautiously, because they may be incomplete. Much of the literature on home hazards and falls focuses on very obvious, major hazards that would be dangerous for anyone, yet many falls involve environmental elements that are less obvious because they pose a threat only to certain individuals or in specific situations (Connell, 1996). For example, a piece of furniture might be placed in such a way that it helps a person navigate the path from bed to bathroom at night. Yet a slight alteration in personal or situational factors one night (e.g., onset of illness causing dizziness, new floor covering or footwear, thunderstorm causing emotional distress) could transform that piece of furniture from an effective adaptation into a fall hazard. A careful evaluation of exactly how individuals interact with and use the elements of their environment is essential in identifying these less obvious home hazards and in discerning whether a hazard is truly environmental (e.g., furniture) or behavioral (e.g., inattention).

Occupational therapists who recommend home modifications should be prepared to address a variety of potential barriers to compliance. A holistic understanding of person-environment relationships helps to overcome these barriers and maximizes the client's likelihood of success in following through on recommendations. When making recommendations for home modifications, remember that respect for the client's values and a collaborative, client-centered approach are paramount. For many clients, options that they suggest or choose for themselves carry a greater sense of ownership and therefore a greater likelihood of being implemented (Clemson, Cusick, & Fozzard, 1999). Sometimes a balance must be achieved between ideal safety and personal taste, such as selecting nonskid rugs to replace slippery throw rugs. Whenever possible, the stigmatizing qualities of a modification should be minimized by choosing devices and equipment that are attractive and stylish rather than those with an institutional appearance (Aminzadeh & Edwards, 1998; Connell, 1996). Stigmas associated with aging and disability can also be combated by emphasizing a universal design perspective on such devices—for instance, understanding that grab bars make bathing safer and more convenient for people of all ages (El-Faizy & Reinsch, 1994).

Risk-reduction education is also valuable in enhancing compliance. The client's knowledge, perceptions, and beliefs about falls and fall risks will greatly influence his or her motivation to follow through on recommendations. Readiness for change is another important factor in this area. Research using the Transtheoretical Model (described in Chapter 3 of this text) found that community-dwelling older adults were more likely to follow through with home modification recommendations if they were in either the action or maintenance stages (McNulty, Johnson, Poole, & Winkle, 2004). Education efforts may help move older adults to the action stage, where they may be more likely to implement recommendations. In order to be convinced of the need for certain modifications, the client may first require precise education as to why a particular modification will reduce the risk of falls (Clemson et al., 1999). Education and counseling may be less threatening and more readily accepted when delivered by a "peer counselor," someone close in age to the client (Connell, 1996). Often, firsthand experience is the best form of education, so be prepared to show clients how much safer, more comfortable, and more convenient a certain modification can be. If possible, consider arranging for the client to go on an "inspiration home visit" to another home that has already been modified, or have the individual view a Web-based virtual tour of homes exhibiting universal design principles (go to http://www.udll.com/ for one such example).

Financial and legal barriers may also contribute to noncompliance. Take time to identify community resources that provide free or reduced-cost home modifications. For clients living in rental properties, make sure the client and the landlord are familiar with the Fair Housing Amendments Act. Landlords are required to make "reasonable accommodations" in procedures, such as taking out the trash, and tenants are allowed to make "reasonable modifications" at their own expense, such as installing grab bars (Connell, 1996).

Finally, plan for adequate monitoring and follow-up to ensure correct, safe, and continued compliance with recommendations. A follow-up phone call or home visit is an ideal opportunity to evaluate the immediate impact of any modifications on the client's day-to-day performance, self-efficacy, and fear of falling. If individuals have not followed through on one or more recommendations, they may benefit from a discussion of barriers to implementation, including their underlying feelings and motivations. Additional education about fall risks may also be indicated. Clients should be engaged in the problem-solving process to identify alternative modifications that would be more acceptable and effective.

Educational Interventions

Effective fall prevention programs should include an educational component to promote behavioral changes, because most older adults live independently and must assume responsibility for reducing their own risk of falling (Desai et al., 1999). Education can raise awareness about one's risk of falling and appropriate risk-reduction behaviors. Yet the intervention should strive to create the "just right" level of awareness; insufficient awareness will not instigate behavior changes to reduce risk, but excessive awareness "results in a hypervigilance that can paradoxically lead to increased risk of falling" (Clemson, Manor, et al., 2003, p. 114). Therefore, educational interventions must go beyond merely naming the various risk factors for falling and must provide constructive, empowering information that will result in healthy behavior change.

Educational interventions taking a cognitive-behavioral approach may be effective in addressing many of the behavioral risk factors associated with falls, especially among highly active older adults. For instance, clients can be instructed in risk-reduction behaviors such as actively looking for environmental hazards in community settings (Reinsch et al., 1992) and adopting time-management strategies to avoid unnecessary rushing. Education and role-playing about what to do when one falls may help increase self-efficacy and reduce the fear of falling, especially for clients who have experienced a long wait before being assisted after a fall. Content Box 24-3 outlines several steps for getting up after a fall. This type of intervention has good potential for use but must be tailored to individuals and their occupational profiles and must also include information on personal alarms.

Older adults who compensate for their deficits with inappropriate behavioral adaptations can benefit from individualized education to refine those adaptations (Clemson, Cumming, et al. 2003; Clemson, Manor, et al., 2003) in order to more effectively avoid falls. For instance, persons who wear glasses may incorporate them into an inappropriate adaptive behavior such as tilting the head down to look at the ground, which would result in reduced scanning of the path ahead. The behavior is deliberate, because these individuals mistakenly believe that looking down will decrease their risk of falling and do not realize that looking down prevents them from fully benefiting from the

Strategies for Recovering From a Fall

1. Remain calm. Assess yourself for injuries. Do not attempt to get up if you have sustained a serious injury. Stay calm, warm, and use your personal alarm or phone if in reach to get help.
2. Look around for a way to help yourself up. Stable furniture can be used for support to climb up off the floor.
3. If you cannot help yourself up, find a way to call for help.
   a. Make a loud noise to alert a neighbor.
   b. Crawl or slide to the front door or telephone.
   c. If you have a personal alarm device, use it.
4. If you have to wait for help, make yourself comfortable and warm, and remain calm until help arrives.
5. When you have recovered, talk to your health-care provider about the fall. Try to recall as many details as possible about what happened the day you fell (writing them down may help). For example, how you were feeling that day, any medications you were taking, what you were doing when you fell, whether you lost consciousness, any obstacles that made you trip, and so on. Even if you weren't injured, you may be at risk for falling again in the future. Ask what you can do to reduce your risk for future falls.

vision correction provided by the glasses. Individualized education will reinforce the person's appropriate adaptive behaviors, such as wearing glasses, and will raise awareness about the risks posed by the inappropriate adaptive behaviors, such as looking down.

Assertiveness training is a valuable educational intervention for fall prevention. To implement some risk-reduction strategies, older adults may need to request help, such as asking a landlord or family member to repair loose carpet or make other home modifications (Walker & Howland, 1991). Occupational therapists can incorporate assertiveness training into fall prevention programs to ensure that clients have the self-advocacy skills to obtain whatever assistance they need and thereby improve compliance with recommendations.

Education also can affect clients' perceived risk for falling. The success of any intervention relies on the client's level of compliance, which is strongly influenced by whether the recommendations make sense to the client in light of his or her perceived risk (Clemson et al., 1999). Therefore, the occupational therapist should carefully assess the client's perceived risk of falling and integrate those findings throughout the educational components of the intervention plan in order to ensure that any recommendations are meaningful to the client. This approach is critical to maximizing compliance with the recommendations and interventions.

Many older adults are able to reduce their perceived risk by adopting specific protective behaviors for risk management, especially in environments they perceive to be more hazardous or unfamiliar. Examples include taking one's time, scanning the path ahead, and concentrating on where one is going. Considering that many of the physical changes related to aging and illness may be perceived as being beyond one's control, these protective strategies provide the important added benefit of a greater sense of control over one's risk of falling (Clemson et al., 1999), which may then help to decrease one's fear of falling. Educational interventions can tap into this natural desire for control by providing additional strategies that "engender . . . a sense of personal control that will stimulate subsequent learning and action" (Walker & Howland, 1991, p. 121) and by providing a reality check as to the accuracy of clients' perceptions and the appropriateness (i.e., safety) of their chosen protective behaviors. A thorough understanding of these psychological processes for each individual is the key to designing successful, personalized, client-centered interventions.

There are many resources available to customize education interventions directed toward older adults, their caregivers, or the broader community. These include fact sheets and printed material produced by the AOTA (2004) as well as a variety of governmental and other organizations identified in the Web resources listed at the end of this chapter. Newer technology, such as podcasts (Morbidity and Mortality Weekly Report, 2008), may provide quick, cost-effective means to provide education, especially as "baby boomers" are fond of "tech toys" (Iconoculture, 2008, ¶ 1–2) and need to begin addressing fall prevention for their aging relatives and themselves.

Other Intervention Strategies

Some clients who have recently experienced a fall may benefit from an intellectual analysis of the fall through a narrative process and reenactment of the event. This type of exercise, guided by an occupational therapist, facilitates reflection on the circumstances surrounding the fall to improve self-awareness of risk factors and to empower the client to prevent future falls. For individuals who initially point to a single environmental factor that caused the fall (e.g., "I fell on the stairs"), this intervention facilitates an opportunity for the client to identify multiple other factors that may have contributed to the event (Clemson, Manor, et al., 2003). This approach also may be useful to combat fear of falling and enhance self-efficacy.

Many intervention trials use a falls diary or calendar to document the circumstances surrounding each fall (Woodland & Hobson, 2003). This is a simple, convenient, and low-cost technique that can be an integral part of both evaluation and intervention. Evidence suggests that the simple daily act of recording the occurrence of falls and near-falls can in itself contribute to a reduction in falls, probably by increasing awareness of one's risk for falling (Steinberg et al., 2000). Additional documentation and interpretation of the circumstances surrounding the fall can also become the basis for narrative occupation-based interventions aimed at raising awareness, combating fear of falling, and increasing self-efficacy for fall prevention (Clemson, Manor, et al., 2003).

Medication monitoring should be considered whenever possible to reduce the risk of falling. Interventions aimed at minimizing the total number of prescription medications have been shown to significantly reduce the risk of falling (Moreland et al., 2003). Specifically, withdrawal of psychotropic medications has been shown to be effective, including benzodiazepines, hypnotics, antidepressants, and major tranquilizers (Campbell, Robertson, et al., 1999).

Pharmacists can also assist with interventions such as participating in interdisciplinary falls teams and fall prevention programs or offering individual client medication management. These professionals can be very helpful in providing and updating information needed to monitor medication use. In addition, they can provide consultation regarding the positive and negative attributes of drugs used to treat vertigo and other conditions linked to falls. Some drugs that are effective for treating motion sickness may also be prescribed for vertigo. However, these drugs, such as meclizine (Antivert), are often labeled "possibly effective" for vertigo and share a common side effect of drowsiness (MedicineNet, 1997; Thomson PDR, 2004), which can be an intrinsic fall risk factor. Another issue is the delayed referral to and use of potentially more efficacious interventions, such as vestibular rehabilitation, resulting from the use of these medications. Vestibular rehabilitation and numerous other intervention types have been shown to be less effective when referral is delayed (Bamiou et al., 2000).

Finally, occupational therapists should consider recommending a mobility device such as a cane or walker while acknowledging that to be convincing, this recommendation may need to be reinforced by the client's physician. Although the association between use of mobility devices and falls is not clearly understood, evidence suggests that they do enhance functional mobility by increasing the feeling of stability and reducing the fear of falling. Yet, mobility devices may be underutilized by those who need them, in part because outside the context of a rehabilitation setting, older adults are rarely evaluated for their need for these

devices (Aminzadeh & Edwards, 2000). Another reason for the poor acceptance of assistive devices among older adults is the stigma and symbolic meaning of canes and walkers. A capable therapist, as part of a comprehensive fall prevention plan, should include mobility devices in the repertoire of possible interventions. Proper fitting and training are essential to ensure that the device is helpful rather than hazardous. If the device is to be used at home, the client should be trained in how to maneuver it throughout the home. Sensitivity and creativity are critical in fostering acceptance of the device. For example, provide peer testimony; adopt a nonmedical, nondisability approach; and look for attractive and convenient designs (Aminzadeh & Edwards, 2000). Keep in mind that some older adults are more open to equipment such as grab bars than to mobility devices (Aminzadeh & Edwards, 1998).

The Occupational Therapy Practitioners' Role in Fall Prevention

Occupational therapists and occupational therapy assistants can be integral members of injury and prevention teams (AOTA, 2004). In medical and rehabilitation settings, occupational therapy interventions often emphasize ADLs such as bathing and dressing. Interventions usually include considerable time spent training the patient and caregivers about safe transfer techniques and the use of safety devices such as grab bars and shower chairs. While falls in the bathroom are sometimes implicated in serious injuries in this population, some studies have found that only a small proportion of falls occur here (Gill et al., 2000; Mackenzie, Byles, & Higginbotham, 2002; Reinsch et al., 1992). Furthermore, much of the literature on fall prevention among older adults focuses on avoidance of hip fractures. To be sure, hip fractures are a severe and costly outcome in every way, but other less severe injuries are far more frequent (Mackenzie et al., 2002; Reinsch et al., 1992) and should not be ignored. For example, when a fall results in minor bruising and cuts, the psychological effects may be very significant, especially in light of the ensuing lifestyle changes that may occur. Outcomes of this nature are not traditionally emphasized in the medical model, yet they represent critical opportunities for health promotion interventions aimed at preventing the downward spiral into reduced physical activity and social participation, and the associated increases in risk for future falls and injuries.

With a holistic understanding of human behavior and function, occupational therapists can analyze the complex interaction of factors involved in falls. In the medical and rehabilitation model, fall prevention interventions emphasize physical activity to improve strength and balance, sometimes coupled with modifications to the home environment. Both occupational therapists and occupational therapy assistants can be instrumental in the enhancement of body structures and functions within these practice contexts. Yet occupational therapists can offer much more through a broader health promotion approach. The evaluation process can go beyond the traditional checklists of mobility issues, medical history, and environmental hazards by addressing subtler factors such as attitudes about falling and the roles and habits that influence behavioral risks. Interventions can also be comprehensive and personalized. With an eye for facilitating adaptive behaviors, the occupational therapy practitioner can support individuals in refining their behaviors to optimize safety within the context of meaningful occupations.

The interdisciplinary nature of fall prevention requires occupational therapists to define their roles within a coordinated team effort. See Table 24-2 for contributions of other disciplines to an interdisciplinary fall prevention team. Occupational therapy expertise is valued for preventive interventions such as assertiveness training, exercise programs, home evaluations and modifications, functional assessments, assistive device training, and risk-reduction education (Woodland & Hobson, 2003) and for fear reduction and return to physical activity and community participation (AOTA, 2004).

Perhaps the most valuable contribution of the occupational therapist to fall prevention, as in other areas, is the ability to provide occupation-based evaluation and intervention, which has been largely ignored in the literature on fall prevention (Woodland & Hobson, 2003). Part of the occupational therapist's expertise is an essentially global view of the individual's occupational performance in terms of all the component assets, deficits, and contextual features that affect the individual's overall wellbeing. This perspective allows the occupational therapist to function as a pseudo "fall prevention case manager" by identifying a wide range of risk factors and making appropriate referrals to other disciplines as needed. For example, a comprehensive occupational therapy evaluation might detect potential risks such as gait abnormalities, possible medication side effects, depression, fear of falling, and visual impairments. Depending on severity and etiology, further evaluation and intervention may be required by physicians, physical therapists, ophthalmologists, social workers, psychologists, or others to adequately address these various deficits. In consultation with other disciplines, the occupational therapist can then focus on an occupation-based approach to each problem. For example, taking medications properly is an occupation that can influence medication side effects. Gait abnormalities can be addressed in the context of occupations such as home maintenance and grocery shopping. Analysis of occupational performance is an important step in addressing depression. Many simple home modifications can provide effective adaptations for visual impairments.

Another benefit of the interdisciplinary approach may be better compliance with recommendations. By communicating with the physician and other health professionals, the occupational therapist can draw attention to the concerns raised in the falls risk assessment and can enlist the support of those other professionals in implementing specific fall prevention interventions. For instance, a physician's opinion is held in very high regard by many older adults (Aminzadeh & Edwards, 1998, 2000) and can therefore be very influential in persuading a client to adopt certain home modifications and other behavioral changes.

Table 24–2   Interdisciplinary Contributions to the Fall Prevention Team

Discipline	Role
Dietitians	Diet review and instruction to promote strong bones and flexibility
Nursing	Monitor hospital, nursing home, rehabilitation center for extrinsic risk factors and monitor patients for intrinsic risk factors
Pharmacy	Medication management
Respiratory therapy	Teach breathing exercises to promote physical activity and body awareness
Occupational therapy	Complete home and community fall assessments and occupational profiles with individualized risk-reduction intervention
Physical therapy	Teach exercises and stretching techniques to promote balance and flexibility
Physician	Review risk factors and fall history with patients

Conclusion

Preventing falls among older adults is an important goal, especially in light of the high fall-related morbidity and mortality and the growing population of older adults at risk for falls. In order for occupational therapists and occupational therapy assistants to contribute to discipline-specific or interdisciplinary fall prevention program development and interventions, they must actively review current research on risk factors and evidence-based practice guidelines. For example, suggesting that the elderly slow their walking pattern may seem at first an appropriate suggestion. However, research results have indicated that this may not be the best recommendation for healthy older adults (van den Bogert, Pavol, & Grabiner, 2002). With current knowledge, occupational therapy practitioners can effectively engage in primary prevention through fall prevention based on evidence.

Preventive health promotion activities can take place at various levels. At the individual level, occu-pational therapists and occupational therapy assistants can help clients modify intrinsic, extrinsic, and behavioral risk factors that can lead to falls. This assistance can be provided by completing a thorough occupational profile and then tailoring education and occupation-based interventions to individual context, needs, and preferences. At the population level, many falls can be prevented through the promotion of overall health and wellbeing among older adults. Many of the components of a multifactorial approach to fall prevention (e.g., exercise, nutrition, vision, medication monitoring, and psychosocial wellbeing) are essential to any general health-promotion program for older adults. The greatest impact on fall prevention usually results from a focused intervention targeting high-risk populations. This type of program must integrate a variety of familiar health promotion approaches with a specific understanding of the complex interaction of factors that contribute to falls.

Case Study 24-1

While aging in place is a popular choice, it may not always be the best option to minimize falls and maximize occupational engagement in older adults. Mrs. Tea had been living with a dog in a two-story split rambler since her husband's unexpected death at age 60. At age 70, she started to sustain falls. The first two were caused by slipping when retrieving mail in wintry conditions. The third fall, also weather related, was due to dehydration from warm weather, which resulted in her collapsing while on a walking trip in Arizona. The fourth fall was also on a walking trip and occurred when she tripped on the ramparts of an old castle during a visit to her homeland, the United Kingdom. With this fall, she sustained her third concussion and severe face injuries. Memory issues, which had begun after the first fall, intensified.

After her first fall, Mrs. Tea received a home evaluation by one of her daughters, an occupational therapist. The other daughter, who had a background in finance, reviewed her financial assets. Subsequent safety modifications were made in her kitchen (e.g., removal of scatter rugs, readjustment of dog's water bowl). Mrs. Tea decided to remain in her current home since the falls occurred outside her home, she had supportive younger neighbors, she was concerned about the cost of a new home, and she felt safe in her present home.

However, after the fourth fall, her daughters became increasingly concerned for her safety and wellbeing. The two daughters and a son-in-law reentered into discussions regarding the current house and its incompatibility with her present and future IADL performance. Mrs. Tea admitted that she no longer wished to cope with wintry weather and its impact on her ability to walk her dog (her most important daily occupation) or drive to her daily swim. The challenge for the older daughter was to find a retirement community that permitted pets and included a pool and covered walkways—within Mrs. Tea's budget. Even though Mrs. Tea and her daughters lived near two large metropolitan areas, limited options were available. One facility, however, seemed to be the perfect match. It satisfied all three requirements, was located halfway between the two daughters' homes, and was close to her granddaughters. In addition, the facility offered regular shuttle rides to the grocery store and two different shopping malls. These amenities allowed her to sell her car, which was helpful in meeting the expenses of the move.

It has been almost 6 years since her move to the retirement community. While the actual processes of selling the house and moving were traumatic for all, the final outcome has been successful. No additional falls have occurred, and the memory issues that developed after the series of falls have diminished and are currently being managed through the use of lists, reminders, and other strategies. Mrs. Tea adapted quickly to her new environment and increased her occupational engagement. Her very social dog, Misty, loved the change in location. The fact that Misty was a social animal and attracted people to stop and talk facilitated Mrs. Tea's ability to meet people and helped her overall adjustment to the new community. While she previously relied on her family for the majority of her social occupations, she now also has a circle of close friends. She is an active member of the community and walks Misty three times a day in all types of weather. She participates in group outings, including culturally relevant activities that allow her to feel connected to her homeland and rekindle memories of her honeymoon in Scotland. She is more active both physically and socially and is more independent than if she had remained in her previous house.

It is important to recognize the positive impact on the successful relocation caused by the unique match between Mrs. Tea's occupational profile and her choice of home. Mrs. Tea was a military wife, so while it was difficult downsizing, sorting through, and prioritizing possessions, her attachment to place was not as strong as it may have been if she had lived in one place all her married life. She was also fortunate that she and her husband had lived frugally, since it allowed her the financial freedom to make the best choice for her health and wellbeing.

An appreciation of temporal context was also important. She had lived alone for 10 years since the death of her husband and was ready to move on to begin a new chapter in her life. She needed this time in her house with her garden and previous dog to first grieve and then start building her own life. Although this was not the future her husband and she had saved and sacrificed for, it was a future she was ready to embrace, in which she was independent, in control, and with her beloved dog.

As one of Mrs. Tea's granddaughters remarked, every family needs an occupational therapist and a financial advisor. Mrs. Tea was fortunate to have two daughters, one in each of these professions. Occupational therapists and occupational therapy assistants can help individuals and families examine the various personal and contextual factors related to falls, as well as options for home modification or relocation.

Questions

1. What is the relationship between falls and memory loss?
2. What issues and factors do families need to consider when caring for an elderly person who repeatedly falls?
3. What additional home modifications might you suggest for this client?
4. For elderly persons, what are the positive and negative aspects of living in their own home versus relocating to a retirement community or assisted-living facility?
5. How does temporal context impact an elderly person's decision to stay at home or relocate?

▶ For Discussion and Review

1. What partnerships could be fostered in your community to increase awareness about fall prevention?
2. How does fear of falling interact with locus of control, environmental press, perceived risk, and self-efficacy?
3. Describe an occupation-based intervention addressing balance impairments in someone who has recently experienced a fall.

▶ Research Questions

1. What percentage of older adults using mobility devices (e.g., walkers, canes) use them incorrectly? Can device-training interventions during natural occupations increase correct device use? If so, can correct device use be shown to reduce the risk of falling among those who use devices? Among those who have not used devices previously?
2. What forms of physical activity and exercise are most appealing, motivating, and acceptable to older adults? How do these preferences vary along sociocultural or gender lines?
3. What concrete standards can be developed to operationalize some of the more subjective risk factors?

For example, when is lighting considered inadequate? How much clutter constitutes a hazard?

Acknowledgments

The authors wish to thank Elizabeth Frey and Alexander Stroup for their invaluable assistance in compiling literature for this chapter while they were graduate assistants at Towson University, and Mary Becker-Omvig, OTR/L, for providing access to an extensive library of resources for community-based fall prevention programs.

References

Alagiakrishnan, K., Masaki, K., Schatz, I., Curb, J. D., & Blanchette, P. L. (2001). Blood pressure dysregulation syndrome: The case for control throughout the circadian cycle. *Geriatrics, 56*(3), 50–60.

American Occupational Therapy Association. (2004). *Occupational therapy and prevention of falls: Education for older adults, families, caregivers, and healthcare providers.* AOTA Fact Sheet. Bethesda, MD: Author.

American Occupational Therapy Association. (2008). Occupational therapy practice framework: Domain and process. *American Journal of Occupational Therapy, 62,* 625–83.

Aminzadeh, F., & Edwards, N. (1998). Exploring seniors' views on the use of assistive devices in fall prevention. *Public Health Nursing, 15*(4), 297–304.

Aminzadeh, F., & Edwards, N. (2000). Factors associated with cane use among community dwelling older adults. *Public Health Nursing, 17*(6), 474–83.

Arfken, C. L., Lack, H. W., Birge, S. J., & Miller, J. P. (1994). The prevalence and correlates of fear of falling in elderly persons living in the community. *American Journal of Public Health, 84*(4), 565–70.

Bamiou, D. E., Davies, R. A., McKee, M., & Luxon, L. M. (2000). Symptoms, disability and handicap in unilateral peripheral vestibular disorders: Effects of early presentation and initiation of balance exercises. *Scandinavian Audiology, 29*(4), 238–44.

Beers, M. H., & Berkow, R. (Eds.). (2005). Falls. In *Merck manual of geriatrics* (3d ed.). Whitehouse Station, NJ; Merck & Co. Retrieved Whitehouse Station, NJ: Merck & Co. March 25, 2006, from http://www.merck.com/mrkshared/mmg/sec2/ch20/ch20a.jsp.

Brouwer, B. J., Walker, C., Rydahl, S. J., & Culham, E. G. (2003). Reducing fear of falling in seniors through education and activity programs: A randomized trial. *Journal of the American Geriatrics Society, 51*, 829–34.

Buchner, D. M., Cress, M. E., de Lateur, B. J., Esselman, P. C., Margherita, A. J., Price, R., & Wagner, E. H. (1997). The effect of strength and endurance training on gait, balance, fall risk, and health services use in community-living older adults. *Journal of Gerontology, 52A*(4), M218–M224.

Campbell, A. J., Borrie, M. J., & Spears, G. F. (1989). Risk factors for falls in a community-based prospective study of people 70 years and older. *Journal of Gerontology, 44*(4), 112–17.

Campbell, A. J., Robertson, M. C., Gardner, M. M., Norton, R. N., & Buchner, D. M. (1999). Psychotropic medication withdrawal and a home-based exercise program to prevent falls: A randomized, controlled trial. *Journal of the American Geriatrics Society, 47*, 850–53.

Campbell, A. J., Robertson, M. C., Gardner, M. M., Norton, R. N., Tilyard, M. W., & Buchner, D. M. (1997). Randomized controlled trial of a general practice programme of home based exercise to prevent falls in elderly women. *British Medical Journal, 315*(7115), 1065–69.

Campbell, V. A., Crews, J. E., Moriarty, D. G., Zack, M. M., & Blackman, D. K. (1999, December 17). Surveillance for sensory impairment, activity limitation, and health-related quality of life among older adults—United States, 1993–1997. *CDC Surveillance Summaries, Mortality and Morbidity Weekly Report 48*(SS-8), 131–56.

Carter, N. D., Kannus, P., & Khan, K. M. (2001). Exercise in the prevention of falls in older people: A systematic literature review examining the rationale and the evidence. *Sports Medicine, 31*(6), 427–38.

Cawthorne, T. (1945). The physiological basis for head exercises. *Journal of the Chartered Society Physiotherapy, 29*, 106–07.

Centers for Disease Control and Prevention. (2008). *Costs of falls among older adults*. Retrieved February 15, 2008, from http://www.cdc.gov/ncipc/factsheets/fallcost.htm.

Clemson, L., Cumming, R. G., & Roland, M. (1996). Case-control study of hazards in the home and risk of falls and hip fractures. *Age and Ageing, 25*, 97–101.

Clemson, L., Cumming, R. G., & Heard, R. (2003). The development of an assessment to evaluate behavioral factors associated with falling. *American Journal of Occupational Therapy, 57*(4), 380–88.

Clemson, L., Cusick, A., & Fozzard, C. (1999). Managing risk and exerting control: Determining follow through with falls prevention. *Disability and Rehabilitation, 21*(12), 531–41.

Clemson, L., Manor, D., & Fitzgerald, M. H. (2003). Behavioral factors contributing to older adults falling in public places. *OTJR: Occupation, Participation and Health, 23*(3), 107–17.

Close, J., Ellis, M., Hooper, R., Glucksman, E., Jackson, S., & Swift, C. (1999). Prevention of falls in the elderly trial (PROFET): A randomised controlled trial. *Lancet, 353*, 93–97.

Cohen, H. S. (2006). Disability and rehabilitation in the dizzy patient. *Current Opinion in Neurology, 19*, 49–54.

Cole, M. H., Ryan, L., Adrean, C., & Silver, J. (2001, November). Fighting against falls. *Rehab Management: The Interdisciplinary Journal of Rehabilitation*. Retrieved March 25, 2006, from http://www.rehabpub.com/ltrehab/112001/3.asp.

Connell, B. R. (1996). Role of the environment in falls prevention. *Clinics in Geriatric Medicine, 12*(4), 859–80.

Cooksey, F. S. (1946). Rehabilitation in vestibular injuries. *Proceedings of the Royal Society of Medicine, 39*, 273–78.

Corna, S., Nardone, A., Prestinari, A., Gatante, M., Grasso, M., & Schieppati, M. (2003). Comparison of Cawthorne-Cooksey exercises and sinusoidal support surface translations to improve balance in patients with unilateral vestibular deficit. *Archives of Physical Medicine and Rehabilitation, 84*(8), 1173–84.

Cumming, R. G. (2002). Intervention strategies and risk-factor modification for falls prevention: A review of recent intervention studies. *Clinics in Geriatric Medicine, 18*(2), 175–89.

Cumming, R. G., Miller, J. P., Kelsey, J. L., Davis, P., Arfken, C. L., Birge, S. J., & Peck, W. A. (1991). Medications and multiple falls in elderly people: The St. Louis OASIS study. *Age and Ageing, 20*, 455–61.

Cumming, R. G., Thomas, M., Szonyi, G., Salkeld, G., O'Neill, E., Westbury, C., & Frampton, G. (1999). Home visits by an occupational therapist for assessment and modification of environmental hazards: A randomized trial of falls prevention. *Journal of the American Geriatrics Society, 47*, 1397–1402.

Davison, J., Bond, J., Dawson, P., Steen, I. N., & Kenny, R. (2005). Patients with recurrent falls attending accident in emergency benefit from multifactorial intervention—A randomized control trial. *Age and Ageing, 34*(2), 162–68.

Day, L., Fildes, B., Gordon, I., Fitzharris, M., Flamer, H., & Lord, S. (2002). Randomised factorial trial of falls prevention among older people living in their own homes. *British Medical Journal, 325*, 128–31.

Desai, M. M., Zhang, P., & Hennessy, C. H. (1999). Surveillance for morbidity and mortality among older adults—United States, 1995–1996. *CDC Surveillance Summaries, MMWR, 48*(SS-8), 7–25.

El-Faizy, M., & Reinsch, S. (1994). Home safety intervention for the prevention of falls. *Physical & Occupational Therapy in Geriatrics, 12*(3), 33–49.

Enevold, G., & Courts, N. F. (2000). Fall prevention program for community-dwelling older adults and their caregivers. *Home Healthcare Nurse Manager, 4*(4), 22–28.

Englander, F., Hodson, T. J., & Terregrossa, R. A. (1996). Economic dimensions of slip and fall injuries. *Journal of Forensic Sciences, 41*(5), 733–46.

Fletcher, P. C., & Hirdes, J. P. (2002). Risk factors for falling among community-based seniors using home care services. *Journal of Gerontology: Medical Sciences, 57A*(8), M504–M510.

Fortin, J. D., Yeaw, E. M. J., Campbell, S., & Jameson, S. (1998). An analysis of risk assessment tools for falls in the elderly. *Home Healthcare Nurse, 16*(9), 624–29.

Gallagher, B., Corbett, E., Freeman, L., Riddoch-Kennedy, A., Miller, S., Smith, C., Radensky, L, & Zarrow, A. (2001). A fall prevention program for the home environment. *Home Care Provider, 6*(5), 157–63.

Gardner, M. M., Robertson, M. C., & Campbell, A. J. (2000). Exercise in preventing falls and fall related injuries in older people: A review of randomized controlled trials. *British Journal of Sports Medicine, 34*(1), 7–17.

Gardner, M. M., Robertson, M. C., McGee, R., & Campbell, A. J. (2002). Application of a falls prevention program for older people to primary health care practice. *Preventive Medicine, 34*, 546–53.

Gill, T. M., Williams, C. S., & Tinetti, M. E. (2000). Environmental hazards and the risk of nonsyncopal falls in the homes of community-living older persons. *Medical Care, 38*(12), 1174–83.

Graham, J. E., & Rockwood, K. (1997). Prevalence and severity of cognitive impairment with and without dementia in an elderly population. *Lancet, 349*(9068), 1793–96.

Herdman, S. J., Blatt, P. J., & Schubert, M. C. (2000). Vestibular rehabilitation of patients with vestibular hypofunction or with benign paroxysmal positional vertigo. *Current Opinion in Neurology, 19*, 49–54.

Hong, Q., & Robinovitch, S. N. (2003, Spring). *Ability to recover balance depends on base of support size.* Poster session presented at the meeting of the International Society for Posture and Gait Research, Sydney, Australia. Retrieved March 26, 2006, from www.powmri.edu.au/ispg2003 /ISPG2003/abstract%20PDFs/Postural%20perturbation% 20posters/Hong_Q_1.pdf.

Iconoculture. (2008). *Boomers today.* Retrieved May 17, 2008, from http://www.iconoculture.com/microsites/boomers/ ?-kk=baby%20boomers&-kt=275f0ad0-7730-4591-9dbc -69fd30a12b65&gclid=CJ7M-IrwrZMCFQx_Hgod7Uaw5A.

Kelley, S. D. M. (2003). Prevalent mental health disorders in the aging population: Issues of comorbidity and functional disability. *Journal of Rehabilitation, 69*(2), 19–25.

Kessenich, C. R. (1998). Tai chi as a method of fall prevention in the elderly. *Orthopaedic Nursing, 17*(4), 27–29.

King, M. B., & Tinetti, M. E. (1995). Falls in community-dwelling older persons. *Journal of the American Geriatrics Society, 43*, 1146–54.

Kochera, A. (2002). Falls among older persons and the role of the home: An analysis of cost, incidence, and potential savings from home modification. *Public Policy Institute Issue Brief.* Washington, DC: American Association of Retired Persons.

Lawton, M. P. (1980). *Environment and aging.* Monterey, CA: Brooks/Cole.

Lever, J. A. (2005). A multifactorial intervention reduced the mean number of falls but not the proportion who fell in older people with recurrent falls. *Evidence Based Nursing, 8*, 120.

Liu-Ambrose, T., Khan, K. M., Eng, J. J., Lord, S. R., & McKay, H. A. (2003, March). *Strength or agility training significantly reduces fall risk compared to posture training in 75 to 85 year old women with low bone density: A six month RCT.* Poster session presented at the meeting of the International Society for Posture and Gait Research, Sydney, Australia. Retrieved April 1, 2006, from http://www.powmri .edu.au/ispg2003/ISPG2003/abstract%20PDFs/Falls%20in %20the%20elderly/LiuAmbrose_T_2.pdf.

Mackenzie, L., Byles, J., & Higginbotham, N. (2002). A prospective community-based study of falls among older people in Australia: Frequency, circumstances and consequences. *OTJR: Occupation, Participation and Health, 22*(4), 143–52.

Mathias, C. J., Deguchi, K., & Schatz, I. (2001). Observations on recurrent syncope and presyncope in 641 patients. *Lancet, 357*(9253), 348–53.

McGee, M. (2000, Summer). Vestibular rehabilitation. *British Acoustic Neuroma Association Headline News.* Retrieved on March 28, 2006, from http://www.ukan.co.uk/archive/ content4/vestib.htm. [Transcript of talk provided at Derby/Nottingham Branch on May 13, 2000.]

McNulty, M. C., Johnson, J., Poole, J. L., & Winkle, M. (2004). Using the transtheoretical method of change to implement home safety modifications with community-dwelling older adults: An exploratory study. *Physical & Occupational Therapy in Geriatrics, 21*(4), 53–66.

MedicineNet. (1997). *Meclizine.* Retrieved March 31, 2006, from http://www.medicinenet.com/meclizine/article.htm.

Merkelj, I. (2001). Urinary incontinence in the elderly. *Southern Medical Journal, 94*(10), 952–57.

Moreland, J., Richardson, J., Chan, D. H., O'Neill, J., Bellissimo, A., Grum, R. M., & Shanks, L. (2003). Evidence-based guidelines for the secondary prevention of falls in older adults. *Gerontology, 49*(2), 93–116.

Morbidity and Mortality Weekly Report. (2008, March 31). *A cup of health with CDC: Falls among older adults.* Retrieved May 17, 2008, from http://www2a.cdc.gov/ podcasts/player.asp?f=5813.

Mosley, A., Galindo-Ciocon, D., Peak, N., & West, M. J. (1998). Initiation and evaluation of a research-based fall prevention program. *Journal of Nursing Care Quality, 13*(2), 38–44.

Plautz, B., Beck, D. E., Selmar, C., & Radetsky, M. (1996). Modifying the environment: A community-based injury-reduction program for elderly residents. *American Journal of Preventive Medicine, 12*(Suppl 1), 33–38.

Reinsch, S., MacRae, P., Lachenbruch, P. A., & Tobis, J. S. (1992). Why do healthy older adults fall? Behavioral and environmental risks. *Physical & Occupational Therapy in Geriatrics, 11*(1), 1–15.

Resende, C. R., Taguchi, C. K., de Almeida, J. G., & Fujita, R. R. (2003). Vestibular rehabilitation in elderly patients with benign paroxysmal positional vertigo. *Brazilian Journal of Otorhinolaryngology, 69*(4), 535–40.

Ribeiro, A. S. B., & Pereira, J. S. (2005). Balance improvement and reduction of likelihood of falls in older women after Cawthorne and Cooksey exercises. *Revista Brasileria De Otorrinolaringologia, 71*(1), 38–46.

Robertson, M. C., Campbell, A. J., Gardner, M. M., & Devlin, N. (2002). Prevention injuries in older people by preventing falls: A meta-analysis of individual-level data. *Journal of the American Geriatrics Society, 50*(5), 905–11.

Rosedale, M. (2001). Catching falls: A synthesis of recent research. *Caring, 20*(1), 14–19.

Rubenstein, L. Z., & Josephson, K. R. (2002). The epidemiology of falls and syncope. *Clinics in Geriatric Medicine, .18,* 141–58.

Salkeld, G., Cumming, R. G., O'Neill, E., Thomas, M., Szonyi, G., & Westbury, C. (2000). The cost effectiveness of a home hazard reduction program to reduce falls among older persons. *Australian and New Zealand Journal of Public Health, 24*(3), 265–71.

Sattin, R. W., Huber, D. A. L., DeVito, C. A., Rodriguez, J. G., Ros, A., Bacchelli, S., Stevens, J. A., & Waxweiler, R. J. (1990). The incidence of fall injury events among the elderly in a defined population. *American Journal of Epidemiology, 131*(6), 1028–37.

Schmucker, D. L. (2001). Liver function and phase I drug metabolism in the elderly. *Drugs and Aging, 18*(11), 837–51.

Shaw, F. E. (2002). Falls in cognitive impairment and dementia. *Clinics in Geriatric Medicine, 18,* 159–73.

Shaw, F. E., Bond, J., Richardson, D. A., Dawson, P., Steen, I. N., McKeith, I. G., & Kenny, R. A. (2003). Multifactorial intervention after a fall in older people with cognitive impairment and dementia presenting to the accident and emergency department: Randomised controlled trial. *British Medical Journal, 326,* 73–75.

Steinberg, M., Cartwright, C., Peel, N., & Williams, G. (2000). A sustainable programme to prevent falls and near falls in community dwelling older people: Results of a randomised trial. *Journal of Epidemiology and Community Health, 54,* 227–32.

Steinmetz, H. M., & Hobson, S. J. G. (1994). Prevention of falls among the community-dwelling elderly: An overview. *Physical & Occupational Therapy in Geriatrics, 12*(4), 13–29.

Stevens, J. A., Ryan, G., & Kresnow, M. (2006, November 17). Fatalities and injuries from falls among older adults— United States, 1993–2003 and 2001–2005. *Mortality and Morbidity Weekly Report, 55*(45), 1221–24.

Texas Department of Aging and Disability Services, Quality Matters Web. (2003). *Managing fall risk.* Retrieved March 25, 2006, from http://mqa.dhs.state.tx.us/qmweb/Falls .htm#Eval.

Thompson, P. G. (1996). Preventing falls in the elderly at home: A community-based program. *Medical Journal of Australia, 164*(9), 530–32.

Thomson PDR (2004). Antivert. In *Physician's desk reference* (58th ed., p. 2570). Montvale, NJ: Author.

Tideiksaar, R. (2002). *Falls in older people: Prevention and management* (3d ed.). Baltimore: Health Professions Press.

Tinetti, M. E., Baker, D. I., McAvay, G., Claus, E. B., Garrett, P., Gottschalk, M., Kock, M. L., Trainor, K., & Horwitz, R. I. (1994). A multifactorial intervention to reduce the risk of falling among elderly people living in the community. *New England Journal of Medicine, 331*(13), 821–27.

Tinetti, M. E., Speechley, M., & Ginter, S. F. (1988). Risk factors for falls among elderly persons living in the community. *New England Journal of Medicine, 319,* 1701–07.

U.S. Department of Health and Human Services. (2000). *Healthy People 2010* (2d ed.). With understanding and improving health and objectives for improving health. 2 vols. Washington, DC: U.S. Government Printing Office.

U.S. Department of Health and Human Services. (2004). *The effect of reducing falls on long-term care expenses: Literature review.* Retrieved March 25, 2006, from http://aspe.hhs.gov/daltcp/reports/fallexplr.htm#table1.

van den Bogert A. J., Pavol, M. J., & Grabiner, M. D. (2002). Response time is more important than walking speed for the ability of older adults to avoid a fall after a trip. *Journal of Biomechanics, 35*(2), 199–205.

Walker, J. E., & Howland, J. (1991). Falls and fear of falling among elderly persons living in the community: Occupational therapy interventions. *American Journal of Occupational Therapy, 45*(2), 119–22.

Wolf, S. L., Barnhart, H. X., Kutner, N. G., McNeely, E., Coogler, C., Xu, T., & the Atlanta FICSIT Group. (1996). Reducing frailty and falls in older persons: An investigation of tai chi and computerized balance training. *Journal of the American Geriatrics Society, 44,* 489–97.

Woodland, J. E., & Hobson, S. J. G. (2003). An occupational therapy perspective on falls prevention among community-dwelling older adults. *Canadian Journal of Occupational Therapy, 70*(3), 174–82.

World Health Organization. (2001). *International classification of functioning, disability, and health.* Geneva, Switzerland: Author.

World Health Organization. (2006). *Injuries and violence prevention: Falls.* Retrieved March 26, 2006, from http://www.who.int/violence_injury_prevention/other _injury/falls/en/.

Wu, G. (2002). Evaluation of the effectiveness of tai chi for improving balance and preventing falls in the older population—A review. *Journal of the American Geriatrics Society, 50,* 746–54.

Chapter 25

Promoting Wellness in End-of-Life Care

Michael A. Pizzi

> Our failure to face our own fear of death is an important reason why we find it so difficult to help the dying and the bereaved . . . Our hectic style of life owes much to the suppressed fear of death and the unexamined notion that the faster we live, the more we shall get out of this short life . . . [there are] places where we can experience and experiment with a different way of healthy living and healthy dying . . . medical intervention is subservient to exploring the potential in dying for health [with] health defined as the sustaining and development of a personal identity nourished by the resources and challenges of the environment and, most importantly, our multidimensional relationships.
>
> —Neuberger, 2003, p. 207

Learning Objectives

This chapter is designed to enable the reader to:

- Discuss the history of occupational therapy relative to end-of-life care (ELC) within the United States, including occupational therapy palliative care research.
- Distinguish between quality of life, quality of care, and quality of dying.
- Describe the different contexts of care and identify the role of occupational therapy in each.
- Apply principles of health, health promotion, and wellbeing to palliative care.
- Describe the concept of a good death and identify strategies for facilitating a good death through occupational engagement.
- Assess occupational needs for people at the end of life and develop appropriate ELC occupational therapy interventions.

Key Terms

Client-centered care

Dignified death

End-of-life care

Good death

Health-related quality of life

Hospice

Palliative care

Quality of care

Quality of dying

Therapeutic use of self

Introduction

End-of-life care (ELC), also known as *terminal care,* is care provided at the final stage of human development. Occupational therapists and occupational therapy assistants can effect change in a person's wellbeing by acknowledging the power of occupation in people's lives, even at the end of those lives. Occupation may even be more potent when a person is keenly focused on fully experiencing the life remaining, the quality of that life, and the quality of the dying process. Meaning and quality of life (QOL) can be optimized for people at the end of life, thus positively affecting their state of wellbeing. Wellbeing and wellness can be goals for people with terminal illnesses. These goals can be facilitated by occupational therapists and occupational therapy assistants through a conscious change in thinking, or a reframing of practice regarding the dying trajectory and the importance of occupational engagement for enhancing meaning, spiritual connectedness, and QOL (Bye, Llewellyn, & Christl, 2001; Pizzi & Briggs, 2004; Pizzi & Chromiak, 2001).

The facilitation of meaning at the end of life can be assisted by creating a positive philosophy of care. This philosophy, which supports the process of living, including being, doing, and becoming (Lyons, Orozovic, Davis, & Newman, 2002; Wilcock, 1999), and values dignity and self-respect, is the foundation of occupational therapy in ELC and hospice care. Interventions based on this philosophy promote wellbeing for those with life-threatening illness through adaptation and engagement in occupations of the person's interest and choice. In collaboration with the patient, occupational therapists and occupational therapy assistants investigate possibilities for life and living, being and doing until death.

In this chapter the author will

1. provide an overview of occupational therapy in hospice care within the United States;
2. describe the contexts for palliative care occupational therapy;
3. discuss the research in palliative care and occupational therapy;
4. detail several assessments and principles to guide interventions for dying persons and their families; and
5. develop the construct of a good death through occupational engagement.

The main purpose of this chapter is to continue development of theory and practice for occupational therapy in ELC that integrates constructs and values of health promotion with palliative care. Through the integration of these approaches, the outcome of the dying process can be more positive and classified as healthy dying or a **good death,** where QOL and wellbeing of the patient and family is maximized through improved care. The author uses the term *patient* interchangeably with *client,* which is consistent with the 2008 version of the American Occupational Therapy Association's (AOTA) *Occupational Therapy Practice Framework: Domain and Process* (referred to as the *Framework*). There is support for the use of both terms, depending on the therapist's work environment.

History of Occupational Therapy in ELC

Oelrich (1974) was the first to openly discuss death and dying in the occupational therapy literature within the United States and to examine the potential role for occupational therapists in ELC. According to Oelrich,

It is important to know the patient's life style before the illness, his role, and personal satisfactions in order to assist the patient to cope with the disease. The patient needs to continue to feel useful, worthwhile, and to be as active as his condition permits. Self-care and independence, if physically possible, contribute to a feeling of worth. In planning the treatment program, the physical limitations, psychological behavior, mental attitude, family and social problems, the patient's interests, work role, and motivation are all important factors. Goals to be achieved with the patient may

include the building of self-esteem, reduction of anxiety and depression, and *promotion of the feeling of being useful* [italics added]. An atmosphere in which the patient can accept the illness and death, yet remain as independent as possible, is part of the overall goal. Activity that is consistent with the patient's physical potential serves to prevent undue regression and promotes self-esteem. Generally suitable tasks or work promotes a feeling of usefulness. As the disease progresses, the patient's ability to assimilate unfamiliar activities declines and the tasks become those which are familiar and structured. (p. 431)

Oelrich (1974) presented a holistic and health-promoting perspective for occupational therapy and palliative care. Others have reflected and built on this foundation, which also included the promotion of health through participation (Flanigan, 1982; Gammage, McMahon & Shanahan, 1976; Holland & Tigges, 1981; Pizzi, 1984, 1992a, 1992d; Pizzi & Briggs, 2004; Tigges, 1993, 1998; Tigges & Marcil, 1988). Occupational engagement of mind, body, and spirit has also been emphasized in a variety of activities and occupations, including arts and crafts and play for children involved with palliative care (Bewley, 1985; Dawson, 1982; Pizzi, 1992c, 1993). Kubler-Ross, who is credited with breaking through societal anxiety regarding death and dying, stated that "occupational therapists have helped many of our patients with arts and crafts projects as a means of showing them that they can still function on some level" (1977, p. 225). Despite many occupational therapy practitioners's disengagement from arts and crafts, the fundamental human values of feeling useful, being productive, and participating in meaningful occupations, all of which are historically linked to the profession, are applicable in enhancing the QOL of individuals at the end of life. Not until the 1980s did the literature reflect use of a frame of reference or theory base from which evaluation and intervention were implemented. Tigges and Sherman (1983) and Pizzi (1983, 1984, 1992a) began to emphasize the need to utilize a theory, namely occupational behavior, to begin framing palliative care in occupational therapy, especially in hospice care. "Occupational behavior . . . provides not only a holistic basis under which one may practice, but also includes a humanistic perspective which is vital to practice with the terminally ill" (Pizzi, 1983, p. 50). Theory continues to be crucial to ground assessment and intervention in both palliative care in general and specifically for the care of the person with cancer or HIV/AIDS (Marcil & Tigges, 1992; Pizzi, 1990a, 1992a, 1993; Pizzi & Burkhardt, 2003; Pizzi & Chromiak, 2001).

In 1986, an AOTA position paper on occupational therapy and hospice was approved by the Representative

Assembly (Evans et al., 1986). That same year, the AOTA created a task force to discuss ELC and develop working guidelines on hospice care and the roles of occupational therapy. This was a monumental project that aligned with the Medicare Hospice Benefit, which allows for occupational therapy services to be contracted and utilized as needed. The guidelines covered all aspects of occupational therapy and hospice care, including history of occupational therapy in hospice care, policy, assessment, interventions, and the need for future research (AOTA, 1987). In the AOTA (2005) official document on hospice, the authors make an excellent case for the use of both adaptation and prevention, citing the role of occupational therapy as exploring the multidimensional aspects of living and dying to facilitate wellbeing. Examples of adaptation strategies identified in the document include adjusting the physical environment to enable continued participation in social activities, employing assistive devices in daily activities, and modifying daily routines based on client's activity tolerance. Prevention goals in ELC may include preventing

- social isolation;
- injury to client and caregiver;
- exacerbation of symptoms during activity; and
- complications from immobility (AOTA, 2005).

The promotion of wellbeing has been the focus of some of the palliative care occupational therapy literature. It has been discussed as a focus for women with HIV (Pizzi, 1992d), as a basis for occupational therapy programming for adults with HIV and AIDS (Galantino, Pizzi, & Lehmann, 1993; Gutterman, 1990; Pizzi & Burkhardt, 2003), in cancer care (Pizzi & Burkhardt, 2003), and in community-based practice (Pizzi & Chromiak, 2001).

Utilizing the *Ottawa Charter for Health Promotion,* sanctioned by the World Health Organization (WHO), vanderPloeg (2001) makes a clear case for the integration of palliative care and health promotion. This guide states that health promotion is

> the process of enabling people to increase control over and to improve health. To reach a state of complete physical, mental and social wellbeing, an individual or group must be able to identify and realize aspirations, to satisfy needs, and to change and cope with the environment. Health is therefore seen as a resource for everyday living, not the object of living. Health is a positive concept emphasizing social and personal resources, as well as physical capabilities. Therefore health promotion is not just the responsibility of the health sector, but goes beyond healthy lifestyles to wellbeing. (WHO, 1986, p. 5)

To best define this natural integration of palliative care and health promotion, vanderPloeg (2001) states that the philosophies of both hold the following:

1. Health and illness are fluctuating conditions.
2. Individuals are integrated organisms in which the elements of mind, body, spirit, emotions and environment are interrelated.
3. Individuals are not only adaptive but also have the potential to transcend difficulties and create new patterns of behaviour enabling continuation of a meaningful and satisfying existence.
4. A humanistic approach to health care is directed to the quality and dignity of life, not necessarily its prolongation. (p. 46)

These are also principles of practice and beliefs upon which the profession of occupational therapy was founded. These beliefs can guide and support practice in occupational therapy palliative care.

It is evident that the role of occupational therapy in palliative care continues to evolve. As more occupational therapists and occupational therapy assistants engage in this work, the need for occupational therapy services that promote a good death will become more visible. The lack of current substantive evidence for the integration of health promotion principles in palliative care demonstrates a professional need for practice and research. The transformation of the dying process can be made evident by the application and integration of these principles in order to facilitate wellness, QOL, and participation in life until death.

Definitions and Meanings in ELC

The term **end-of-life care** has essentially replaced the phrase *terminal care.* The use of *ELC* connotes a more positive and developmental perspective than the word *terminal,* although their meanings are the same. The new term also symbolizes that humans have lives to live until they die, and it is in that living that occupational therapists and occupational therapy assistants can make a difference in effecting purpose and meaning.

Palliative care is the term being used to describe a total program of care designed for people for whom cure cannot be achieved. The Institute of Medicine (IOM) report on ELC (Field & Cassel, 1997) was one of the first documents to extensively discuss the subject. This report elucidated terms and constructs and developed many recommendations for practitioners' adoption of strategies for enabling a good death.

The IOM report stated that hospice and palliative care are responses to perceived inadequacies in the prevention and relief of symptoms and distress in people approaching death. The term **hospice** has at least three somewhat different uses. First, a hospice may be a freestanding facility, inpatient hospital, or nursing home unit. In the United States, the client's home is the most common location to provide care, usually by family caregivers. Second, hospice may also be an organization that provides the necessary services to ensure a good death. This use of the term *hospice* also implies insurance coverage (there is a hospice benefit through Medicare) and an overall affiliation with a hospice program. Third, *hospice* implies an approach to care based on holistic principles of best practice that incorporate the clinical, social, metaphysical, and spiritual arenas of care (Field & Cassel, 1997). There is an abundance of literature that discusses the psychospiritual issues related to suffering (Byock, 1997; Field & Cassel, 1997; Kaut, 2002); some of which is discussed later in this chapter.

This third meaning of hospice is generally regarded as palliative care versus hospice programs or organizations. In a broad sense, palliative care seeks to prevent, relieve, reduce, or soothe the symptoms of disease or disorder without effecting a cure. Palliative care in this broad sense is not restricted to those who are dying or enrolled in hospice programs. Sometimes palliation is used adjunctively to life-saving measures for purposes of preserving the QOL of individuals and to help prevent or relieve pain (MacDonald, 1991, as cited in Field & Cassel, 1997). For people with chronic pain, palliative care can help manage discomfort while it holistically helps them meet their needs and goals and those of their loved ones.

Palliative care is also needed for children and adolescents dealing with life-threatening illness. The American Academy of Pediatrics (AAP) clearly illustrates this point by noting that QOL and relief of symptoms are the primary goals of palliative care so that children may continue to experience and enjoy life to its fullest despite a terminal diagnosis (AAP, 2000). These goals underscore two important realities: (1) death is the end point to living while dying, and (2) helping people live well while dying requires "strategies and tools for measuring and monitoring symptoms, functional status, emotional well-being, and burdens associated with terminal illness and treatment" (Field & Cassel, 1997, ¶ 3).

The concept of a **dignified death** implies skilled caregiving and respect for the person who is dying.

> Even excellent patient care may not always prevent . . . pain, incontinence, vomiting, delirium, or traumatic but sometimes appropriate medical interventions. A worthy and more achievable goal is death dignified by care that honors, protects, and cherishes those who are dying.

The goal of a dignified death would be conveyed by word and action that dignity resides in people, not physical attributes, and that helps people to preserve their integrity while coping with unavoidable physical insults and losses. (Field & Cassel, 1997, p. 25)

A good death can be restored and promoted, enabling people to experience dignity by providing control in daily living, by promoting occupational choice for occupational engagement, or by making the physical environment more homelike (Pizzi, 1984; Pizzi & Chromiak, 2001).

The construct of **quality of dying** focuses on "a person's experience of living while terminally ill or imminently dying" (Field & Cassel, 1997, p. 25). The outcomes are defined from the special world of the dying patient; for example, some physical outcomes become less realistic while other outcomes (e.g., spiritual wellbeing or sense of peace) may become more meaningful (Field & Cassel, 1997, p. 25). This construct parallels that of experiencing a good death through occupational engagement, which will be explored in more depth.

Quality of care stresses the link between the structure and processes of health care and outcomes for individuals and populations. High-quality care should contribute to the quality of living and the quality of dying but is not synonymous with them (Field & Cassel, 1997, p. 25). Yee (2003) discusses a framework for measuring quality in health care. The framework refers to dimensions of structure (i.e., where the care is provided), process (i.e., how the care occurs), and outcomes. Quality of life and death have many factors that need to be attended to in order to facilitate a good death. Promoting health through occupational engagement until death can ensure quality is preserved on all levels. Most people wish for a long, satisfying life—that is, they value both how long they live *and* how well they live. The construct of **health-related quality of life** (HRQOL) emphasizes health that is self-perceived and valued rather than as seen by experts (Cohen, Mount, Strobel, & Bui, 1995; Gold, Franks, & Erickson, 1996). Health-related QOL outcomes include physical, mental, social, and role functioning; a sense of wellbeing; freedom from bodily pain; satisfaction with health care; and an overall sense of general health (Field & Cassel, 1997, p. 25). For occupational therapists and occupational therapy assistants in ELC, this construct is more fully explained by Pizzi (1992b):

> Quality of life is not simply about pain control and keeping people comfortable—it is about enhancing the ability to perform activity important to the person and family system, helping those we serve develop competence, mastery, and control when life-threatening

illness takes control, creating opportunities to live fully and productively until death. (p. 1)

Client-Centered Care and Therapeutic Use of Self in ELC

Meaning is derived by a person's life choices, experiences and beliefs, and occupations. Meaningful occupations that are client-centered and engage the mind, body, and spirit can enhance the dying person's and their family's QOL and spirituality. **Client-centered care** is care that engages the person in helping to define what is most relevant and meaningful to do and to be as one approaches the end of life. As Peloquin (1997) so eloquently states, "Occupation . . . animates and extends the human spirit; we participate in that animation. Gazing past the details of practice while led by their design to the point beyond, we discern a deeper aim. The discovery is awesome" (p. 168).

The Sulmasy (2002) model, depicted in Figure 25-1, appears to be an open systems model of care that is client-centered and incorporates occupational engagement. This open system examines the interrelationships between the person's spiritual state and biopsychosocial state. Either state of being can influence the other, and the composite state of how one is feeling physically, psychologically, interpersonally, and spiritually is the construct called QOL. In occupational therapy, if optimizing QOL is a primary outcome in ELC, then practice must incorporate the principles of health promotion that include spiritual wellbeing and client-centeredness.

An example of the Sulmasy model's use and its components is represented in the case of Maria, an elderly Italian woman who could not participate in her favorite pastime of cooking due to end-stage chronic obstructive pulmonary disease (COPD). This occupation provided great meaning to her life, as she enjoyed making others happy with her skills, particularly her family. When the family would visit, Maria withdrew from them, until the occupational therapist explored interventions to enable her to cook from the bedside (by giving instructions and watching others engage in the occupation) and, finally, from a wheelchair, which she said she felt compelled to try because "people just weren't doing it right!" Her physical and mental health improved, albeit for a short time, due to the effects of participating once again in her favorite occupation.

Peloquin (1993) examined phenomenological narratives and identified several themes regarding the client-practitioner relationship. These themes included the practitioner failing to see the personal consequences of illness or disability, distance, harmful withholdings, discouraging words, brusque behaviors, and the misuse of power.

> The voices within these narratives send out a steady plea. The central complaint is that when practitioners depersonalize, they are not inclined to care, and their behaviors sap a patient's courage. Helpers rarely listen when patients ask them to attend; patients then reason that practitioners lack the required sensitivity. (Peloquin, 1993, p. 835)

For hospice work, it is imperative to utilize the strength of presence and professionalism to enhance dignity and wellbeing that promotes a healthy life until death. "Practitioners must see that they can step into their patients' worlds with compassion. Any small part of the pain that helpers share makes room in which patients can then turn to their own courage" (Peloquin, 1993, p. 836).

Therapeutic use of self refers to therapists' ability to perceive what actions and behaviors on their part would be helpful or therapeutic to the client, as opposed

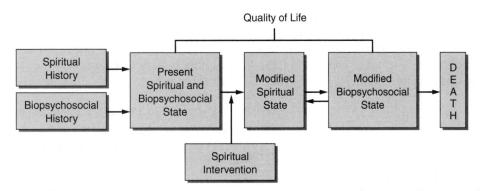

Figure 25-1   Biopsychosocial-spiritual model for ELC.

*Re-created from Figure 2 in "A biopsychosocial-spiritual model for the care of patients at the end of life," by D. S. Sulmasy, 2002, Gerontologist, 42, 29. Copyright ©
2002 by the Gerontological Society of America.*

to actions that would be insignificant, disruptive, or even harmful to the client and the therapeutic relationship (Fidler & Fidler, 1963). Pizzi (1996) developed strategies that enhance therapeutic use of self to engage the person in the therapy process so positive mental, physical, social, and spiritual health can be revitalized. These include recognizing the following:

- that the practitioner is the most important therapeutic modality;
- the need to be authentic in the process of intervention and be present;
- the need to be self-aware of judgments, biases, prejudices, beliefs, values, and joys that contribute to the therapy process and functional outcomes; and
- the need to engage in therapeutic and effective communications that can foster a higher level of wellbeing for the dying and their loved ones.

Simply listening, as opposed to explaining, doing, or fixing, can be an important support the occupational therapy practitioner offers the dying. By being fully present and listening without judgment, therapists bear witness to the person's struggle (Sharp, 1996).

Research suggests that older patients receiving hospice care may benefit from interventions directed to issues related to family, spirituality, outlook on mortality, and meaningful physical activity (Mackey & Sparling, 2000). Suffering is commonly experienced by people with an incurable illness as they struggle with discomfort, disability, and inevitable death (Byock, 1997). A large part of the unnecessary suffering of dying comes from not feeling safe to acknowledge or express natural fears and sadness, not feeling as if time is being provided for them to communicate honestly, or not feeling appreciated as a living person (Longaker, 1997).

The quality of occupational living incorporates all aspects of human functioning but also incorporates the existential domains of life. The occupational therapy process focuses on optimizing life quality and wellbeing through occupational engagement. When occupational therapists and occupational therapy assistants really know those whom they serve, then the holistic needs of the dying and their families can be more readily met, thus preserving dignity and quality living while dying.

ELC and Health Promotion: A Natural Fit

Rehabilitation in palliative care is a paradox (Thorpe, 1993). Bye (1998) and Bye and colleagues (2001) discussed occupational therapists' perceptions of pallia-

tive care practice and suggested strategies to reframe practice. Pizzi (1983, 1984, 1990b, 1993), Pizzi and Briggs (2004), and Pizzi and Chromiak (2001) provide guidance through an innovative paradigm based on the *Framework* (AOTA, 2008) for examining the occupational therapy evaluation process in ELC. This guidance is both conceptual and pragmatic, and comes from a health promotion perspective. Additional discussions in the above works review open systems approaches and environmental influences on care, the design of occupation-based interventions following specific intervention principles, and various assumptions of occupational therapy and occupational science relevant to work with the terminally ill. Pizzi (1993) also emphasized the need for guiding principles for the development and selection of appropriate assessments in hospice that are unique for the terminally ill yet incorporate basic constructs and principles from occupational therapy. It is also essential that practitioners examine the community culture from which a hospice practice can be developed and understand that hospice is not necessarily a physical place but a context and attitude of care (Pizzi & Chromiak, 2001).

Palliative care can be described as a reaffirmation of living with dignity and hope (Doyle, Hanks, & MacDonald, 1998). Practitioners must negotiate both the goals of safe and comfortable dying with maximized living and QOL. Continuous reexamination of goals and adapting the plan of care during the dying process is a crucial element in the provision of hospice therapy services. In hospice and ELC, intervention planning and goal-setting must be done collaboratively with the client and family with an understanding of the limited time frame. Realistic short- and long-term goals need to be individualized (Fulton & Else, 1998; Pizzi 1984, 1993).

The approaches taken by occupational therapists and occupational therapy assistants in palliative care, ELC, and hospice can be viewed not only through the lens of occupational therapy models but also through health promotion models (examples of these models are described in Chapter 3). With a foundation of health promotion knowledge, occupational therapists can adapt their skills and talents for the terminally ill and can explore more deeply the concept of facilitating a good death.

Early discussions with patients and significant others will allow for the opportunity to consider improvement, maintenance, or decline in occupational participation in a way that may be less threatening. The dying trajectory is individual; thus, people can optimize function and participation within the limits of the disease process. This client-centered approach empowers the client and family system to reorganize and reprioritize life goals (Pizzi & Chromiak, 2001). The changes do not reflect a failure of the patient, family, or therapist but rather a natural process at the end of life. This needs to be discussed openly with the patient and significant others. Hope is discovered and renewed by the patient in the living of each day (Pizzi & Briggs, 2004). Children and youth coping with the harsh realities of a life cut short are also entitled to having a goal of hope through developmentally appropriate assessments and interventions that reflect their preferences and choices (AAP, 2000).

> Engagement with the human, the vulnerable, is the central source of meaning and healing at the end of life. The awareness that ELC includes—in fact demands—a human relationship between the health professional and the dying person is an important step in providing dignity to those who are dying. (Kaufman, 2002, p. 34)

There is an apparent natural fit for occupational therapists and occupational therapy assistants to work with people experiencing life-threatening and terminal illness.

> The AAP strongly supports an integrated model of both palliative and curative treatment. It is difficult to determine which children may benefit from palliative care. If palliative care is reserved for children who are dying or have a terminal condition, other patients who may benefit from these services may not receive them. Time of death is often difficult to predict. If the nearness of death is used to determine if children receive palliative care, some children may die without the benefits of individualized family-centered palliative care. With a broader definition that includes children living with a life-threatening condition, all children who need palliative care may benefit. In addition, aspects of an integrated palliative care approach, including symptom management and counseling, may prove beneficial when provided early in the course of a child's illness. (AAP, 2000, p. 352)

The AAP is committed to client- and family-centered care and the availability of occupational choices of dying children and adolescents, which supports improved mental and emotional health of children and their overall wellbeing. Developmentally appropriate communication about death with children and adolescents is an important aspect of this type of care.

The training of occupational therapists and occupational therapy assistants who view health outcomes that include wellbeing and QOL supports the appropriateness of membership on the palliative care team. Content Box 25-1 displays the six elements that promote quality ELC, which are all within the scope of occupational therapy

Content Box 25-1

Six Elements of Quality End-of-Life Care

- Overall quality of life
- Physical wellbeing and functioning
- Psychosocial wellbeing and functioning
- Spiritual wellbeing
- Patient perceptions of care
- Family wellbeing and perceptions

Adapted from Table 5.3 in *Approaching death: Improving care at the end of life* (p. 142), by M. J. Field & C. K. Cassel (Eds.), 1997, Washington, DC: Institute of Medicine. Copyright © 1997 by National Academy of Sciences.

practice (Field & Cassel, 1997). The *Framework* provides examples of some of the potential outcomes of occupational therapy interventions: occupational performance, adaptation, role competence, self-advocacy, participation, occupational justice, QOL, and prevention, as well as health and wellness (AOTA, 2008 pp. 662–63). All of these outcomes can be achieved through occupational therapy practice in ELC.

Health professionals are viewed as experts who utilize clinical reasoning to select appropriate assessments and interventions. Singer, Martin, and Kelner (1999) outlined five aspects of ELC from the patients' perspective: receiving adequate pain and symptom management, avoiding inappropriate prolongation of dying, achieving a sense of control, relieving the burden on loved ones, and strengthening relationships with loved ones. Through surveys of dying patients, physicians, and other health-care providers, Steinhauser, Christakis, and colleagues (2000) further elaborated and elucidated the differences and similarities in the perspectives of each of these groups. They concluded that the health-care provider's sensitivity to the varied and diverse perceptions and roles of patients and their families can result in more positive experiences in ELC. This is important over and above the usual goals of hospice care, which include the control of pain and symptoms, the ability to communicate with one's physician, the emotional preparation for death, and the opportunity to achieve a sense of completion (Steinhauser, Christakis, et al., 2000).

The occupational therapy client-centered approach is a natural fit for work in palliative care. Table 25-1 outlines the basic values of hospice and corresponding occupational and physical therapy approaches. This table describes many strategies for involvement with terminally ill clients and their loved ones (Koff, 1980; Pizzi & Briggs, 2004).

Table 25–1 **Hospice and Occupational Therapy Values and Approaches to Care**

Hospice Values and Approaches (Koff, 1980)	Occupational and Physical Therapy and Approaches
The basic regard for the recipient of care	Client-centered
Acceptance of death as a natural part of living	Awareness of human development and temporal context
Consideration of the entire family as the unit of care	Family dynamics and systems thinking
Maintenance of the patient at home for as long as possible	Environments of care; environmental modifications and adaptations; caregiver training
Assistance for the patient attempting to assume control over his or her own life	Psychosocial and psychospiritual enhancement via provision of improvements or adaptations in function
Reduction or removal of pain and other distressing symptoms	Pain management, strengthen when possible; energy conservation; work simplification; complementary techniques
Comprehensive provision of services by an interdisciplinary team	Team approach
Total, not fragmented, care	Holistic thinking and clinical reasoning
Continuity of services after death	Grief, bereavement, and planning for more positive physical and mental health for survivors; family/significant other–oriented approaches

From "Occupational and physical therapy in hospice: The facilitation of meaning, quality of life and wellbeing," by M. Pizzi & R. Briggs, 2004, *Topics in Geriatric Rehabilitation, 20*(2), p. 121. Copyright © 2004 by Lippincott, Williams & Wilkins. Adapted with permission.

Contexts for ELC and Palliative Care

At the end of life, people die in diverse ways and in a variety of contexts. While the context may often dictate the type of care provided, possibly secondary to reimbursement issues, principles of health promotion and palliative care that can promote a good death can be applied in all contexts. The following provides an overview of various contexts in which people at the end of life receive care.

Hospitals

Hospital culture often regards death as a failure. Modern medicine has been very successful in rescuing, stabilizing, or curing people with serious medical problems, possibly because a small percentage of people die before the end of a normal life span. Every hospital's goal should be to optimize conditions for a good death to occur. A continuing challenge is to find better ways to maintain curative efforts while also preventing needless emotional and physical harm for clients and their families (Field & Cassel, 1997).

In acute care occupational therapy, life-and-death issues are commonplace. Yet, there appears to be little to no training in educational programs or in hospitals to prepare for work with the dying. For example, in a study of spirituality and its place in occupational therapy palliative care, Rose (1999) investigated the attitudes of 44 occupational therapists. Responses to a mailed questionnaire indicated that spirituality was an important part of life for 35 respondents (80%), that it helped 33 respondents (75%) cope with daily job responsibilities, and that it was viewed as an important dimension of health and rehabilitation by 39 respondents (89%). Spiritual issues were considered to be within the scope of occupational therapy by 33 respondents (75%). However, only 8 respondents (18%) stated that they consistently addressed spirituality within assessment. The respondents described several activities that addressed clients' spirituality, including open-ended discussion, facilitation of activities of daily living (ADLs) that contribute to maximizing quality of life, and creative activities. Thirty-two respondents (73%) considered that their education had not prepared them to meet clients' spiritual needs, and 28 respondents (64%) wanted further training in this area. Although this is only one study with a small sample, the results do provide some insights about the attitudes, values, and needs of some occupational therapists working in ELC.

While working as a staff therapist in a major research hospital with children with HIV and AIDS, the author discovered that children who received clear communication about their diagnosis and comprehended it were more likely to have higher levels of self-esteem and self-confidence than those from whom the diagnosis was hidden. The implication for caregivers was to slowly introduce the construct of life-threatening illness to the child based on their chronological and developmental age. Occupational therapists can help families develop a plan for this communication using verbal, nonverbal, and play strategies.

The growth of hospice, combined with pressures to minimize hospital use, is shifting care to other settings, more often the home or sometimes a nursing home. These other contexts for dying might afford a more supportive arena for occupational therapy palliative care.

Nursing Homes

Nursing homes differ from hospitals in many respects, including the lower level of physician involvement, relatively low ratios of registered nurses to patients, and the amount of care provided by nursing assistants or aides (Feasley, 1996). Staff may not be trained in caring for dying patients and may not provide adequate palliative care. A home setting may have limited resources to adequately manage the dying moments; thus, people may be transferred to hospitals, and their dying hours or days are spent in an unfamiliar place with unfamiliar people. "The experience of nursing home patients who die is not well documented" (Field & Cassel, 1997, p. 100). Pain management in nursing homes is often a major problem for residents, particularly for those at the end of life (Ferrell, Ferrell, & Osterwell, 1990; Morley, Kraenzle, Bible, & Bundren, 1995; Sengstaken & King, 1993).

There is an increase in nursing home admissions due to managed care plans minimizing hospital stays and the "graying of America" phenomena. Nursing homes are not well prepared to care for dying patients, despite the fact that most residents are functionally impaired (Field & Cassel, 1997; Mezey, Dubler, Mitty, & Brody, 2002). Most require attentive personal care. Some may be anxious, depressed, or fearful. Most who enter a nursing home for reasons other than rehabilitation and stay for more than a few months will either die there or transfer to a hospital. They will often not live at home again (Mezey et al., 2002).

Jones, Ackerud, and Boyle (1997) examined differences in rates of use of hospice services between nursing homes owned by the same company. Percentages of hospice use varied from 2% to 39% among 23 nursing homes. Administrators most sympathetic to hospice care had hospice utilization rates three times higher than in homes with administrators who were least sympathetic. Kitzes, Schmoll, and Dixon (2003) state that residential and nursing home facilities are obligated to make adaptations to ensure ongoing quality care and appropriate services when patients are involved with hospice care. These adaptations are listed in Content Box 25-2.

Hospice at Home

The National Hospice and Palliative Care Organization (NHPCO) standards state that home is a person's place of residence (NHPCO, 1997). Given this definition, a residence can be a personal home, a group home, a shelter, or a jail. The designation of someone as terminally ill and likely to benefit from primarily palliative rather than life-prolonging care is more difficult to determine for some diseases than others (e.g., AIDS versus metastatic lung cancer). The National Hospice Organization (NHO) developed guidelines for hospices (NHO, 1996) that can help with both prognosis and the context in which a person may receive care. This kind of policy guidance may contribute to improved care for the nonterminal chronically ill. Hospices put palliative care principles into practice. For example, hospices should back up their commitment to "be there" for patients.

Homecare Without Hospice Services

Homecare is important for people who do not qualify for hospice programs. This group includes many people with serious chronic illness (e.g., congestive heart failure, COPD). These are persons who traditionally may not be perceived as dying; however, they are

---

Content Box 25-2

Adaptations in Nursing Homes for End-of-Life Care

- Ensure privacy and space for family gathering
- Allow 24-hour visiting and overnight stays
- Provide for religious activity and spiritual worship
- Provide flexibility in scheduling care, accommodating individual needs
- Permit family to prepare meals
- Allow patient choice in food and timing of meals
- Provide a comfortable, homelike atmosphere
- Ensure access to services required by plan of care
- Ensure safety, comfort, and patient satisfaction
- Maintain coordination of care by hospice team member

Adapted From Table 4-3 of "Hospice/palliative care settings," by J. Kitzes, B. Schmoll, & C. Dixon, 2003, in *Hospice and palliative care: Concepts and practice* (2d ed., p. 52), W. B. Forman, J. A. Kitzes, R. P. Anderson, & D. K. Sheehan (Eds.). Sudbury, MA: Jones and Bartlett.

coping with a long-term illness that will likely end in death. Another option for keeping people at home involves the use of day-care services designed specifically for people who are able, with or without special assistance, to leave their homes for supportive care. Homecare services, though differing in quality and availability, can reduce distress, provide respite, and work extensively with families requiring psychosocial care as they deal with instability during the dying process (Thorpe, 1993). Often, in the case of occupational therapy, an attachment may form quickly with the therapist; however, if functional progress is not seen, a discontinuation of services occurs, leaving the client and family feeling abandoned by the system.

The Medicare hospice benefit is limited to those with a prognosis of 6 months or less to live (AOTA, 1987). However, it is not applicable to many patients with uncertain prognoses living with serious illnesses. For these individuals, coverage for home health services can help them secure important supportive services, such as medical social services and home health aide services. A major limitation of the home health benefit is that beneficiaries must be homebound and need part-time or intermittent skilled nursing care, physical therapy, or speech therapy. Some dying patients would be able to benefit significantly from home palliative care before they become completely homebound. (*Note:* At the time of this writing, occupational therapy was not considered a primary provider under Medicare.)

In Great Britain, where the hospice movement began and where a socialized medical system prevails, there are numerous hospice day-care programs. There, hospice day care is a program that provides "a day out and a day off." The person afflicted with a chronic or terminal illness has the opportunity for a day out while the relatives or friends providing the care in the home get a day off. A day out for those coping with a life-threatening illness or other serious disability has two primary benefits: It is both a health-care experience and—in many ways even more important—a psychosocial or personal experience (Holland, 1984). Adult hospice day care makes available medical, nursing, social work, spiritual guidance, and therapy. It brings people together primarily for social support among those at the end of life, although that does not preclude its offering ancillary services for caregivers and other concerned individuals (Dawson, 1993).

Community Programming

Broader and more intensive community education may help patients, families, and providers become more aware of the range of health care and other resources available to patients approaching death, including those for whom hospital care is not appropriate and who do not qualify for hospice care. These resources may be valuable, especially if potential for integrating them into the care processes and contextual transitions are identified. Thus, community groups, occupational therapists, and occupational therapy assistants can develop inventories of resources available to dying patients. These resources can include health-care institutions, religious institutions, other charitable organizations, support groups, and agencies serving special populations, such as older individuals, children, or people with disabilities.

One very successful community program is ART Is the HeART (Rollins & Riccio, 2002). This child and youth community-based program matches artists expert in a variety of media (e.g., drama, dance, music, art) with children and youth coping with life-threatening illness and who are involved with hospice care. The overarching goal of the program is to have children learn to use the arts as a healthy and effective coping strategy to deal with illness, death, or dying—their own or that of a family member. The program has three aims:

1. To develop artists to be effective members of the hospice and home health-care teams
2. To help children cope more effectively with illness, disability, dying, and death in the home or hospice care setting
3. To promote replication of ART Is the HeART in communities throughout the United States and abroad (Rollins & Riccio, 2002)

This type of community-based program can be established by occupational therapists, occupational therapy assistants, or occupational therapy or occupational science academic departments. Whether developing their own program or collaborating with a community-based organization, occupational therapy practitioners can be a tremendous asset to the success of such a program.

Summary of Contexts for ELC

The contexts in which people live while dying have been described. Occupational therapists and occupational therapy assistants can work in all of these contexts. However, they are rarely called upon, as they are still viewed as part of a rehabilitation team, with rehabilitation rarely seen as compatible with care for the dying. In hospitals, nursing homes, homecare, hospice care, and the many contexts where children, adolescents, and adults live and die, it is imperative that occupational therapy practitioners begin to define themselves as health professionals possessing knowledge and skills to optimize a person's health while dying to promote a good death. Clients who are dying require an affirmation of living until they die (Bye, 1998), despite the context in which they are receiving care. Occupational engagement for persons who are dying can be facilitated in any care setting. Health promotion principles of care can be integrated through the reframing of service provision.

Interventions Across Contexts

Bye and colleagues (2001) outlined therapy interventions for advancing terminal illness that can be applied across contexts. In the early stages of dying, therapy is designed to maintain function or make small improvements (e.g., decrease painful active range to reach into cupboards for meal preparation). The midstage includes use of compensatory techniques to maintain function and increase safety and safety awareness. Efforts are made to maintain QOL despite declining functional status. The final or end stage involves palliative care, including supportive care from the health team and family system.

Therapists work toward enhancing QOL throughout the dying process. A person may fluctuate between the above stages; thus, it is important for therapists to be vigilant about constant reassessment of occupational performance. These stages of the dying process can occur in any context. Current and future occupational needs can be addressed with the dying and their loved ones in these contexts, from an acute care hospital setting to a hospice or home setting. Basic occupational principles and knowledge of the dying process can be applied across contexts and is supported by the *Framework* (AOTA, 2008).

> A useful strategy for health professionals concerned with making death "better" is to seek meaning in its multiple end-of-life locations, which include the life course and cultural world of the patient, the hopes and moral understandings of the family, the convictions of health professionals about comfort care, and the institutional pathways of treatment through which decision making is conceived. (Kaufman, 2002, p. 39)

Occupational Therapy Research in ELC

A body of research exists in the area of hospice, terminal care, and ELC related to occupational therapy. One of the first research studies analyzing the role of the occupational therapist in palliative care was undertaken by Dawson (1982). This phenomenological study explored the role of the occupational therapist through interviews with three therapists and four terminally ill clients. Although there was support for occupational therapy in palliative care, the role was ill-defined and unclear to both professionals and patients. Occupa-

tional therapy creates an environment in which occupational engagement is client-centered and easily facilitated for people at the end of life (Dawson, 1982).

Rahman (2000) conducted an exploratory study of the perspectives of occupational therapists with regard to their role in hospice and whether they experienced a conflict in the dual status of living and dying for individuals with terminal illness. The qualitative analysis revealed themes of tuning in and comfort care, coping with loss, working toward death, journeying with patients, being a team player, using values and principles of occupational therapy, and experiencing a dichotomous role. It was found that occupational therapists used a holistic approach in their work and addressed issues of care within the physical, social, emotional, and spiritual domains. Hasselkuss (1993) completed a qualitative single case study and reports the view of caregiving for someone with a terminal illness. She notes that caring for someone with a terminal illness presents a paradox between facilitating comfort and QOL while simultaneously supporting approaching death. This appears to be a dilemma hospice therapists face daily. There is also research that indicates that the more fully a therapy program is discussed with the patient, the more effective the terminal care received via rehabilitation approaches will be considered by the surviving family (Yoshioka, 1994). Bye (1998) analyzed data gathered by 10 occupational therapists working in hospice care. The core theme developed through the qualitative analysis was "affirming life preparing for death." Bye concluded that

> the outcome is not about independence or permanent rehabilitation to a normal life—hallmarks of traditional occupational therapy. It is about occupational therapists helping clients to realize their goals to connect with life, and people in their life, on a level beyond illness and receipt of care. The achievement of this outcome affirms clients' lives. (1998, p. 19)

Similarly, Prochnau, Liu, and Boman (2003) performed a qualitative study that examined the experiences of palliative care occupational therapists. Engaging in a thematic analysis, the authors discovered themes of satisfaction (i.e., feeling like one was making a difference), hardship (i.e., dealing with grief when patients died), coping (i.e., developing self-nurturance and refining current coping mechanisms), spirituality (i.e., developing a deeper appreciation for meaningful interactions and changing perceptions about death and dying), and growth (i.e., feeling enriched and inspired by the experience).

Through qualitative analysis of 12 transcripts of hospice professionals (i.e., nurses, social workers, occupational and physical therapists) Pizzi (2004) found that there are common threads of facilitating meaning and wellbeing among team members, although the means by which meaning and wellness until death is created differs in discipline-specific ways. The content thematic analysis revealed themes of

- being holistic;
- framing and reframing practice;
- client- and family-centered care;
- being with dying; and
- interdisciplinary teaming.

Lyons and colleagues (2002) engaged several participants in a qualitative study of dying persons' occupational experiences. Recognized themes of doing, being, and becoming were identified in a study grounded in the work of Wilcock (1998, 1999). The theme of *doing* refers to maintaining valued occupations and striving to preserve physical and mental functioning. The theme of *being* refers to social connectedness and self-exploration that enhance feelings of self-worth. The theme of *becoming* refers to engagement in new and altruistic occupations that offer personal growth opportunities and facilitate a sense of contributing to others.

Jacques and Hasselkuss (2004) described an ethnographic approach used with caregivers (professional and informal), clients, and staff at a small Midwestern hospice. They studied the complexity of occupation in ELC. Their findings were distilled into four types of occupation: engaging in meaningful occupations which continue life, putting things in order in preparation for death, waiting for death, and the "gentle goodbye." While these were presented to demonstrate an understanding of occupation as the good death, Jacques and Hasselkuss (2004) continued by stating,

> The conclusions drawn from this study of occupation at the end of life are that occupation is the good death experience and that enabling occupation in an ELC environment, such as a residential hospice, can help bring about a good death experience for all involved in the dying process. (pp. 52–53)

Outcomes such as quality of care; QOL, including quality of death; and the best resolution of bereavement are hard to measure, especially when patients are frail and ill. Thus, many studies exclude QOL as an outcome variable or include only patients who can complete questionnaires. The challenge is to ensure that those aspects of care that are harder to measure do not become a lower priority than aspects such as survival or function that are easier to measure (Higginson, 1999).

Research in ELC is vital to produce sufficient evidence for occupational therapy practice. Occupational therapy studies with this population, most of which is strongly based in practice, vary in terms of research rigor. Ongoing qualitative and quantitative research in occupational therapy ELC will assist future generations of practitioners to develop a solid theoretical foundation and strong evidence for the role of occupational therapy in ELC. Research to identify best practices should be continued to further validate the many contributions made by occupational therapy to ELC.

Occupational Therapy Evaluation

Evaluation in ELC and palliative care is an ongoing process due to the nature of the illness trajectory. The process, which should include both an occupational interview and data from observation, can uncover a great many occupational needs, problems, and concerns for both clients and their loved ones. Appropriate client-centered evaluation in ELC includes an occupational profile (AOTA, 2008) that assists in the discovery of factors that are essential and meaningful in a person's life. This then assists the occupational therapist in developing a specific intervention plan that can promote health and wellbeing for people at the end of life.

From initial evaluation through to regular reevaluation, the illness trajectory can be transformed into a wellness trajectory until death. Facilitating an individual's occupational engagement in meaningful activities will enhance the QOL of the dying person and their loved ones. This promotes a healthy or good death (Content Box 25-3).

There are a variety of assessments that can be used by occupational therapists working in ELC settings. Some of these assessments are specific to hospice, others are specific to occupational therapy, and some are generic and appropriate for use with persons who are dying and their families.

Assessments Specific to ELC

The Brief Hospice Inventory (Guo, Fine, Mendoza, & Cleeland, 2001) was developed to cover four dimensions that relate to the dying person in hospice: physical symptoms (i.e., pain, nausea, tiredness, loss of appetite, and shortness of breath), psychological symptoms (i.e., depression, anxiety, and distress related to changes in self-care ability), the dying person's perception of hospice care (i.e., overall symptom management, sense of being cared for, and helpfulness of hospice care), and QOL (i.e., pertaining to comfort and feelings of life as a gift). Occupational therapists could utilize this measure to screen for information and use it to develop appropriate occupation-based interventions that address identified issues. The information could also be helpful to other team members. This inventory

Guiding Principles for Assessment and Intervention for End-of-Life Care

- Be client-centered. Assess the goals, dreams, aspirations, occupational needs, and wishes of the client and make those the priority.
- Utilize open systems thinking. Occupational reasoning skills need to focus on the patient NOT living in a vacuum but as part of many systems, including the family and significant others. All of these systems interact with the client and need to have their impact on the client considered in assessment and intervention.
- Occupational adaptation in life to accommodate new changes that occur in health contributes to wellbeing and life satisfaction.
- A person can transform their illness trajectory to a wellness trajectory through engagement in self-chosen meaningful and productive occupations.
- Occupation must be of a person's interest and have meaning to the individual to promote wellness and a "good death."
- Life-affirming and self-affirming actions and words promote positive healthful living and wellness until death.
- Quality of life is the ultimate outcome when one's body, mind, and spiritual needs are met, given the occupational choices of the individual and that of their loved ones being served.
- Palliative care clinical reasoning incorporates the philosophy and themes of occupational therapy in hospice, knowledge of the dying process, and an understanding of loss, grief, and bereavement issues.

can be adapted for all dying persons, even if they are not in hospice care.

An occupational therapy assessment specific for use with the dying is the Hospice Assessment of Occupational Function (HAOF), which can be obtained by e-mailing the author through his website at www.michaelpizzi.com. This assessment was developed using principles of open systems and occupational science. It is a holistic assessment for therapists to gather data on the physical, psychosocial, emotional, and spiritual aspects of the client's life. The resultant data are synthesized using the practitioner's clinical reasoning skills, which then results in client-centered, collaborative intervention and program planning.

There are also several QOL instruments designed specifically for ELC and hospice (see Chapter 7). Occupational therapists can utilize these instruments to complement the HAOF or other holistic and relevant assessments used for people with a terminal illness. No assessments currently exist for children and adolescents specific to ELC and occupational therapy. Devel-

opmental and play assessments for children and youth already utilized in occupational therapy can be adapted for this population relative to ELC.

Generic Assessments Appropriate for ELC

There are many generic QOL assessments that can assist therapists working in ELC (Cohen & Mount, 1992; McMillan & Mahon, 1994; Spitzer, Dobson, & Hall, 1981). Notably, the McGill Quality of Life Questionnaire (Cohen et al., 1995; Cohen, Mount, Bruera, Rowe, & Tong, 1997), which measures QOL and wellbeing, supports health promotion in palliative care. This questionnaire is a brief interview that covers four domains: physical, psychological, existential, and perceived support. The interview is semi-structured, thus allowing for the therapy process to be more client-centered, beginning with the initial assessment. Interventions can be adapted based on the narrative evoked from the interview items.

The Occupational Loss Assessment (OLA) was developed by Pizzi (1994) to assess the client's subjective sense of loss and the extent of that loss in areas of self-care, work, leisure, home management, connecting with people, and mobility. (This can be obtained by e-mailing the author through his website at www.michaelpizzi.com.) Interventions can be established based on the perceived level of loss and clients' need to restore or adapt occupational abilities in specific areas. If ability cannot be reestablished, then occupational therapists can facilitate engagement in occupations that help the client compensate for or work through the loss. Another section of the assessment asks clients to review other losses in their lives, the age at which the loss occurred, and if the loss was positive or negative.

In Western society, loss is often seen as negative; however, it can be a positive loss that enhances growth and QOL (e.g., leaving an abusive relationship). Working through occupational loss is often an important end-of-life task for people. Reframing the losses for the dying, using principles of health and wellbeing, along with spiritual and existential views of life, can assist dying clients in re-creating and reframing themselves as occupational beings engaged in moving on with their lives through to their death. Loss, grief, and bereavement are health issues that most occupational therapy practitioners are not well prepared to address and that deserve much more attention both in and outside of palliative care.

An occupational therapy assessment specifically designed as a client-centered, health promotion tool is the Pizzi Holistic Wellness Assessment (PHWA; Pizzi, 2001), described in Chapter 10 (also available at www.michaelpizzi.com). The PHWA is a self-assessment designed to assist individuals to become aware of the most important health issues impacting their daily occupational performance. The assessment also addresses self-responsibility for health by exploring self-determined strategies to optimize health. Therapists do not do things to or for people; rather, they suggest ways to optimize healthy living and facilitate the process of health and healing by increasing awareness to issues (e.g., physical, psychosocial, and contextual) that need to be addressed. Due to the qualitative nature of this assessment, practitioners are encouraged to utilize it to help dying clients identify meaningful occupations. The holism inherent in the assessment is of vital importance, as clients are often more motivated in therapy when intervention is initiated using at least one valued occupation defined by the client.

Other assessments described in Chapter 10 are health promotion based; however, several can be adapted for occupational therapy ELC. There are no holistic, occupation-based assessments, except perhaps for the HAOF, designed specifically for ELC. The guiding principles (Content Box 25-5) will help occupational therapists and occupational therapy assistants assess people and facilitate their clients' choices for occupational engagement at the end of life.

Occupational Interventions to Promote a Good Death

The concept of a good death is primarily noted in the palliative care medicine and nursing literature. Emmanuel and Emmanuel (1998) proposed a framework for a good death that is supported in the literature. Dimensions of a good death that could be addressed by health professionals included physical symptoms, social relationships and support, hopes and expectations, psychological and cognitive symptoms, economic demands, caregiving needs, and spiritual and existential beliefs. A good death is often described as encompassing elements such as having family or significant others present, being without pain, being physically comfortable, and maintaining dignity through privacy and caring (Thompson & McClement, 2002).

Steinhauser, Clipp, and colleagues (2000) studied components of a good death from the perspective of clients, families, and health-care providers, and they identified six elements of a good death: effective pain and symptom management, clear decision-making, preparation for death, completion (e.g., life review, time spent with loved ones), contributing to others, and affirmation of the whole person. From an occupational perspective, occupational therapy practitioners could engage clients in any of these areas through occupation, thus promoting a good death.

Although the concept of a dying child is difficult to accept, a good death is possible for children and youth as well. Beaune and Newman (2003) enumerated several elements that can contribute to a good death for dying children and their families (Content Box 25-4) while the AAP developed some guidelines for communication with children about death.

Mak and Clinton (1999) highlighted the need for clear communication between health providers and clients and their families by examining outcomes desired by clients at the end of life. They identified elements of a good death from the perspectives of nurses and hospice patients that included comfort or relief from pain, being aware of dying, accepting the timing of one's death, preparing for departure, living with one's choice about where to die, having partnerships in decision-making, and maintaining a sense of hope throughout the dying process. Field and Cassel (1997) in the IOM report made another distinction between a good and bad death:

> [A] good death is free of avoidable distress and suffering for patients, families and caregivers; in general accord with patients' and families' wishes; and reasonably consistent with clinical, cultural, and ethical standards. A bad death, in turn, is characterized by needless suffering, dishonoring of patient and family wishes or values, and a sense among those participating [in the end of life process] that norms of decency have been offended. Bad deaths include those resulting from or accompanied by neglect, violence, or unwanted and senseless medical treatments. (p. 24)

Amella (2003) identified nursing interventions that can promote healthier living throughout the dying process and can help facilitate a good death especially

---

Content Box 25-4

Elements That Contribute to a Good Death for Dying Children and Their Families

- Open and frequent communication between child, parents, and team members
- Client-centered care throughout the dying process, including bereavement services for survivors
- Culturally competent, compassionate care
- Freedom of choice for child and family regarding care settings and individuals to attend final moments

From "In search of a good death: Can children with life threatening illness and their families experience a good death? [Letter to the editor], by L. Beaune & C. Newman, 2003, *British Medical Journal, 327*(7408), p. 223. Copyright 2003 by BMJ Publishing Group.

among the elderly involved with palliative care. Despite the obvious medical nature of some of these approaches, many are within the scope of occupational therapy using principles of prevention and health promotion. All of these interventions relate directly or indirectly with the promotion of health and a good death for people at the end of life. These include the following:

- "Monitoring of vital signs including weight (if able)"
- Providing "Influenza and Pneumovax vaccine"
- Recommending "aspirin if at risk for cardiovascular disease" and if not contraindicated
- Conducting "visual, hearing and oral health screening"
- Monitoring for signs of abuse
- Evaluating "ADLs and instrumental ADLs assessments to provide appropriate assistance and referrals"
- Evaluating "etiology of incontinence"
- "Monitoring of blood glucose if diabetic"
- Conducting "depression and cognitive screening"
- Completing "pain assessment"
- Conducting "medication review"
- Reviewing "advance directives"
- Providing "caregiver support" (Amella, 2003, p. 47)

A holistic view of people and well-designed, occupation-based intervention can prevent needless suffering of the dying and their loved ones. These help to lessen pain and increase comfort. Occupations should include one or more of the following requirements:

1. Be of interest to the person and inspire confidence and courage to cope with circumstances
2. Be applied systematically based on assessment data
3. Be adaptable according to client/family needs and capabilities
4. Deemphasize pathology and focus on the health of clients
5. Emphasize positive healthy emotional expression
6. Provide a holistic program of care (Pizzi, 1984; Pizzi & Chromiak, 2001) Reductionistic interventions (e.g., range of motion, strengthening, cognitive retraining) are ideally incorporated into meaningful occupation rather than addressed separately.

Even when it appears that a specific intervention positively changes occupational performance, the person experiences wellness through the self-discovery of how to best manage his or her being. After self-discovery, the therapy process unfolds collaboratively between the client and therapist. (Pizzi, 2001, p. 57)

It is important to attend primarily to the most meaningful and important occupations of each day, adapting the occupation as needed. Engagement in favored occupations and activities can evoke joy and a deep spiritual sense of peace. Occupation-based interventions can immediately assist clients in creating their own QOL and wellbeing. The occupational therapy process can help clients unfold their life story. In ELC, occupational therapy practitioners assist in creating closure of a life through occupational engagement. Collaboration among the occupational therapist, the client, and the family is essential. This sense of completion for a client and family assists them to better cope with their grief and subsequent bereavement after death. Occupational engagement of the dying person permits a good death with improved QOL as the outcome. If occupational therapists and occupational therapy assistants follow a client-centered approach, use solid clinical reasoning, and have a deep respect for and understanding of the complex nature of the dying process, they will be able to promote a good death.

Conclusion

Occupational engagement and the promotion of a good death has been introduced and discussed as a possible framework for occupational therapy practice in palliative care and ELC. The following points were emphasized:

- The promotion of health and wellbeing is applicable and appropriate for people at the end of life.
- A holistic view and well-designed, occupation-based intervention can prevent needless suffering of the dying and their loved ones.
- Occupational therapists do not do things to or for people, but rather suggest ways to optimize healthy living and enhance the process of health and healing by facilitating occupational participation and by increasing awareness to issues (e.g., physical, psychosocial, and contextual) that need to be addressed.
- Engagement in favored occupations, adapted to a healthy level of participation, can evoke joy and a deep spiritual sense of peace for people at the end of life.
- Research in ELC is preliminary and needs to be expanded to ensure appropriate evidence to build theory and best practice in occupational therapy.
- Occupational engagement in life for the dying person and caregivers until death permits a good death with improved QOL as the outcome.

Occupational therapists, occupational therapy assistants, and students can be empowered to facilitate a good death through appropriate and holistic evaluation and occupation-based interventions. These interventions can be powerfully transformative, replete with meaning and purpose, and can add a dimension of living that effectively enhances QOL and wellbeing until death. Occupational therapy students must be educated to ELC issues, including loss, grief, and bereavement to help students develop *best practice* strategies. These best practices need to include prevention, health promotion, and lifestyle evaluation as well as interventions that are focused on individuals, populations, and communities.

Everyone has a right to the best health, even those who are dying. In the trajectory of chronic illness, as the individual comes closer to death, actions that advance health continue to promote a better quality of life, and finally a better death. . . . Health promotion may allow the older person and the caregiver to be free of avoidable stress and suffering, and to have a more active role in treatment. (Amella, 2003, p. 47)

Case Study 25-1

Howie is a 55-year-old who was married to Gwen for many years before her sudden death 10 years earlier. He has a strong work ethic and worked for the railroad and at assorted odd jobs. After his wife's death, from which he never fully emotionally recovered, he worked with his brother-in-law, Al, in masonry. They had an excellent rapport and everyone liked Howie.

When he was diagnosed with metastatic lung cancer with a prognosis of 6 months to live, there was no question that his sister Jeanne and Al would care for him in their bi-level home. Jeanne and Al had three children, ages 6, 10, and 14. They always liked Uncle Howie because he always brought a case of apple butter for them after he visited his stepchildren in North Carolina. He was also a kind and generous man who had little but gave a lot.

Howie initially had much difficulty breathing, often needing to take a break after ascending two to three steps to climb the 12 steps up the second floor of the bi-level home. He became physically weaker from both his cancer and the radiation. His physical body and body image changed weekly. Howie loved to fish, go crabbing at the Jersey shore, bowl (he had a 190 average), and play cards. However, all of these occupations diminished over time, compounded by a deepening depression. His physical and cognitive capacities waned, decreasing his occupational participation even more.

The children began to withdraw from him despite encouragement from their mother. Jeanne began to feel extremely helpless as she watched her beloved brother deteriorate. As he came closer to death, he brought the family close to him and said, "Thank you for being my family, for taking an interest in me and loving me during this tough time. I will never forget you." Three days later, he died in the hospital, with his family around him.

Questions

1. Do you think Howie was experiencing a good quality of life and a "good death"? If so, what is the evidence? Identify and discuss at what point in the dying trajectory an occupational therapist could have intervened.
2. Could hospice care have helped this family? If so, in what ways?
3. Discuss at least two ELC assessments that could be applicable to Howie and to the caregivers.
4. List and discuss at least five health promotion interventions that could be implemented in this case.
5. How else might have occupational therapy worked with both Howie and the family to help them experience a good death? Should the children have been more involved? If so, in what ways? If not, why not?

▶ For Discussion and Review

1. How would you define a good death and a bad death?
2. Do you think occupational therapy can make a significant contribution to people and caregivers at the end of life? Consider the AOTA *Framework* as you develop your answers.
3. What are the contributions of occupational therapists and occupational therapy assistants to promoting healthier living for caregivers involved with end-of-life care?
4. Describe a research method that can be used to quantify occupational dimensions of quality of life at the end of life.
5. Does the occupational process of facilitating meaning and purpose for someone at the end of life differ compared to that of someone with an acute illness? A chronic illness?

▶ Research Questions

1. How might clients at the end of life and their caregivers define and characterize quality of life and wellbeing at the end of life?
2. Do occupation-based interventions actually facilitate a good death? More than other interventions?
3. How does the PHWA compare with other ELC assessments in being a client-centered and health- and occupation-related assessment when used with people at the end of life or their caregivers? Are the interventional and QOL outcomes different for individuals when using the PHWA and other assessments in ELC?
4. Do caregivers of people at the end of life have different occupational needs than those caring for people with acute illness? With chronic illness?

References

Amella, E. (2003). Geriatrics and palliative care: Collaboration for quality of life until death. *Journal of Hospice and Palliative Nursing, 5*(1), 40–48.

American Academy of Pediatrics, Committee on Bioethics and Committee on Hospital Care. (2000). Palliative care for children: Policy statement. *Pediatrics, 106*(2), 351–57.

American Occupational Therapy Association. (2008). Occupational therapy practice framework: Domain and process (2d ed.). *American Journal of Occupational Therapy, 62,* 625–83.

American Occupational Therapy Association. (2005). Occupational therapy and hospice. *American Journal of Occupational Therapy, 59*(6), 671–75.

American Occupational Therapy Association, Commission on Practice, Hospice Task Force. (1987). *Guidelines for occupational therapy services in hospice.* Rockville, MD: Author.

Beaune, L., & Newman, C. (2003). In search of a good death. *British Medical Journal, 327,* 222–23.

Bewley, R. (1985). Occupational therapy for children with renal failure. *Australian Occupational Therapy Journal, 32,* 10–16.

Bye, R. (1998). When clients are dying: Occupational therapy perspectives. *Occupational Therapy Journal of Research, 18*(1), 3–24.

Bye, R., Llewellyn, G., & Christl, K. (2001). The end of life. In B. Bonder & M. Wagner (Eds.), *Functional performance in older adults* (2d ed., pp. 500–19). Philadelphia: F. A. Davis.

Byock, I. (1997). *Dying well.* New York: Riverhead Books.

Cohen, S. R., & Mount, B. M. (1992). Quality of life in terminal illness: Defining and measuring subjective wellbeing in the dying. *Journal of Palliative Care, 8*(3), 40–45.

Cohen, S. R., Mount, B. M., Bruera, E., Rowe, J., & Tong, K. (1997). Validity of the McGill Quality of Life Questionnaire in the palliative care setting. A multi-center Canadian study demonstrating the importance of the existential domain. *Palliative Medicine, 11,* 3–20.

Cohen, S. R., Mount, B. M., Strobel, M. G., & Bui, F. (1995). The McGill Quality of Life Questionnaire: A measure of quality of life appropriate for people with advanced disease. A preliminary study of validity and acceptability. *Palliative Medicine, 9,* 207–19.

Dawson, S. (1982). The role of occupational therapy in palliative care. *Australian Occupational Therapy Journal, 29,* 119–24.

Dawson, S. (1993). Day hospice: A study of the benefits of day hospice for a person with terminal illness. *New Zealand Journal of Occupational Therapy, 44,* 10–13.

Doyle D., Hanks, G. W. C., & MacDonald, N. (1998). *Oxford textbook of palliative medicine* (2d ed.). New York: Oxford University Press.

Emmanuel E. J., & Emmanuel, L. L. (1998). The promise of a good death. *Lancet, 351,* 21–29.

Evans, K. A., Lund, N. W., Pizzi, M., Thompson, B., Tigges, K. N., Bell, E., & Epstein, C. F. (1986). Occupational therapy and hospice (position paper). *American Journal of Occupational Therapy, 40,* 839–40.

Feasley, J. C. (Ed.). (1996). *Best at home: Assuring quality long-term care in home and community-based settings* [Institute of Medicine Report]. Washington, DC: National Academy Press.

Ferrell, B. A., Ferrell, B. R., & Osterwell, D. (1990). Pain in the nursing home. *American Journal of Nursing, 95*(7), 43–45.

Fidler, G. S., & Fidler, J. W. (1963). *Occupational therapy: A communication process in psychiatry.* New York: Macmillan.

Field, M. J., & Cassel, C. K. (Eds.). (1997). *Approaching death: Improving care at the end of life.* Washington, DC: Institute of Medicine.

Flanigan, K. (1982). The art of the possible: Occupational therapy in terminal care. *British Journal of Occupational Therapy, 45,* 274–76.

Fulton, C. L., & Else, R. (1998). Physiotherapy. In D. Doyle, G. W. C. Hanks, & N. MacDonald (Eds.), *Oxford textbook of palliative medicine* (2d ed., pp. 819–28). New York: Oxford University Press.

Galantino, M. L., Pizzi, M., & Lehmann, M. D. (1993). Interdisciplinary management of disability in HIV infection. In M. O'Dell (Ed.), *Physical medicine and rehabilitation: State of the art reviews* (pp. 155–74). Philadelphia: Hanley and Belfus.

Gammage, S. L., McMahon, P. S., & Shanahan, P. M. (1976). The occupational therapist and terminal illness: Learning to cope with death. *American Journal of Occupational Therapy, 30,* 294–99.

Gold, M., Franks, P., & Erickson, P. (1996). Assessing the health of the nation: The predictive validity of a preference-based measure and self-rated health. *Medical Care, 34*(2), 163–77.

Guo, H., Fine P. G., Mendoza T. R., & Cleeland, C. S. (2001). A preliminary study of the utility of the brief hospice inventory. *Journal of Pain Symptom Management, 22,* 637–48.

Gutterman, L. (1990). A day treatment program for people with AIDS. *American Journal of Occupational Therapy, 44*(3), 234–42.

Hasselkus, B. (1993). Death in very old age: A personal journey of caregiving. *American Journal of Occupational Therapy, 47*(8), 717–23.

Higginson, I. J. (1999). Evidence based palliative care. *British Medical Journal, 319*, 462–63.

Holland, A. E. (1984). Occupational therapy and day care for the terminally ill. *British Journal of Occupational Therapy, 47*, 345–48.

Holland, A. E., & Tigges, K. N. (1981). The hospice movement: A time for professional action and commitment. *British Journal of Occupational Therapy, 44*, 373–76.

Jacques, N. D., & Hasselkuss, B. R. (2004). The nature of occupation surrounding death and dying. *OTJR: Occupation, Participation and Health, 24*(2), 44–53.

Jones, B., Ackerud, L. N., & Boyle, D. (1997). Differential utilization of hospice services in nursing homes. *Hospice Journal, 12*(3), 41–57.

Kaufman, S. R. (2002). A commentary: Hospital experience and meaning at the end of life. *Gerontologist, 42*, 34–39.

Kaut, K. P. (2002). Religion, spirituality and existentialism: Implications for assessment and application. *American Behavioral Scientist, 46*(2), 220–34.

Kitzes, J., Schmoll, B., & Dixon C. (2003). Hospice/palliative care settings. In W. B. Forman, J. A. Kitzes, R. P. Anderson, & D. K. Sheehan (Eds.), *Hospice and palliative care: Concepts and practice* (2d ed., pp. 47–55). Sudbury, MA: Jones and Bartlett.

Koff, T. (Ed.). (1980). *Hospice: A caring community.* Cambridge, MA: Winthrop.

Kubler-Ross, E. (1977). *On death and dying.* London: Tavistock.

Longaker C. (1997). *Facing death and finding hope.* New York: Doubleday.

Lyons, M., Orozovic, N., Davis, J., & Newman, J. (2002). Doing-being-becoming: Occupational experiences of persons with life threatening illness. *American Journal of Occupational Therapy, 56*(3), 285–95.

Mackey, K. M., & Sparling, J. W. (2000). Experiences of older women with cancer receiving hospice care: Significance for physical therapy. *Physical Therapy, 80*(5), 459–68.

Mak, J. M. H., & Clinton, M. (1999). Promoting a good death: An agenda for outcomes research—A review of the literature. *Nursing Ethics, 6*, 97–106.

Marcil, W. M., & Tigges, K. N. (1992). *The person with AIDS: A personal and professional perspective.* Thorofare, NJ: SLACK.

McMillan, S. C., & Mahon, M. (1994). Measuring quality of life in hospice patients using a newly developed hospice quality of life index. *Quality of Life Research, 3*, 437–44.

Mezey, M., Dubler, N. N., Mitty, E., & Brody, A. A. (2002). What impact do setting and transitions have on the quality of life at the ELC and the quality of the dying process. *Gerontologist, 42*(3), 54–67.

Morley, J. E., Kraenzle, D. M., Bible, B., & Bundren, B. (1995). Perception of quality of life by nursing home residents. *Nursing Home Medicine, 3*(8), 191–94.

National Hospice Organization. (1996). *Hospice fact sheet.* Arlington, VA: Author.

National Hospice and Palliative Care Organization. (1997). *Standards of a hospice program of care.* Arlington, VA: National Hospice Organization.

Neuberger, J. (2003). A healthy view of dying. *British Medical Journal, 327*, 207–20.

Oelrich, M. (1974). The patient with a fatal illness. *American Journal of Occupational Therapy, 28*, 429–32.

Peloquin, S. (1993). The depersonalization of patients: A profile gleaned from narratives. *American Journal of Occupational Therapy, 47*(9), 830–37.

Peloquin, S. (1997). Nationally speaking: The spiritual depth of occupation: Making worlds and making lives. *American Journal of Occupational Therapy, 3*, 167–68.

Pizzi, M. (1983). Hospice and the terminally ill geriatric patient. *Occupational and Physical Therapy in Geriatrics, 3*(1), 45–54.

Pizzi, M. (1984). Occupational therapy in hospice care. *American Journal of Occupational Therapy, 38*(4), 252–57.

Pizzi, M. (1990a). The model of human occupation and adults with HIV infection and AIDS. *American Journal of Occupational Therapy, 44*(3), 257–64.

Pizzi, M. (1990b). Nationally speaking. The transformation of HIV infection and AIDS in occupational therapy: Beginning the conversation. *American Journal of Occupational Therapy, 44*(3), 199–204.

Pizzi, M. (1992a). Adaptive human performance and HIV infection: Considerations for therapists. In M. L. Galantino (Ed.), *Clinical assessment and treatment in HIV: Rehabilitation of a chronic illness* (pp. 31–42). Thorofare, NJ: SLACK.

Pizzi, M. (1992b). Hospice: The creation of meaning for people with life-threatening illness. *Occupational Therapy Practice, 4*(1), 1–7.

Pizzi, M. (1992c). Rehabilitation of the pediatric population. In M. L. Galantino (Ed.), *Clinical assessment and treatment in HIV: Rehabilitation of a chronic illness* (pp. 127–35). Thorofare, NJ: SLACK

Pizzi, M. (1992d). Women, HIV infection, and AIDS: Tapestries of life, death, and empowerment. *American Journal of Occupational Therapy, 46*, 1021–27.

Pizzi, M. (1993). Environments of care: Hospice. In H. Hopkins & H. Smith (Eds.), *Willard and Spackman's occupational therapy* (8th ed., pp. 853–64). Philadelphia: Lippincott.

Pizzi, M. (1994). Occupational Loss Assessment. In M. Pizzi, *HIV infection and AIDS: A professional's guide to wellness, health and productive living* (pp. 89–91). Silver Spring, MD: Positive Images and Wellness. [Contact the author for reprint requests at www.michaelpizzi.com.]

Pizzi, M. (1996). *Geriatric wellness workshop handouts.* Silver Spring, MD: Positive Images and Wellness.

Pizzi, M. (2001). The Pizzi Holistic Wellness Assessment. In B. Velde & P. Wittman (Eds.), *Occupational therapy in health care* [special issue on community based practice], *13*(3/4), 51–66.

Pizzi, M. (2004). *Promoting a good death: Perspectives of hospice professionals.* Unpublished doctoral dissertation.

Pizzi, M., & Briggs, R. (2004). Occupational and physical therapy in hospice: The facilitation of meaning, quality of life and wellbeing. *Topics in Geriatric Rehabilitation, 20*(2), 120–30.

Pizzi, M., & Burkhardt, A. (2003). Occupational therapy for adults with immunological disorders. In E. B. Crepeau, E. S. Cohn, & B. A. B. Schell (Eds.), *Willard and Spackman's occupational therapy* (10th ed., pp. 821–34). Philadelphia: Lippincott, Williams & Wilkins.

Pizzi, M., & Chromiak, S. B. (2001). Hospice: Creating meaningful environments of care. In M. Scaffa (Ed.), *Occupational therapy in community-based practice settings* (pp. 253–70). Philadelphia: F. A. Davis.

Prochnau, C., Liu, L., & Boman, J. (2003). Personal-professional connections in palliative care occupational therapy. *American Journal of Occupational Therapy, 57*(2), 196–204.

Rahman, H. (2000). Journey of providing care in hospice: Perspectives of occupational therapists. *Qualitative Health Research, 10*(6), 806–18.

Rollins, J. A., & Riccio, L. L. (2002). ART Is the HeART: A palette of possibilities for hospice care. *Pediatric Nursing, 28*(4), 355–62.

Rose, A. (1999). Spirituality and palliative care: The attitudes of occupational therapists. *British Journal of Occupational Therapy, 62,* 307–12.

Sengstaken, E. A., & King, S. A. (1993). The problems of pain and its detection among geriatric nursing home residents. *Journal of American Geriatric Society, 41*(5), 541–44.

Sharp J. (1996). *Living our dying.* New York: Hyperion.

Singer, P. A., Martin, D. K., & Kelner, M. (1999). Quality end of life care: Patients' perspectives. *Journal of the American Medical Association, 281,* 163–68.

Spitzer, W. O., Dobson, A. J., & Hall, J. (1981). Measuring the quality of life of cancer patients: A concise QL-index for use by physicians. *Journal of Chronic Disease, 34,* 585–97.

Steinhauser, K. E., Christakis, N. A., Clipp, E. C., McNeilly, M., McIntyre, L., & Tulsky, J. A. (2000). Factors considered important at the end of life by patients, family, physicians and other care providers. *Journal of the American Medical Association, 284*(19), 2476–82.

Steinhauser, K. E., Clipp, E. C., McNeilly, M., Christakis, N. A. M., McIntyre, L., & Tulsky, J. A. (2000). In search of a good death: Observations of patients, families, and providers. *Annals of Internal Medicine, 132,* 825–32.

Sulmasy, D. P. (2002). Biopsychosocial-spiritual model for the care of patients at the end of life. *Gerontologist, 42,* 24–33.

Thompson, G., & McClement, S. (2002). Defining and determining quality in end of life care. *International Journal of Palliative Nursing, 8*(6), 288–93.

Thorpe, G. (1993). Enabling more dying people to remain at home. *British Medical Journal 307,* 915–18.

Tigges, K. N. (1993). Rehabilitation in palliative care: Occupational therapy. In D. Doyle, G. Hanks, & N. Macdonald (Eds.), *Oxford textbook of palliative medicine* (pp. 535–43). Oxford, UK: Oxford University Press.

Tigges, K. N. (1998). Occupational therapy. In D. Doyle, G. Hanks, & N. Macdonald (Eds.), *Oxford textbook of palliative medicine* (2d ed., pp. 829–37). New York: Oxford University Press.

Tigges, K. N., & Marcil, W. M. (1988). *Terminal and life-threatening illness: An occupational behavior perspective.* Thorofare, NJ: SLACK.

Tigges, K. N., & Sherman, L. M. (1983). The treatment of the hospice patient: From occupational history to occupational role. *American Journal of Occupational Therapy, 37,* 235–38.

vanderPloeg, W. (2001). Viewpoint, health promotion in palliative care: An occupational perspective. *Australian Occupational Therapy Journal, 48,* 45–48.

Wilcock, A. A. (1998). *An occupational perspective of health.* Thorofare, NJ: SLACK.

Wilcock, A. A. (1999). Reflections on doing, being, and becoming. *Australian Journal of Occupational Therapy, 46,* 1–11.

World Health Organization. (1986). *The Ottawa charter for health promotion.* Geneva, Switzerland: Author.

Yee, M. Y. (2003). Continuous Quality Improvement (CQI) in hospice. In W. B. Forman, J. A. Kitzes, R. P. Anderson, & D. K. Sheehan (Eds.), *Hospice and palliative care: Concepts and practice* (2d ed., pp. 57–65). Sudbury, MA: Jones and Bartlett.

Yoshioka, H. (1994). Rehabilitation for the terminal cancer patient. *American Journal of Physical Medicine, 73*(3), 199–206.

Educating Practitioners for Health Promotion Practice

Regina Michael Campbell, Patricia Atwell Rhynders, Marlene Riley, M. Beth Merryman, and Marjorie E. Scaffa

> In order to meet current health care challenges, . . . we must redefine how we educate our future healthcare professionals. As Surgeon General, my job is to protect and advance the health of the nation. To accomplish that mission, we must move our society and our health professions from the current treatment-oriented focus to a prevention-oriented focus.
>
> —Carmona, 2004, p. 482

Learning Objectives

This chapter is designed to enable the reader to:

- Relate the curricular standards on prevention and health promotion in occupational therapy to service learning.
- Discuss the compatibility of service learning with the philosophy of occupational therapy.
- Discuss the differences between community service and service learning.
- Identify the differences between service learning and traditional Level I fieldwork.
- List the 10 principles of good practice in service-learning pedagogy.
- Describe the four elements of service learning.
- Explain the importance of an environmental scan in identifying potential service-learning fieldwork sites.

Key Terms

Clinical Prevention and Population Health Curriculum Framework

Community service
Environmental scan
Lifestyle Redesign

Service learning
Synergy

Introduction

There is a national movement in the health professions toward adding a prevention and health promotion orientation to the traditional treatment-focused approach. This is, in part, a response to an objective in *Healthy People 2010: Understanding and Improving Health* that states, "Increase the proportion of schools of medicine, schools of nursing, and other health professionals training schools whose basic curriculum for healthcare providers includes the core competencies in health promotion and disease prevention" (U.S. Department of Health and Human Services [USDHHS], 2000, p. 1-24). With this objective in mind, the Association of Teachers of Preventive Medicine and the Association of Academic Health Centers convened a task force to develop a curriculum framework that could be used by a variety of health professions educational programs.

The work of the task force was financially supported by the USDHHS Office of Disease Prevention and Health Promotion, and the Health Resources and Services Administration (Riegelman, Evans, & Garr, 2004). Originally, the task force represented only seven disciplines; however, recently several allied health disciplines were added, including occupational therapy.

The **Clinical Prevention and Population Health Curriculum Framework** consists of four components: evidence-based practice, clinical preventive services and health promotion, health systems and health policy, and population health and community aspects of practice. In addition, the curriculum includes 18 domains under the four components. The name "Clinical Prevention and Population Health" was chosen specifically so the curriculum framework reflected a dual emphasis on individual-focused and population-focused health promotion efforts and reflected the interaction of the two (Riegelman et al., 2004). The task force encourages health professional educational programs to explore innovative methods of incorporating clinical prevention and population health content—for example, service-learning and problem-based case studies.

Increasingly, prevention and health promotion are being seen as appropriate areas for occupational therapy intervention and as an essential part of practice. The Accreditation Council for Occupational Therapy Education (ACOTE) has recognized the need for occupational therapy graduates to be educated and skilled in prevention and health promotion strategies as they relate to the profession's core construct of occupation. In 2006, ACOTE approved a new set of accreditation standards for master's programs that include five competencies related directly to prevention and health promotion (ACOTE, 2007):

B.1.9 Demonstrate knowledge of global social issues and prevailing health and welfare needs

B.2.4 Articulate the importance of balancing areas of occupation to the achievement of health and wellness.

B.2.5 Explain the role of occupation in the promotion of health and the prevention of disease and disability for the individual, family, and society

B.2.9 Express support for the quality of life, well-being, and occupation of the individual, group, or population to promote physical and mental health and prevention of injury and disease considering the context (e.g., cultural, physical, social, personal, spiritual, temporal, virtual)

B.5.2 Select and provide direct occupational therapy interventions and procedures to enhance safety, wellness, and performance in activities of daily living (ADLs), instrumental activities of daily living (IADLs), work, play, leisure and social participation

The historical roots of occupational therapy are grounded in the experiential learning theories of John Dewey. His philosophy of education was directed toward pragmatism, reflection, and interest in community and democracy. Dewey was a proponent of creating a learning environment that would engage learners in a world outside the classroom and challenge them to work in a collaborative learning process (Chambliss, 1996). These themes can be seen throughout occupational therapy history, beginning with Jane Addams and Eleanor Clarke Slagle and the early settlement Hull House days (Addams, 2004).

In keeping with this philosophy, occupational therapists have long acknowledged the need for occupational therapy education to provide educational learning that extends beyond theory and the classroom (Fidler, 1966). *Student affiliation, student internships,* and *fieldwork learning experiences* are terms commonly used to denote occupational therapy's commitment to experiential learning theory. Service learning is a contemporary educational methodology that embraces the experiential learning constructs of Dewey and occupational therapy's educational philosophy. This chapter will describe two programs and their use of service-learning experiences to educate students about the role of occupational therapy in prevention and health promotion.

Service Learning

Service learning has been defined as "a teaching and learning strategy that integrates meaningful community service with instruction and reflection to enrich the learning experience, teach civic responsibility and strengthen communities" (National Service Learning Clearinghouse [NSLC], 2004b, ¶ 1). It is an adaptation of clinical practice or experiential education whose hallmark is an edict to benefit not only the learner, but also the community. Although community service is an element of service learning, it differs by definition. **Community service** can be defined as "volunteerism that occurs in the community, action taken to meet the needs of others and better the community as a whole" (NSLC, 2004a, ¶ 14). Too often, academic fieldwork serves the needs of the students and the academic institution, without sufficient regard for the needs of the community. Integrating service learning throughout the health professional's preparatory experiences can nullify this effect by reinforcing the values of respect and reciprocity, with consideration of the community's benefit. In service learning, the curriculum must encourage contemplation and consideration of the community's viewpoints. The cognitive benefits to students relate to their ability to critically think about complex concepts, apply those concepts to real-life environments, and share in the real consequences of their actions (Astin & Sax, 1998).

Service learning is consistent with occupational therapy philosophy in that it advocates learning by doing and learning in context. In collaborative learning, a by-product of service learning, the learner enters into a partnership with those living and working in the community. The learner's experience, rather than that of the teacher, directs the classroom experience. The linking of didactic and laboratory education with service learning meets the needs of adult learners, allows them to gain appreciation for the core constructs of occupational therapy, and promotes practice that meets societal needs.

One limitation of conventional fieldwork and practice can be that each discipline tends to work in parallel, isolating their contributions within that paradigm. As a result, each may be unprepared to view health promotion from any perspective but their own. Another limitation is that academic research often remains separate from its practical application in terms of meeting the perceived needs of the community.

Learning by Doing in Context

The role of professionals in the community differs from their role in the medical setting, moving from that of the expert to that of equal partner and collaborator. Consequently, professionals must develop skills to interact with people in a way that allows them to discover the values and perceived needs of the community, while respecting the community's wisdom and prerogative to choose interventions they believe will work. There is a need to modify traditional models of educating health professionals to give teams competence in transdisciplinary collaboration. Service learning shows promise in achieving this competence. It provides opportunities to serve the needs of communities, expand knowledge, examine market needs, and make meaning of the value of occupation in promoting health.

Restructuring occupational therapy Fieldwork I to include service-learning principles and goals provides the educational methodology needed to help students develop a basic comfort level with and an understanding of the needs of individuals and populations while engaging the learner in an active learning process. The experiences are intended to complement the didactic content and to broaden students' awareness of the health promotion needs of the community and the roles of community organizations in community health. The

educational experience can be structured in a variety of ways, depending on the climate in which the services are to be offered. In fact, it is critical to structure service learning after careful analysis of the community climate.

Service learning also yields affective domain advantages of improved academic performance, clarification of personal values, development of leadership characteristics, interpersonal and conflict-resolution skills, and a lifelong commitment to community service (Astin & Sax, 1998). Community partners benefit from enhanced service quality, quantity, and variety (Astin & Sax 1998). In the long-term, the community benefits from having these professionals develop cognitive, affective, and action skills to translate theory into practice to support partnerships and to recognize the merit of including a variety of stakeholders. Students benefit from observing and teaching in the type of environment in which they will practice the skills learned while providing a service to the community.

Serving to Learn—Learning to Serve

Often the health-care needs of a community can exceed the availability of resources. Therefore, a clear, systematic plan of Fieldwork I service-learning intervention with a realistic analysis to balance needs with current and future resources is essential to achieve curriculum objectives and to support effective, efficient community educational partnerships.

Throughout the course of occupational therapy history, service has been one of the profession's stellar ideas (Peloquin, 1991), with caring for and caring about the patient being as implicit as occupation (King, 1980). Sharing of educational strategies that incorporate service learning into occupational therapy curriculum designs can increase awareness and open channels of communication that are needed to speed the rate of diffusion of health promotion into occupational therapy practice. Although service is directed outwardly to address the needs of both the learner and the community—rather than inwardly without regard for the community—academic rigor should not be compromised (Harkavy, 1998). Howard (1993) recommends 10 principles of good practice for service-learning pedagogy (Content Box 26-1).

Infusing Health Promotion and Wellness Into Occupational Therapy Education

Two examples, from Texas Woman's University and Towson University, of infusing health promotion and wellness into occupational therapy education will be

Content Box 26-1

10 Principles of Good Practice for Service-Learning Pedagogy

Principle 1: Academic credit is for learning, not service

Principle 2: Do not compromise academic rigor

Principle 3: Establish learning objectives

Principle 4: Establish criteria for selection of service placements

Principle 5: Provide educationally sound learning strategies to harvest community learning and realize course learning objectives

Principle 6: Prepare students for learning from the community

Principle 7: Minimize the distinction between students' community learning role and classroom learning role

Principle 8: Rethink the faculty instructional role

Principle 9: Be prepared for variation in, and some loss of control with, student learning objectives

Principle 10: Maximize the community responsibility orientation of the course to promote purposeful civic learning

From "Principles of good practice for service learning pedagogy," by J. Howard, 1993, retrieved April 20, 2009, from http://www.ginsberg .umich.edu/resources/for_faculty.html pedagogical.

described. Both of these examples focus on service learning and developing community partnerships, but each has unique features.

Texas Woman's University

Woven into Texas Woman's University (TWU) School of Occupational Therapy's (OT) (2001) vision, philosophy, mission, strategic goals, and curriculum design is a view of humanity that embraces the humanitarian heritage of the profession and supports the educational methodology of service learning. The school's vision is to provide an integrated curriculum that prepares graduates for new roles within an evolving health-care system. The School of Occupational Therapy mission, which supports the university's mission, is to accept the responsibility of educating students, primarily women, of different ages and cultures to become occupational therapists who integrate and exemplify the philosophies, ethics, and standards of TWU and the American Occupational Therapy Association (AOTA).

The school's philosophy of occupational therapy is grounded in beliefs about the "occupational nature of humankind." Unity of the mind and the body, purposeful interaction with the environment, the human capacity to integrate and adapt, and the right to a meaningful existence are core beliefs that guide the curriculum.

Occupation is the means through which adaptation occurs and the end for which adaptation is desired. Adaptation is seen as a continuous and essential human process for the promotion of survival and self-actualization (TWU School of OT, 2001, p. VI-12).

The curriculum design integrates contemporary views of health and occupation with the changing paradigms of service delivery and the values of the profession. Across four semester modules, the concepts and constructs of occupation, wellness, and adaptation objectives are integrated into each of TWU's five curriculum strands: occupational adaptation, principles of intervention, scholarly inquiry, tools and modalities, and Fieldwork I and II. The educational strategies employed to infuse wellness and health promotion into occupational therapy course and fieldwork objectives depend on faculty expertise and lines of research, community alliances, and the contexts and resources available at each of the program's three locations in Denton, Dallas, and Houston. Service learning Fieldwork I experiences can play an integral role in promoting the innovative spirit believed needed to gain access to primary prevention and health promotion practice.

In order to identify service-learning opportunities in the community that were congruent with the curriculum design, an environmental scan was conducted. An **environmental scan** is defined as "a systematic and ongoing process used to identify essential cues about how the world is changing and how the changes will affect individuals, associations and society" (American Society of Association Executives [ASAE], 2003). Generally, an environmental scan consists of four primary characteristics:

1. Broad examination of holistic, economic, global, political, technological, and social trends
2. Collection of data from a variety of sources, including, but not limited to, literature review, surveys, interviews, focus groups, and site visits
3. Awareness of innovative thinking and methods being employed by those within and outside of the organization to address change
4. Study of trends and changes occurring in unrelated industries and professions (ASAE, 2003; Dalton, Jarratt, & Mahaffie, 2003)

Health Promotion Trends and Emerging Service Markets

The Fieldwork I service-learning placements developed on the TWU Dallas campus illustrate how health promotion can be infused into occupational therapy education. Environmental scan data for Vickery Meadow and the surrounding community identified four emerging health promotion service markets:

1. After-school
2. Immigrants and refugees
3. Intentional and unintentional injury prevention
4. Community-dwelling well elderly

These markets were targeted for Fieldwork I development because they provide contexts needed to meet ACOTE health promotion education standards regarding development across the life span. They also support TWU's curriculum learner outcome for occupational therapy entry-level professional master's graduates to develop knowledge and skills needed to practice creatively, adaptively, and proactively in accordance with occupational therapy standards and with social and health-care trends and to assume leadership roles within a variety of settings (TWU School of OT, 2001). National trend data suggests that these emerging health promotion markets extend beyond the Dallas community.

After-School Programs. Research has identified that children left unsupervised during after-school hours are more likely to be involved in violence, substance abuse, and other risk-taking behaviors. With some 15 million children left unsupervised and alone on a regular basis during nonschool hours, communities, families, and the nation are turning to after-school programming to meet health-care needs of children. The Harvard Graduate School 1999 *Program in After School Research* report found significant growth and political support for after-school programs. Government funding, through the 21st Century Community Learning Centers, has increased from $1 million in 1997 to $1 billion in 2002 (Noam, 2002).

Nonprofit and faith-based agencies are developing after-school programs to meet the wellbeing and safety needs of children and youth. In recent years, the federal government's attitude toward funding faith-based programming directed toward promoting health and wellbeing has changed. The USDHHS has developed the Center for Faith-Based and Community Initiatives to make federal funding more accessible to faith-based organizations striving to address the social needs of their community. The TWU–Dallas Center After-School Health Promotion Service Learning Fieldwork I placements have included Girls, Incorporated; HOSTS (Helping One Student to Succeed); Heart House; Project Transformation; and Vickery Meadow Wellness Center. Descriptions of these sites can be found in Content Box 26-2.

Refugee and Immigrant Services. Since 1990 there has been a 33% increase in the number of immigrants living in the United States, the largest number reported in the nation's history. Approximately 26.3 million immigrants currently reside in the United States. Thirty-nine percent of foreign-born children live in

---

Content Box 26-2

After-School Program Fieldwork Sites

- *Girls, Incorporated:* A national youth organization dedicated to inspiring high-risk underserved girls between the ages of 6 to 18 to be strong, smart, and bold. Services provided include research, education, and direct advocacy.
  http://www.girlsincdallas.org
- *HOSTS (Helping One Student to Succeed):* A national intervention system designed to accelerate learning and build a strong foundation for student achievement in reading and math. HOSTS uses a structured mentoring model to provide individualized academic intervention in readiness, language arts, math, Spanish readiness, and English language development.
  http://www.hosts.com
- *Heart House:* A nonprofit, free, after-school program dedicated to providing a safe haven and academic support to low-income children and encouraging them to become good citizens.
  http://www.hearthouse.org
- *Project Transformation:* A nonprofit faith-based supported program designed to connect the energy of young adults, the strength of church-supported institutions, and the untapped resources of urban neighborhoods with the evolving needs of urban children and youth.
  http://www.projecttransformation.org
- *Vickery Wellness Center:* An apartment clubhouse program developed in partnership with Buckner Children and Family Services of North Texas, Melody Village Apartment, Southwest Housing Authority, and Presbyterian Healthcare System dedicated to providing restoration and healing social services for individuals and families.
  http://www.bucknerchildren.org/dallas/community-programs/vickery.asp

---

poverty (Grantmakers Concerned with Immigrants and Refugees, 2006). TWU's Refugee and Immigrant Service Learning Fieldwork I placements have included Vickery Meadow Learning Center and the International Rescue Committee. See Content Box 26-3 for descriptions of these sites.

Injury Prevention. Injury prevention is an objective for the nation as presented in *Healthy People 2010* (USDHHS, 2000). According to the National Center for Health Statistics (NCHS), 101,537 people in the United States died of unintentional injuries in 2002, and another 26.6 million were treated in emergency departments (NCHS, 2004). Approximately 6 million people per year visit hospital outpatient departments for care of their injuries (NCHS, 2004). Injuries rank fifth as a cause of death for all Americans and are the leading cause of death and disability for children and young adults, with approximately 20 children dying each day (Mercy, Sleet, & Doll, 2003).

Refugee and Immigrant Services Fieldwork Sites

- *Vickery Meadow Learning Center (VMLC)* is dedicated to improving English literacy levels among non-English-speaking adults by providing programs in communication and life skills. VMLC believes that the ability to understand, read, write, and speak English contributes to independence, productivity, and overall wellbeing of adult learners, their families, and the greater community. http://www.vmlc.org
- *International Rescue Committee (IRC)* is among the world's largest nonprofit, nonsectarian, voluntary agencies providing assistance to refugees, displaced persons, and others fleeing persecution and violent conflict. http://www.theirc.org/about

Leading the list of causes of injury are motor vehicle collisions, drowning, homicide, suicide, falls, fires, suffocation, and poisoning. In fact, injuries rival the common cold in terms of frequency and account for 15% of childhood medical expenses (Miller, Romano, & Spicer, 2000). Falls are a major source of injury that kill more than 15,000 Americans of all ages each year (NCHS, 2004). The economic impact for fatal and non-fatal injuries in this country is estimated to be $66 billion in present and future work losses, due to premature death or long-term disability, $14 billion in lifetime medical spending, and $1 billion in other resource costs (Deal, Gomby, Zippiroli, & Behrman, 2000).

TWU Intentional and Unintentional Injury Prevention Service Learning Fieldwork I placements have included the Family Place of Dallas, Injury Free Coalition for Kids, Injury Prevention Center of Dallas, New Beginnings Center, Presbyterian Healthcare System–Dallas, and SafeKids. Descriptions of these placements appear in Content Box 26-4.

Community Dwelling Well Elderly. According to Macfayden, "Every month the net balance of the world population aged 55 years and older increases by 1.2 million persons" (as cited in Bonder, 1994, p. 8). The TWU community-dwelling well-elderly service-learning Fieldwork I placements have included the Jewish Community Center of Dallas, Visiting Nurse Association of Texas—Elder Care Program, and the Alzheimer's Association Greater Dallas Chapter (Content Box 26-5).

Service Learning Curriculum Plan

Contemporary educational processes that use service learning to integrate didactic and laboratory learning consist of four basic elements:

1. Preparation
2. Service
3. Reflection
4. Celebration (Fertman, 1994)

Element 1: Preparation.   TWU School of Occupational Therapy's innovative curriculum design integrates content for each course within and across four semester modules to achieve curriculum goals and learning outcomes. The didactic material, linked with Fieldwork I experiential learning, provides an ideal community laboratory for learning by doing, learning in context, and service.

First semester Module I coursework is designed to increase the learner's understanding of the value of the

Injury-Prevention Fieldwork Sites

- *The Family Place of Dallas* provides programming to eliminate family violence through intervention and proactive prevention, extensive community education, advocacy, and assistance for victims and their families. http://www.familyplace.org/Page.aspx?pid=216
- *The Injury Free Coalition for Kids* is a national program of the Robert Wood Johnson Foundation comprised of hospital-based, community-oriented programs whose coalition efforts are anchored in research, education, and advocacy. Currently, the coalition includes 27 sites located in 24 cities, each housed in hospital trauma centers. http://www.injuryfree.org
- *Injury Prevention Center of Dallas (IPC)* is the first of its kind in Texas and the Southwest. The IPC fosters community-based injury-prevention efforts within Dallas County. The IPC has participated in, directed, and helped develop several injury-prevention initiatives throughout Dallas County that address motor vehicle injuries, violence, falls, burns/scalds, poisonings, occupational injuries, and recreational injuries. http://www.injurypreventioncenter.org
- *New Beginning Center* fosters an environment of safety, support, and respect for families affected by domestic violence through advocacy and diverse community partnerships. http://www.newbeginningcenter.org/
- *Presbyterian Healthcare System–Dallas* supports its not-for-profit mission by providing outreach programs, charity care, and other initiatives to improve the health of the people in the community in partnership with schools and other social service organizations. http://www.presbyterian .org/about_us/hospital_information/community _involvement/index.html
- *SafeKids* is a national nonprofit network of partners, including public health experts, corporations, foundations, and government agencies committed to preventing the foremost killer of children—unintentional childhood injury. http://www.safekids.org

Community-Dwelling Well Elderly Fieldwork Sites

- *Jewish Community Center of Dallas* builds a dynamic Jewish community by promoting the interests and welfare of that community; furthering an appreciation and understanding of shared Jewish heritage; fostering personal growth of members through cultural, educational, social, recreation, and civic activities; strengthening and enriching Jewish family life; and promoting understanding and contributing to common good of the general community. Services and programs are open to those outside the Jewish community. http://www.jccdallas.org
- *Visiting Nurse Association of Texas—Elder Care Program* provides high-quality, efficient health and health-related social services in the least restrictive environment—primarily the residence— in order to promote wellness, dignity, mobility, and independence for citizens in the service area. http://www.vnatexas.org/eldercare.htm
- *Alzheimer's Association Greater Dallas Chapter* is dedicated to eliminating Alzheimer's disease through the advancement of research and to enhance care and support for individuals, their families, and caregivers. http://www.alz.org/greaterdallas/

profession's foundational beliefs; the standards, language, domains, processes, and concepts of the profession; and the profession's official documents (Content Box 26-6). In Module I course work, students gain an appreciation for the importance of analysis of self, person, occupation, context, and their resultant impact on health and wellbeing; of the function of research in enhancing interventions; and of sustaining and advancing the profession (TWU School of OT, 2001). Interwoven into the curriculum design are elements, domains, and learner outcomes that are instrumental to the design and implementation of health promotion and primary-prevention intervention.

Two cornerstone courses in Module I serve to infuse ACOTE's health promotion standards into the curriculum:

- A didactic course entitled "Occupation, Wellness and Adaptation"
- A Fieldwork I course entitled "Adaptation Within the Community"

In the Occupation, Wellness and Adaptation course, a series of lectures by occupational therapy faculty and other health promotion professionals are provided over a 15-week semester (Content Box 26-7). Having public health professionals or injury-prevention specialists on the teaching team can serve to illustrate by example the

collaborative partnership needed for the promotion of health through occupation. A team-teaching approach to instruction is preferred over a guest lecture approach in order to increase understanding and appreciation of the knowledge, skills, and expertise needed to foster interdisciplinary partnerships in education and practice, as they are necessary for building healthier communities. In a small evaluation of this format's effectiveness, students reported positive measures of knowledge, attitudes, skills, behaviors, and self-efficacy. The attitudes and self-efficacy measures were particularly positive (Rhynders & Salvaggio, 2002).

TWU's Fieldwork I course Adaptation Within the Community is structured to include a weekly 1-hour seminar and 25 hours of service learning over the course of the semester. Course goals are detailed in Content Box 26-8. Fieldwork I students are encouraged

Module I Course Descriptions

TWU School of Occupational Therapy course offerings and descriptions:

- *Occupation, Wellness & Adaptation:* Exploration of development of occupational self and occupational performance and adaptation in variety of contexts. Model of examining adaptation through occupation in time and space. Two lecture hours a week. Two credit hours.
- *Adaptation Within the Community:* Placement in community settings under supervision of a qualified professional other than occupational therapists. Analyze functions of individuals engaged in a variety of occupations. Two laboratory and 1 seminar hours a week. Credit: 1 hour.
- *Person, Tools, & Occupations:* Exploration of purpose and meaning of activities with emphasis on play, games, and crafts. Experience the process of activity analysis, including documentation of observations.
- *Scholarly Inquiry Seminar:* Exploration of nature and process of scholarly inquiry. Application of critical thinking to the domains of knowledge in the practice of occupational therapy.
- *Occupational Therapy Process:* History of occupational therapy practice. Survey of current practice, including scope and standards and ethics. Includes aspects of occupational therapy process and language of health care and community areas of practice.
- *Evaluation Process:* The evaluation process of problems seen in occupational performance areas, components, and contexts. Includes principles of tests and measurements and use of assessment instruments commonly used in occupational therapy practice. One lecture and 2 laboratory hours; 2 hours credit.

Occupation, Wellness and Adaptation Course Goals and Lecture Topics

Course Goals

- Examine occupations related to specific age, life course, gender, and cultural groups
- Identify activities, tasks, and roles commonly related to these occupations and recognize the influence of occupational components performance upon these occupations and roles
- Identify places and points in the social and health-care systems where such problems might be referred to occupational therapy
- Select appropriate practice models or frames of reference to guide occupational therapy intervention in wellness, health, and preventive programs

Lecture Topics

- Overview of occupation, OT philosophy, practices and language related to primary, secondary, and tertiary occupational therapy intervention
- Constructs and concepts of wellness and health promotion
- AOTA and external documents relevant to occupation, health, wellness, and primary prevention
- Role of occupational therapy in health promotion and wellness—historical overview
- Functions of occupational therapy in community-based and built health promotion practices
- Interdisciplinary models of health promotion
  - Public Health Model, Health Belief Model, social cognitive theory
  - Injury Prevention Model/Frame of Reference
  - Surveillance Strategies—Haddon Matrix
- Relationship of the three Es in prevention—education, environment, and enforcement—to occupational therapy constructs of person, occupation, and environment
- Adaptation—historical overview of adaptation in occupational therapy practice
- Cultural issues in primary prevention
- Individual versus population intervention strategies
- Action research—goals and relevance to emerging practice markets
- Health promotion Lifestyle Redesign student demonstration projects

Fieldwork I Course Goals

- Explore the need of the setting in terms of personal skills, use of self as tool
- Identify own response to community and treatment settings and assess impact of relationship with individuals, clients, staff, and supervisor on own behavior
- Explore the supervisor-supervisee relationship and learn to share responsibility for it
- Demonstrate understanding of the meaning of occupational engagement to individual client, and impact of culture on meaningful occupations
- Compare and contrast the occupational performance and adaptation and the impact upon such component strengths and limitations, age, life stage, and life skills and context
- Know and practice professional work behaviors

would expand their understanding of self, occupation, adaptation, and wellness.

Element 2: Service.   The congruency of the missions of the university and the School of Occupational Therapy, the educational standards of the profession, and the health-care needs of the community across each of the three campuses provided the infrastructure needed to direct TWU's curriculum design. In 1997, TWU adopted a strategic plan called "Pioneering of the Future," which sought to expand outreach and partnership, increase sources of funding, and develop student service and volunteerism. Additionally, the inclusion of health promotion objectives in occupational therapy educational and practice standards provided the impetus needed to expand occupational therapy Fieldwork I placements to include primary prevention, injury prevention, and health promotion.

University and Dallas community environmental scan data serve to illustrate how health promotion, injury prevention, and wellness goals can be incorporated into didactic and service-learning course objectives. TWU School of Occupational Therapy Dallas–Presbyterian Campus is located in a geographic area of Dallas, Texas, known as Vickery Meadow. In the 1980s, the Vickery Meadow community was a model apartment/town-house community built to attract young, single, upwardly mobile professionals. A Supreme Court ruling, changes in fair housing practices, and expansion of businesses north of the city brought a dramatic shift in Vickery's demographics. In 1991, the Vickery Meadow community was viewed as one of the unhealthiest communities in the city, with a high rate of crime and poverty, overutilization of emergency room services for nonemergency ailments, and a distinct lack of community infrastructure that would support families.

to view their community as an educational experiential laboratory on which to reflect; to understand self, occupation, wellness, and adaptation; and to broaden their perspectives of roles and functions of occupational therapy across diverse systems of intervention.

The Fieldwork I course utilizes a wide spectrum of health delivery systems to broaden the learner's perspective of occupation and utilizes community services designed to facilitate health and wellness for individuals and populations. Students are encouraged to select, from a list of available service-learning options, a placement they believe would be meaningful and

The Vickery Meadow community has been considered one of the most ethnically diverse and densely populated communities in the Dallas metroplex. Over 53,000 predominately low-income residents reside in the community's 15,000 apartment units and 2300 condominiums located within a 3-mile square radius. The typical Vickery Meadow household averages 5.3 people, with 39% of households identified as living below the poverty level on an annual salary of less than $24,000. The Vickery community is a popular resettlement community for immigrants and refugees. The cultural representation of the community is 60% Hispanic, 18% African American, 22% white, and 6% others. More than 20 different languages are spoken by residents, and more than 7000 adults are reported to speak no English (Ricon & Associates, 2000).

In 1993, in an effort to improve the health of the community, Presbyterian Healthcare Systems (PHS), the largest employer in the Vickery Meadow area; the Presbyterian Foundation; and a group of property owners formed a public improvement district partnership called Vickery Meadow Improvement District (VMID). As a public improvement district authorized by Chapter 372 of the Texas Local Government Code, VMID levies and collects special assessments on property and retail establishments in the Vickery Meadow district. The mission of the Vickery Meadow Improvement District (VMID) is as follows:

> to provide a safe, appealing neighborhood for families, businesses, and property owners; thereby, improving the quality of life for everyone in Vickery Meadow. The District is committed to providing special supplemental services relating to advertising, promotion, health and sanitation, public safety, security, business recruitment, economic development, and recreation. (VMID, 2008, ¶ 4)

The VMID, as a public improvement district, is governed by trustees and an executive board that consists of volunteers from diverse vocational backgrounds. The Vickery Community Action Team (VCAT), a coalition under the Community Health Committee of VMID, consists of representatives from more than 50 businesses, government agencies, interactive community police, social services agencies, schools, universities, and faith-based agencies. The VCAT meets monthly to share information and coordinate services to improve the health and quality of life of the community where people live, work, and play.

Although significant improvements in the community's health have been made with the reduction of crime and provision of health care and social services, the work of VMID and its partners remains unfinished. The infrastructure of the neighborhood was built for singles, not families, and overcrowding of schools, access to preventive care and health-care services, resettlement of immigrants and refugees, an excessive high school dropout rate, poverty, and a high incidence of domestic violence continue to challenge the health of the community.

Data collected from environmental scans, interaction with health promotion leaders, and active engagement of faculty in community health promotion initiatives are essential in laying the foundation for innovative, effective, and efficient Fieldwork I service-learning placements that promote the advancement of occupational therapy health promotion practices.

Element 3: Reflection. A contemporary model of health promotion recognizes that promoting health is a complex process that is not equal to health education. Students have the opportunity to experience and reflect on the interaction across diverse systems, services, and disciplines needed to comprehensively address desired healthy lifestyles, access to services, safe environments, social conditions, behavioral intentions, self-efficacy, social norms, legislative regulation, education, communication, community development, and activism. Learners also have opportunities to participate in the social action and advocacy needed to build healthy communities. Reflection is a critical part of the service-learning process. As Bruner states, "Meaning making involves situating encounters with the world in their appropriate cultural contexts" (as cited by Woods et al., 2000, p. 590).

Course learning assignments challenge students to reflect on and apply person, occupation, and contextual data collected through service learning. They are encouraged to experiment with assessment and planning tools such as the Haddon Matrix (Haddon, 1968) to examine how the "3 Es" of prevention (i.e., education, environmental modification, enforcement) interface with occupational therapy models, constructs, and concepts and to develop innovative culturally and contextually sensitive marketing strategies for the advancement of occupational therapy in health promotion.

Fieldwork I student seminar discussion groups are constructed to demonstrate the diversity of health promotion service markets across the life span, systems of service, cultures, and socioeconomic groups. Weekly 1-hour discussion groups examine occupational performance in context with focus on health promotion, injury prevention, and wellness across each of the eight areas of occupation—ADLs, IADLs, rest and sleep, education, work, play, leisure, and social participation (AOTA, 2008, p. 628). In a weekly e-mail journal submitted to the course instructor, students document self-reflection, occupational health issues, and observation questions related to individual and populations' performance, and the role of occupation and functions of occupational therapy in the context of the fieldwork site.

In collaboration with occupational therapy faculty and Fieldwork I supervisors, students are also required to apply first-semester assessment course knowledge and skills to formulate evaluation plans based on the needs of the Fieldwork I agency, individuals, and populations being served. Community residents act as "client educators" by allowing problem-based teams of students, under the supervision of faculty, to gain competency in administering, scoring, and interpreting health promotion and injury-prevention assessments that address diverse areas of occupation. Examples of assessments that have been used by first-semester graduate occupational therapy students include COPM; SAFE; Geriatric Depression Scale and Falls Self Efficacy Scale; COPES; CAPS; COPS; Caregiver Stress Inventory; and the Walkability Checklist, a nationally developed pedestrian safety assessment and educational tool.

Element 4: Celebration. When health promotion educational strategies are innovatively linked to occupational therapy curriculum design, in partnership with needs of the community, value is added to the curriculum, and learners are actively engaged in meaningful and purposeful occupations. In addition, the power of occupation, the value of diversity, the promotion of occupational therapy in health promotion, and community-based scholarly inquiry are celebrated.

To examine the power of occupation and the role occupational therapy plays in health promotion partnerships, TWU students are challenged to view themselves as "lifestyle redesigners" as they prepare innovative marketing strategies to promote awareness of the role of occupational therapy in health promotion and wellness. The University of Southern California's (USC) **Lifestyle Redesign** is described as the process of facilitating the client's ability to "select and perform an individually tailored blend of activities" in order to achieve "a healthy and personally satisfying" lifestyle (Clark, Carlson, Jackson, & Mandel, 2003, p. 10). Lifestyle Redesign's core concepts are used to provide a framework by which to examine the impact of occupational therapy in the promotion of health and wellbeing across a broad range of health-delivery systems and services. The four core concepts of USC's Lifestyle Redesign approach are

1. Occupation is life itself.
2. Occupation can create new visions of possible selves.
3. Occupation has a curative effect on physical and mental health and on a sense of life order and routine.
4. Occupation has a place in preventive care. (Mandel, Jackson, Zemke, Nelson, & Clark, 1999, p. 13)

The project in the course *Occupation, Wellness and Adaptation* has students work in teams to develop a

Lifestyle Redesign marketing project that serves to demonstrate to Fieldwork I service-learning agencies the power of occupation and the role of occupational therapy in health promotion (Content Box 26-9).

Diversity, with regard to age and health promotion contexts being served on Fieldwork I, challenges learners to value diversity and use clinical reasoning skills to identify client-centered adaptive strategies that are culturally appropriate and meaningful to those being served. Students select a culture and ethnic group they would like to learn more about. Throughout the course of the semester, they research the attitudes and values of the population across six performance areas of occupation. At the end of the course, a cultural festival is held so the students can celebrate cultural diversity and the potential impact that culture can have on delivery of occupational therapy services.

By promoting occupational therapy in the community, opportunities for employment and paid internships can evolve as a result of service-learning partnerships. Increased involvement of occupational therapy faculty and students in community health promotion programming provided an increase in financial support opportunities for students. In gaining an awareness of and appreciation for the contributions occupational therapy service-learning students bring to community-based programming, the Jewish Community Center of Dallas has made available to TWU Dallas Center occupational therapy students a paid graduate student internship. In addition, service-learning students have discovered part-time social service employment opportunities with service-learning agencies and have gained access to community-funded academic scholarship funds.

Content Box 26-9

Learning Outcomes for the Lifestyle Redesign Assignment

1. Experience the process needed to establish new areas of practice
2. Develop skill in preparing a community and service profile (Fazio, 2001)
3. Identify literature that supports role of occupational therapy in primary prevention
4. Apply concepts, constructs, and principles of occupation to promote health and wellness and adaptation
5. Use innovation and creativity to explore potential roles and functions for occupational therapy in primary prevention, health promotion, and wellness
6. Articulate the contributions occupational therapy can make in primary prevention and the power of occupation in promoting health and preventing illness

Scholarly inquiry can also be celebrated. As a result of the Fieldwork I service-learning experiences and reflections, some students have developed an interest in health promotion as a potential area of future employment in occupational therapy. In partial fulfillment of graduation requirements, TWU entry-level master's degree students, working in partnership with faculty, health promotion, and injury-prevention specialists, have established new lines of research directed to injury prevention, health promotion, and wellness.

Reviews of literature, survey, and surveillance data, and critical analysis studies have been conducted to examine drowning prevention, child passenger safety education of families with special-needs children, low-income families' perceptions of home-safety needs and interventions, pedestrian safety rules and their cultural implications, play with wheeled objects, service-learning after-school partnerships, prevention of unintentional injuries in immigrants and refugees, health promotion needs, prevention of falls in elderly, and the role of occupational therapy in school-based primary-care centers. Students have also contributed to the development of intervention plans and advocacy campaigns to formulate legislative policy to support graduated licensing laws for teenage drivers.

Towson University

As a result of a grant award from the Shriver Center, the Department of Occupational Therapy and Occupational Science at Towson University (in Towson, Maryland) applied a service-learning philosophy to health promotion coursework. This shifted the original focus of the course from community-based fieldwork to service learning. Unlike traditional didactic methods, service learning encompasses three components—academic preparation, action, and ongoing reflection (Rudmann, Ward, & Varekojis, 1999). The academic preparation includes developing the skills to conduct a needs assessment and to design a relevant program for a specified population and the strategic skills to facilitate implementation of the program. The action component involves the student's direct service at the community agency and the reciprocal benefits the agency receives from the student's skills and efforts. The reflection component is ongoing and enables the student to record and monitor professional growth, challenges, and development.

The course *Occupational Therapy Health Promotion Initiatives in the Community* meets the service-learning goal by providing a win-win, both for the student (learning) and the site (service). This outcome is different than at a traditional Level I fieldwork setting where the student is learning but the site is gaining a less tangible return. In addition to providing a valuable fieldwork opportunity for students, there are other benefits, including opportunities for faculty development, identification of partnerships with community agencies, and expanded health promotion services for at-risk individuals in the community.

Initially the required course was two credits and sequenced in the last semester of the undergraduate program, concurrent with the pediatric Level I clinical experience and prior to beginning Level II fieldwork. Prerequisites included completion of mental health and physical dysfunction Level I fieldwork. Acknowledging the complexity of skills needed for success, the course was modified to become a required three-credit graduate-level course in 2003. The prerequisites were changed to include completion of three Level I fieldworks and the first Level II fieldwork. The content was also expanded to include additional training in developing a budget and obtaining funding for community programs. Greater emphasis was placed on participation in the context of the family and terminology consistent with the *International Classification of Functioning* (World Health Organization, 2001). In addition, the *Occupational Therapy Practice Framework: Domain and Process* (AOTA, 2008) was incorporated into the course.

The use of a service-learning paradigm for health promotion course work provides contextual learning opportunities for students, potential for faculty development, and access to occupational therapy services through partnerships with community agencies. Each of these benefits will be described below.

Contextual Learning Opportunities

This course provides students the opportunity to apply occupational therapy theory to health promotion practices in the community with particular emphasis on the multiple and varied contexts in which such practice occurs. Course content integrates knowledge and skills for the practice of occupational therapy services that foster healthy development; prevent health problems; maintain optimal function; and develop occupational performance skills of individuals, families, and communities (Reitz, 1998). Students are introduced to program development models such as the Generic Health Fitness Delivery System (GHFDS), the Comprehensive Health Education Model (CHEM), and the Model for Health Education Planning (MHEP), as described by McKenzie and Smeltzer (1997). An outline of the health promotion course using a service-learning model can be found in Content Box 26-10.

Students are challenged to examine and choose a project that involves consultative, direct, or advocacy services (Dungeon & Greenberg, 1998). In this manner,

Content Box 26-10

Outline of Health Promotion Course Using a Service-Learning Model

Preparation (25%)
- Six weeks classroom instruction in health promotion and community program development
- Needs assessment
- Program proposal

Action (50%)
- Six weeks implementation
  - Direct service
  - Consultative
  - Advocacy

Reflection (25%)
- Journal with reflective paper
- Group presentations to classmates

the model of delivery is congruent with nonmedical models of community practice. Sites have various organizational structures, cultures, and needs, so options include either initiating a new site through consultative or needs assessment, or building on a program at an agency where students have designed or implemented programs in previous semesters. Programmatic focus varies, but fully addressing the community context is a course requirement. Regardless of the population, students are required to apply knowledge and skills relative to individuals served by the program, family members, and agency staff. This requires a broader awareness of multiple areas, including developmental tasks and roles across the life span (Murray, 1997).

In most sites, a professional other than an occupational therapist provides the on-site supervision. This supervision includes providing a management-level contact who can help students appropriately navigate the agency by enabling access or suggesting alternatives for conducting the needs assessment if access is not feasible. Supervisors have included master's-level social workers, educators, and paraprofessional staff. One of the more complex tasks for the course instructor is the coordination and clarification of student supervision. Faculty frequently need to take on greater oversight than a traditional Level I site due to the overwhelming demands and lack of regular availability of site supervisors, the need for role clarification of the occupational therapy students, and the high turnover rate of management-level staff in nonprofit agencies.

Students repeatedly report that the community work provides them an opportunity to apply leadership skills that they have experienced only in more contrived classroom situations until taking the course. A higher level of autonomy, judgment, and decision-making is required when interacting with the agency leadership. Students have commented on areas specific to the domain of occupational therapy that benefited their community experience, including occupational performance analysis, group dynamics, occupation-based program development, therapeutic use of self, and communication skills. This directly contrasts the medical model Level I fieldwork experience, where there is often a more passive role of observation for the student.

Community sites offer direct experience with alternative roles for occupational therapy practitioners, such as consultation and advocacy (Bossers, Cook, Polatajako, & Laine, 1997). In addition, students are presented with the myriad social and economic challenges that poverty imposes on daily life. They achieve a better understanding of context, especially cultural influences on various populations. For example, students working with 3- and 4-year-olds in a Head Start program located near an X-rated movie theater gained an awareness of the multiple challenges faced by parents and children in such settings. In another example, students addressed real-life barriers to employment when they discussed time-management concerns with residents at a women's shelter.

Community sites can also provide a staging opportunity for students to participate in the development of a future Level II site. One student was able to develop a Level II site as a direct result of a service-learning project in a county department of aging, which in turn led to a full-time position upon graduation. The development of partnerships between academic departments and community agencies has been successful in expanding occupational therapy presence in the community (Scaffa, 2001).

Potential for Faculty Development

Teaching health promotion in a service-learning format has provided unique opportunities for the faculty and the students. Due to the service component of the health promotion service-learning course, more sites are seeking student placements. Faculty members have expanded the service-learning model to other courses, which has strengthened the commitment between fieldwork sites, the department, and the university. Adopting a service-learning orientation has bolstered the potential for grant funding, as many that provide funds for health promotion and community intervention specifically require such a focus. There are many grant opportunities for programs that serve the community, for partnerships/collaboration efforts between university and nonprofit agencies, and for funding interdisciplinary projects. There appear to be synergies between the inclusion of service-learning in fieldwork, grant funding, and the development of paid employment opportunities in community-based practice. **Synergy** in this context refers to multiple people or systems interacting or collaborating with an end result much greater than additive.

Occupational therapists look for ways to meet the needs of individuals in the community where the need to function in meaningful occupations is most authentic. The medical model, which adheres to strict medical necessity requirements for payment, lacks the structure to support community health promotion. There is a need to develop alternative models and delivery methods to ensure access to health promotion services that enable client function. The health promotion course provides a means to establish partnerships with nonprofit agencies that evolve to support other opportunities, such as paid consultation (Merryman, 2002).

Access to Occupational Therapy Services Through Partnerships With Community Agencies

Collaboration with nonprofit agencies promotes increased access to occupational therapy services by creating part-time positions. These are significantly less costly than private consultation with an occupational therapist. Agencies are able to "try on" occupational therapy, and students are able to experience firsthand a nonmedical model approach to health promotion freed from the constraints of reimbursement issues (Smillie, 1992). For example, occupational therapy students developed a peer mediation program in an urban middle school. Using a health-planning model as a structural framework and using occupational therapy principles to guide the development of session plans, students used funds from a service-learning grant to take their participants to an outdoor ropes and team-building program. The middle-school students received additional training during school hours on implementation of the peer mediation model to aid in its continuation. This provided an expanded role beyond the typical health promotion services a school is able to provide students. Another example involved occupational therapy students who were hired to present their training program on strategies for interaction and motivation of individuals with serious mental illness for a state-sponsored workshop for line-staff in assisted-living environments. In another instance, students who designed environmental adaptations for a religious teaching setting were hired to train staff and oversee implementation of changes.

Sample Partnerships and Programs

As an example of a service-learning partnership, a program in collaboration with the Arthritis Foundation will be described. The Maryland Chapter of the Arthritis Foundation awarded the Engalitcheff Quality of Life grant for development of a health promotion program on living with arthritis. The program was developed to address quality-of-life issues for individuals with arthritis. Since this population typically engages in few leisure pursuits due to limited mobility and resources (Zimmer, Hickey, & Searle, 1995), the funding was used to directly serve them. The target population included females over the age of 65 with symptoms of osteoarthritis. Many participants presented with multiple comorbidities that impacted function. A leisure skill inventory was administered to identify potential areas of interest.

The program sessions incorporated adapted methods and application of joint-protection techniques to identified leisure activities. The Well-Elderly study (Clark et al., 1997) found that specialized training in the importance of meaningful activities and how to select and perform activities to live a healthy and satisfying lifestyle showed significant benefits across various health, function, and quality-of-life domains. The program built on those results but emphasized performing leisure activities in a manner that was appropriate for joint preservation.

The 10 students who participated in the program's development and implementation were able to meet individualized learning goals. Two graduate students enrolled in their senior research course developed training session outlines. These students worked with three undergraduate students who implemented the sessions with a total of 18 participants in three sites. The graduate students were able to gain experience as program facilitators and to carry out research on the program's effectiveness and satisfaction of the participants. Information from the initial implementation phase was then shared with five students enrolled in the Health Promotion Initiatives course in the subsequent semester, who were able to build on the program and offer it in an additional five sites with 47 new participants. As a result of this single program, 65 individuals received a health program in eight different sites.

Funding for health promotion programs with aging adults with osteoarthritis can be requested from a variety of sources, including local Arthritis Foundation chapters, local departments of aging, interdisciplinary sources, and service-learning community funding sources. A service-learning award from the Shriver Center funded another health promotion program for this population. Funds were used to provide People with Arthritis Can Exercise (PACE) instructor training for six students, one faculty member, and two staff from the University Wellness Center. Students were then able to begin their Level II Fieldwork and ultimately their entry-level positions with the added credentials to provide the PACE program.

Additional program settings for older adults have included adult day-care centers, an elder hostel, and senior apartment buildings. Program sites for adults have included the University Wellness Center, stress management, homeless and domestic violence shelters, and welfare-to-work settings. Program sites for children and youth have included schools, Head Start, YMCA, and Girl Scouts.

Future Directions

As a result of this model, the students are better equipped for health promotion service provision, especially for underserved populations. Students are better prepared to seek positions in community-based practice areas. They demonstrate and report improved knowledge of program development, increased confidence, strengthened communication skills, and increased awareness of nonmedical model roles for occupational therapists.

In 2001, a University System of Maryland faculty development grant was awarded for Interdisciplinary Collaboration in Service-Learning Health Promotion Initiatives in the Community. The purpose of the project was to develop a Web resource to enhance coordination of health promotion initiatives with other disciplines. The Web resource provides an ongoing means of disseminating information and sharing with other occupational therapy faculty and faculty from other disciplines who may be interested in identifying a potential project for collaboration. Faculty can browse existing health promotion sites and can forward information on their own partnerships. Categories of information found on the website are listed in Content Box 26-11.

Content Box 26-11

Interdisciplinary Collaboration in Service Learning

Health Promotion Initiatives Website Resources

Program categories include

* child and adolescent programs/services;
* community-based living programs/services;
* day programs/services;
* older adult programs/services; and
* vocational and work programs/services.

The website also includes links to information on topics such as

* service-learning resources;
* funding sources;
* occupational therapy emerging practice areas; and
* interdisciplinary teams.

Information can be found at http://pages.towson.edu/mriley/usm/Index.htm.

Conclusion

Despite competing orientations among and between occupational therapy educators and practitioners over the years, members of the profession never lost sight of the important link between education and practice in sustaining and expanding occupational therapy practice parameters. The range of educational methodologies employed to implement curriculum plans is varied and closely linked to the climate of innovation and the innovative spirit of those designing the educational experience. Service-learning health promotion Fieldwork I experiences, inventively linked with didactic course content, provides the opportunity to examine in context the health needs of individuals and populations; it also helps to facilitate the development of interdisciplinary community partnerships while gaining an appreciation for the knowledge and skills necessary to create change.

Occupational therapy curriculum and practitioners' professional development plans must be congruent with professional standards, institutional missions, and the needs of their nation, while addressing differences in geographic needs, demographic representation, and availability of resources in service areas. Diversity in educational institutions' missions, program resources, and infrastructure of the communities in which the educational program resides will determine the educational strategies used to infuse health promotion into a curriculum.

As a profession, occupational therapy is acutely aware of the need to anticipate trends and to develop action plans accordingly (Fazio, 2001; Finn, 1972; Johnson, 1973). The rate at which trends and emerging practice markets are identified, innovations are disseminated, and policies are adopted depends on innovation leadership and on a climate favorable to supporting and maintaining the innovation. To incorporate health promotion into occupational therapy, educators and practitioners must be perceptive to environmental conditions and the value of interdisciplinary alliances in implementing and maintaining health promotion innovation; this can facilitate the diffusion of innovation. See Chapter 3 for more information on diffusion of innovations. In order to continue meeting the needs and demands of society, educators and practitioners must employ inventive academic and clinical strategies that facilitate the infusion of health promotion throughout occupational therapy services across the continuum of care.

Learning does not occur merely because the service is carried out. In service learning, a partnership is formed and the needs of the student are balanced with the needs of the community. Service-learning objectives and outcomes must be linked to the course content and must include a mechanism for reflection, reciprocity, and sustainability. Current fieldwork education practices can be transitioned to service learning with some work on the part of the academic faculty, the community partners, and the students.

Curriculum designs that include Fieldwork Level I service-learning placements promote partnerships with diverse groups of community residents and health promotion specialists across a wide range of health promotion organizations/systems. They also afford a unique educational opportunity and innovative means by which to reflect on and demonstrate the power of occupation in promoting health and wellbeing.

The integration of health promotion in occupational therapy curriculum design, course objectives, and learning assignments provides a multitude of learning possibilities and means by which to actively engage the learner in the occupational adaptation process. Throughout didactic and service-learning Fieldwork I courses, students are challenged to apply language, domains, processes, and constructs of occupational therapy; to practice skills in interpersonal relations, clinical reasoning, assessment, and task analysis; and to explore with their interdisciplinary partners the value of occupational therapy in achieving health promotion and injury-prevention outcomes.

▶ For Discussion and Review

1. What factors would you use to persuade occupational therapists to address the prevention and health promotion needs of their clients?
2. How does service-learning differ from community service?
3. Compare and contrast service learning with traditional fieldwork.
4. Describe how you might conduct an environmental scan in your community to identify health promotion needs.
5. How can principles of Lifestyle Redesign be applied to health promotion practice in occupational therapy?
6. Explain the concept of synergy and how it relates to community-based health promotion.
7. Discuss how the accreditation standards regarding prevention, health promotion, and wellness are addressed in your occupational therapy program's curriculum.

▶ Research Questions

1. What are the basic skills students need to provide occupation-based health promotion services in community settings?

2. Do students who participate in service learning have a better understanding of health promotion than students who participate in traditional fieldwork?
3. What are the unique contributions occupational therapy can make to prevention and health promotion efforts?
4. What are the most effective ways to meet the competencies related to health promotion described in the ACOTE accreditation standards?
5. How do the ACOTE accreditation standards relate to the *Healthy People 2010* objectives?

References

Accreditation Council for Occupational Therapy Education. (2007, April). *Accreditation Council for Occupational Therapy Education (ACOTE®) standards and interpretive guidelines.* Retrieved October 29, 2007, from http://www .aota.org/Educate/Accredit/StandardsReview/40601.aspx.

Addams, J. (2004). *Twenty years at Hull House.* Whitefish, MT: Kessinger.

American Occupational Therapy Association. (2008). *Occupational therapy practice framework: Domain and process* (2d ed.). Bethesda, MD: Author.

American Society of Association Executives. (2003). *Newsletter.* Retrieved September 2, 2006, from http://www .asaecenter.org.

Astin, A. W., & Sax L. J. (1998). How undergraduates are affected by service participation. *Journal of College Student Development, 39,* 251–63.

Bonder, R. (1994). Growing old in the United States. In R. Bonder & M. Wagner (Eds.), *Functional performance in older adults.* Philadelphia: F. A. Davis.

Bossers, A., Cook, J., Polatajko, H., & Laine, C. (1997). Understanding the role-emerging fieldwork placement. *Canadian Journal of Occupational Therapy, 64,* 2.

Carmona, R. H. (2004). Healthy people curriculum task force: A commentary by the Surgeon General. *American Journal of Preventive Medicine, 27*(5), 482–83.

Chambliss, J. J. (1996). *Philosophy of education: An encyclopedia.* New York: Routledge.

Clark, F., Azen, S. P., Zemke, R., Jackson, J., Carlson, M., Mandel, D., Hay, J., Josephson, K., Cherry, B., Hessel, C., Palmer, J., & Lipson, L. (1997). Occupational therapy for independent-living older adults. *Journal of the American Medical Association, 278*(16), 1321–26.

Clark, F. A., Carlson, M., Jackson, J., & Mandel, D. (2003). Lifestyle Redesign improves health and is cost-effective. *OT Practice, 8*(January 29), 9–13.

Dalton, J. G., Jarratt, J., & Mahaffie, J. B. (2003). *From scan to plan: Integrating trends into the strategy-making process. Executive summary.* Washington, DC: Foundation of the American Society of Association Executives.

Deal, L. W., Gomby, D. S., Zippiroli, L., & Behrman, R. E. (2000). Unintentional injuries in childhood: Analysis and recommendations. In R. Behrman (Ed.), *The future of children—Unintentional injuries in childhood.* Los Altos, CA: The David and Lucille Packard Foundation.

Dungeon, B. J., & Greenberg, S. L. (1998). Preparing students for consultation roles and systems. *American Journal of Occupational Therapy, 52*(10), 801–09.

Fazio, L. (2001). *Developing occupation-centered programs for the community: A workbook for students and professionals.* Upper Saddle River, NJ: Prentice Hall.

Fertman, C. I. (1994). *Service learning for all students.* Bloomington, IN: Phi Delta Kappa Educational Foundation.

Fidler, G. S. (1966). Learning as a growth process: A conceptual framework for professional education. *American Journal of Occupational Therapy, 20,* 1–8.

Finn, G. (1972). The occupational therapist in preventive programs. *American Journal of Occupational Therapy, 26,* 59–66.

Grantmakers Concerned with Immigrants and Refugees. (2006). *About immigration: Immigration fact sheets, immigration—Demographics.* Retrieved October 31, 2007, from http://www.gcir.org/about_immigration/fact_sheets/demographics.htm.

Haddon, W. (1968). The changing approach to the epidemiology, prevention, and amelioration of trauma: The transition to approaches etiologically rather than descriptively based. *American Journal of Public Health, 58,* 1431–38.

Harkavy, I. (January 29, 1998). *The First John Dewey Lecture.* Retrieved April 19, 2004, from http://www.umich.edu/~mserve/faculty/ resources/Dewey-Harkavy.doc.

Howard, J. (1993). *Principles of good practice for service learning pedagogy.* Retrieved April 19, 2004, from http://www.morgridge.wisc.edu/manual/pdf/principles.pdf.

Johnson, J. (1973). Occupational therapy: A model for the future. *American Journal of Occupational Therapy, 27,* 229–45.

King, L. J. (1980). Creative caring. *American Journal of Occupational Therapy, 34*(5), 522–28.

Mandel, D., Jackson, J., Zemke, R., Nelson, L., & Clark, F. (1999). *Lifestyle Redesign: Implementing the Well Elderly Program.* Bethesda, MD: American Occupational Therapy Association.

McKenzie, J. F., & Smeltzer, J. L. (1997). *Planning, implementing, and evaluating health promotion programs.* Boston: Allyn & Bacon.

Mercy, J. A., Sleet, D. A., & Doll, L. S. (2003). Applying a developmental approach to injury prevention. *American Journal of Health Education (Supplement), 34*(5), 6–12.

Merryman, M. B. (2002, May 13). Networking as an entrée to paid community practice. *OT Practice,* 10–13

Miller, T., Romano, E., & Spicer, R. (2000). The cost of childhood unintentional injuries and the value of prevention. In R. Behrman (Ed.), *The future of children—Unintentional injuries in childhood.* Los Altos, CA: The David and Lucille Packard Foundation.

Murray, R. B. (1997). *Health assessment and promotion strategies through the lifespan* (6th ed.). East Norwalk, CT: Appleton & Lange.

National Center for Health Statistics. (2004). *Fast stats: Accidents/unintentional injuries.* Retrieved April 19, 2004, from http://www.cdc.gov/nchs/fastats/acc-inj.htm.

National Service Learning Clearinghouse. (2004a). *Glossary.* Retrieved September 2, 2007, from http://www.servicelearning.org/what_is_service-learning/glossary/index.php.

National Service Learning Clearinghouse. (2004b). *Service learning is . . .* Retrieved September 2, 2007, from http://www.servicelearning.org/what_is_service-learning/.

Noam, G. (2002). *Afterschool education: A new ally for education reform.* Retrieved April 18, 2004, from http://www.edletter.org/past/issues/2002-nd/afterschool.shtml.

Peloquin, S. M. (1991). Occupational therapy service: Individual and collective understandings of the founders, part 1. *American Journal of Occupational Therapy, 45,* 352–60.

Reitz, S. M. (1998). *Health promotion initiatives in the community syllabus.* Towson University, Towson, MD.

Rhynders, P., & Salvaggio, S. (2002). *The role of service learning in preparing occupational therapists for community-based injury prevention.* Unpublished manuscript. Texas Woman's University, School of Occupational Therapy, Dallas.

Ricon & Associates. (2000). *Vickery Meadows Survey.* Unpublished market survey report. Dallas, Texas. For more information, see http://www.riconassoc.com/demoinfo.html.

Riegelman, R. K., Evans, C. H., & Garr, D. R. (2004). Why a clinical prevention and population health curriculum framework? *American Journal of Preventive Medicine, 27*(5), 481.

Rudmann, S. V., Ward, K. M., & Varekojis, S. M. (1999). University-community partnerships for health: A model interdisciplinary service-learning project. *Journal of Allied Health, 28*(2), 109–12.

Scaffa, M. (Ed.). (2001). *Occupational therapy in community-based practice settings.* Philadelphia: F. A. Davis.

Smillie, C. (1992). Preparing health professionals for a collaborative health promotion role. *Canadian Journal of Public Health, 83*(4), 279–82.

Texas Woman's University School of Occupational Therapy. (2001). *Self study.* Unpublished document, Texas Woman's University, School of Occupational Therapy, Dallas.

U.S. Department of Health and Human Services. (2000). *Healthy People 2010: Understanding and improving health* (2d ed.). Washington, DC: Government Printing Office.

Vickery Meadow Improvement District. (2008). *Who is VMID?* Retrieved February 24, 2009 from http://www.vickerymeadow.org/whois.php.

Woods, W., Nielson, C., Humphry, R., Coppola, S., Baranek, G., & Rourk, J. (2000). A curriculum renaissance: Graduate education centered on occupation. *American Journal of Occupational Therapy, 54,* 586–97.

World Health Organization. (2001). *Internal classification of functioning, disability and health.* Geneva, Switzerland: Author.

Zimmer, Z., Hickey, T., & Searle, M. (1995). Activity participation and well-being among people with arthritis. *Gerontologist, 35*(4), 463–71.

Chapter 27

Health Promotion Research in Occupational Therapy

Charles H. Christiansen and Kathleen M. Matuska

> It is often necessary to make a decision on the basis of information sufficient for action but insufficient to satisfy the intellect.
> —Immanuel Kant

Learning Objectives

This chapter is designed to enable the reader to:

- Describe the importance of research to the health promotion process.
- Identify different approaches to health promotion research and the types of information each approach provides.
- Identify the strengths and limitations of information provided by various types of research.

- Describe the challenges to conducting research in community-based health promotion.
- Discuss results of health promotion research conducted within and outside of occupational therapy.
- Identify areas for future research in health promotion that are especially germane to occupational therapy.

Key Terms

Critical knowledge

Disability adjusted life years (DALYs)

Instrumental knowledge

Interactive knowledge

Participatory research

Qualitative research

Quality adjusted life years (QALYs)

Quantitative research

Randomized controlled trial (RTC)

Introduction

Health promotion is a complex process involving various types of approaches and interventions, each aimed at fostering lives that provide for optimal health. Some health promotion strategies engender policies or environmental conditions aimed at avoiding or preventing health conditions, while others seek to influence personal beliefs and behaviors related to health. Occupational therapy practitioners are involved in providing many of these services (American Occupational Therapy Association [AOTA], 2008).

Because interventions must be carried out within communities in order to achieve their goals (Scaffa, 2001), the selection and implementation of strategies is greatly influenced by the characteristics of the professionals and people living there. As a result, the delivery of health promotion programs is nearly always influenced by factors other than scientific evidence, such as traditions, values, and beliefs. Yet, if the benefits of health promotion are to be fully realized,

empirical evidence must be sought, the effectiveness of new approaches must be demonstrated, and information about new practices and innovations must be accepted and adopted by community members and professionals. Each of these necessary actions identifies an important area of focus in health promotion research.

In this chapter, the authors intend to

1. describe the importance of research to the health promotion process;
2. identify different approaches to health promotion research and the types of information each approach provides;
3. discuss the strengths and limitations of information provided by various types of research;
4. review some examples of health promotion research conducted within and outside of occupational therapy; and
5. describe barriers and opportunities related to research efforts.

The authors conclude by identifying areas for future research in health promotion that are viewed as especially germane to occupational therapy.

The Need for Health Promotion Research

Perhaps the most compelling reason for conducting research in health promotion is an ethical one. It is often not recognized that any clinical decision regarding an intervention for a patient or a population constitutes an ethical decision. Rogers (1983) pointed out that because health-care providers have a moral duty to do what is best for a given recipient of care at the time a service is delivered, awareness of the relative effectiveness of a given intervention choice is necessary, especially when several options are available. This implies that the professional must be fully informed about the evidence supporting a given strategy if decisions about interventions are to be ethical.

In earlier decades, much clinical intervention—and most community health strategies—had not been proven effective through empirical research (Smith, 1991). In fact, most practices, both in medicine and public health, were based on anecdotal clinical experience, expert opinion, tradition, and subjective choices made by provider preference. Nowadays, however, expectations have changed dramatically. Funding agencies, accrediting agencies, and patients expect that decisions about interventions will be supported by empirical study. Society now expects that objective evidence of effectiveness will underlie all treatment or intervention programs. These shifting sentiments are behind the evidence-based practice movement of the new millennium (Institute of Medicine [IOM], 1997; Sackett & Rosenberg, 1995; Sackett, Rosenberg, Muir-Gray, Haynes, & Richardson, 1996).

Demographic and Economic Imperatives of Health Promotion Research

Changes in the demographics of the population also underscore the importance of research in health promotion. As a greater proportion of the population in North America becomes older, the incidence of chronic disease and disability increases, placing demands on the health-care system. Secondary and tertiary prevention programs become important with this age group in order to reduce the consequences of morbidity and prevent more serious disability. Moreover, with a larger elderly population, the proportion of adults in traditional working age groups is smaller.

With fewer workers, the importance of preventing illness and promoting health becomes more important in the workplace, because any nation's economy depends upon a dependable and productive workforce. Both dependability and productivity are related to workforce health.

Trends in the diversity of the population are also a factor driving research. The United States, and North America in general, is experiencing dramatic changes in the cultural and racial/ethnic diversity of its populations. Studies have indicated that cultural and ethnic differences influence health practices and create disparities in access to care and the type and quality of care delivered (Kuzbansky et al., 2001). These phenomena argue convincingly for research that provides a better understanding of the factors influencing the delivery of services that can appropriately and equitably benefit the entire population.

Perhaps most importantly, encouraging healthy lifestyles can result in the adoption of habits and behaviors that reduce risks for injury and disease, or prevent or reduce the disabling effects of chronic disease. Such efforts targeted at younger people can result in less morbidity as they reach middle age and maturity. Exercise; proper body mechanics; the use of seat belts and other safety equipment; healthy nutritional practices; and the reduction or avoidance of risks associated with smoking, drugs, and sexually transmitted infections are examples of lifestyle-related practices that influence optimal health.

Taken together, these demographic, health, safety, and lifestyle-related issues point to the potential economic benefits of health promotion programs. However, since such efforts often involve the expenditure of public funds, it becomes doubly important to ensure that community health programs produce their expected results. Stated in another way, once the case for implementing health promotion programs on theoretical grounds is made, it must then be defended on economic grounds as measured by some indicator of public benefit, such as increased life expectancy, increased quality of life, and decreased disability.

Because of the economic issues involved in determining programmatic options, economists and program analysts have developed measures of effectiveness and presumed benefit called *summary measures of population health* (SMPH). These have been developed to estimate the benefit of implementing a particular intervention program (Field & Gold, 1998). Examples of such measures include **quality adjusted life years** (QALYs) and **disability adjusted life years** (DALYs; see Content Box 27-1 for a brief description of these measures).

Content Box 27-1

QALYs and DALYs: Preference-Based Measures for Community Health Intervention Decision-Making

Quality Adjusted Life Years (QALYs)

A QALY is a measure of the value of a specific health outcome. It is an indicator of both the length of life and quality of life. QALYs are used to assess the cost-effectiveness of various interventions. Weights, or utility values, are assigned to various levels of health, from 1 (perfect health) to 0 (death). QALYs are calculated by multiplying the change in utility value acquired through the intervention by the duration of the treatment effect in years. For example, if an intervention improves a person's health status (utility value) from 0.5 to 0.8 and the effect lasts for 10 years, then the QALY is 3.

Disability Adjusted Life Years (DALYs)

The DALY is a measure of disease burden and is calculated as the years of healthy life lost due to disease or disability. One DALY indicates the loss of 1 year of healthy life due to disability. It is an indication of the cap between current health status of a population and the ideal health status where everyone lives to advanced age with no disease or disability. DALYs are calculated by summing the years of life lost due to premature death and the years lost due to disability. This calculation takes into consideration life expectancy by weighting age at onset of disease or disability. Disability status is also weighted to account for differences in severity.

From *Problems and solutions in calculating quality-adjusted life years (QALYS)* by L. Prieto & J. A. Sacristan, 2003. Retrieved May 25, 2009, from http://www.pubmedcentral.nih.gov/articlerender.fcgi?artid =317370.
Metrics: Disability-adjusted life year (DALY) by World Health Organization, 2009. Retrieved May 25, 2009, from http://www.who.int/ healthinfo/global_burden_disease/metrics_daly/en/index.html.

The Special Challenge of Health Promotion Research

Some experts in the field of health promotion assert that the traditional modes of health-care inquiry are not the best way to understand the community and societal influences on health (Raphael, 2000). Health promotion addresses group or community concerns that go beyond individual health practices and addresses the multiple social, cultural, and physical factors that impact the health of a community. Community-based research has emerged as a legitimate way to help communities understand and solve their own health problems. Although community-based research can take different forms, the most important element is the active involvement of the community members. Research that is done in the community is not necessarily community-based; it often involves explaining the research to community members and gaining their support or assistance but does not allow the community members an opportunity to influence the research question, design, or methods (Schultz, Israel, Selig, Bayer, & Griffin, 2000). Community-based research is more of a partnership that involves community members at all levels.

There continues to be some tension with traditional research, in that tightly designed trials are considered the gold standard of research but may not serve the community's specific needs. Understanding the complexities of behaviors within communities requires a balance among scientific rigor and a working, ethical relationship with its members. When community members participate in the process, the research can take many forms and can contribute different kinds of new knowledge relevant to their specific needs that will ultimately improve their lives.

Evaluating Community-Based Research

Communities are complex and dynamic and are influenced by multiple social, cultural, economic, and political systems; all these affect the health and wellbeing of the people in them. Consequently, studying the important variables affecting the health of community members and the effectiveness of health promotion programs can be a daunting task. Nevertheless, community-based research needs to be conducted in a way that ultimately provides useful, credible knowledge through carefully planned methods. Hancock and colleagues (1997) have suggested criteria for reviewing the rigor of community research involving interventions. Their four domains are

1. design, including the randomization of communities to condition, and the use of sampling methods that assure representation of the entire population;
2. measures, including the use of outcome measures with demonstrated validity and reliability and process measures that describe the extent to which the intervention was delivered to the intended audience;
3. analysis, including consideration of "both individual variation within each community and community-level variation within each treatment" (p. 232) condition; and
4. specification of the intervention, including sufficient detail to enable replication.

The extent to which a report of community-based research addresses these criteria can be used as a guide to the level of confidence one may place in the findings. Table 27-1 lists questions appropriate for evaluating each of these areas.

Table 27–1 **Some Criteria for Reviewing Intervention Research in Communities**

Criterion (Threat to Validity)	Relevant Questions
Subject selection and design	Are communities randomized to condition (type of intervention)?
	Are sampling methods used that ensure representativeness of the entire population?
Measures	Are outcome measures used that have adequate reliability and validity?
	Are process measures in place to describe the extent to which the intervention was delivered to the target population?
Data analysis	Are differences measured both within and across communities for each treatment condition?
Description of the independent variable (intervention)	Is the intervention described with sufficient detail to enable replication in other studies?

Adapted from "Community action for health promotion: A review of methods and outcomes 1990–1995" by L. Hancock et al., 1997, *American Journal of Preventive Medicine, 13*(4), 229–39.

Ideas That Influence Health Promotion Research

Because the structures influencing health are so complex and interrelated, it is important for health promotion research efforts to address these structures and clearly identify ideas about how they relate to each other and influence health. Such collections of underlying beliefs and principles can be called *approaches, paradigms, traditions, ideologies, conceptual frameworks, models,* or *constructs*. In this section, the authors will refer to them as *ideologies*. An ideology is simply a particular way of thinking about phenomena.

There are many different ideologies that guide the focus of health promotion interventions, each with its own body of evidence. Traditionally, health promotion efforts fall under one of three main categories:

1. Interventions that promote changes in the social/environmental aspects of communities
2. Education to promote healthy lifestyle choices
3. Health screenings or health-care delivery focused on prevention and intervention of biomechanical problems (Raphael, 2000)

The particular ideology to which one ascribes will determine the outcomes desired and the research methodology chosen. For example, if the prevailing belief is that personal behavior or lifestyle determines overall health, then the health promotion strategies will take the form of encouraging healthy behaviors. Related outcomes research will focus on the impact of behavior changes. If, however, the prevailing belief is that social/political or environmental structures are the strongest determinants of health, then health promotion activities will focus on changing social and political structures, and research will study the impact of these changes (Wilkinson & Marmot, 1998). Finally, more traditional biomedical approaches to health promotion will focus efforts on disease prevention. Outcomes of interest in this tradition will consider disease incidence and prevalence along with measures of the effectiveness of symptom management.

Types of Research in Health Promotion

What is learned about health and health promotion with research can be categorized according to three types of knowledge: *instrumental knowledge, interactive knowledge,* or *critical knowledge* (Raphael, 2000). These three types of knowledge, each providing distinct and important information to guide health promotion practices, are explained and illustrated in the following sections.

Instrumental Knowledge

Instrumental knowledge is developed through traditional scientific approaches. It is currently the dominant approach in public health for tracking community health status and determining intervention effectiveness. Traditional, scientific approaches value experimental, quantitative evidence of outcomes and assigns credibility of the findings based on the rigor of the research design. This approach is concerned with controlling physical and social environments (Raphael, 2000).

It is generally agreed that the effectiveness of interventions can only be determined by appropriately designed empirical studies. Of the types of research designs typically used, **randomized controlled trials (RCTs)** provide the most convincing evidence, because they control for the possibility of alternate hypotheses, or other explanations for outcomes. RCTs are prospective research studies that employ random selection and random assignment of participants to intervention and control groups, that have safeguards against bias, that use pre- and post-testing to determine effects of intervention, and that generate outcomes that demonstrate practical significance (Kielhofner, Hammel, Finlayson, Helfrich, & Taylor, 2004; Nelson & Mathiowetz, 2004). Unfortunately, RCTs are often difficult to implement, particularly in community settings, where it is hard to control conditions and to assign participants randomly to intervention and nonintervention groups. Consequently, other types of empirical studies are sometimes employed, with varying levels of confidence in the results based on their varying levels of control.

For example, in outcomes research designed to determine the effectiveness of interventions, the highest level of rigor provides the greatest amount of certainty and confidence in the findings. Research designs are classified into three levels of "evidence," ranging from controlled trials, having the highest level of rigor and constituting Level I evidence; to uncontrolled designs, constituting Level II evidence; to case studies and expert opinion based on anecdotal reports, which constitute Level III evidence (see Fig. 27-1).

Quantitative evidence has provided a great deal of support for the risk factors associated with health problems and the effectiveness of some health promotion activities in reducing these risk factors. For example, health promotion in the work site is common, and evidence supporting its effectiveness is growing. With rising health-care costs and competition, employers have a great deal of incentive to keep their employees healthy by encouraging lifestyles that reduce health risk factors. In a 6-year study of six major private and public employers, researchers found that overall health-care expenditures were substantially influenced by modifiable risk factors such as exercise, alcohol use, eating habits, tobacco use, depression, and stress (Anderson et al., 2000). Risk factors such as obesity have been found to increase absenteeism (Tucker & Friedman, 1998) and represent approximately 5% of the total medical costs (Thompson, Edelsberg, Kinsey, & Oster, 1998). Based on a meta-analysis of qualifying research, Pelletier (2001) concluded that comprehensive health promotion and disease-management programs aimed at modifying these risk factors at the work site were found to be cost-effective and resulted in positive clinical outcomes.

Other quantitative data may provide information about the effects of lifestyle on health. For example, mass media campaigns about healthy lifestyles are increasing overall awareness but not necessarily changing behaviors. Approximately 60% of adults are inactive, and nearly half of 12- to 21-year-olds are inactive (Marcus & Forsyth, 1999). The most significant predictor of health-care costs in young adults is health risks, particularly obesity, stress, and general lifestyle (Tucker & Clegg, 2002). Epidemiological studies and clinical trials of adults aged 60 and older showed that active and fit individuals are at a much lower risk for morbidity, mortality, and loss of function when compared with sedentary and unfit persons (Blair & Wei, 2000).

One of the criticisms of traditional, quantitative methods of inquiry is that it does not consider the unique experience of community members nor account for the complex patterns of interactions and situations (Raphael, 2000). It may also be overly focused on individual medical and behavioral variables and may not consider the strong influence of social and environmental influences. Finally, in an effort to control variables and adhere to accepted research protocol, basic science runs the risk of manipulating people in the community or being so reductionistic that the results are hardly useful to the community in terms of improving their health and quality of life.

Level I	Level II				Level III	
Randomized controlled trial (RCT)	Controlled trial without randomization	Cohort or case control analysis study	Multiple time series study	Uncontrolled experiment with dramatic results	Case study	Expert opinion

More rigor and higher confidence → Less rigor and lower confidence

Figure 27-1 Levels of rigor in outcomes research.

Adapted from A dictionary of epidemiology *by J. M. Last, 1995, New York: Oxford University Press. With permission.*

Interactive Knowledge

The second category, **interactive knowledge,** is gained by interactions with people, where their ideas and stories are exchanged and the interaction results in deeper understanding of the perceptions of their health concerns or issues (Letts, 2003). Qualitative methods are used that seek insights based on subjective reports of personal lived experiences, a perspective that is often missed with quantitative data.

Qualitative research concerns itself with the meanings and interpretations of events by individuals and groups. For example, it is often not enough to track prevalence rates and other demographic data to understand the trends in teenage drinking in order to plan drinking-prevention programs. It is more helpful to understand the meanings and functions of alcohol consumption and abuse when planning prevention programs. For example, Beccaria and Guidoni (2002) analyzed data from three qualitative studies on young people and alcohol in Italy. Through in-depth interviews and focus groups with teenagers, the researchers learned the strength of the social and cultural rewards of drinking and concluded that traditional health promotion efforts emphasizing the health damages caused by drinking will probably have little effect.

Similarly, even with extensive health promotion activities aimed at preventing teenage smoking, the prevalence of smoking is increasing, particularly for girls (Seguire & Chalmers, 2000). In a qualitative ethnographic study of 25 adolescent girls who smoked, Seguire and Chalmers (2000) concluded that smoking for these girls could be identified as adaptive or functional. Smoking served such functions as fitting in with a peer group, maintaining friendships, and coping with stress and family conflict. Even though these girls expressed some regret and seemed to underestimate the power of nicotine (only two had quit at the time of the study), the immediate reward of their smoking behavior was stronger (Sequire & Chalmers, 2000). Understanding the multiple influences on health behavior through qualitative research will ultimately create more effective health promotion activities.

Many health promotion programs at the work site promote lifestyle changes and risk-factor modification as a way to improve health and quality of life. Interestingly, in a qualitative research project using semistructured interviews of 29 white-collar employees from a large banking organization, Dugdill (2000) found that they identified psychosocial factors such as job design, ability to make decisions, and control over their work as a more relevant contributor to health in the work setting than individual lifestyle issues. Based on these findings, Dugdill recommended a more comprehensive approach to health promotion in the workplace with equal consideration of the workplace environment and collaboration with the workforce.

The interactive knowledge gained from qualitative research is useful in health promotion, because it may help occupational therapy practitioners understand the values, attitudes, perceptions, biases, and concerns of people in communities related to their health behaviors. People rarely make health-related behavioral changes unless they believe they are at risk for a health problem and believe in the ultimate health benefit of the behavioral change (Rosenstock, 1974). Qualitative research is an effective way to discover some of these attitudes so that health promotion efforts can focus on the most important variables affecting health behaviors.

Critical Knowledge

The third category, **critical knowledge,** is developed through discussion and reflection of issues that disenfranchise or disenable people and includes an action component meant to right the societal structures that were discovered to be wrong (Raphael, 2000). Participatory research is an example of a methodology that develops critical knowledge. This is discussed below, with attention on special implications for implementing health promotion programs in communities.

Participatory Research

The primary concern of **participatory research** is finding the solution for a particular community health problem by determining the role that societal structures and power relations play in promoting that problem and by acting to change those disenabling roles. In this approach, the researcher assumes a role as partner with the aim of developing the research capacity in the participants (Gibbon, 2002).

Participatory research is a useful and effective way of gaining an understanding of community problems and facilitating solutions to those problems. It involves both the researcher and clients or consumers in defining their own health concerns, beliefs, and values in a collaborative process (Cornwall & Jewkes, 1995). This leads to a process that allows participants to explore, identify, and reflect on possibilities or opportunities that let them implement changes in their lives (Soltis-Jarrett, 1997). This type of research is consistent with community-based models in which community participation, shared decision-making, and a shared ownership of solutions are critical. If the process is executed well, the outcome can be predicted to serve the specific needs of the community by helping them understand and overcome oppressive social situations that affect their health (Gibbon, 2002). There are perceived benefits of this approach

(Content Box 27-2) the most important of which is the improved likelihood of translating findings into community practices that achieve relevant health-related goals.

Participatory research is also consistent with occupational therapy concepts of client-centered practice and occupation because of the importance placed on equal relationships among all participants and the expectation that some kind of action (occupation) will result from the research (Letts, 2003). Letts suggests that participatory research is an appropriate way for occupational therapy to understand the occupational and health-related needs of the community and to be most effective in addressing those needs. Much as in client-centered therapy, when the issues directly concern the participants and they are invested in the problem-solving process, they are likely to follow through on actions to address the problem.

Because of its very nature, the participatory research process has its challenges. The researcher has no idea how the research will evolve, even with a vague end point in mind. Letts (2003) became involved with only

a general idea to explore health promotion, environments, and aging, and it emerged as a community organizing effort. Thus it is difficult to plan and prepare for emerging process and logistical challenges. It is time-consuming and effortful to create a process where all participants' values and concerns are equally represented and where a collective commitment to action is undertaken. Finally, the researcher must have skills and knowledge of group process and must consider ethical issues in working with people, such as relinquishing control and supporting self-sufficiency upon exiting from the process.

There are several different approaches to participatory research. These have been described as action research, action learning, participatory action research, and feminist participatory research (Letts, 2003). Although each term is slightly different, the phrases are frequently used interchangeably, thus creating additional confusion.

| Content Box 27-2 |

Some Benefits of Community-Based Participatory Research

- Community partners perceive the relevance of the research and are more likely to apply findings.
- Brings to bear a diverse group of participants with different skills, knowledge, expertise, and interests to address difficult problems.
- Improves the validity and relevance of research by using local knowledge and theory-base drawn from the experience of the people involved.
- Results can be used by all partners involved to allocate resources and influence policies that will benefit the community.
- Reduces the distrust of research sometimes displayed by communities that have historically been "subjects" of such research.
- May assist in bringing together partners involved who may otherwise be unlikely to cooperate.
- May reduce the fragmentation and separation of individual from culture and context that is sometimes observed in more narrowly defined, categorical approaches.
- Provides funding, training, and possible employment opportunities to the communities involved.
- May improve health and wellbeing of communities involved, both directly through the identification of needs and indirectly through increasing power and control over the research process.

Adapted from "Review of community-based research: Assessing partnership approaches to improve public health" by B. A. Israel, A. J. Schulz, E. A. Parker, & A. B. Becker, 1998, *Annual Review of Public Health, 19,* 173–202.

Health Promotion Research in Occupational Therapy

Occupational therapy has embraced the idea that environmental influences and lifestyle choices affect health and wellness and that health promotion aimed at creating positive changes in these factors is effective (AOTA, 2008). This set of beliefs influenced research aimed at addressing questions such as What are the personal and environmental factors that influence occupational competence and quality of life? What health promotion activities are most effective in improving occupational competence and quality of life? How do occupational choices, patterns, and routines affect wellbeing and health? In the following sections, examples of health promotion research in the occupational therapy literature are provided. The examples are organized according to the types of research that have been previously introduced in this chapter.

Quantitative Health Promotion Studies in Occupational Therapy

There are many examples of **quantitative research** methods used in occupational therapy for health promotion. The Well Elderly study (Clark et al., 1997) is perhaps the best example of a randomized, controlled research design supporting the effectiveness of occupational therapy health promotion services with older adults. The researchers demonstrated that occupational therapy services for well elderly adults slowed the health declines of aging relative to matched controls and that these gains were maintained over a year (Clark et al., 2001). Health promotion by occupational therapy to reduce or prevent the secondary problems associated with an existing disease has also been found effective with quantitative research. In a controlled, repeated measures design, Mathiowetz, Matuska, and Murphy (2001) found that individuals with multiple sclerosis living independently in the community who participated in a 6-week course on energy conservation significantly reduced their fatigue impact, improved their quality of life in several domains, and maintained those gains after 6 weeks. These positive changes were not found following a control period that consisted of a support group only. Christiansen, Backman, Little, and Nguye (1999) used quantitative methods to explore the relationship between occupation and subjective wellbeing and concluded that attributes of meaningful occupation are related to perceived wellbeing. Their research supports the idea that health promotion activities should encourage health-related behaviors such as diet and exercise, and that meaningful occupations need to be included in our lives for optimal health. Quantitative research has been used by occupational therapy to demonstrate outcomes of specific community-based interventions and to further knowledge about the important factors contributing to health and wellbeing. This research provides an evidence base for occupational therapists to use in their health promotion work.

Qualitative Health Promotion Studies in Occupational Science and Occupational Therapy

Occupational science has contributed significantly to the research and research methods used in understanding human occupation. **Qualitative research** (providing interactive knowledge) is frequently the method of choice used in occupational science due to its flexible nature and suitability in measuring complex interactions typical in human behavior. Qualitative research about what, when, why, and how people engage in occupation and the relationships with health and wellbeing is slowly growing. For example, researchers have described the occupational opportunities, challenges, and adaptive strategies used by mothers of children with disabilities (Kellegrew, 2000; Larson, 2000; Olson & Esdaile, 2000; Segal, 2000), relocated refugees experiencing drastic environmental changes (Connor Schisler & Polatajko, 2002), and low-income older adults (Clark et al., 1995). The traditional medical model often overlooks the wellbeing of these groups and others, because they are considered "well" until they enter the system with a health-related problem. Preventative health promotion is needed to support the wellbeing of these groups, and the increased understanding of their lived experiences will help occupational therapists deliver preventative services in a way most beneficial to them.

A greater understanding of the occupational opportunities, challenges, and adaptive strategies of people with disabilities has been gained through qualitative research. Farber (2000) conducted in-depth interviews with eight mothers with disabilities and found that the quality of their experiences varied relative to how much they saw themselves as like or unlike other mothers and how much environmental support they had. Farber suggested that although many mothers with disabilities make the necessary adaptations on their own, occupational therapists can assist those who struggle with coping or adapting by offering family and community education and advocacy for community accessibility.

After the child-rearing years, women with disabilities face the same midlife and aging challenges as other women but with the double burden of a disability. Pentland and colleagues (2003) conducted focus groups and interviewed 29 midlife women with spinal cord injuries and found that the additional issues of dealing with a disability in midlife made them feel unlike other groups of women and that the loss of roles and occupations created feelings of isolation and contributed to fears of future losses. They reported concerns with gynecological problems and fatigue that interfered with their daily occupations and were frustrated with the limited support or information available to them for these issues. One disturbing finding was that many of the women felt that the focus of rehabilitation was not on what was important or needed for living with a disability. They reported several things they considered important, such as relying on their own positive attitude, pursuing a goal or project that energized and motivated them, better assistive technology and accessibility, and flexible formal and informal support (Pentland et al., 2003). If improving quality of life is the goal of health promotion, then occupational therapists need to focus intervention on these types of expressed needs rather than overemphasizing personal independence.

Other qualitative studies have contributed to an understanding of mental illness and how it affects quality of life and occupational choices. Information from 35 persons with schizophrenia suggests that in addition to other confirmed quality-of-life factors such as finance, activity, and social interaction, factors associated with quality of life include occupational engagement as a means to connect and belong with others, the provision of choices and a sense of control, and assistance with managing time (Laliberte-Rudman, Yu, Scott, & Pajouhandeh, 2000). Additionally, the occupational choices made by individuals with mental illness are frequently an attempt to balance what they do, with whom they do it, and how they feel about it (Nagle, Valiant, Cook, & Polatajko, 2002). Nagle and others

(2002) discovered through in-depth interviews with eight persons with mental illness that their occupational choices such as not maintaining paid employment were not because they lacked motivation; they were active choices within the options available and were attempts to keep their lives balanced and manageable. Interventions aimed at teaching work and community-living skills without considering these factors may not be effective.

With the growing elderly population, occupational therapists will be serving increasingly more retired or preretired communities. Expected life spans are increasing such that an individual could conceivably be retired for 25 to 35 years. Health promotion for this group should include healthy lifestyle education but perhaps more importantly should provide information and support about coping and adapting to the occupational transition of retirement. Through qualitative methods, Jonsson, Borell, and Sadlo (2000) found that retirees went from the imbalance of too much work to the imbalance of not enough regular commitments. They found managing time and changes in the meaning of occupations to be challenging. Other qualitative studies support the idea that retirees need to do careful planning to fill the void with meaningful occupations to maintain a sense of balance and wellbeing (Jonsson, 1993; Jonsson, Josephsson, & Kielhofner, 2001; Osgood, 1993). These studies showed that engaging occupations seemed to be the main determinant of positive experiences during retirement and that the occupations most satisfying were those that provided regular challenge and engagement with others and that proved satisfying earlier in their lives. Health promotion should educate and support older adults as they maneuver through this transition.

Finally, other notable qualitative studies in the occupational therapy literature have studied injured workers (Stone, 2003), injured farmers (Molyneaux-Smith, Townsend, & Guernsey, 2003), and women survivors of childhood abuse (Ratcliff, Farnsworth, & Lentin, 2002). The research was designed to understand how the participants cope, adapt, or adjust to their situations and how this impacts their health and wellbeing.

Participatory Research in Occupational Therapy

Unfortunately, there are very few examples of participatory research in the occupational therapy literature. This is surprising, given how the field values both community approaches and client-centered values. In several studies conducted by occupational therapists, community members were involved in a process after the research question was identified, but they were not involved with framing the research question itself, one of the key elements of participatory research (Letts, 2003).

Letts (2003) was a member of a participatory research team whose efforts resulted in the Toronto Seniors Council, an organization concerned with issues of importance for older adults in Toronto. This group originally formed because of concerns about the recent restructuring of local government, and they wanted to ensure that important services affecting their health and wellbeing were considered when funding decisions were made. Outcomes such as this are anticipated with well-executed participatory research, where effective action naturally follows the process.

More recently, Suarez-Balcazar (2003) reported on a project to empower community members through use of technology. A group of citizen leaders in an urban community of primarily minority residents was provided assistance in organizing a Web TV approach to using the Internet to gain information on health information related to disease prevention and access to services. The researchers used Web stories, provided by community members on the project's home page, as a form of information sharing and project evaluation. By evaluating the content of the stories, the researchers (and the participants) could evaluate the project's success. Suarez-Balcazar highlighted the implications of this approach for occupational therapists in the community, noting that occupational therapy has multiple roles, including facilitating positive change in health practices, assisting the identification of appropriate services for recognized problems, and working with community-based organizations (CBOs) to empower marginalized populations and document and evaluate the effectiveness of change-related programs.

There are many examples of occupational therapists working with communities that seem to fit the components of participatory research, such as facilitating self-reliance and involving members in all aspects of the programs (Scaffa, 2001), yet they are considered services to the community and not adequately researched. Occupational therapists working in communities need to consider participatory research as a method to benefit community members and for the advancement of evidenced-based practice.

Barriers and Challenges in Health Promotion Research

As discussed previously, research in health promotion follows many of the same principles as research in other areas of health care. Moreover, it has similar goals, aimed at translating science into practices that result in the improvement of health within communities and populations. Perhaps because of this, health promotion research has its own particular set of challenges.

First, its interventions often involve human behavior, values, attitudes, beliefs, and habits that are influenced by cultural and social values (Green & Kreuter, 1991; Poss, 1999). These variables are often difficult to define and measure. Second, because health promotion research is done in communities, logistical challenges associated with selecting, recruiting, and retaining subjects are often encountered. Unlike clinical trials, which often motivate subject participation based on an individual's need to reduce the symptoms associated with a condition, health promotion research often deals with conditions that are asymptomatic.

For example, cholesterol and high blood pressure may not produce symptoms that motivate behavior change. Additionally, the interventions employed in health promotion may be subject to the political and social influences present in any organization, community, or neighborhood at a given time. Traditions, beliefs, attitudes, and experiences can work individually or in combination to reduce participation and compliance. Examples here would include social attitudes toward breastfeeding, fears of complications associated with immunization programs, or religious misgivings about the use of birth control or devices to control for sexually transmitted infections (STIs).

Conclusion

Health promotion research in occupational therapy is in its infancy. As the profession recognizes its opportunities in promoting health in communities and populations through emphasis on activity selection and lifestyle design, more research will be forthcoming. Baum and Law (1998) urge research related to occupational therapy community-based practice to determine factors and conditions that influence successful participation in community living for the able-bodied and disabled. Occupational therapy interventions in the community need to follow a public health model of service that focuses on prevention of disability in individuals and communities (Scaffa, Desmond, & Brownson, 2001). Prevention efforts are categorized as primary, secondary, or tertiary.

Primary prevention is targeted to persons who are free of illness, disease, or impairment with the purpose of preventing the development of illness, disease, or injury. Secondary prevention targets individuals at risk for illness, disease, or injury and frequently involves screening or education to minimize complications of an existing illness. Tertiary prevention aims to prevent secondary complications or to reduce the disabling impact of the illness, disease, or injury.

Of the three types of prevention, tertiary prevention is most typically used for individuals with disabilities; here, the focus is on helping them regain maximal function or training them to manage secondary conditions or symptoms. Although the evidence of effectiveness of occupational therapy rehabilitation for people with disabilities is growing (Mathiowetz & Matuska, 1998; Trombly & Ma, 2002), there is less known about occupational therapy's effectiveness in primary and secondary prevention for people with and without disabilities. Individuals with disabilities have the same need for healthy lifestyles as able-bodied persons. Healthy behaviors such as exercise, improving diet, controlling weight, screening for diseases, and staying actively engaged in meaningful occupations is equally important for persons with disabilities yet is often overlooked in favor of management of the disease or disability (Patrick, 1997; Patrick, Richardson, Starks, Rose, & Kinne, 1997). Occupational therapy needs to focus on the lived experiences of individuals with disabilities long after they have left rehabilitation or other traditional types of intervention to promote improved physical and mental health, with the overall goal of improving quality of life. For more information on wellness and people with disabilities, refer to Chapter 19.

In addition, the concept that certain lifestyles are more health promoting than others is gaining empirical support (Baum, 1998). Lifestyles consisting of certain healthy behaviors, such as maintaining fitness, practicing good nutrition, being safe, reducing stress, and avoiding STIs and habit-forming drugs or alcohol, are seen as optimal for health and wellness. There is increasing interest in various disciplines about the types and configurations of lifestyles that lend themselves to higher levels of satisfaction and general wellbeing; this, in turn, is health promoting through their opportunities for enjoyment, socialization, challenge, rest and recreation, personal growth, and self-expression. Over the decades, publications in the popular press have also demonstrated a widespread acceptance of the notion that a balanced lifestyle is good for health.

Often, the idea of lifestyle balance has been discussed in the context of perceptions that the time available for recreation and relaxation has diminished as the pace and intensity of demands for work and everyday life have increased. This is evident in a large study of how people in the United States use time and how they derive satisfaction from it (Robinson & Godbey, 1999). Results from this study show that people are not concerned about the amount of leisure time available to them, but rather the pace of their lives—most of their free time comes during the week and is in small amounts, which doesn't allow a person to undertake more satisfying uses of leisure.

While the idea of a balanced lifestyle has intuitive appeal, the challenge of explicitly describing such a lifestyle in operational terms has not been documented in the literature, nor has the concept otherwise been validated. A few writers in occupational science and occupational therapy have addressed the topic in conceptual terms, but few empirical studies have been completed. Christiansen observed that there were many possible ways to characterize lifestyle balance and that because of differences in how various lifestyle pursuits are classified and experienced, it was likely that time use would be an inadequate approach to studying lifestyle balance (Christiansen, 1996).

In this chapter, the authors have attempted to provide an overview of the need for research in health promotion, traditional categories and approaches for such research, and barriers and challenges associated with community-based approaches. Research in health promotion was described as contributing to three types of knowledge—instrumental, interactive, and critical—each derived through particular types of studies. Because of the special characteristics and challenges associated with studying and implementing health promotion programs in communities, the value of community-based research was discussed, with particular emphasis on participatory research. Examples of health promotion research in occupational science and occupational therapy were provided, and promising areas for future health promotion research relevant to occupational therapy were identified.

▶ For Discussion and Review

1. What are the differences between qualitative research and quantitative research?
2. What are the benefits and limitations of participatory research?
3. What are the challenges to conducting health promotion research in the community?
4. Define *instrumental knowledge, interactive knowledge,* and *critical knowledge* and how they are used in research.
5. What types of research have been done in occupational therapy health promotion? What are the lessons learned from these studies?
6. Identify topics and research questions for future occupational therapy health promotion research.

▶ Research Questions

1. What are clients' lives like years after participating in occupational therapy? Are they happy? Healthy?
2. How does disability affect opportunities to engage in healthy behaviors?
3. What factors in the person or environment contribute to quality of life for persons with disabilities?

4. What is effective in helping individuals with disabilities achieve health and quality of life?
5. What is lifestyle balance? How do people know if they have it? How does one achieve it?
6. What impact does lifestyle balance have on health and quality of life?
7. What personal or environmental factors support or hinder lifestyle balance?

References

American Occupational Therapy Association. (2008). Occupational therapy services in the promotion of health and the prevention of disease and disability. *American Journal of Occupational Therapy, 62*(6), 694–703.

Anderson, D. R., Whitmer, W.W., Goetzel, R. Z., Ozminkowski, R. J., Wasserman, J., & Serxner, S. HERO Research Committee. (2000). The relationship between modifiable health risks and group level health care expenditures. *American Journal of Health Promotion, 15*(1), 45–52.

Baum, C., & Law, M. (1998). Nationally speaking: Community health: A responsibility, an opportunity, and a fit for occupational therapy. *American Journal of Occupational Therapy, 52*(1), 7–10.

Beccaria, F., & Guidoni, O. V. (2002). Young people in a wet culture: Functions and patterns of drinking. *Contemporary Drug Problems, 29*(2), 305–30.

Blair, S. N., & Wei, M. (2000). Sedentary habits, health, and function in older women and men. *American Journal of Health Promotion, 15*(1), 1–8.

Christiansen, C. H. (1996). Three perspectives on balance in occupation. In R. Zemke & F. Clark (Eds.), *Occupational science: The evolving discipline* (pp. 181–91). Philadelphia: F. A. Davis.

Christiansen, C. H., Backman, C., Little, B., & Nguyen, A. (1999). Occupation well being: A study of personal projects. *American Journal of Occupational Therapy, 53*(1), 25–34.

Clark, F., Azen, S., Carlson, M., Mandel, D., LaBree, L., Hay, J., Zemke, R., Jackson, J., & Lipson, L. (2001). Embedding health-promoting changes into the daily lives of independent-living older adults: Long-term follow-up of occupational therapy intervention. *Journal of Gerontology, 56B,* 60–63.

Clark, F., Azen, S., Zemke, R., Jackson, J., Carlson, M., Mandel, D., Hay, J., Josephson, K., Cherry, B., Hessel, C., Palmer, J., & Lipson, L. (1997). Occupational therapy for older adults: A randomized controlled trial. *Journal of the American Medical Association, 278,* 1321–26.

Clark, F., Carlson, M., Zemke, R., Frank, G., Patterson, K., Larson Ennevor, B., Rankin-Martinez, A., Hobson, L., Crandall, J., Mandel, D., & Lipson, L. (1995). Life domains and adaptive strategies of a group of low-income, well older adults. *American Journal of Occupational Therapy, 50,* 99–108.

Connor Schisler, A. M., & Polatajko, H. J. (2002). The individual as mediator of the person-occupation-environment interaction: Learning from the experience of refugees. *Journal of Occupational Science, 9*(2), 82–92.

Cornwall, A., & Jewkes, R. (1995). What is participatory research? *Social Science and Medicine, 41*(11), 1667–76.

Dugdill, L. (2000). Developing a holistic understanding of workplace health: The case of bank workers. *Ergonomics, 43*(10), 1738–50.

Farber, R. S. (2000). Mothers with disabilities: In their own voice. *American Journal of Occupational Therapy, 54,* 260–68.

Field, M. J., & Gold, G. M. (Eds.). (1998). *Summarizing population health: Directions for the development and application of population metrics.* Institute of Medicine, Washington, DC: National Academy Press.

Gibbon, M. (2002). Doing a doctorate using a participatory action research framework in the context of community health. *Qualitative Health Research, 12*(4), 546–58.

Green, L. W., & Kreuter, M. W. (1991). *Health promotion planning: An educational and environmental approach* (2nd ed.). Mountain View, CA: Mayfield.

Hancock, L., Sanson-Fisher, R., et al. (1997). Community action for health promotion: A review of methods and outcomes, 1990–1995. *American Journal of Preventive Medicine, 13*(4), 229–39.

Institute of Medicine. (1997). *Linking research and public health practice: A review of CDC's program of centers for research and demonstration of health promotion and disease prevention.* Washington, DC: National Academy Press.

Israel, B. A., Schulz, A. J., Parker, E. A., & Becker, A. B. (1998). Review of community-based research: Assessing partnership approaches to improve public health. *Annual Review of Public Health, 19,* 173–202.

Jonsson, H. (1993). The retirement process in an occupational perspective: A review of literature and theories. *Physical and Occupational Therapy in Geriatrics, 11*(4), 424–32.

Jonsson, H., Borell, L., & Sadlo, G. (2000). Retirement: An occupational transition with consequences for temporality, balance, and meaning of occupations. *Journal of Occupational Science, 7,* 29–37.

Jonsson, H., Josephsson, S., & Kielhofner, G. (2001). Narratives and experience in an occupational transition: A longitudinal study of the retirement process. *American Journal of Occupational Therapy, 55*(4), 424–32.

Kellegrew, D. H. (2000). Constructing daily routines: A qualitative examination of mothers with young children with disabilities. *American Journal of Occupational Therapy, 54,* 252–59.

Kielhofner, G., Hammel, J., Finlayson, M., Helfrich, C., & Taylor, R. R. (2004). Documenting outcomes of occupational therapy: The Center for Outcomes Research and Education. *American Journal of Occupational Therapy, 58*(1), 15–23.

Kuzbansky, L. D., Krieger, N., Kawachi, I., Rockhill, B., Steel, G. K., & Berkman, L. F. (2001). United States: Social inequality and the burden of poor health. In T. Evans, M. Whitehead, F. Diderichsen, A. Bhuiya, & M. Wirth (Eds.). *Challenging inequities in health: From ethics to action* (pp. 104–21). Oxford, UK: Oxford University Press.

Laliberte-Rudman, D., Yu, B., Scott, E., & Pajouhandeh, P. (2000). Exploration of the perspectives of persons with schizophrenia regarding quality of life. *American Journal of Occupational Therapy, 54,* 137–47.

Larson, E. A. (2000). The orchestration of occupation: The dance of mothers. *American Journal of Occupational Therapy, 54,* 269–80.

Last, J. M. (1995). *A dictionary of epidemiology.* New York: Oxford University Press.

Letts, L. (2003). Occupational therapy and participatory research: A partnership worth pursuing. *American Journal of Occupational Therapy, 57,* 77–87.

Marcus, B. H., & Forsyth, L. H. (1999). How are we doing with physical activity? *American Journal of Health Promotion, 14*(2), 118–24.

Mathiowetz, V., & Matuska, K. M. (1998). Effectiveness of occupational therapy with multiple sclerosis. *Neuro Rehab, 11,* 141–51.

Mathiowetz, V., Matuska, K., & Murphy, M. (2001). Effectiveness of an energy conservation program for fatigue in multiple sclerosis. *Archives of Physical Medicine and Rehabilitation, 82,* 449–56.

Molyneaux-Smith, L., Townsend, E., & Guernsey, J. (2003). Occupation disrupted: Impacts, challenges, and coping strategies for farmers with disabilities. *Journal of Occupational Science, 10,* 14–20.

Murray, C., & Lopez, A. (1996). *The global burden of disease.* Cambridge, MA: Harvard University Press.

Nagle, S., Valiant Cook, J., & Polatajko, H. (2002). I'm doing as much as I can: Occupational choices of persons with severe and persistent mental illness. *Journal of Occupational Science, 9,* 72–81.

Nelson, D. L., & Mathiowetz, V. (2004). Randomized controlled trials to investigate occupational therapy research questions. *American Journal of Occupational Therapy, 58*(1), 24–34.

Olson, J., & Esdaile, S. (2000). Mothering young children with disabilities in a challenging urban environment. *American Journal of Occupational Therapy, 54,* 307–14.

Osgood, N. (1993). Creative activity and the arts. In J. R. Kelly (Ed.), *Activity and aging, staying involved in later life* (pp. 174–86). Newbury Park, CA: Sage.

Patrick, D. L. (1997). Rethinking prevention for people with disabilities part I: A conceptual model for promoting health. *American Journal of Health Promotion, 11*(4), 257–60.

Patrick, D. L., Richardson, M., Starks, H. E., Rose, M. A., & Kinne, S. (1997). Rethinking prevention for people with disabilities part II: A framework for designing interventions. *American Journal of Health Promotion, 11*(4), 261–63.

Pelletier, K. R. (2001). A review update. *American Journal of Health Promotion, 16*(2), 107–16.

Pentland, W., Walker, J., Minnes, P., Tremblay, M., Brouwer, B., & Gould, M. (2003). Occupational responses to mid-life and aging in women with disabilities. *Journal of Occupational Science, 10,* 21–30.

Poss, J. E. (1999). Providing culturally competent care: Is there a role for health promoters? *Nursing Outlook, 47*(1), 30–36.

Prieto, L., & Sacristan, J. A. (2003). *Problems and solutions in calculating quality-adjusted life years (QALYS).* Retrieved May 25, 2009, from http://www.pubmedcentral.nih.gov/articlerender.fcgi?artid=3147370.

Raphael, D. (2000). The question of evidence in health promotion. *Health Promotion International, 15,* 355–67.

Ratcliff, E., Farnworth, L., & Lentin, P. (2002). Journey to wholeness: The experience of engaging in physical occupation for women survivors of childhood abuse. *Journal of Occupational Science, 9,* 65–71.

Robinson, J., & Godbey, G. (1999). *Time for life: The surprising ways Americans use their time* (2nd ed.). University Park, PA: Penn State Press.

Rogers, J. (1983). Eleanor Clark Slagle lecture—1983. Clinical reasoning: The ethics, science and art. *American Journal of Occupational Therapy, 37,* 601–16.

Rosenstock, I. (1974). Historical origins of the health belief model. In M. Becker (Ed.), *The health belief model and personal behavior.* Thorofare, NJ: SLACK.

Sackett, D. L., & Rosenberg ,W. M. (1995). On the need for evidence-based medicine. *Health Economics, 4*(4), 249–55.

Sackett, D., Rosenberg, W. M. C., Muir Gray, J. C., Haynes, R. B., & Richardson, W. (1996). Evidence-based medicine: What it is and what it isn't. *British Medical Journal, 312,* 71–72.

Scaffa, M. E. (2001). *Occupational therapy in community-based practice settings.* Philadelphia: F. A. Davis.

Scaffa, M., Desmond, S., & Brownson, C. (2001). Public health, community health, and occupational therapy. In M. E. Scaffa (Ed.), *Occupational therapy in community-based practice settings.* Philadelphia: F. A. Davis.

Schultz, A., Israel, B., Selig, S., Bayer, I., & Griffin, C. (2000). The research perspective: Development and implementation of principles for community-based research in public health. In T. Bruce & S. McKane (Eds.), *Community-based public health: A partnership model.* Washington, DC: American Public Health Association.

Segal, R. (2000). Adaptive strategies of mothers with children with attention deficit hyperactivity disorder: Enfolding and unfolding occupations. *American Journal of Occupational Therapy, 54,* 300–06.

Seguire, M., & Chalmers, K. (2000). Late adolescent female smoking. *Journal of Advanced Nursing, 31*(6), 1422–30.

Smith R. (1991). Where is the wisdom? The poverty of medical evidence. *British Medical Journal, 303,* 987–99.

Soltis-Jarrett, V. (1997, December). The facilitator in participatory action research: Les raisons d'etre. *Advances in Nursing Science, 20*(2), 45–54.

Stone, S. D. (2003). Workers without work: Injured workers and wellbeing. *Journal of Occupational Science, 10,* 7–13.

Suarez-Balcazar, Y. (2003). *Empowerment and participatory evaluation of community interventions: Implications for occupational therapy.* Paper given at the 2003 Annual Conference of the American Occupational Therapy Association, June 2003.

Thompson, D., Edelsberg, J., Kinsey, K., & Oster, G. (1998). Estimated economic costs of obesity to U.S. business. *American Journal of Health Promotion, 13*(2), 120–27.

Trombly, C., & Ma, H. (2002). A synthesis of the effects of occupational therapy for persons with stroke, part I: Restoration of roles, tasks, and activities. *American Journal of Occupational Therapy, 56,* 250–59.

Tucker, L. A., & Clegg, A. G. (2002). An analysis of the clinical-and-cost-effectiveness studies of comprehensive health promotion and disease management programs at the worksite: 1998–2000. Differences in health care costs and utilization among adults with selected lifestyle-related risk factors. *American Journal of Health Promotion, 16*(4), 225–33.

Tucker, L. A., & Friedman, G. M. (1998). Obesity and absenteeism: An epidemiologic study of 10,825 employed adults. *American Journal of Health Promotion, 12*(3), 202–07.

Wilkinson, R., & Marmot, M. (Eds.) (1998). *Social determinants of health: Solid facts.* Geneva, Switzerland: World Health Organization.

World Health Organization. (2009). *Metrics: Disability-adjusted life year (DALY).* Retrieved May 25, 2009, from http://www.who.int/healthinfo/global_burden_disease/metrics_daly/en/index.html.

Selection of Key Historical Highlights in Public Health*

Year	Event	Reference
1752	The first voluntary hospital in the United States was established in Philadelphia.	(Institute of Medicine [IOM], 1988)
1773	The first public mental health hospital in the United States was established in Williamsburg, Virginia.	(IOM, 1988; Zwelling, 1985)
1798	U.S. Public Health Service founded.	(Timmreck, 1995)
1798	Pinel removes the chains from insane in Bicetre Asylum.	(Tulchinsky & Varavikova, 2000)
Early to mid-1800s	"Health was perceived as an ongoing process . . . community activities . . . were associated with health (integration of mind, body, and spirit). Illness was perceived to be an imbalance between the individual and the world health; as such it was part of a collective experience in a particular historical, cultural, and social setting."	(Berliner & Salmon, 1980, as cited by Johnson, 1986, p. 2)
1848	The Public Health Act of 1848 passes in Great Britain; this act was the result of two studies by Chadwick of the "life and health of the working class in 1838 and that of the entire country in 1842" and influenced sanitation and public health in both that country and the United States.	(IOM, 1988, p. 59).
1855	First state health departments are instituted.	(Timmreck, 1995)
1872	American Public Health Association (APHA) founded.	(APHA, 2003)
1882	Germ theory substantiated by Koch (Life online, n.d.) leads to "scientific medicine," and individuals began to shift responsibility for their health to the physician and the health-care system.	(Johnson, 1986)
1900s	Social activists such as Addams and Meyer, Pragmatism, and Hull House used the concepts of empowerment and self-determination to combat the ills of industrialization and other social issues.	(Breines, 1986)
1920	Public health definition included the concepts of promotion, prevention, and maintenance of health.	(Winslow, 1920)
1948	World Health Organization (WHO) founded.	(Lyons & Petrucelli, 1987, p. 586)
1953	Creation of the U.S. Department of Health, Education, and Welfare, now known as the U.S. Department of Health and Human Services (USDHHS).	(USDHHS, 2005)

Continued

Year	Event	Reference
1963	Enactment of the Mental Retardation Facilities and Community Mental Health Centers Act of 1963 (P.L. 88-164).	(Geller, 2000)
1973	Health Maintenance Organization Act of 1973 "provided incentives for the medical system to practice preventive medicine to keep patients out of expensive hospital beds."	(Green & Kreuter, 1991, p. 7)
1974	Publication of Lalonde's *A New Perspective on the Health of Canadians.* This was a "landmark document" in the trend to focus attention on lifestyle diseases.	(Best & Cameron, 1986)
1975	Passage of "Public Law 94-317 Promotion gave policy support to health promotion in the U.S. with the Health Information and Promotion Act and the creation of the federal Office of Disease Prevention and Health Promotion."	(Green & Kreuter, 1991, p. xvii)
1979	Publication of *Healthy People: Surgeon General's Report on Health Promotion and Disease Prevention.*	(USDHHS, 1979)
1980	Publication of *Promoting Health/Preventing Disease: Objectives for the Nation.* Established health policy agenda for the next 10 years.	(USDHHS, 1980)
1982	Planned Approach to Community Health (PATCH) begins.	(Timmreck, 1995)
1986	*Ottawa Charter for Health Promotion* is produced.	(WHO, 1986)
1987	WHO's Healthy Cities Project Phase I is initiated.	(WHO, 2004a)
1990	Publication of *Healthy People 2000: National Health Promotion and Disease Prevention Objectives,* which outlined health policy for the next decade.	(USDHHS, 1990)
1990	Americans with Disabilities Act is signed.	(USDOJ, 2006)
1992	PATCH, which designates the community health promotion agenda for the 1990s, begins.	(Timmreck, 1995)
1993–1994	Failure of federal health reform.	(Lasker et al., 1997)
1997	*Jakarta Declaration on Leading Health Promotion into the 21st Century* is signed.	(WHO, 1997)
2000	Publication online of *Healthy People 2010,* which details the health policy agenda for the next decade.	(USDHHS, 2000)
2001	Release of *Healthy People in Healthy Communities.*	(USDHHS, 2001)
2002	Release of *Healthy Campus 2010: Making It Happen.*	(American College Health Association, 2002)

*Modified and updated from S. M. Reitz, *Rural interdisciplinary health promotion service learning training,* June 22–23, 2003, Western Maryland Area Health Education Center, Cumberland, MD.

References

American College Health Association. (2002). *Healthy Campus 2010: Making it happen*. Baltimore: Author.

American Public Health Association. (2003). *Growth of international health: An analysis and history*. Retrieved March 13, 2006, from http://www.apha.org/wfpha/pdf/InternationalHealthBook1.pdf.

Best, J., & Cameron, R. (1986). Health behavior and health promotion. *American Journal of Health Promotion, 1*, 48–56.

Breines, E. (1986). *Origins and adaptations*. Lebanon, NJ: Geri-Rehab.

Geller, J. L. (2000). The last half-century of psychiatric services as reflected in Psychiatric Services. *Psychiatric Services, 51*(1), 41–67.

Green, L. W., & Kreuter, M. W. (1991). *Health promotion planning: An educational and environmental approach* (2d ed.). Mountainview, CA: Mayfield.

Institute of Medicine. (1988). *The future of public health*. Washington, DC: National Academy Press.

Johnson, J. (1986). *Wellness: A context for living*. Thorofare, NJ: SLACK.

Lasker, R. D., & the Committee on Medicine and Public Health. (1997). *Medicine & public health: The power of collaboration*. New York: New York Academy of Medicine.

Lyons, A., & Petrucelli, R. (1987). *Medicine: An illustrated history*. New York: Abradale.

Reitz, S. M. (2003, June 22–23). *Rural interdisciplinary health promotion service learning training*. Lecture presented at the Western Maryland Area Health Education Center, Cumberland, MD.

Timmreck, T. C. (1995). *Planning, program development, and evaluation: A handbook for health promotion, aging, and health services*. Boston: Jones and Bartlett.

Tulchinsky, T. H., & Varavikova, E. A. (2000). *The new public health: An introduction for the 21st century*. San Diego, CA: Academic.

U.S. Department of Health and Human Services. (1979). *Healthy People: Surgeon General's report on health promotion and disease prevention*. Washington, DC: Government Printing Office.

U.S. Department of Health and Human Services. (1980). *Promoting health/preventing disease: Objectives for the nation*. Washington, DC: Government Printing Office.

U.S. Department of Health and Human Services. (2000). *Healthy People 2010: Understanding and improving health* (2d ed.). Washington, DC: Government Printing Office.

U.S. Department of Health and Human Services. (2001). *Healthy people in healthy communities: A community planning guide using Healthy People 2010*. Retrieved November 27, 2004, from http://www.healthypeople.gov/Publications/HealthyCommunities2001/healthycom01hk.pdf.

U.S. Department of Health and Human Services. (2005). *Historical highlights*. Retrieved September 8, 2006, from http://www.hhs.gov/about/hhshist.html.

U.S. Department of Justice. (2006). *ADA signing ceremony*. Retrieved September 10, 2006, from http://www.usdoj.gov/crt/ada/videogallery.htm.

Winslow CEA. (1920). The untilled field of public health. (originally published in *Science, 51*, p. 23) in B.J. Turnock (1997). *Public health, what it is and how it works*. Gaithersburg, MD: Aspen.

World Health Organization. (1986). *Ottawa charter for health promotion*. Retrieved December 4, 2004, from http://www.who.int/hpr/NPH/docs/ottawa_charter_hp.pdf.

World Health Organization. (1997). *Jakarta declaration on leading health promotion into the 21st century*. Retrieved May 29, 2005, from www.who.int/hpr/NPH/docs/jakarta_declaration_en.pdf.

World Health Organization. (2004). *Background for healthy cities network*. Retrieved November 27, 2004, from http://www.euro.who.int/healthy-cities/CitiesAndNetworks/20020111_1.

Zwelling, S. S. (1985). *Quest for a cure: The public hospital in Williamsburg, Virginia, 1773–1885*. Williamsburg, VA: Colonial Williamsburg Foundation.

Summary of Recommendations of Institute of Medicine (IOM) Report*

General Recommendations

- Recommendation 2-1: Increase awareness of racial and ethnic disparities in health care among the general public and key stakeholders.
- Recommendation 2-2: Increase healthcare provider's awareness of disparities.

Legal, Regulatory, and Policy Interventions

- Recommendation 5-1: Avoid fragmentation of health plans along socioeconomic lines.
- Recommendation 5-2: Strengthen the stability of patient-provider relationships in publicly funded health plans.
- Recommendation 5-3: Increase the proportion of underrepresented U.S. racial and ethnic minorities among health professionals.
- Recommendation 5-4: Apply the same managed care protections to publicly funded HMO enrollees that apply to private HMO enrollees.
- Recommendation 5-5: Provide greater resources to the U.S. DHHS Office for Civil Rights to enforce civil rights laws.

Health Systems Interventions

- Recommendation 5-6: Promote the consistency and equity of care through the use of evidence-based guidelines.
- Recommendation 5-7: Structure payment systems to ensure an adequate supply of services to minority patients, and limit provider incentives that may promote disparities.
- Recommendation 5-8: Enhance patient-provided communication and trust by providing financial incentives for practices that reduce barriers and encourage evidence-based practice.

- Recommendation 5-9: Support the use of interpretation services where community need exists.
- Recommendation 5-10: Support the use of community health workers.
- Recommendation 5-11: Implement patient education programs to increase patients' knowledge of how to best access care and participate in treatment decisions.

Cross-Cultural Education in the Health Professions

- Recommendation 6-1: Integrate cross-cultural education into the training of all current and future health professionals.

Data Collection and Monitoring

- Recommendation 7-1: Collect and report data on health care access and utilization by patients' race, ethnicity, socioeconomic status, and where possible, primary language.
- Recommendation 7-2: Include measure of racial and ethnic disparities in performance measurement.
- Recommendation 7-3: Monitor progress toward the elimination of healthcare disparities.
- Recommendation 7-4: Report racial and ethnic data by OMB categories, but use subpopulation groups where possible.

Research Needs

- Recommendation 8-1: Conduct further research to identify sources of racial and ethnic disparities and assess promising intervention strategies.
- Recommendation 8-2: Conduct research on ethical issues and other barriers to eliminating disparities.

---

*From *Unequal treatment: Confronting racial and ethnic disparities in healthcare* (pp. 20-21), by Institute of Medicine, 2003, Washington, DC: National Academies Press.

Dietary Guidelines for Americans, 2005 (USDA & USDHHS)

Adequate Nutrients Within Calorie Needs

- Consume a variety of nutrient-dense foods and beverages within and among the basic food groups while choosing foods that limit the intake of saturated and trans fats, cholesterol, added sugars, salt, and alcohol.
- Meet recommended intakes within energy needs by adopting a balanced eating pattern such as the USDA Food Guide (MyPyramid) or the DASH Eating Plan.

Weight Management

- To maintain body weight in a healthy range, balance calories from foods and beverages with calories expended.
- To prevent gradual weight gain over time, make small decreases in food and beverage calories and increase physical activity.

Physical Activity

- Engage in regular physical activity and reduce sedentary activities to promote health, psychological wellbeing, and a healthy body weight.
  - To reduce the risk of chronic disease in adulthood: Engage in at least 30 minutes of moderate-intensity physical activity, above usual activity, at work or home on most days of the week.
  - For most people, greater health benefits can be obtained by engaging in physical activity of more vigorous intensity or longer duration.
  - To help manage body weight and prevent gradual, unhealthy body weight gain in adulthood: Engage in approximately 60 minutes of moderate- to vigorous-intensity activity on most days of the week while not exceeding caloric intake requirements.
  - To sustain weight loss in adulthood: Participate in at least 60 to 90 minutes of daily moderate-intensity physical activity while not exceeding caloric intake requirements. Some people may need to consult with a health-care provider before participating in this level of activity.
- Achieve physical fitness by including cardiovascular conditioning, stretching exercises for flexibility, and resistance exercises or calisthenics for muscle strength and endurance.

Food Groups to Encourage

- Consume a sufficient amount of fruits and vegetables while staying within energy needs. Two cups of fruit and 2½ cups of vegetables per day are recommended for a reference 2000-calorie intake, with higher or lower amounts depending on the calorie level.
- Choose a variety of fruits and vegetables each day. In particular, select from all five vegetable subgroups (dark green, orange, legumes, starchy vegetables, and other vegetables) several times a week.
- Consume 3-plus ounces (or equivalent) of whole-grain products per day, with the rest of the recommended grains coming from enriched or whole-grain products. In general, at least half the grains should come from whole grains.
- Consume 3 cups per day of fat-free or low-fat milk or equivalent milk products.

Fats

- Consume less than 10% of calories from saturated fatty acids and less than 300 mg/day of cholesterol, and keep trans fatty acid consumption as low as possible.
- Keep total fat intake between 20% to 35% of calories, with most fats coming from sources of polyunsaturated and monounsaturated fatty acids, such as fish, nuts, and vegetable oils.
- When selecting and preparing meat, poultry, dry beans, and milk or milk products, make choices that are lean, low-fat, or fat-free.
- Limit intake of fats and oils high in saturated and/or trans fatty acids, and choose products low in such fats and oils.

Carbohydrates

- Choose fiber-rich fruits, vegetables, and whole grains often.
- Choose and prepare foods and beverages with little added sugars or caloric sweeteners, such as amounts suggested by the USDA Food Guide and the DASH Eating Plan.
- Reduce the incidence of dental caries by practicing good oral hygiene and consuming sugar- and starch-containing foods and beverages less frequently.

Sodium and Potassium

- Consume less than 2300 mg (approximately 1 tsp of salt) of sodium per day.
- Choose and prepare foods with little salt. At the same time, consume potassium-rich foods, such as fruits and vegetables.

Alcoholic Beverages

- Drink alcoholic beverages sensibly and in moderation—defined as the consumption of up to one drink per day for women and up to two drinks per day for men.
- Alcoholic beverages should not be consumed by some individuals, including those who cannot restrict their alcohol intake, women of childbearing age who may become pregnant, pregnant and lactating women, children and adolescents, individuals taking medications that can interact with alcohol, and those with specific medical conditions.
- Alcoholic beverages should be avoided by individuals engaging in activities that require attention, skill, or coordination, such as driving or operating machinery.

Food Safety

- To avoid microbial foodborne illness:
  - Clean hands, food contact surfaces, and fruits and vegetables. Meat and poultry should not be washed or rinsed.
  - Separate raw, cooked, and ready-to-eat foods while shopping, preparing, or storing foods.
  - Cook foods to a safe temperature to kill microorganisms.
  - Chill (refrigerate) perishable food promptly and defrost foods properly.
  - Avoid raw (unpasteurized) milk or any products made from unpasteurized milk, raw or partially cooked eggs or foods containing raw eggs, raw or undercooked meat and poultry, unpasteurized juices, and raw sprouts.

Recommended Computer Workstation Guidelines

For any computer workstation, some basic guidelines can reduce the worker's risk of discomfort or injury. The head should be held erect, and the monitor should be placed directly in front of the user, about an arm's length away (estimated at 20 to 30 inches; Jacobs, 1999, p. 231). Flat monitors have made this configuration possible even on small desks and tabletops. Printed material should be placed to the immediate side of the monitor or on the tabletop in front of the monitor, if space permits. The key position to avoid for prolonged amounts of time is a twisted neck. The worker's shoulders should be relaxed, with the upper arms close to the side of the body and relaxed. Elbows should be flexed or bent to approximately 90 degrees to reach the keyboard, and forearms should be in a pronated or "hands-down" position (Jacobs, 1999, p. 231). Keeping the wrists in a neutral position for keyboard use can reduce the risk of some common cumulative trauma injuries, including carpal tunnel syndrome. In order to ensure that this neutral position is maintained, the keyboard should be positioned directly in front of the worker and in a flat, not angled, position. The small tabs on the back of a standard computer keyboard that can angle the keyboard should not be used in most cases, again to promote the neutral wrist position. A mouse or other input device should be placed directly beside the keyboard to facilitate easy and comfortable movement between these two devices, and it should fit comfortably in the user's hand. A variety of keyboard and mouse trays are available that can be installed under the desk or tabletop to better fit the user. These trays are highly recommended to prevent static postures and promote varying positions of the upper extremities throughout the workday. Ideally, a tray should be large enough to accommodate both the keyboard and the mouse (or other input device), and both height and tilt should be easily adjustable.

In recommending back and lower extremity positioning, consideration must be given to the office chair. Back support should be provided at the lumbar spine, or low back, in order to facilitate biomechanically stable back positions (Jacobs, 1999, p. 227). Higher chairs, often used for executives, frequently support the thoracic or middle portion of the back, which encourages slouched sitting postures and shoulder positions that can promote discomfort and stiffness. To ensure that lumbar support is possible for a variety of users, the chair backrest should be adjustable in height. The seat pan should be wide enough for the individual and should have a rounded or waterfall front to avoid compressing the back of the worker's knees. The hips and knees should be supported in approximately 90 degrees of flexion. The floor or some type of footrest should support the feet. Armrests on chairs are generally not recommended for workers who use their computers for extended periods of time. They often promote elevated or abducted shoulders, which in turn discourages neutral wrist postures. Although some workers prefer armrests, they should be adjustable in both height and lateral distance away from the seat pan to allow proper arm positioning.

Many types of equipment are available that claim to be ergonomically correct. A wide variety of wrist supports, split keyboards, input devices, desks, and chairs may be used at the discretion of the user. There is no standard solution for every worker, or else there would be no need for the study of ergonomics. However, it is vital that workers be aware of their own optimal working position and the need to avoid any one prolonged position for the majority of the workday. Some type of break or stretch should be performed periodically; even a position that may appear to be the perfect ergonomic fit can be uncomfortable without intermittent movement and stretch.

Acknowledgment

The editors wish to express their appreciation to Lynne Murphy, who prepared this appendix.

Reference

Jacobs, K. (1999). *Ergonomics for therapists* (2d ed.). Boston: Butterworth-Heinemann.

Family Self-Analysis*

Part I: The Individuals

1. Identify the members in your family. Write a brief description about each member. Include a short biography about each individual's life. The following information should be included:
   a. First Name
   b. Age
   c. Interests
   d. Meaningful Activities Engaged/Involved In
   e. Personality Characteristics
   f. Values
   g. Life Goals

Part II: Family History

1. Describe the family as a unit. Identify any significant events that have made an impact on the family as a unit. Include recent and decades old events that are meaningful.

Part III: Understanding the Relationships

1. Identify the family roles of each member.

   • Who is the leader?
   • Is there a gatekeeper?
   • Is there an attention seeker?
   • Who is the stabilizer?

2. Identify and discuss significant relationships between family members.

3. Describe the following processes among family members:
   a. How do members communicate with each other?
   b. How are decisions made?
   c. Are conflicts dealt with? If so, what process is followed?
   d. Who has the power in the family?
   e. What types of events are stressful?
   f. Describe a meaningful memory. Why is it meaningful?

4. Identify and discuss significant relationships between family members and significant others outside the family of origin unit.

5. What are four descriptors that you would use to help identify your family unit?

6. Describe the home with details. What would a visitor see when he walks in the door and around the home? What does the home say about the family?

7. Identify three challenges that the family has faced and how they were dealt with.

Part IV: Summary

1. Based on the information above, describe the family system in one page. Is there a theme to your family that helps tell your story?

2. In conclusion, discuss what this experience was like for you? What did you learn?

*From *Family self analysis,* by K. G. Eskow, 2001, unpublished manuscript, Family Studies Department, Towson University, Towson, MD. Reprinted with permission of the author.

Parent Tips for Child Success*

Nova Southeastern University, Department of Occupational Therapy, Ft. Lauderdale, Florida 33328

Parent Tip	How to Do the Activity	Skills Developed by the Activity
1. Create a game	Decorate a paper plate as a target or Frisbee, set rules.	Problem-solving; following rules; motor skills; creativity
2. Hopscotch	Draw and number connected squares for child to jump in sequence.	Motor skills; turn-taking
3. Memory	Display familiar objects, cover, see how many objects are remembered.	Memory; helps make connections about relationships between objects
4. Coins in a sock	Place various numbers or sizes of coins in a sock, find the biggest/smallest, count #.	Problem-solving; motor skills
5. Objects in a sock	Choose small objects with various characteristics, find specific objects/something hard/something soft.	Problem-solving; sense of touch; critical thinking
6. Dough art	Make bread or cookie dough, create shapes by hand, bake, and eat!	Math skills of measurement and volume; motor skills; allows creative thinking; sharing
7. Necklaces of cereal	Use "O" cereals to string together after sorting by color, counting.	Math skills; motor skills; problem-solving
8. Sock puppets	Use an old sock to decorate with eyes and hair, fold to create a mouth. Tell a story with your puppet.	Creativity; critical thinking; motor skills
9. Sock toss	Fold an old sock into a soft ball to play catch.	Motor skills; eye-hand coordination
10. Make a book	Sew or staple folded paper to make a book. Write a story and illustrate it.	Creativity; problem-solving; critical thinking; motor skills
11. Guessing game	Parent gives a clue that isn't too specific, child guesses, parent adds clues. Example: (1) "I'm thinking of an animal with four legs"; (2) "It lives in people's houses"; (3) "It says meow."	Critical thinking; comparison of information; problem-solving
12. Alike and different	Take any two objects and ask your child to say how they are alike and how they are different.	Critical thinking; comparison of information
13. Rhyming games	Start out easy—"What rhymes with cat?" (Hat, bat, mat, fat, etc.).	Listening skills; critical thinking
14. How many?	Depending on the age of your child, ask him how many legs does a dog have, a person. To make this harder, ask, "How many legs do two people have?"	Critical thinking; problem-solving; math skills

Continued

Parent Tip	How to Do the Activity	Skills Developed by the Activity
15. Stacking games	Encourage child to stack like and unlike objects such as coins or pieces of vegetables	Problem-solving; eye-hand coordination; awareness of cause and effect
16. "What would you rather be?" game	Ask your child silly things like, "Would you rather be a car or a bus?" "A cat or a dog?" Ask him why he chose his answer.	Self-expression; presenting a logical argument

*Offered in English, Spanish, and Creole translations.

Falls Prevention Assessment Checklist

SUBJECTIVE AND HISTORY

☐ Previous falls — Identify contributing risk factors in any previous falls

☐ Medications — Psychotropics

Antihypertensives

Polypharmacy

☐ Use of alcohol

☐ Level of physical activity

☐ Social network

☐ Urinary incontinence

☐ Fear of falling

OBJECTIVE

Screen and Refer as Appropriate

☐ Cognitive status — Mini Mental State Exam

☐ Depression — Geriatric Depression Scale

☐ Balance

☐ Strength, coordination — Five chair stands in 30 seconds

☐ Grip strength

☐ Range of motion

☐ Gait unsteadiness

☐ Use of mobility device

☐ Postural hypotension

☐ Foot problems — Sensory impairment

Wounds

Bunions, etc.

☐ Vision

☐ Hearing

Observe and Evaluate

☐ Ability to perform ADLs

☐ Functional mobility, transfers

☐ Environmental hazards — Observe person-environment interactions

☐ Footwear — Proper fit, cushioning, sole/tread

Appropriateness for specific floor coverings and gait pattern

Continued

551

☐	Medication management	Takes meds as prescribed
		Notifies provider of OTC meds
☐	Behavioral risks	Pace (rushing)
		Attention to potential hazards

Adapted for use in occupational therapy from evidence-based guidelines provided by: Moreland, J., Richardson, J., Chan, D. H., O'Neill, J., Bellissimo, A., Grum, R. M., & Shanks, L. (2003). Evidence-based guidelines for the secondary prevention of falls in older adults. *Gerontology, 49*(2), 93–116.

Index